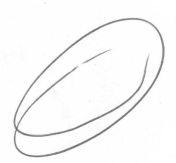

Breastfeeding and Human Lactation

BREASTFEEDING AND HUMAN LACTATION

LACTATION   SECOND EDITION

Jan Riordan, EdD, RN, IBCLC, FAAN
Associate Professor, School of Nursing
Wichita State University
Wichita, Kansas

Kathleen Auerbach, PhD, IBCLC
Adjunct Professor, School of Nursing
University of British Columbia
Vancouver, BC, Canada

JONES AND BARTLETT PUBLISHERS
Sudbury, Massachusetts
BOSTON   TORONTO   LONDON   SINGAPORE

World Headquarters

Jones and Bartlett Publishers
40 Tall Pine Drive
Sudbury, MA 01776
800-832-0034
978-443-5000
info@jbpub.com
www.jbpub.com

Jones and Bartlett Publishers Canada
P.O. Box 19020
Toronto, ON M551X1
Canada

Jones and Bartlett Publishers International
Barb House, Barb Mews
London W6 7PA
UK

Production Credits

Acquisitions Editor: Karen McClure
Developmental Editor: Dean DeChambeau
Senior Production Editor: Lianne Ames
Manufacturing Buyer: Jane Bromback
Design: Publicom, Inc.
Editorial Production Service: Publicom, Inc.
Illustration: Publicom, Inc.
Typesetting: Publicom, Inc.
Cover Design: Dick Hannus
Printing and Binding: Hamilton Printing
Cover Printing: Hamilton Printing
Cover Illustrator: Marcia Smith

Chief Executive Officer: Clayton Jones
Chief Operating Officer: Don Jones, Jr.
Publisher: Tom Walker
VP, Sales & Marketing: Rob McCarry
Senior Managing Editor: Judith H. Hauck
Marketing Director: Rich Pirozzi
Production Manager: Anne Spencer

Section-Opener Photo Credits:
p. 1: Sergei Vasiliev; p. 91: WHO/PAHO (19834);
p. 239: Sergei Vasiliev; p. 513: WHO (20532); p. 707:
St. Joseph Medical Center.

Library of Congress Cataloging-in-Publication Data

Breastfeeding and human lactation / [edited by] Jan Riordan, Kathleen
   G. Auerbach -- 2nd ed.
       p.   cm.
   Includes bibliographical references and index.
   ISBN 0-7637-0545-4
   1. Breast feeding. 2. Lactation.   I. Riordan, Jan.
   II. Auerbach, Kathleen G.
RJ216.B775 1998
6491.33--dc21   98-3502
                                                   CIP

Printed in the United States of America
02 01 00 99 98   10 9 8 7 6 5 4 3 2 1

*To the breastfeeding women and their babies
around the globe, who have taught us and who
continue to allow us to learn from them*

TABLE OF CONTENTS

Preface   xix   Chapter Authors   xxii

SECTION 1
THE HISTORICAL AND SOCIOCULTURAL CONTEXT OF INFANT FEEDING

CHAPTER 1

Tides in Breastfeeding Practice   3

Evidence About Breastfeeding Practices   3
- Large-Scale Surveys   3
- Small Surveys   4
- Other Evidence   4

The Biological Norm in Infant Feeding   4
- Early Human Evolution   4
- Early Breastfeeding Practices   5

The Replacement of Maternal Breastfeeding   5
- Wet-Nursing   5
- Hand-Fed Foods   6
- Timing of the Introduction of Hand Feeding   7

Technological Innovations in Infant Feeding   8
- The Social Context   8
- The Technological Context   9
- The Role of the Medical Community   10

The Prevalence of Breastfeeding   12
- United States, England, and Europe   12
- Developing Regions   12

The Cost of Not Breastfeeding   14
- Health Risks of Using Manufactured Infant Milks   14
- Economic Costs of Using Manufactured Infant Milks   15

The Promotion of Breastfeeding   16
- Characteristics of Breastfeeding Women   17
- Promotion Efforts   18

Summary   22

References   23

CHAPTER 2

The Cultural Context of Breastfeeding   29

Definitions and Characteristics   29

The Dominant Culture   29

Ethnocentrism Versus Relativism   31

Assessing Culture   32

Language Barriers   34

The Effects of Culture on Breastfeeding   35
- Rituals and Meaning   36
- Colostrum   37
- Resuming Sexual Relations   37
- Wet-Nursing   37

Childbirth Practices   38

Infant Care   38

Maternal Foods   40
- Foods That Increase Breastmilk   40
- Food Restrictions   42
- "Hot" and "Cold" Foods   43
- Vegetarians   44
- Religious Influences   44

The Doula   44

Weaning   44

Implications for Practice   47

Summary   49

References   50

CHAPTER 3

Families   53

Family Forms and Functions   53

The Effect of a Baby on a Family   56

Family Theory   57

Fathers   58
  Attachment to the Baby   58
  Breastfeeding   59

Levels of Family Functioning   61
  The Teenage Mother   62
  The Low-Income Family   64
  Obstacles to Breastfeeling Among Low-
    Income Families   64
  The Down Side of Family Experiences   68
  The Importance of Peer Counselors   71
  Social Support   72

Breastfeeding Promotion   73
  Advocacy and Counseling   73
  Breastfeeding Programs That Work   81

Summary   83

References   84

SECTION 2

ANATOMICAL AND BIOLOGICAL IMPERATIVES

CHAPTER 4

Anatomy and Physiology   93

The Mother   93
  Mammogenesis   93
  Structure   94
  Variations   97
  Pregnancy   98
  Lactogenesis   98
  Hormonal Influences   98
  Milk Production   102
  Galactopoiesis   102
  Oxytocin   103
  Galactorrhea   104

Clinical Implications: Mother   104
  Breast Assessment   104
  Classification of Nipple Function   106
  Early Frequent feedings   106

The Infant   107
  Newborn Oral Development   107
  Suckling   108
  Breathing and Suckling   113

Clinical Implications: Infant   113
  Breastfeeding Assessment   113
  Suckling Assessment   113

Summary   115

References   115

CHAPTER 5

The Biological Specificity of Breastmilk   121

Maturational Changes   121

Energy, Volume, and Growth   123
  Caloric Density   123
  Milk Volume and Storage Capacity   123
  Infant Growth   126

Nutritional Values   126
  Fat   127
  Lactose   128
  Protein   129
  Vitamins and Micronutrients   130
  Minerals   131
  Renal Solute Load   133

Antiinfective Properties 133
   Respiratory Illness 135
   Otitis Media 135

The Immune System 137
   Cells 138
   Antibodies and Other Immunoglobulins 138
   Nonantibody Antibacterial Protection 141
   Fecal Flora 142
   Antiinflammatory Components 142

Bioactive Components 142
   Enzymes 143
   Growth factors 145
   Hormones 146
   Taurine 147

Antiallergenic Properties 147

Implications for Clinical Practice 149

Summary 151

References 151

CHAPTER 6

Drugs and Breastfeeding 163

The Passage of Maternal Drugs into Breastfeeding Infants 164
   Drug Factors 164
   Maternal Factors 165
   Infant Factors 165
   Breast and Milk Factors 166
   Routes of Transport 166

Drugs That Affect Milk Volume 167

Drug Safety 167
   Nonsteroidal Antiinflammatory Drugs 170
   Analgesics and Narcotics 170
   Anesthetics 170
   Anticoagulants 170
   Anticonvulsants 170
   Antidepressants 172
   Antihistamines 173
   Antimicrobials 173
   Antifungals 174
   Bronchodilators 174
   Beta-Blockers and Antihypertensives 174
   Calcium Channel Blockers 174

   Contraceptives 175
   Diuretics 175
   Laxatives 175
   Herbs 175
   Scabicides and Pediculicides 176
   Steroids 176
   Clinical Implications 176

Maternal Substance Abuse and Addiction 180
   Marijuana 180
   Cocaine 180
   Amphetamines 181
   Alcohol 181
   Clinical Implications 181

Environmental Contaminants 182

Summary 184

References 185

Appendix 6-A: The Transfer of Drugs and Other Chemicals into Human Milk 190

CHAPTER 7

Viruses in Human Milk 221

Human Immunodeficiency Virus 221
   Laboratory Tests 222
   What We Know in the Late 1990s 222
   Clinical Implications 223
   U.S. Public Health Service Recommendations 226
   Counseling 227

Herpes Simplex 227

Chickenpox 229

Cytomegalovirus 229

Rubella 231

Hepatitis B 231

Hepatitis C 232

Human T-Lymphotropic Virus 233

Implications for Practice 234

Summary 234

References 235

SECTION 3

PRENATAL, PERINATAL, AND POSTNATAL PERIODS

CHAPTER 8

Breastfeeding Education   241

Learning Principles   242

Adult Education   242

Curriculum Development   244

The Change Process   244

Parent Education   246
Prenatal Education   248
Early Breastfeeding Education   249
Continuing Support for Breastfeeding Families   249

How Effective Is Breastfeeding Education?   253

Teaching Strategies   255

Therapeutic Communication   255

Small-Group Dynamics   258

Multimedia Presentations   258
Slides   259
Transparencies   259
Videotapes   259
CD ROMs   260

Educational Materials   260

Education for At-Risk Populations   262

Educational Needs and Early Discharge   264

Health Care Provider Education   265
Continuing Education   265
Objectives and Outcomes   269

The Team Approach   270

Lactation Consultants   271

Summary   272

References   273

CHAPTER 9

The Breastfeeding Process: The Perinatal and Intrapartum Period   279

Breastfeeding Preparation   279

Breast and Nipple Preparation   280

The Birth Plan and Feeding Plan   281

Early Feedings   281

Cup-Feeding the Neonate   287

Nipple Shields   287

Hypoglycemia   288

Cesarean Births   291

Breast Fullness Versus Engorgement   294

Hand Expression   295

Clinical Implications   298
Discharge Planning   300
Feeding Positions   301
Basic Feeding Techniques   301
Signs That Intervention Is Needed   303

Summary   304

References   305

CHAPTER 10

The Breastfeeding Process: The Postpartum Period   311

Adequate Hydration and Nutrition of the Neonate   312

Insufficient Milk Supply (IMS)   312
Perceived Insufficient Milk Supply   312
Actual or Primary Insufficient Milk Supply   314

Breast Massage 315

Sore Nipples 315

Neonatal Physiological Jaundice 321

Crying and Colic 321

Stooling Patterns 324
Changes Over Time 324
Stooling as an Indication of a Problem 325

Multiple Infants 326

Refusing the Breast 328

Too Much Milk 329

Leaking and Breast Pads 330

Clothing 331

Breastfeeding During Pregnancy 331

Clinical Implications 332

Summary 335

References 336

CHAPTER 11

Slow Weight Gain and Failure to Thrive 341

Normal Growth 341

Growth Charts: How Good Are They? 343

The Slow-Gaining Infant 344

Failure to Thrive 347

Factors Associated with Inadequate
Caloric Intake 349
Red Flags 349
Infant Factors 355
Maternal Factors 358
Clinical Implications 359

Supplementation 359
Devices 359
Other Methods 362

Summary 364

References 364

Appendix 11-A: Maternal-Infant
History Form 368

CHAPTER 12

Jaundice and the Breastfeeding Baby 375

Early-Onset (Neonatal) Jaundice 375

Pathological Jaundice 377

Factors Associated with Early-Onset
Jaundice 377
Infant Characteristics 377
Hospital Routines 378

Routine Therapy for Early-Onset
Jaundice 380

Incipient Vulnerable Child Syndrome:
One Cost of Overdiagnosis 381

Late-Onset Jaundice 382

Clinical Implications 384

Summary 389

References 389

CHAPTER 13

Breast Pumps and Other Technologies 393

Concerns of Mothers 393

Stimulating the Milk-Ejection Reflex 394

Hormonal Considerations 396
Prolactin 396
Oxytocin 398

Pumps 399
Mechanical Milk Removal 399
The Evolution of Pumps 399

Hand Pumps 399

Battery-Operated Pumps 402

Electric Pumps 402

Product Effectiveness and Safety   408

Miscellaneous Pumps   408
Juice-Jar Breast Pump   408
Ora'lac   408
Venturi Breast Pump   408
Medela Pedal Pump   408

Clinical Implications Regarding Breast
Pumps   409

Sample Guidelines for Pump
Recommendations and Pumping
Techniques   418

Common Pumping Problems   419

Nipple Shields   427
Review of the Literature   428
Risks   428
Responsibilities of Health Care Professionals   430
Weaning from a Shield   431

Breast Shells   432
Recommendations on Breast Shells   432

Feeding-Tube Devices   433
Description   433
Situations for Use   434

Clinical Implications   435

Summary   438

References   439

Appendix 13-A: Manufacturers and
Distributors of Breastfeeding Devices   444

CHAPTER 14

Breastfeeding the Preterm Infant   449

Preterm Infants   449

Mothers of Preterm Infants   450

Rates of Breastfeeding Initiation and
Duration   450

Providing Research-Based Breastfeeding
Services   452

The Decision to Breastfeed   452
Facilitating an Informed Decision   452
Alternatives to Exclusive, Long-Term
Breastfeeding   452

Milk Expression and Collection   456
Principles of Milk Expression   456
Selecting a Breast Pump   456
Reimbursement   456
Milk-Expression Technique   457
Milk-Expression Schedule   458
Preventing Low Milk Volume   458

Skin-to-Skin Care   459

Nonnutritive Suckling   459

Management of Low Milk Volume   460

Gavage Feeding of Mothers' Milk   460

Fortifying and Modifying EMM   462
Commercial Additives   462
Hindmilk Feeding   463

Maternal Medications and Small Preterm
Infants   464

Standards for Storing and Handling Milk
in the NICU   465

Feeding at Breast in the NICU   465
The Science of Early Breastfeeding   465
Initiating Early Breastfeeding   466
Positions for Early Breastfeeding   466
Milk Transfer for Preterm Infants   467
Test Weighing   468
Facilitating Milk Transfer   469
Milk Ejection   469
Infant Suckling   470
Breastfeeding Devices   471

Postdischarge Breastfeeding Management   472
Getting Enough: Milk-Transfer Problems   472
Practice Implications   472

Summary   473

References   474

CHAPTER 15

Breast-Related Problems 483

Nipple Variations 483
   Inverted or Flat Nipples 483
   Large or Elongated Nipples 484

Plugged Ducts 484

Mastitis 485

Skin Rashes, Lesions, and Eczema 487

Candidiasis (Thrush) 488

Breast Pain 492

Vasospasm 492

Milk Blister 493

Mammoplasty 490
   Breast Reduction 493
   Mastopexy 494
   Augmentation 494

Breast Lumps and Surgery 496
   Galactoceles 497
   Fibrocystic Disease 497
   Bleeding from the Breast 498
   Breast Cancer 499

Clinical Implications 502
   Mastitis 502
   Breast Surgery and Abscess 504

Summary 507

References 507

SECTION 4 — BEYOND POSTPARTUM

CHAPTER 16

Maternal Nutrition During Lactation 515

Maternal Caloric Needs 515

Maternal Fluid Needs 517

Weight Loss During Lactation 518

Exercise 519

Calcium Needs and Bone Loss 519

Vegetarian Diets 521

Dietary Supplements 521

Foods That Pass Through Milk 522
   Caffeine 521
   Food Flavorings 522

Goal of the Maternal Diet During Lactation 522

Nutrition Basics 524
   Energy 524
   Macronutrients 524
   Micronutrients 527

Clinical Implications 528

Summary 536

References 536

CHAPTER 17

Women's Health and Breastfeeding 541

Alterations in Endocrine and Metabolic Functioning 541
   Type 1 Diabetes 541
   Thyroid Disease 543
   Pituitary Dysfunction 549
   Cystic Fibrosis 550

Acute Illness and Infections 550

Dysfunctional Uterine Bleeding 551

Surgery 552

Relactation 553

Induced Lactation 555

Autoimmune Diseases 557
Systemic Lupus Erythematosus 557
Multiple Sclerosis 558
Rheumatoid Arthritis 558

Disabilities and Impairments 559
Clinical Implications 559

Seizure Disorders 562

Headaches 563

Postpartum Depression 564
Clinical Implications 565

Asthma 569

Smoking 569

Diagnostic Studies Using Radioisotopes 570

The Impact of Maternal Illness and
Hospitalization 570

Summary 572

References 572

CHAPTER 18

Maternal Employment and Breastfeeding 577

Why Women Work 577

Number of Women Who Work 577

Prenatal Planning and Preparation 578

The Puerperium 579

Returning to Work 579

Hand-Expressing or Breast Pumping? 581

Storage 583

Feeding Options 585

Loss of Sleep 586

The Triple Breeder-Feeder-Producer 586

The Continuing "War" Between Work
and Home 587

The Importance of Social Support 588

Lactation Programs at Work 590

Health Care Workers: A Special Case? 591

The Day-Care Dilemma 592

Clinical Implications 593

Summary 597

References 598

CHAPTER 19

Child Health 601

Developmental Outcomes and
Infant Feeding 601

Growth and Development 602
Physical growth 602
Weight and Length 604
Senses 604
Reflexes 606
Levels of arousal 606

Theories of Development 606
Nature Versus Nurture 606
Erikson's Psychosocial Theory 606
Piaget's Cognitive Theory 607

Social Development 608
Language and Communication 608
Attachment and Bonding 613
Temperament 616
Stranger Distress 618
Separation Anxiety 619
Clinical Implications 619

Immunizations 620

Dental Health 621

Solid Foods 624
Introducing Solid Foods 624
Choosing the Diet 625

Choosing Feeding Location   627
Delaying Solid Foods   628

Obesity   **628**

Weaning   **629**

Clinical Implications   **630**

Summary   **631**

References   **631**

CHAPTER 20

The Ill Breastfeeding Child   637

Infections   **637**
Gastrointestinal Infections   638
Respiratory Infections   640
Meningitis   641
Otitis Media   642

Alteration in Neurological Functioning **642**
Down Syndrome   642
Neural-Tube Defects   643
Hydrocephalus   643
Clinical Implications   644

Congenital Defects   **644**
Congenital Heart Defects   644
Oral and Gastrointestinal Defects   644
Clinical Implications   651

Metabolic Dysfunction   **653**
Phenylketonuria   653
Galactosemia   653
Congenital Hypothyroidism   654
Celiac Disease   654
Cystic Fibrosis   655

Allergies and Food Tolerance   **655**
Allergies While Breastfeeding   656

Hypoglycemia   **658**

Sudden Infant Death Syndrome   **659**

Hospitalization   **661**
Parental Stresses   662
Coping with Siblings   663
Emergency Admission   663
Home: The Rebound Effect   664

Chronic Grief and Loss   **664**
The Magic-Milk Syndrome   664
The Empty Cradle   665

Clinical Implications   **665**

Summary   **667**

References   **668**

CHAPTER 21

Fertility, Sexuality, and Contraception During Lactation   675

Fertility   **675**
The Demographic Impact of Breastfeeding   675
Mechanisms of Action   676
Lactational Amenorrhea   677
The Suckling Stimulus   678
Breastfeeding Frequency and Duration   679
Supplemental Feeding   680
The Repetitive Nature of the Recovery
   of Fertility   681
The Bellagio Consensus   683

Sexuality   **685**
Libido   685
Sexual Behavior During Lactation   689

Contraception   **691**
Contraceptive Methods   692
Clinical Implications   698

Summary   **700**

References   **701**

SECTION 5

CONTEMPORARY ISSUES

CHAPTER 22

Work Strategies and the Lactation Consultant 709

History	709
Certification	710
Educational Offerings	711
Hospital Lactation Programs	712
Playing Politics	715
The Unique Characteristics of Breast-feeding Counseling	718
Assertiveness	718
Roles and Responsibilities	723
Lactation Consultants and Voluntary Counselors	724
Marketing	726
Networking	726
Reporting and Charting	727
Nursing Diagnosis	728
Methods for Charting	728
Clinical Care Plans	729
Legal Considerations	730
Reimbursements	731
The LC in Hospital-Based Practice	731
The LC in Private Practice	732
The Business of Doing Business	735
Collaboration with Other Health Care Workers	737
Partnerships	738
Burnout	739
Do's and Don'ts of Lactation Consulting	741
Summary	743
References	744

CHAPTER 23

Research and Breastfeeding 747

Approaches to Research Methods	747
Qualitative Approaches	747
Types of Qualitative Methods	748
Quantitative Approaches	749
Types of Quantitative Methods	749
Additional Approaches	751
Multiple Approaches	751
Elements of Research	752
Research Problem and Purpose	752
Variables, Hypotheses, and Operational Definitions	753
Review of the Literature	756
Protection of the Rights of Human Subjects	756
Method	757
Data Analysis	758
Results, Discussion, and Conclusions	758
Application of Methods to Qualitative Approaches	759
Reliability and Validity	759
Sampling and Sample Size	760
Data Collection	760
Data Analysis	760
Application of Methods to Quantitative Approaches	761
Sampling and Sample Size	761
Data Collection	762
Reliability and Validity	764
Data Analysis	765
The Evaluation of Research Reports and Articles for Use in Practice	768

Using Research in Clinical Practice 770

Summary 770

References 772

Related Readings 774

CHAPTER 24

Donor Human Milk Banking: More Than Nutrition 775

The History of Human Milk Banking 775

Current Trends in the United States and Canada 776

Donor Milk Banking Outside North America 777

Cultural Issues 779

The Benefits of Donor Milk 779
Species Specificity 779
Ease of Digestion 779
Promotion of Growth, Maturation, and
  Development of Organ Systems 779
Allergy Prophylaxis 780
Immunological Benefits 780

Clinical Uses of Donor Milk 780
Distribution of Donor Milk: Neonates
  Versus the Older Infants 780
Nutrition 780
Nutrition and Disease Prevention for
  Premature Infants 784
Milk Fortification 784
Medicinal Therapy 785

Current Practice 786
Donor Selection and Screening 786
Heat Treatment 787
Collection, Handling, and Storage 789
Packaging and Transport 789
Quality Assurance 789
Environmental Contaminants 794
Policies and Procedures 794
Costs of Donor Milk 794

Summary 795

References 795

Appendixes 801
A. Composition of Human Colostrum and
   Mature Breast Milk 803
B. Via Christi Health System, St. Joseph
   Campus Breastfeeding Policies 805
C. Via Christi Health System, St. Joseph
   Campus Breastfeeding Education Protocol 810
D. Nursing Diagnosis Related to Breastfeeding 819
E. New York State Code in Support of
   Breastfeeding (Added 1984) 820
F. American Academy of Pediatrics: Breast-
   feeding and the Use of Human Milk 821
G. Prototype Lactation Consultant Job
   Proposal or Description 826
H. ILCA Standards of Practice for Lactation
   Consultants 829
I. Tables of Equivalencies and Methods of
   Conversion 833
J. Wellstart International Patient History 834
K. Conversion Tables 842
L. Standardized Height and Weight
   Growth Charts 843

Glossary 845

Index 857

PREFACE

Since the first edition of this book was published in 1993, breastfeeding rates across the U.S. have risen to about 60 percent. Most of this increase has been in the population served by WIC–the result of more interest in and funding for breastfeeding promotion programs. Other exciting developments have changed the field. Research studies now verify that breastfed children are more intelligent and that *not* breastfeeding costs the health care system billions of dollars annually. The United States finally became a signatory to the WHO Code in 1994. The insurance industry now drives the health care system, reversing the reward system, so that disease prevention and less expensive health care is profitable rather than the other way around. The percentage of women employed outside the home was only 33 percent in 1950. By 1997, this figure has nearly doubled for women who have preschoolers or younger children. Some milk banks have closed because of the fear of spreading AIDS through breastfeeding.

The length of the hospital stay after normal birth is now two days or less in the U.S.; while breastfeeding mothers and babies return home less likely to be exposed to hospital infections and to supplementary feedings as a result of these short stays, this brief time allows almost no opportunity to ensure that the baby is breastfeeding effectively. Mothers still needing care themselves return home to assume full-time child care before they feel physically able to do so. Follow-up care of a new family in their home should be universal, yet newspapers and journals report cases of dehydrated babies, because no one seems to care that parents have neither the knowledge nor the support for breastfeeding that could help them.

The number and influence of lactation consultants continues to grow. More than 5,000 health care workers from 36 countries have been certified by the International Board of Lactation Consultants. Many hospitals, large and small, offer lactation services of some type and employ lactation consultants.

This text represents more than 60 years of the authors' combined clinical experience. It brings together in a single resource clinical techniques, research findings, and the varied roles of the lactation consultant. The relationship between daily clinical practice and concepts is reciprocal–just as clinical practice improves as a result of research outcomes, clinical observations point the way to research studies. Over 2,000 research studies support our clinical recommendations. Readers will note that many of the research studies discussed in this text give credence to information that observant clinicians have known for years.

As this book goes to press we are entering a new millennium as witnesses to an historic shift in the dominant social paradigm that is redefining the roles of women. Women activists for birthing and breastfeeding rights have been at the forefront of the consumer movement of this last quarter-century. They will be no less needed in the twenty-first century than they were in the last half of the twentieth century. The rights of women include their right to be fully, not partially, informed; to take fully active, not institutionally constrained, roles in childbearing and childrearing. We view this book as our contribution to empowering women to gain their rights.

The second edition of our text has a clear clinical focus. The expansion of knowledge and continuing research studies required that Chapter 9, The Breastfeeding Process, in the first edition become two chapters, Chapters 9 and 10, which are the key twin chapters on the breastfeeding process. In each, we present the most current, research-based clinical knowledge and techniques. If the reader must choose what to read first in order to gain the "basics" of clinical expertise in breastfeeding, we recommend these two chapters.

We also have added a chapter on maternal nutrition. Nearly every chapter contains a clinical implications section. Throughout the book are new references deemed by the authors to be the most important from the vastly expanded research and clinical literature. New color visuals that depict anatomical and immunological concepts have been added. Readers will be pleased to see that the section including clinical color photographs has been expanded and is now found in the center of the book.

Section 1 sets the stage on which the information in later chapters can be placed. This section focuses on "the big picture," placing lactation and breastfeeding in historical and sociocultural context and identifying different ways in which the breastfeeding family functions within that context.

Section 2 focuses on another kind of "big picture": basic anatomic and biologic imperatives. Clinical application of techniques must be based on a clear understanding of the relationships between form, function, and biological constructs. Thus this section, too, provides the background upon which to build other aspects of lactation and breastfeeding behavior.

Breastfeeding skills are not necessarily instinctive in humans. Thus teaching the basics of *what* to do, *when* to do it, and *how* is a primary caregiving goal when assisting the new lactating mother. Ideally, the mother learns about breastfeeding before her baby's birth; her learning continues when she puts her baby to breast during the early postpartum period. Section 3 thus concerns itself with the early perinatal period, paying particular attention to the importance of prenatal education of the pregnant family, to the need for assistance and support for breastfeeding after birth, and following the family's return home. In spite of mounting evidence to the contrary, neonatal physiological jaundice still leads to clinical decisions that interfere with breastfeeding. In this section, we also consider the implications of the infant who fails to gain weight appropriately and how to assist the baby to grow as expected. It addresses preterm babies' special needs and how to support their mothers as they express milk and later feed directly. Also discussed are breast-related problems. In addition, we critically evaluate breastfeeding devices and recommend how and when they are most appropriately used.

Section 4 focuses on the importance of maternal nutrition, the mother's and baby's health status, and the ill breastfeeding child, followed by an examination of the effect of the mother's employment on lactation, and concludes with a discussion of maternal sexuality and fertility and their relationship to one another and to lactation.

Section 5 examines the field of lactation consulting and carefully looks at research—how it is conducted, why ongoing research is needed, and how research findings can be applied in clinical settings. It concludes with a review of the development and current activities of human milk banking.

An extensive glossary of key terms relating to lactation can be found in the *Study Guide* to this text. To avoid confusion between the word *nursing*—meaning the profession—and nursing, meaning breastfeeding, *nursing* in the text refers to the profession. The masculine pronoun has been used to denote the infant or child throughout the text as a matter of convenience to distinguish the child from the breastfeeding mother. Nurses, lactation consultants, and other health care workers are referred to in the feminine gender, recognizing that males serve in various health care professions.

Acknowledgments

We gratefully acknowledge the people who helped and supported us during the writing of this book, in particular

Anne Andrianos, Syracuse, New York
Jan and Jill Barger, Wheaton, Illinois
Virginia Brackett, Evanston, Illinois
Jane Bradshaw, Lynchburg, Virginia
Pat Bucknell, Avon Lake, Ohio
Ann Calandro, Waxhaw, North Carolina
Vicki Carlson, Lancaster, New Hampshire
Roger Clark, Wichita, Kansas
Paula Conning, Orangeville, Ontario, Canada
Donna Corrieri, Boca Raton, Florida
Fritzi Drosten, Oakland, California
Karen Foard, State College, Pennsylvania
Catherine Watson Genna, Woodhaven, New York
Jacki Glover, Lethbridge, Alberta, Canada
Terri Hazen, Willoughby, Ohio
Susan Hilton, Lexington, North Carolina
Elisa Hirsch, Westlake Village, California
Vicki Honer, Roanoke, Virginia
Kay Hoover, Morton, Pennsylvania
Angela Jacobi, Chicago, Illinois
Debby Kearney, Casselberry, Florida
Linda Kutner, Mooresville, North Carolina
Lisa Marasco, Santa Maria, California
Margaret Marquardt, Long Beach, California
Pamela Morrison, Harare, Zimbabwe
Amy Mueller, Traverse City, Michigan
Chris Mulford, Swarthmore, Pennsylvania

Audrey Naylor, San Diego, California
Elizabeth Novelo Puzar, San Jose, California
Ellen Petok, Los Angeles, California
Faith Ploude, Miami, Florida
Jeanne Rago, Morristown, New Jersey
Shirley Riordan, Wichita, Kansas
Quinn and Rika Riordan, Tokyo, Japan
Deborah Shinskie, Summerville, South Carolina
Calayne Stanton, Spring Hill, Kansas
Ruth Solomon, Harrisburg, Pennsylvania
Linda Stewart, San Diego, California
Arnold L. Tanis, Florida
Peggy Toman, Oskosh, Wisconsin
Gina Woodley, San Antonio, Texas
Lorna Weixelman, Wichita, Kansas
Ruth Wester, San Diego, California
Barbara Wilson-Clay, Manchaca, Texas
Karen Zeretzke, Baton Rouge, Louisiana
Linda Zielinski, Boise, Idaho

Reviewers who improved the text include

Judy Angeron, Via Christi Health System, Wichita, Kansas
Helen Armstrong, UNICEF Baby Friendly Project, Tufts University, Boston, Massachusetts
Jan Barger, Wheaton, Illinois
Roberta Baven, Wichita State University, School of Nursing, Wichita, Kansas
Fred Chang, University of Kansas, School of Medicine, Wichita, Kansas
Mary Margaret Coates, TechEdit, Wheat Ridge, Colorado
Sarah Danner, U.S. Baby Friendly, Peterborough, New Hampshire
Ros Escott, South Hobart, Tasmania, Australia
Ann Flores, Via Christi Health System, Wichita, Kansas
Eileen Hawkins, Wichita State University, School of Nursing, Wichita, Kansas
Vergie Hughes, Lactation Education Resources, Fairfax, Virginia
Heather Hull, Wichita State University, School of Nursing, Wichita, Kansas
Miriam Labbok, Nutrition & Maternal/Infant Health, Agency for International Development, Washington, DC
Verity Livingstone, University of British Columbia School of Medicine, Vancouver, BC, Canada
Chele Marmet, Lactation Institute and Breastfeeding Clinic, Encino, California
Joan Melzer, Kansas Newman College, Wichita Kansas
Maureen Minichin, Armadale, Victoria, Australia
Gerald Nelson, The University of Kansas, School of Medicine, Wichita, Kansas
Rosanne Orlando, Brookhaven Memorial Hospital Medical Center, New York
Virginia Phillips, Brisbane, Queensland, Australia
Ellen Shell, Lactation Institute and Breastfeeding Clinic, Encino, California
JoAnne Scott, International Board of Lactation Consultant Examiners, Falls Church, Virginia

We extend special thanks to La Leche League International for providing the foundation for our breastfeeding education as La Leche League leaders and to those institutions that welcomed us to their libraries to explore their treasures: Via Christi Health System, The University of Kansas School of Medicine, both of Wichita, Kansas; Rush-Presbyterian-St. Luke's Medical Center and John Crerar Medical Library, both of Chicago, Illinois, and St. Joseph's Hospital Library, Bellingham, Washington.

Last, we lovingly acknowledge our families, who encourage and nurture us: Hugh, Michael, Neil, Shirley, Brian, Quinn, and Rika Riordan, Teresa and Richard Chenoweth, Renee and Don Olmstead, and Doug Auerbach.

Jan Riordan

Kathleen G. Auerbach

CHAPTER AUTHORS

Lois Arnold, MPH, IBCLC
Executive Director
Human Milk Banking Association of North
    America, Inc.
Sandwich, Massachusetts

Debi Leslie Bocar, RN, MS, MEd, IBCLC
Lactation Consultant
Mercy Health Center
Oklahoma City, Oklahoma

Yvonne Bronner, ScD, RD, LD
Assistant Professor
Department of Maternal and Child Health
Johns Hopkins University School of Hygiene and
    Public Health
Baltimore, Maryland

Linda P. Brown, PhD, RN, FAAN
Associate Professor
University of Pennsylvania
School of Nursing
Philadelphia, Pennsylvania

Mary Margaret Coates, MS, IBCLC
TechEdit
Wheat Ridge, Colorado

Richard Guthrie, MD
Professor, Department of Pediatrics
University of Kansas School of Medicine at
    Wichita
Wichita, Kansas

Roberta Hewat, RN, PhD, IBCLC
Assistant Professor, School of Nursing
University of British Columbia
Vancouver, British Columbia, Canada

Nancy Hurst, RN, MSN, IBCLC
Director, Lactation Support Program and Milk
    Bank
Texas Children's Hospital
Houston, Texas

Kathy I. Kennedy, MA, DrPH
Adjunct Faculty
University of Denver
Denver, Colorado

Paula P. Meier, DNSc, RN, FAAN
NICU Lactation Program Director, Department
    of Maternal-Child Nursing
Associate Director for Clinical Research, Section
    of Neonatology
Rush-Presbyterian-St. Luke's Medical Center
Chicago, Illinois

Marsha Walker, RN, IBCLC
Lactation Associates
Weston, Massachusetts

THE HISTORICAL AND SOCIOCULTURAL CONTEXT OF INFANT FEEDING

Lactation and breastfeeding exist within the constraints of each culture in which the physical function and the behavior are practiced. Just as the breastfeeding course flows and ebbs in a mother's life, so it has experienced flows and ebbs in different cultures through the years. Though clearly playing a beneficial role in women's and infants' health, breastfeeding as a human behavior reflects its importance in society over time by how, when, where, and for how long it is practiced. The theoretical constructs that allow us to examine the family—identifying its members, their unique roles, their relationships, and how each contributes to a sum greater than its parts—also enable us to identify issues specific to the breastfeeding family, regardless of race, parental age, or socioeconomic status.

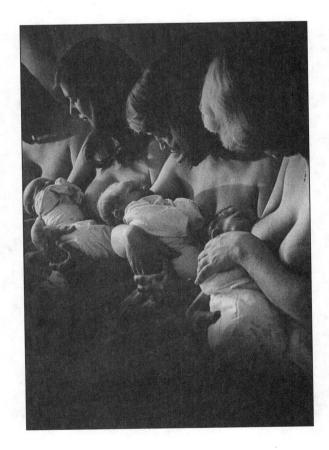

Tides in Breastfeeding Practice

Mary-Margaret Coates

Throughout the world today, an infant is apt to receive less breastmilk than at any time in the past. Until the 1940s, the prevalence of breastfeeding was high in nearly all societies. Although the feeding of manufactured milks and baby milks had begun before the turn of the century in parts of Europe and North America, the practice spread slowly during the next decades. It was still generally limited to segments of population elites, and it involved only a small percentage of the world's people. During the post–World War II era, however, the way in which most mothers in industrialized regions fed their infants began to change, and the export of these new practices to developing nations was under way.

Evidence About Breastfeeding Practices

How do we know what we "know" about the prevalence of breastfeeding? (*Prevalence* is used here to mean the combined effect of breastfeeding initiation rates and breastfeeding continuance rates.) Before attempting to trace trends in infant-feeding practices, let us consider the nature of the evidence.

Large-Scale Surveys

National surveys that produced the kind of representative data that allow statistical evaluation have been available only since 1955. These surveys consist primarily of national fertility or natality surveys and of marketing surveys conducted by manufacturers of artificial baby milk. In the United States, the National Fertility Studies of 1965 and 1970 (sponsored by the National Institute of Child Health and Human Development), and the National Surveys of Family Growth of 1973 and 1976 (sponsored by the National Center for Health Statistics), included questions about breastfeeding (Hendershot, 1980; Hirschman & Butler, 1981). National Natality Surveys, which collected data in 1969 and 1980 about how newborns were fed, were conducted by the National Center for Health Statistics (Forman et al., 1985). Results of several market surveys conducted between 1955 and 1995 have also been published (Martinez & Nalezienski, 1979; Ryan et al., 1991; Ryan, 1997).

Outside the United States, representative data for countries in Latin America, Asia, Africa, and the Middle East are derived from three sources. World Fertility Surveys conducted from 1972 to 1984 were sponsored by the Office of Population within the United States Agency for International Development (USAID), the United Nations Fund for Population Activities, and the United Kingdom Office of Development Assistance (Lightbourne & Singh, 1982). The World Health Organization began ongoing surveys on infant feeding in the mid-1970s. Its Global Data Bank on Breast-Feeding pools information garnered from well-designed, variously sized nutrition and breastfeeding surveys around the world; on the basis of these data, breastfeeding practices are periodically summarized (WHO, 1996; Saadeh et al., 1993). Finally, demographic and health surveys were initiated in 1984; these ongoing surveys are sponsored jointly by the USAID and governments of host countries in which the surveys are made.

Small Surveys

Local or special-purpose studies document the variety of practices within smaller regions or population segments. Before 1955, such studies provided the only quantitative information available on breastfeeding. Bain's (1948) compilation of the incidence of breastfeeding in U.S. hospitals was the first study of such practices published in this country.

Other Evidence

Until the last several decades, breastfeeding was the unremarkable norm. Thus what we "know" about breastfeeding from much earlier times often must be inferred from evidence of other methods of feeding infants. Most historical material available in English-language literature derives from a rather limited geographical area: Western Europe, Asia Minor, the Middle East, and North Africa. Written materials, which include verses, legal statutes, religious tracts, personal correspondence, inscriptions, and medical literature, extend back to before 2000 BC.

Some of the earliest existing medical literature deals at least in passing with infant feeding. An Egyptian medical encyclopedia, the *Papyrus Ebers* (c. 1500 BC), contains recommendations for increasing a mother's milk supply (Fildes, 1986). The first writings to discuss infant feeding in detail are those of the physician Soranus, who practiced in Rome around AD 100; his views were widely repeated by other writers of the mid-1700s. It is not immediately apparent to what degree these early exhortations either reflected or influenced actual practices. Many writings before AD 1800 deal primarily with wet nurses or with how to hand-feed infants.

Archeological evidence provides some information about infant feeding prior to 2000 BC.

Some of the earliest artifacts are Middle Eastern pottery figurines that depict lactating goddesses, such as Ishtar of Babylon and Isis of Egypt. The abundance of this evidence suggests that lactation was held in high regard (Fildes, 1986). Such artifacts first appear in sites about 3000 BC, when pottery making first became widespread in that region. Information about infant feeding may also be derived from paintings, inscriptions, and infant-feeding implements.

Modern ethnography has a place of special importance. By documenting the infant-feeding practices of present-day nontechnological hunting-gathering, herding, and farming societies, ethnographers expand our knowledge of the range of "normal" breastfeeding practices. At the same time, they provide a richer appreciation of cultural practices that enhance the prevalence of breastfeeding. Such studies are also our best window onto breastfeeding practices that may be the biological norm for *Homo sapiens sapiens*.

In summary, the historical aspect of this chapter deals with data from limited social strata in a limited geographical region. However, the common threads of these data provide a useful context within which we may better understand modern breastfeeding practices, especially in Western cultures.

The Biological Norm in Infant Feeding

Early Human Evolution

The class Mammalia is characterized principally by the presence of breasts (mammae) which secrete and release a fluid that for a time is the sole nourishment of the young. This manner of sustaining newborns is extremely ancient; it dates back to the late Mesozoic era, some 100 million years ago. (See Fig. 1–1.) Hominid precursors first appeared about 4 million years ago; the genus *Homo* has existed for some 2 million years. The currently dominant human species, *Homo sapiens sapiens,* has existed for only perhaps 40,000 years. Information about breastfeeding practices among our earliest ancestors is uncertain, though other information about Paleolithic societies that existed 10,000 or more years ago sheds light on this subject.

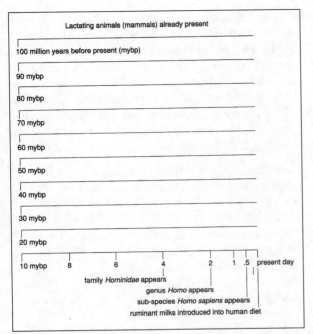

FIGURE 1–1. The antiquity of lactation. *The bottom line shows the approximate times of first appearances of lactating precursors of modern humans and of regular use of nonhuman animal milks by humans.*

Early Breastfeeding Practices

Diets reconstructed by archeological methods reveal that the Late Paleolithic era, roughly 40,000 to 10,000 years ago, was populated by preagricultural peoples who ate a wide variety of fruits, nuts, vegetables, meat (commonly small game), fish, and shellfish. This diet closely resembles that of twentieth-century hunter-gatherer societies (Eaton & Konner, 1985). Therefore, the infant-feeding practices of societies today may reflect breastfeeding practices of much earlier (prehistoric) times. Consider the breastfeeding practices of the iKung of the Kalahari Desert in southern Africa (Konner & Worthman, 1980) and hunter-gatherer societies of Papua New Guinea and elsewhere (Short, 1984). Among these people, breastfeeding of young infants is frequent (averaging four feeds per hour) and short (about two minutes per feed). It is equally distributed over a 24-hour period and continues, tapering off gradually, for two to six years. These breastfeeding patterns are considered a direct continuation of practices that prevailed at the end of a long, dietetically stable, evolutionary period ending about 10,000 BC. This assumption is supported by observations of the human's closest primate relative, the chimpanzee, which secretes a milk quite similar to that of humans, suckles several times per hour, and sleeps with and nurses its young at night (Short, 1984).

The Replacement of Maternal Breastfeeding

However, the practice of giving foods other than maternal breastmilk is deeply rooted. Both written and archeological records show that by 2000 BC, some babies were wet-nursed or fed animal milks. Considering the biological impetus for mothers to breastfeed, why have some mothers sought other foods for their infants? Mothers acclimate to the idea of feeding their infants foods other than their own breastmilk under many economic, social, familial, and personal circumstances. Alternatives become acceptable when maternal breastfeeding is impossible or when it appears to provide no social or health advantage to either the mother or the infant, whereas the alternative food or method of feeding does appear to offer such an advantage. Women choose other than breastmilk foods for their infants when two conditions are met: alternative foods are available, and the use of these alternative foods is socially acceptable (Zeitlyn & Rowshan, 1997).

Wet-Nursing

Wet-nursing may not have been the earliest alternative to maternal breastfeeding, but it was the only one likely to enable the infant to survive. Wet-nursing is common, although not universal, in today's traditional societies and (by inference) among ancient human societies. An already lactating woman may have been the most obvious choice for a wet nurse, but women who stimulate lactation without a recent pregnancy have been described in many traditional societies (Slome, 1976; Wieschhoff, 1940).

Wet-nursing for hire is mentioned in some of the oldest surviving texts, which implies that the practice was well established, even in ancient times. The Babylonian Code of Hammurabi

(c. 1700 BC) forbade a wet nurse to substitute a new infant for one who had died. The Old Testament Book of Exodus (c. 1250 BC) records the hiring of a wet nurse for the foundling Moses; the fact that the wet nurse was Moses's own mother is incidental. The epic poems of Homer, written down around 900 BC, contain references to wet nurses. A treatise on pediatric care in India, written during the second century AD, contains instructions on how to qualify a wet nurse when the mother could not provide milk. The Koran, written about AD 500, also permits parents to "give your children out to nurse."

Although the history of wet-nursing has continued virtually uninterrupted from the earliest times to the present, the popularity of the practice among the elite classes who used it most has waxed and waned. In England during the 1600s and 1700s and elsewhere in Europe, the middle classes began to employ wet nurses. The use of less attentive nurses and the sending of infants greater distances from home diminished maternal supervision of either nurse or infant. Often infants were not seen by their parents from the time they were given to the nurse until they were returned home after weaning (provided they lived). However, by the latter part of the 1700s, wet-nursing (except in foundling hospitals) was on the decline in North America and England, owing to increased public concern regarding the moral character of wet nurses and the quality of the care they provided. Throughout this long period, wet nurses were used sometimes because of maternal debility but more often because of the social expectation of the class of women who could afford to hire them. Thus the use of wet nurses by social elites foreshadows the demographic pattern seen later in the use of manufactured baby milks.

Hand-Fed Foods

The Agricultural Revolution. The idea that animal milks are suitable foods for human infants is reflected in such myths as that of Romulus and Remus, the mythical founders of Rome, who are usually depicted as being suckled by a wolf. Surprisingly, the currently most popular hand-fed infant foods—animal milks and cereals—did not become part of the human diet until well along in the evolutionary history of *Homo sapiens sapiens.*

Cereal grains first appeared only about 10,000 years ago, and animal milks somewhat later (McCracken, 1971). The widespread adoption of these foods was made possible by the development of agriculture and (later) animal husbandry. Perhaps because of the availability of new weaning foods, periods of lactation normally lasting for three to four years were shortened to about two years in farming and herding societies (Schaefer, 1986).

Gruels. In much of the world, the soft foods added most commonly to the infant diet have been gruels containing a liquid, a cereal, and other substances that added variety or nutritional value. The cereal might be rice, wheat, or corn. It might be boiled and mashed; ground and boiled; or, as in the case of bread crumbs, ground, baked, crushed, and heated. The liquid might be animal milk, meat broth, or water; eggs or butter might also be added. Where grains are not commonly eaten, similar soft infant foods are based on starchy plants, such as taro, cassava, or plantain.

Animal Milks. Animal milks are a relatively recent addition to the human diet; this is implied genetically, because children beyond weaning age commonly do not produce lactase, an enzyme needed to digest the milk sugar lactose. In cultures that do not use animal milks, such as those in Bangladesh or Thailand, some children may be lactose-intolerant before age one; in those cultures that *do* use animal milks, the onset of lactose intolerance occurs considerably later—after age 10 in Finland (Simoons, 1980). Adult lactose tolerance is common only in cultures in which animal milks have traditionally been an important part of the diet, such as those of northern Europe and western Asia (McCracken, 1971).

Feeding Vessels. The earliest "vessel" used to hand-feed an infant was undoubtedly the human hand, and the foods so fed were probably soft or mashed rather than liquid. The earliest crafted vessels for feeding liquids were probably animal horns pierced by holes in the tips; such horns continued to be used into the 1900s in parts of Europe. The oldest pottery vessel thought to have been used for infant feeding, a small spouted bowl found in an infant's grave in France, is dated c. 2000–1500 BC (Lacaille, 1950). Small spouted or football-shaped bowls have been found in infant burial sites in

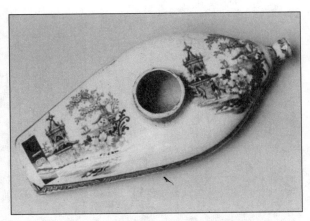

FIGURE 1–2. Photograph of English Staffordshire Spode nursing bottle c. 1825. *(Courtesy V. H. Brackett.)*

Germany (c. 900 BC) and in the Sudan in North Africa (c. 400 BC) (Lacaille, 1950). These utensils suggest that hand feeding of infants has been attempted for more than three millennia. (Fig. 1–2.)

Timing of the Introduction of Hand Feeding

What archeological evidence cannot tell us is why or how much these infants were hand-fed. Neonates may temporarily be offered certain foods as prelacteal feeds; young infants may be offered occasional tastes of other foods, and they will be offered increasing amounts of soft foods as they make the transition to the adult diet (mixed feeds). Finally, infants may be reared from birth on other foods (artificial feeding).

Prelacteal Feeds. Many of the world's infants, even those who later will be fully breastfed, receive other foods as newborns. Of 120 traditional societies (and, by inference, in many ancient preliterate societies) whose neonatal feeding practices have been described, 50 delay the initial breastfeeding more than two days, and some 50 more delay it from one to two days. The reason is to avoid the feeding of colostrum, which is described as being dirty, contaminated, bad, bitter, constipating, insufficient, or stale (Morse et al., 1990).

Early medical writers in the eastern Mediterranean region (Greece, Rome, Asia Minor, and Arabia) and later in Europe–from Soranus through those of the 1600s–also discouraged the use of colostrum for feeding. These writers recommended avoiding breastfeeding for periods as short as one day (Avicenna, c. AD 1000) to as long as three weeks (Soranus, c. AD 100). Commonly, to promote passage of meconium, the newborn was first given a "cleansing" food: most often, honey, sweet oils (such as almond), or sweetened water or wine.

In Europe, the fear of feeding an infant colostrum may have contributed to the undermining of maternal breastfeeding, at least among the upper classes, and to the spread of wet-nursing (Deruisseau, 1940). A similar charge has been leveled at the prelacteal bottle feeds commonly given in Western (or Western-style) hospital nurseries; many studies show that early bottle feeds undermine breastfeeding and increase the use of manufactured baby milk (Bloomquist et al., 1994; Verronen et al., 1980; Winikoff et al., 1986; Wright et al., 1996). One can only wonder whether routine Western hospital practices, which include delayed first breastfeeding and prelacteal feeds of water or artificial baby milk, are technological vestiges of this widespread traditional "taboo."

Not all published work supports the idea that prelacteal feeds and a delay in initiating breastfeeding reduce the likelihood of continued lactation (Richards, 1986). Some believe that ensuing breastfeeding is associated with the maternal perception that prelacteal feeds are appropriate. They hold that a particular set of culturally approved maternal behaviors follows the commencement of breastfeeding: nearly constant contact with or close proximity to the infant, ad lib breastfeeding day and night, and no further use of feeding bottles (Nga & Weissner, 1986; Woolridge et al., 1985).

Mixed Feeds. On the basis of current practices of many traditional societies, early mixed feedings may be the most common infant-feeding regimen (Dimond & Ashworth, 1987; Kusin et al., 1985; Latham et al., 1986; Wieschhoff, 1940).

Mixed feeding is widely practiced, even during the time when breastmilk forms the foundation of the infant diet. In many regions, such as Africa and Latin America, breastfeeding continues into the second or third year of life. In non-Western cultures, hand-fed foods include tea infusions, mashed fruits, and a variety of starchy gruels or pastes. Where the use of a particular food dominates a culture (e.g., rice in many parts of Asia), that food is usually the principal family food fed to an infant (Jelliffe, 1962). In some (mostly non-Western) cultures, such foods are offered to weaning infants in such a way that they supplement, rather than replace, breastmilk (Greiner, 1996; Whitehead, 1985) and thus do not appreciably hasten cessation of breastfeeding. The use of feeding bottles, however, can shorten the weaning interval, the period between full sustenance by breastmilk and full sustenance by family foods (Winikoff & Laukaran, 1989).

Hand Feeding from Birth. In a few regions of northern Europe (e.g., Switzerland, Finland, and Iceland), a cool, dry climate and a tradition of dairy farming permitted the survival of at least some infants who were fed cow milk nearly from birth. From at least the 1400s in Switzerland and Finland, breastfeeding was actively discouraged (Fildes, 1986). However, even in climatically optimum areas, hand feeding was hazardous. In Iceland, infants were hand-fed during the 1600s and 1700s despite disastrous results; married women bore as many as 30 infants because so few newborns survived (Hastrup, 1992). In France, some foundlings and infants with syphilis were fed directly from goats; this practice was first described in writing in the 1500s, and it persisted until the early 1800s (Wickes, 1953a). Of necessity, foundling hospitals of the 1700s and 1800s in Europe and the United States hand-fed infants but with appalling mortality rates: up to 100 percent died. (See Fig. 1–3.) However, by the mid-1900s, hand feeding from birth had become the norm in industrialized countries, and hand-fed infants survived and grew.

Technological Innovations in Infant Feeding

The Social Context

During the late 1800s and the early 1900s, high infant mortality, even among infants cared for at home, was a major public concern. Both physicians and parents recognized that poorly nourished children were more susceptible to illness. Between 1910 and 1915, the newly created United States Children's Bureau sponsored several studies of infant mortality in major cities. Each study showed that babies fed artificial (i.e., anything other than

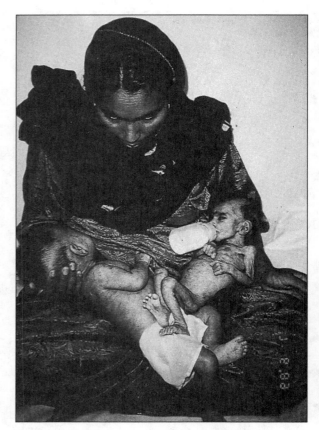

FIGURE 1–3. UNICEF photograph of thriving, three-month-old breastfed twin and his dying bottle-fed sister. *(Courtesy of Children's Hospital, Islamabad, Pakistan.)*

mother's) milks were three to five times as likely to die as those who were breastfed. The studies also documented that the rates of breastfeeding and infant mortality were linked: each increased steadily as family income decreased. In summarizing these results, Williamson (1915) commented that "the disadvantages of a low income were sufficient to offset the greater prevalence of breast feeding among the babies of the poorer families." During this same period, a similar observation was made in England, where high infant mortality prevailed among poor, working-class mothers, 80 percent of whom breastfed their infants (Levenstein, 1983).

As women's aspirations for community service and commercial involvement were rising, Victorian beliefs about modesty discouraged breastfeeding in public. Advertising, which promoted bodily cleanliness, may have led to associating breastmilk with body fluids that were unclean or noxious, a notion that persists to this day, at least in North America (Morse, 1989). Advances in the prevention of disease, largely through public health measures related to sanitation, extended an expanding faith in "modern science" to the field of "modern medicine." Women's magazines developed a wide audience of readers interested in female accomplishments outside the home, in modern attitudes, and in technological innovations; these same magazines reinforced concerns about infant health. An 1880 issue of the *Ladies' Home Journal* contained this statement (Apple, 1986):

If fed from your breast, be sure that the quantity and quality supply his demands. If you are weak or worn out, your milk cannot contain the nourishment a babe needs . . .

The Technological Context

Between about 1860 and 1910, scientific advances and technological innovations created many new options in infant feeding that appeared to enhance infant survival. The upright feeding bottle and rubber nipple, each of which could be cleaned thoroughly, made artificial feeding easier and safer. New foods to be used with this equipment appeared. Large-scale dairy farming produced abundant supplies of cow milk, which was marketed first as canned evaporated milk and later in condensed form (i.e., highly sweetened to retard spoilage) or in dried form.

This technological ferment, fueled both by the need for improved infant health care and by a popular belief in the ability of science and technology to provide answers, attracted analytical chemists. Around 1850, chemists had begun to turn their attention to food products. Now viewed as rudimentary, early investigations into the composition of human and cow milk convinced them that ". . . the combined efforts of the cow and the ingenuity of man" could construct a food the equal of human milk (Gerrard, 1974). Patented foods, such as Liebig's Food and Nestlé's Milk Food, were first marketed in Europe and the United States in the 1860s. The Nestlé's product was a mixture of flour, cow milk, and sugar, and was meant to be dis-

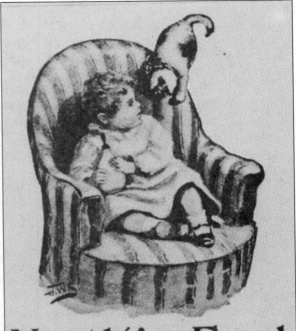

Nestlé's Food

Nestlé's Food is a complete and entire diet for babies. Over all the world Nestlé's Food has been recognized for more than thirty years as possessing great value as a protection against Cholera Infantum and all other forms of Summer Complaint.

Nestlé's Food is safe. It requires only the addition of water to prepare it for use. The great danger always attendant on the use of cow's milk is thus avoided.

Consult your doctor about Nestlé's Food, and send to us for a large sample can and our book, " The Baby," both of which will be sent free on application.

THOMAS LEEMING & CO.
73 Warren Street, New York

FIGURE 1–4. Advertisement for artificial infant milk, *which appeared in the* Ladies' Home Journal *12:26, 1895.*

solved in milk or water before feeding. Milk modifiers, such as Mellin's Food, and milk foods, such as Horlick's Malted Milk, were popular in the United States by the 1880s.

Extravagant claims for these foods–Liebig's Food was called "the most perfect substitute for mother's milk"—were combined with artful advertising that played on fears for the health of the infant and on faith in modern science (Apple, 1986). (See Fig. 1–4.) One hundred years later, we see these advertising themes played out again and again.

In the 1890s, physician Thomas Rotch developed a complex system of modifying cow milk so that it more closely resembled human milk. Rotch observed that the composition of human milk varies, as do the digestive capacities of infants. He devised mathematical formulas to denote the proportions of fat, sugar, and protein in cow milk, ingredients that some infants required at a specific age (Rotch, 1907). The result was an exceedingly complex system of feeding that required constant intervention by the physician, who often changed the "formula" weekly. Supervising infant feeding then became a principal focus of the newly emerging specialty of pediatrics.

Commercial advertising promoted the use of manufactured infant milks to both mothers and physicians. The basic themes—a mother's concern for her infant's health, the perfection of the manufactured product, and the difficulty of breastfeeding—have persisted over the years (Apple, 1986).

The Role of the Medical Community

Regulation of Childbirth. During the early part of this century, childbirth moved from home or midwife-attended births to hospitals, where a birthing woman was separated from her family and attended by a physician. During the middle part of this century, hospital routines and the use of general anesthesia during labor and delivery separated mother and infant much of the time in the early postpartum period. Bottle-feedings by nursery staff became increasingly common. Normal postpartum hospital stays in the United States lengthened; during the 1930s and 1940s, they were sometimes as long as two weeks. This period, intended to permit the mother to recuperate from (an often highly medicated) childbirth, resulted as well in a return home with an impaired breastmilk supply and a baby who was accustomed to bottle-feedings. Bain (1948) notes that babies who were older than eight days at discharge were less apt to be breastfed than were younger ones.

Regulation of Breastfeeding. Underlying many changes in the feeding of infants was a "regulatory"

frame of mind, the seeds of which had been sown in Europe as early as the 1500s. The advent of book printing about that time permitted a much wider dissemination of works regarding infant care. Their authors shared a concern for the high incidence of gastrointestinal illness in infants and for high infant-mortality rates. For reasons not at all clear today, overfeeding was deemed a central factor in both. Writers concerned with child care responded by advocating the regulation of feeding to prevent presumed overfeeding.

Writing in the mid-1600s, Ettmuller (1703) was not the first to recommend infrequent feedings: "Nothing is more apt to disorder the child than suckling it too often, since large quantities of milk stagnating in the stomach, must needs corrupt . . . especially if fresh milk be pour'd in before the preceeding be digested."

Some 200 years later in 1900, French obstetrician Pierre Budin (1907), famous for his early interest in premature infants and for his advocacy of breastfeeding, was nonetheless typical of many others in recommending small feedings: ". . . [I]t is better at first to give too little than too much, (for an underfed infant failed to gain weight but it was free from digestive troubles). . . ."

Even medical writers who strongly recommended breastfeeding also recommended highly regulated times for feedings—a fixed number of feedings at fixed times. William Cadogan (1749), whose firm endorsement of breastfeeding and largely sound advice prompted many privileged English women to breastfeed, advocated only four feeds per day at equal intervals and eschewed night feeds! A prototype mothercraft manual by Hugh Smith (1774) contains excellent advice: to feed colostrum and to allow the newborn to suckle frequently to stimulate lactation. However, it then instructs mothers to limit feedings (beginning at one month), to five per day timed at 7 and 10 AM and 1, 6, and 11 PM. About 50 years later, after recommending ad lib feedings for the first 10 days, Thomas Bull (1849) instructed mothers to feed the infant for the rest of the first month at regular four-hour intervals day and night, because he also believed that irregular feeding harmed the infant. After one month, the night feeding was to be eliminated.

These influential publications began the process of removing the management of infant feeding from the mother (or from the realm of women in general) and placing it in the hands of (usually) male "authorities." Cadogan (1749) commended this change that put "men of sense rather than foolish unlearned women" in charge, and Rotch a century and a half later (1907) deplored that "mothers and nurses . . . dominated the physicians."

Regulation and Industrialization. This "regulatory" frame of mind fit nicely with the needs of the growing industrial sector of the economy, which relied on efficiency and schedules governed by the clock. Societal perceptions of infants' innate characteristics and needs were interpreted in this light (Millard, 1990). Early in the twentieth century, infants were seen as needing order imposed on their characters from the outside (Rossiter, 1908):

. . . [A]n infant two days old may be forming either a good or a bad habit. A child that is taken up whenever it cries is trained into a bad habit; the same principle is true in reference to nursing a baby to stop its crying. Both these habits cultivate self-indulgence and a lack of self-control . . .

"Good" mothering thus drifted toward meeting the letter of schedules often imposed by the medical profession rather than toward meeting the mutual needs of mother and infant as expressed by and interpreted within the dyad.

Although rigid, externally imposed schedules diminished after the 1960s, it is still assumed in most literature that lactation functions better when mother and baby together develop feeding routines. The lack of some routine is usually perceived as abnormal by both mother and physician (Millard, 1990). However, employment skills, such as an awareness of time and responsiveness within a hierarchical authority structure, are those least apt to enable a mother or a pediatrician to accommodate the irregularities of early breastfeeding.

Regulation of Contraception. During the late 1950s and early 1960s, the widespread acceptance of oral contraceptives may have reinforced the decline in breastfeeding (Meyer, 1968). Contraceptives containing estrogen and progestin reduce breastmilk volume and thus contribute to lactation insufficiency, early supplementation, and early weaning from the breast. Moreover, women who planned to use combined estrogen and progestin

oral contraceptives were discouraged from breast-feeding to avoid passing those hormones to the infant. During this period, several million women per year in the United States alone were thereby removed from the pool of potential breastfeeders. Currently marketed low-progestin contraceptives pose fewer hazards to the maternal milk supply and the baby, and often they are routinely recommended to mothers nursing young infants (Kelsey, 1996).

Accommodation Between Physicians and Infant Milk Manufacturers. The relationship between physicians and infant food manufacturers has in general promoted mothers' dependency on either the manufacturer or the physician for information on infant feeding. In the late 1800s, as proprietary infant foods were being developed, manufacturers advertised to both groups. By the 1920s, some preparations were advertised to mothers but could be purchased only by prescription or used only after consulting a physician; the package contained no instructions for use. By 1932, the American Medical Association essentially required baby-milk manufacturers to advertise only to the medical profession (Greer & Apple, 1991). The mutual economic benefits of this policy were clearly spelled out in many advertisements placed by such formula manufacturers as Mead Johnson (1930) in medical journals in the 1930s:

When mothers in America feed their babies by lay advice, the control of your pediatric cases passes out of your hands, Doctor. Our interest in this important phase of medical economics springs, not from any motives of altruism, philanthropy or paternalism, but rather from a spirit of enlightened self-interest and co-operation because (our) infant diet materials are advertised only to you, never to the public.

Despite several early studies that showed breastfed infants to be healthier than those bottle-fed (Grulee et al., 1934; Howarth, 1905; Woodbury, 1922), many physicians acted for years as if there were little advantage to breastfeeding. This persistent view was expressed through the 1960s. For instance, Aitken and Hytten (1960) reported that ". . . with modern standards of hygiene artificial feeding on simple mixtures of cow's milk, water and sugar is a satisfactory substitute for breast feeding . . ."

Likewise, Hill (1968) noted that ". . . formula feeding has become so simple, safe, and uniformly successful that breast-feeding no longer seems worth the bother."

Advertising came full circle in 1988 when Nestlé Food Company sought to enter the United States market for infant formula by advertising directly to consumers. Although medical societies opposed this move on the grounds of protecting the public, direct advertising has continued.

The Prevalence of Breastfeeding

United States, England, and Europe

The Recent Past. The net result of these shifts in technology and attitudes has been a rapid decline in the prevalence of breastfeeding in Western nations since the 1940s. In the United States, the proportion of newborns receiving any breastmilk at one week postpartum declined steadily to a low of 25 percent in 1970 (Martinez & Krieger, 1985). The proportion of newborns exclusively breastfed at hospital discharge was even lower: It declined from 38 percent in 1946 (Bain, 1948) to 21 percent in 1956 and only 18 percent by 1966 (Meyer, 1968). The period of most dramatic decline of breastfeeding coincided with U.S. economic factors that encouraged major migrations from rural to urban areas. For example, between 1945 and 1970, approximately five million African-Americans moved from the rural South to the urban North. The association between internal migration from rural to urban areas and a decline in breastfeeding also has been noted in developing countries (Jelliffe & Jelliffe, 1978). The trend reversed in the 1970s and peaked in the mid-1980s, when 52 percent of women initiated exclusive breastfeeding in hospital, and 17 percent persisted in exclusive breastfeeding at six months postpartum (Fig. 1–5). Breastfeeding prevalence plateaued and has fluctuated since that time.

Current Breastfeeding Practices. One marketing study made in the United States in 1995 showed that only 60 percent of hospital-born infants received any breastmilk in the hospital; of those, only 18 percent were still receiving any breastmilk by six months of age (Ryan, 1997). These figures compare with 63 percent and 24 percent for 1984, respectively (Ryan et al., 1991).

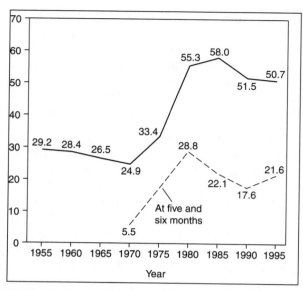

FIGURE 1–5. Percentage of infants in the United States receiving any breastmilk at birth (upper curve) and at five and six months (lower curve), 1955–1995. *Based on data from Martinez and Krieger (1985), Ryan et al. (1991), and Ryan (1997).*

Developing Regions

The Role of Colonial Empires. Declines in the prevalence of breastfeeding were noted in non-Western regions somewhat later than in the West. Between World Wars I and II, British, French, and German colonial empires controlled fully one-fourth of the inhabited globe and one-fourth of the world's population. These empires served as vehicles for the expansion of markets for artificial baby milks.

Colonial ruling elites who followed the practices of their social class in their country of origin (which, moreover, placed social distance between themselves and the nationals of their adopted country) were much more likely to feed their infants artificial milks than to breastfeed. That most of these infants survived resulted in large part from the higher levels of sanitation and medical care that their position in life afforded them. To some degree, these colonial elites served as unwitting role models for indigenous peoples.

Concern for the health of indigenous peoples led many health care workers to transmit Western attitudes regarding infant feeding to the populations they served: by example, by direct recommendations, and by the training provided to indigenous health care providers. Westerners have traditionally assumed that the foods good for them must be good for all people and have passed these prejudices on to foreign nationals trained in Western schools (McCracken, 1971). Perhaps because Western medical personnel were successful at treating many other health problems, local populations were prepared to accept attitudes that encouraged the use of artificial baby milks. Health care personnel in hospitals helped to introduce the use of manufactured baby milks and contributed to undermining breastfeeding (Winikoff & Laukaran, 1989).

Colonial transportation and communication networks, and health care clinics and hospitals aided the advertisement and sale of artificial baby milks to this huge population. The decline in breastfeeding accelerated after World War II, in part because of greater contact between Western health care personnel and populations in developing countries, and in part because relief projects shipped to war-torn countries the surplus skim milk produced in abundance by the large dairy industry in the United States (Wade, 1974). Between 1976 and 1977, 42 transnational companies manufactured, distributed, and marketed infant-milk products in four countries surveyed: Ethiopia, Nigeria, India, and the Philippines (World Health Organization [WHO], 1981).

Infant Feeding and Infant Mortality. The relation between infant feeding and mortality is complex. Infant mortality has tended to be highest among populations in which breastfeeding was most common: the poor. Rural mothers in Ethiopia and Zaire reported that at least 30 percent of their infants died, although 97 percent of mothers were breastfeeding at 18 months postpartum, as were 80 percent of a similar group of mothers in rural Zaire (WHO, 1981). The same relationship held in the United States during the early 1900s (see p. 8).

Although widespread artificial feeding has been associated with poorer infant survival, both in Western nations early in this century and in developing nations in the mid-1900s, the reverse is not always the case. The advent of primary health care for a large portion of a population may explain decreases in infant mortality in the face of a decline in breastfeeding. In Nicaragua, the proportion of infants breastfed at six months declined 25 per-

centage points (from 58 percent to 33 percent) between 1977 and 1988. During this same period, infant mortality declined from about 10 percent to about 6.5 percent (Sandiford et al., 1991). It seems clear that the pervasive problems of poverty, in both Western and non-Western locales, were at the root of the appalling infant mortality in impoverished populations.

The Recent Past. During the 1970s, when breastfeeding rates were generally increasing in Western nations, they continued to decline in the more populous developing regions. Between the late 1970s and the mid- to late-1980s, however, trends in developing nations varied (Fig. 1–6). During this period, breastfeeding initiation rates stayed about the same or increased slightly in 15 Asian, African, and Latin American countries (Indonesia, Sri Lanka, Thailand, Kenya, Ghana, Senegal, Tunisia, Morocco, Colombia, Dominican Republic, Ecuador, Mexico, Peru, and Trinidad/Tobago).

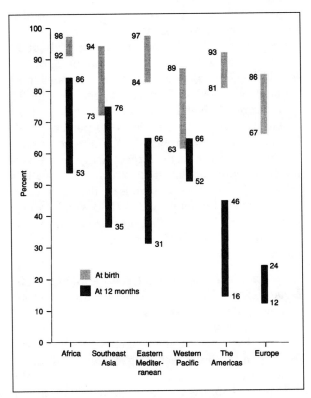

FIGURE 1–6. Range of percentages of infants breastfed during the 1980s at birth (upper bar) and at 12 months (lower bar) in six regions of the world. *(Based on data from the World Health Organization [1989a].)*

However, the median duration of any breastfeeding decreased in twice as many countries (10) as those in which it increased (5), and the greatest decline (five and a half months in Thailand) was twice the greatest increase (two and a half months in Ghana and Trinidad/Tobago) (Dr. R. K. Sharma, personal communication, 1991).

Current breastfeeding practices. In 1996, the World Health Organization estimated that worldwide, about one-third of all infants younger than four months are exclusively breastfed and that any breastfeeding continues for a median duration of about 18 months. However, initiation and continuance rates differ among regions. Southeast Asian infants are most likely to be exclusively breastfed (49 percent) and have the longest median duration of breastfeeding (25 months). In three other regions –the Americas, Eastern Mediterranean, and Western Pacific–about one-third of young infants are exclusively breastfed, but the median duration of breastfeeding ranges from almost 20 months in the Eastern Mediterranean to only half that (10 months) in the Americas. African investigators report a relatively low rate of exclusive breastfeeding (about 20 percent), but a relatively long median duration (21 months). Generalizing breastfeeding rates and duration reported in Europe (16 percent and 11 months, respectively) is difficult as only 4 of 50 countries, representing perhaps 20 percent of all European infants, provided WHO with survey results. On the whole, the foregoing figures are estimated to represent almost 60 percent of the world's infants. However, it is surmised that infants in countries that did not provide WHO with information regarding breastfeeding practices are even less likely to be exclusively breastfed and are breastfed for even shorter periods.

Characteristics of Breastfeeding Women in Developing Regions. Generalizations about demographic characteristics most likely to predict who will breastfeed have many exceptions. In general, rural women are more likely to begin breastfeeding and to breastfeed longer than are those of urban areas; poorer mothers are more likely to breastfeed than are the more affluent. The urban poor, often recent immigrants from more rural areas, are the mothers among whom breastfeeding rates are declining most rapidly. However, in Kenya and Trinidad/Tobago, increases in median duration during the 1980s occurred in a broad range of socioeconomic and educational levels. During this same period in the Dominican Republic, the median duration of breastfeeding rose among urban and employed mothers, although the overall median duration dropped 15 percent (Dr R. K. Sharma, personal communication, 1991).

The Cost of Not Breastfeeding

To see a world in a grain of sand and a heaven in a wild flower, / Hold infinity in the palm of your hand and eternity in an hour.

—William Blake, "Auguries of Innocence," c. 1803

Although isolated voices championed breastfeeding throughout its years of steady decline, not until the 1970s did the trend toward artificial feeding reverse (see Fig. 1–5). The reasons that prompted this change are not clear (Eckhardt & Hendershot, 1984) but seem to reflect a widespread desire by many to include simpler, more natural practices in their lives. Basic, clinical, and demographic research increasingly demonstrated the benefits of breastmilk and breastfeeding to the infant, and of lactation and breastfeeding to the mother. Later still, it has come to be recognized that there is a cost to not breastfeeding.

Health Risks of Using Manufactured Infant Milks

Risks to the Infant. It has been recognized since the advent of manufactured infant milks that infants fed these products suffered more illness (Grulee et al., 1934; Howarth, 1905; Woodbury, 1922). This observation is confirmed by more recent studies (Chen et al., 1988; Cunningham et al., 1991; Fallot et al., 1980). At the time of the earlier studies, the immunological role of breastmilk was unclear; most deleterious effects of manufactured milks were attributed to contamination. In more recent decades, it has become established that artificial baby milk increases the risk of ill health by many pathways (Walker, 1993). Not only can these foods be (or easily become) contaminated (Aksit et al., 1997), but they lack the immunological and other health-promoting factors present in human milk. In addition, they contain nutrients that are foreign or are mixed in nonphysiological proportions (Minchin, 1987). Furthermore, the act of bottle-feeding differs from that of breastfeeding in ways that may contribute to health problems in some infants (Mathew & Bhatia, 1989). Artificially fed infants are denied the benefits of "autoimmunization," whereby the breast produces antibodies to organisms to which the infant has been exposed (Fishaut et al., 1981). Immunization may be less effective in artificially fed infants, because manufactured milks do not enhance the immune response to vaccination (Pabst & Spady, 1990).

Recent research shows that artificially fed infants are more susceptible to gastrointestinal infections caused by *Campylobacter* (Ruiz-Palacios et al., 1990), cholera (Glass et al., 1983), *Shigella* (Cleary et al., 1989), and to inguinal hernia (Pisacane et al., 1995) and urinary-tract infections (Marild et al., 1990; Pisacane et al., 1990). Artificial infant milk may enable respiratory pathogens to become established (Andersson et al., 1986), and infants so fed are more likely to develop ear infections (Forman et al., 1984; Kero & Piekkala, 1987). Grulee et al. (1934) noted that infants fed cow milk were more likely to have eczema; infants fed manufactured infant milk are also more likely to manifest allergic signs (Chandra et al., 1989; Working Group on Cow's Milk Protein Allergy, 1988). One of these signs may be disturbed sleep (Kahn et al., 1987). In premature infants, artificial feeds are a significant risk factor for the potentially fatal condition of necrotizing enterocolitis (Lucas & Cole, 1990). Bottle feeds are associated with poorer oxygenation during feedings in both premature infants (Meier & Anderson, 1987) and term neonates (Mathew & Bhatia, 1989).

Risks to the Child and Adult. The effects of artificial feeding may extend well beyond infancy. Artificial feeding is implicated in some diseases that develop in childhood, such as tonsilitis (Pisacane et al., 1996), celiac disease (Greco et al., 1988; Kelly et al., 1989), diabetes (Mayer et al., 1988; Scott, 1990), juvenile rheumatoid arthritis (Mason et al., 1995), and lymphoma (Davis et al.,

1988). They are also more apt to show neurological abnormalities (Lanting et al., 1994) and to suffer atopic disease (Saarinen & Kajosaari, 1995). Adults afflicted by inflammatory bowel disease (Calkins & Mendeloff, 1986) or Crohn's disease (Bergstrand & Hellers, 1983) or those with multiple sclerosis (Pisacane et al., 1994) are more likely to have been fed artificially as infants. Bottle-feeding is also associated with oral malocclusion (Labbok & Hendershot, 1987).

Risks to the Mother. Artificial feeding is also detrimental to maternal health. In the absence of lactational amenorrhea, additional pregnancies may adversely affect her health. Mothers who artificially feed their infants are more likely than are breastfeeding mothers to develop osteoporosis (Cummings et al., 1985; Hoffman et al., 1993), premenopausal breast cancer (McTiernan & Thomas, 1986; Newcomb et al., 1994; Thomas & Noonan, 1993), ovarian cancer (Schneider, 1987), and other dangers of the reproductive system (Gwinn et al., 1990; Rosenblatt & Thomas, 1995). Bottle-feeding mothers who have diabetes will not enjoy the amelioration of symptoms that may be experienced by breastfeeding mothers who have diabetes (Butte et al., 1987).

Economic Costs of Using Manufactured Infant Milks

The presence or absence of breastfeeding affects the economics of the family, the community, and the nation. Some of these effects are more pronounced in less developed regions, but to a degree they affect both elite and poor populations in technologically advanced regions.

Costs to the Family. Although lactation imposes some demands on the mother's body stores, these demands are moderated by gastric changes that allow lactating women to metabolize foods more efficiently while lactating (Illingworth et al., 1986; Uvnas-Moberg et al., 1987) and by the water-conserving effect of prolactin (Dearlove & Dearlove, 1981). Moreover, the contraceptive effect of full, unrestricted breastfeeding reduces a woman's physical and economic costs of childbearing (Jackson, 1988; Kennedy et al., 1989).

The direct monetary costs of rearing a breastfeeding infant are markedly lower than those of rearing one who is artificially fed. In industrial nations, the cost of manufactured baby milk may exceed the cost of additional food for the lactating mother by two or three times (Jarosz, 1993); in developing nations, the ratio is many times higher. In regions where one-third to one-half of those in large urban areas live in poverty, the cost of manufactured products required to provide adequate nutrition (and implements with which to feed them) is a significant portion of the family income (Serva et al., 1986). Other family members may eat more poorly because the baby is artificially fed.

An equally important consideration is the reduced need for medical care by breastfed infants (particularly those who are exclusively breastfed). The frequency and severity of illnesses in young infants are often inversely related to the proportion of their diet that comes from breastmilk (Chen et al., 1988). More breastfeeding increases infant intake of high-quality protein and a variety of other needed nutrients, and it decreases infant exposure to potential pathogens in other foodstuffs (Habicht et al., 1988).

Because full breastfeeding, which includes frequent feedings throughout a 24-hour period, tends to delay resumption of ovulation (Lewis et al., 1991), spacing between births tends to increase. Births spaced less than two years apart may increase the mortality risk of both the older and the younger infant (Retherford et al., 1989). Especially in families living at subsistence level, the older a child is when displaced from the breast and the fewer the number of children in a family, the more likely each is to be healthy. In malnourished communities, breastfeeding may substantially increase child survival up to three years of age (Briend et al., 1988).

Thus the breastfed infant stands a significantly greater likelihood of surviving. The mother's physical and emotional investment in pregnancy and lactation and the familial investment in time and money are repaid by the survival of a child; they are lost to the family when that child dies.

Costs to the Community and State. Community or national units that provide health care must respond to the local epidemiology of infant illness, in which feeding may play a major role. Morbidity is more prevalent in artificially fed infants (Jason et al., 1984; Kovar et al., 1984) regardless of location.

The increase of the infant population resulting from the loss of the contraceptive effect of breastfeeding also serves to increase the need for pediatric health care.

A little-discussed aspect of the decline of breastfeeding is that certain sectors of an economy can become economically dependent on the payrolls met and taxes paid by infant milk manufacturers, especially if capital funds are obtained from outside the country. Once they become a financial presence in a country, dislodging those manufacturers may be politically and economically difficult, despite increases in health costs elsewhere in the economy.

Nonetheless, manufactured milk products widely used for infant feeding are subsidized by the diversion of resources (land, dairy cattle, and people to manage both) and by manufacturing capacity pulled from other possible uses. Alternatively, manufactured milk products must be purchased on the international market, and such purchases may markedly affect a nation's balance of trade. Jelliffe and Jelliffe (1978) estimate that 150 cans of ready-to-feed manufactured baby milk are used during the first six months of artificial feeding. When one considers that more than 20 million babies are born annually in Africa alone, it becomes apparent that providing adequate volumes of manufactured milks represents a staggering burden and a largely unnecessary diversion of human and monetary resources from other, more beneficial programs. At a time when environmental issues have become paramount, these unnecessary uses of power and raw material, not to mention the disposal of discarded packaging, is an increasing concern.

The Promotion of Breastfeeding

Many studies in North America and Europe have attempted to define the relative characteristics of women who do and who do not breastfeed. This information then gives direction to efforts for promoting breastfeeding. A flaw of many studies is the lack of a clear definition of what behavior was termed "breastfeeding." Breastfeeding behaviors of interest include (1) initiation of any breastfeeding with the newborn, (2) initiation of exclusive breastfeeding, (3) duration of exclusive breastfeeding, and (4) duration of any breastfeeding. The adoption by researchers of a consistent terminology, such as that proposed by Labbok and Krasovec (1990), will aid in interpreting and comparing study results.

Characteristics of Breastfeeding Women

Initiation of Lactation. Consistently since the 1970s, breastfeeding in North America and Western Europe has been more likely to be initiated by older white women of a higher social class: these mothers are more likely to be affluent, to have more years of formal education, to be nonsmokers, to have attended childbirth classes, to have more social support, and to intend to breastfeed. By contrast, the exclusive feeding of manufactured infant milk is more likely among lower income, nonwhite women who smoke and have fewer years of formal education. The conclusion of Grossman et al. (1990) that low-income women who chose to breastfeed were more likely to be similar in several respects (such as age, education, and most sources of support) to high-income women who breastfeed is important. Regional differences impinge on women in both the United States and Canada. In general, the incidence of breastfeeding increases from east to west in both countries; in the United States it increases also from south to north. Breastfeeding is little practiced among indigenous peoples of either country.

Infants who are larger at birth are more likely to be breastfed at one week (Forman et al., 1985; Ryan et al., 1990). Houston and Field (1988) note that smaller babies are more apt to be fed on a routine schedule, which perhaps increases the difficulty of establishing breastfeeding.

Role of the Health Care System. The role of the health care system in both undermining and enhancing the initiation of breastfeeding is widely debated. The usual division of care of the breastfeeding dyad—between a gynecologist/obstetrician and a pediatrician—renders the identification and resolution of breastfeeding problems more difficult. Many studies show that few physicians discuss breastfeeding with their patients (although pediatricians are more likely to do so). In any case, few

mothers rely on a physician's advice when deciding whether to breastfeed (Mansbach et al., 1984).

Many hospital practices have been implicated in undermining breastfeeding. In an attempt to increase breastfeeding initiation rates, the changes outlined in the following paragraphs have been recommended (Wright et al., 1996). The most basic recommendations have been incorporated by the WHO as the "Ten Steps to Successful Breast-feeding" (see Box 1–2 on p. 21).

Continuance of Lactation. The *duration* (as opposed to *initiation*) of lactation is strongly affected by the mother's determination to continue breastfeeding in a predominantly bottle-feeding society (Bottorff, 1990; Coreil & Murphy, 1988; Mulford, 1995). It may be adversely affected by additional factors, including admission of the neonate into a special-care nursery, even if the reason for admission was minor and transient (Kemper et al., 1989; Persson, 1985). Early supplementation of breastfeeding with manufactured infant milk is strongly implicated in shortening the duration of breastfeeding both in the United States (Kurinij et al., 1988) and in developing nations (Winikoff & Laukaran, 1989).

Mothers who are physically able to lactate and nurse healthy infants may perceive that their baby requires more milk than they are able to provide. The volume of breastmilk made available to the infant may reflect any or a combination of three factors: (1) intrinsic maternal lactational capacity, (2) the effectiveness of infant suckling, and (3) the mother's "socially determined" capacity (i.e., the amount of milk she produces as a function of cultural attitudes toward breastfeeding and cultural constraints on breastfeeding behavior).

A mother's attentiveness to her infant also has a strong socially determined component. A mother may also seek other foods when she perceives that her breastfed infant needs more maternal attention than she feels she can (or should need to) provide. Infant nursing patterns, general contentedness, or sleeping behavior that differ markedly from maternal expectations may prompt the use of supplements. Although the relative role played by each factor may vary among individuals, cultural constraints on breastfeeding behavior are always important determinants of breastmilk transfer.

Promotion Efforts

The many ways of encouraging mothers to breast-feed their own infants–"breastfeeding promotion"–may be considered to lie on a continuum. At one end, in societies where breastfeeding is the cultural norm, promotion consists of assuming that mother and infant will breastfeed. This is combined with social arrangements, such as special foods or lightened duties for the mother, especially for the first few weeks after birth, to ensure that breastfeeding becomes well established. At the other end, in societies in which artificial feeding is the norm, promotion often consists of encouragement, sometimes by government officials and often by health care professionals or members of elite population groups, to others to breastfeed, without at the same time removing cultural barriers to breastfeeding.

Exhortation. Perhaps the commonest form of breastfeeding promotion has been exhortation. Caesar (in 48 BC) ridiculed–and Tacitus (c. AD 100) deplored–Roman mothers who left their children in the care of wet nurses (Hymanson, 1934). During the 1500s in Europe, when breastfeeding was infrequently practiced among the aristocracy, long poems addressed to this class attempted to convince mothers of the cruelty of not breastfeeding (Davidson, 1953). Stricter Protestant sects of that era considered breastfeeding to be a religious duty and, by the early 1600s, women who did not breastfeed were condemned by Puritan clergy, both from the pulpit and in religious tracts (Fildes, 1986).

Statements by Health Organizations. In 1978, the American Academy of Pediatrics (Committee on Nutrition, 1978) and the Canadian Paediatric Society jointly issued a statement endorsing breastfeeding–as part of the WHO's program to identify 1979 as the International Year of the Child. Similar public endorsements by other professional organizations of physicians, nurses, and nutritionists appeared several years later (Coates, 1990).

Governmental Support: the United States. In 1978, the U.S. Public Health Service defined National Health Objectives for 1990. One stated that 75 percent of women should breastfeed at hospital discharge and 35 percent at six months, as opposed to the actual 1978 figures of 45 percent and 21 percent (U.S. Department of Health and Human Services, 1980). Because these goals were not met by 1990, they were reasserted as goals for the year 2000. To help to find ways to work toward these goals, the Surgeon General convened a Workshop on Breastfeeding and Human Lactation in 1984.

Although other government agencies in the United States also work to improve infant nutrition, the Special Supplemental Food Program for Women, Infants, and Children (WIC) program probably directly affects the greatest number of people. This program, established in 1972, provides free nutrition counseling and food supplements, including manufactured baby milk, to low-income mothers and their infants. This clientele comes from the population segment in the United States least likely to breastfeed (MacGowan et al., 1991).

The WIC program follows in the footsteps of infant welfare programs of the 1890s and early 1900s in France, England, and the United States, which provided centers where infants could be weighed and examined weekly. These centers also provided cow milk ("fresh and clean" in some, sterilized in others) to nonbreastfeeding mothers in an effort to reduce infant illness and death caused by the use of contaminated milks. By 1903, such milk dispensaries were already being accused of discouraging breastfeeding because they seemed to endorse the use of other infant milks (Wickes, 1953b). Even today, government-sponsored distribution of free milk (as has occurred in Nicaragua since 1970) has been seen as one reason for the decline of breastfeeding there (Sandiford et al., 1991).

WIC has become the largest purchaser of manufactured infant milk, with 40 percent of all formula sold in the United States sold to the WIC program. For years, WIC paid the full retail price; by 1991, when by law WIC was required to purchase manufactured infant milks from the lowest bidder (usually in the form of a rebate from the manufacturer), bids typically came in less than a penny apart in unit price. It has been estimated that in 1988, the purchase of artificial milks for WIC infants' first month of life amounted to more than $30 million (Lazarov, 1989).

Formula manufacturers traditionally have maintained close ties with this important customer in additional ways. A large U.S. artificial baby milk

BOX 1–1

WHO/UNICEF Code for Marketing Breast-Milk Substitutes

- No advertising of these products to the public.
- No free samples to mothers.
- No promotion of products in health-care facilities.
- No company "mothercraft" nurses to advise mothers.
- No gifts or personal samples to health workers.
- No words or pictures idealizing artificial feeding, including pictures of infants, on the products.

- Information to health workers should be scientific and factual.
- All information on artificial feeding, including the labels, should explain the benefits of breastfeeding and the costs and hazards associated with artificial feeding.
- Unsuitable products, such as condensed milk, should not be promoted for babies.
- All products should be of a high quality and take into account the climatic and storage conditions of the country where they are used.

manufacturer that bids on WIC contracts also publishes WIC's house newsletter, *WIC Currents.* Formula manufacturers have provided clinics with informational pamphlets on breastfeeding and posters of breastfeeding women; the company logo is prominently displayed on both.

However, in the latter half of the 1980s, the promotion of breastfeeding became an important goal of WIC. Compared with nonbreastfeeding mothers, breastfeeding women now have a higher priority for enrollment in WIC programs: they are provided more, increasingly varied foods, and their benefits persist longer—one year, as opposed to six months for nonbreastfeeders.

During the 1980s, WIC obtained funds that allowed improved training of WIC nutritionists with respect to breastfeeding, permitted research on how to encourage low-income women to breastfeed, and enabled demonstration projects through which breastfeeding rates have in fact been increased. Reinforcing this commitment is a 1991 directive that bans formula advertising on any item used or displayed in WIC clinics and requires that the formula itself be stored out of sight of clients.

The World Health Organization. In the 1970s, the deleterious effects of manufactured baby milks on infant health and survival became better appreciated, and the role of advertising in spreading the use of such milks became increasingly suspect. In 1981, the WHO, by a vote of 118 to 1 (the United States being the dissenting country), approved the International Code of Marketing of Breast-Milk Substitutes. The Code provides a model of marketing practices that permits the availability of manufactured baby milk but forbids their advertisement or free distribution directly to consumers. (See Box 1–1.) It also seeks to balance the information provided by infant-milk manufacturers in both written "educational" material and in the text or pictures on containers of the product (Armstrong, 1988; IBFAN/IOCU, 1985). In 1996, the World Health Assembly passed six resolutions that further clarified the intent of the Code. Of these six resolutions, one reaffirms the use of local family foods to complement the diet of breastfeeding infants beyond about six months of age. Another reaffirms the need to end the free or low-cost (subsidized) distribution of artificial baby milks to newly parturient women in hospital. Two other resolutions proscribe receipt of funds from manufacturers or distributors of artificial baby milks or feeding supplies to be used for professional training in infant and child health or for financial support of any organization that monitors compliance with the international code (United Nations Children's Fund, 1996a).

An individual country may adopt the international code in the manner that best fits the needs of that country. In some, as in the United States, no action has been taken, and formula manufacturers are bound only by voluntary adherence to the industry-written "codes of ethics." A few other countries have adopted and enforce various aspects of the Code.

The Code focuses attention on ways in which the infant formula industry influences both consumers and professionals to support the use of their products. Direct advertising to consumers may be the most obvious ploy, but what Jelliffe and Jelliffe (1978) called "manipulation by assistance" is also effective. For example, formula manufacturers not only provide free formula to hospital nurseries but assist in the design of those nurseries (to promote separation of mother and infant), donate equipment to hospitals (e.g., gowns for premature infants) and to individual physicians, and support conferences (including some dealing with breastfeeding). They may even entertain hospital staff at company-sponsored events; in 1990 in one midwestern U.S. city, hospital staff were taken on an outing to the dog races. These "gifts" are treated by the companies as marketing expenses. Lactation consultants also can be the targets of "manipulation by assistance" provided by manufacturers of artificial baby milks and of other feeding products banned by the Code.

As individuals and institutions become financially dependent on such gifts and are enmeshed in social relationships with company salespersons, they are more likely to tacitly endorse, or even recommend, artificial baby milks. By highlighting such practices as marketing ploys, the Code may make health care professionals more aware of the intent behind them and thus perhaps more resistant to their allure.

In 1990, the WHO and United Nations International Children's Emergency Fund (UNICEF) were instrumental in the development of the Innocenti Declaration, which restated the importance of breastfeeding for maternal and child health. It set forth four goals to be met by 1995:

1. the establishment of national breastfeeding co-ordinators

2. the practice of "Ten Steps to Successful Breast-Feeding" by maternity services (see Box 1–2)

3. the implementation of the WHO code

4. enactment of enforceable laws for protecting the breastfeeding rights of employed women (UNICEF, 1990)

Some 140 countries now have national breastfeeding committees, and about 185 offer maternity leaves of at least 12 weeks, usually only to those formally employed (UNICEF 1996a). The World Alliance for Breastfeeding Action (WABA), a multinational coalition of individuals and private organizations involved in research and promotion of breastfeeding, works to ensure that the goals of the Innocenti Declaration are met, and annually supports activities presented in connection with World Breastfeeding Week.

The Baby-Friendly Hospital Initiative (BFHI) was launched in 1992 to encourage in all countries specific hospital practices that promote exclusive breastfeeding. To be designated *baby-friendly,* hospitals must demonstrate to an external review board that it practices each of the Ten Steps to Successful Breast-Feeding. In 1992, 290 hospitals in 12 countries achieved baby-friendly status. Studies are now beginning to be published that examine the degree to which the "Ten Steps" are being implemented (Karra et al., 1993; Kovach, 1997; Wright et al., 1996). By early 1998, 12,931 hospitals in 117 countries had achieved this status (UNICEF, 1996a). With the principal exception of the Scandinavian countries, industrialized nations have moved more slowly than have developing nations. East Asia and the Pacific region accounted for more than half of the designations; South Asia accounted for another 12 percent.

Breastfeeding advocates in the industrialized world labor against three impediments: an artificial milk industry that is powerful enough, both financially and politically, to avoid regulation; a pervasive bottle-feeding culture that does not consider

BOX 1–2

Ten Steps to Successful Breast-Feeding

Every facility providing maternity services and care for newborn infants should:

1. Have a written breastfeeding policy that is routinely communicated to all health-care staff.

2. Train all health-care staff in skills necessary to implement this policy.

3. Inform all pregnant women about the benefits and management of breast-feeding.

4. Help mothers initiate breastfeeding within 30 minutes after birth.

5. Show mothers how to breastfeed and how to maintain lactation even if they should be separated from their infants.

6. Give newborn infants no food or drink other than breastmilk, unless medically indicated.

7. Practice rooming-in—allow mothers and infants to remain together—24 hours a day.

8. Encourage breastfeeding on demand.

9. Give no artificial teats or pacifiers (also called *dummies* or *soothers*) to breastfeeding infants.

10. Foster the establishment of breastfeeding support groups and refer mothers to them on discharge from the hospital or clinic.

Source: Protecting, promoting and supporting breastfeeding: The special role of maternity services. A joint WHO/UNICEF statement. Geneva: World Health Organization, 1989.

Note: These steps and the complete elimination of free and low-cost supplies of breastmilk substitution, bottles, and teats from health care facilities form the basis of the Baby Friendly Hospital Initiative.

breastfeeding important to child or maternal health; and the lack of much precedence for government-mandated health programs. As a result, all industrialized nations together can claim less than 3 percent of all baby-friendly hospitals (UNICEF, 1996b); in Australia, 2 hospitals have been so designated, and in the United States, 11. However, by early 1997, almost 300 hospitals and 20 birth centers in the United States had signed certificates of intent to seek baby-friendly designation according to the global BFHI criteria.

Legislation. Legislation intended to increase the prevalence of breastfeeding may mandate actions that encourage breastfeeding or discourage feeding of artificial baby milk (or use of wet nurses) or both. Lycurgus, king of Sparta about 350 BC, set an

early example: he required not only that mothers nurse their own infants but that nursing mothers be shown kindness and respect (Hymanson, 1934).

A more modern example is legislation following the model of the WHO Code of Marketing of Breast-Milk Substitutes. The advertising of infant-feeding bottles and artificial infant milks was forbidden by law in the mid-1970s in Papua New Guinea; both are still available but only by prescription. The benefits of breastfeeding were publicized to the general population and to health workers. This dual approach increased the prevalence of breastfeeding among children who were less than two years of age by 23 percent (from 65 percent in 1976 to 88 percent in 1979 (Biddulph, 1981). In 1986, the government of the Philippines banned the distribution of free and subsidized artificial infant milks to hospitals, and it imposed fines or prison sentences on violators of the ban. The distribution of such milks intended for young infants declined by 95 percent between 1986 and 1988. Although it remains to be seen whether this policy will result in an increase in breastfeeding, the policy now makes it less convenient and more expensive for mothers to use artificial infant milks in the hospital (Popkin et al., 1990).

Private Support Movements. During the 1970s, the trend to artificial feeding reversed (see Fig. 1–5). The reasons are not clear (Eckhardt & Hendershot, 1984) but seem to have been part of a widespread desire of many to include simpler, more natural practices in their lives. In the 1950s and 1960s, when breastfeeding was becoming less prevalent, individuals interested in breastfeeding and sharing information about breastfeeding found each other and formed mutual-support groups. La Leche League was founded in the United States in 1956, Nursing Mothers' Association of Australia began in 1965, and Ammenhjelpen of Sweden in 1968. Such groups assist individual women and focus national attention on the benefits of breast-feeding.

La Leche League now has more than 3,000 groups in 66 countries around the world. Its manual is translated into 8 languages, and it provides some information in 19 others. Members of groups such as these, by their demonstration that even "modern" mothers can breastfeed and by their requests to medical personnel for information about medical practices that support breastfeeding, have been a major force behind the dissemination of technical information concerning lactation, human milk, and breastfeeding. To better reach low-income women who are not commonly La Leche League members, the organization has begun training peer counselors. These counselors, low-income women who have breastfed and have completed a training program, offer breastfeeding advice and support in clinics serving low-income populations. Such counselors can be very effective: a Chicago WIC clinic reported an eightfold increase in breastfeeding during a six-month period in which peer counselors were available (Heiser, 1990). La Leche League is officially recognized as a nongovernmental organization qualified to consult on breastfeeding to organizations such as the United Nations and the U.S. Agency for International Development.

S U M M A R Y

Humans evolved within the mammalian lineage, which has provided a species-specific milk for the nourishment and protection of the young of each species. For millennia, the staple of the human infant's diet has been human milk obtained directly from the human breast, commonly in situations where no other food was suitable. Within the last century or so, as breastfeeding became associated with more restrictive aspects of women's lives, as breastmilk was thought by some to be inferior to increasingly available manufactured infant milks, and as use of manufactured milks became a hallmark of privileged segments of society, large portions of both lay and health care populations came to believe that there was little reason to persist in traditional breastfeeding practices.

In the 1990s, however, it has become increasingly clear that breastfeeding confers health and psychological advantages on the breastfeeding infant and to the child and adult into which that infant will grow. Breastfeeding enhances aspects of maternal health as well. Breastfeeding is economically frugal, ecologically sound, and important. Most mothers and most health care providers now recognize these benefits.

The promotion efforts outlined in this chapter are needed because, to some degree in most countries (and particularly in industrialized ones), the most important requirement is missing: acceptance by society of the need for a mother and child to be together and the right of the breastfeeding dyad to participate in social, civic, and commercial activities outside the home. For many women, the ultimate barrier to breastfeeding is not sore nipples, nighttime nursing, or employment outside the home. It is the disapproval they encounter for "wasting" their education and career skills by staying home with their breastfeeding infants or for being considered disruptive or even obscene for taking their breastfeeding infant with them to work or worship, perhaps to a city council or parent-teacher meeting, or simply to a restaurant or to a park. A goal for women should be to empower all mothers so that they are able to attend to all their duties, maternal as well as civic, religious, and professional.

Those who breastfeed or who promote the reestablishment of breastfeeding as the norm in infant feeding do so not because there are no alternatives but because the alternatives are inferior. Unfortunately, the belief that breastfeeding is the optimal way to nourish an infant may not be enough to empower a woman to breastfeed. Knowledge of beneficial breastfeeding practices and the social acceptance of those practices is also required. Currently, the prevalence of breastfeeding reflects the importance that society places on it, as measured by the degree to which breastfeeding mothers and infants are accepted in the life of the community at large. Returning breastfeeding wisdom to the public domain and reintegrating it into the social fabric so that women who wish to breastfeed may do so without hindrance is the challenge that awaits.

REFERENCES

Aitken FC, Hytten FE: Infant feeding: comparison of breast and artificial feeding. *Nutr Abstr Rev* 30:341–71, 1960.

Aksit S, et al: Aflatoxin: is it a neglected threat for formula-fed infants? *Acta Paediatr Japon* 39:34–6, 1997.

American Academy of Pediatrics Committee on Nutrition, and the Nutrition Committee of the Canadian Paediatric Society: Breast-feeding: a commentary in celebration of the International Year of the Child. *Pediatrics* 62:591–601, 1978.

Andersson B, et al: Inhibition of attachment of *Streptococcus pneumoniae* and *Haemophilus influenzae* by human milk and receptor oligosaccharides. *J Infect Dis* 153:232–7, 1986.

Apple RD: "Advertised by our loving friends": the infant formula industry and the creation of new pharmaceutical markets, 1870–1910, *J Hist Med Allied Sci* 41:3–23, 1986.

Armstrong H: The International Code of Marketing of Breast-Milk Substitutes (Part two of a series). *J Hum Lact* 4:194–9, 1988.

Bain K: The incidence of breast feeding in hospitals in the United States. *Pediatrics* 2:313–20, 1948.

Bergstrand O, Hellers G: Breast-feeding during infancy in patients who later develop Crohn's disease. *Scand J Gastroenterol* 18:903–6, 1983.

Biddulph J: Promotion of breast-feeding: experience in Papua New Guinea. In: Jelliffe DB, Jelliffe EF, eds. *Advances in international maternal and child health,* vol. 1. Oxford: Oxford Press, 1981. (Cited in Huffman, 1984.)

Bloomquist HK, et al: Supplementary feeding in the maternity ward shortens the duration of breast feeding. *Acta Paediatr* 83:1122–6, 1994.

Bottorff, JL: Persistence in breastfeeding: a phenomenological investigation. *J Adv Nurs* 15:201–9, 1990.

Briend A, Wojtyniak B, Rowland MGM: Breast feeding, nutritional state, and child survival in rural Bangladesh. *Br Med J* 296:879–82, 1988.

Budin P: *The nursling* (WJ Maloney, trans.). London: 1907. (Cited in Wickes, 1953b.)

Bull T: *Hints to mothers,* 6th ed. London: 1849. (Cited in Wickes, 1953a.)

Butte NF, et al: Milk composition of insulin-dependent diabetic women. *J Pediatr Gastroenterol Nutr* 6:936–41, 1987.

Cadogan W: *An essay on nursing and the management of children from their birth to three years of age,* 3rd ed. London: J Roberts, 1749. (Cited in Kessen, 1965, pp. 10–30.)

Calkins BM, Mendeloff AI: Epidemiology of inflammatory bowel disease. *Epidemiol Rev* 8:60–91, 1986.

Chandra RK, Pusi S, Hamed A: Influence of maternal diet during lactation and use of formula feeds on development of atopic eczema in high-risk infants. *Br Med J* 299:228–30, 1989.

Chen Y, Yu S, Li W: Artificial feeding and hospitalization in the first 18 months of life. *Pediatrics* 81:58–62, 1988.

Cleary TG, et al: Human milk immunoglobulin A antibodies to *Shigella* virulence determinants. *Infect Immunol* 57:1675–9, 1989.

Coates MM, ed: Policy statements. In: *The lactation consultant's topical review and bibliography of the literature on breastfeeding.* Franklin Park, IL: La Leche League International, 1990.

Coreil J, Murphy JE: Maternal commitment, lactation practices, and breastfeeding duration. *JOGNN* 17:273–8, 1988.

Cummings SR, Kelsey JL, Nevitt MC: Epidemiology of osteoporosis and osteoporotic fractures. *Epidemiol Rev* 7:178–208, 1985.

Cunningham AS, Jelliffe DB, Jelliffe EFP: Breastfeeding and health in the 1980s: a global epidemiologic review. *J Pediatr* 118:659–66, 1991.

Davidson WD: A brief history of infant feeding. *J Pediatr* 43:74–87, 1953.

Davis MK, Savitz DA, Graubard BI: Infant feeding and childhood cancer. *Lancet* 2(8607):365–8, 1988.

Dearlove JC, Dearlove BM: Prolactin, fluid balance, and lactation. *Br J Obstet Gynaecol* 88:652–4, 1981.

Deruisseau LG: Infant hygiene in the older medical literature. *Ciba Symposia* 2:530–60, 1940.

Dimond HJ, Ashworth A: Infant feeding practices in Kenya, Mexico and Malaysia: the rarity of the exclusively breastfed infant. *Hum Nutr Appl Nutr* 41A:51–64, 1987.

Eaton SB, Konner M: Paleolithic nutrition: a consideration of its nature and current implications. *N Engl J Med* 312:283–89, 1985.

Erkhardt KW, Hendershot GE: Analysis of the reversal in breast feeding trends in the early 1970s. *Public Health Rep* 99:410–5, 1984.

Ettmuller M: *Etmullerus Abrig'd,* 2nd ed. London, 1703. (Cited in Wickes, 1953a.)

Fallot ME, Boyd JL III, Oski FA: Breastfeeding reduces incidence of hospital admissions for infection in infants. *Pediatrics* 65:1121–4, 1980.

Fildes VA: *Breasts, bottles, and babies: a history of infant feeding.* Edinburgh: Edinburgh University Press, 1986.

Fishaut M, et al: Bronchomammary axis in the immune response to respiratory syncytial virus. *J Pediatr* 99:186–9, 1981.

Forman MR, et al: The PIMA infant feeding study: breast feeding and respiratory infections during the first year of life. *Int J Epidemiol* 13:447–53, 1984.

Forman MR, et al: Exclusive breast-feeding of newborns among married women in the United States: the National Natality Surveys of 1969 and 1980. *Am J Clin Nutr* 42:864–9, 1985.

Gerrard JW: Breast-feeding: second thoughts. *Pediatrics* 54:757–64, 1974.

Glass RI, et al: Protection against cholera in breastfed children by antibodies in breast milk. *N Engl J Med* 308:1389–92, 1983.

Greco L, et al: Case control study on nutritional risk factors in celiac disease. *J Pediatr Gastroenterol Nutr* 7:395–9, 1988.

Greer FR, Apple RD: Physicians, formula companies, and advertising: a historical perspective. *Am J Dis Child* 145:282–6, 1991.

Greiner T: The concept of weaning: definitions and their implications. *J Hum Lact* 12:123–8, 1996.

Grossman LK, et al: The infant feeding decision in low and upper income women. *Clin Pediatr* 29:30–7, 1990.

Grulee CG, Sanford HN, Herron PH: Breast and artificial feeding: influence on morbidity and mortality of twenty thousand infants. *JAMA* 103:735–9, 1934.

Gwinn ML, et al: Pregnancy, breast feeding and oral contraceptives and the risk of epithelial ovarian cancer. *Int J Epidemiol* 43:559–68, 1990.

Habicht J-P, DaVanzo J, Butz WP: Mother's milk and sewage: their interactive effect on infant mortality. *Pediatrics* 88:456–61, 1988.

Hastrup K: A question of reason: breastfeeding patterns in seventeenth and eighteenth-century Iceland. In: Maher V, ed. *The anthropology of breast-feeding–natural law or social construct.* Oxford: Berg Publishers, 1992: 91–108.

Heiser B: Reaching out to all. *Breastfeed Abstr* 9:19–20, 1990.

Hendershot GE: *Trends in breast feeding,* United States Department of Health and Human Services, no. 80–1250. Hyattsville, MD: National Center for Health Statistics, 1980.

Hill LF: A salute to La Leche League International. *J Pediatr* 73:161–62, 1968.

Hirschman C, Butler M: Trends and differentials in breast feeding: an update. *Demography* 18:39–54, 1981.

Hoffman S, et al: Parity, lactation and hip fracture. *Osteoporosis Int* 3:171–6, 1993.

Houston MJR, Field PA: Practices and policies in the initiation of breastfeeding. *JOGNN* 17: 418–24, 1988.

Howarth WJ: The influence of feeding on the mortality of infants. *Lancet* 2 (July 22):210–3, 1905.

Hymanson A: A short review of the history of infant feeding. *Arch Pediatr* 51:1–10, 1934.

IBFAN/IOCU: *Protecting infant health: a health worker's guide to the International Code of Marketing of Breast-milk Substitutes.* Penang, Malasia: IBFAN/IOCU, 1985.

Illingworth PJ, et al: Diminution in energy expenditure during lactation. *Br Med J* 292:437–41, 1986.

Jackson RI: Ecological breastfeeding and child spacing. *Clin Pediatr* 27:373–7, 1988.

Jarosz LA: Breast-feeding versus formula: cost comparison. *Hawaii Med J* 52:14–16 passim, 1993.

Jason JM, Nieburg P, Marks JS: Mortality and disease associated with infant-feeding practices in developing countries. *Pediatrics* 74:702–27, 1984.

Jelliffe DB: Culture, social change and infant feeding: current trends in tropical regions. *Am J Clin Nutr* 10:19–45, 1962.

Jelliffe DB, Jelliffe EFP: *Human milk in the modern world.* Oxford: Oxford University, 1978.

Kahn A, et al: Difficulty in initiating and maintaining sleep associated with cow's milk allergy in infants. *Sleep* 19:116–21, 1987.

Karra MV, et al: Hospital infant feeding practices in metropolitan Chicago: an evaluation of five of the "Ten Steps to Successful Breast-feeding." *J Am Diet Assoc* 93:1437–39, 1993.

Kelly DW, et al: Rise and fall of coeliac disease, 1960–1985. *Arch Dis Child* 64:1157–60, 1989.

Kelsey JJ: Hormonal contraception and lactation. *J Hum Lact* 12:315–8, 1996.

Kemper K, Forsyth B, McCarthy P: Jaundice, terminating breast-feeding, and the vulnerable child. *Pediatrics* 84:773–8, 1989.

Kennedy K, et al: Consensus statement on the use of breastfeeding as a family planning method. *Contraception* 39:477–96, 1989.

Kero P, Piekkala P: Factors affecting the occurrence of acute otitis media during the first year of life. *Acta Paediatr Scand* 76:618–23, 1987.

Konner M, Worthman C: Nursing frequency, gonadal function, and birth spacing among iKung hunter-gatherers. *Science* 207:788–91, 1980.

Kovach AC: Hospital breastfeeding policies in the Philadelphia area: a comparison with the ten steps to successful breastfeeding. *Birth* 24:41–48, 1997.

Kovar MG, et al: Review of the epidemiologic evidence for an association between infant feeding and infant health. *Pediatrics* 74:615–38, 1984.

Kurinij N, Shiono PH, Rhoads GG: Breast-feeding incidence and duration in black and white women. *Pediatrics* 81:365–71, 1988.

Kusin JA, Kardjati S, van Steenbergen W: Traditional infant feeding practices: right or wrong? *Soc Sci Med* 21:283–6, 1985.

Labbok M, Hendershot GE: Does breast-feeding protect against malocclusion? An analysis of the 1981 Child Health Supplement to the National Health Interview survey. *Am J Prev Med* 3:227–32, 1987.

Labbok M, Krasovec K: Toward consistency in breastfeeding definitions. *Stud Fam Plann* 21: 226–30, 1990.

Lacaille AD: Infant feeding-bottles in prehistoric times. *Proc R Soc Med* 43:565–8, 1950.

Lanting CI, et al: Neurological differences between 9-year-old children fed breast-milk or formula-milk as babies. *Lancet* 344:1319–22, 1994.

Latham MC, et al: Infant feeding in urban Kenya: a pattern of early triple nipple feeding. *J Trop Pediatr* 32:276–80, 1986.

Lazarov M: Testimony of Minda Lazarov, Director, Tennessee Breastfeeding Promotion Project, before the Subcommittee on Nutrition and Investigations of the Senate Committee on Agriculture, Nutrition and Forestry, June 15, 1989. Available from the Tennessee Department of Health and Environment.

Levenstein H: "Best for babies" or "Preventable infanticide"? The controversy over artificial feeding of infants in America, 1880–1920, *J Am Hist* 70:75–94, 1983.

Lewis PR, et al: The resumption of ovulation and menstruation in a well-nourished population of women breastfeeding for an extended period of time. *Fertil Steril* 55:529–36, 1991.

Lightbourne R, Singh S, Green CP: The World Fertility Survey: charting global childbearing. *Popul Bull* 37:7–55, 1982.

Lucas A, Cole TJ: Breast milk and neonatal necrotising enterocolitis. *Lancet* 336(8730):1519–23, 1990.

MacGowan RJ, et al: Breast-feeding among women attending Women, Infants, and Children clinics in Georgia, 1987. *Pediatrics* 87:361–6, 1991.

Mansbach IL, et al: Advice from the obstetrician and other sources: do they affect women's breast-feeding practices? A study among different Jewish groups in Jerusalem. *Soc Sci Med* 19:157–62, 1984.

Marild S, Jodal U, Hanson LA: Breastfeeding and urinary-tract infection. *Lancet* 336(8720):942, 1990.

Martinez GA, Krieger FW: 1984 Milk-feeding patterns in the United States. *Pediatrics* 76:1004–8, 1985.

Martinez GA, Nalezienski JP: The recent trend in breast-feeding. *Pediatrics* 64:686–92, 1979.

Mason T, et al: Breast feeding and the development of juvenile rheumatoid arthritis. *J Rheumatol* 22:1166–70, 1995.

Mathew OP, Bhatia J: Sucking and breathing patterns during breast- and bottle-feeding in term neonates: effects of nutrient delivery and composition. *Am J Dis Child* 143:588–92, 1989.

Mayer EJ, Hamman RF, Gay EC: Reduced risk of IDDM among breast-fed children: The Colorado IDDM Registry. *Diabetes* 37:1625–32, 1988.

McCracken RD: Lactase deficiency: an example of dietary evolution. *Curr Anthrop* 12:479–517, 1971.

McTiernan A, Thomas DB: Evidence for a protective effect of lactation on risk of breast cancer in young women: results from a case-control study. *Am J Epidemiol* 124:353–8, 1986.

Mead Johnson (advertisement). *JAMA* 95:22, 1930.

Meier P, Anderson GC: Responses of small preterm infants to bottle- and breast-feeding. *MCN* 12:97–105, 1987.

Meyer HF: Breast feeding in the United States. Report of a 1966 national survey with comparable 1946 and 1956 data. *Clin Pediatr* 7:708–15, 1968.

Millard AV: The place of the clock in pediatric advice: rationales, cultural themes, and impediments to breastfeeding. *Soc Sci Med* 31:211–21, 1990.

Minchin M: Infant formula: a mass, uncontrolled trial in perinatal care. *Birth* 14:25–35, 1987.

Morse JM: "Euch, those are for your husband!" Examination of cultural values and assumptions associated with breast-feeding. *Health Care Women Int* 11:223–32, 1989.

Morse JM, Jehle C, Gamble D: Initiating breast-feeding: a world survey of the timing of postpartum breastfeeding. *Int J Nurs Stud* 27:303–13, 1990.

Mulford C: Swimming upstream: breastfeeding care in a non-breastfeeding culture. *JOGNN* 24:464–74, 1995.

Nestlé's Food (advertisement): *The Ladies' Home Journal* 9:26, 1892.

Newcomb PA, et al: Lactation and reduced risk of premenopausal breast cancer. *N Engl J Med* 330:81–7, 1994.

Nga NT, Weissner P: Breast-feeding and young child nutrition in Uong Bi, Quang Ninh province, Vietnam. *J Trop Pediatr* 32:137–9, 1986.

Pabst HF, Spady DW: Effect of breast-feeding on antibody response to conjugate vaccine. *Lancet* 336(8710):269–70, 1990.

Persson LA: Multivariate approaches to the analysis of breast-feeding habits. *Bull WHO* 63:1129–36, 1985.

Pisacane A, et al: Breast feeding and inguinal hernia. *J Pediatr* 127:109–11, 1995.

Pisacane A, et al: Breast feeding and multiple sclerosis. *Br Med J* 308(6941):1411–2, 1994.

Pisacane A, et al: Breast feeding and tonsillectomy. *Br Med J* 312:746–7, 1996.

Pisacane A, Graziano L, Zona G: Breastfeeding and urinary tract infection. *Lancet* 336(8706):50, 1990.

Popkin BM, Fernandez ME, Avila JL: Infant formula promotion and the health sector in the Philippines. *Am J Public Health* 80:74–75, 1990.

Retherford RD, et al: To what extent does breast-feeding explain birth-interval effects on early childhood mortality? *Demography* 26:439–50, 1989.

Richards B: Early suckling and prolonged breast-feeding [letter]. *Am J Dis Child* 141:741, 1986. Taylor PM, Maloni JA, Brown DR [reply]. *Am J Dis Child* 141:741, 1986.

Rosenblatt KA, Thomas DT, the WHO Collaborative Study of Neoplasia and Steroid Contraceptives: Prolonged lactation and endometrial cancer. *Int J Epidemiol* 24:499–503, 1995.

Rossiter FM: The practical guide to health, a popular treatise on anatomy, physiology, and hygiene, with a scientific description of diseases, their causes and treatment, designed for nurses and home use. Pacific Press Publishing, 1908. (Reprinted in part in *J Hum Lact* 7:89–91, 1991.)

Rotch TM: An historical sketch of the development of percentage feeding. *NY Med J* 85:532–7, 1907.

Ruiz-Palacios GM, et al: Protection of breast-fed infants against *Campylobacter* bacteria by antibodies in human milk. *J Pediatr* 116:707–13, 1990.

Ryan AS: The resurgence of breastfeeding in the United States. *Pediatrics* electronic pages 99(4):April 1997. (To read or download, go to http://www.pediatrics.org/cgi/content/full/99/4/e12.)

Ryan AS, et al: Duration of breast-feeding patterns established in hospital: influencing factors. Results from a national survey. *Clin Pediatr* 29:99–107, 1990.

Ryan AS, et al: Recent declines in breast-feeding in the United States, 1984–1989. *Pediatrics* 88:719–27, 1991.

Saadeh R, et al: *Breastfeeding: the technical basis and recommendations for action*. Geneva: World Health Organization, 1993.

Saarinen UM, Kajosaari M: Breastfeeding as prophylaxis against atopic disease: prospective follow-up study until 17 years old. *Lancet* 346(8982): 1065–9, 1995.

Sandiford P, et al: Why do child mortality rates fall? An analysis of the Nicaraguan experience. *Am J Public Health* 81:30–37, 1991.

Schaefer O: The impact of culture on breastfeeding patterns. *J Perinatol* 6:62–5, 1986.

Schneider AP III: Risk factor for ovarian cancer. *N Engl J Med* 317:508–9, 1987.

Scott FW: Cow milk and insulin-dependent diabetes mellitus: is there a relationship? *Am J Clin Nutr* 51:489–91, 1990.

Serva V, Karim H, Ebrahim GJ: Breast-feeding and the urban poor in developing countries. *J Trop Pediatr* 32:127–9, 1986.

Short RV: Breast feeding. *Sci Am* 250:35–41, 1984.

Simoons FJ: Age of onset of lactose malabsorption. *Pediatrics* 66:646–8, 1980.

Slome C: Nonpuerperal lactation in grandmothers. *J Pediatr* 49:550–2, 1976.

Smith H: *Letters to married women on nursing and the management of children,* 3rd ed. London: 1774. (Cited in Fildes, 1986.)

Thomas DB, Noonan EA: Breast cancer and prolonged lactation. *Int J Epidemiol* 22:619–26, 1993.

UNICEF: Breastfeeding/Baby-Friendly Hospital Initiative, Update on Progress. 1996. BFHI, Nutrition Section. New York: UNICEF, November 1996a.

United Nations Children's Fund: Breastfeeding/ Baby-Friendly Hospital Initiative, Update on progress, 1996. BFHI, Nutrition Section, New York: UNICEF, November 1996a.

United Nations Children's Fund: Innocenti Declaration on the Protection, Promotion and Support of Breastfeeding, Florence, Italy, 1 August 1990. UNICEF, Nutrition Cluster (H-8F), 3 United Nations Plaza, New York, NY 10017.

United Nations Children's Fund: 1995 Progress Report, Baby-Friendly Hospital Initiative, Nutrition Section with BFHI team and UNICEF Field Offices. New York: UNICEF, 1996b.

United States Department of Health and Human Services, Public Health Service: *Promoting health/preventing disease: objectives for the nation.* Washington: US Government Printing Office, 1980.

Uvnas-Moberg K, et al: Release of GI hormones in mother and infant by sensory stimulation. *Acta Paediatr Scand* 76:851–60, 1987.

Verronen P, et al: Promotion of breastfeeding: effect on neonates of change of feeding routine at a maternity unit. *Acta Paediatr Scand* 69:279–82, 1980.

Wade N: Bottle-feeding: adverse effects of a Western technology. *Science* 184:45–8, 1974.

Walker M: A fresh look at the risks of artificial infant feeding. *J Hum Lact* 9:97–107, 1993.

Whitehead RG: The human weaning process, *Pediatrics* 75(suppl 1):189–93, 1985.

Wickes IG: A history of infant feeding: III. Eighteenth and nineteenth century writers. *Arch Dis Child* 28:332–40, 1953a.

Wickes IG: A history of infant feeding: V. Nineteenth century concluded and twentieth century. *Arch Dis Child* 28:495–502, 1953b.

Wieschhoff HA: Artificial stimulation of lactation in primitive cultures. *Bull Hist Med* 8:1403–15, 1940.

Williamson MA: *Infant mortality: Montclair, NJ. A study of infant mortality in a suburban community.* Washington, DC: United States Department of Labor, Children's Bureau, 1915.

Winikoff B, et al: Dynamics of infant feeding: mothers, professionals, and the institutional context in a large urban hospital. *Pediatrics* 77:357–65, 1986.

Winikoff B, Laukaran VH: Breast feeding and bottle feeding controversies in the developing world: evidence from a study in four countries. *Soc Sci Med* 29:859–68, 1989.

Woodbury RM: The relation between breast and artificial feeding and infant mortality. *Am J Hyg* 2:668–87, 1922.

Woolridge MW, Greasley V, Silpisornkosol S: The initiation of lactation: the effect of early versus delayed contact for suckling on milk intake in the first week postpartum. A study in Chiang Mai, northern Thailand. *Early Hum Dev* 12:269–78, 1985.

Working Group on Cow's Milk Protein Allergy. Cow's milk allergy in the first year of life. *Acta Paediatr Scand* Suppl 348:2–14, 1988.

World Health Organization: *Contemporary patterns of breast-feeding.* Geneva: World Health Organization, 1981.

——: WHO Global Data Bank on Breast-Feeding, Nutrition Unit of the World Health Organization, Geneva, 1996.

World Health Organization: The prevalence and duration of breast-feeding: updated information, 1980–1989. *Wkly Epidemiol Rec* 42:321–23, 1989.

Wright A, Rice S, Wells S: Changing hospital practices to increase the duration of breastfeeding. *Pediatrics* 97:669–75, 1996.

Zeitlyn S, Rowshan R: Privileged knowledge and mothers' "perceptions": the care of breast-feeding and insufficient milk in Bangladesh. *Med Anthrop Q* 11:56–58, 1997.

THE CULTURAL CONTEXT OF BREASTFEEDING

Jan Riordan

Definitions and Characteristics

Culture exerts a major influence on a mother's attitude toward breastfeeding and on how she decides to feed her baby, an activity that crosses the boundary between private and public. Thus attitudes and patterns of infant feeding cannot be understood without placing them in their specific cultural context. This chapter looks at breastfeeding as a human behavior that is sensitive to cultural influence and social change.

Culture is defined as the values, beliefs, norms, and practices of a particular group, which are learned and shared and guide thinking, decisions, and actions in a patterned way (Leininger, 1985). Culture provides implicit and explicit codes of behavior. Culture is:

- learned both through language and socialization
- shared, often unconsciously, by all members of a cultural group who are then bound together under one identity
- an adaptation to specific conditions related to environmental and technical factors and to the availability of natural resources
- a dynamic, ongoing process

From a practical standpoint, a society's culture consists of whatever one has to know or believe to operate in a manner acceptable to its members (van Esterik, 1988). Culture is a blueprint for human behavior, one that helps us to gain a clearer understanding of individual behaviors. The new mother is the product of all of her history: what she has learned about infants and infant feeding, and what she has seen. If she grows up in a breastfeeding culture, she has many opportunities to observe how infants are fed and knows that her female relatives and neighbors with breastfeeding experience, will support her when she becomes a mother (Mulford, 1995). Women and their families have a right to expect that their cultural needs will be met as they are helped with breastfeeding and lactation. Without understanding the mother's cultural practices, our care and intervention could do more harm than good (Fig. 2–1).

The Dominant Culture

The United States and the entire Western hemisphere are peopled by immigrants and their descendants. Almost 60 million people immigrated to the United State between 1820 and 1990. With each new wave, anxiety grew among those

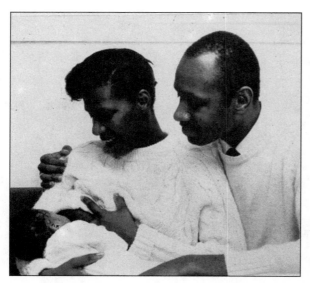

FIGURE 2–1. *Each family has its own expectations about breastfeeding that are based in part on culture.*

already entrenched, and steps were taken to resist the newcomers, a process that continues even today.

Every society has a dominant culture, the values of which are shared by the majority of its members as a result of early common experiences. Although there are approximately 100 ethnic groups in the United States (Spector, 1985), the dominant cultural group is that of white, middle-class Protestants, descendants of northern Europeans who immigrated to the United States several generations ago. Norms characteristic of this group are a conservative value system, family orientation, commitment to higher education for one's children, a work ethic, materialism, a personal faith in God, the quest for physical beauty, cleanliness, high technology, punctuality, independence, and free enterprise. Given these prevailing values, it may be relevant to consider women's roles, their contribution to the economy, and the extent to which breastfeeding is perceived to hinder this. Has economic independence and the need for women to have some power within a male-dominated society contributed to a decline in breastfeeding rates (Kendall, 1995)? See Table 2–1.

The dominant health culture in the United States views birth as dangerous for the mother and neonate. Breastfeeding is seen as the optimal method of infant feeding but difficult to accomplish and a private act not to be practiced in public. These norms are slowly changing as waves of immigrating Asians and Hispanics, from 1970 to the present time, become the "new" Americans. In the United States, Western allopathic medicine is viewed by many as "professional" health care; any medical tradition outside this system is considered traditional folk medicine with its accompanying connotations of primitive, "useless," "lay," and "outdated" (Boyle & Andrews, 1989). The dominant U.S. health system marketplace is composed of the hospital, the health worker's office, and the community health department. The folk belief–system marketplace centers around the home of the clients or of their extended kin (Scott & Stern, 1985). These authors identify three types of health care consumers:

- the corporate buyer, who buys the dominant health care system completely
- the careful shopper, who balances between the folk health system and the dominant health system
- the cultural buyer, who buys only the folk health system

Folk health beliefs may be combined with health care beliefs of the dominant culture (Zeitlyn & Rowshan, 1997). For instance, Scott and Stern (1985) found that black women in northern Louisiana selected bicultural elements from the influences of folk treatments offered by older women in their culture and from influences of scientific Western-style remedies.

The role of women in a culture may also define the experience of breastfeeding. In some societies, male control over breastfeeding serves to weaken the woman's role as mother and to emphasize her role as wife. Rather than viewing insufficient milk supply and early weaning as problems in themselves, these factors could be interpreted as reflecting insecurity about the abilities of women's bodies and the precariousness of women's lives and as a symptom of broader self-questioning (Obermeyer & Castle, 1997). Maher (1992) suggests that women in Morocco turn to formula-feeding as a way of gaining some control for themselves within a male-dominated society. For these women, breastfeeding

Table 2-1

POSSIBLE CULTURAL BELIEFS AND PRACTICES

	Asian	American Black	Hispanic, Chicano
Beliefs about health	Seen as a balance of energy—*yin* vs. *yang*	Ability to be productive, a state of harmony with the universe	Health is a state of equilibrium; disease is due to an imbalance
Support or resource person for a new mother	Mother, mother-in-law	Older woman with experience; peers	Mother is often cared for by her own mother
Infant feeding	Mother prefers to formula-feed; sees formula as "superfood" that will make baby grow larger; may bottle-feed in hospital and both breastfeed and bottle-feed at home; does not use breast pump	Most mothers are in low socioeconomic group, choose formula-feeding; breastfeeding may be seen as embarrassing; early introduction of solids	Mother is likely to breastfeed; may wait three days if she considers colostrum to be "dirty"; gives baby small amounts of family foods
Family and parenting	Male babies are preferred; father is head of household	Fears "spoiling" baby; grandmother (mother of mother) helps parent	Mother is a homemaker, father is provider
Infant care	Hot-cold foods to treat illnesses; feels responsible for baby's behavior; brings baby to social events, church	May put excess clothing on baby to keep infant warm; abundant use of oil on baby's scalp and skin	Infant must be protected from the "evil eye" (*mal de ojo*); various remedies are used to treat fallen (depressed) fontanel; female ears are pierced; male may not be circumcised

and not working represent loss of earning power and a lack of control over their lives.

Ethnocentrism Versus Relativism

Ethnocentrism may be defined as being centered in one's ethnic or cultural system (i.e., judging the world by one's standards or, in the vernacular, believing that "my group is best"). When caring for culturally diverse groups, nurses and health care workers at first tend to ethnocentricity, believing that their professional, scientifically based practices are superior. Many health care workers reading this book have been socialized into their profession within the framework of a Western health care system that emphasizes the biomedical model and is based on the white, working- and middle-class value system. If this system is the only model used to evaluate and implement care, the nurse or lactation consultant is ethnocentric. When health care workers are exposed to other cultures, they may begin to appreciate why certain behaviors and values are effective in that culture and may move beyond ethnocentric behaviors (Tripp-Reimer et al., 1984).

The opposite of ethnocentrism is *cultural relativism,* in which the care provider recognizes and appreciates cultural differences and therefore treats

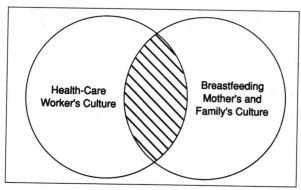

FIGURE 2–2. Shared values and beliefs. *(From MS Orque, B Block, & LS Monrroy: Ethnic nursing care: a multicultural approach. St Louis: Mosby, 1983:19.)*

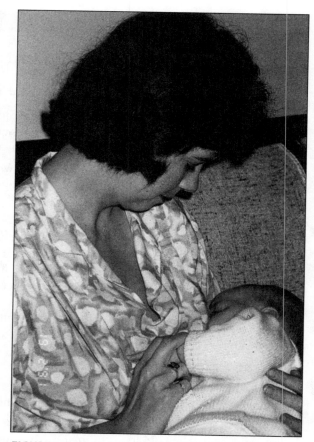

FIGURE 2–3. Canadian physician breastfeeding. *Recognizing one's own cultural values is the basis of appreciating cultural diversity. (Courtesy G. Arsenault.)*

individual clients with deference to their cultural backgrounds. The health worker builds on and uses cultural variations rather than seeing them as obstacles. To provide optimal assistance, caregivers must first understand their personal reactions to cultural differences and then appreciate how these cultural values affect the lives of their clients. By discovering areas of commonality between themselves and their patients, nurses or care providers will be better able to recognize and deal with cultural similarities and variations between the clients and themselves (Orque et al., 1983). This process is illustrated in Figures 2–2 and 2–3.

Cultural relativism likewise recognizes variation within cultures, such as the diverse ethnic groups in the United States. At one time, people expected and hoped that these ethnic and cultural groups would blend into one common whole: the melting-pot approach. It has not worked out that way; many third- and fourth-generation Americans proudly claim and identify with their original ethnic heritage. The tendency to label subpopulations to explain behaviors is responsible for many myths about new Americans. Brownlee (1978) describes a clinic worker in Boston who was annoyed at the way local residents generalized about the city's many cultural groups: "Haitian is like this, Hispanic is like that, you know those Italians all lie . . . and oh, those Puerto Ricans, they never ever . . ."

Assessing Culture

To provide culturally appropriate care, health workers must first systematically gather informa-

tion about a culture. Ethnographic fieldwork is vital to obtain data about the components of a given culture. Cultural elements that require assessment include language, foodways, dress, patterns of social behavior, religious customs, rituals, use of time and space, nonverbal communication, health and illness belief systems, and economic and political systems. Collecting cultural data is a skill that must be studied, learned, and practiced in order to suggest the appropriate questions to ask and the proper way in which to ask those questions. The health care worker should collect data sufficient to compile as complete a picture as possible without becoming overwhelmed with excessive raw data and information.

Cultural information can be gathered by conducting focus groups, interviewing key informants, and reviewing current literature. Focus groups are interviews in which information is collected from a group of four to ten participants who discuss their thoughts and experiences about breastfeeding or other selected topics.

In a focus group, women are more likely to share ideas with other group members; this interaction triggers additional thought and in-depth discussion not possible in a one-to-one interview. The following techniques can provide other rich sources of cultural data:

- finding a close confidant and other knowledgeable informants to help "bridge the gap" between cultures
- talking with family members (mothers, fathers, grandmothers, older children) who can alert the care provider to divergent cultural beliefs among the family members
- visiting hospitals and clinics and talking with nurses and physicians
- getting to know local leaders and residents of the community who are widely respected
- learning through formal, in-depth interviews and informal conversations
- learning through both participating in and observing behaviors
- gathering clues from overheard conversations and unsolicited comments

Surveys may not be useful because people tend to say what they think the investigator wants them to say, regardless of their real feelings and attitudes. Cultural assessment tools (Brownlee, 1978; Giger & Davidhizar, 1991; Orque et al., 1983) may be easily adapted to gather information on childbearing and infant feeding practices within a given culture. Such a guide is given in Box 2–1.

It is essential to assess and understand infant feeding practices and styles when choosing culturally appropriate policy and breastfeeding promotion strategies. For example, people living in Kenya consider formula a product and consider breastfeeding an activity or process. These beliefs will likely influence any infant feeding programs or policies developed in that country (van Esterik & Elliott, 1986). Also helpful are demographic data that show breastfeeding trends within a certain area. For example, data that show rural women as more likely to breastfeed and to do so longer than urban mothers may influence how one might plan a breastfeeding promotion program to reach both urban and rural mothers. Rural people are also more likely to continue traditional rituals than are urban families who may not have even heard of these practices.

A simple but effective method for evaluating the value of a cultural practice (Williams & Jelliffe, 1972) is to consider whether the practice is beneficial, harmless, harmful, or uncertain to a particular outcome:

- *Is it beneficial?* Several cultures prohibit the lactating mother from having intercourse because it is believed that semen poisons her breastmilk (Counts, 1984); a side benefit of this practice is enhanced fertility control. Such beliefs ensure that infants continue to be breastfed and are well nourished and nurtured, as many cultures proscribe breastfeeding when a woman becomes pregnant again. Such cultural practices as carrying a baby close, breastfeeding on demand, and spacing children by long-term breastfeeding are likewise considered beneficial.

- *Is it harmless?* Placing an amulet or garlic charm around the baby's neck to protect him from "the evil eye" or pinning a belly band around his abdomen to prevent an umbilical hernia are harmless practices. If the mother eats garlic to prevent illness, the practice is harmless to her baby, even though her milk will be garlic-flavored (Mennella & Beauchamp, 1991).

- *Is it harmful?* Colostrum is considered poisonous and unfit for the infant in many cultures (Baumslag, 1987; Counts, 1984; Davies-Adetugbo, 1997; Fernandez & Popkin, 1988). The newborn is fed by a lactating relative or is given gruel until the "true" milk begins to flow, thereby depriving the baby of the concentrated immune properties of colostrum. Another harmful belief is that breastmilk causes diarrhea and that breastfeeding must be stopped when diarrhea occurs (Guthrie et al., 1983).

BOX 2–1

Elements Useful for Assessing Culture

GENERAL

- History and origins of the cultural group
- Customs, values
- Behaviors and attitudes

COMMUNICATION

- Language patterns (verbal and non-verbal)
- Language barriers
- Use of time and space
- Art and literature

FAMILY

- Childbearing and child-rearing practices
- Family organization, roles, decision making
- Kinship patterns
- Housing
- Food habits

HEALTH PRACTICES

- Healing systems (folk or cultural healers versus biomedical)
- Health beliefs

- Effect of illness on family
- Biological variations

RELIGION

- Tenets and practices
- Rituals and restrictions

SOCIOPOLITICAL SYSTEMS

- Type of political system governing health and welfare
- Educational system
- Economic role of women
- Income levels per capita
- Degree of technology in use

INFANT CARE AND FEEDING PRACTICES

- Input from family and support persons
- Level of knowledge
- Traditions, rituals, and taboos
- Values concerning breastmilk and other infant foods
- Attitude toward breastfeeding (process versus product)

- *Is it uncertain?* Some practices fall into this "gray" area. Until more information is gathered, they cannot be evaluated. For example, while working as a part of a nursing team in the Dominican Republic, I noted that women avoided eating fresh fruits for two weeks after delivery. This cultural restriction is common in Hispanic cultures.

Language Barriers

When working with families who speak a different language, the care provider ideally can understand and speak that language. If she cannot, she should study the language spoken by the breastfeeding families that she frequently serves. Rapport is difficult when language differences form a barrier.

When it is necessary to use a translator, a trained interpreter is able to rephrase words so they are understandable and more acceptable to the member of the culture. When using a translator, care providers should speak slowly, avoid using slang and subjectives (e.g., *would* and *if*), and use a normal voice. It also may be wise to tape-record the discussion with the mother, so that the taped discussion may be used again. Even with a translator, there may be problems, because many languages have many different dialects. Vietnamese, for example, is a language with many regional dialects. Also, a word may have different shades of meaning in different regions of the country. In preparing a flip chart and audiocassette for encouraging breastfeeding among mothers in the Dominican Republic, the author used the word *amamantar* to mean *breastfeeding,* as it is used in many Spanish-speaking countries. This provided much amusement to the Dominican mothers, to whom it meant "milk the cow."

Most people who are new to a culture are shy. Out of respect for the people with whom they are dealing, they may nod their head and say yes even though they may disagree or not understand what is being said. An example of this is described by Bowles (1987): A student nurse on a postpartum unit cared for an East Indian woman who spoke very little English. Whenever the doctor or nurse asked whether she was going to breastfeed or bottle-feed, she would say "bottle"; consequently, she was given a lactation suppressant. After the woman was discharged, the student and her instructor made a home visit and found the mother and baby happily breastfeeding under the safe supervision of the child's grandmother. They had failed to recognize that the mother's bottle-feeding reply was a cultural masquerade in response to being in a "bottle culture." Whenever possible, printed materials regarding breastfeeding should be written in the family's language. Information sheets on breastfeeding in many different languages may be ordered from La Leche League International.

The Effects of Culture on Breastfeeding

In the United States, care providers work increasingly with Asian families who have immigrated in search of a new life and opportunities. Immigrants tend to adopt the cultural practices of the new country; for these newcomers, adaptation means bottle-feeding instead of breastfeeding. For many of them, breastfeeding becomes a choice, neither a cultural norm nor an economic necessity. The women may be wrongly told that it is the custom in the United States to bottle-feed babies. A local community health nurse asked a Vietnamese mother, "But didn't your mother breastfeed you?" The woman replied, "Yes, but that's the old way. We're in a new land now."

Very few Southeast Asian women living in the United States (Rasbridge & Kulig, 1995; Serdula et al., 1991) or in Australia (Rossiter, 1992, 1994) breastfeed. These mothers were breastfed as infants, and they breastfed those children born in their native land. However, in their eagerness to acculturate, these women turn away from their cultural heritage of breastfeeding. Hmong women living in Wisconsin stated that they bottle-fed rather than breastfed for the following reasons: "not enough milk in breasts"; "can go someplace without taking a baby"; "going back to school"; "stale milk in breasts" (Jambunathan & Stewart, 1995). The father of the baby is likely to agree with his wife, especially if their baby is a boy, in the belief that their son will grow to be physically larger (and more like American men) and to have "harder bones" if he is fed formula.

Consider the influences of a new culture when a mother receives a formula discharge pack from the hospital and free formula through the WIC program in the land "where babies don't die." The WIC office in a Dallas Cambodian community was universally referred to as the *kinlaeng baek tuk dah ko,* "the place to get formula" (Rasbridge & Kulig, 1995). Consider, too, the messages the mother receives when she sees the stacks of formula in the supermarket and the magazine pictures of attractive mothers bottle-feeding their babies.

Rossiter (1994) noted that when breastfeeding classes in Australia are language- and culture-specific, Vietnamese women have more positive attitudes toward breastfeeding and are more likely to breastfeed. The author suggested that lack of continuous support was a possible explanation for the relatively short duration of breastfeeding. One problem is that Vietnamese immigrant women often are the sole breadwinners and work away from the home. Schooling to learn the language is reserved for the men.

The U.S. view of the breast as erotic and society's notion that motherhood is incompatible with sexuality also have negative ramifications for breastfeeding among Asian immigrants, who initially feel comfortable with breastfeeding but cannot reconcile this behavior with what they see in their new environment. They worry about how others will perceive them if they do breastfeed (Rodriguez-Garcia & Frazier, 1995).

The overwhelming influence of environment on breastfeeding in suppressing the practice is not limited to Southeast Asian immigrants to the United States. Chinese who immigrated to Glasgow, U.K., likewise gave up breastfeeding after arriving in that country. Only 2 percent of the Chinese babies born in Glasgow were breastfed, although 81 percent of those born in Hong Kong of the same mother had been breastfed (Koh, 1981).

Well-meaning efforts to acculturate recent immigrants can also disrupt breastfeeding by separating mothers from their babies. For example, new Vietnamese-Americans are encouraged to attend government-sponsored English classes. Because these classes are important, and breast pumping is unacceptable to many Indochinese mothers (La Du, 1985), formula is given instead. These breastfeeding mothers should be allowed to keep their babies with them in class.

Breastfeeding in a public place or in the presence of friends is an activity that is extremely sensitive to cultural norms (Fig. 2–4). For instance, in Saudi Arabia it is not uncommon to see a totally veiled woman baring her breast to feed her infant in public with no one taking notice—except, perhaps, a foreigner. In France, women in topless swimming suits on certain beaches are perfectly acceptable. However, a French woman would hesitate, or at least cover herself carefully, while breastfeeding in public, even in a restaurant near the "topless" beach. Modesty is important for the Mexican-American mother and may be viewed as inconsistent with breastfeeding in public (Wright et al., 1988).

Cultural attitudes toward modesty and breastfeeding may be compared to attitudes about the degree of difficulty of breastfeeding. In Kenya, breastfeeding is not considered a particularly difficult or problematic activity, although it is thought to be time consuming. Women do not worry or complain about breastfeeding; in a survey by van Esterik and Elliot (1986), most women reported no problems associated with it. Because breastfeeding is viewed as a natural process, medical personnel in that country were less aware that mothers might need help with breastfeeding; as a result, there are

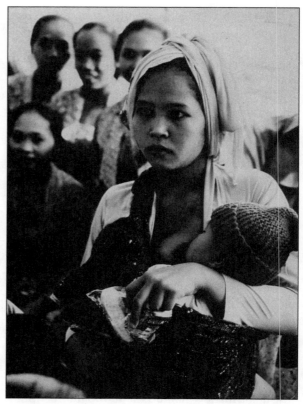

FIGURE 2–4. Well-nourished woman and breastfeeding infant in Searo, *where breastfeeding is a basic part of the life process. (Courtesy World Health Organization.)*

few instructions or rules for effectively managing breastfeeding problems.

Rituals and Meaning

Rituals and cultural meanings associated with infant feeding are critical elements in assessing the culture's infant-feeding practices. Unfortunately, the word *ritual* has come to connote a meaningless ceremonial act. Actually, rituals can have a significant effect if the individual believes in them. Eating a special food or praying to a patron saint to increase the milk supply are cultural rituals that work for some people, just as taking a pill on the advice of a Western-trained doctor may have a positive effect, even if the medicine is a sugar pill. Researchers call this the *placebo effect,* which is based on the observation that if one believes that a particular action will have a desired effect, it will.

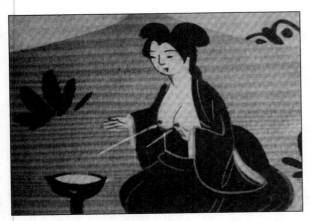

FIGURE 2–5. Votive picture *(ema in Japanese). This wooden plaque is given to the breastfeeding mother by the temple. She, in turn, prays to the plaque for sufficient milk. If her wish is fulfilled, she writes her name and age on the plaque and dedicates it to the temple. (Courtesy K. Sawada.)*

In the Philippines, the ritual of *lihi* assures a good flow of rich milk. The ceremony involves stroking the mother's breasts with broken papaya leaves and stalks of sugar cane. The white sap of the papaya ensures that the mother's milk will be copious, thick, and white, whereas the cane guarantees that it will be sweet (Guthrie et al., 1983). In certain rural areas of Japan, figurines and paintings depicting a woman with a bounteous milk supply are displayed in the belief that they increase the mother's milk (Fig. 2–5). A picture of a breastfeeding mother seated in front of a waterfall has been used in the United States for similar effect. The use of nipple creams, popular in some Western countries, could be considered a ritual that is a comfort measure, even if it is not necessary from a physiological point of view.

Colostrum

In many cultures throughout the world, colostrum is accepted and encouraged as the first food for infants. Others believe that colostrum is "old" milk that has been in the breasts for months and is unfit for the newborn and thus should be expressed and thrown away until the "true" milk appears on the second or third day (Conton, 1985; Fishman et al., 1988). In many developing countries, mothers do not give their babies this first milk because they fear it to be "pus" or "poison" Davies-Adetugbo, 1997). This belief exists among people in countries thousands of miles apart, including the native peoples of Guatemala and Korea, and Africans in Sierra Leone and Lesotho. On Vanatinai Island in the Coral Sea, the mother feeds her baby about one hour after birth, but she must first drink mwaoli tea and then express the contents of her breasts in the belief that she must rid them of the residue of fats, coconut, fish, wild game, or pig that she ate during her pregnancy (Lepowsky, 1985).

Resuming Sexual Relations

The notion that semen contaminates breastmilk, a vestige of medieval European thought, is widespread in many developing countries (Conton, 1985; Counts, 1984). It assumes that there is a physiological connection between the uterus and the breast and that the mother's milk may become contaminated by sexual contact and thereby make a baby sick. The Lusi people in Papua New Guinea, for example, believe that new parents should refrain from sexual activity lest the semen contaminate the breastmilk through "cords" that are thought to link the uterus and breast. This is especially true if the semen comes from a man other than the baby's father. Refraining from sexual relations should continue until the child is old enough to tell its parents of its dreams or when it is old enough to gather shellfish (about three years of age) (Counts, 1984). One negative result of a taboo against having sexual intercourse while lactating is that men pressure women to shorten breastfeeding so they can resume sexual relations and that women, concerned that their milk may be "contaminated" by sperm, are more likely to wean early (Maher, 1992).

Wet-Nursing

Wet-nursing is a long-established practice in many developing countries. Traditionally, a child whose mother has died or who was otherwise unable to breastfeed is either passed around among breastfeeding women or is adopted by a lactating mother whose child has recently died (Counts, 1984). Among Japanese and Thai mothers of Chinese ancestry, breastmilk can be shared between infants of the same gender but not those of the opposite gender. In cultures in which breastmilk is viewed as a conduit for ancestral power, it is not unusual for wet nurses to be restricted to women from the mother or father's clan or lineage (Lepowsky, 1985; van Esterik, 1988). Meanings attached to breastfeeding vary across cultures.

In Mali, children are thought to be of the same blood as the mother not through birth but through breastfeeding (Dettwyler, 1988). Thus two children who have been breastfed by the same woman cannot marry, even if they are not related. Similarly, Fijians believe that when a woman breastfeeds a child who is not her own, a special bond and a concomitant sense of responsibility develop (Morse, 1985).

In the United States, cross-nursing (Krantz & Kupper, 1981) used to be practiced but rarely discussed. In more recent years, cross-nursing is discouraged because of concerns about infection from the human immunodeficiency virus (HIV) or other viruses and because of the availability of artificial baby milk. However, mothers still cross-nurse. For example, mothers in Northwest Indian tribes, especially sisters, regularly cross-nurse secretly.

Childbirth Practices

Like breastfeeding, childbirth is heavily influenced by culture. Mercer and Stainton (1984) clarify the role of culture in childbirth as providing norms that influence attitudes, values, and interpretations of personal and interpersonal experience. The "fire rest" is a ritual carried out after childbirth in Southeast Asian and Caribbean cultures (Fishman et al., 1988). To restore a new mother's reproductive organs, traditional Filipino childbirth practices, for example, expect her to sit in a special slotted chair over hot coals for one hour each day for nine days after giving birth. This procedure is called *drying* or *roasting* and also involves restricting the mother's diet to certain "hot" and "cold" foods. The mother is not allowed to bathe for two weeks after delivery, until the "fresh uterus" returns to its normal shape with the help of massages administered by a midwife. A special bath is given at this time to remove unclean substances from the body through perspiration (McKenzie & Chrisman, 1977).

In Melanesia and Polynesia, the mother lies beside a coconut fire while her women friends massage her with oil (Kitzinger, 1990). To involute the uterus and to prevent vaginal discharge later, a Vietnamese woman may squat over a small coal fire or a cauldron of steaming water filled with alcohol, lemon grass, or Chinese medicine (Mathews & Manderson, 1981). The Haitian version of this postpartum warming is known as the *three baths*–two baths in water boiled with special leaves and later a cold bath followed by a cleansing purge (Harris, 1987).

A seclusion period of about 40 days is common in many cultures. This time of support from female kin and seclusion for the mother and baby varies according to the culture. Generally, it permits a mother to become acquainted with her baby, to establish her milk supply, and to reduce both her and her infant's exposure to infectious disease. In Bedouin Arab society, besides resting from routine chores during the 40 days, the mother is visited by female relatives who bring small gifts of money to mark the birth of the baby (Forman et al., 1990).

In Korea, the mother's mother-in-law traditionally takes care of her after the child's birth and serves as her "doula." During pregnancy, Korean women undergo *Thae Kyo* or education-teaching of the fetus. In this ancient tradition a mother-in-law trains her daughter-in-law to be a mother (M. Pope, personal communication, Seoul, Korea, 1989). *Thae Kyo* instructs the expectant mother that to avoid bad luck in having her baby, she should not see fires or fights, she must think pure thoughts and eat "pretty" foods, and she must always walk in a straight line. During the postpartum period, which lasts about three to four weeks, the woman is also cared for by her own mother and her husband. This perception that the mother is "sick" and requires care runs counter to the expectations of U.S.-trained nurses and to early discharge from the hospital.

Infant Care

Swaddling or bundling is an ancient practice still used today to soothe the infant and maintain his body temperature. Swaddling and carrying the baby on the mother's side or back also frees her hands for other tasks. In many parts of rural Nigeria, an infant is wrapped on the mother's back all day and sleeps with her at night. During the first 40 days, the baby is snugly wrapped, a practice that ensures that the infant stays warm and reduces his energy requirements (Omuloulu, 1982).

In Bogota, Colombia, and other parts of the world that do not have intensive care nurseries, premature infants who are clinically stable go directly to the mother as early as two to three hours after birth. By being held in an upright position, skin-to-skin between their mother's beasts, they are kept warm (Anderson et al., 1986, 1992) (Fig. 2–6). This practice served as the beginning of what is now known as *kangaroo care.*

In any culture, swaddling and carrying the baby close typifies mothers who practice unrestricted breastfeeding. As early as 24 hours after delivery, the Zambian infant is secured to his mother's body with a *dashica,* or long piece of cloth. The baby rides on the mother's hip in the *dashica,* and his head is not supported. As a result, the Zambian infant maintains a strong shoulder girdle to keep his head steady and thereby develops early head control. The *aquawo*–a specially woven, strong cotton cloth folded in a special way–is the infant carrier in Bolivia. The *aquawo* can be turned around to several positions to facilitate breastfeeding. In Mexico, a woman uses a long, wide shawl called a *rebozo* for carrying her infant while she goes about her daily activities.

Many different types of baby carriers are seen in the United States. Their use suggests that mothers and fathers, regardless of their cultural backgrounds, recognize and enjoy the convenience these carriers afford. Women who work in the fields use a cradleboard device that functions much like swaddling. Carrying the infant swaddled to his mother's body develops the child's muscle tone and seems to encourage alertness. Being carried about during daily activities offers many opportunities for tactile, visual, and social stimulation.

Babies in the Dominican Republic are not secured to their mother in any fashion but are carried in their arms in a horizontal position until they are old enough to sit up by themselves. Because it is believed that a baby can break his or her neck easily if the head is not held, a mother will become visibly anxious when the nurse assesses her baby's head control.

An infant may be affected by diseases recognized only in that culture. In Spanish-speaking cultures, the most common is *mollera caida* (fallen fontanel). The health professional interprets a depressed fontanel in the baby as a symptom of

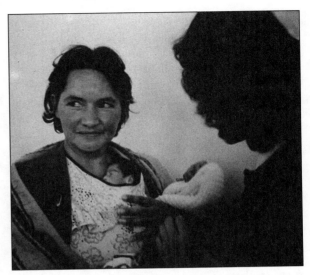

FIGURE 2–6. A premature infant in Bogota goes home *12 hours after birth, cradled skin-to-skin with his mother. (Courtesy G. C. Anderson.)*

dehydration, whereas a Hispanic mother may see it as curable illness caused by removing her nipple while the baby is still suckling, or by the baby falling. One mother explained that her baby's fontanel had fallen in church after the baby was accidentally knocked over in her baby seat: "My mother-in-law diagnosed her right away as having *mollera caida.* She could tell because when the baby sucked, there was a different sound to it and there was no grip to it. She was then taken to the *curandera* (healer) who cured her by applying pressure on the infant's palate with her thumbs" (Ehling, 1981).

Another Hispanic and Puerto Rican folk disease is *mal de ojo,* or evil eye, which is presumably caused by someone who admired the baby but did not touch him. It is also thought to be caused by people casting very strong glances. Symptoms of *mal de ojo* are sometimes vague, but the baby is usually very unhappy, cries continuously, cannot sleep, and may even die (Lacay, 1981). The cure is effected by finding the person who is thought to have given the infant the evil eye and having her or him touch the baby. Lactation consultants (LCs) working with such clients should take care to touch the baby when admiring him or her to avoid being thought of as the cause of a later case of *mal de ojo.*

Babies often are outfitted with special ornaments or bands that have a specific purpose. Hispanic grandmothers often worry a great deal about the infant's umbilicus and may insist that the baby wear a belly band (*fajita*) to prevent an umbilical hernia. Haitian babies may wear a band of cloth around the abdomen to develop a strong body and a sense of balance (Harris, 1987). A traditional necklace protects the Laotian newborn (La Du, 1985). Babies in Papua New Guinea are protected from disease by special rituals, such as blackening the top of the baby's head with burnt coconut husk (Lepowsky, 1985). In the Philippines, applying charred chicken gizzard to the baby's lips is believed to prevent diarrhea (Guthrie, 1983).

In most cultures, infants sleep with or close to their mothers. Chinese infants frequently sleep in their parents' bed or in the same room with them at night. The first year is characterized by warmth and security, and infants are showered with attention by everyone in the family. Extended family members who live nearby are close to the infant. Traditionally, Chinese infants are not allowed to cry but are immediately picked up and rocked or carried by a member of the family in a back sling (Char, 1981).

Maternal Foods

Whether she lives on a mountaintop in remote Tibet, in a dusty Mexican village, or in an American suburb or urban high-rise apartment, the lactating woman produces milk that is amazingly homogeneous in composition, despite the wide diversity of foods she consumes. Only the milk of a woman who is severely malnourished will be measurably diminished in its nutrient content and volume because body nutrients are depleted before the milk suffers.

Part of understanding a culture involves becoming acquainted with its foodways–the way in which a distinct group selects, prepares, consumes, and otherwise uses portions of the available food supply. *Food behavior* denotes and describes the foodways of an individual. The list of various ethnic foods in Table 2–2 gives an overview of the wide variety of food patterns followed by lactating women.

For more than half the inhabitants of this planet, including lactating women, beans, rice, and grains are daily fare. Fruits and vegetables appear seasonally, and meat is found in the family cooking pot only on special occasions. When it does appear, it is usually poultry, goat, horse, or dog, rather than beef. In most cultures, meat plays a minor part in flavoring rice, beans, and vegetables, not the major role it has served in affluent Western industrialized countries.

The daily food pattern of a breastfeeding Mexican mother who eats very little meat might concern us if we did not have a basic knowledge of amino acids and complementary proteins. Beans, a staple item in Mexican foodways, provide an incomplete protein when served alone, because they are low in methionine, an essential amino acid. This deficiency, however, is completely corrected when beans are served with a food high in methionine, such as whole-grain breads or cereals. Complementary proteins can be obtained by numerous combinations. For example, eggs or a milk product will balance the protein and amino acids of a meal consisting primarily of plant proteins. However, two protein foods cannot complement each other if they have similar amino acids in their composition. For this reason, nuts and black-eyed peas are not complementary proteins, because both legumes lack the same amino acids.

Foods That Increase Breastmilk

Almost all cultures abound with an array of prescriptive foods for lactating women. In the United States, beer and brewer's yeast have been touted as galactogogues (i.e., foods that are thought to increase milk secretion and to improve let-down). Parturient mothers in a number of countries gratefully accept the chicken soup given to them. In addition to its fluid value, chicken soup (a perennially favorite medicinal food) contains calcium and sodium to maintain electrolyte balance.

In Mexico, the use of a wide variety of galactagogues was a common practice until recent times. The herbalist's "bible" in Mexico recommends anise and cotton seeds to increase breastmilk (Vargas, 1979). In traditional Japan, a low-calorie diet (rice, gruel, soup, vegetables) for mothers during the immediate postpartum period was believed

Table 2-2

BRIEF DESCRIPTIONS OF AN ASSORTMENT OF ETHNIC AND REGIONAL FOODS

Grain group

Anadama: Cornmeal-molasses yeast bread (New England)

Bagels: Bread dough shaped like a donut, cooked in water, then baked; chewy (Jewish-American)

Bulgur: Granular wheat product with nutlike flavor, served like rice (Middle Eastern)

Brioche: Type of egg-rich French roll, often served at breakfast

Challah: Braided eggbread

Chapatis: Unleavened bread used by Indians

Croissants: Flaky crescent-shaped rolls (French)

Crumpets: Muffinlike product cooked on griddle; often served toasted (British)

Grits: Coarsely ground hominy (corn product) (Southern USA)

Johnnycake: Cornbread (New England)

Kasha: Coarsely ground grain toasted before cooking in liquid

Latkes: Pancakes

Limpa: Rye bread (Swedish)

Mush: Cooked cereal (often cornmeal)

Pasta: Macaroni, spaghetti, noodles in variety of forms (Italian)

Polenta: Cornmeal (Italian)

Scones: Round, flat, unleavened, unsweetened bread product (British)

Sopapillas: Fried bread (rich dough) (Mexican)

Tortillas: thin rounds of leathery dough made from lime-treated corn or from wheat flour, often fried until crisp (Mexican)

Fruit and vegetable group

Bok choy: Green leafy, stalklike vegetable (Oriental)

Chayote: Green or white squash-like vegetable eaten raw, cooked, or pickled (Mexican)

Dandelion greens: Young leaves from wild dandelion plants, eaten raw or cooked

Greens in "pot liquor" ("likor"): Green leafy vegetables such as kale or turnip, mustard or collard greens, cooked with salt pork, served with cooking liquid (Southern USA)

Jalapeños: Hot peppers

Kelp: Seaweed

Papaya: Large, yellow, melonlike tropical fruit

Prickly pear: Fruit of a cactus

Viandas: Starchy tropical vegetables such as sweet potato, cassava, plantain (banana-like in appearance) (Puerto Rican)

Meat group

Adobo: Meat, soy sauce (Filipino)

Chitterlings: Pork intestine, tripe ("soul food")

Chorizo: Sausage (Mexican)

Escargots: Snails (French)

Falafel: Mashed chick peas mixed with other ingredients and fried (Israeli)

Feijoada: Black beans, meat (Brazilian)

Finnan haddie: Smoked haddock

Frijoles refritas: refried pinto or calico beans (Mexican)

Gefilte fish: Ground or flaked fish seasoned and shaped into balls (Jewish-American)

Hog maw: Stomach of pig (Southern USA)

Jerky: Dried meat strips

Kibee: Fresh raw lamb, ground, seasoned; eaten uncooked (Middle Eastern)

Kielbasa: Polish sausage

Miso: Soybean paste

Pepperoni: Italian hot sausage

Sauerbrauten: Pot roast marinated in acidic sauce (German

Sashimi: Raw fish (Japanese)

Teriyaki: Broiled beef marinated in sweet soy sauce (Hawaiian)

Table 2-2 *(cont.)*

BRIEF DESCRIPTIONS OF AN ASSORTMENT OF ETHNIC AND REGIONAL FOODS

Mixed dishes

Couscous: Semolina, meat stew (North African)

Goulash: Stew usually seasoned with paprika (Hungarian)

Gumbo: Okra and meat stew, thickened with filé (pulverized sassafras leaves) (Louisiana Creole)

Hoppin John: Blackeyed peas and rice (Southern USA)

Jambalaya: Rice, ham, and seafood (Louisiana Creole)

Moussaka: Eggplant casserole (Greek)

Scrapple: Pork and cornmeal (Pennsylvania Dutch)

Tacos: Fried tortillas filled with meat or beans, vegetables, hot sauce (Mexican)

Wonton: Stuffed dough, fried or cooked in broth (Chinese)

Others

Baklava: A layered pastry rich in honey (Greek)

Butterhorns: Sweet pastry

Cracklins: Crispy pieces left after pork fat is rendered (Southern)

Fatback: Fat from belly of pig

Kuchen: Cake

Lard: Pork fat rendered to be used as shortening

Salt pork: Salted pork fat, sometimes with bit of meat

Sofrito: Specially seasoned tomato sauce used by Puerto Ricans

Spumoni: Fruit ice cream (Italian)

Strickle sheets: Coffee cake (Pennsylvania Dutch)

Strudel: Paper-thin pastry with fruit filling or cheese (German)

Tzimmes: Carrot-prune dessert (Jewish-American)

Source: Suitor CW, Hunter MF: Nutrition: principles and application in health promotion. *Philadelphia: Lippincott, 1980.*

to help the secretion of milk; in Korea, *miyuk gup,* a seaweed soup, is believed to cleanse the body of lochia ("bad blood") and to increase breastmilk. Lactating women in Japan were also encouraged to eat lotus roots. Because the root has many holes, it was thought to prevent plugged milk ducts. Another Japanese tradition was to wrap rice or red beans in a cotton cloth made to look like a small breast. A woman who wished to have enough milk for her coming baby offered one of these breast models to Buddha as she prayed. Later, she cooked and ate the rice or beans (Sawada, 1981).

Ethnographic records show that the Navajo woman's milk supply was believed to increase if she drank broth made from blue cornmeal (Moore, 1969). The Ojibwa encouraged the eating of wild rice, lake trout, and white fish. In the Philippines, soups containing marungay leaves and papayas are supposed to make the milk flow; sour foods, however, are believed to decrease milk and to increase lochia (Affonso, 1978). Pakistani galactogogues include cumin, cotton seeds, and goat's stomach; in India, fried ginger and black pepper are recommended (Baumslag, 1987).

Food Restrictions

Food restrictions or taboos regarding the postpartum diet are common; many restrictions result in diets that are similar to those for sick people. Currently, we have no good evidence that the common maternal food restrictions found in many cultures help the infant, nor can we say that they harm the mother. Despite the absence of proof of such a relationship, many people in the United States still believe that hot, spicy foods have a deleterious effect on milk supply.

Restricting fruit in the postpartum diet is a common practice in many Spanish-speaking cultures, including that encompassing some Mexican-Americans. After the baby is born, Haitian women avoid foods that are white because they are thought to increase vaginal discharge; one way to get around this taboo is to add another food (for instance, coffee to milk) to color it (Harris, 1987).

"Hot" and "Cold" Foods

For many cultural groups, foodways involve a balance that must be maintained to sustain health or be restored when illness occurs. Balance between opposing energy forces is based on the Greek theory of body humors. After centuries of dissemination throughout the world, this theory now appears as the hot (*caliente*) and cold (*frio* or *fresco*) system in Hispanic cultures. Other people, such as the Vietnamese, Chinese, East Indians, and Arabs, also use a hot-cold designation to some extent. Classifying foods as "hot" or "cold" in a given culture has little to do with their form, color, texture, or temperature, although "hot" foods are believed to be more easily digested than are "cold" foods. Instead, the classification is based on the food's effect on an illness or condition, which is itself categorized as "hot" or "cold." During the last trimester of pregnancy, the unborn child is believed to be "hot"; therefore, the mother is in a hot state. Once the child is born, accompanied by a loss of blood, a "cold" condition exists for both. To correct this imbalance, women believe that they need humorally warming foods; to replace heat and energy, extra blankets and warm clothes are necessary. Failure to observe these puerperal prescriptions is thought to have serious long-term medical implications (Fishman et al., 1988; Mathews & Manderson, 1981).

Traditional Chinese consider chicken, squash, and broccoli to be "hot." "Cold" foods include melon, fruits, soybean sprouts, and bamboo shoots. In India, milk may be "hot" or "cold," depending on where a person lives. In Hispanic cultures, "cold" foods include most fresh vegetables, tropical fruits, dairy products, beans, squash, and some meats. "Hot" foods—cereal grains, chili peppers, temperate-zone fruits, goat's milk, oils, and beef—

serve to balance the "cold" foods. Because the potential listing of "hot" and "cold" foods in any particular culture is almost endless, health providers must do their ethnographic homework regarding the belief system of the cultures with whose members they are working. Among Vietnamese women who delivered infants in Australia in the early 1980s, foods restricted after childbirth included raw vegetables and all fruit. Among Vietnamese-Chinese mothers, bananas, cabbage, soy-milk soft drinks and unboiled water were also prohibited (Mathews & Manderson, 1981).

Another belief system concerning food balance is the Chinese *yin-yang* theory. In America, the system is practiced by people who use macrobiotics. Like the hot-cold theory, the basis of the *yin-yang* belief rests on a proper balance between opposing energy forces. On one side, yin represents "female," a negative force (cold, emptiness, darkness); on the other side, yang represents "male," a positive force (warmth, fullness, light). Too much of either yin or yang food is considered threatening to health. Whether a food is considered yin or yang depends on the effect it is thought to have on the body; the designation is not associated with color, texture, or other obvious characteristics. Without an extensive orientation for things Chinese, it is difficult to understand the "yin-ness" or "yang-ness" of food.

Traditional cultures have used medicinal herbs extensively. For instance, Cambodian mothers who have immigrated to the United States still use tiger balm and ginger root to treat their children's illnesses (Rosenberg, 1986). Northern Mexicans make special teas from so-called "hot" plants, such as sesame and absinthe, and in some parts of Latin America, herb teas are drunk in the evening to stimulate milk for the morning (Baumslag, 1987). Herbs taken by the breastfeeding mother may have pharmacological effects on her baby, including irritation of the mucosal lining of the intestine and an increase in the release of flatus. As a result, some breastfed infants of mothers who regularly consume herbs may experience increased gas and loose stools. Unless these gastrointestinal symptoms become troublesome and an allergic response occurs, it is more important for the mother to continue enjoying her favorite herbs than to stop using them because of her baby's minor stool changes.

Vegetarians

For reasons of health, religion, ethnic values, or economy, many people worldwide are vegetarians. Two general classifications are recognized: *lacto-ovo-vegetarians,* who use eggs and dairy products in addition to plant foods, and *vegans,* who use only plant foods. A lactating vegetarian who eats a wide variety of grains, legumes, nuts, fruits, vegetables, and dairy products has a nutritionally sound diet. Frequently, industrial nation families who practice vegetarianism by choice are quite knowledgeable about nutrition. They are rarely obese and have superior diet patterns because they conscientiously avoid processed, empty-calorie foods. Concerns about breastfeeding usually center on whether the mother is consuming adequate protein and vitamin B_{12}, because this vitamin is not found in vegetable protein. Even a strict vegan diet can be carefully planned and supplemented, if need be. Supplemental vitamins, fortified soy milk, and fortified yeast are all good sources of B_{12}. (See Chapter 16 for a detailed discussion of vegetarian diets.)

Women who consume large amounts of green vegetables sometimes produce milk that has a greenish tint. This also can occur among women taking advantage of large quantities of certain foods when they are in season. "Green" milk, although not at all harmful to the infant, can be rather unnerving at first to the unwary until they understand the cause.

A basic diet guide for balanced vegetarian meals includes

- *Grains, legumes, nuts, and seeds:* six or more servings including several slices of whole grain bread, beans, and some nuts or seeds
- *Vegetables:* three servings or more, including one or more servings of dark, leafy greens
- *Fruit:* one to four pieces, including citrus fruits for a raw source of vitamin
- *Milk and eggs:* dairy products (if the baby does not show an allergic response) and eggs to meet basic protein requirements.

Religious Influences

Religion also influences the foodways of the breastfeeding woman, her breastfeeding practices, and how long she breastfeeds (Ineichen et al, 1997). If she is a Seventh-Day Adventist or a member of certain Eastern religious sects, she very likely practices vegetarianism. Orthodox Muslim and Black Muslim women are expected to breastfeed their babies according to religious teachings, and Islamic dietary regulations prohibit pork, animal shortening, products containing gelatin, and alcoholic beverages. No animal meat can be eaten unless it has been slaughtered in a prescribed manner. During the month-long Ramadan fast, Muslims are not allowed to eat or drink anything between sunrise and sunset. If they are not exempt, this practice imposes a hardship on pregnant and lactating women who require a regular intake of fluid and calories (Prentice et al., 1983).

Orthodox Jewish mothers closely observe dietary laws that prohibit pork products and shellfish. According to these laws, meat and milk cannot be eaten at the same meal. After meat is eaten, she must wait before consuming milk products. Dietary counseling must include planning her daily meals so that she takes in adequate calcium and phosphorus from milk products or substitute foods.

The Doula

Much has been written about the importance of social support of the breastfeeding woman. Raphael (1973), who coined the word *doula,* explained the characteristics of such a person as one who is knowledgeable in the breastfeeding process and who "mothers the mother." To undertake this important task, different cultures designate one or more specific people to this role. Usually, but not always, this person is an older woman, often the mother's mother, mother-in-law, or aunt with breastfeeding experience that she passes on to the mother. At the same time, she assists the mother with her household work and protects her from the stresses of the outside world. The doula role has taken new forms and has gained greater popularity in the United States in the past few years. Doulas, who are trained in childbirth procedures, are being hired by families to stay with the mother and family during childbirth in a birth center or hospital and to assist them in the days immediately following their return to the home.

Weaning

Weaning is a time when childhood illness and death are more likely in developing countries; thus it is a key issue in studies of cross-cultural child-care practices. Cultural assessment includes the timing of feeding, types of foods given to infants, and weaning practices. When a substantial proportion of dietary intake comes from food other than breastmilk, growth rates falter, and the effects of morbidity come into play. Woolridge (1991) suggests, as a rule of thumb, that when 25 to 50 percent of a baby's kilocalories come from breastmilk, the milk will protect the baby from environmental pathogens. At the same time, every breastfed infant reaches a point at which breastmilk alone can no longer meet its nutritional needs and solid foods are necessary.

Early solid and semisolid infant foods given by mothers vary widely across cultures, as does the timing of their introduction. Worldwide, there is a high rate of both the initiation of breastfeeding and early supplementation with other foods. Although infants in Papua New Guinea are not introduced to supplemental foods until six months (Lepowsky, 1985) (an optimal age), this is not the usual pattern. In a comparison study of how mothers feed their infants in four diverse countries, Winikoff et al. (1988) noted that early introduction of other foods is common. The majority of Kenyan babies are given foods other than breastmilk before they are four months old (Dimond & Ashworth, 1987; van Esterik & Elliott, 1986); in East Java, force-feeding by hand is a common practice from as early as a few days after birth (van Steenbergen et al., 1991).

What implications can we derive from these diverse practices in infant feedings? Van Esterik (1988) suggests looking at a culture's breastfeeding "style" (i.e., the cultural assumptions underlying infant feeding practices) to distinguish between breastfeeding as a process and breastmilk as product. According to this model, a given culture will tend to emphasize breastfeeding style as either a process or a means to obtain a product (Auerbach, 1991). When breastfeeding is considered a process, supplements are small in amount and are not given to replace breastfeeding. For example, mothers in Kenya perceive breastfeeding as a process, something that mothers and infants do and not solely as food for the infant. As such, finger-feeding the baby small amounts of food from the family cooking pot is part of the socialization of the infant, and meals consist of several foods.

In the United States, breastfeeding is considered primarily as a product that can be closely approximated, although not completely replaced, by formula. Emphasis is on its nutritional and immunological properties as opposed to nonproduct issues, such as fertility, maternal satisfaction, and feelings of closeness to the baby. If breastfeeding is seen primarily as a product in a given culture, it is seldom considered an integral part of the maternal experience. For example, when a mother in southern Senegal speaks of her children, whether they are toddlers or grown women working alongside her in the rice fields, she often grasps one of her breasts, lifts it outward and says, "First I gave the breast to 'Fatu' who held it and gave it to 'Seku'" and so on, naming her way through the ordinal sequence of her offspring. Her breasts define her role as mother and also temporarily "belong" to the nursling whose milk they contain (Whittemore & Beverly, 1996).

Weaning from the breast is a process during which mothers gradually introduce their babies to culturally assigned foods as they continue to breastfeed. According to Raphael (1984), mothers worry as much about the availability of additional foods as they do about the amount of milk they produce. Weaning begins with the introduction of sources of food other than breastmilk and ends with the last breastfeeding. Three types of weaning have been described:

- Gradual weaning that takes place over several weeks or months

- Deliberate weaning, a conscious effort initiated by the mother to end breastfeeding at a particular point

- Abrupt weaning, an immediate cessation of breastfeeding, which may be forced on the baby by the mother or on mother and baby by others

Examples of gradual, deliberate, or abrupt weaning may be found in any culture. Gradual weaning, however, is the least traumatic, to both the infant and the mother.

Weaning practice can affect infant health, particularly in developing countries or in inner-city areas in which weaning diarrhea is prevalent. In cultures in which food is available sporadically or is meager, kwashiorkor, a severe form of protein deficiency, appears during the transition from breastmilk to other foods. In Ga, the language of Ghana, the term *kwashiorkor* means "the disease of the deposed baby." Identifying the reasons for women weaning early sheds considerable light on the beliefs and attitudes that influence the continuation of breastfeeding.

Reasons given for early weaning are similar in many cultures. For example, the following reasons given by poor Filipino mothers for early termination of breastfeeding are similar to those of women living in North America (Guthrie et al., 1983): insufficient milk; mother returning to work (selling foods on the street requires that the mother be exposed to the hot sun, causing milk to lie in the breast for many hours, after which time it is not fit for the baby); mother becoming sick with Bughat, a culture-bound vague illness that only women who have borne children can develop; milk that is salty or not good (one mother raised six children on one breast because she decided that the milk of the other was salty at her first pregnancy).

Particular solid foods are meant to initiate gradual weaning. Specially prepared rice, the major infant food in East Java, is hand-fed in small amounts to almost all infants, and all babies breastfeed (van Steenbergen et al., 1991). Rice, finger-fed in small amounts, initiates the Thai baby to a rice culture and helps to stave off spiritual parents who might come to take the baby away (Woolridge, 1991). Before putting children to sleep, grandmothers in Senegal feed the children finely ground peanuts sweetened with sugar while holding them in their lap near the fire. This practice is so common that a mother who is asked whether her child is weaned will respond simply, "His grandmother is roasting peanuts" (Whittemore & Beverly, 1996).

Various stages in infant development are sometimes used as cues to begin deliberate weaning. A common belief among African cultures is that the child should be walking before weaning is attempted. Some kind of independence is implicit in the concept of weaning, so it seems reasonable that the child be self-sufficient in locomotion before leaving the dependency of its mother's breast. In many Western cultures, teething is a developmental reference point thought to signal readiness to wean. In others, subsequent pregnancy signals the time to wean (Bohler & Ingstad, 1996). Usually a toddler or child will spontaneously wean with a new pregnancy. The reasons for this behavior include a diminished milk supply, changes in the milk composition, and a less desirable taste.

For mammals, the length of lactation is positively correlated with adult female mass. Generally, larger mammals have long lactation periods (Hayssen, 1993). What is the "natural" age for weaning in humans? Dettwyler (1995) suggests four criteria associated with age at weaning in primates that range from 27 months to 7 years:

- *Weaning according to tripling or quadrupling of birth weight:* Using U.S. data, male infants quadruple their birth weight by about 27 months and female infants by around 30 months.

- *Weaning according to attainment of one-third adult weight:* Weaning for the human would be predicted at between 4 and 7 years of age.

- *Weaning according to adult body size:* Using this comparison predicts the age for weaning in humans at between 2.8 and 3.7 years, with larger-bodied populations breastfeeding for the longest time.

- *Weaning according to time of dental eruption of permanent molars:* Modern humans' first molar eruption occurs around 5.5 to 6.0 years of age (the same time as that for adult immune competence).

Some rather harsh techniques have been used to bring about abrupt weaning. One time-honored method calls for pepper, garlic, ginger, or onion to be applied to the mother's breasts to discourage the baby from breastfeeding (Aquino, 1981). In the Fiji Islands, weaning of *kali* ("to separate") is a four-day period during which the breast is denied to the infant and the baby's food is specially cooked in a separate pot. The infant is not allowed to sleep with the mother until after weaning and is sometimes cared for by one of the mother's female relatives in another household for this period (Katz, 1984).

In cultures in which early weaning from bottle or breast is a common practice, long-term breastfeeding is accepted by a minority of people within the culture. The sight of a walking child calmly sliding onto the mother's lap for milk and deftly opening her buttons to gain access to her breasts is considered shocking and subject to ridicule in

BOX 2–2

Specific Folkways and Methods for Handling Them

- Touching a Spanish-speaking family's baby while admiring him helps avoid giving the baby *mal de ojo*.

- An anemic breastfeeding mother is not vegetarian and she believes anemia is a *yin* condition. Suggest that she consume more meat, a *yang* food, to improve her iron status (Suitor & Hunter, 1980).

- The Korean mother refuses a cold pack for engorged breasts or for pain resulting from an episiotomy (Schneiderman, 1996). Offer her cool water from a washcloth or from a peri bottle.

- The mother expects a 40-day period of special care postpartum. Respect the tradition and help her through early discharge with one or more home visits.

- The baby burps during feedings. According to some Hispanic mothers, this air goes to the breast and stops the flow of milk, causing her milk duct to become plugged. Ask her to switch to the other breast and then back to the first breast to release the "air."

- The mother believes that colostrum is "bad." Suggest that she express the first few drops of "impure" milk and discard it before putting the baby to breast, then say, "The sooner you breastfeed, the better the milk" (Skeel & Good, 1988; van Esterik, 1988).

- Another Mexican-American belief is that the milk in the breast will sour if a woman is upset or angry. Sour milk, of course, should never be fed to the baby. If the mother's husband or partner is angry with her, she can avoid an argument by pleading that her milk will become sour, thereby avoiding the problem (K. Frantz, personal communication, 1981).

some cultures. The term *closet nursing* describes a practice that has evolved in the United States in response to criticism of breastfeeding that extends beyond the dominant culture's expectations (Avery, 1977; Morse & Harrison, 1987). In closet nursing, breastfeeding continues by mutual consent of mother and child, but only in secret. The mother and baby usually have a code word for breastfeeding that can be used in public (Wrigley & Hutchinson, 1990). In the United States, the main reason given by mothers for breastfeeding longer than 12 months can be summarized thus: "Breastfeeding was a special time for me and my baby, and I wasn't ready to give that up"; also, mothers wanted to let the baby choose the time for weaning (Hills-Bonczyk et al., 1994).

Implications for Practice

Every culture has its visible elements (housing, clothing, food) and its invisible elements (attitudes, tradition, values); an understanding of both contributes significantly to communication between the breastfeeding client and the health care provider (Haider et al, 1997; see Box 2–2).

Immigrant mothers may be served foods that traditionally are forbidden to postpartum women, such as raw vegetables and fruit for Vietnamese mothers. If the dietary department of an institution is aware of this, it can provide alternate foods to these women.

Many Indochinese women living in the United States formula-feed their infant, at least while in the hospital, and then both breastfeed and bottle-feed after leaving the hospital; therefore, formula discharge packs are not appropriate. It is advisable to have women health workers care for these mothers, because they regard it improper for men to touch a woman's body (especially the breasts). If mothers in any culture believe that certain foods can promote lactation, these women should be encouraged to bring these foods to the postpartum unit. This practice will enhance breastfeeding and provide a clear signal that the health care system supports breastfeeding and is respectful of these cultural beliefs (Chan-Yip & Kramer, 1983).

Regardless of the culture, weaning is ideally a collaborative effort in which both the mother and baby reach a state of readiness to begin weaning. In a culture in which unrestricted breastfeeding is practiced and in which the child breastfeeds for a prolonged period, the mother has very little ambivalence when she decides to wean and says, "You, child, have had enough milk!" (Mead & Newton, 1967).

Although weaning practices vary from culture to culture, weaning is thought to be the least traumatic when it is slow, gradual and related to the needs of the child. It is essential to identify factors that influence continuation or early termination of breastfeeding so as to develop appropriate programs to assist the mother who wishes to maintain breastfeeding. Women involved in long-term breastfeeding develop a special bond with their baby. The mother's choice of how long she wishes to breastfeed is an individual right that may not mesh with others' expectations. All breastfeeding families deserve to be treated in a nonjudgmental manner that accepts the cultural diversity that they represent (see Box 2–3).

BOX 2–3

Breastfeeding in Specific Countries

RUSSIA

In economically troubled Russia, increasing numbers of Russian women, influenced by advertising of German formula companies, are formula-feeding their babies. Russian physicians are attempting to reverse this trend by warning such mothers about infant health problems that are caused by lack of breastfeeding. New mothers remain in the hospital for 7 to 14 days, have paid maternity leave for 18 months, and are assured of returning to their previous job. Children are considered a "privileged class": maternity care, education, and health care are free. Additionally, Russian families are financially rewarded by the government for having children; yet Russian women are reluctant to have children and limit their offspring to one or two (personal communication with Russian women in Leningrad, summer, 1989).

JAPAN

Almost all women give birth to their infants in a hospital or clinic. Unmedicated childbirth is the norm, because Japanese physicians believe the newborn is healthier without analgesia. Japanese women grow up believing that breastfeeding is natural and advantageous for the baby. At three months, almost half the mothers are still breastfeeding; by six months, the percentage drops to one-third. The Ministry of Health in Japan actively promotes breastfeeding. Japanese mothers are inclined to follow "doctor's orders" and are reluctant to challenge their (mostly male) physicians' opinions. Many young Japanese women experience a dissonance between their culture's old-world values (staying home, raising children, breastfeeding) and the values of the new world (working, career, bottle-feeding) (M. Hasegawa, personal communication, 1991; R. Riordan, personal communication, 1996).

KOREA

Postpartum Korean mothers are tended by their mothers-in-law and look to them for advice about feeding and caring for their babies; therefore, breastfeeding promotion efforts should include these relatives. About half of Korean babies are formula-fed with manufactured milks imported from the West and advertised as "the second kind of mother's milk" (M. Pope, personal communication, 1988).

SWEDEN

Swedish culture supports breastfeeding as the norm and formula-feeding as the exception. Most Swedish births (90–95 percent) are attended by midwives, and almost all new mothers (98 percent) begin breastfeeding. New mothers are followed by the midwife for the first six days. After that, follow-up care is given by district health nurses, who are child health nurses. Swedish women receive a year's leave with pay following their baby's birth. Leave time can be split and shared by the baby's father. Midwives use acupuncture in some births and take a course in acupuncture as a part of their training. Swedish students learn the benefits of breastfeeding in secondary education along with fertility control. The Baby-Friendly Hospital Initiative is very active and effective in Sweden.

SUMMARY

The study of child-rearing patterns of a given culture is crucial to all health care professionals who work with new and growing families. The seeds of a culture are planted, grow, and thrive in child-rearing patterns. Cultural awareness provides liberation from egocentric views in which one looks at the universe and sees only one's beliefs in the center. The study of any culture begins with critical self-reflection and awareness of the differences between one's cultural values and those of other people. By becoming aware of these differences, we begin a process of partnership in which all groups have something to contribute and something to learn.

Analysis of infant feeding within its cultural context is critically linked to social action and policy decisions regarding breastfeeding promotion and teaching. Curtailment of breastfeeding is common in a society in which male control over breastfeeding is considered latent or overt conflict between men and women.

For those who examine cultural issues carefully, so-called cultural obstacles to solving problems usually include the solutions, too. Within the cultural context of underlying infant-feeding problems, solutions must ultimately emerge. Changes, if they are to last, must originate from within a culture, rather than being imposed from without.

REFERENCES

Affonso DO: The Filipino American. In: Clark A, ed. *Culture, childbearing, health professionals.* Philadelphia: Davis, 1978:128–53.

Anderson GC: Current knowledge about skin-to-skin (Kangaroo) care for preterm infants. *J Perinatol* 11:216–26, 1992.

Anderson GC, Marks EA, Wahlberg V: Kangaroo care for premature infants. *AJN* 86:807–9, 1986.

Aquino CJ: The Filipino in America. In: Clark A, ed. *Culture and childrearing.* Philadelphia: Davis: 1981: 166–90.

Auerbach K: Breastmilk versus breastfeeding: product vs process [editorial], *J Hum Lact* 7:115–16, 1991.

Avery JL: Closet nursing: a symptom of intolerance and a forerunner of social change? *Keep Abreast J* 2:212–26, 1977.

Baumslag N: Breastfeeding: cultural practices and variations. *Adv Int Matern Child Health* 7:36–50, 1987.

Bohler E, Ingstad, B: The struggle of weaning: factors determining breastfeeding duration in East Bhutan. *Soc Sci Med* 43:1805–15, 1996.

Bowles BC: Cultural masquerade [letter]. *J Hum Lact* 3:157, 1987.

Boyle JS, Andrews MM: *Transcultural concepts in nursing care.* Glenview, IL: Scott, Foresman, 1989.

Brownlee AT: *Community, culture and care: a cross-cultural guide for health workers.* St Louis: Mosby, 1978.

Chan-Yip AM, Kramer MS: Promotion of breastfeeding in a Chinese community in Montreal. *Can Med Assoc J* 129:955–8, 1983.

Char EL: The Chinese American. In Clark A, ed. *Culture and childrearing.* Philadelphia: Davis, 1981:141–64.

Conton L: Social, economic and ecological parameters of infant feeding in Usino, Papua New Guinea. *Ecol Food Nutr* 16:39–54, 1985.

Counts DA: Infant care and feeding in Kaliai, West New Britain, Papua New Guinea. *Ecol Food Nutr* 15:49–59, 1984.

Davies-Adetugbo AA: Sociocultural factors and the promotion of exclusive breastfeeding in rural Yoruba communities on Osun State, Nigeria. *Soc Sci Med* 45:113–25, 1997.

Dettwyler KA: A time to wean: the hominid blueprint for the natural age of weaning in modern human populations. In: Stuart-Macadam P, Dettwyler KA, eds. *Biocultural perspectives.* New York: Aldine De Gruyter, 1995.

Dettwyler KA: More than nutrition: breastfeeding in urban Mali. *Med Anthropol Q* 2:172–83, 1988.

Dimond HJ, Ashworth A: Infant feeding practices in Kenya, Mexico and Malaysia: the rarity of the exclusively breast-fed infant. *Hum Nutr Appl Nutr* 41A:51–64, 1987.

Ehling MB: The Mexican American (El Chicano). In: Clark A, ed. *Culture and childrearing.* Philadelphia: Davis, 1981:193–209.

Fernandez MA, Popkin BM: Prelacteal feeding patterns in the Philippines. *Ecol Food Nutr* 21:303–14, 1988.

Fishman C, Evans R, Jenks E: Warm bodies, cool milk: conflicts in post partum food choice for Indochinese women in California. *Soc Sci Med* 26:1125–32, 1988.

Forman MR, et al: The forty-day rest period and infant feeding practices among Negev Bedouin Arab women in Israel. *Med Anthropol* 12:207–16, 1990.

Giger JN, Davidhizar RE: *Transcultural nursing.* St Louis: Mosby, 1991:5.

Guthrie GM, et al: Early termination of breastfeeding among Philippine urban poor. *Ecol Food Nutr* 12:195–202, 1983.

Haider R, et al: Reasons for failure of breast-feeding counseling: others' perspectives in Bangladesh. *Bull WHO* 75:191–96, 1997.

Harris K: Beliefs and practices among Haitian American women in relation to childbearing. *J Nurse Midwif* 32:150–5, 1987.

Hayssen V: Empirical and theoretical constraints on the evolution of lactation. *J Dairy Sci* 76: 3213–33, 1993.

Hills-Bonczyk SG, et al: Women's experiences with breastfeeding longer than 12 months. *Birth* 21:206–12, 1994.

Ineichen B, Pierce M, Lawrenson R: Jewish and Celtic attitudes to breast feeding compared. *Midwifery* 13:40–43, 1997.

Jambunathan J, Stewart S: Hmong women in Wisconsin: what are their concerns in pregnancy and childbirth. *Birth* 22:204–10, 1995.

Katz MM: Infant care in a group of outer Fiji Islands. *Ecol Food Nutr* 15:323–39, 1984.

Kendall S: Cross-cultural aspects and breastfeeding promotion. *Health Visitor* 68:450–1, 1995.

Kitzinger S: *The crying baby.* London: Penguin, 1990.

Koh THHG: Breastfeeding among the Chinese in four countries. *J Trop Pediatr* 27:88–91, 1981.

Krantz JZ, and Kupper NS: Cross-nursing: wet-nursing in a contemporary culture. *Pediatrics* 67:715–17, 1981.

Lacay GI: The Puerto Rican in mainland America. In: Clark A ed: *Culture and childrearing.* Philadelphia: Davis, 1981:211–27.

La Du EB: Childbirth care for Hmong families. *MCN* 10:382–5, 1985.

Leininger M: *Qualitative research methods in nursing.* Orlando: Grune & Stratton, 1985.

Lepowsky MA: Food taboos, malaria and dietary change: infant feeding and cultural adaptation of a Papua New Guinea Island. *Ecol Food Nutr* 16:105–26, 1985.

Maher V: Breastfeeding in cross-cultural perspectives, paradoxes and proposals. In: Maher V, ed. *The anthropology of breastfeeding.* Oxford: Berg, 1992.

Mathews M, Manderson L: Vietnamese behavioral and dietary precautions during confinement. *Ecol Food Nutr* 11:9–16, 1981.

McKenzie JL, Chrisman NJ: Healing, herbs, gods and magic: folk health beliefs among Filipino-Americans. *Nurs Outlook* 25:326–9, 1977.

Mead M, Newton N: Cultural patterning of perinatal behavior. In: Richardson SA, Buttmacher AF, eds. *Childbearing: its social and psychological aspects.* Baltimore: Williams & Wilkins, 1967:142–3.

Mennella JS, Beauchamp GK: Maternal diet alters the sensory qualities of human milk and the nursling's behavior. *Pediatrics* 88:737–44, 1991.

Mercer RT, Stainton MC: Perceptions of the birth experience: a cross-cultural comparison. *Health Care Women Int* 5:29–47, 1984.

Moore WH, ed: *Nutrition, growth and development of North American Indian children.* Department of Health, Education, and Welfare publ. no. 72-76. Washington, DC: National Institutes of Health, 1969.

Morse JM: The cultural context of infant feeding in Fiji. In: Marshall LB ed. *Infant care and feeding in the South Pacific.* New York: Gordon & Breach, 1985: 255–68.

Morse JM, Harrison MJ: Social coercion for weaning. *J Nurse Midwif* 32:205–10, 1987.

Mulford C: Swimming upstream: breastfeeding care in a nonbreastfeeding culture. *JOGNN* 24:464–73, 1995.

Obermeyer CM, Castle S: Back to nature? Historical and cross-cultural perspectives on barriers to optimal breastfeeding. *Med Anthropol* 17:39–63, 1997.

Omuloulu A: Breastfeeding practice and breast-milk intake in rural Nigeria. *Hum Nutr Appl Nutr* 36A:445–51, 1982.

Orque MS, Bloch B, Monrroy LSA: *Ethnic nursing care: a multicultural approach.* St Louis: Mosby, 1983.

Prentice AM, et al: Metabolic consequences of fasting during Ramadan in pregnant and lactating women. *Hum Nutr Clin Nutr* a37c:283–94, 1983.

Raphael D: *The tender gift: breastfeeding.* Englewood Cliffs, NJ: Prentice-Hall, 1973.

Raphael D: Weaning is always: the anthropology of breast feeding behavior. *Ecol Food Nutr* 15:203–13, 1984.

Rasbridge LA, Kulig JC: Infant feeding among Cambodian refugees. *MCN* 20:213–8, 1995.

Rodriguez-Garcia R, Frazier L: Cultural paradoxes relating to sexuality and breastfeeding. *J Hum Lact* 11:111–15, 1995.

Rosenberg JA: Health care for Cambodian children: integrating treatment plans. *Pediatr Nurs* 12:118–25, 1986.

Rossiter JC: The effect of a culture-specific education program to promote breastfeeding among Vietnamese women in Sydney. *Int J Nurs Stud* 31:369–79, 1994.

Rossiter JC: Attitudes of Vietnamese women to baby feeding practices before and after immigration to Sydney, Australia. *Midwifery* 8:103–12, 1992.

Sawada K: Breastfeeding customs in Japan. Proceedings of the Eighth International Conference of La Leche League, International. Chicago, 1981.

Schneiderman JU: Postpartum nursing for Korean mothers. *MCN* 21:155–8, 1996.

Scott MDS, Stern PN: The ethno-market theory: factors influencing childbearing health practices of northern Louisiana Black women. *Health Care Women Int* 6:45–61, 1985.

Serdula MK, et al: Correlates of breast-feeding in a low-income population of whites, blacks, and Southeast Asians. *J Am Diet Assoc* 91:41–5, 1991.

Skeel LS, Good ME: Mexican cultural beliefs and breastfeeding: a model for assessment and intervention. *J Hum Lact* 4:160–63, 1988.

Spector RE: *Cultural diversity in health and illness,* 2nd ed. New York: Appleton-Century-Crofts, 1985:3.

Suitor CW, Hunter MF: *Nutrition: principles and application in health promotion,* Philadelphia: Lippincott, 1980:53–64.

Tripp-Reimer T, Brink P, Saunders JM: Cultural assessment: content and process. *Nurs Outlook* 32:78–82, 1984.

van Esterik P: The cultural context of infant feeding. In: Winikoff B, Castle MA, Laukaran VH, eds. *Feeding infants in four societies: causes and consequences of mothers' choices.* New York: Greenwood Press, 1988:187–201.

van Esterik P, Elliott T: Infant feeding style in urban Kenya. *Ecol Food Nutr* 18:183–95, 1986.

van Steenbergen WM, et al: Nutritional transition during infancy in East Java, Indonesia: 1. A longitudinal study of feeding pattern, breast milk intake and the consumption of additional foods. *Eur J Clin Nutr* 45:67–75, 1991.

Vargas LA: Traditional breastfeeding methods in Mexico. In: Rapheal D, ed. *Breastfeeding and food policy in a hungry world.* New York: Academic, 1979.

Whittemore RD, Beverly EA: Mandinka mothers and nurslings: power and reproduction. *Med Anthropol Q* 10:45–62, 1996.

Williams C, Jeliffe D: *Mother and child health: delivering the services.* Oxford: Oxford University, 1972.

Winikoff B: Summary. In: Winikoff B, Castle MA, Laukaran VH, eds. *Feeding infants in four societies: causes and consequences of mothers' choices.* New York: Greenwood Press, 1988.

Woolridge M: Breastfeeding in the US and Thailand (presentation). Miami: International Lactation Consultant Association, 1991.

Wright AL, et al: Infant feeding practices among middle-class Anglos and Hispanics. *Pediatrics* 82:496–503, 1988.

Wrigley EA, Hutchinson S: Long-term breastfeeding: the secret bond. *J Nurse Midwifery* 35:35–41, 1990.

Zeitlyn S, Rowshan R: Privileged knowledge and mothers' "perceptions": the case of breast-feeding and insufficient milk in Bangladesh. *Med Anthrop Q* 11:56–8, 1997.

FAMILIES

Kathleen G. Auerbach

When we as lactation consultants help a breast-feeding mother and baby, we help a family. The breastfeeding family exists in a social context; therefore, the care provider must recognize that "family" is a group that is variously defined and experienced. We need to know about the family from which the mother comes and into which her child will be born and reared. Although every family is expected to perform similar functions, the ways in which those functions are recognized and accomplished will vary.

Certain families need special attention. A case in point is the single pregnant adolescent, who may not have others on whom she can depend and whose needs are greater than they would be were she married or part of a well-established support network. The family living in poverty may need to breastfeed to provide the baby with protections that are available only in human milk; however, in most settings in the developed world, the poorest mothers are least likely to breastfeed. Care providers need to be cognizant of breastfeeding promotion programs developed with particular families in mind.

This chapter examines the family from a developmental perspective. The birth of a baby has rightly been described as a crisis because it forces new ways of behavior on all family members. The chapter also discusses issues pertaining to the development of spousal and parent-child attach-ment, paying particular attention to the father's role as a helpmate and supporter of his partner's role as mother and as breastfeeder. It also address-es the special needs of the adolescent mother and of women living in poverty.

Family Forms and Functions

In a lifetime, an individual experiences many family forms. Each form meets different needs and serves different functions. Some include children; others do not. Some forms will be experienced only at certain times in the life cycle, whereas others may occur at several different times. A *traditional family* is defined as one in which the mother is a full-time homemaker and primarily responsible for rearing the children, while her husband is a full-time worker outside the home. Although he is committed to seeing that the children are raised to adulthood, his role in child rearing is secondary to that of his wife. Although this form has often been viewed as ideal, it is experienced by only a small percentage of families, usually for a minority of the life of that family. A *nuclear family* is composed of one or both parents and their children, who are either born to or adopted by them. An *extended family* usually contains lateral kin (such as aunts, uncles, or cousins), who occupy the same generational status as the parents and children in a nuclear family, or vertical kin (such as grandparents or grandchildren), who represent generations different from the parents and children in the nuclear family. In some cases, an extended family may include "fictive" kin, individuals who cannot trace lineage through blood or marriage ties to the nuclear family members but who act, and are treated, as if they were related.

Examining how different family forms are likely to be experienced throughout an individual's lifetime can provide insight into the stresses that an individual is likely to encounter. It also reveals the people on whom an individual will lean as he or she attempts to cope with those stresses. Consider, for example, a hypothetical individual whom we shall call Marsha.

Marsha began life in her *family of orientation* (the family into which she was born or adopted). This family is considered traditional because Marsha's mother has remained home since the birth of Marsha's older brother, and Marsha's father is the sole breadwinner. Marsha also has a younger sister and a younger brother, providing her with both same-gender and opposite-gender sibling relationships.

In her late teens, Marsha went away to college. After she graduated and began her first job as a commercial artist for a local public relations firm, she moved into her own apartment, reveling for the first time in her very own space.

Four years later, Marsha met John, an architect. After a whirlwind courtship, and against the advice of their parents, the two married and moved into John's apartment. Two years later, they bought a house in the hope of filling some of the upstairs bedrooms with children. Just before their third wedding anniversary, Marsha gave birth to John, Jr., thus creating her *family of procreation*. Three years later, Mary Jane (MJ) was born. At the end of her pregnancy with John, Marsha quit her job. Until Mary Jane was one year old, Marsha remained a full-time homemaker while John was the family's breadwinner; Marsha thus cared for their two children in a pattern much like that of both grandmothers.

Time away from work became increasingly difficult for Marsha; she decided to go back to work when Mary Jane reached her first birthday. "After all, MJ will be only one floor away from me.

I called and there is space for her at the new day-care center in the same building as my old job, and Bernie said he'd take me back," she explained to John. For the next three years, both spouses worked full-time.

As sometimes happens, neither spouse found their increasingly busy life conducive to maintaining communication. After 10 years of marriage, John and Marsha experimented with a trial separation and finally divorced. Marsha maintained physical custody of the children as they continued to live with her. John found a small co-op apartment near Marsha and the children so that under the joint custody arrangement they had worked out, he would be able to see the children with minimal difficulty.

For the first two years after the divorce, Marsha found single life difficult, but she felt that she and the children had never been closer. Then she met Joe, whose ex-wife lived out-of-state with their three children (Luci, Adam, and Marie), ages four to seven. Shortly after Marsha and Joe were wed, Marsha's children, now ages 14 and 11, decided to live with John. Marsha became a non-custodial parent, although she continued to see the children frequently. Six months after Marsha's children left her home, Joe's children returned to him for a visit; while there, Joe's ex-wife was killed in a car accident. Hence, Joe and Marsha assumed full-time custody of Joe's children.

A year later, Marsha's own children asked to return to live with Joe and Marsha when their father's job took him out of state. At this point, Marsha was a mother in a "blended" family that included a preschooler, school-age, and high school–aged children.

A year after MJ left home for college, Joe was injured in the San Francisco earthquake. He took early retirement. Marsha was secretly relieved that the work of caring for Joe's teenage children fell more heavily on Joe's shoulders now that he was a full-time house-husband. This arrangement continued until Luci joined the Marines and Joe, Jr., received a scholarship to Harvard. Ten months later, while visiting a travel agent's office to plan a special fifteenth-anniversary cruise, Joe suffered a fatal massive heart attack.

Marsha took the cruise alone and returned to a home empty of people but echoing with memories.

A year after Joe's death, she was awakened in the middle of the night by a telephone call from a weeping Mary Jane, asking whether she could come home. She explained that she and her husband Jason had had a terrible fight, and Mary Jane was afraid that he might become violent. Marsha put on the front porch light, set the tea kettle over a tiny flame, and made up the bed in MJ's old room.

For two years, MJ and her son, Jason, Jr., lived with Grandma Marsha. As Marsha was preparing to ask MJ to "get a grip" on her life and move out, Jason completed his drug-and-alcohol-rehabilitation program, rejoined a health-and-fitness club, won the intraclub weight-lifting championship, and appeared on Marsha's doorstep to reclaim his family and "begin life anew." Marsha kissed them all good-bye and returned to the quiet of her very own space. She contemplated taking early retirement at 62 and signing up for a photographic safari.

Since leaving her family of orientation, Marsha experienced ten different family configurations. If she moves in with her sister after selling her home, she may experience yet another form, that of a single-generation kin network. She experienced what is often called a *traditional nuclear family* for only 4 of the 10 years that she was married to John—and for less than one-tenth of her entire adult life since leaving her own family of orientation. Although this example is hypothetical, the life experiences that it represents are typical of those experienced by many people in developed nations today.

Although the forms may vary, each group of individuals who consider themselves to be part of a family is characterized by five universal tenets (Spradley, 1985):

1. It is a small social system.
2. It has its own culture and rules.
3. It has structure.
4. It has certain basic functions.
5. It moves through stages in its life cycle.

The existence of these universal features means that, regardless of its composition, a family pro-vides certain elements to its members. These generally consist of affection, security, identity, affiliation, socialization, and controls (Spradley, 1985).

From the standpoint of a mother and infant or a mother and young child, *affection* is important. It affirms for the child that he is loved and appreciated for his own sake. *Security* derives from the physical and social restrictions that, along with other controls, set the boundaries by which appropriate behavior is identified and rewarded.

The family's *identity* is most often recognized by outsiders through a shared surname, which often places the members of that family within a larger social context, such as a neighborhood or community. Particularly in small towns, the members of a family may share a status established many generations earlier.

Affiliation is a recognition by its members that they relate to one another in ways that differ from the ways they interact with other individuals who are not family. The jokes made about first meeting the parents or siblings of a future spouse are an acknowledgment that not being a member of the family sets one apart as different from its members.

Socialization refers to how older family members teach younger members appropriate behavior and what to value. A child who "minds his manners" when at a restaurant with grandparents has been socialized to behave in this manner by the members of his or her family, who have served as role models for acceptable decorum in public. Unacceptable behavior is corrected in practice settings, such as around the dinner table at home.

Finally, *controls* involve not only a recognition of appropriate behavior but a mechanism for identifying and correcting inappropriate behavior. In cases in which gender-role-specific behavior is expected, the boy who offers to wash dishes may be viewed as engaging in inappropriate behavior by some, although in his family no such gender-specific division of labor is made. In many ways, identifying appropriate, inappropriate, or deviant behavior is a recognition of subcultural norms or values. In a pluralistic society in which many different subcultures and ethnic groups abound, the way in which behavior is structured and controlled may vary markedly from one family group to the next. Thus breastfeeding in the living room in the presence of friends, male and female, may be viewed as completely acceptable in some families and as clearly incorrect behavior in others. For some mothers, breastfeeding requires draping a shawl around her shoulders and the baby's upper torso. The health care worker assisting the breastfeeding mother is well advised to ask for guidance about what the mother's family expects of her in order to provide advice that will be viewed as appropriate within that family setting.

Today's families increasingly recognize that child rearing will occupy only a portion of the entire life experience of a couple (regardless of the number of relationships experienced). Although a baby may be the outcome and reflection of the love its parents feel for one another, the presence of a baby nearly always adds stress to the new family unit.

One way to identify how babies represent potential and ongoing stress for the young couple is to recognize how family interaction patterns are affected by the addition of a new member. The couple relationship is easy to understand. Each member of the couple relates to the other in a spousal relationship. Add one child and two new relationships are added: one linking mother to child and one linking father to child. In addition, the couple is now not only husband and wife but mother and father. In assuming these roles, each partner may view the other in new ways that are not always supportive of a continued spousal role (Majewski, 1986). When another child is added, the relationships become even more complex. Both the mother and the father have new relationships with the new baby. A sibling relationship also is added. Thus, in a two-person household, two relationships exist. In a three-person household, three relationships exist; in a four-person household, though only four people live in the house, six relationships exist (Fig. 3–1). With each new person added to the family, more than one new relationship is also added, because each person interacts with all other family members.

How families interact with health care workers in a hospital or clinic setting often is related to the structure of the family in its own environment. If the husband/father makes all decisions relating to the family's role with the outside world, it may not be surprising that when the woman is asked when she will register at the hospital, her husband

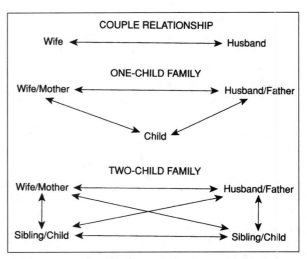

FIGURE 3-1. How family relationships change with the addition of a new member.

answers! This may not reflect the woman's dependency on her partner so much as the couple's established way of organizing their life. Likewise, if one were to ask the husband something that is the responsibility of the wife/mother, he would expect her to answer, for that is part of her role in their family.

The Effect of a Baby on a Family

People have babies for many reasons. For some, having a baby meets their desire to nurture. A baby links its parents to the future. Some seek to assert their adult status or their sexuality through parenthood. Parenting can fulfill cultural expectations, provide a sense of security regarding later life, or serve as an outlet for personal creativity.

Meeting a Desire to Nurture. Sometimes it is the young wife who is the first to state explicitly her need to nurture; sometimes it is her husband. Before agreeing to have a baby, some young couples adopt a kitten or a puppy, which serves as a kind of surrogate baby. In some couples, the decision to become pregnant may be tinged with a good deal of concern about a pet's feelings of rejection after the baby comes. Will the pet be jealous and, if so, what can the couple do to help it accept the baby? Health care workers who laugh at these concerns will be viewed as insensitive to genuine concerns about established relationships between owner and pet.

Linking Oneself to the Future.
Especially for men, a child becomes their tangible link to immortality. In families practicing patrilineage, a male heir is especially valued in order to pass on the family name. In an unpublished study that the author conducted in the mid-1980s, nearly three-fourths of young adults in their early twenties preferred a firstborn male to a firstborn female child. For at least 40 percent of these young adults, the desire for a female child did not predominate until the fourth child.

Asserting Adult Status Through Parenthood.
Many teenage parents view the ability to impregnate or to become pregnant as an indication of their adulthood. The product of that ability is not the primary concern during the pregnancy, when a great deal of attention is often paid to the expectant mother.

Fulfilling Cultural Expectations.
In some of her classic work, Margaret Mead describes cultures in which having a baby does not necessarily follow marriage; it may precede it. In many cases, in fact, having a baby as a result of casual sexual activity may enhance the young woman's "marriageability" (Mead, 1928). Certain cultural expectations, such as having a baby, promote an individual's establishment of a home apart from his or her parents. In different subcultures in the United States, once one has been married a certain number of years, one is expected to have children.

Asserting One's Sexuality.
In some cases, establishing oneself as an adult requires that one make clear one's adult sexual ability. Often this is linked to gaining adult status through parenthood, for one must be sexually active and prove one's sexual ability in order to impregnate or to become pregnant.

Seeking Security for Later Life.
In most postindustrial societies, children are no longer viewed as a kind of social security for the aged. However, this view is often maintained, especially among recent immigrant groups from developing countries in which government old-age security programs do not exist.

Serving as an Outlet for Personal Creativity.
Having a baby can be viewed as the ultimate expression of one's creativity. The degree of satisfaction that new parents feel when others exclaim over the beauty of their baby and its "perfection" is verification of their success in producing such a winning creation.

The desire to nurture is but one of many reasons that propel young couples and young single women into pregnancy and parenthood. The health care worker who assists these clients must be aware that the client's reasons for a pregnancy may not be the same as those the consultant might have chosen. In addition, the value of the baby may differ from the value of the pregnancy. All of these elements play a role in the new mother's decisions regarding how to feed her baby.

Family Theory

Numerous theories have been applied to understanding how families work, what influences them to work effectively, and how best to offer assistance when they don't. One approach that seems particularly appropriate to health care providers assisting young families is to recognize that they expand and contract at different times. Thus, over time, a given family is likely to experience a couple stage, an expansion stage, a stable stage, and a contracting stage.

Most families begin as *couples*. The *expansion* stage begins with the first pregnancy and continues until the birth of the last child. In some families, this stage may be very brief, the duration of one pregnancy only; in other families, it might last more than two decades as new infants are added to the family. The *stable* stage occurs when members are neither added nor taken away. This stage is followed by the *contracting* stage, which begins when the oldest child leaves home and continues until the only individuals remaining in the home are the original couple or their replacements in the family (if one or both of the original couple has remarried). However one views the family from a developmental perspective, the number of stages identified is not nearly as important as are the tasks expected of the family at different times in the life cycle.

The health care worker assisting breastfeeding mothers is most likely to interact with members of families during the expansion phase of the family's life cycle. It is important to recognize that varying tasks characterize this phase of the family, in order to identify how those tasks will influence decision making and behavior related to infant feeding and other aspects of the early mother-child relationship.

Fathers

Attachment to the Baby

Some investigators have emphasized the degree of similarity between mother-infant and father-infant behaviors in the attachment process in parents (Lamb, 1977) (Fig. 3–2). Classic among them is the observation of Greenberg and Morris (1974) that fathers present at the birth of the baby seemed to become more comfortable handling the baby sooner than did those who were not present. Additionally, these investigators described a sequence of touching remarkably similar to that engaged in by mothers. The fingertips are used first to make tentative contact with the extremities of the newborn; this is followed by a gradual movement of the hand until the entire palm is in contact with the baby's chest, face, or head.

Peterson, Mehl, and Leiderman (1979) found that the father who participated at the birth by providing support to the mother was more likely to feel attached to his child than if he was not present at the birth. The authors recommend prenatal education and structuring the birth environment to enhance father participation. Likewise, Bowen and Miller (1980) showed that being at the baby's birth was important to paternal attachment behavior; those fathers who were present looked and talked to their infants more than did fathers who did not attend the birth.

Fathers tend to progress from gazing to touching in the first 15 minutes after birth. Enthusiastic reactions to the neonate were more likely when the father was not anxious about the mother's condition (Tomlinson, Rothenberg & Carver, 1991). Jones (1981) reported that fathers who held their newborns within the first hour postpartum engaged in more nonverbal behavior with their one-month-

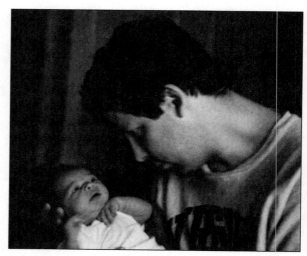

FIGURE 3-2. A father attaches to his baby in much the same way as does the mother.

old infants than did fathers who did not hold the baby soon after birth. Additionally, the fathers who were quick to hold their newborns seemed less put off by infant irritability, often providing more care during such periods than was observed in other fathers. When fathers enter into caregiving roles from the first with their infants, they are more likely to feel that they are an important part of the baby's life (Fein, 1976; Lamb, 1976). Investigators who have examined the male parenting role have noted that the "emergent" role of the participative father has begun to be emphasized with greater frequency as an appropriate role in all social classes (Fein, 1978).

Recent examinations of the ways in which men evolve into fathers suggests that the role remains relatively invisible to others; it is a passive reflection of what is happening to the pregnant wife until after the baby's birth. When the baby begins to interact with the father directly, the father's role becomes more explicit—in his own mind as well as in the awarenesses of others (Jordan, 1990; Jordan & Wall, 1993). In settings in which men are heavily involved in child care, as when the father provides daily care of his children for many hours while the mother works away from home, or when the father assumes a house-husband role, boys and girls tend to grow up with more flexible views of what is "man's work" and "woman's work"

(Robinson, 1979). The degree to which such flexibility is retained in the face of assumptions of stricter, more traditional gender-role behaviors as portrayed in children's literature, and reflected in the comments of others with whom the child interacts in school and elsewhere remains to be seen. According to Levine (1977), nurturing is a fundamental human quality that need not be gender-specific. That it is viewed as feminine by many must be seen as a cultural artifact rather than a reflection of inherent differences between males and females.

When a baby is born prematurely, the frequency of the father's visiting predicted later positive fathering behavior after the baby's discharge from the hospital (Levy-Shiff et al., 1990). When the fathers visited frequently, the baby's weight gain was more rapid, and the father's involvement with the baby at 8 and 18 months after birth was more intensive, regardless of the mother's visiting patterns during the period when the baby was in the premature care unit.

However, in one study of Australian fathers considered "highly participant" (Russell, 1982), fathers actually spent little time with their children. Kunst-Wilson and Cronenwett (1981) measured the amount of time fathers talked to their babies in the first three months and discovered that they did so fewer than three times per day, averaging only 37.5 seconds each time! Compared with the mothers, fathers spent very little time engaged in child-care tasks or in taking responsibility for children, nor were they simply available to their children in the same sense as were the mothers. Ironically, these same fathers placed a high value on sharing in caregiving and reported deriving satisfaction from their interactions with their children.

Breastfeeding

The role of the father as a supporter of breastfeeding is frequently mentioned in the lay literature. Particularly when he has a positive mind-set relating to breastfeeding, it is thought that he can play an important role (Littman et al., 1994). Discussions of infant feeding are most effective in allaying concerns and dispelling myths if they occur prenatally. In addition, informing a father of how he can help his breastfeeding wife without having to feed the baby is viewed as particularly helpful (Voss et al., 1993). Rustia and Abbott (1993) note, however, that the culture of fatherhood (including the expectations of others about how new fathers *will* respond) has changed more rapidly than the conduct of fathers (men's behaviors once they become fathers). These behaviors often evolve out of the observations of other fathers and their own experiences (Freed et al., 1992). If a previous baby was bottle-fed, the father is likely to harbor numerous misconceptions about breastfeeding that may interfere with his decision to support breastfeeding (Giugliani et al., 1994). His negative feelings about breastfeeding can also have a major effect (Lerner, 1979). Although the negative aspects of the father's role relative to breastfeeding are less recognized, Jordan (1986) and Jordan and Wall (1990) discuss the father's (potential) negative feelings. Breastfeeding is sometimes viewed as a means by which the mother denies the father access to the baby by making exclusive the early infant feeding experience (Jordan, 1986). Women's own fears about lack of support for breastfeeding by their partners may contribute to the misconceptions and negative attitudes that each has but does not express. Here, too, prenatal education and information sharing can dispel unvoiced misconceptions and promote breastfeeding as a healthful *family* activity (Freed, Fraley, & Schanler, 1993).

The early days of fathering can be as stressful and disruptive to the father as mothering is to the mother; it is not at all unusual for a father to become disenchanted with his marriage after the first baby's birth (Wandersman, 1980). Jealousy of the mother's and infant's physical and emotional closeness, feelings of uselessness during breastfeeding, sexual frustration, and repulsion from the sight of full, dripping breasts are all reported by some fathers (Hangsleben, 1983). Some fathers feel ashamed of these emotions and tend not to talk about them; or they may joke about being jealous of the new baby.

The most comfortable place for fathers to express these socially unacceptable but very real feelings is with other new fathers, many of whom may harbor the same feelings. Childbirth education classes and La Leche League groups often offer fathers-only classes, in which new fathers can openly share their feelings and perceptions about the realities of parenthood in an atmosphere of unconditional acceptance. Experienced fathers can help one another realize that they are not alone in having ambivalent feelings about the closeness between their breastfeeding wives and babies and about giving up certain pleasures in exchange for new responsibilities (Freed & Fraley, 1993). One such father reported (Riordan, 1983, p. 101):

If I'd been more prepared that they would be this complete unit unto themselves, it would have been easier. For a while I felt left out, like I was around only to bring home the money and wasn't a part of it. I felt bad, then guilty about feeling bad. Before the baby came, my wife really spoiled me, you know, really adored and lavished attention on me. Then, whammo, she was pregnant three months after we were married and I wasn't getting that kind of treatment anymore. I resented it. Things really broke loose and we had a showdown; I finally had to open up and let her know how I really felt. After that, when it was all in the open, things got better. With the next baby, I don't think I'll go through those feelings again.

Support groups for new fathers validate a commitment to recognize the needs of new fathers, to help them develop coping strategies for optimal parenting of their breastfed baby. These father groups tend to attract men who are having more difficulty or who are more open in admitting to feeling stressed by making adjustments. These actions can potentially strengthen family relationships in the years ahead (Taubenheim & Silbernagel, 1988).

Implicit in the notion that breastfeeding prevents father-child closeness is acceptance of the assumption that the most (perhaps the only) significant way in which a father can interact with his child is by feeding her or him. The health care worker can encourage the father to consider the many ways in which he can interact with the baby, particularly during the very early period when artificial feeding may increase the risk of breastfeeding failure (Fig. 3–3). Some of these options are:

- *Burping the baby after a feeding:* The necessity of burping is less an issue than is the opportunity to frequently hold the baby when the infant is

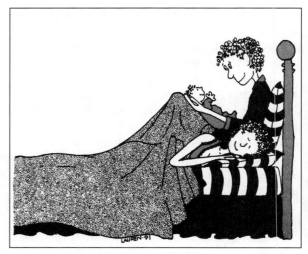

FIGURE 3-3. One of the many ways a dad helps with the care of his baby.

likely to be relaxed and somnolent; if a burp is obtained, the father also gains a sense of having accomplished something tangible that can be translated to mean, "I am a good father."

- *Changing the baby's wet diapers:* This activity occurs frequently.

- *Changing the baby's soiled diapers:* This, too, occurs frequently and, in breastfed infants, is far less unpleasant because the odor is less noxious than are the feces of an artificially fed baby.

- *Giving the baby a massage:* Fathers who massage their babies often find that they can put a baby to sleep with little effort; such activity can assist an overstimulated or colicky baby to relax sufficiently to fall asleep.

- *Bathing the baby:* Assisting with baby's bath is usually most happily accomplished after the baby begins to enjoy the bath.

- *Rocking the baby:* The father's involvement with the baby frees the mother to engage in other activities.

- *Singing or reading to the baby:* This activity can begin as soon after birth as the father wishes. Often, repeating the same songs that were played during the pregnancy will result in clear signals of recognition by the baby. The parents often view this recognition as a sign of their child's intelligence and receptivity to their efforts.

- *Playing with the baby:* Although the last item in this list, playing is usually the first thing that mothers will say fathers do best. Often, babies quickly identify fathers as "playthings" and mothers as "caregivers" because fathers spend far more time tickling or playing with an infant and less time in caregiving activity, such as changing, feeding, and cleaning. Such patterns are most likely to emerge in families in which clearly different gender roles are exhibited by mothers and fathers.

Levels of Family Functioning

To provide the most appropriate assistance for the young family, health care workers must be able to determine how well the family is functioning. In so doing, help can be planned and provided in such a way that the family moves from a less effective to a more effective level of self-care. Tapia (1986) has identified different levels of functioning and the behaviors characteristic of each level.

In Tapia's functioning hierarchy, families are not defined according to the age of the parent but rather according to the maturity of their social action. A family in which the parents are adolescents, for example, may function at any one of five levels identified by Tapia. In short, just as a family contains members of different ages and capabilities, each family functions at different levels. During stressful periods, a family that had previously functioned well may be so affected by stress factors that its ability to function is seriously impaired; this results in its characterization as an adolescent rather than an adult family. In cases of extreme stress, some previously functioning families become chaotic, thereby failing to meet any of its members' needs and threatening its own ability to survive as a unit.

Families at different levels of functioning require different levels of assistance from the health care worker (Tapia, 1986). In level 1, Infancy or Chaotic Family Functioning, members tend to live day to day without a future orientation. Outsiders are distrusted; rarely are community resources and services used, and the adult family members tend to be hostile or to resist offers of help. The parents tend to be immature and may be confused regarding their roles within the family. A family in its *infancy,* whose organization is chaotic, will need to view the health care provider as an active partner as it moves through the health care system. In some cases, this may mean that the nurse accompanies the pregnant mother through the corridors of a large hospital (much like a mother would lead her offspring) to ensure that the pregnant woman finds her way through what must surely seem like an impenetrable maze. In other cases, it may mean that the nurse or LC must sit through the client's labor and assist her each time she breastfeeds her newborn throughout her hospital stay. This role is like that of an older sibling who has been through the experience before and whose calm, reassuring presence is highly valued. Honest answers to questions are most helpful as the new family attempts to understand its experience.

In level 2, Childhood Family Functioning, the family members are more likely to trust themselves and others and to harbor hope for a better life. Although the parents may show some confusion about their respective roles, they are willing to work together to benefit the family unit, but dealing with change is difficult. Thus a family in its *childhood* needs somewhat less assistance. Instead, active teaching works well. If the baby needs to be diapered, the health care provider may need to demonstrate this procedure more than once while the new parents observe. The health care provider will then ask one of the parents to perform the task. When the new parent does so, assistance at each juncture in the procedure may be necessary.

At level 3, Adolescent Family Functioning, the family may experience more than the usual number of conflicts and problems. As a result, survival and physical needs may be met, but emotional conflicts can create difficulties. One parent may be functioning at an adult level to a greater degree than is the other parent. On the positive side, however, solutions to problems can be identified and there is usually a clear future orientation. The family that is moving through its own *adolescence* needs a helper who points out the family members' abilities to cope. In this case, the health care worker serves as an adult assistant to the family and allows the new parents to take care of their own baby, seeking help at their own pace. Something as simple as offering to teach the parents how to diaper their baby for the first time works well with this family.

With level 4, Adult Family Functioning, the family has fewer conflicts and problems and appears to be stable, healthy, and happy. Both physical and emotional needs are being met. Although there may be problems relating to certain developmental tasks, the members are both willing and able to seek assistance from others to resolve problems. The family that is functioning at an *adult* level views the health care providers with whom the members have contact as experts and as outside partners. These family members usually are adept at seeking information and are eager to engage in new activities on their own. They eagerly seek new knowledge even as they are practicing new skills. The new breastfeeding mother who is operating at the adult level is ready to take in additional information related to what she is doing. For example, if she remarks that she feels sleepy shortly after she puts the baby to her breast, an explanation that this is one of the normal effects of the milk let-down response (Mulford, 1990) can help her to understand that she is responding normally to breastfeeding.

Finally, at level 5, a *mature* family that is functioning optimally uses the health care worker only sporadically. When questions arise, the family member will seek information; however, the mother will not lean on the nurse or the lactation consultant and expect the consultant to make decisions.

Knowing where the family falls in this continuum of functioning assists the provider in determining how little or how much assistance the family needs. In situations where the needs of the family exceed the ability, time available, or skill level of the care provider, referral to other professionals may be the most appropriate action.

The Teenage Mother

Few situations are fraught with more difficulties than that in which a child has a child. The younger the mother when her first baby is born, the more likely she is to encounter problems that will impede her ability to care for herself or her baby.

Wherever young women are expected to complete a high school education before they embark on adult roles, such as marriage and raising children, the teenage mother is a visible reminder that society has failed to protect her from too early parenthood and that she has failed her society, which expects that parenthood comes after marriage and at least minimal schooling. For such young women, schooling may not be resumed or may be delayed for several years, and marriage—if it occurs—comes after, rather than before, the birth of her child. Subsequent pregnancies are likely to occur within two years of the first birth (Polit & Kahn, 1986).

Many caregivers assume that the young mother is neither interested in giving nor ready to give to another person by breastfeeding (Stotland & Peterson, 1985). As a result, the pregnant teen may not be encouraged to plan how she will feed her baby. What her older sister or friends have done is what she assumes she will do, and often they have bottle-fed their infants.

Yoos (1985) explored the infant-feeding choices of 50 teenage mothers. She found striking differences between those who chose bottle-feeding and those who chose breastfeeding. Bottle-feeders were more likely to live in an extended family setting (60 percent) rather than in a nuclear family headed by two adults of the opposite gender, as did the breastfeeders (41 percent). Even more striking were the reasons given for bottle-feeding, which the author described as "self-oriented" (79 percent); breastfeeding teens were much more likely to mention infant-oriented reasons (88 percent). Only among the bottle-feeders was breastfeeding equated with a sexual act and therefore found to be inappropriate between mother and infant. Yoos suggests that because adolescence is a period when self-centeredness is normal, it is difficult for the young woman to set aside concerns about herself in order to care for the needs of someone else. When parenthood impinges on adolescence, breastfeeding is a less likely choice because the mother has difficulty setting aside her own needs for her baby's.

The attitudes of teenage boys and girls reflect the attitudes of their elders as well as their peers. Pascoe and Berger (1985) compared high school girls' attitudes about breastfeeding in the United States and Israel and found that Israeli girls were more likely to plan to breastfeed when they had children (68 percent vs. 42 percent) than were their counterparts in the United States. Most of the Israeli girls were breastfed as infants, compared with only one-third of the U.S. teens. Neither group, however, had discussed breastfeeding with their teenage friends; in both groups, breastfeeding was considered less expensive than bottle-feeding, but it was also considered old-fashioned. These attitudes, combined with the lack of understanding of the physiology of lactation, support the contention that many teenage girls need information about breastfeeding before they can be expected to make an informed choice, even in the face of another family member's experience with breastfeeding.

Another study of U.S. high school students' attitudes about breastfeeding revealed that the greater their exposure to breastfeeding in the family or among friends, the more positive were these students' attitudes and the more knowledgeable were they about lactation. The students' age at the time of the survey also influenced how knowledgeable they were; students in grades 11 and 12 were more likely than those in grades 9 and 10 to have read or heard about breastfeeding in a course. The authors concluded that early introduction of breastfeeding in a classroom setting can stimulate later discussion and increase the knowledge base on which later decisions will be made (Cusson, 1985).

An Australian study (Wolinski, 1989) looked at teens' attitudes about breastfeeding. Most of these students had seen a close relative or friend breastfeed, knew that they had been breastfed, and had seen a sibling at the breast (63–80 percent). Nevertheless, 31 percent of the students felt that women did not breastfeed because it was inconvenient to do so, because they had no milk (25 percent), because it was painful (24 percent), or because it was embarrassing (18 percent). Almost all of the students, male and female, agreed that any infant, including their own future infants, should be breastfed at home, with only family or females present. More than 50 percent believed that it was inappropriate to breastfeed outside the home or when boys or men were present. This suggests that even in a society in which most infants are breastfed, privacy and modesty are concerns of teenage girls and boys.

Another study of teens in Liverpool, U.K., revealed that 75 percent of the students thought breastfeeding was healthier than bottle-feeding, but 8 percent perceived it as "rude" (Gregg, 1989). Both boys and girls felt that breastfeeding should be done in private, either alone or with just the baby's father or a female family member present. Almost none of these teens felt that breastfeeding should occur outside the mother's home. Students who had been breastfed themselves or who had seen a baby breastfeed were more likely to say that they intended for their child to be breastfed. The investigator recommended discussing breastfeeding as soon as possible to reduce the likelihood that it would be viewed as an embarrassing behavior and to "modify society's acceptance of the breast as a purely sexual organ," another factor very likely to have influenced the students' preference that breastfeeding occur only in the mother's home (Gregg, 1989).

A more recent study involving high school and college-age students also found that "embarrassment" was a major barrier to breastfeeding, again inferring that it should be considered a private behavior. Also important was the students' reported sources of breastfeeding information: from home, school, and television (Forrester et al., 1997).

Teen mothers, when asked to identify their needs after the birth of their baby, identified the infant's medical needs first, followed by daily physical care of the infant, psychosocial needs of mothers and babies and, finally, the mother's physical care (Howard & Sater, 1985). Mothers rated information about how to breastfeed and care for the breasts as important or very important. This high level of interest in meeting their baby's needs suggests that teen mothers are likely to be motivated to follow advice when it is offered. However, because many teenage mothers often share social characteristics that are linked with the choice not to breastfeed—such as lower educational attainment, low income, and unmarried status—fewer of these young women will choose to breastfeed (Peterson & Da Vanzo, 1992).

In this author's experience of working with teens who have become mothers, the teens' questions were no different from those of older, more experienced women. Most new mothers are concerned about how to help a baby grasp the breast, how to avoid sore nipples, and how to provide sufficient milk. In contrast, the kind of assistance offered to teens depends on their life situation. The teen mother living alone may need more assistance and referral to a breastfeeding support group in her local community. The teen mother living with her own mother, who may be caring for the baby while the teen is in school, may need to know about resources on which she can draw for additional information and support about breastfeeding. The teen mother living with the baby's father or another male adult needs to know how to balance her baby's needs and other people's plans for her. For example, if her friends want her to go to a school dance, she needs help in recognizing that the baby cannot be abandoned until she returns. A happy breastfeeding experience, of whatever duration, helps the young mother to progress toward adulthood with a stronger and more positive sense of self and of what she wants for her children in the future.

The Low-Income Family

Families in an affluent society are expected to reflect the wealth of that society. When families are not affluent, they are confronted with daily reminders that they have failed to live up to the expectations of others. This is especially true in developed countries with a strong work ethic in which any degree of underemployment or unemployment may be interpreted as personal failure or refusal to accept a basic tenet of that society. Children may not always know they are poor unless this is pointed out. Too often, however, particularly in urban neighborhoods located near affluent areas, the comparison of the "haves" and the "have nots" is overt and never-ending.

The cost of feeding an infant artificially is often invisible—both to mothers, who must buy the substitutes, and to governments, which may provide the food. In part, this cost derives from lack of inclusion of mother's milk as a food source for babies. Although the 1973 World Food Conference proposed that human milk should be included in food-production statistics, this has not occurred. Oshaug and Botten (1994, p. 481) note that "human milk is a substantial resource not only in food terms but also in economic terms." They estimated that the total value of human milk production (calculated by examining studies on breast-milk production during that year for all babies who

were breastfed) in Norway in 1992 was more than $400 million (U.S.). Were human milk to be considered in food production statistics, its value–and, conversely, the costs of artificial milk products– would suddenly be made visible to the public in a way that could not be ignored.

The relative costs of infant feeding choices is important because the cost in health care dollars required to restore infants to health after illnesses related to artificial feeding and the cost to provide a more expensive, if inferior, food substitute for human milk, is more than many families and nations can afford. In the United States and other developed countries, fewer low-income mothers than their more affluent countrywomen choose to breastfeed (Lowe, 1993). Poor women whose babies most need the benefits of human milk, including its far lower production cost and its marked safety as compared to artificial baby milk, are least likely to breastfeed. As more women in the developing world seek to emulate women in the developed world, the cost to these women and the countries in which they live will be even higher.

Obstacles to Breastfeeding Among Low-Income Families

Background variables can predict whether a low-income woman will breastfeed. Grossman et al. (1989) found that if a poor woman was married, if she had at least a high school education, if she began prenatal care in the first trimester, and if she was white or Hispanic, she was more likely to breastfeed than if she had less than a high school education, if she began prenatal care in the second or third trimester, and if she was black. Libbus and Kolostov (1994) report that if the maternal grandmother breastfed and if the male partner endorsed breastfeeding, the low-income women in their study were more likely to intend to breastfeed and to view it as a positive experience.

Lack of Support. The availability of an outside source of support in the first six weeks postpartum nearly doubled the mean breastfeeding duration in a group of low-income women (Barron et al., 1988). In addition, the more breastfeeding friends the mother had, the longer was she likely to breastfeed ($p < .05$). The involvement of WIC in promoting breastfeeding among their low-income clients has been discussed with increasing frequency, because funds within the WIC allotment have been specifically earmarked for breastfeeding promotion. Kramer's discussion (1991) highlights the need for continuing work, particularly in the area of prenatal information and early postpartum support and assistance. He notes that too many WIC programs continue to accept and distribute materials from the infant-formula companies. Training WIC personnel in how to assist breastfeeding women also may render this supplemental food program more effective in increasing the breastfeeding rate among the nation's low-income families.

Support from family members also makes a difference, according to Scrimshaw et al. (1987). In her study of more than 500 Mexican-American women in the Los Angeles area, she found that the influence of the mother's own mother, her husband, and other relatives or friends was much more important than that of doctors or nurses with whom they came into contact. In addition, rooming-in opportunities influenced breastfeeding behavior, presumably through an increase in the number of hours per day in which mother and baby were housed together (see Table 3–1).

Support of a woman's decision to breastfeed by important members of the mother's support system (Rassin et al., 1986) may help to explain the strong influence of ethnicity on infant-feeding choice. Additionally, the assumption by health care workers that only certain women (e.g., white, middle-class, well-educated, first-time mothers) are interested in breastfeeding effectively shuts the door on future opportunities to reach women for whom breastfeeding could be a deliberate choice, if only they knew it existed as an option for them (Manstead et al., 1984). Williams and Pan (1994) found that discussion of infant feeding with a physician who was supportive of breastfeeding was more likely to lead low-income African-American, Anglo-American, Asian-American, and Latina women to breastfeed.

Related to social support is the mother's own perception of the importance of breastfeeding. Through a series of in-depth interviews, Locklin (1995) found that the perception of having succeeded at something–in this case, breastfeeding–

empowered her sample of low-income women of color to view themselves more positively.

Lack of Information. Sometimes the reasons for not breastfeeding are related to lack of information. Kistin et al. (1990) studied low-income black women in the United States and found that prenatal education sessions that included far-ranging discussions about breastfeeding not only increased the likelihood that the women would choose to breastfeed but also the likelihood that they would act on their choice when the baby was born. These sessions also positively influenced the duration of breastfeeding. The investigators concluded that "greater educational efforts in institutions and offices serving black, low-income, urban women might yield significant changes in breastfeeding rates" (Kistin et al., 1990).

In Hill's study (1988), attendance at classes designed to inform low-income mothers about breastfeeding significantly increased the likelihood that these women would choose breastfeeding, if they attended two or more classes. Recognizing the benefits of breastfeeding and acknowledging a desire to breastfeed may come only after being informed of the differences between artificial feeding and human milk feeding. Therefore, simply adding to childbirth-preparation classes a session on infant feeding or offering a one-time-only class on breastfeeding may be insufficient to break down the barriers protecting the passive bottle-feeding choice so that breastfeeding can be considered and then implemented.

Long et al. (1995) reported that in their Native American WIC population in Utah, initiation of breastfeeding (84 percent versus 70 percent) was more likely when contact with a peer counselor was part of the ongoing services available to their clientele. In addition, continuation of breastfeeding was more likely among those women seeing a peer counselor for the first three months postpartum.

Brent et al. (1995) found that prenatal and postpartum instruction from a lactation consultant also made a difference. In their study, not only did more low-income women begin breastfeeding (61 percent, as compared to 32 percent in the control group not seen by the lactation consultant), but they breastfed longer (median 84 versus 33 days; $p < .005$).

Table 3–1

RACE OR ETHNIC GROUP AND WHOSE ADVICE THE MOTHER CONSIDERS IMPORTANT

Ethnic Group	Influential Person Regarding Breastfeeding
Anglo-American	Male partner, baby's father Grandmother (maternal and paternal) Mother's best friend
Mexican-American	Male partner, baby's father Grandmother (maternal and paternal)
Black American	Peers Maternal grandmother

Source: Derived from T Baranowski et al: Social support, social influence, ethnicity and the breastfeeding decision. Soc Sci Med 17:1599–1611, 1983; Cronenwett & Reinhardt: Support and breastfeeding: a review. Birth 14:199–203, 1987.

Hospital Practices. Sometimes, the reasons for choosing not to breastfeed are related to hospital factors. In Brazil, if the baby of a low-income mother received the breast first, that child was more likely to continue to breastfeed past six months. However, if something other than the breast was offered in the hospital, the mother was less likely to nurse as long. Often, the first feeding in the hospital was followed later by supplementary water feedings, which reduced the duration of breastfeeding. It takes but a small leap of the imagination to understand why so many of the women who breastfed for short periods thought they had inadequate milk before their babies were four months old (Martines, Ashworth, & Kirkwood, 1989).

The only variable that predicted shortened duration of breastfeeding among Romero-Gwynn's (1989) sample of Cambodian and Laotian immigrants was the use of formula giveaways in the hospital where the birth occurred. These women viewed such products as high-status items because of their extreme high cost and lack of availability in their home country. Their explanation of "insufficient milk" may simply have been a convenient hook–easily accepted without question by others–on which to hang their decision not to breastfeed, even though they had successfully breastfed older children prior to their emigration to the United States.

Perez-Escamilla et al. (1992) found that rooming-in positively affected breastfeeding duration among primiparas (but not multiparas) in her sample of low-income urban Mexican women. Additionally, those women who were rooming-in and who received breastfeeding guidance during the hospital stay also breastfed longer than those women who did not room-in and/or who did not receive additional assistance before they went home.

Hospital-Based Formula Marketing. The use of formula in the hospital has also been found to reduce the duration of breastfeeding (Samuels, Margen, & Schoen, 1985). In this study, mothers in three different ethnic groups received care from a health maintenance organization (HMO). Formula use at that time was the single largest avoidable impediment to breastfeeding and appeared to have both a direct effect on very early weaning in the first four weeks as well as an increasingly cumulative effect through the first two months postpartum.

Scrimshaw et al. (1987; see also Snell et al., 1992; and Wright, Rice, & Wells, 1996) found that the use of hospital formula negatively affected the duration of breastfeeding among Hispanic women in Los Angeles. Only one ounce of formula per day contributed to early weaning, even in the face of long duration of breastfeeding in which the baby spent most of his or her time with the mother and she received both verbal and direct assistance to begin breastfeeding soon after birth. This finding may highlight the "valued" nature of formula feeding, particularly when this practice is introduced by authority figures in a hospital, in which the mother feels that she must emulate nurses' practices and follow doctors' recommendations.

Timing of Solid Food Introduction. In addition to formula use, the timing of solid food introduction also influences the duration of breastfeeding. In their low-income population, Hawkins, Nichols, and Tanner (1987) reported that the introduction of solid foods explained 32 percent of the variance in the duration of breastfeeding. Of interest in their sample were the additional findings that among short-term breastfeeders (4 weeks or less) and moderate breastfeeders (5–24 weeks), inadequate milk supply or the baby's poor weight gain were cited in 50 percent and 37 percent of cases respectively, to explain weaning the baby. All of the short-term breastfeeders and nearly one-half of the moderate breastfeeders claimed that inadequate milk supply was a problem. What we do not know is how the timing of the introduction of solids related to an awareness of this problem or to the decision to terminate breastfeeding. Might the problem have been secondary to early solid feedings and subsequent reduced breastfeeding frequency, or might the solids have been introduced in an effort to counter an inadequate milk supply that was reflected in poor infant weight gain?

High-income and low-income breastfeeding and bottle-feeding women are more similar when one compares them according to feeding choice rather than income status. Grossman et al. (1990a) found that breastfeeding women, whatever their income, were more like one another than were the low-income breastfeeding women and their bottle-feeding counterparts, particularly with regard to such variables as where they obtained support for their infant-feeding choice, when they began prenatal care, when they decided to breastfeed, whether they had attempted to breastfeed a previous infant, and whether they viewed positively their previous breastfeeding experience. The same concerns are likely to affect all women, regardless of income; therefore, it is inappropriate to assume, simply on the basis of presumed maternal finances or social

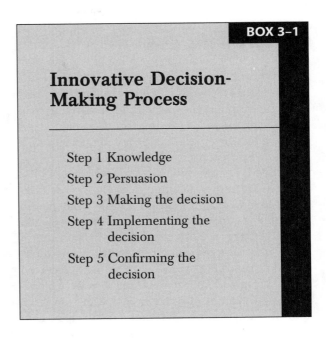

BOX 3–1

Innovative Decision-Making Process

Step 1 Knowledge

Step 2 Persuasion

Step 3 Making the decision

Step 4 Implementing the decision

Step 5 Confirming the decision

status, that a mother will not be interested in learning about, and later practicing, breastfeeding.

Sullivan and Jones (1986) present an innovation-decision-making process model to explain why some low-income women choose to breastfeed and why others do not (see the five-step checklist in Box 3–1).

In this model, knowledge is an important first step to the innovative behavior. Before breastfeeding is likely to be chosen, the mother needs information on which to base her decision. Such knowledge is followed by persuasion, often in the form of discussions, video materials about breastfeeding that show other women engaged in breastfeeding, and the experiences of other women, including friends and family members. Making the decision to breastfeed follows persuasion, and implementing the decision occurs after the baby's birth. Postdelivery support of a mother's decision to breastfeed leads to confirmation that hers was the right decision for her. When confirmation does not occur, or other factors interfere with the opportunity to have her decision confirmed, the mother is likely to stop nursing. In their study sample, Sullivan and Jones found that maternal or infant complications that interfered with the opportunity to put breastfeeding into practice soon after delivery occurred in the confirmation process and contributed to the decision making in a majority of those who later chose to bottle-feed.

Confirming a mother's choice is another way of providing her with positive feedback. Low-income Hispanic women who were part of a WIC program responded positively to a hospital visit, phone call, letter, or group support at two weeks postpartum: they breastfed longer compared with a group who received no such confirmation of breastfeeding (Saunders & Carroll, 1988). Differences in breastfeeding rates were most striking at four weeks postpartum: Of the women who had all four interventions, 95 percent were still breastfeeding, as compared with 80 percent of those who received some but not all of the interventions, and 70 percent of those who received none. Early and repeated postpartum breastfeeding support can be effective in increasing the duration of breastfeeding. Repeated contact may help to explain why other studies involving only one contact—in the hospital (Lynch et al., 1986) or after the mother and baby go home (Grossman et al., 1990b)—have not shown similar positive results.

The Down Side of Family Experiences

Not all families meander into the sunset "happily ever after." When a marriage dies, the death of that relationship affects not only the spouses but also any children they may have as well as other relatives and friends. When the mother is breastfeeding, issues surrounding custody may be colored by the fact that she feels (rightly or wrongly) that the court should take her feeding method into consideration in deciding on custody arrangements and contacts of her children with her soon-to-be former husband.

The role of the lactation consultant in such a situation must necessarily be limited to advocacy for breastfeeding. Unless the LC is an attorney, points of law are not her concern. Instead, she can perform a valuable service by educating the judge and the mother's (and perhaps the father's) attorney about the importance of breastfeeding for the child's continued physical and psychological health (Baldwin & Friedman, 1993; Smith, 1991; Suhler, Bornmann, & Scott, 1991). Questions may surface pertaining to how the father's attachment to the child is enhanced when breastfeeding is protected.

Questions relating to the frequency of breastfeeding may not arise. In most cases, if the child is older than a few months, short periods of time with the father (away from the mother) are unlikely to place the breastfeeding relationship at risk. In addition, maintaining the child's attachment with both parents requires that child and parent be together often (as much as possible), as they would have been if the marriage and joint parenting experience had remained intact.

When the mother is seeking to maintain breastfeeding beyond the time when most people in her society—including the judge and the attorneys—are likely to find it acceptable, the lactation consultant can provide information that again focuses on the health-preserving aspects of breastfeeding (Wilson-Clay, 1990). Such longer-term breastfeeding does not necessarily limit reasonable visitation periods with the noncustodial parent, nor does it prevent periods of separation of the child from the mother. It does place the issue squarely where it must remain: preserving the best interests of the child. Summarized in Box 3–2 are guidelines for appearing in court if asked to testify in a case in which custody includes consideration of the ongoing breastfeeding relationship.

The lactation consultant may become involved if a woman wishes to breastfeed or is breastfeeding and living in a situation in which she or her children are being threatened or assaulted. Whenever the lactation consultant believes that such violence is occurring, she has a responsibility to report this to relevant authorities who are in a position to intervene and to provide a safe haven for the mother and her children if she chooses to use it. Assisting with breastfeeding in abusive households need not be any different from assisting any other woman, although sensitivity to the abuse situation is necessary. In one case, the author had to resort to sitting on the floor by an abused woman's hospital bed so that she could make eye contact. The severity and duration of the abuse that this woman had suffered was such that she could not communicate with anyone who assumed a position of authority over her (Simkin, 1992). Only when the other party was physically inferior to (or smaller than) her did she feel safe enough to interact.

The number of breastfeeding women who are in homes in which they are being abused is not known. Acheson (1995) reported that lack of breast-feeding was associated with physical and sexual abuse of the woman or her children or both. In her retrospective review of 800 pregnancies and births in one family practice, Acheson noted that postpartum depression occurred more frequently in the absence of breastfeeding, as did marital problems and domestic violence. The author suggested that the striking 38-fold decrease in frequency of violence against women or their children (or both) when breastfeeding is practiced warrants careful scrutiny. One must ask the question: what is it about the decision to breastfeed, or its practice, that is related to nonviolent households? In other words, is the social dynamic in families in which violence occurs such that breastfeeding is also unlikely and, if so, what factors compose that social dynamic?

A history of childhood abuse, including sexual abuse, is likely to result in a variety of reactions to the breastfeeding experience that may present the lactation consultant with unique challenges. For example, if a mother wishes to breastfeed but cannot bring herself to allow the baby to latch onto the breast, and if issues such as breast tenderness are not immediately evident, the consultant must consider the possibility that the breast area was involved in the sexual abuse that the mother may have suffered years earlier. In many such instances, expressing milk (sometimes for many months) may be the most comfortable way for the mother to provide her milk to her baby while protecting herself from what she perceives emotionally (consciously or unconsciously) as an assault on her person.

The incidence of child abuse worldwide is unknown. Depending on one's definition and the country in which such statistics are extrapolated from reported cases, ratios such as 1:3 to 1:5 for girls and 1:8 to 1:10 for boys have been cited (Finkelhor, 1994; Gorey & Leslie, 1997). Given such a high incidence of abuse, beliefs surrounding the breasts' function and emotions pertaining to these beliefs are very likely to include fears that stem from experiences outside the realm of most lactation consultants' field of expertise.

Sexual abuse can have both short-term and long-term effects on the victim. Those effects may be expressed in various ways, including symptoms of posttraumatic stress disorder, cognitive distortions, emotional distress, impaired sense of self,

interpersonal difficulties, health problems, and numerous kinds of avoidance behavior (including amnesia for the abuse-related events, dissociation, and self-destructive behaviors such as drug abuse). Sometimes pregnancy (Grant, 1992), childbirth (Courtois & Riley, 1992; Kitzinger, 1992; Rose, 1992), or breastfeeding can trigger recall that has previously been suppressed. Coping mechanisms will vary from one woman to the next and may or may not be manifested during pregnancy, childbirth, or breastfeeding (K. Kendall-Tackett, personal communication, 1997).

When she has established rapport with the lactation consultant and feels safe, the mother may admit that she has been a victim of childhood abuse. In many cases, however, she may be unaware of the reason for her extreme discomfort, owing to brain changes that occur as a result of abuse and the coping mechanisms, including amnesia relating to the abusive events, that she may have practiced for years in order to maintain a facade of normalcy (Mukerjee, 1995). In addition, if the mother recalls the abuse, she may or may not view it as being connected in any way with her current situation, including difficulties she may be having with breastfeeding.

If breastfeeding triggers sudden recall, nurturing her baby in this manner may be extremely frightening to her. The mother may fear her own actions relating to her baby. One mother with whom the author worked said she had no recall of being abused until she put her baby to her breast for the first time. This action triggered a flashback so frightening to her that she screamed and immediately dropped the baby onto her bed. By the time hospital staff reached her, she was weeping and begged them to take the baby to the nursery. When she was discharged, her husband had no idea why she cried uncontrollably each time she attempted to put her baby to her breast. This woman desperately wanted to breastfeed, but she feared that she would hurt the baby if he "bit" her, and his wide gape when approaching the breast made her want to "run for cover," as she put it. The staff began helping her by giving her permission to pump her breasts to give her baby her milk. This action was something she could completely control. Being able to determine the degree of suction the pump exerted was important to her. After a week of

Suggestions for Testifying at a Deposition or at Trial

In most cases, the role of the lactation consultant will be limited to providing testimony pertaining to the breastfeeding process and the value of human milk as a primary (or sole) nutriment for the baby. It is unwise to make comments about the merits of the case. That is not your job; more importantly, you may not have all the facts relating to the case. Thus any such statements you might choose to make could reduce your credibility as a breastfeeding expert.

You may be asked to serve as an expert witness for one party or as a friend of the court. Whatever the terms under which you have been asked to testify, talk about what you know. Leave the rest of the case alone.

APPEARANCE AND DEMEANOR ARE IMPORTANT

- Face the jury when responding to questions. How you testify is as important as what you say. You want the judge, counsel, and jury to remember the testimony, not your nervous tics.
- Respond politely and respectfully to the questions and the questioner, in keeping with customary courtroom formality. Avoid jargon, street language, or slang. Words that are not understood will alienate the listeners. Remain calm if you are asked questions designed to anger or fluster you. If you maintain equanimity under fire, you will impress the jurors and gain credibility for your statements. Avoid making jokes; humor can be misunderstood.
- Dress to inform the court that you are a professional; avoid short skirts, work clothes, and gaudy jewelry.

DO'S AND DON'TS WHEN RESPONDING TO QUESTIONS

Do . . .
- Provide background information succinctly. This may include your address, number of years that you have been in practice, and the like.
- Answer all questions honestly, completely, and accurately. If you do not remember something, say so. If you are dishonest, the jury will sense it.
- Answer questions dispassionately. Do not debate the issues. Simply present the facts about lactation and breastfeeding as you know them.
- Answer only those questions asked of you. Avoid anticipating other questions or digressing into areas not called for by the question. Do not give unsolicited opinions.
- If you are asked to estimate something (such as how long each episode of breastfeeding is likely to take, or how often most babies breastfeed), answer as accurately as you can but ensure that the persons hearing your answer understand that you are providing an estimate only.
- Wait until the entire question has been asked before attempting to answer. Pause briefly before doing so. This will allow counsel to make an objection.
- Ask the judge for permission to provide an explanation (if an explanation is required) before answering a yes-no question.
- Answer each part of a compound question separately. Sometimes a compound question will be asked to confuse you. It is always appropriate to ask counsel to rephrase a question if you do not

understand what has been asked or if it is not possible for you to respond to the question as it was originally asked.
- Confine your answers to what you know, what you did, or what you observed. Avoid hearsay answers. Do not volunteer what others have told you unless you are asked to do so.
- If you are interrupted, stop, collect yourself, and complete your answer to the first question. After doing so, ask that the next question, which had interrupted your previous answer, be repeated.

Do not . . .
- Answer a question with a question. If you have a question, direct it to the judge.
- Guess. If you do not recall something, say so.
- Place your stamp of approval on what you have said in words that are not your own. If counsel paraphrases what you have said and the paraphrase is not accurate, say so.

Source: Derived from information provided by Priscilla G. Bornmann, JD, McKinley & Bornmann, PLC, Alexandria, VA.

pumping, during which time she gradually increased the pump pressure, she was willing to "try the baby again." She began with occasional feedings and gradually was able to tolerate frequent, cue-based feedings without fearing that she would harm her baby.

Acceptance of each woman's decision to breastfeed—however that is defined at a given time—may enable her to move closer to a full breastfeeding relationship with her baby and to further cement a healthy ongoing relationship with all of her children, something she may not have enjoyed in her family of origin.

The Importance of Peer Counselors

In their population of low-income women, most of whom were African-American or Hispanic, Kistin et al. (1994) found that contact with a peer counselor was positively related to breastfeeding initiation, duration, and exclusivity. Specifically, 93 percent of those intending to breastfeed who had contact with the peer counselor actually began breastfeeding, as compared with only 70 percent of the group who had intended to breastfeed but who did not see a peer counselor prenatally. In addition, 77 percent (versus 40 percent) of those with peer counselor contact and support were exclusively breastfeeding at the time of hospital discharge, and

44 percent (versus 16 percent) were still doing so at 6 weeks postpartum. In addition, among the first group, mean duration of breastfeeding was nearly twice as long (15 weeks versus 8 weeks). This study makes clear that intention to breastfeed may be insufficient to sustain women in low-income circumstances unless they also have identified someone who is knowledgeable about breastfeeding and available to offer them support and encouragement. The empowerment gained from the breastfeeding experience, as discussed by Locklin and Naber (1993), may be an overlooked secondary effect of breastfeeding that has potentially long-term impacts on other aspects of these women's lives.

Sciacca et al. (1995) included incentives as well as contact with a peer role model in their study and found that the rate of exclusive breastfeeding at hospital discharge (88.5 percent versus 55.2 percent), 2 weeks (80.8 percent versus 34.5 percent), 6 weeks (50 percent versus 24.1 percent), and 3 months postpartum (42.3 percent versus 17.2 percent) was significantly higher when the mothers had peer role modeling and received a variety of incentives to choose to breastfeed and to continue doing so. The authors concluded that educational interventions prenatally and postpartum effectively promoted breastfeeding, particularly when both the women and their male partners were involved.

Social Support

As is true of peer counselors, the role of supportive significant others in the breastfeeding mother's life cannot be overemphasized. Freedom of choice regarding infant-feeding decisions is always couched within the social context in which it occurs. Thus, in a family in which extended breastfeeding is viewed as aberrant behavior, it is unlikely that the mother will choose to continue breastfeeding unless she receives a preponderance of positive, or at least neutral, reactions from her significant others. In another family in which breastfeeding is viewed as just another activity of two- or three-year-olds, extended breastfeeding is far more likely to occur. Insofar as the mother and her baby interact with significant others, these people's acceptance of such breastfeeding behavior must be taken into account when assessing how best to assist her.

Woollett (1987) and Kessler et al. (1995) note that most women choose to breastfeed or not to breastfeed and that support systems, real or perceived, influence those choices. In their study, Kaufman and Hall (1989) found that women who gave birth to preterm babies and who identified no source of support were six times more likely to stop breastfeeding than were women with a support system. Those most likely to continue breastfeeding could identify several persons who supported their feeding decision. As with mothers of preterm infants, teenage mothers also tend to breastfeed longer when they have a support system whose members affirm, aid, and affect in specific practical ways their mothering behavior, including breastfeeding (Dormire, Strauss, & Clark 1989).

Social support also influences the timing of weaning the baby from the breast. Usually pressure to wean, from family members and others, is more likely as the baby approaches or exceeds his or her twelfth month (Rogers, Morris, & Taper, 1987). Morse and Harrison (1987) suggest that others' support moves gradually from actively supporting breastfeeding (often manifested in the first few months of the baby's life), to tolerating breastfeeding, to ignoring breastfeeding (sometimes interpreted as passive support for breastfeeding insofar as no negative statements are heard or negative action is taken), to actively encouraging weaning. This last stage usually is manifested sometime after the baby's sixth month and may grow markedly stronger after the baby's twelfth month in the developed world, when others view the baby as too old to breastfeed. Among Hong Kong families, bottle-feeders received support from their physicians, failed breastfeeders received no support for breastfeeding and were influenced by advertisements to use formula, and breastfeeders reported receiving a preponderance of support for breastfeeding. In addition, the successful breastfeeders were more aware of the risks of bottle-feeding than were the other groups (Hung, Ling, & Ong, 1985).

Social support is especially important in the period immediately following any life stress. One such stress, insofar as it necessitates changes in relationships and life patterns, is childbirth. Another is breastfeeding, particularly if the mother has not breastfed an older child or if she is the first in her family or group of friends to do so. Very often, mothers and others assume that the mode of feeding is the cause of other infant behaviors (Forsyth, Leventhal, & McCarthy, 1985). If mothers receive advice that is inappropriate or that is based on faulty or incorrect assumptions (Anlar, Anlar, & Tonyali, 1988; Auerbach, 1990a), subsequent breastfeeding difficulty and even unnecessary weaning is more likely. In a group of working-class, first-time mothers, breastfeeding was more likely to occur, and to remain the only feeding method for the baby's first three months, when the mothers received support and information before, during, and after the baby's birth (Jenner, 1988). However, in a group of disadvantaged American mothers, McLorg and Bryant (1989) found that the advice of health care workers was far less likely to be followed than was that of grandmothers, many of whom lived in the same house with the new mother. These researchers recommended that health care workers recognize the grandmother as a key informant and network person and involve her in health care and advice giving.

It is unfortunate when health care workers are not viewed as support resources. In one article, the author (1979) reiterates how nurses in five different but related roles can assist the breastfeeding mother, providing her both information and specific assistance at various points in her childbearing and child-rearing career. Such assistance can help the mother to feel that she is not going it alone but rather has a wealth of assistance that she can tap should the need arise.

The racial or ethnic group with which the mother identifies influences whom she seeks out for advice and assistance relating to childbearing and breastfeeding. Baranowski et al. (1983) found that those who are supportive of breastfeeding vary by ethnic group. For example, among their low-income Anglo-American sample, the male partner, the mother's own mother, the grandmother, and the best friend all supported breastfeeding. This pattern, with the exception of the best friend, was found among Mexican-Americans as well. However, among African-American respondents, fewer than half of these potential support individuals was found to be supportive of breastfeeding. Additionally, the percentage of individuals who were clearly not supportive was higher; this was particularly true of the best friend, who might have served as a role model for the mother if she were among the first in her group of friends to have a baby and to choose a method of infant feeding for the child (Table 3–1).

In another study of WIC clients, Saunders and Carroll (1988) found that the more support the mother had for breastfeeding, the more likely she was to continue breastfeeding. They recommended that health care workers make clear their support of breastfeeding and encourage other family members to support this choice as well. Pridham (1987) found that books, friends, and relatives were more likely to be cited as support resources than were clinicians in the first three months of breastfeeding. Perhaps these mothers were looking to books as objective sources of information rather than advice, which they freely received from friends and relatives, often more frequently than through visits to the health care worker.

After early discharge from the hospital, the degree of support that new mothers have at home is critical. It is imperative that the health care provider learn whether the new mother will have someone to whom she can turn once she is at home. If she does not, steps need to be taken to provide follow-up support or to arrange for home visitation by one of the many social-service organizations that provide such assistance. In addition, much of the teaching that is viewed as appropriate during the postpartum period may have to be shifted to a prenatal setting in order to free what little time is available at discharge for key planning issues. (See Chapter 9 for additional discussion of teaching elements that should be addressed at hospital discharge.)

How men support women varies. Reversion to traditional gender-roles is more likely shortly after the birth of a baby, when the infant's and mother's individual and related physical needs may require that she depend more on her partner than she has previously (Pleck, 1977). How the new family restructures its life to take into account previous patterns of behavior and newly recognized needs, short-term as well as long-term, will determine how readily the family, as a unit, continues to function effectively (Box 3–3).

Breastfeeding Promotion

Advocacy and Counseling

Breastfeeding promotion can take several forms. For some people, it means the statements of support for breastfeeding by leaders in the health care community: the American Academy of Pediatrics (AAP, 1982; AAP, 1997; AAP Committee on Nutrition, 1980; American Dietetic Association (ADA, 1986); Canadian Dietetic Association (CDA, 1989); International Pediatric Association (IPA, 1976); United States Public Health Service (Arango, 1984); the International Lactation Consultant Association (ILCA, 1991); and the American College of Nurse-Midwives (ACNM, 1993). But words are cheap: actions count. Breastfeeding promotion can be viewed as one leg of a three-legged stool; without the other two legs–support and protection–promotion will not succeed (Auerbach, 1990b). The implications of this analogy are clear: breastfeeding promotion is more complex than simply putting up posters, wearing buttons that identify the wearer as supportive of breastfeeding, or eliminating advertising copy for artificial baby milk.

Advocacy requires knowledge of the goals of the client for whom one provides active support. Being an advocate, then, necessitates that the caregiving professional be willing to stick her neck out. Assuming the posture of an ostrich with its head in

BOX 3–3

Variables That Influence Mothers' Decisions to Initiate and to Continue Breastfeeding

VARIABLES OVER WHICH HEALTH CARE PROVIDERS HAVE NO INFLUENCE OR CONTROL

Race of the mother or family	Balcazar et al., 1995
Social class or status	Sciacca et al., 1995
	Baranowski et al., 1983
Level of maternal education	Nolan & Goel, 1995
Mother's attendance at prenatal class	Kistin et al., 1990
	Wiles, 1984
Mother's marital status	Peterson & Da Vanzo, 1992
Mother's parity	O'Campo, 1992
Mother's plan to return to work or school	O'Campo, 1992
Mother's age	Peterson & Da Vanzo, 1992
Mother's sources of information (prenatally) about infant feeding	Sciacca et al., 1995
	Pugin et al., 1996
Mother's smoking status	Hill & Aldag, 1996
Health of mother during pregnancy, birthing, postpartum period	Dillon & Totten, 1989
Gender of the baby	Crowell et al., 1994
Health of baby at birth	Novotny et al., 1994
Previous breastfeeding experience	Piu et al., 1984
	Wylie & Verber, 1994

VARIABLES THAT HEALTH CARE PROVIDERS AND THEIR PRACTICES MAY INFLUENCE

Mother's intention to breastfeed	Balcazar et al., 1995
	O'Campo et al., 1992
	Wambaugh, 1997
Mother's anticipated length of breastfeeding	O'Campo et al., 1992
Maternal confidence	O'Campo et al., 1992
Use, timing, and dose of analgesia or anesthesia	Thorp & Breedlove, 1996
	Crowell et al., 1994
Time of the first feeding	Endresen & Helsing, 1995
	Wright et al., 1996
Mother's discomfort with breastfeeding in hospital	Duckett et al., 1993

Problems encountered in the hospital and at home	Duckett et al., 1993
	Forsyth et al., 1985
	Wright et al., 1996
Mother's commitment to breastfeed	Coreil & Murphy, 1988
	Wambaugh, 1997
Mother's sources of information (postpartum) about infant feeding	Kistin et al., 1994
	O'Campo et al., 1992
Support and assistance offered to the mother	O'Campo et al., 1992
	Baranowski et al., 1983
	Kessler et al., 1995
Use of supplemental or complemental feeds	Duckett et al., 1993
	Perez-Escamilla et al., 1992
	Wright et al., 1996
Staff attitudes toward breastfeeding (mothers)	Lazzaro et al., 1995
Health providers' advice regarding breastfeeding	Balcazar et al., 1995

References

Balcazar H, et al: What predicts breastfeeding intention in Mexican-American and non-Hispanic white women? Evidence from a national survey. *Birth* 22:74–80, 1995.

Baranowski T, et al: Social support, social influence, ethnicity and the breastfeeding decision. *Soc Sci Med* 17:1599–1611, 1983.

Coreil J, Murphy JE: Maternal commitment, lactation practices, and breastfeeding duration. *JOGNN* 17:273–8, 1988.

Crowell MK, Hill PD, Humenick SS: Relationship between obstetric analgesia and time of effective breast feeding. *J Nurse Midwif* 39:150–6, 1994.

Dillon KM, Totten MC: Psychological factors, immunocompetence, and health of breast-feeding mothers and their infants. *J Gen Psychol* 150:155–62, 1989.

Duckett L, Henly SJ, Garvis M: Predicting breast-feeding duration during the postpartum hospitalization. *West J Nurs Res* 15:177–98, 1993.

Endresen EH, Helsing E: Changes in breastfeeding practices in Norwegian maternity wards: national surveys 1973, 1982, and 1991. *Acta Paediatr* 84:719–24, 1995.

Forsyth BW, Leventhal JM, McCarthy PL: Mothers' perceptions of problems of feeding and crying behaviors. *Am J Dis Child* 139:269–72, 1985.

Hill PD, Aldag JC: Smoking and breastfeeding status. *Res Nurs Health* 19:125–32, 1996.

Kessler LA, et al: The effect of a woman's significant other on her breastfeeding decision. *J Hum Lact* 11:103–9, 1995.

Kistin N, et al: Breast-feeding rates among black urban low-income women: effect of prenatal education. *Pediatrics* 86:741–6, 1990.

Kistin N, Abramson R, Dublin P: Effect of peer counselors on breastfeeding initiation, exclusivity, and duration among low-income urban women. *J Hum Lact* 10:11–5, 1994.

Lazzaro DE, Anderson J, Auld G: Medical professionals' attitudes toward breastfeeding. *J Hum Lact* 11:97–101, 1995.

Nolan L, Goel V: Sociodemographic factors related to breastfeeding in Ontario: results from the Ontario health survey. *Can J Public Health* 86:309–12, 1995.

Novotny R, et al: Health of infant is the main reason for breast-feeding in a WIC population in Hawaii. *J Am Diet Assoc* 94:293–7, 1994.

O'Campo P, et al: Prenatal factors associated with breast-feeding duration: recommendations for prenatal interventions. *Birth* 19:195–201, 1992.

Perez-Escamilla R, et al: Effect of the maternity ward system on the lactation success of low-income urban Mexican women. *Early Hum Dev* 31:25–40, 1992.

Peterson CE, Da Vanzo J: Why are teenagers in the United States less likely to breastfeed than older women? *Demography* 29:431–50, 1992.

Piu M, et al: Incidence and duration of breast-feeding in a group of primiparae after physiological delivery. *Clin Exp Obstet Gynecol* 11:55–9, 1984.

Thorp JA, Breedlove G: Epidural analgesia in labor: an evaluation of risks and benefits. *Birth* 23:63–83, 1996.

| BOX 3–3 | **(cont.)** |

Wambaugh KA: Breastfeeding intention and outcome: a test of the theory of planned behavior. *Res Nurs Health* 20:51–9, 1997.

Wiles LS: The effect of prenatal breastfeeding education on breastfeeding success and maternal perception of the infant. *JOGN Nurs* 13:253–7, 1984.

Wright A, et al: Changing hospital practices to increase the duration of breastfeeding. *Pediatrics* 97:669–75, 1996.

Wylie J, Verber I: Why women fail to breast-feed: a prospective study from booking to 28 days post-partum. *J Hum Nutr Diet* 7:115–20, 1994.

Source: Derived in part from Janke JR: The incidence, benefits and variables associated with breastfeeding: implications for practice. Nurse Pract *18:22–32, 1993.*

the sand to avoid the challenges that are going to be leveled at the advocate, particularly for behavior requiring change on the part of others, will fail. Being an advocate requires one to identify:

- the client for whom the advocacy is directed
- the purpose of the advocacy
- the resources of the advocate
- the persons in power who must be contacted and those who will be affected by the advocacy actions
- the receptivity of persons in powerful positions to the planned advocacy actions
- the actions that will need to be altered on the basis of an evaluation of the advocacy action that is effected

Breastfeeding promotion works best when it involves family and key community members, coupled with training and supervision of the primary health care workers (Habicht, 1979; Lutter et al., 1997). Chandler and Roush (1982) have suggested that such individuals can serve as physician-extenders, reserving the physician's time for crisis management rather than uneventful ongoing assistance. Clift (1989), noting how artificial formula is advertised on the radio in many developing countries, suggests that preventive health-behavior campaigns, of which breastfeeding promotion is an often overlooked example, can use the same media. If farm workers in China can be given messages extolling the appropriateness of family planning by electric megaphone from an all-terrain vehicle, why not a message about the importance of breastfeeding? Figure 3–4 illustrates one method of breastfeeding promotion; it depicts the health care worker incorporating her skills and advocacy role into helping a mother to reach her breastfeeding goal.

The care provider needs to use a deliberative approach that requires direct interaction between herself and the mother and encourages two-way communication to assure that the information provided is not only understood but is relevant to the mother and her needs (Princeton, 1986). This notion is based on the assumption that the mother is able to identify what she needs and that she is an active player in the relationship between herself and the care provider. The deliberative approach encompasses three phases (Table 3–2). Phases 1 and 2 may occur in the hospital, but they also might have to be dealt with if the mother is seen for the first time in her home or at a community health center. Phase 3 is specific to a noninstitutional setting and will, perhaps more than the previous phases, require recognition and acceptance of the legitimacy of cultural and social values and family concerns related to the baby.

Providing meaningful care to the mother as she ministers to her baby must be a value of the health care worker. If the worker sees high-tech care as the epitome of assistance but the mother is fearful of it, neither will be very happy with the other. Unless the health care worker in the community accepts as legitimate the notion that it is as appropriate for her to provide preventive care as curative care (Hanvey, 1990), the most needed kind of maternal and newborn care will not be given.

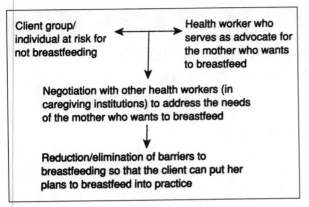

FIGURE 3-4. The importance of assuming a partner-ship role with the client *when promoting, supporting, and protecting the mother who wants to breastfeed.*

Whereas the WHO Code has stimulated some governments to design programs that promote breastfeeding (Kocturk & Zetterstrom, 1988; Rea & Berquo, 1990), the United States did not ratify an affirmative vote for the WHO Code until 1995. Members of the health care community in the United States remain relatively uninformed about the existence of the WHO Code or its significance for hospital routines and the activities of health care workers relating to breastfeeding. Positive atti-tudes, knowledge, and perceptions concerning breastfeeding are not enough (Burkhalter & Marin, 1991; Cadwallader & Olson, 1986). Training in how to assist the mother and ongoing support of her efforts is also necessary if breastfeeding pro-motion is to result in a change in breastfeeding behavior. In a study by Cunningham and Segree (1990) and in a report by Soysa, Fernando, and Abeywickrama (1988), the health care profession-als who had contact with the women were found to impede rather than to positively reinforce the sub-jects' breastfeeding activities. Breastfeeding promo-tion requires that the practices of health care professionals must be changed so that they support early initiation of breastfeeding (Wright, Rice, & Wells, 1996). These practices should include opportunities for early breastfeeding, immediate postpartum contact between mother and infant, rooming-in, breastfeeding according to maternal or infant need, and eliminating formula feeding in the hospital, by the nurses as well as the mothers. Sharing the findings of studies that reveal how

breastfeeding, both in hospital and after discharge, is influenced by these modifications in hospital practices is important in changing attitudes and in maintaining optimal care patterns. Perhaps the most important change involves altering the atti-tudes of the health care professionals who talk about the breast being best but who foster maternal doubts by their actions, which often impede breast-feeding practice.

As noted in Chapter 1, the Baby-Friendly Hospital Initiative highlights ten steps by which any institution caring for new postpartum mothers and their neonates can assist the initiation of breast-feeding. When the "Ten Steps to Successful Breast-Feeding" are part of the caregiving offered in a given institution, the mothers who give birth and begin breastfeeding there are more likely to have an optimal experience and to provide their baby's birthright for a longer period than women who must struggle to maintain contact with their baby and who must obtain help after they have been dis-charged. Two studies in particular have identified the ways in which implementation (or the failure of implementation) of these ten steps has influenced the breastfeeding experiences of the mothers who gave birth and subsequently received care in the hospitals whose care patterns were examined.

By comparing duration rates of breastfeeding, Endresen and Helsing (1995) noted how the "Ten Steps to Successful Breast-Feeding" have influ-enced the practice. In 1973, fewer than 30 percent of women were still breastfeeding at 12 weeks post-partum. By 1991, more than 80 percent of Norwegian mothers were breastfeeding 12 weeks after giving birth. The authors suggest that changes in Norwegian maternity ward care patterns con-tributed to this change. Those changes included:

- All of the wards in the 1991 study initiated breastfeeding within the first 2 hours of birth (Step 4).

- In 1973, 40 percent of the babies received cow's-milk mixtures as supplements; by 1991, 25 percent of the babies received no supple-ments at all, and none received cow's-milk mixtures (Step 6).

- The amount of time mothers spent with their babies (rooming-in) substantially increased. In

---

Table 3–2

THE DELIBERATIVE NURSING APPROACH TO ENSURE COMMUNICATION AND UNDERSTANDING BY THE BREASTFEEDING MOTHER

	Focus of Encounter	Elements of Encounter
Phase 1	The mother	Observe nonverbal behavior Encourage mother to discuss her needs
Phase 2	The mother-infant dyad	Teach the art and science of breastfeeding, including specific skills relating to the mother's needs and the baby's behavior
Phase 3	The mother-infant dyad	Review issues that are still an issue for the mother; praise any evidence of her own and the baby's learning; relate her needs to community resources on which she can call

Source: Derived from JC Princeton: Incorporating a deliberative nursing care approach with breastfeeding mothers. Health Care Women Int 7:277–93, 1986.

1973, 58 percent of mothers spent 5 hours or less with their babies. In 1991, 64 percent spent between 5.5 and 16 hours with their babies. Even if the mother did not have her baby with her at night, it was "common practice to bring the baby to the mother for breastfeeding in the course of the night" (Step 7).

- Breastfeeding on demand was more widely practiced. Only 3 percent of mothers breastfed on demand in 1973, but 80 percent of new mothers did so in 1991 (Step 8).

In the United States, a similar study was conducted (Wright, Rice, & Wells, 1996) by comparing experiences of mothers in 1990 and 1993. The following findings were reported:

- Breastfeeding was discussed by health care providers with two-thirds of the pregnant mothers in each of the years studied (Step 3).
- The baby was nearly three times more likely (63 percent versus 25 percent) to be put to the breast within the first hour after birth in 1993 than in 1990, prior to incorporation of the "Ten

Steps to Successful Breast-Feeding" into staff in-services and training (Step 4).

- In 1990, 61 percent of the mothers received help with breastfeeding. By 1993, 82 percent of the mothers reported receiving help while they were in the hospital (Step 5).
- In 1990, 61 percent of the babies of women who said they planned to breastfeed exclusively for at least 2 months received no formula supplements. By 1993, this percentage had increased to 88 percent (Step 6).

In addition, Wright et al. examined the effects of five of the Ten Steps on the likelihood that the women were fully breastfeeding at one month and at four months postpartum (Table 3–3). The findings reveal that four of the five steps contributed to nearly two-thirds of the mothers exclusively breastfeeding at one month postpartum. Although slightly fewer than 50 percent of these mothers had roomed-in with their babies at least 60 percent of the time, this finding suggests that such access to their babies may have helped mothers learn to breastfeed and to breastfeed frequently and without the potential interference of such practices as separating neonate from mother (Elander & Lindberg, 1984), giving artificial milk foods to the baby instead of breastfeedings (Newman, 1990; Perez-Escamilla et al., 1996), distributing gift packs to mothers that infer that formula will be needed after the mother's and baby's departure from the hospital (Frank et al., 1987; Snell et al., 1992), giving the baby a pacifier by which to achieve comfort, in lieu of the mother's breast (Victora et al., 1993; Barros et al., 1995), and providing the mother with the name of a support group in the community from whom she might obtain additional support and information about breastfeeding (McNatt & Freston, 1992; Ridler, 1988).

It is likely that other studies examining the effects of the Baby-Friendly Hospital Initiative will be conducted and will lend additional support to those seeking to make similar changes in other institutions.

One community-based breastfeeding promotion program included training of health care providers, educational opportunities for the mothers, and mass-media efforts (Rodriguez-Garcia, Aumack, & Ramos, 1990). The curriculum for health care workers included recognition of the effect of cultural beliefs and myths on breastfeeding, and instruction in ways to work with mothers for effective counseling. Continuing supervision and evaluation of the health care workers' actions increased the likelihood that these workers offered consistent information. The active involvement of administrative personnel assured that the health care workers believed that their efforts were important and were supported by those in supervisory positions. The results were impressive: prior to the intervention program, breastfeeding initiation rates averaged 73 percent; after the intervention program was begun, nearly 90 percent of the women in the target communities began breastfeeding. Breastfeeding duration rates also increased.

Jelliffe (1975) is not the first to note that inclusion in any course of instruction on the physiology of lactation and breast structure, and the practical application of that knowledge through instruction in breastfeeding management, is essential if health care workers are to be effective promoters of breastfeeding. The lack of such instruction in most medical and nursing schools helps us to understand why so few physicians and nurses feel adequately prepared to assist the mother who wants to breastfeed or who is attempting to do so despite the impediments placed in her way (often unwittingly) by these same health care providers.

Lazzaro et al. (1995) reported that most physicians and nurses in their sample encouraged breastfeeding when the mother had not yet decided how she would feed her baby but that fewer than half of these individuals advocated breastfeeding when a mother said she was going to bottle-feed her new baby. Furthermore, most of these same respondents reported recommending the use of commercial milk supplements for breastfeeding babies.

Perhaps even more telling are the differences in perception relating to breastfeeding counseling offered by health professionals. When Coreil et al. (1995) compared what providers offered to what mothers were seeking, a chasm of miscommunication was revealed. For example, the providers tended to use technical language that the patients could not understand and to offer information that conflicted with what other professionals said. Although the mothers sought practical information, theory was more often provided by the professionals—a telling outcome. Client respondents identified health care professionals as the "weak link" in the chain of breastfeeding information.

Freed's siren call (1993) to "teach what we preach" was followed up by a study that pointed out how poorly most health care providers are trained to assist breastfeeding women beyond exhorting them to feed naturally. Whether reporting the results of surveys of residents or practicing physicians, Freed et al. (1995a,b) found that most providers depended on personal experience (or their spouse's) rather than the few didactic lectures they had received to help them assist patients. Although more than 90 percent of those surveyed agreed that physicians should be involved in promoting breastfeeding, most could not provide appropriate recommendations related to breastfeeding. A similar survey of nursing students revealed nearly identical findings (Freed et al., 1996). These study outcomes may not be surprising, but they surely beg the question that Freed originally posed. If health care providers are going to preach breastfeeding, they must be trained to

---

Table 3–3

BABY-FRIENDLY HOSPITAL INITIATIVE RECOMMENDATIONS AND THEIR EFFECT WHEN INCORPORATED INTO HOSPITAL PRACTICE

		Babies Fully Breastfeeding	
		At 1 mo	At 4 mo
Baby given formula in hospital (Step 6)			
	Yes	37% [b]	8% [a]
	No	68%	22%
Mother given gift pack with formula, coupons (Step 6)			
	Yes	49%	17%
	No	61%	15%
Baby rooms-in with mother (Step 7)			
	Yes (≥ 60% of time)	62%	22%
	No (< 60% of time)	48% [a]	9% [b]
Baby given pacifier in hospital (Step 9)			
	Yes	46% [b]	12%
	No	62%	20%
Mother given name of support group (Step 10)			
	Yes	63%	22%
	No	51%	12% [a]

[b] $p < .01.$

[a] $p < .05.$

Source: Derived from A Wright et al: Changing hospital practices to increase the duration of breastfeeding. Pediatrics *97:669–75, 1996.*

teach breastfeeding as well, and to do so, they must be provided with more knowledge than mere personal experience.

Kocturk and Zetterstrom (1989, p. 817) note that most promotional programs appear to be based on an assumption that all mothers have the same needs regarding infant feeding and that a single message (e.g., the breast is best for baby) will be effective in motivating all mothers in the world, regardless of socioeconomic and cultural differences. Yet, women in different ethnic groups, mothers of different ages, and women from different socioeconomic settings do not always respond in the same way to the opportunity to breastfeed. Moving beyond such assumptions is essential if

specific groups of women are to be reached. One program used a structured approach that incorporated continuing training and motivation of the health care workers who were in contact with the mothers. The authors found that motivation of the staff was not enough to change their behavior; specific implementation practices were needed (Palti et al., 1988).

The activities of a prenatal clinic run by the Santa Cruz County (California) Health Services Agency is one example of breastfeeding promotion in the United States. The agency offered information about breastfeeding as part of the prenatal clinic beginning early in the third trimester, provided a group meeting once a month at the local

WIC office, and made follow-up phone calls or home visits at 6, 12, and 24 weeks postpartum. This combination of activities increased breastfeeding rates substantially as compared with the preproject patterns (Skeel, McCarty, & Pierce, 1986).

In a migrant health clinic, mothers were given baby layettes if they attended a prenatal class on breastfeeding. Of those Hispanic or black mothers who attended the class, 52 percent were breastfeeding at the time of hospital discharge, as compared with only 10 percent of those women of the same ethnic group who did not attend the prenatal class (Young & Kaufman, 1988).

In one study, both television commercials and print advertisements were used. The attitudes of teenage girls toward breastfeeding were evaluated before and after the running of the print and video commercials. Only the television commercial was found to have influenced attitudes about breastfeeding. Sadly, knowledge scores about breastfeeding were unchanged by the commercial advertising campaign, suggesting that the visual medium may influence attitudes but is unlikely to increase recall of specific facts about breastfeeding (Friel et al., 1989). Such social marketing does influence behavior, including infant-feeding behavior. The billboards that used to festoon the sides of roads in developing countries were there for a reason: since the adoption of the WHO Code, pictures of presumably healthy infants on formula tins are no longer seen. Instead, those advertisements have been replaced by billboards touting the wonders of infant foods, such as pureed solids and infant juices. Such advertising would not proliferate if it were not effective (Clift, 1989).

Not all breastfeeding promotion programs work, however. When administrators neither supervise nor actively support a program, the likelihood of staff involvement in practices designed to assist breastfeeding is reduced, for, as Stokamer (1990) notes, "If breastfeeding is important to the administration, it will be important to the staff." Also important is the manner in which that "importance" is conveyed to the staff. Simply expecting staff to "carry on," without providing them with the means to do so, is not only self-defeating but very likely will result in failure of the staff to share the administration's message that breastfeeding is important.

Breastfeeding Programs That Work

Every cultural setting requires that a breastfeeding promotion program be geared to the specific needs of the target population, with due consideration given to those cultural elements that form the social boundaries. (See the checklist of factors in Box 3–4.) In Santiago, Chile, one such breastfeeding promotion program has demonstrated that breastfeeding duration can be increased when a multifaceted program is put into place. In this case, six different interventions were attempted:

1. Training the health team so that providers were knowledgeable about breastfeeding

2. Offering information and encouragement regarding breastfeeding when mothers attended the prenatal clinic

3. Providing prenatal breastfeeding skills education in a group setting

4. Offering information, support, and encouragement to new mothers while they were in the hospital

5. Creating an outpatient lactation clinic for mothers

6. Offering the Lactational Amenorrhea Method (LAM) as a first form of family planning (Pugin et al., 1996)

In this setting, a goal was to increase the percentage of women who were fully breastfeeding six months after their baby's birth. Comparing the intervention group with a control group for whom these interventions were not available revealed that nearly three times as many women (61 percent versus 27 percent) were fully breastfeeding at 6 months if all six elements were in place. Although all women appeared to benefit, regardless of their parity and mothering experience, the more complete program was particularly effective if the mother participated in anticipation of her first birth (94 percent versus 67 percent). The authors concluded that breastfeeding support, when it is part of a multipronged program that includes training of health care workers and other assistance for mothers, can create measurable change in the direction desired at relatively low cost.

BOX 3–4

Checklist of Factors Contained in an Optimal Multifaceted Breastfeeding Promotion Program

- A clearly identified, measurable outcome variable
- Media campaign that stimulates public support for the program
- Ongoing active involvement of administrators and supervisory personnel at all levels of the health care system
- Training and ongoing continuing education of health care workers at all levels
- Identification of specific hospital routines that are targeted for change

- Specific techniques for informing women prenatally about breastfeeding
- Specific techniques for assisting women with breastfeeding immediately after birth
- Specific techniques for assisting women with breastfeeding throughout the lactation course
- Means of comparing the outcome variable prior to initiation of the program and at various times after the program has been implemented

---

In the United States, another program takes a different approach and is based on the premise that the attitude of one's friends and support people about breastfeeding will strongly influence whether one chooses to breastfeed and how one does so (Bryant, 1982; McLorg & Bryant, 1989). Based on a series of focused interviews with low-income women in the southeastern United States, the Best Start program was developed. This program is aimed at reaching women who are least likely to breastfeed: low-income, often nonwhite, generally not well educated women. The training program includes four clearly defined objectives:

1. To identify the most common factors that deter low-income women from breastfeeding (which requires that the trainee know something about the women with whom she expects to be working)

2. To develop strategies for helping women overcome identified barriers to breastfeeding (barriers that may vary in different parts of the country and for different ethnic groups and subcultures)

3. To identify those factors that attract low-income women to breastfeeding (requiring that the trainee know something about the population of women with whom she will be working)

4. To develop strategies for building on those appealing elements (which will vary in different parts of the country and for different ethnic groups and subcultures) so that women will be encouraged to breastfeed.

Evaluation of the Best Start program (Hartley and O'Connor, 1996) reveals that more women involved in the program were breastfeeding at hospital discharge (31 percent versus 15 percent) and at two weeks postpartum (21 percent versus 13 percent) as compared to a control group of women not involved in the program. In this study, these findings were most marked in mothers who were 19 years of age or younger. The authors concluded that this program represents a simple, low-cost educational intervention that is effective in increasing breastfeeding initiation and duration rates, particularly among low-income mothers and especially teenage low-income mothers.

Once the effective elements of a multifaceted breastfeeding promotion program have been identified, information is provided that will help the trainee to expand her understanding of appropriate and inappropriate ways of discussing breastfeeding. One typical example is the practice of asking a pregnant woman how she plans to feed her baby. If such a question is asked in advance of the mother having any information about breastfeeding other than what a neighbor, friend, or relative may have told her, and if she lives in an environment where bottle-feeding is highly visible, she is very likely to answer, "Bottle-feeding," without giving the subject much thought. Such a response effectively shuts the door on any future discussion about breastfeeding that might have taken place had the original question not been asked. Alternatives to such an approach should be discussed so that health care workers will be better equipped to offer information that may encourage women to choose breastfeeding when they may not have considered such an option previously.

Specific barriers are then identified, and role playing is used to assist those in the training program to practice how they might answer a prospective client's concerns. Among these barriers are lack of confidence, embarrassment, loss of freedom, the influence of family and friends, and dietary and health practices.

Dietary and health practices can be a major stumbling block if a woman attending a WIC clinic understands that she has qualified for the supplemental food program because she is nutritionally at risk. She may silently fear that if she has not been eating well enough to create a healthy baby without WIC food supplements, she is very likely unable to make good milk either. Workers in such clinics may need to revise the ways in which they emphasize nutritional risk, to assist mothers in understanding that milk production is far less dependent on food choices than is pregnancy (see Chapter 16 for additional discussion).

Finally, issues that attract women to breastfeeding—taking advantage of the unique health benefits to the baby that breastfeeding provides, enhancing the lifelong mother-infant bond, and providing a special time between mother and baby—are discussed with trainees. Also addressed are ways to use the Best Start program to cement these positive messages about breastfeeding. Originally designed for use in WIC offices, the Best Start program includes posters, informational pamphlets designed for a low-literacy audience, and video presentations that are designed to be used as public-service announcements and to spark discussion in client focus groups. In some cases, WIC offices use selected segments of the video presentations to help mothers see that women like themselves, with similar concerns, think breastfeeding is best for both them and their babies. The pamphlets speak directly to the concerns women have and then offer alternative views to help women see that such fears need not prevent them from breastfeeding. Such an honest approach legitimizes the concerns but does not accept them as justifications for not breastfeeding; rather, they become the topic of serious consideration regarding ways to reduce their power as barriers. Yet to be performed is a carefully controlled study in different settings to determine how effective these social marketing tools are in improving breastfeeding initiation and duration in low-income U.S. populations in which breastfeeding is least likely to occur.

SUMMARY

Different family forms reflect different members' needs. Family developmental theories enable the health care worker to identify specific family functions throughout the life cycle. The goal of the health care provider should be to help the family to meet its own needs without her or his assistance. Key issues related to family functioning are the family's place within the support system and larger community. The early parenting period is characterized by patterns of attachment behavior and ways that these reflect the growing competence of the parents as parents. In some cases, the father may be the mother's single and most constant supporter; in other situations, he may be less involved in the family and unlikely to support breastfeeding.

Effective breastfeeding promotion goes beyond words and slogans. It requires tools for health care providers, who will have contact with the breastfeeding father as well as the mother.

Promotion programs must be structured so that they take into consideration the cultural and social context within which the program and its participants function. Two such programs, one in a developing country and one designed to reach low-income women in the United States, serve as examples of elements that must be considered.

Awareness of the social support system that the mother can tap, in addition to any health care providers to whom she might look for assistance, is imperative for the caregiver who is attempting to provide ongoing information and help, particularly when that help is provided outside an institutional setting.

REFERENCES

Acheson L: Family violence and breastfeeding. *Arch Fam Med* 4:650–2, 1995.

American Academy of Pediatrics (Work Group on Breastfeeding): Breastfeeding and the use of human milk. *Pediatrics* 100:1035–9, 1997.

American Academy of Pediatrics: The promotion of breast-feeding. *Pediatrics* 69:654–61, 1982.

American Academy of Pediatrics Committee on Nutrition: Encouraging breast-feeding. *Pediatrics* 65:657–8, 1980.

American College of Nurse-Midwives: Policy statement on breast-feeding (see Appendix A). *J Nurse Midwif* 38:1–4, 1993.

American Dietetic Association: Position of the American Dietetic Association: promotion of breast feeding. *J Am Diet Assoc* 86:1580, 1986.

Anlar Y, Anlar B, Tonyali A: Some factors influencing the time of lactation. *J Trop Pediatr* 34:198, 1988.

Arango JO: Promoting breast feeding: a national perspective. *Public Health Rep* 99:559–65, 1984.

Auerbach KG: The role of the nurse in support of breast feeding. *J Adv Nurs* 4:263–85, 1979.

Auerbach KG: Breastfeeding fallacies: their relationship to understanding lactation. *Birth* 17:44–9, 1990a.

Auerbach KG: Breastfeeding promotion: why it doesn't work [editorial]. *J Hum Lact* 6:45–6, 1990b.

Balcazar H, Trier CM, Cobas JA: What predicts breastfeeding intention in Mexican-American and non-Hispanic white women? Evidence from a national survey. *Birth* 22:74–80, 1995.

Baldwin EN, Friedman KA: Is breastfeeding really a visitation issue? *Mothering* 68:84–8, 1993.

Baranowski T, et al: Social support, social influence, ethnicity and the breastfeeding decision. *Soc Sci Med* 17:1599–1611, 1983.

Barron SP, et al: Factors influencing duration of breast feeding among low-income women. *J Am Diet Assoc* 88:1557–61, 1988.

Barros FC, et al: Use of pacifiers associated with decreased breastfeeding duration. *Pediatrics* 95:497–9, 1995.

Bowen SM, Miller BC: Paternal attachment behavior as related to presence at delivery and preparenthood classes: a pilot study. *Nurs Res* 29:307–11, 1980.

Brent NB, Redd B, Dworetz A, et al: Breast-feeding in a low-income population: program to increase incidence and duration. *Arch Pediatr Adolesc Med* 149:798–803, 1995.

Bryant CA: The impact of kin, friend and neighbor networks on infant feeding practices: Cuban, Puerto Rican and Anglo families in Florida. *Soc Sci Med* 16:1757–65, 1982.

Burkhalter BR, Marin PS: A demonstration of increased exclusive breastfeeding in Chile. *Int J Gynaecol Obstet* 34:353–59, 1991.

Cadwallader AA, Olson CM: Use of a breastfeeding intervention by nutrition paraprofessionals. *J Nutr Educ* 18:117–22, 1986.

Canadian Dietetic Association: Promoting breast-feeding: a role for the dietician/nutritionist: official position of the Canadian Dietetic Association. *J Can Diet Assoc* 50:211–14, 1989.

Chandler CG, Roush RE: Training allied health professionals to deliver breast-feeding services to women in the pre- and postnatal periods. *J Allied Health* 11:124–30, 1982.

Clift E: Social marketing and communication: changing health behavior in the Third World. *Am J Heath Prom* 3:17–24, 1989.

Coreil J, et al: Health professionals and breastfeeding counseling: client and provider views. *J Hum Lact* 11:265–71, 1995.

Courtois CA, Riley CC: Pregnancy and childbirth as triggers for abuse memories: implications for care. *Birth* 19:222–3, 1992.

Cronenwett LR, Reinhardt R: Support and breast-feeding: a review. *Birth* 14:199–203, 1987.

Cunningham WE, Segree W: Breast feeding promotion in an urban and a rural Jamaican hospital. *Soc Sci Med* 30:341–8, 1990.

Cusson RM: Attitudes toward breast-feeding among female high-school students. *Pediatr Nurs* 10:189–91, 1985.

Dormire SL, Strauss SS, Clarke BA: Social support and adaptation to the parent role in first-time adolescent mothers. *JOGNN* 18:327–37, 1989.

Duckett L, Henly SJ, Garvis M: Predicting breast-feeding duration during the postpartum hospitalization. *West J Nurs Res* 15:177–98, 1993.

Elander G, Lindberg T: Short mother-infant separation during first week of life influences the duration of breastfeeding. *Acta Paediatr Scand* 73:237–40, 1984.

Endresen EH, Helsing E: Changes in breastfeeding practices in Norwegian maternity wards: national surveys 1973, 1982, and 1991. *Acta Paediatr* 84:719–24, 1995.

Fein RA: The first weeks of fathering: the importance of choices and supports for new parents. *Birth Fam J* 3:53–8, 1976.

Fein RA: Research on fathering: social policy and an emergent perspective. *J Soc Issues* 34:122–35, 1978.

Finkelhor D: Current information on the scope and nature of child sexual abuse. *Future Child* 4:31–53, 1994.

Forrester IT, Wheelock G, Warren AP: Assessment of students' attitudes toward breastfeeding. *J Hum Lact* 13:33–7, 1997.

Forsyth BW, Leventhal JM, McCarthy PL: Mothers' perceptions of problems of feeding and crying behaviors. *Am J Dis Child* 139:269–72, 1985.

Frank DA, et al: Commercial discharge packs and breast-feeding counseling: effects on infant-feeding practices in a randomized trial. *Pediatrics* 80:845–54, 1987.

Freed GL: Breast-feeding: time to teach what we preach. *JAMA* 269:243–5, 1993.

Freed GL, et al: National assessment of physicians' breast-feeding knowledge, attitudes, training, and experience. *JAMA* 273:472–6, 1995a.

Freed GL, et al: Pediatrician involvement in breast-feeding promotion: a national study of residents and practitioners. *Pediatrics* 96:490–4, 1995b.

Freed GL, et al: Methods and outcomes of breast-feeding instruction for nursing students. *J Hum Lact* 12:105–10, 1996.

Freed GL, Fraley JK: Effect of expectant mothers' feeding plan on prediction of fathers' attitudes regarding breast-feeding. *Am J Perinatol* 10:300–3, 1993.

Freed GL, Fraley JK, Schanler RJ: Accuracy of expectant mothers' predictions of fathers' attitudes regarding breast-feeding. *J Fam Pract* 37:148–52, 1993.

Freed GL, Fraley JK, Schanler RJ: Attitudes of expectant fathers regarding breast-feeding. *Pediatrics* 90:224–7, 1992.

Friel JK, et al: The effect of a promotion campaign on attitudes of adolescent females towards breast-feeding. *Can J Public Health* 80:195–9, 1989.

Giugliani ERJ, et al: Are fathers prepared to encourage their partners to breastfeed? A study about fathers' knowledge of breastfeeding. *Acta Paediatr* 83:1127–31, 1994.

Gorey KM, Leslie DR: The prevalence of child sexual abuse: integrative review adjustment for potential response and measurement biases. *Child Abuse Negl* 21:391–8, 1997.

Grant LJ: Effects of childhood sexual abuse: issues for obstetric caregivers. *Birth* 19:220–1, 1992.

Greenberg M, Morris N: Engrossment: the new-born's impact upon the father. *Am J Orthopsychiatry* 44:520–31, 1974.

Gregg JEM: Attitudes of teenagers in Liverpool to breast feeding. *Br Med J* 299:147–8, 1989.

Grossman LK, et al: Breastfeeding among low-income, high-risk women. *Clin Pediatr* 28:38–42, 1989.

Grossman LK, et al: The infant feeding decision in low and upper income women. *Clin Pediatr* 29:30–7, 1990a.

Grossman LK, et al: The effect of postpartum lactation counseling on the duration of breast-feeding in low-income women. *Am J Dis Child* 144:471–4, 1990b.

Habicht J-P: Assurance of quality of the provision of primary medical care by non-professionals. *Soc Sci Med* 13:67–75, 1979.

Hangsleben KL: Transition to fatherhood: An exploratory study. *JOGN Nurs* 12:265–70, 1983.

Hanvey L: Values in maternal and newborn care. *Can Nurse* 86:22–4, 1990.

Hartley BM, O'Connor ME: Evaluation of the 'Best Start' breast-feeding education program. *Arch Pediatr Adolesc Med* 150:868–71, 1996.

Hawkins LM, Nichols FH, Tanner JL: Predictors of the duration of breastfeeding in low-income women. *Birth* 14:204–9, 1987.

Hill PD: Maternal attitudes and infant feeding among low-income mothers. *J Hum Lact* 4:7–11, 1988.

Howard JS, Sater J: Adolescent mothers: self-perceived health education needs. *JOGN Nurs* 14:399–404, 1985.

Hung BKM, Ling L, Ong SG: Sources of influence on infant feeding practices in Hong Kong. *Soc Sci Med* 20:1143–50, 1985.

International Lactation Consultant Association: Position paper on infant feeding. Evanston, Ill: ILCA, 1991.

International Pediatric Association: Recommendations for action programmes to encourage breast feeding. *Acta Paediatr Scand* 65:275–7, 1976.

Janke JR: The incidence, benefits and variables associated with breastfeeding: implications for practice. *Nurse Pract* 18:22–32, 1993.

Jelliffe EFP: Introducing breast-feeding into modern health services. *J Trop Pediatr Environ Health* 21:280–83, 1975.

Jenner S: The influence of additional information, advice and support on the success of breast feeding in working class primiparas. *Child Care Health Dev* 14:319–28, 1988.

Jones C: Father to infant attachment: effects of early contact and characteristics of the infant. *Res Nurs Health* 4:193–200, 1981.

Jordan PL: Breastfeeding as a risk factor for fathers. *JOGNN* 15:94–7, 1986.

Jordan PL: Laboring for relevance: expectant and new fatherhood. *Nurs Res* 39:11–6, 1990.

Jordan PL, Wall VR: Breastfeeding and fathers: illuminating the darker side. *Birth* 17:210–3, 1990.

Jordan PL, Wall VR: Supporting the father when an infant is breastfed. *J Hum Lact* 9:31–4, 1993.

Kaufman KJ, Hall LA: Influences of the social network on choice and duration of breast-feeding in mothers of pre-term infants. *Res Nurs Health* 12:149–59, 1989.

Kessler LA, et al: The effect of a woman's significant other on her breastfeeding decision. *J Hum Lact* 11:103–9, 1995.

Kistin N, et al: Breast-feeding rates among black urban low-income women: effect of prenatal education, *Pediatrics* 86:741–6, 1990.

Kistin N, Abramson R, Dublin P: Effect of peer counselors on breastfeeding initiation, exclusivity, and duration among low-income urban women. *J Hum Lact* 10:11–5, 1994.

Kitzinger JV: Counteracting, not reenacting, the violation of women's bodies: the challenge for perinatal caregivers. *Birth* 19:219–20, 1992.

Kocturk T, Zetterstrom R: Breast-feeding and its promotion. *Acta Paediatr Scand* 77:183–90, 1988.

Kocturk T, Zetterstrom R: The promotion of breastfeeding and maternal attitudes. *Acta Paediatr Scand* 78:817–23, 1989.

Kramer MS: Poverty, WIC, promotion of breast-feeding. *Pediatrics* 87:399–400, 1991.

Kunst-Wilson W, Cronenwett L: Nursing care for the emerging family: promoting paternal behavior. *Res Nurs Health* 4:201–11, 1981.

Lamb ME: Father-infant and mother-infant interaction in the first year of life. *Child Dev* 48:167–81, 1977.

Lamb ME, ed: *The role of the father in child development.* New York: Wiley, 1976.

Lazzaro DE, Anderson J, Auld G: Medical professionals' attitudes toward breastfeeding. *J Hum Lact* 11:97–101, 1995.

Lerner HE: Effects of the nursing mother-infant dyad on the family. *Am J Orthopsychiatry* 49:339–48, 1979.

Levine JA: Redefining the child care 'problem': men as child nurturers. *Child Educ* 54:55–61, 1977.

Levy-Shiff R, et al: Fathers' hospital visits to their preterm infants as a predictor of father-infant relationship and infant development. *Pediatrics* 86:289–93, 1990.

Libbus MK, Kolostov LS: Perceptions of breast-feeding and infant feeding choice in a group of low-income mid-Missouri women. *J Hum Lact* 10:17–23, 1994.

Littman H, et al: The decision to breastfeed: the importance of fathers' approval. *Clin Pediatr* 33:214–9, 1994

Locklin MP: Telling the world: low income women and their breastfeeding experiences. *J Hum Lact* 11:285–91, 1995.

Locklin MP, Naber SJ: Does breastfeeding empower women? Insights from a select group of educated, low-income, minority women. *Birth* 20:30–5, 1993.

Long DG, et al: Peer counselor program increases breastfeeding rates in Utah Native American WIC population. *J Hum Lact* 11:279–84, 1995.

Lowe T: Regional and socio-economic variations in the duration of breastfeeding in Victoria. *Breastfeed Rev* 11:312–15, 1993.

Lutter CK, et al: The effectiveness of a hospital-based program to promote exclusive breast-feeding among low-income women in Brazil. *Am J Public Health* 87:659–63, 1997.

Lynch SA, et al: Evaluating effect of a breastfeeding consultant on the duration of breastfeeding. *Can J Public Health* 77:190–5, 1986.

Majewski JL: Conflicts, satisfactions and attitudes during transition to the maternal role. *Nurs Res* 35:10–4, 1986.

Manstead ASR, Plevin CE, Smart JL: Predicting mothers' choice of infant feeding method. *Br J Soc Psychol* 23:223–31, 1984.

Martines JC, Ashworth A, Kirkwood B: Breast-feeding among the urban poor in southern Brazil: reasons for termination in the first 6 months of life, *Bull WHO* 67:151–61, 1989.

McLorg PA, Bryant CA: Influence of social network members and health care professionals on infant feeding practices of economically disadvantaged mothers. *Med Anthrop* 10:265–78, 1989.

McNatt MH, Freston MS: Social support and lactation outcomes in postpartum women. *J Hum Lact* 8:73–77, 1992.

Mead M: *Coming of Age in Samoa.* New York: Morrow Quill, 192:147–57.

Morse JM, Harrison MJ: Social coercion for weaning. *J Nurse Midwif* 32:205–10, 1987.

Mukerjee M: Hidden scars: sexual and other abuse may alter a brain region. *Sci Amer* (Oct): 14–15, 1995.

Mulford C: Subtle signs and symptoms of the milk ejection reflex. *J Hum Lact* 6:177–8, 1990.

Newman J: Breastfeeding problems associated with the early introduction of bottles and pacifiers. *J Hum Lact* 6:59–63, 1990.

Oshaug A, Botten G: Human milk in food supply statistics. *Food Policy* 19:479–82, 1994.

Palti H, et al: Evaluation of the effectiveness of a structured breast-feeding promotion program integrated into a maternal and child health service in Jerusalem. *Isr J Med Sci* 24:342–8, 1988.

Pascoe JM, Berger A: Attitudes of high school girls in Israel and the United States toward breast feeding. *J Adoles Health Care* 6:28–30, 1985.

Perez-Escamilla R, et al: Effect of the maternity ward system on the lactation success of low-income urban Mexican women. *Early Hum Dev* 31:25–40, 1992.

Perez-Escamilla R, et al: Prelacteal feeds are negatively associated with breast-feeding outcomes in Honduras. *J Nutr* 126:2769–73, 1996.

Peterson CE, Da Vanzo J: Why are teenagers in the United States less likely to breast-feed than older women? *Demography* 29:431–50, 1992.

Peterson GH, Mehl LE, Leiderman PH: The role of some birth-related variables in father attachment. *Am J Orthopsychiatry* 49:330–8, 1979.

Pleck JH: The work-family role system. *Soc Prob* 24:417–27, 1977.

Polit DF, Kahn JR: Early subsequent pregnancy among economically disadvantaged teenage mothers. *Am J Public Health* 76:167–71, 1986.

Pridham KF: Meaning of infant feeding issues and mothers' use of help, *J Reprod Inf Psychol* 5:145–52, 1987.

Princeton JC: Incorporating a deliberative nursing care approach with breastfeeding mothers. *Health Care Women Int* 7:277–93, 1986.

Pugin E, et al: Does prenatal breastfeeding skills group education increase the effectiveness of a comprehensive breastfeeding promotion program? *J Hum Lact* 12:15–9, 1996.

Rassin DK, Richardson CJ, Baranowski T: Ethnic determinants of lactation in a population of mothers in the United States. In: Hamosh M, Goldman AS, eds. *Human lactation* 2. New York: Plenum 1986:69–81.

Rea MF, Berquo ES: Impact of the Brazilian national breast-feeding programme on mothers in Greater Sao Paulo. *Bull WHO* 68:365–71, 1990.

Ridler J: The importance of breast-feeding support groups [editorial]. *So Afr Med J* 74:384, 1988.

Riordan J: *A practical guide to breastfeeding*, St Louis: Mosby, 1983.

Robinson BE: Men caring for the young: an androgynous perspective. *Fam Coord* 28:553–9, 1979.

Rodriguez-Garcia R, Aumack KJ, Ramos A: A community-based approach to the promotion of breastfeeding in Mexico. *JOGNN* 19:431–8, 1990.

Rogers CS, Morris S, Taper LJ: Weaning from the breast: influences on maternal decisions. *Pediatr Nurs* 13:341–5, 1987.

Romero-Gwynn E: Breast-feeding pattern among Indochinese immigrants in Northern California. *Am J Dis Child* 143:804–8, 1989.

Rose A: Effects of childhood sexual abuse on childbirth: one woman's story. *Birth* 19:214–8, 1992.

Russell G: High participant Australian fathers: some preliminary findings. *Merrill Palmer Q* 28:137–56, 1982.

Rustia JG, Abbott D: Father involvement in infant care: two longitudinal studies. *Int J Nurs Stud* 30:467–76, 1993

Samuels SE, Margen S, Schoen EJ: Incidence and duration of breast-feeding in a health maintenance organization population. *Am J Clin Nutr* 42:504–10, 1985.

Saunders SE, Carroll J: Post-partum breast feeding support: impact on duration. *J Am Diet Assoc* 88:213–5, 1988.

Sciacca JP, et al: Influences on breast-feeding by lower-income women: an incentive-based, partner-supported educational program. *J Am Diet Assoc* 95:323–8, 1995.

Scrimshaw SCM, et al: Factors affecting breast-feeding among women of Mexican origin or descent in Los Angeles. *Am J Public Health* 77:467–70, 1987.

Simkin P: Overcoming the legacy of childhood sexual abuse: the role of caregivers and childbirth educators. *Birth* 19:224–5, 1992.

Skeel L, McCarty E, Pierce S: Promoting breast feeding among Hispanic women in Santa Cruz county. *Public Health Rep* 101:661–2, 1986.

Smith LJ: Expert witness: what to emphasize. *J Hum Lact* 7:141, 1991.

Snell BJ, et al: The association of formula samples given at hospital discharge with the early duration of breastfeeding. *J Hum Lact* 8:67–72, 1992.

Soysa PE, Fernando DN, Abeywickrama K: Role of health personnel in the promotion of breast feeding practices. *J Trop Pediatr* 34:75–8, 1988.

Spradley BW: *Community health nursing: concepts and practice*, 2nd ed. Boston: Little, Brown, 1985.

Stokamer CL: Breastfeeding promotion efforts: why some do not work. *Int J Gynaecol Obstet* 31(suppl):61–5, 1990.

Stotland NL, Peterson CH: A modest proposal: breastfeeding for the infants of adolescent mothers. *Adv Psychosom Med* 12:81–90, 1985.

Suhler A, Bornmann PG, Scott JW: The lactation consultant as expert witness. *J Hum Lact* 7:129–40, 1991.

Sullivan J, Jones LC: Breastfeeding adoption by low-income black women. *Health Care Women Int* 7:295–309, 1986.

Tapia JA: Fractionalization of the family unit. In: Schuster CS, Ashburn SS, eds. *The process of human development*. Boston: Little, Brown, 1986.

Taubenheim AM, Silbernagel T: Meeting the needs of expectant fathers. *MCN* 13:110–3, 1988.

Tomlinson PS, Rothenberg MA, Carver LD: Behavioral interaction of fathers with infants and mothers in the immediate postpartum period. *J Nurse Midwifery* 36:232–9, 1991.

Victora CG, et al: Use of pacifiers & breastfeeding duration. *Lancet* 341(8842):404–6, 1993.

Voss S, et al: Fathers and breastfeeding: a pilot observational study. *J R Soc Health* 113:176–8, 1993

Wandersman LP: The adjustment of father to their first baby: the roles of parenting groups and marital relationship. *Birth Fam J* 7:155–61, 1980.

Williams EL, Pan E: Breastfeeding initiation among a low income multiethnic population in Northern California: an exploratory study. *J Hum Lact* 11:245–51, 1994.

Wilson-Clay B: Extended breastfeeding as a legal issue: an annotated bibliography. *J Hum Lact* 6:68–71, 1990.

Wolinski M: Adolescent views on breastfeeding: a descriptive survey. *Breastfeeding Rev* 14:9–12, 1989.

Woollett A: Who breastfeeds? The family and cultural context. *J Reprod Inf Psychol* 5:127–31, 1987.

Wright A, Rice S, Wells S: Changing hospital practices to increase the duration of breastfeeding. *Pediatrics* 97:669–75, 1996.

Yoos L: Developmental issues and the choice of feeding method of adolescent mothers. *JOGN Nurs* 14:68–72, 1985.

Young SA, Kaufman M: Promoting breastfeeding at a migrant health center. *Am J Public Health* 78:523–5, 1988.

ANATOMICAL AND BIOLOGICAL IMPERATIVES

After pregnancy, the mother's endocrine and digestive systems continue to provide nourishment for her child through breastfeeding. However, the mother now synthesizes and stores energy in a special organ–the breast–and the child now receives its nourishment in the form of milk rather than from nutrients passing through the umbilical cord. Breastmilk, a "living fluid" and nutriment, meets most closely the needs of the human infant for whom the milk was produced. No human-made substitute has yet been devised that nourishes the infant as well

Viruses and bacteria stimulate particular protective reactions in the mother's body, which in turn provide important protection to the vulnerable infant through mother's milk. However, environmental contaminants and drugs also can be found in human milk. The question arises: if such contaminants and drugs can be found in the breast and in the milk it creates, to what degree do these elements represent acceptable and unacceptable risks when ingested by the breastfeeding infant?

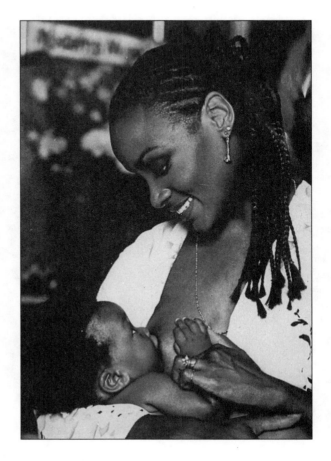

CHAPTER 4

ANATOMY AND PHYSIOLOGY

Jan Riordan

It is essential that health care providers understand the anatomy of the human female breast and the physiological mechanisms of milk production. It is equally necessary to recognize the unique anatomy of the infant's oral structures and the physiological mechanisms of suckling. This chapter is divided into two parts; the first focuses on the mother, the second on the infant. In lactation, as in all human biological systems, there is a working relationship between anatomy (form) and physiology (function). Although function changes as form changes, the functional capacity of the human breast is not wholly dictated by form. Breast size, for instance, is a poor predictor of lactational capability. It is the infant's appetite that determines milk yield, rather than the mother's capacity to produce milk. *Psychophysiology* as used here reflects the sensitivity of breastfeeding to psychogenic influences. For example, for both the mother and the suckling infant, stress and fear can inhibit breastfeeding.

Throughout this text, the developmental cycle of the mammary gland has four phases: mammogenesis, lactogenesis, galactopoiesis, and involution (Table 4–1).

The Mother

Mammogenesis

The mammary system is unlike other organ systems. From birth through puberty, pregnancy, and lactation, no other human organ displays such dramatic changes in size, shape, and function as does the breast. In some cultures, female breasts serve more than one function: they attract the sexual attentions of the male adult and then give nourishment and nurturing to the suckling infant. This first part of the chapter, which focuses on the mother, describes breast development from embryo to adulthood, breast anatomy, changes during pregnancy and lactation, and hormones that influence the course of lactogenesis.

Breast development begins during the fourth week of gestation when a primitive milk streak develops from axilla to groin on the trunk of the embryo. This streak becomes the mammary ridge or milk line by the fifth week of embryonic life. The ridge or line is actually a thickening of epithelial cells in a localized ventrolateral area on the embryo (the "milk hill" stage) that continues through weeks seven and eight and is accompanied by inward growth into the chest wall. Between 12 and 16 weeks' gestation, these specialized cells differentiate further into the smooth muscle of the nipple and areola. Also during this period, epithelial cells continue to develop into mammary buds and then proliferate to form 15 to 25 epithelial branches that eventually become alveoli (Dawson, 1934; Vorherr, 1974).

Placental sex hormones enter fetal circulation and stimulate formation of channels (canalization) of the branched epithelial tissue. This process

Table 4–1

STAGES OF LACTATION

Mammogenesis	• Mammary (breast) growth; increased size and weight of breast • Proliferation of ducts and glandular system under estrogen and progesterone
Lactogenesis, stage 1 (late pregnancy)	• Initiation of milk synthesis in late pregnancy • Differentiation of alveolar cells from secretory cells
Lactogenesis, stage 2 (day two or three to day eight)	• Closure of tight junctions in alveolar cell • Onset of copious secretion of milk • Fullness and warmth in breasts • Switch from endocrine to autocrine control
Galactopoesis (later than day nine to beginning of involution)	• Maintenance of established secretion • Control by autocrine system (supply-demand)
Involution (average 40 days after last breastfeeding)	• Additions of regular supplementation • Decreased milk secretion from build-up of inhibiting peptides

continues until the fetus is 32 weeks old. From 32 to 40 weeks' gestation, lobular-alveolar structures containing colostrum develop. During this time, the fetal mammary gland mass increases four times over its original mass, and the nipple and areola develop further and become pigmented. After birth, the neonate's mammary tissue may secrete colostral milk (so-called witches milk).

Mammary gland development during childhood is limited to general growth. However, at puberty, estrogen becomes the major influence on breast growth in a girl when, at 10 to 12 years of age, primary and secondary ducts grow and divide and form club-shaped terminal end buds that are associated with beginning function of the hypothalamus-pituitary-ovarian axis. The buds develop into new branches and small ductules of areolar buds, which later become the acini or alveoli in the mature female breast. During each menstrual cycle, proliferation and active growth of duct tissue occurs during the follicular and ovulatory phases, reaching a maximum in the late luteal phase and then regressing. During each ovulatory cycle,

peaks of ovarian steroids, primarily progesterone, foster further mammary development that never regresses to its former state of the preceding cycle. Complete development of mammary function occurs only in pregnancy. At the same time, new budding of structures continues until about age 35 (Dabelow, 1957; Vorherr, 1974). In addition to estrogen and progesterone, prolactin and an epidermal growth factor or a specific mammary growth factor are other hormones believed to be required for mammary growth (Tonelli & Sorof, 1980).

Structure

The basic units of the mature glandular tissue are the *alveoli*, which are composed of secretory acinar units in which the ductules terminate. Each cluster of secretory cells of an alveolus is surrounded by a contractile unit of *myoepithelial cells* responsible for ejecting milk into the *ductules*. Each ductule then merges, without communicating with its neighbors, into a larger collecting *lactiferous* or *mammary duct*.

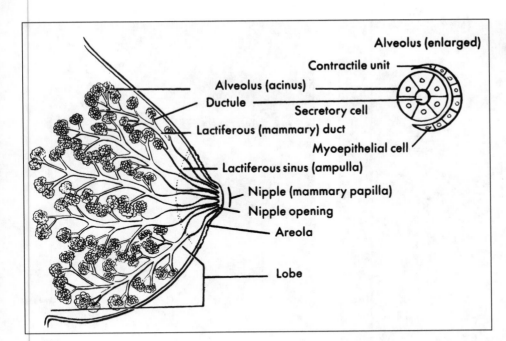

FIGURE 4–1.
Schematic diagram of breast.

Alveolus (enlarged)

Contractile unit

Alveolus (acinus)

Ductule

Secretory cell

Lactiferous (mammary) duct

Myoepithelial cell

Lactiferous sinus (ampulla)

Nipple (mammary papilla)

Nipple opening

Areola

Lobe

The ducts are surrounded by myoepithelial cells and highly vascular connective tissue. Mammary ducts then widen into the *ampullae* or *lactiferous sinuses* located behind the nipple and the areola, the surrounding pigmented area of the breast. In each breast are 15 to 20 subdivided *lobes* (Figs. 4–1, 4–2).

Between and around the uneven edges of the lobes is a thick layer of fat. As seen in Figure 4–3, running vertically through the breast and attaching the deep layer of the subcutaneous tissue to the dermis of the skin are the *suspensory ligaments* or *Cooper's ligaments*. The breast's structure is mainly the result of fibrous tissues that surround and course through it. Glandular tissue that extends toward the axilla partly under the lateral border of the pectoralis majora is known as the *axillary tail* (Fig. 4–4). Each breast of an adult woman weighs, on average, 150 to 200 gm and increases to 400 to 500 gm (about one pound) during lactation.

The breast is highly vascularized. Blood is supplied to the breast through the internal mammary (60 percent) and lateral thoracic (30 percent) arteries. The lymph vessels of the breast are numerous and, for the most part, join the lymph nodes of the axilla. The majority of lymph vessels follow the lactiferous ducts and thus converge toward the nipple, where they join a plexus situated beneath the areola (subareolar plexus).

The nerve supply of the breast is derived from the intercostal nerves of the fourth, fifth, and sixth intercostal spaces. The fourth intercostal nerve penetrates the posterior aspect of the breast (left breast at four o'clock, right breast eight o'clock) and supplies the greatest amount of sensation to the nipple and to the areola. The breast has uneven patterns of sensation: the areola is the most sensitive part of the breast, the skin adjacent to the areola is less sensitive, and the nipple itself is the least sensitive. Women with larger breasts report less sensation than women with smaller breasts. Of women with small or moderate-sized breasts, those who have never been pregnant report greater sensation in their nipples and areolae. Midway to the nipple and areola, the fourth intercostal nerve becomes more superficial. As it reaches the areola, it divides into five branches: one central, two upper, and two lower. The lowermost branch consistently pierces the areola at five o'clock on the left side and seven o'clock on the right side. Any trauma to this nerve will cause some loss of sensation in the breast (Courtiss & Goldwyn, 1976; Edgerton & McClary, 1958). If the lowermost nerve branch

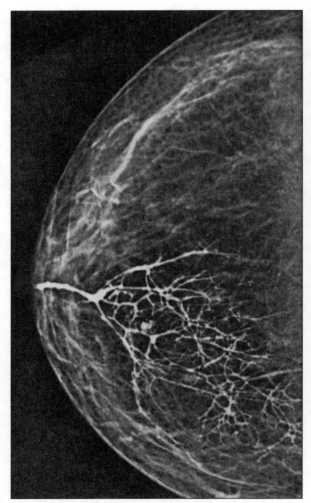

FIGURE 4–2. Contrast opacification of a single lactiferous duct *demonstrates a branching network that defines a single lobe of the breast. (From DB Kopans:* Breast imaging. *Philadelphia: Lippincott, 1989:20.)*

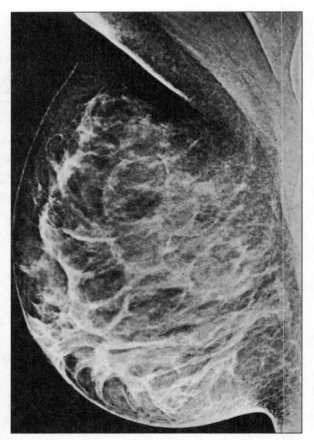

FIGURE 4–3. Curvilinear densities represent Cooper's ligaments. *(From DB Kopans:* Breast imaging. *Philadelphia: Lippincott, 1989:20.)*

is severed, the mother loses sensation to the nipple and areola (Farina, Newby, & Alani, 1980).

The covering smooth skin is modified at the center of each breast to form a *mammary papilla* or nipple into which the lactiferous sinuses open. Some of these ducts join so that 5 to 10 openings appear on the nipple surface. There are 15 to 20 openings (pores) in the nipple. The nipple projects as a small, cylindrical body with pigmented wrinkled skin slightly below the center of each breast at about the level of the fourth intercostal space. Surrounding the nipple is the *areola*, within which lie the Tubercles of

Montgomery, small sebaceous glands with intertwining lactiferous ducts that enlarge during pregnancy (Smith, 1982). The Tubercles of Montgomery range in number from 4 to 28 on each breast. It is widely held that these tubercles provide nipple lubrication and antisepsis, but no evidence or documentation of this function exists. The nipple and areola contain erectile smooth muscles. Hair follicles surround the nipple; most women have at least some nipple hair. In a lactating mother, the average diameter of the areola is 6.4 cm, and the average diameter of the erectile portion of the nipple is 1.6 cm and the length 0.7 cm (Ziemer, 1993). Contraction of bundles of smooth muscles beneath the nipple and areola cause the nipple to be firm and protruding. These structures are seen in Figures 4–5 through 4–7 on the first two pages of the color insert.

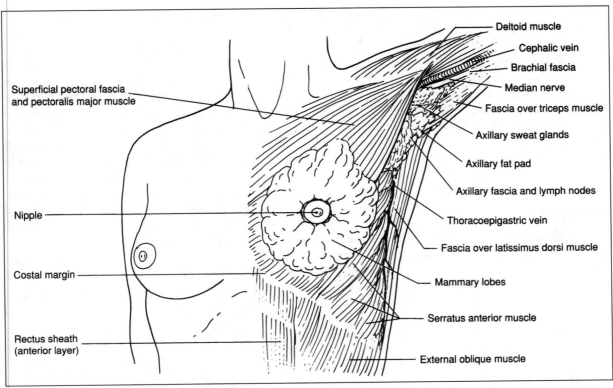

FIGURE 4–4. Anterior pectoral dissection *showing the lobular nature of the mammary gland extending toward the axilla and its location anterior to the pectoralis major muscle. Includes the superficial axillary lymph and sweat glands. (Adapted from CD Clemente:* Anatomy: a regional atlas of the human body. *Philadelphia: Lea & Febiger, 1978.)*

Variations

From woman to woman, breasts vary in color, size, shape, function, and placement on the chest wall. Lobular size varies within a single breast, from one breast to another, and from woman to woman. Moreover, some breast asymmetry is common: the left breast is often larger than the right. Areola and nipple color vary according to complexion: pink in blonds, browner in brunettes, and black in dark-skinned women (Love & Lindsey, 1990). *Supernumerary* nipple tissue or an *accessory* nipple may occur at any point along the milk line from the axilla to the groin (polymastia) and may be associated with renal anomalies (Berman & Davis, 1994). Only rarely does a true or complete accessory mammary gland develop. The most common areas in which an accessory breast might develop are in the axilla and on the thorax (See Color Plate 17).

Lack of full protraction of the nipple on the common pinch test (Fig. 4–8) is fairly common in primigravid women. Poor nipple protractility in women during their first pregnancy has been reported to range from 28 to 35 percent (Blaikeley et al., 1953; Hytten & Baird, 1958; Waller, 1946). Protractility of the nipple gradually improves during pregnancy and, by puerperium, most women have good nipple protraction. Generally, nipple protraction continues to improve with each subsequent pregnancy and lactation experience. The relationship between protractility and subsequent breastfeeding difficulty is minimal. Because the infant makes a teat not from the nipple alone but from the surrounding breast tissue, the actual shape of the nipple may be a secondary consideration.

Alexander found that about 10 percent of pregnant women who intend to breastfeed have inverted or nonprotractile nipples (Alexander et al., 1992). Although true inversion appears to be rare, its treatment can be difficult. Usually the inversion is on one breast only and the mother may breastfeed from a single breast. When the inversion is bilateral, feedings at the breast may have to be supplemented. In some cases, a mother's first breastfeeding experience may be more difficult than subsequent ones—after frequent suckling by the infant, which exerts negative pressure and helps to evert the previously inverted tissue.

Pregnancy

During pregnancy, the breasts grow larger, the skin appears thinner, and the veins become more prominent. The diameter of the areola increases from about 34 mm in early pregnancy to 50 mm postpartum (Hytten, 1954), although there is a wide range of areolar width in any population. As the nipples become more erect, pigmentation of the areola increases and the glands of Montgomery enlarge. Estrogen and progesterone exert their specific effect on the breast during pregnancy; the ductal system proliferates and differentiates under the influence of estrogen, whereas progesterone promotes an increase in size of the lobes, lobules, and alveoli. Adrenocorticotropic hormone (ACTH) and growth hormone combine synergistically with prolactin and progesterone to promote mammary growth.

Lactogenesis

The first half of pregnancy is characterized by growth and proliferation of the ductal tree and further formation of lobules. During the second half of pregnancy, secretory activity accelerates and the acini or alveoli become distended by accumulating colostrum (Russo & Russo, 1987). After 16 weeks of pregnancy, lactation occurs even if the pregnancy does not progress. An accessory breast may also swell. Just before and during childbirth, a new wave of mitotic activity increases the total DNA of the gland (Salazar & Tobon, 1974; Vorherr, 1974).

The capacity of the mammary gland to secrete milk during later pregnancy is called *lactogenesis, stage 1* (or lactogenesis 1). During lactogenesis 1, breast size increases as epithelial cells of the alveoli differentiate into secretory cells for milk production. Fat droplets accumulate in these cells. The onset of copious milk secretion after birth is *lactogenesis, stage 2* (days two or three to eight postpartum). During lactogenesis 2, milk volume increases rapidly from 36 to 96 hours postpartum and then abruptly levels off. Lactogenesis 2 is accompanied by a significant fall in breastmilk levels of sodium, chloride, and protein and a rise in lactose and milk lipids. Humenick (1987) refers to these changes in the milk as its "maturation." These changes in cellular metabolism are a result of closure of junction complexes between alveolar cells. The closure of these "tight junctions" precedes the onset of copious milk secretion (Neville et al., 1991).

Hormonal Influences

Lactogenesis is triggered following the expulsion of the placenta by a fall in progesterone and estrogen levels and the continued presence of prolactin. A great deal of information about these hormonal functions during lactation is now known through radioimmunoassay studies. The postpartum period is characterized hormonally by elevated levels of prolactin, which acts synergistically with cortisol, insulin, growth hormone, and thyrotropin-releasing hormone (TRH). The principal hormone in milk biosynthesis is prolactin.

Prolactin. Without prolactin, lactation does not occur. During pregnancy, prolactin, which is secreted by the anterior pituitary gland, has an important role in increasing breast mass. A group of peptides, including angiotensin II, gonadotropin-releasing hormone (GnRH), and vasopressin, stimulate the release of prolactin. The mammary ducts and alveoli mature and proliferate as prolactin levels steadily rise from the normal nonpregnancy level of 10 to 25 ng/ml to a peak of 200 to 400 ng/ml at term (Tyson et al., 1972). Lactation during pregnancy is inhibited by high levels of progesterone, which interfere with prolactin action at the alveolar cell receptor level. The inhibiting influence of progesterone is so powerful that lactation is delayed if placental fragments are retained after birth.

As progesterone and estrogen levels abruptly drop after a woman gives birth, the anterior pituitary gland, no longer inhibited by these two hormones, releases very large amounts of prolactin.

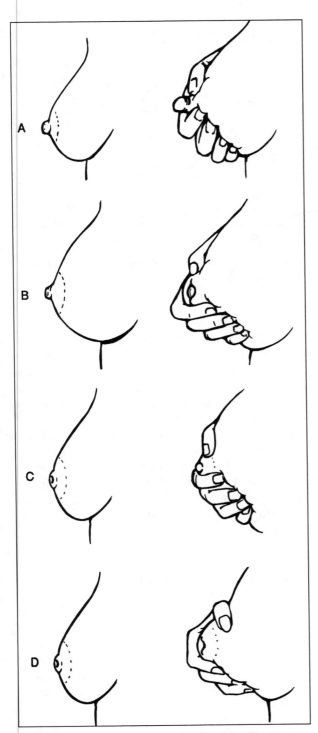

FIGURE 4–8. A. Protracting normal nipple. B. Moderate to severe retraction. C. Inverted-appearing nipple, which, when compressed using pinch test, will either invert further inward or will protract forward (upper right). D. True inversion; nipple inverts further (lower right).

Because human placental lactogen (HPL) competes with prolactin for breast receptors, the decline of HPL after delivery of the placenta also promotes prolactin action. Figure 4–9 describes the rise and fall of hormones during pregnancy and lactation.

Following lactogenesis 2, milk secretion shifts from endocrine to autocrine control. Prolactin secretion continues to be controlled by the hypothalamus. This control is largely inhibitory; that is, whenever the pathway between the hypothalamus and the pituitary is disrupted, prolactin levels rise. During galactopoiesis, the hypothalamus is dependent upon nipple stimulation and withdrawal of milk in order for lactation to continue. When the nipple is stimulated and milk is removed from the breast, the hypothalamus inhibits the release of dopamine; this lower level of dopamine stimulates the release of prolactin and causes milk production (Chao, 1987). Stimulation of the nipple is reported to be sufficiently potent to cause the synthesis of breastmilk even in nonparturient individuals (Newton & Newton, 1962).

Plasma prolactin levels rise and fall in proportion to the frequency, intensity, and duration of nipple stimulation and the suckling stimulus (Noel et al., 1974; Tyson et al., 1972). Prolactin concentration in blood usually doubles in response to suckling and peaks approximately 45 minutes after the beginning of a breastfeeding session (Noel, Suh, & Frantz, 1974). During the first week after birth, prolactin levels in breastfeeding women fall about 50 percent. If a mother does not breastfeed, prolactin levels usually reach nonpregnant levels by seven days postpartum (Tyson et al., 1972) (Fig. 4–10).

Research on prolactin during lactation reveals the following findings about maternal serum prolactin levels:

- They decline slowly over the course of lactation (Battin et al., 1985; Cox et al., 1996; Noel et al., 1974; Tyson et al., 1972) but remain elevated for as long as the mother breastfeeds, even if she breastfeeds for years (Gross & Eastman, 1979; Stallings et al., 1996).

- They are associated with the frequency of suckling: the more feedings, the higher the level of serum prolactin. More than eight breastfeedings per 24 hours prevents decline of the concentration of prolactin before the next breastfeeding (Cox et al., 1996; Gross et al., 1980).

- They are not related to the short-term rate of milk synthesis or milk yield after lactation becomes established (after one month). Instead, the short-term rate of milk synthesis is higher when most of the available milk has been removed from the breast (Cox et al., 1996; Daly et al., 1993).

- They are higher in amenorrheic than in cycling women during the first year postpartum (Battin et al., 1985; Stallings et al., 1996). The role of prolactin in the delay of fertility is well known. Prolactin delays the return of ovulation by inhibiting ovarian response to follicle-stimulating hormone (Bonnar et al., 1975).

- They are not related to the degree of postpartum breast engorgement (West, 1979).

- They may be affected by smoking and beer: a mother who smokes cigarettes has lower prolactin levels (Baron et al., 1986). A mother who drinks beer may conclude that her prolactin levels are higher (Mennella & Beauchamp, 1993).

Battin et al. (1985) studied serum prolactin levels in eight breastfeeding women for 180 days postpartum. The infants of these mothers obtained almost all of their daily nutriment from breastmilk. Mean baseline prolactin levels were 90 ng/ml at 10 days postpartum; afterward, these levels slowly declined but remained elevated at 180 days postpartum (44.3 ng/ml). At 10 days postpartum, four women in the study who remained amenorrheic throughout the study had higher (about 110.0 ng/ml) baseline prolactin levels as compared to the remaining four women (about 70.1 ng/ml) who spontaneously menstruated prior to 180 days. Gross and Eastman (1979) found that breastfeeding women whom they studied in Australia had elevated prolactin levels at 66 weeks postpartum. An overview of prolactin serum levels during pregnancy and breastfeeding is shown in Figure 4–10. Prolactin reportedly has a relaxing effect, causing the breastfeeding woman to feel calm, even euphoric, during the feeding.

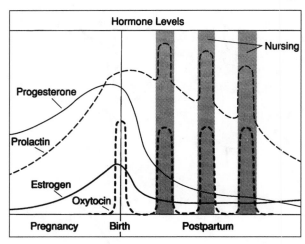

FIGURE 4–9. Hormone levels during pregnancy and lactation. *(Adapted from S Love:* Dr. Susan Love's breast book. *Boston: Addison-Wesley, 1990:34.)*

Prolactin also is present in breastmilk. The release of prolactin into intraalveolar secretions of the breast plays a role in establishing and maintaining lactation. Milk prolactin concentration is lower than its concentration in blood plasma and is highest in early transitional milk (about 43 ng/ml) and the foremilk rather than the hindmilk (Cox et al., 1996). This early transmission of prolactin in the aqueous foremilk is thought to have an effect on intestinal fluid and electrolyte exchange in the newborn (Yuen, 1988). Breastmilk prolactin steadily declines but remains detectable in mature milk (about 11 ng/ml) until weaning up to 40 weeks postpartum (Yuen, 1988).

The Prolactin Receptor Theory. DeCarvalho et al. (1983) suggested that frequent feeding in early lactation stimulates a faster increase in milk output because suckling stimulates the development of receptors to prolactin in the mammary gland. According to DeCarvalho's group, the number of these receptors per cell increases in early lactation and remains constant thereafter. This framework is supported by animal studies (Hinds & Tyndale-Biscoe, 1982; Sernia & Tyndale-Biscoe, 1979).

DeCarvalho et al. (1983) demonstrated that infants gained more weight by their fifteenth day when they were breastfed an average of 9.9 times per day as compared with infants in the control group who were breastfed an average of 7.3 times

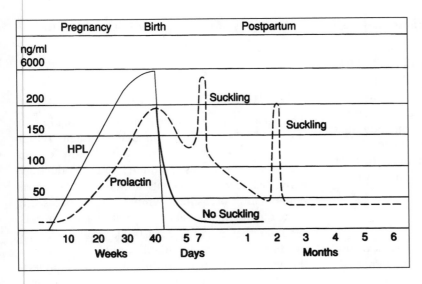

FIGURE 4–10. Fluctuation of human placental lactogen and prolactin serum levels in pregnancy and lactation. *(Adapted from DA Battin, et al: Effect of suckling on serum prolactin, luteinizing hormone, follicle-stimulating hormone, and estradiol during prolonged lactation.* Obstet Gynecol 65:785–88, 1985; JE Tyson, et al: Am J Obstet Gynecol 113:14–20, 1972; L Speroff, RH Glass, NG Kase: Clinical gynecology, endocrinology and infertility, *4th ed. Baltimore: Williams & Wilkins, 1989:283.)*

per day. By the thirty-fifth day, however, postpartum milk intake and weight gain from birth were not significantly different between the two groups. This suggests that frequent feeding in early lactation stimulates a faster increase in milk output but that this output later slows despite frequent breastfeedings. DeCarvalho's theory is partially consistent with findings by Cox, Owens, and Hartmann (1996) that show that after one month there is no relationship between the basal or suckling-stimulated concentration of prolactin in plasma and the short-term rate of milk synthesis.

Zuppa et al. (1988) found that although serum prolactin levels were slightly lower in multiparous mothers as compared with primiparous mothers in the first four postpartum days, the volume of milk obtained by the infants of the multiparous mothers was significantly higher. They concluded that multiparous women had a greater number of mammary gland receptors for prolactin. The implication here is that the controlling factor in breastmilk output is the number of prolactin receptors rather than the amount of prolactin in serum. More receptors may result in more than adequate milk production, even in the presence of lower prolactin levels. This finding helps to explain why the infants of multiparous mothers begin gaining weight somewhat faster than do those of primiparous mothers.

Human Placental Lactogen (HPL). HPL is made by the placenta and is actively secreted into the maternal circulation from the second month of pregnancy. HPL reaches its maximum level (6,000 ng/ml) at term (Speroff, Glass, & Kase, 1989). As yet, the role of HPL in lactogenesis is not clear (Neville & Berga, 1983); because it is produced in such large amounts, it may have a lactogenic effect.

Cortisol. Cortisol, a main glucocorticoid, acts synergistically on the mammary system in the presence of prolactin (Neville & Berga, 1983). The final differentiation of the alveolar epithelial cell in a mature milk cell takes place because prolactin is present but only after prior exposure to cortisol and insulin. Glucocorticoids are hormones secreted by the adrenal glands and help to regulate water transport across the cell membranes during lactation.

Thyroid-Stimulating Hormone (TSH). Thyroid hormones promote mammary growth and lactation through a permissive rather than a regulatory role. Dawood et al. (1981) established a marked and significant increase in plasma TSH level on the third to fifth postpartum days.

Prolactin-Inhibiting Factor (PIF). PIF, a hypothalamic substance, either dopamine itself or mediated by dopamine, inhibits prolactin secretions (Diefenbach et al., 1976). Nipple stimulation suppresses PIF and dopamine, causing prolactin levels to rise and the breast to produce milk. Some drugs, such as phenothiazines and reserpine derivatives, increase breastmilk production because they also inhibit PIF (Bohnet & Kato, 1985).

Thyrotropin-Releasing Hormone (TRH). TRH is believed to increase TSH and prolactin levels. Therefore, TRH may play a role in the control of prolactin secretion. However, Gehlbach, Bayliss, and Rosa (1989) were unable to conclude that TRH had any role in the release of prolactin when they measured plasma prolactin and TSH responses to breastfeeding during the first postpartum month.

Milk Production

With closure of tight junctions in the cells of the alveoli and through the mediation of the hypothalamus, the alveolar cells respond with milk secretion at the base of the alveolar cell, where small droplets form and migrate through the cell membrane and into the alveolar ducts for storage, as shown by the ultrasound image in Figure 4–11. The rate of milk synthesis after each breastfeeding episode varies, ranging from 17 ml/hr to 33 ml/hr in one study (Arthur et al., 1989).

The highly vascularized secretory cells extract water, lactose, amino acids, fats, vitamins, minerals, and numerous other substances from the mother's blood, converting them to milk for her infant. Stores of adipose tissue laid down during pregnancy are drawn upon to provide substrate for milk synthesis (Agius & Williamson, 1980). When the milk "comes in" or rapidly increases in volume, creating breast fullness three to four days after birth, closure of the junctional complexes between the mammary alveolar cells prevents direct access of extracellular space to the lumen of the mammary alveoli (Neville et al., 1991). Thus sodium, chloride, and lactose concentrations are altered. At this point, lactation shifts from endocrine (hormone-driven) control to autocrine (milk removal–driven) control (Prentice et al., 1989).

Before this switch-over occurs, lactation is driven hormonally; after it occurs, lactation is driven by suckling and milk removal. It follows, then, that the amount of colostrum secreted by nonbreastfeeding women during the first few days postpartum is similar to that of breastfeeding women; however, this reverses abruptly after the first few days. Thus breastfeeding is not a major factor for the *initiation* of lactation, but it is essential for the *continuation* of lactation.

Galactopoiesis

The breast is not a passive container of milk but an organ of active production that is infant, rather than hormone-, driven. The removal of milk from the breasts facilitates continued milk production; conversely, lack of adequate milk removal or stasis tends to limit breastmilk synthesis in the breasts. It is the quantity and quality of infant suckling or milk removal that governs breastmilk synthesis. Milk production reflects the infant's appetite rather than the woman's ability to produce milk, which, in fact, can be severalfold higher (Daly & Hartmann, 1995). As long as milk is removed regularly from the breast, the alveolar cells will continue to secrete milk almost indefinitely (Vorherr, 1974). Conversely, women who had weaned their babies by eight weeks were much more likely than were mothers who were still breastfeeding at that time to report having experienced longer periods between each breastfeeding episode, to have used more supplements per day, and to have perceived that feedings (despite their lesser frequency) occurred "too often" (Humenick & Van Steenkiste, 1983).

This phenomenon, the *supply-demand response,* is a feedback control that regulates the production of milk to match the intake of the infant. A common adage that expresses this response is, "The more the mother breastfeeds, the more milk there will be" (La Leche League International, 1997, p. 70). Because lactation is an energy-intensive process, it makes teleological sense that there should be safeguards against wasteful overproduction as well as mechanisms for a prompt response to the infant's need.

A case of a new mother who became pregnant three months after having a pituitary resection supports the concept of autocrine control (De Coopman, 1993). After delivering a healthy infant, this mother had sufficient milk to completely sustain her baby by breastfeeding without supplementation. This unusual situation was attributable to the pituitary abscess which caused milk production to continue through her pregnancy after she weaned her first child; thus her milk yield postpar-

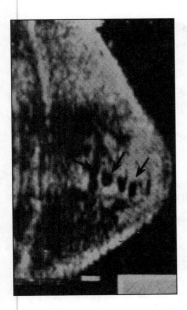

**FIGURE 4–11.
Ultrasound image
showing milk-filled
ducts.** *Mother lactating 10 months.
(From Division of
Ultrasound, Department of Radiology
and Department of
Pathology:* Atlas of
breast ultrasound.
*Philadelphia:
Thomas Jefferson
University Medical
College and Hospital,
1980:121.)*

tum was based on milk removal as much as on hormonal stimulation.

Oxytocin

In response to suckling, the posterior pituitary hormone oxytocin causes the milk-ejection reflex or *let-down,* a contraction of the myoepithelial cells surrounding the alveoli. Some women feel pressure and a tingling, warm sensation during milk ejection. Others, whose milk production is adequate, may not experience this sensation. The secreted milk is then ejected into the ductules and moved along to the lactiferous sinuses, where it becomes available to the newborn through the nipple openings.

Oxytocin plays a major role in the continuance of lactation. Oxytocin levels in the blood rise within one minute of breast stimulation, remain elevated during stimulation, and return to baseline levels within six minutes after cessation of nipple stimulation. This rise and fall of oxytocin levels continues at each feeding throughout the lactation course, even when the mother breastfeeds for an extended period (Leake et al., 1983). The posterior pituitary contains a surprisingly large store of oxytocin (3,000–9,000 mU) when compared with the amount required to elicit the ejection reflex (50–100 mU) (Lincoln & Paisley, 1982).

Oxytocin has another important function—to contract the mother's uterus. Uterine contractions help to control postpartum bleeding and to aid in uterine involution. The uterus not only contracts during breastfeeding but continues to contract rhythmically for as long as 20 minutes after the feeding. These cramps may be painful during the first few days postpartum. After involution is complete, however, these rhythmical pulsations may be a source of pleasure to the mother (Riordan & Rapp, 1980). Oxytocin also has peripheral effects, notably dilation of peripheral vascular beds and increased blood flow without increased systemic arterial pressure. As a result, breastfeeding is accompanied by increased skin temperature not unlike that of a menopausal hot flash (Marshall, Cumming, & Fitzsimmons, 1992). New mothers often report an increase in thirst while breastfeeding, which appears to be closely related to the increase in plasma oxytocin (James et al., 1995).

Through oxytocin mediation, these afferent pathways become so well established that let-down can occur even when the mother merely thinks of her baby. There are many anecdotal reports of spontaneous lactation in mothers who have weaned or who have never breastfed. In contrast, stress or emotional upheaval can potentially inhibit the let-down reflex and prolactin levels, making less milk available to the infant (Newton & Newton, 1948). Milk synthesis is a complex interplay of the hypothalamic-pituitary-gonadal axis that is susceptible to stress. Chemically, stress and fear release adrenaline at the level of the mammary gland and noradrenaline within the central nervous system. Both can potentially inhibit the milk-ejection reflex (Lincoln & Paisley, 1982).

Whitworth's (1988) review emphasizes that prolactin is essential for both initiating and maintaining milk production. Although oxytocin appears to be keyed more closely to milk ejection, in the absence of prolactin, milk is not made. Whitworth's discussion ends (p. 183) with the simple observation that "lactation . . . is controlled by the young, who in turn receive the benefits of milk secretion" (Fig. 4–12).

The influence of supplemental feedings on oxytocin and prolactin peaks was measured by Johnstone and Amico (1986). These investigators found that mothers who were not providing additional formula feedings to their infants had higher oxytocin levels over time than did women who were giving their babies supplemental feedings. The nonsupplementing women's oxytocin levels not only remained higher but also tended to climb over time, so that their oxytocin levels were higher at 15–24 weeks than they were at earlier periods (2–4 weeks and 5–14 weeks). In sharp contrast, the oxytocin levels of the mothers who were supplementing were lower at all times examined, and no rise in oxytocin peaks was noted over time. In both of these groups of women, prolactin levels tended to decline over time. Among mothers who were not supplementing, however, prolactin levels were consistently higher at all times examined. These data suggest that over time prolactin levels can be expected to fall, but oxytocin levels will continue to climb. However, when a mother supplements with formula-feedings, prolactin levels decline markedly and fall even further over time, and oxytocin levels remain depressed and do not climb.

Galactorrhea

Galactorrhea is the spontaneous secretion of milk from the breast under nonphysiological circumstances. Small amounts of milk or serous fluid commonly are expressed for weeks, months, or years from women who have previously been pregnant or lactating. Many anecdotal reports of spontaneous lactation present an intriguing enigma. For example, one pediatrician suddenly began lactating after the death of her six-week-old infant whom she had not breastfed. Along with full breasts and dripping milk, she experienced uterine cramping. Thyrotoxicosis (Lawrence, 1994), certain drugs (reserpine, methlydopa, phenothiazines), and the use of intrauterine devices containing copper (Horn & Scott, 1969) can trigger abnormal milk secretion.

Surprisingly, only 30 percent of women with galactorrhea have higher-than-normal prolactin levels (Frantz, Kleinberg, & Noel, 1972); these women are otherwise healthy and have no history of menstrual irregularity or infertility. It is suggested that these women may be overly sensitive to normal circulating prolactin levels (Friesen &

Cowden, 1989). For other women, galactorrhea is a symptom of a larger problem of hyperprolactinemia; in addition to a spontaneous milk secretion, they may also complain of amenorrhea, difficulty in becoming pregnant, and lack of libido. Any woman with persistent galactorrhea should be referred to a physician for a thorough physical examination and biochemical assessment.

Clinical Implications: Mother

Breast Assessment

Usually little attention is given to prenatal assessment of the breast and nipples because of Western cultural inhibitions about the breast and physicians' lack of recognition of its importance. As a consequence, after giving birth, mothers may experience feeding difficulties that could have been prevented. Nurses and lactation consultants practicing as primary caregivers are the ideal people to perform a prenatal breast assessment, particularly because physicians (especially males) are often reluctant to do so.

Ideal for teaching as well as for data gathering, physical assessment of the breast and nipples includes both inspection and palpation. While one is assessing the breasts, the following observations and questions are relevant.

Inspection. Size, symmetry, and shape of the breasts proper have minimal effect on lactation. The assessment provides the opportunity to reassure the woman with small breasts that she will be able to breastfeed and have a sufficient supply of milk. Asymmetry of breast size is usually normal, but *marked* asymmetry may be an indication of inadequate glandular tissue in a small minority of women. Inadequate glandular tissue might prevent the mother from exclusively breastfeeding her baby; however, she can continue to enjoy the breastfeeding relationship if she provides the baby with additional nutrition while feeding from the breast (Neifert, Seacat, & Jobe, 1985).

For the woman with large breasts, discussing the importance of a support bra and where such a bra may be obtained is helpful. Holding and feed-

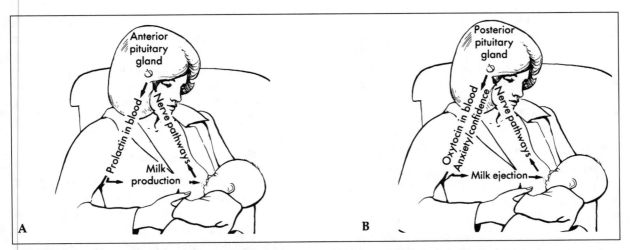

FIGURE 4–12. (A) Release and effect of prolactin on milk ejection. (B) Release and effect of oxytocin.

ing her infant will not be the same for the large-breasted woman as for mothers with average-sized breasts. Instead of simply holding the breast, the mother with large breasts may need to lift her breast and to hold or push part of the breast back to permit her infant to grasp the nipple and maintain an adequate airway. During this prenatal discussion, the mother may talk about some of her deeper feelings about having large breasts and her decision to breastfeed.

The skin of the breast should be inspected for any deviations. Skin turgor and elasticity can be assessed by gently pinching the skin, although the effect of elasticity on lactation is questionable: women who have been pregnant before have more elastic skin because it has been stretched from a previous pregnancy; women pregnant for the first time have firmer tissue.

A lateral incision in the vicinity of the cutaneous branch of the fourth intercostal nerve (left breast, five o'clock position; right breast, seven o'clock position) made during breast augmentation or reduction surgery may mean severed innervation of the nipple and areola (Farina et al., 1980). Surgery on the breast, especially if it involves an incision at the areolar margin, is likely to interfere to some degree with milk production. However, even having undergone such surgery, most mothers still can breastfeed. Breast-reduction surgery, because of the greater likelihood of the movement and replacement of nipple tissue, is more likely

than augmentation surgery (Hurst, 1996) to negatively influence later lactation performance (Neifert et al., 1990). Scar tissue from injury should be evaluated for its effect on skin elasticity and the degree to which nerve reactivity may have been affected.

Note should also be taken of any skin thickening and dimpling of the breast or nipple tissue. Although rare in a woman of childbearing age, such a change could be an early sign of a tumor and should be referred promptly to a physician for evaluation.

Now is the time to ask, "Have your breasts grown during pregnancy?" Also inquire, "Have you experienced any tenderness and soreness?" An increase in breast size, swelling, and tenderness usually indicates adequately functioning breast tissue responsive to hormonal changes.

Next, the nipple should be carefully inspected. (For the purpose of this discussion, *nipple* will refer to the areola as well as the nipple shaft and pores.) If the nipples appear small, explain that the size of a woman's nipples is of secondary importance to their functional ability. Likewise, any nipple structural abnormality such as inversion should be assessed only in terms of its function.

The look of the breast does not dictate its ability to function. A case in point may be women who have sustained significant scarring from burns (see Color Plate 21) Second- and third-degree burns rarely extend so deeply into the parenchyma that they destroy the glandular tissue of the breast, even when the burns have occurred in adulthood. Significant scarring of the dermis and epidermis, however, may result in (1) reduced maternal sensation when the infant suckles, (2) minimal tissue elasticity, thus requiring the mother to alter the baby's position at the breast; and (3) reduced milk ejection if a nipple has been surgically reconstructed. Nevertheless, scar tissue on the breast or nipple does not, by itself, preclude breastfeeding.

Palpation. After thorough hand washing, the nurse or lactation consultant should assess the nipple by compressing or palpating the areola between the forefinger and the thumb just behind the base of the nipple (the pinch test). This action simulates the compression that occurs when the infant is at the breast. Because of possible nipple adhesions within the underlying connective tissue, a nipple that initially appears everted may retract inwardly on stimulation. Conversely, a nipple that appears flattened or inverted may, on palpation, evert; therefore, differentiation must be made between structure and function in assessing the nipples.

The classification of nipple function in Table 4–2 is suggested as a standard terminology. It must be emphasized that although many primigravidas (Hytten, 1954; Waller, 1957) have nipples that tend to retract during pregnancy, most evert easily by the end of pregnancy and do not interfere with breastfeeding. Thus nipple assessment should be performed periodically through the pregnancy to track changes and to inform the mother how her body is preparing to feed her baby.

Classification of Nipple Function

When the nipple is compressed using the pinch test, it responds in one of the ways identified in Figure 4–8. This response may reflect degree of function.

Flat or retracted nipples rarely cause breastfeeding problems because they may be treatable during pregnancy. Dysfunction may be present in one nipple while the other is perfectly normal, or it may be present in both nipples. Retraction or inversion can prevent the infant from effectively milking the lactiferous sinuses that lie beneath the areola. Retraction or simple inversion identified in early pregnancy, however, does not necessarily foretell later difficulty. The infant forms a teat not only from the nipple but from the surrounding breast tissue. When inversion is noted early in pregnancy, time is on the mother's side. As pregnancy progresses, hormonal changes increase the size and protractility of the nipples. The mother also has time to use interventions that help prevent subsequent feeding problems.

Early Frequent Feedings

Encouraging early and frequent breastfeeding is a simple, low-cost recommendation for breastfeeding initiation. If the infant is able to suckle effectively at the breast soon after birth, there is a direct relationship between the frequency and strength of suckling and subsequent availability of breastmilk. There appears to be an early window of opportunity for the infant's suckling to stimulate prolactin receptors (discussed earlier in this chapter), which in turn enhances milk production.

Salariya, Easton, and Cater (1978) found that both early initiation of breastfeeding and frequent feedings thereafter contributed to longer breastfeeding duration. In their study, the group most likely to be breastfeeding at 6 weeks and at 12 weeks had begun breastfeeding within 10 minutes of the baby's birth and continued to do so at 2-hourly intervals. The group least likely to be breastfeeding first breastfed 4 to 6 hours after delivery and continued breastfeeding thereafter only every 4 hours. The authors concluded that early suckling had a stronger influence than did increased frequency of suckling but that feeding every 2 hours helped to establish lactation sooner and to reduce the need for complementary feedings. They recommended putting the baby to the breast as soon as possible after delivery, followed by feedings every 2 hours thereafter until lactation was well established, after which feedings on demand should continue.

Finally, a basic knowledge of anatomy and physiology is put to valuable use when the lactation consultant or nurse translates basic concepts into easily understandable teaching materials. If a client understands that the reason for placing her baby as far back onto her areola as possible is because her milk is stored behind the nipple in "holding" containers (called *lactiferous sinuses*), then she will be more likely to do so. If a client realizes a stressful

Table 4–2

CLASSIFICATION OF NIPPLE FUNCTION

Protraction	Nipple moves forward; considered a normal functional response. No special interventions are needed.
Retraction	Instead of protracting, the nipple moves inward.
Minimal	An infant with a strong suck exerts sufficient pressure to pull the nipple forward. A weak or premature infant may have difficulties at first.
Moderate to severe	Nipple retracts to a level even with or behind the surrounding areola. Intervention is helpful to stretch the nipple outward and improve protractility.
Inversion	On visual inspection, all or part of the nipple is drawn inward within the folds of the areola.
Simple	The nipple moves outward to protraction with manual pressure or when cold (pseudoinversion).
Complete	The nipple does not respond to manual pressure because adhesions bind the nipple inward; very rarely there is congenital absence of the nipple.

environment may inhibit her milk supply, she may take action to reduce stressful situations over which she has control. If a woman understands that the reason she needs less covering when she breast-feeds is that she literally has hot flashes during feedings, she will take measures to "keep cool." Examples of the application of basic biological principles of maternal lactation are legion and form the basis of many of the chapters that follow.

The Infant

Infants perform a series of complex oral movements to obtain sufficient nutriment from their mother's breast to meet daily nutritional requirements and to support rapid growth, especially during the first few months of life. Suckling is a dynamic process, as the infant is continually adjusting to a changing anatomy. The act of suckling is far more than simply obtaining food. Bosma (1982) contends that "the infant's earliest autonomous functions are focused about his mouth and pharynx area, which is the principal site of interaction with his environment. The mouth is the cockpit of his awareness and of his most discriminate responses."

Newborn Oral Development

In the embryo, facial and pharyngeal regions develop from neural-crest cells at about the time of neural-tube closure. Further development is due to tissue differentiation from the endoderm, which later forms the digestive tract. During gestation, the fetus is able to swallow fluid as early as 11 weeks (Miller, 1982) and has a suck reflex at 24 weeks (Herbst, 1981). The rooting response and the link between sucking and swallowing is established by 32 weeks (Amiel-Tison, 1967; Bu'Lock et al., 1990). Although these abilities are present relatively early in fetal development, the combination of sucking, swallowing, and breathing is not well coordinated until about 37 weeks (Bu'Lock et al., 1990).

At birth, the infant's mouth is vertically short in comparison with that of the adult. There is so little room that when the newborn's mouth is closed, the tongue is in lateral contact with the gums and with the roof of the mouth. There are other proportional differences in size and shape between the infant and the adult skull (Figs. 4–13 and 4–14). The infant's lower jaw (mandible) is small and somewhat receded. Whereas the adult's hard palate is deeply arched and situated on a higher plane relative to the base of the skull, the infant's is short, wide, and only slightly arched at birth. Corrugated transverse folds (rugae) on the hard palate assist the newborn in holding the breast during suckling.

Because the infant's tongue fills the small oral cavity, the extent and the direction of tongue movement is limited. Taste buds on the tongue (mostly on the tongue tip) are present at birth, but the newborn has an increased suckling response only to sweet taste. The entire surface of the tongue is within the oral cavity. The infant's lips are well adapted to effect an airtight closure around the breast. The lips are partially everted so that the oral mucosa presents slightly externally; they have tiny swellings on the inner surface (eminences of the pars villosa) that facilitate holding the breast and areola in place (Ardran, Kemp, & Lind, 1958; Bosma & Showacre, 1975).

During the first year after birth, the lower jaw grows downward, creating a larger intraoral space. The tongue also gradually descends. By the fourth or fifth year of age, the tongue is attached directly to the epiglottis of the larynx. The frenulum is a fold of mucous membrane midline on the undersurface of the tongue that helps to anchor the tongue to the floor of the mouth. If the frenulum is too short to allow freedom of tongue movement or is placed too far forward to permit tongue extension upward or forward, it can interfere with an infant's ability to suckle (Notestine, 1990).

The infant's epiglottis lies just below the soft palate, unlike the adult's, as seen in Figure 4–14. This makes it possible for food to move laterally on the outside of the epiglottis and to pass directly into the esophagus. The epiglottis plays an important role by closing off the pathway to the lungs when the infant swallows. Such closure ensures that the milk will travel into the esophagus rather than into the trachea. Relative to an adult larynx, the infant larynx is much higher in the oral cavity and occupies a larger space. It is short and funnel-shaped (Crelin, 1973). As fluid passes through the mouth, the larynx elevates so that fluid can move easily into the pharynx. Because the larynx is high and elevated during swallowing, it depends much less on the action of the epiglottis and on closure of the vocal folds to protect the airway (Morris, 1982).The shape of the pharynx gradually changes as the child grows. At birth, the pharynx curves very gradually downward to join the oral cavity. This curvature would prevent articulate speech even if the necessary central nervous system linkage were present. By puberty, the posterior walls of the nasal and oral segments join almost at a right angle.

The infant has pads of fat on both cheeks to assist with suckling. Each pad is a circumscribed layer of fat enclosed within its own capsule of fibrous connective tissue. It lies between the buccinator and masseter muscles. It is thought that buccal fat pads provide stability for suckling and reduce the likelihood of collapsing of the cheeks and buccinator muscles between the gums. When babies suck their own tongues, the degree of negative pressure is such that drawing in of the cheeks occurs, creating a characteristic dimpling. Collapsing of the cheeks is more likely in a premature baby who lacks the layer of fat (including that in the cheeks) that gives full-term infants their characteristic plump facial appearance.

Suckling

The precise way in which infants use their oral and facial muscles to efficiently take in nourishment from their mothers' breasts is vital information for health professionals, because some breastfeeding infants have initial difficulty getting on the breast, and a few continue to have suckling dysfunction. In a remarkable study of spontaneous feeding behavior, infants were placed in a prone position between their mother's breasts after an unmedicated delivery. The infants began licking, suckling, and rooting movements after about 15 minutes, began hand-to-mouth movements after about 34 minutes, and spontaneously began to suckle after 55 minutes. Licking movements both precede and follow the rooting reflex in alert infants (Widstrom et al., 1987).

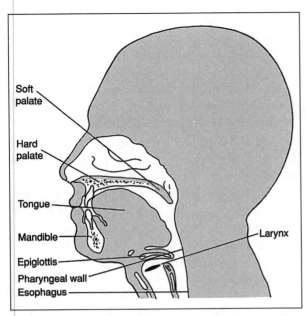

FIGURE 4–13. Midsagittal section of cranial and oral anatomy of an adult while swallowing.

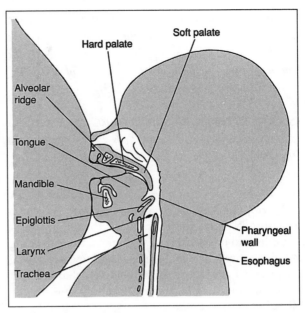

FIGURE 4–14. Midsagittal section of cranial and oral anatomy of an infant while swallowing.

The position of the neonate's tongue is critical to feeding. After the rooting stimulus, the infant opens the mouth wide (the *gape*), keeping the tongue at the bottom of the mouth. This tongue position enables the infant to "catch" the mother's nipple and attach to the breast without help. It is important to note that an infant places the tongue in the palate when crying, which might be a security reflex, to prevent obstruction of the trachea during the inspiration phase. Widstrom and Thingstrom-Paulsson (1993) postulate that forcing a crying baby to the breast might cause the infant to place the tongue in his or her palate, a defensive response that inhibits suckling and disturbs the rooting-tongue reflex system.

In the literature *sucking* and *suckling* are not distinguished, both terms being used interchangeably to refer to suckling. In this text, we too use these terms interchangeably, though some individuals feel strongly about the distinction (Montagu, 1979, pp. 190–191):

The baby is said to "suck" at its mother's nipple. The baby knows better than to do anything so foolish, for were he to "suck" the nipple all he would, for the most part, succeed in achieving would be to pro- *duce a partial vacuum in his mouth and fail to develop the ability to suckle properly. A baby sucks at the nozzle on the top of a bottle, but at the mother's breast a baby suckles.*

Does the infant suckle or suck at the breast? Traditionally, the baby sucked and the mother suckled. When breastfeeding fell out of favor in the United States, so did the word *suckle* because mothers were no longer suckling. Yet the word has not been out of use for so long that we have completely forgotten it. It lingers at the fringes of our collective memory, although we are not quite sure of its meaning. Now that breastfeeding is a more visible activity, and we have discovered that the mechanism by which babies extract milk from the breast differs considerably from the method that they use on a bottle teat, we urge adoption of separate words to differentiate the two acts. The word *suckle* seems ideal for breastfeeding, and it has come to be used in this sense in modern American breastfeeding literature. However, this term still retains its original meaning in the breastfeeding literature of many of the British Commonwealth countries. *The Oxford English Dictionary* (1961) defines the two terms thus:

Suck: *(1) the action or an act of sucking milk from the breast; the milk or other fluid sucked at one time (p. 89); (2) to apply the lips to a teat, breast, the mother, nurse, or dam, for the purpose of extracting milk from, with the mouth (p. 90).*

Suckle: *(1) transitive. To give suck to; to nurse (a child) at the breast; (2) to cause to take milk from the breast or udder; to put to suck (p. 94).*

Physical therapy literature in the United States has adopted *suckling* to denote action to obtain breastmilk by an infant younger than four to six months and the word *sucking* to mean breastfeeding after that time. The shift in terminology, according to physical therapists, highlights the changes that occur in the infant's use of the mouth and tongue after the early months of life. *Suckling* describes the early stripping action of the areola and breast when tongue peristalsis moves from front to back. Morris (1982) calls it "a lick type of suck." As the first midyear of life approaches, the oral space changes, both structurally and while the infant feeds. The oral cavity elongates vertically so that it is more spacious. The palate and epiglottis are no longer in apposition. The infant's tongue begins to elevate and to acquire a forward-backward movement; it is now possible for the infant to accept solid foods without choking. By six months, the baby's lips become more functional, the neurological system matures, and the infant is able to make a variety of sounds (Morris, 1982).

Some experienced clinicians disagree with this view, arguing that the infant's sucking pattern on the breast does not change over time. Instead, these clinicians believe that as infants develop, they become more versatile and develop a much wider repertoire of oral abilities, including the ability to carry a bolus of food from the front of the mouth to the back and to swallow it, although they suck (or suckle) the same way that they always have.

Babies suckle and swallow at a frequency of about once per second or faster when breastmilk is actively flowing. This rate is similar to that of other primates. If the milk flow lessens or stops, the infant will increase this rate to about two suckles per second (Wolff, 1968). In other words, when the milk flow increases, the rate of suckling decreases.

Conversely, when milk flow is low, the rate of suckling is higher. Inch and Garforth (1989, p. 1362) describe the suckling rhythm as follows:

When the baby first goes to the breast, short fast bursts of sucking can be observed. During this period no milk is flowing and unrelieved suction is applied to the surface of the nipple. Once the milk begins to flow it fills the oral cavity and relieves the negative pressure. As soon as this happens, the sucking pattern changes, and long, slow, continuous, sucking supervenes. Very little milk transfer is necessary to cause the shift away from short, fast, continuous suckling.

Drewett and Woolridge (1979) observed that suckling rates fluctuate at different stages of the feeding and that the suckling rates are greater than that reported by Wolff (1968). These authors reported a rate of 72.4 sucks per minute during the first two minutes of feeding. This rate drops at two to four minutes to 70.8 sucks per minute and increases again to 73.3 and 74.9 sucks per minute at four to seven and seven to ten minutes, respectively.

In addition to yielding milk and calories, suckling facilitates feelings of calm, reduces heart rate and metabolic rate, and elevates the pain threshold (Blass, 1994). Wolff (1968) originally defined two categories of suckling: nutritive (full and continuous milk flow) and nonnutritive (alternating suckling bursts and rests during minimal milk intake). Bowen-Jones, Thompson, and Drewett (1982) challenged the validity of these two categories. The latter study showed that breastfeeding babies *always* suckle in bursts, with resting periods between bursts. If these resting periods are long and only a small amount of milk is transferred, we call it *comfort nursing.* The term *nonnutritive suckling* is now accepted to mean either spontaneous suckling in the absence of anything being introduced into the infant's mouth (common during sleep) or suckling as prompted by something that is not a liquid nutriment (e.g., a pacifier) being introduced into the infant's mouth (McBride & Danner, 1987).

Nonnutritive suckling has important implications for development, especially under special circumstances such as prematurity. Measel and Anderson (1979) examined the effect of nonnutritive suckling in premature infants and discovered that it increases peristalsis, enhances secretion of digestive fluids, and decreases crying in these infants. For more information about premature infant suckling patterns, see Chapter 14.

Several clinicians have examined the suckling process in great detail. With the advent of ultrasonography and other technologies, it is now possible to accurately quantify suckling patterns, replacing earlier descriptions that inferred only what actually occurred. When infants feed from both breasts, milk transfer from the second breast decreases by 58 percent as compared with the first breast, even though there are no significant changes in suckling pressure (Prieto et al., 1996). Detailed descriptions of infant suckling mechanics have been described by Morris (1982), Marmet and Shell (1984), Woolridge (1986), McBride and Danner (1987), and Smith et al. (1985). Figure 4–15 illustrates suckling movements. The following description of functional suckling at the breast is based on the work of these investigators:

1. The nipple and its surrounding areola and underlying breast tissue are drawn deeply into the infant's mouth; then the infant's lips and cheeks form a seal. The infant's lips are flanged outward around the mother's breast and are minimally involved.

2. The tip of the infant's tongue is maintained behind the lower lip and over the lower gum while the rest of the anterior tongue cups the areola of the breast.

3. During the feeding, the mother's highly elastic nipple elongates to two to three times its resting length into a teat by suction created within the baby's mouth. The nipple extends back as far as the posterior tongue junction between the hard and soft palates. At its base, the nipple is held between the upper gum and tongue that covers the lower gum. The mother's nipple and areolar tissue undergo extensive changes during feeding.

4. The jaw moves the tongue up, compressing the maternal areola against the infant's alveolar ridge, which causes milk to be expressed from the lactiferous sinuses into the infant's mouth.

5. As the anterior portion of the tongue is raised, the posterior tongue is depressed and retracted in undulating or peristaltic motions, forming a groove that channels the milk to the back of the oral cavity where it stimulates receptors that initiate the swallowing reflex. This backward movement produces a negative pressure, similar to withdrawing a piston in an airtight syringe.

6. If the volume of milk taken is sufficient to trigger swallowing, the back of the tongue elevates and presses against the posterior pharyngeal wall. The soft palate rises and closes off the nasal passageways. The larynx then moves up and forward to close the trachea, propelling the milk into the esophagus. Afterward, the larynx returns to its previous position.

7. The infant lowers the jaw, the lactiferous sinuses refill, and a new cycle begins. A rhythm is created by this sequence of vertical jaw movements and the depression and elevation of the posterior tongue. Each suck sequence is followed by a swallow. McBride and Danner (1987, pp. 111–112) describe the normal suck-swallow pattern:

As milk in the sinuses is depleted, several sucking sequences may occur before each swallow. The sucking-swallowing sequence is repeated approximately once per second in continuous fashion as long as milk is present and the infant is hungry. If the first one or two sucking sequences do not yield a palatable liquid, the normal infant will open and close his mouth in a tremorlike movement. The rapid jaw movement and the infant's tongue and lips stimulate tactile nerve endings in the mother's areola, initiating the release of oxytocin from her pituitary gland.

There are profound differences between bottle-feeding and breastfeeding, as shown in Table 4–3. Generally, compared with bottle-feeding, breastfeeding infants suckle more times per day and maintain a higher level of oxygen pressure and

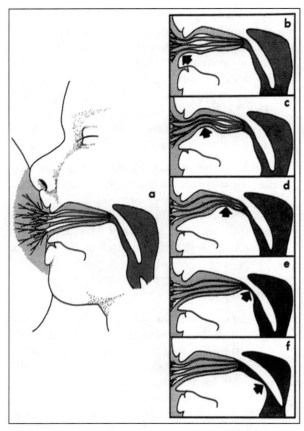

FIGURE 4–15. Complete suck cycle. *The baby is shown in median section. The baby exhibits good feeding technique: the nipple is drawn well into the mouth, extending back to the junction of the hard and soft palate (the lactiferous sinuses are depicted within the teat, although these cannot be visualized on scans).*

a. 'Teat' is formed from the nipple and much of the areola, with the lacteal sinuses, which lie behind the nipple, being drawn into the mouth with the breast tissue. The soft palate is relaxed and the nasopharynx is open for breathing. The shape of the tongue at the back represents its position at rest, cupped around the tip of the nipple.

b. The suck cycle is initiated by a welling up of the anterior tip of the tongue. At the same time, the lower jaw, which has been momentarily relaxed (not shown) is raised to constrict the base of the nipple, thereby 'pinching off' milk within the ducts of the teat (these movements are inferred as they lie outside the sector viewed in ultrasound scans).

c. The wave of compression by the tongue moves along the underside of the nipple in a posterior direction, pushing against the hard palate. This roller-like action squeezes milk from the nipple. The posterior portion of the tongue may be depressed as milk collects in the oropharynx.

d. & e. The wave of compression passes back past the tip of the nipple and pushes against the soft palate. As the tongue impinges on the soft palate, the levator muscles of the palate contract, raising it to seal off the nasal cavity. Milk is pushed into the oropharynx and is swallowed if sufficient has collected.

f. The cycle of compression continues and ends at the posterior base of the tongue. Depression of the back portion of the tongue creates negative pressure, drawing the nipple and its milk contents once more into the mouth. This is accompanied by a lowering of the jaw, which allows milk to flow back into the nipple.

In ultrasound scans it appears that compression by the tongue, and negative pressure within the mouth, maintain the tongue in close conformation to the nipple and palate. Events are portrayed here rather more loosely to aid clarity. (From Woolridge, MW: The 'anatomy' of infant sucking. Midwifery 2:164-71, 1986.)

skin temperature (Mathew, 1988; Meier & Anderson, 1987). The differences between bottle-feeding and breastfeeding of premature infants are even greater. Meier and Pugh (1985, p. 398) describe these differences after viewing videotapes of premature infants nursing at the breast and feeding from a bottle:

For example, the infants had to open their mouths more widely to breastfeed than to bottle feed. Once they became accustomed to making this adjustment during breastfeeding, they attempted to do it while bottle feeding. As a result, wide gaps could be seen between the commercial nipple and an infant's mouth during bottle feedings, and "smacking" sounds could be heard while the infant was sucking.

Suckling patterns of premature infants are described in depth in Chapter 14. Marked differences are also noted in sucking patterns of bottle-fed preterm infants as compared to full-term infants, in terms of the maximum pressure exerted during sucking, the duration of each suck, the number of sucks per burst, and the volume of formula consumed per suck (Medoff-Cooper et al., 1989).

Breathing and Suckling

In a normal, coordinated, nutritive suckling cycle, swallowing does not inhibit respiration, and breathing appears to continue throughout the suckling cycle (Morris, 1982), despite the assertion of Ardran, Kemp, and Lind (1958) that at the onset of the swallow, as the bulk of the bolus enters the pharynx, airflow is momentarily interrupted and then restored. In a perfectly coordinated cycle of suckling, swallowing, and breathing, breathing movements appear to be related in a 1:1:1 sequence (Bu'Lock et al., 1990; Weber et al., 1986; Wolff, 1968). During uncoordinated feedings, however, breathing is interrupted by swallowing and may be subordinate to it (Halverson, 1944; Johnson & Salisbury, 1977; Logan & Bosma, 1976).

Although suckling, swallowing, and breathing are generally well coordinated during a feeding, infant cyanosis is a relatively common event, especially in neonates. The neonate almost always recovers spontaneously (Mathew, 1988) and often continues to suck and swallow despite cyanosis. Oxygen saturation in the feeding infant normally declines. Mean levels drop from 96 percent (during feeding) to 93 percent (postfeeding) in breastfed infants and from 95 percent (during feeding) to 92 percent (postfeeding) in bottle-fed infants (Hammerman & Kaplan, 1995).

Unless hypoxic, the newborn is an obligate nose breather, owing in part to the positioning of the soft palate and to the lack of space in the mouth through which air can travel in and out (Morris, 1982). Although it is true that babies have ventilatory problems when the nasal passages are occluded, an infant is capable of breathing through the mouth when necessary (Rodenstein et al., 1985).

Clinical Implications: Infant

The ability to suckle, even in many full-term infants, is not fully developed at birth or can be inhibited by drugs given to the mother during childbirth. Usually after several attempts, the infant latches onto the breast and begins to suckle vigorously and effectively. These first feedings are critical because they imprint a suckling pattern that tends to be repeated in subsequent feedings. A healthy infant unaffected by labor or birth analgesia or anesthesia should be allowed to demonstrate hunger before being offered the breast. She or he is capable of attaching to the nipple with little assistance. Forcing the infant to the breast might abolish the rooting reflex and disturb placement of the tongue (Widstrom & Thingstrom-Paulsson, 1993).

Breastfeeding Assessment

Consistent assessment of breastfeedings and identification of early problems so that they can be resolved before they worsen are essential in a hospital environment. Breastfeeding assessment tools are only just being developed, and health professionals do not yet agree on the components that compose effective breastfeeding. Not until 1994, with the work of Meier et al. (1994), was it discovered that the use of clinical clues to estimate the amount of breastmilk ingested by an infant did not accurately indicate intake for preterm infants. Riordan and Koehn (1997) tested the reliability of three tools developed by nurses and lactation consultants for systematically assessing and scoring feedings at the breast: the Infant Breastfeeding Assessment Tool (IBFAT), the Mother-Baby Assessment Tool (MBA), and the LATCH. (These tools are available for use with permission from their creators.)* The results of this study showed that these tools are not sufficiently reliable as they are now written and that further work is warranted.

Suckling Assessment

The infant's first few breastfeedings should be observed early in the neonatal period. Such observation enables the health care worker to determine how well the infant roots, fixes or latches on, and suckles the breast. Minor adjustments of maternal position or infant position can be made without interrupting or interfering with the mother and infant as they begin to learn how to breastfeed together.

---

*See assessment tools in Auerbach KG, Riordan J, Resource Guide to Accompany Breastfeeding and Human Lactation, *Boston: Jones & Bartlett, 1996.*

Table 4–3

COMPARISONS BETWEEN BREASTFEEDING AND BOTTLE-FEEDING IN FULL-TERM INFANTS

Breastfeeding	Bottle-feeding	References

More frequent suckling/min
    Continuous suckling = 88
    Intermittent suckling = 80
	Less frequent suckling/min
	    Continuous suckling = 63
	    Intermittent suckling = 58
		Mathew, 1988

Breathing patterns
    Shortening of expiration
    Prolonging of inspiration
	Breathing patterns
	    Prolonged expiration
	    Shortening of inspiration
		Mathew, 1988

Oxygen saturation < 90%
    2 of 10 infants
	Oxygen saturation < 90%
	    5 of 10 infants
		Mathew, 1988

Bradycardia
    0 of 10 infants
	Bradycardia
	    2 of 10 infants
		Mathew, 1988

Extended opening of mouth to grasp mother's nipple	Less extension to grasp rubber teat	Maher, 1988
Infant's lips flanged outward, relaxed and resting against the breast to make a seal	Lips closer together and pursed to maintain contact with rubber teat	McBride & Danner, 1987
Extensive mandibular (jaw) action	Minimal mandibular action	Maher, 1988
Tongue grooved around nipple; remains under nipple throughout feed; moves in peristaltic action from front to back	Tongue upward and thrust forward against end of teat, "piston-like," to control milk flow	Woolridge, 1986; Marmet and Shell, 1984; Weber, Woolridge, and Baum, 1986
Silent, except for soft swallow sounds, and (in older infants), cooing or "singing" sounds of pleasure	High-pitched squeak at end of intake of air prior to new suck	
Duration of feeding varies from short (few minutes) to long (30 minutes or longer)	Duration of feeding is usually 5–10 minutes	Ardran et al., 1958
Includes nutritive and non-nutritive suckling throughout the feeding but less distinct differences	Involves nearly exclusively nutritive suckling	Woolridge, 1986

If the infant cannot suckle the breast at all after several attempts, a visual evaluation and a digital examination of the infant's mouth may be appropriate. The roof of the mouth should be wide and gently domed. The tongue should be long enough to extend over the lower gum line but not so long that it protrudes past the lips. The baby's response to a featherlight stroking of the center of the lower lip should be noted. In most cases, the alert infant will open the mouth wide and the tongue will come forward in response to such stimulation, as if seeking its source. The infant's frenulum (the small tissue tag under the tongue) should be far enough away from the tip of the tongue to prevent stricture during suckling. If the frenulum appears tight, a visual examination should be performed to determine whether the frenulum prevents the tongue from elevating or extending sufficiently to produce the wavelike motion necessary for effective suckling (Marmet et al., 1990).

A finger slid into the baby's mouth should identify the hard palate as being intact. The tongue should groove around the finger. When the pad of the finger lightly touches the palate, the baby usually initiates a suck response that includes stroking by the tongue on the underside of the finger from knuckle to nail edge. In a healthy newborn, the strength of oral negative pressure is such that the examiner will feel as if the nailbed is being pulled deeper into the baby's mouth. The nature of the suckling action should be rhythmic, although some neonates quickly realize that the finger does not reward suckling and so they cease doing so after several attempts. Others, unfortunately, may become "hooked" on receiving nutriment in this manner and refuse the breast.

Because the finger is not a breast, with its soft areolar and nipple tissue, suckling at the breast should be the first experience of the infant. Thereafter, a finger assessment may be attempted, although it is not necessary in most cases and should be used judiciously.

Even if the baby is found to have an anatomical variation, such variation may not interfere with effective suckling. However, any infant with a cleft palate, a high palatal arch, or a short tongue may require interventions, most often provided by a health care team (physician, physical therapist, and speech therapist), before he or she can suckle. Marmet and Shell (1984) and McBride and Danner (1987) describe sequential steps to assist when dysfunctional suckling is identified.

SUMMARY

Knowledge of maternal breast anatomy and the psychophysiology of lactation are necessary antecedents to clinical practice. The fundamental biological principles of lactation discussed in this section are used, although not always consciously, in almost every clinical situation in which lactation is involved. Knowledge of the structure and function of the normal breast and of infant suckling are necessary for appropriate assessment; knowing what is normal must precede recognizing the abnormal and recommending actions designed to support an optimal breastfeeding experience. Enabling the natural physiological mechanisms to function optimally is more likely to lead to an uncomplicated breastfeeding experience; interference with these mechanisms can result in difficulty with breastfeeding for mother and infant.

At the same time, anatomy and physiology are the building blocks in a larger picture of the breastfeeding and lactation experience. Physiologically most women are equipped to produce sufficient milk for their infant or infants. Yet the most commonly cited problem in breastfeeding worldwide is the mother's perception that she has insufficient milk (Hill & Humenick, 1989). Social and cultural influences play a major role in the mother's perceptions of her ability to nourish her infant from her breasts. Succeeding chapters will explore the myriad of social, cultural, and psychological aspects of breastfeeding.

REFERENCES

Agius OL, Williamson DH: Lipogenesis in interscapular brown adipose tissue of virgin, pregnant, and lactating rats. *Biochem J* 190:447, 1980.

Alexander JM, Grant AM, Campbell: Randomized controlled trial of breast shells and Hoffman's exercises for inverted and non-protractile nipples. *Br Med J* 304:1030-2, 1992.

Amiel-Tison C: Neurological evaluation of the maturity of newborn infant. *Arch Dis Child* 43:89, 1967.

Ardran GM, Kemp MB, Lind J: A cineradiographic study of breast feeding. *Br J Radiol* 31:156–62, 1958.

Arthur PG, et al: Measuring short-term rates of milk synthesis in breast-feeding mothers. *Q J Exp Physiol* 74:419–28, 1989.

Baron JA, et al: Cigarette smoking and prolactin in women. *Br Med J* 293:482, 1986.

Battin D, et al: Effect of suckling on serum prolactin, luteinizing hormone, follicle-stimulating hormone, and estradiol during prolonged lactation. *Obstet Gynecol* 65:785–8, 1985.

Berman MA, Davis, GD: Lactation from axillary breast tissue in the absence of a supernummeray nipple: a case report. *J Reprod Med* 39:657–9, 1994.

Blaikeley J, et al: Breastfeeding–factors affecting success. *J Obstet Gynaecol Br Em*p 60:657–9, 1953.

Blass EM: Behavioral and physiological consequences of suckling in rat and human newborns. *Acta Paediatr Suppl* 397:71–6, 1994.

Bohnet HG, Kato K: Prolactin secretion during pregnancy and puerperium: response to metoclopramide and interactions with placental hormones. *Obstet Gynecol* 65:789–92, 1985.

Bonnar J, et al: Effect of breast-feeding on pituitary-ovarian function after childbirth. *Br Med J* 4:82–4, 1975.

Bosma J: Form and function in the infant's mouth and pharynx. In: Bosma J, ed. *Third symposium on oral sensation and perception*. Springfield, IL: Thomas, 1982:3–29.

Bosma J, Showacre J: *Development of upper respiratory anatomy and function*. Rockville, MD: U.S. Department of Health, Education and Welfare, 1975:5–49.

Bowen-Jones A, Thompson C, Drewett RF: Milk flow and sucking rates during breast-feeding. *Dev Med Child Neurol* 24:626–33, 1982.

Bu'Lock F, Woolridge MW, Baum JD: Development of coordination of sucking, swallowing and breathing: ultrasound study of term and preterm infants. *Dev Med Child Neurol* 32:669–78, 1990.

Chao S: The effect of lactation on ovulation and fertility. *Clin Perinatol* 14(1):39–49, 1987.

Clemente CD: *Anatomy: a regional atlas of the human body*. Philadelphia: Lea & Febiger, 1978.

Courtiss EH, Goldwyn RM: Breast sensation before and after plastic surgery. *Plast Reconstr Surg* 58:1–12, 1976.

Cox DB, Owens RA, Hartmann PE: Blood and milk prolactin and the rate of milk synthesis in women. *Exp Physiol* 81:1007–20, 1996.

Crelin ES: *Functional anatomy of the newborn*. New Haven, CT: Yale University Press, 1973:27–33.

Dabelow A: Die Milchdruse. In: Bargmann W, ed. *Handbuch der Mikroskopischen Anatomic des Menschen*, vol. 3, part 3: Haut und sinnes organs. Berlin: Springer-Verlag, 1957:277–85.

Daly SEJ, Hartmann PE: Infant demand and milk supply. Part 1: Infant demand and milk production in lactating women. *J Hum Lact* 11:21–3, 1995.

Daly SEJ, Owens RA, Hartmann PE: The short-term synthesis and infant-regulated removal of milk in lactating women. *Exp Physiol* 78:209–20, 1993.

Dawood MY, et al: Oxytocin release and plasma anterior pituitary and gonadal hormones in women during lactation. *J Clin Endocrinol Metab* 52:678–83, 1981.

Dawson EK: A histological study of the normal mamma in relation to tumour growth: 1. Early development to maturity. *Edinb Med J* 41:653–82, 1934.

DeCarvalho MD, et al: Effect of frequent breast-feeding on early milk production and infant weight gain. *Pediatrics* 72:307–11, 1983.

De Coopman J: Breastfeeding after pituitary resection: support for a theory of autocrine control of milk supply? *J Hum Lact* 9:35–40, 1993.

Diefenbach WP, et al: Suppression of prolactin secretion by L-dopa in the stalk-sectioned rhesus monkey. *J Clin Endocrinol Metab* 43:638, 1976.

Division of Ultrasound, Department of Radiology and Department of Pathology. *Atlas of breast ultrasound*. Philadelphia: Thomas Jefferson University Medical College and Hospital, 1980:121.

Drewett RF, Woolridge M: Sucking patterns of human babies on the breast. *Early Hum Dev* 315:315–21, 1979.

Edgerton MT, McClary AR: Augmentation mammaplasty with special reference to use of polyvinyl alcohol sponge (Ivalon). Psychiatric implications and surgical indications. *Plast Reconstr Surg* 21:279, 1958.

Farina MA, Newby BG, Alani HM: Innervation to the nipple-areola complex. *Plast Reconstr Surg* 66(4):497–501, 1980.

Frantz A, Kleinberg DL, Noel G: Studies on prolactin in man. *Recent Prog Horm Res* 28:527–34, 1972.

Friesen HG, Cowden EA: Lactation and galactorrhea. In: DeGroot LJ: *Endocrinology in pregnancy.* Philadelphia: Saunders, 1989:2074–86.

Gehlbach DL, Bayliss P, and Rosa C: Prolactin and thyrotropin responses to nursing during the early puerperium. *J Reprod Med* 34(4):295–98, 1989.

Gross BA, Eastman DJ: Prolactin secretion during prolonged lactation amenorrhoea. *Aust NZ J Obstet Gynaecol* 19:95–9, 1979.

Gross B, et al: A cross-cultural comparison of prolactin secretion in long-term lactation. *Prog Reprod Biol* 6:179–86, 1980.

Halverson HM: Mechanisms of early infant feeding. *J Genet Psychol* 64:185–223, 1944.

Hammerman C, Kaplan M. Oxygen saturation during and after feeding in healthy term infants. *Biol Neonate* 67:94–9, 1995.

Herbst JJ: Development of suck and swallowing. In: Lebenthal E, ed. *Textbook of gastroenterology and nutrition in infancy,* vol. 1. New York: Plenum, 1981: 97–107.

Hill PD, Humenick SS: Insufficient milk supply. *Image* 21:145–8, 1989.

Hinds LA, Tyndale-Biscoe CH: Prolactin in the marsupial *Macropus engenii* during the estrous cycle, pregnancy, and lactation. *Biol Reprod* 26:391–8, 1982.

Horn HW, Scott JM: IUD insertion and galactorrhea. *Fertil Steril* 20:400–4, 1969.

Humenick SS: the clinical significance of breast-milk maturation rates. *Buth* 14:174–9, 1987.

Humenick SS, Van Steenkiste S: Early indicators of breast-feeding progress. *Issues Comp Pediatr Nurs* 6:205–15, 1983.

Hurst N: Lactation after augmentation mammoplasty. *Obstet Gynecol* 87:30–4, 1996.

Hytten FE: Clinical and chemical studies in lactation: IX. Breastfeeding in hospital. *Br Med J* 18:1447–52, 1954.

Hytten FE, Baird D: The development of the nipple in pregnancy. *Lancet* 1:1201–4, 1958 (June 7).

Inch S, Garforth S: Establishing and maintaining breastfeeding. In: Chalmers I, Enkin M, Keirse M, eds. *Effective care in pregnancy and childbirth.* Oxford: Oxford University Press, 1989:1359–74.

James RJA, et al: Thirst induced by a suckling episode during breast feeding and its relation with plasma vasopressin, oxytocin and osmoregulation. *Clin Endocrinol* 43:277–82, 1995.

Johnson P, Salisbury DM: Preliminary studies on feeding and breathing in the newborn. In: Weiffenbach JM, ed. *Taste and development: the genesis of sweet preference.* Department of Health, Education, and Welfare, publ. no. (NIH)77-1068. Bethesda, MD: National Institutes of Health, 1977.

Johnstone JM, Amico JA: A prospective longitudinal study of the release of oxytocin and prolactin in response to infant suckling in long term lactation. *J Clin Endocrinol Metab* 62:653–7, 1986.

Kopans DB: *Breast imaging.* Philadelphia: Lippincott, 1989:20.

La Leche League International: *The womanly art of breastfeeding,* 6th ed. Schaumberg, IL: La Leche League, 1997.

Lawrence RA: *Breastfeeding: a guide for the medical profession.* St Louis: Mosby, 1994.

Leake R, et al: Oxytocin and prolactin responses in long-term breast-feeding. *Obstet Gynecol* 62:565–8, 1983.

Lincoln DW, Paisley AC: Neuroendocrine control of milk ejection. *J Reprod Fertil* 65:571–86, 1982.

Logan WJ, Bosma JF: Oral and pharyngeal dysphagia in infancy. *Pediatr Clin North Am* 14:47–61, 1976.

Love SM, Lindsey K: *Dr. Susan Love's breast book.* Reading, MA: Addison-Wesley, 1990:3–20.

Marmet C, Shell E: Training neonates to suck correctly. *MCN* 9:401–7, 1984.

Marmet C, Shell E, Marmet R: Neonatal frenotomy may be necessary to correct breastfeeding problems. *J Hum Lact* 6:117–20, 1990.

Marshall WM, Cumming DC, Fitzsimmons GW: Hot flushes during breast feeding? *Fertil and Steril* 57:1349–50, 1992.

Mathew OP: Regulation of breathing patterns during feeding. In: Mathew OP, Sant Ambrogio G, eds. *Respiratory function of the upper airway.* New York: Marcel Dekker, 1988:535–60.

McBride MC, Danner SC: Sucking disorders in neurologically impaired infants: assessment and facilitation of breastfeeding. *Clin Perinatol* 14(1): 109–30, 1987.

Measel CP, Anderson GC: Nonnutritive suckling during tube feedings: effect on clinical course in premature infants. *JOGN Nursing* 8:265–72, 1979.

Medoff-Cooper B, Weininger S, Zukowsky Z: Neonatal sucking as a clinical assessment tool: preliminary findings. *Nurs Res* 38:162–5, 1989.

Meier P, Anderson GC: Responses of small preterm infants to bottle- and breast-feeding, *MCN* 12:97–105, 1987.

Meier P, et al: A new scale for in-home weighing for mothers of preterm and high risk infant. *J Hum Lact* 10:163–8, 1994.

Meier P, Pugh EJ: Breast-feeding behavior in small preterm infants. *MCN* 10:396–401, 1985.

Mennella JA, Beauchamp GK: Beer, breast feeding, and folklore. *Dev Psychobiol* 26:459–66, 1993.

Miller AJ: Deglutition. *Physiol Rev* 62:129–83, 1982.

Montagu A: Breastfeeding and its relation to morphological, behavioral, and psychocultural development. In: Raphael D, ed. *Breastfeeding and food policy in a hungry world.* New York: Academic, 1979: 189–93.

Morris SE: *The normal acquisition of oral feeding skills: implications for assessment and treatment.* New York: Therapeutic Media, 1982:19–29.

Neifert M, et al: The influence of breast surgery, breast appearance, and pregnancy-induced breast changes on lactation sufficiency as measured by infant weight gain. *Birth* 17:31–8, 1990.

Neifert MR, Seacat JM, Jobe WE: Lactation failure due to insufficient glandular development of the breast. *Pediatrics* 76(5):823–8, 1985.

Neville MC et al: Studies in human lactation: milk volume and nutrient composition during weaning and lactogenesis. *Am J Clin Nutr* 54:81–92, 1991.

Neville MC, Berga SE: Cellular and molecular aspects of the hormonal control of mammary function. In: Neville MC, Neifert MR, eds. *Lactation: physiology, nutrition, and breast-feeding.* New York: Plenum, 1983:141–77.

Newton M, Newton N: The let-down reflex in human lactation. *Pediatrics* 33:69–87, 1948.

Newton M, Newton N: The normal course and management of lactation. *Clin Obstet Gynecol* 5:44–63, 1962.

Noel GL, Suh HK, Frantz AG: Prolactin release during nursing and breast stimulation in post partum and non-post-partum subjects. *J Clin Endocrinol Meta* 38:413–23, 1974.

Notestine GE: The importance of the identification of ankyloglossia (short lingual frenulum) as a cause of breastfeeding problems. *J Hum Lact* 6:113–15, 1990.

Oxford English dictionary, volume 10, *"Sole/Sz."* Oxford: Clarendon Press, 1961.

Prentice A, et al: Evidence for local feed-back control of human milk secretion. *Biochem Soc Trans* 17:489–92, 1989.

Prieto CR, et al: Sucking pressure and its relationship to milk transfer during breastfeeding in humans. *J Reprod Fertil* 108:69–74, 1996.

Riordan J, Koehn M: Reliability testing of three breastfeeding assessment tools. *JOGNN* 26:181–7, 1997.

Riordan J, Rapp E: Pleasure and purpose: the sensuousness of breastfeeding. *JOGN Nursing* 9:109–12, 1980.

Rodenstein DO, Perlmutter N, Stanescu DC: Infants are not obligatory nose breathers. *Am Rev Respir Dis* 131:343–47, 1985.

Russo J, Russo IH: Development of the human mammary gland. In: Neville MD, Daniel CW, eds. *The mammary gland: development, regulation, and function.* New York: Plenum, 1987:67–93.

Salariya EM, Easton PM, Cater JI: Duration of breast-feeding after early initiation and frequent feeding. *Lancet* 2:1141–3, 1978.

Salazar H, Tobon H: Morphologic changes of the mammary gland during development, pregnancy and lactation. In: Josimovich J, ed. *Lactogenic hormones, fetal nutrition and lactation.* New York: Academic Press, 1974:1–18.

Sernia C, Tyndale-Biscoe CH: Prolactin receptors in the mammary gland, corpus luteum and other tissues of the Tammar wallaby, *Macropus engenii. J Endocrinol* 26:391–98, 1979.

Smith DM: Montgomery's areolar tubercle: a light microscopic study. *Arch Pathol Lab Med* 106:60–3, 1982.

Smith WL, et al: Physiology of sucking in the normal term infant using real-time ultrasound. *Radiology* 156:379–81, 1985.

Speroff L, Glass RH, Kase NG: *Clinical gynecologic endocrinology and infertility,* 4th ed. Baltimore: Williams & Wilkins, 1989: 283–311.

Stallings JF, et al: Prolactin response to suckling and maintenance of postpartum amenorrhea among intensively breastfeeding Nepali women. *Endocrinol Res* 22:1–28, 1996.

Tonelli QJ, Sorof S: Epidermal growth factor requirement for development of cultured mammary gland. *Nature* 285:250–2, 1980.

Tyson JE, et al: Studies of prolactin in human pregnancy. *Am J Obstet Gynecol* 113:14–20, 1972.

Vorherr H: Development of the female breast. In: Vorherr H, ed. *The breast.* New York: Academic, 1974:1–18.

Waller H: *The breasts and breastfeeding.* London: Heinemann, 1957.

Waller H: The early failure of breastfeeding. *Arch Dis Child* 21:1–12, 1946.

Weber F, Woolridge MW, Baum JD: An ultrasonographic study of the organization of sucking and swallowing by newborn infants. *Dev Med Child Neurol* 28:19–24, 1986.

West CP: Hormonal profiles in lactating and non-lactating women immediately after delivery and their relationship to breast engorgement. *Am J Obstet Gynecol* 86:501–6, 1979.

Whitworth NS: Lactation in humans. *Psychoneuroendocrinology* 13:171–88, 1988.

Widstrom AM, et al: Gastric suction in healthy newborn infants: effects on circulation and developing feeding behaviour. *Acta Paediatr Scand* 76:566–72, 1987.

Widstrom AM, Thingstrom-Paulsson J: The position of the tongue during rooting reflexes elicited in newborn infants before the first suckle. *Acta Paediatr* 82:281–3, 1993.

Wolff PH: The serial organization of sucking in the young infant. *Pediatrics* 42:943–56, 1968.

Woolridge MW: The "anatomy" of infant sucking. *Midwifery* 2:164–71, 1986.

Yuen BH: Prolactin in human milk: the influence of nursing and duration of postpartum lactation. *Am J Obstet Gynecol* 158:583–6, 1988.

Ziemer M: Nipple skin changes and pain during the first week of lactation. *JOGNN* 22:247–56, 1993.

Zuppa AA, et al: Relationship between maternal parity, basal prolactin levels and neonatal breast milk intake. *Biol Neonate* 53:144–7, 1988.

THE BIOLOGICAL SPECIFICITY OF BREASTMILK

Jan Riordan

Breastmilk has been termed "white blood," because it is considered similar to the placental blood of intrauterine life. Indeed, human milk is similar to unstructured living tissue, such as blood, and is capable of transporting nutrients, affecting biochemical systems, enhancing immunity, and destroying pathogens. With the use of sophisticated laboratory techniques, many scientific investigators have substantiated the life-sustaining properties of human milk. Organs themselves provide evidence of the profound influence of breastfeeding. For example, the thymus plays an essential role in the development of the immune system by providing the environment for T-cell differentiation and maturation. At age four months, the thymus is about twice as large in exclusively breastfed infants as in infants fed only infant formula (Hasselbalch et al., 1996).

Breastmilk, like all other animal milks, is species-specific. It has been adapted throughout human existence to meet nutritional and antiinfective requirements of the human infant to ensure optimal growth, development, and survival. Because an infant's birth weight normally requires about four to six months to double, the nutritional needs of the human baby must be substantially dif-

ferent from those of other mammals whose birth weight doubles much more rapidly. In addition, breastmilk enhances brain development: breastfed children may be more intelligent than children not breastfed. In two trials, breastfed children scored from 4.6 to 7 points higher on standardized tests with controlled environmental factors (Johnson et al., 1996; Lucas et al., 1992).

This chapter breaks down these general properties of human milk into specific components and describes for each component species-specific "biochemical messages" that contribute to the well-being of the baby and mother. Knowledge of biological constructs of lactation is critical to the clinician, because it forms the rationale for effective practice in the clinical setting.

Maturational Changes

Factors that influence milk composition include stage of lactation, gestational age of the infant, the stage (beginning or end) of the feeding, the frequency of the baby's demand for milk, and the degree of fullness or emptiness of the breasts. As discussed in Chapter, 4, lactogenesis occurs in two stages. Stage 1 refers to the development, during

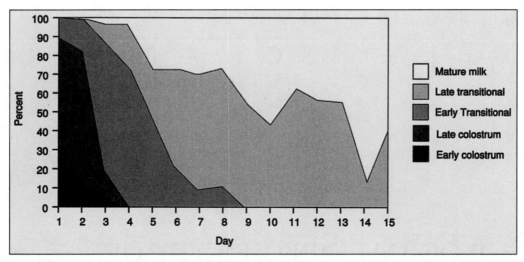

FIGURE 5–1. Milk type by day. *(From SS Humenick: The clinical significance of breast maturation rates.* Birth *14(4):175, 1987. Reprinted by permission of Blackwell Science, Inc.)*

late pregnancy, of the mammary gland's capacity to synthesize milk. Stage 2, traditionally based on postpartum day, refers to the onset of copius milk secretion or the time at which the mother feels her milk "coming in."

Arthur, Smith, and Hartmann (1989) and Humenick (1987, 1994) have proposed two different biological markers as objective measures to define stages of breastmilk maturation. Arthur, Smith, and Hartmann (1989) hold that in the first stage of lactogenesis, average concentrations of lactose, citrate, and glucose are low. However, a sudden and rapid increase in concentrations of these components between 24 to 48 hours after birth heralds the transition from stage 1 to stage 2 lactogenesis.

Humenick (1987, 1994), on the other hand, considers the breakdown of an emulsion dependent on the ratio of sterols plus phospholipids to fat content of milk (maturation index of colostrum and milk [MICAM]) as the biological marker for breastmilk maturation (Fig. 5–1). Both of these methods appear to be valid in that they were positively related to greater milk yield (Casey et al., 1985; Saint et al., 1984), infant weight gain, and lower transcutaneous bilimeter readings

(Humenick, 1987, 1994). These studies also show that breastmilk maturation during lactogenesis proceeds more rapidly in some mothers than in others and is not consistent with the coming in of the milk. The time at which mothers report that their milk comes in is highly variable and ranges from 38 to 98 hours after birth, with an average of 59 hours (Arthur et al., 1989; Kulski & Hartmann, 1981).

Colostrum is thick and creamy yellow, as compared with mature milk, which is thin and bluish-white in color. Compared with mature milk, colostrum is richer in protein and minerals and lower in carbohydrates, fat, and some vitamins. This high concentration of total protein and total ash (minerals) in colostrum gradually changes to reflect the infant's needs over the first two to three weeks as lactation becomes established. The *total dose* of such key components as immunoglobulins, which the infant receives from breastmilk, *remains relatively constant throughout lactation,* regardless of the amount of breastmilk provided by the mother. This happens because concentrations decrease as total volume increases as lactation is established; at weaning, concentration increases as total volume decreases.

Energy, Volume, and Growth

Human milk is rich in nutrient proteins, nonprotein nitrogen compounds, lipids, oligosaccharides, vitamins, and certain minerals. In addition, it contains hormones, enzymes, growth factors, and many types of protective agents. Human milk contains about 10 percent solids for energy and growth; the rest is water, which is vital for maintaining hydration. The pH of early colostrum is 7.45; it falls to a low of 7.0 during the second week of lactation. Thereafter, the pH of milk remains at 7.0 and then rises gradually to 7.4 by 10 months. The significance of these changes is not known (Morriss et al., 1986). Infants can digest breastmilk much more rapidly than formula. The average gastric half-emptying time for breastmilk is 48 minutes, and, for infant formula, 78 minutes (Cavell, 1981).

Caloric Density

The caloric content, or energy density, of human milk is generally considered to be 65 kcal/dl, although published values differ. Garza et al. (1983) reported 57.7/dl, Lepage et al. (1984) reported 66.6, and Lemons et al. (1982) reported 72.2. Using breastmilk as the "gold standard," the American Academy of Pediatrics (AAP, 1976) recommended a calorie content of 67 kcal/dl for commercial formulas.

Energy intakes of breastfed infants beyond the first month are well below those officially recommended by the Committee on Dietary Allowances (1980) and WHO/FAO (1980). These recommendations state that infants should consume 115 kcal/kg/day up to six months and 105 kcal/kg/day between six months and one year. Energy requirements have been overestimated for breastfed infants, because they have been based on volumes of formula required by artificially fed infants. Butte et al. (1984) and Butte et al., (1990) reported that during their first four months, exclusively breastfed infants attained adequate growth with nutrient intakes substantially less than the current dietary recommendation. Likewise, Stuff and Nichols (1989) found that energy intake of human milk-fed infants was about 20 percent below recommended levels. Caloric intake did not increase after solid foods were added to the diet, strongly suggesting that the calorie value of breastmilk feeds was sufficient for the infants' needs.

Wood et al. (1988) studied the breastmilk intake of 21 exclusively breastfed infants during the first five months of life. The kilocalories of breastmilk ingested per kilogram decreased significantly in terms of kilocalories per kilogram. He found that for both genders, study infants were estimated to be receiving 128 kcal/kg at 14 days but only 62.5 kcal/kg at five months. Energy intakes of breastfed infants remained approximately 70 to 75 kcal/kg from the third month on (Garza et al., 1986).

The energy intakes of breastfed and formula-fed infants differs significantly, because their energy expenditure differs greatly. Total daily energy expenditure, minimal rates of energy expenditure, metabolic rates during sleep, rectal temperature, and heart rates are all lower in breastfed infants. Total body water and fat-free mass is lower, and body fat is higher in breastfed infants at four months of age (Butte et al., 1995). By eight months, breastfed infants have consumed about 30,000 kcal less than do bottle-fed infants (Butte, Smith, & Garza, 1990). Although this difference in energy intake should result in about a 2.7-kg mean difference of weight, such is not the case. To explain this discrepancy, Garza, Stuff, and Butte (1986) suggested that (1) differences in intake in the general population are not as great as those found in the babies studied; (2) energy expenditure differs substantially between breastfed and bottle-fed infants; or (3) composition of newly acquired tissue differs between these two groups. A possibility is that the energy density of milk taken by a four-month-old is higher on the average than that taken by the same baby three months earlier. The four-month-old breastfed baby's suckle is more active, leading to a higher fat intake that more than compensates for the volumes needed, because breastmilk is used more completely and with less waste than is artificial milk.

Milk Volume and Storage Capacity

The volume of milk must provide sufficient caloric energy to permit normal growth and development. Small amounts of colostrum—averaging about 37

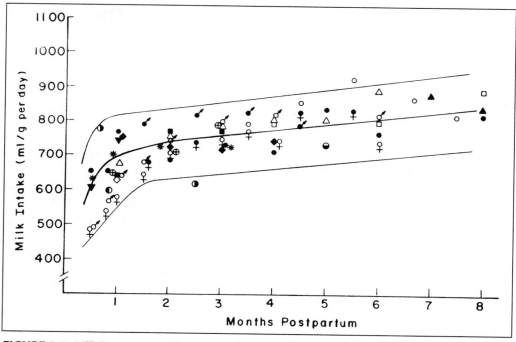

FIGURE 5-2. Milk intakes during established lactation. *The lines show the smoothed mean from this study and ±1 SD. Points are data from the literature obtained by test-weighing of fully breastfed infants. (From MC Neville, et al: Studies in human lactation; milk volumes in lactating women during the onset of lactation and full lactation.* Am J Clin Nutr *48:1381.)*

ml (range, 7–123)–are yielded in the first 24 hours postpartum (Hartmann, 1987; Hartmann & Prosser, 1984); the infant ingests approximately 7 to 14 ml at each feeding (Houston et al., 1983). This milk yield gradually increases for the first 36 hours, followed by a dramatic increase during the next 49 to 96 hours. By day five, volume is about 500 ml/day; it increases more slowly to about 750 ml/day during months three to five of full breastfeeding, and mean intake is about 800 ml/day at six months (Neville et al., 1988). These volumes are similar to others established by test weighing the infant (Dewey & Lonnerdal, 1983; Wood et al., 1988). By using prefeeding and postfeeding infant weighings, Dewey and Lonnerdal (1983) found daily milk intake at one and six months to be 673 and 896 ml, respectively, a difference of 223 ml/day. Likewise, Wood et al. (1988) found that the mean volume of milk intake of 21 study infants increased from 671 (day 15) to 789 ml during the first five months. As seen in Figure 5–2, the volume of milk taken by thriving breastfed infants varies little during the first four months (Butte et al., 1984). Breastmilk intake slowly declines as other foods are added to the baby's diet.

It appears that infants have the capacity to self-regulate their own milk intake. The breast can rapidly change its rate of milk synthesis from one feeding to the next (Daly et al., 1993); previously, it had been assumed that the rate of milk synthesis of a breast needed several days to change significantly. These investigators also found that breasts have the capacity to synthesize much more milk than the infant usually requires, a conclusion consistent with studies of mothers with twins. The amount of milk available to the infant at a single breastfeeding is not an important determinant of the amount of milk consumed by the infant at a breastfeeding. Moreover, infants do not usually obtain all the milk available in a single feeding.

New to lactation science is the concept of breast storage capacity (i.e., the difference between maximum and minimum breast volumes during a 24-hour period). Storage capacity is important in

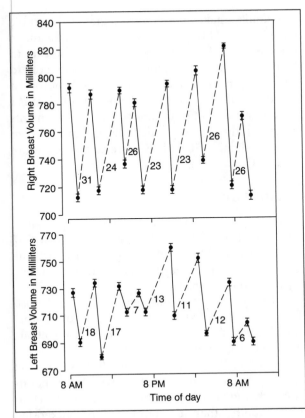

FIGURE 5–3A. Breast-volume changes. *Right and left breast-volume changes of one subject over a period of 24 hours.*

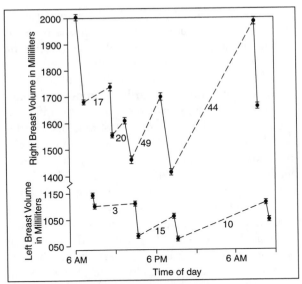

FIGURE 5–3B. Breast-volume changes. *The right and left breast-volume changes of one subject over a period of 28 hours. Each point represents the mean plus or minus the standard error of the mean of replicate breast-volume measurement. Lines link prefeeding and postfeeding mean breast volumes. Dashed lines link postfeeding mean breast volume of a breastfeeding to the prefeeding mean breast volume of the next breast; their slope thus indicates rate of milk synthesis between the two breastfeedings. Rate of milk synthesis also is given by the number (in milliliters per hour) accompanying each dashed line. (From SE Daly, RA Owens, PE Hartmann: The short-term synthesis and infant-regulated removal of milk in lactating women.* Exp Physiol *78:209–20, 1993.)*

determining how the infant's demand for milk is met by the mother. Daly et al. (1993) measured the short-term rates of milk synthesis using a computerized system in which a camera relays video images to a computer that produces a model of the chest by active triangulation. Using this method, these investigators were able to determine the rate of synthesis of human milk. Figure 5–3A shows the volume of milk produced by a small-breasted woman who had a storage capacity of 111 ml for her right breast and a capacity of 81 ml for her left breast. Thus the maximum amount of milk that this woman appeared to be able to store was about 20 percent of her infant's 24-hour milk intake. From her breast volume changes over time, it appears that her infant met its demand for milk by breastfeeding frequently. Conversely, Figure 5–3B displays a larger-breasted woman who produced similar volumes of milk but with larger storage

capacities for her breasts (right breast, 600 ml; left breast, 180 ml), allowing her to store nearly 90 percent of her infant's 24-hour milk intake. Further, there was no relationship between total milk-storage capacity and 24-hour milk production. Thus we can conclude that small breast size does not restrict a woman's ability to provide milk for her infant. On the other hand, mothers with a greater storage capacity do have more flexibility with patterns of breastfeeding.

There appear to be wide differences among women in the rate of milk synthesis which among some women can be double or triple the rate of other women (Arthur et al., 1989; Daly et al., 1992). Milk volume between breasts also differs. Milk yield from right breasts appear to be higher than that from left breasts, clearly demonstrating that the rate of milk synthesis within one breast is independent of the rate of milk synthesis in the other breast (Cox et al., 1996; Daly et al., 1993).

At the same time, the amount of milk available in the breast is not necessarily an important determinant of the amount removed by the infant at feedings. Infant intake of breastmilk also varies widely. For example, at five months, infant intake of breastmilk can range from 200 (partial breastfeeding) to 3,500 ml/day (wet nurse) (Neville & Oliva-Rasbach, 1987). These differences appear to be culturally based. Australian women, for example, have been reported to make more breastmilk than do U.S. women. The average daily yield of well-nourished Australian mothers during the first six months of lactation was found to be in excess of 1,100 ml in one study (Hartmann, 1987) and to range from 535 to 1,078 ml in another (Daly et al., 1993). Mothers breastfeeding twins produce in excess of 2,100 ml/day in the early months. Seasonal changes in breastmilk volume may be influenced by some mothers' need to work during harvest and by their reluctance to introduce supplementary food for fear of diarrheal disease (Serdula, Seward, & Marks, 1986; Whitehead et al., 1978). The nutritional status of the mother does not appear to affect milk volume unless the mother is severely malnourished (Brown et al., 1986a; Forman et al., 1990; Neville & Oliva-Rasbach, 1987; van Steenbergen et al., 1989).

A healthy breastfeeding full-term neonate breastfeeds an average of 4.3 times during the first 24 hours (range, 0–11) and 7.4 times during the next 24 hours (range 1–22) (Yamauchi & Yamanouchi, 1990). Breastmilk intake shows little or no correlation with maternal factors, such as weight-for-height, weight gain, nursing frequency, maternal age, and parity (Dewey & Lönnerdal, 1983). Although birth weight is not a strong predictor of milk intake throughout lactation, infant weight at one month is. Thus lactation performance during the first four weeks postpartum is a strong predictor of milk output during the subsequent period of full lactation (Neville & Oliva-Rasbach, 1987).

Two methodological problems must be addressed in lactation research. Inch and Renfrew (1989) point out the potential for error using prefeeding and postfeeding test weights to calculate

breastmilk intake unless an integrated electronic scale is used. This type of scale calculates the mean value of a number of test weighings during two- to four-second periods; readings are reproducible to within 2 gm even if the baby moves vigorously. Another difficulty is the definition of *breastfed infants* as study subjects. Are all "breastfed" infants in the study receiving all their nutriment from breastfeeding? (These issues are addressed more fully in Chapter 23.)

Infant Growth

Normal human growth is greatest during infancy. The infant gains about 10 g/kg/day (about 5–7 ounces per week) until about four weeks; then the gain drops to 1 g/kg/day (about 3 ounces per week) by the end of the first year.

There are growth differences between breastfed and formula-fed infants. A review of international research (Butte et al., 1984; Fawzi et al., 1997; Jackson et al., 1964; Juex et al., 1983; Motil et al., 1997; Whitehead & Paul, 1981) shows that infants breastfed exclusively have the same or somewhat greater weight gain in the first three to four months than do bottle-fed or mixed-fed infants. After this time, bottle-fed or mixed-fed infants clearly weigh more. The greatest differences are evident between 6 and 20 months of age, when breastfed infants are lighter than bottle-fed or mixed-fed infants (Dewey et al., 1993, 1995; Yoneyama et al., 1994). Increases in length and head circumference growth remain the same for both groups. Length as a reliable indicator for evaluating infant growth and the absence of significant difference in length between breastfed and nonbreastfed infants suggest that formula-fed infants are overfed. This tendency to overfeed with artificial baby milk appears to be greater in girls than in boys (Yoneyama et al., 1994).

Nutritional Values

Around the world, breastmilk is remarkably stable, varying only within a relatively narrow range. Constituents of colostrum and breastmilk are shown in Appendix A, and a profile of lactose protein and lipid concentrations in human milk for the first 30 days of lactation is seen in Figure 5–4. Yet,

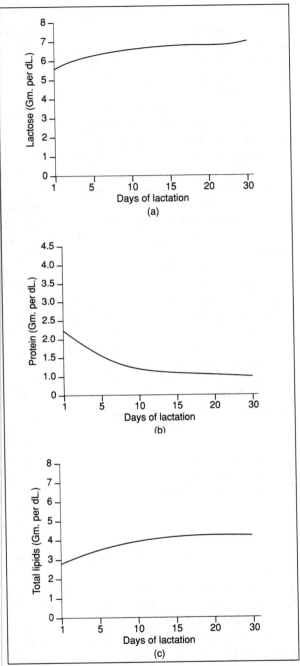

FIGURE 5-4. Lactose, protein, and total lipid concentrations in human milk.

because breastfeeding is an interactive process, the infant helps to determine composition of the feed. During weaning (involution phase), for example, the concentrations of sodium and protein in breast-

milk progressively increase; in contrast, concentrations of potassium, glucose, and lactose gradually decrease (Prosser et al., 1984).

Fat

The fat content of human milk, which provides about one-half of the milk's calories, is its most variable component. The energy density of preterm mother's milk is much greater than that of full-term mother's milk, owing to a 30 percent higher fat concentration (Atkinson, Anderson, & Bryan, 1980). Triglycerides, the main constituent (98–99 percent) of milk fat, are readily broken down into free fatty acids and glycerol by the enzyme lipase, which is found not only in infants' intestines but also in the breastmilk itself (Hamosh, 1985).

The lipid fraction of human milk provides essential fatty acids. The main concern about fatty-acid intake is its effect on brain growth. The rate of brain growth is greatest in the last trimester of pregnancy and continues thoughout the first year of life. Tissues of breastfed and formula-fed infants have distinctly different plasma fatty-acid compositions. Breastmilk contains a wide range of long-chain polyunsaturated fatty acids including docosahexanoic acid (DHA) and arachidonic acid (AA). Infant formula is fortified only with precursor essential fatty acids, linolenic acid, and linoleic acid (Sanjurjo et al., 1988).

Concentrations of DHA are higher in mature milk than in preterm milk (Beijers & Schaafsma, 1996). An essential fatty acid that enhances the developing human visual system, DHA is found in extremely high levels in the photoreceptors and the visual cortex. Breastfed infants accumulate DHA in the cortex, whereas formula-fed infants merely maintain the same amount of DHA present at birth. The neural maturation of preterm breastfed infants is more advanced than that of bottle-fed infants, as assessed by electroretinography, visual evoked potential, and psychometric tests (Birch et al., 1992; Lucas et al., 1992; Uauy et al., 1990).

DHA may cause this greater visual performance (Birch et al., 1993; Carlson et al., 1993; Makrides et al., 1993, 1995). Other studies indicate that formulas containing adequate linoleic and linolenic acids but lacking AA or DHA impose no measurable deficit in performance of visual and cognitive development tests at nine months of age in healthy full-term formula-fed infants (Gale & Martyn, 1996; Innis et al., 1996). Does the infant depend on an exogenous supply of long-chain polyunsaturated fatty acids available only in human milk as Kohn et al. (1994) suggest? Or would supplementation of formula-fed infants with DHA adequately fill this need? The issue remains to be settled. At the time of this writing, DHA "supplements" for pregnant and lactating mothers are being marketed; plans are also under way to add DHA to commercial formula.

Breastfed infants also have a higher proportion of acetic acid in the short-chain fatty-acid spectra than do formula-fed infants. These, along with monoglycerides generated by milk lipases, also act against envelope viruses, bacteria, and fungi (Garza et al., 1987; Siigur et al., 1993). The paler color, softer consistency, and milder odor of breastmilk stools, as compared with formula stools, are due in part to a higher concentration of fatty acid soap content (Quinlan et al., 1995).

Although maternal dietary fat intake does not affect the total amount of fat in human milk, the types of fat in the diet do influence the composition of fatty acids in milk. For example, black mothers in South Africa consuming a traditional maize diet have higher levels of monounsaturated fatty acid in their milk than do their urban counterparts who eat more animal fats (van der Westhuyzen et al., 1988). If the mother eats a high-carbohydrate, energy-replete diet, the proportion of triglycerides of medium-chain fatty acid increases (Garza et al., 1987).

Because cholesterol levels (10–20 mg/dl) in human milk are considerably higher than those of formulas derived from bovine milk (Wagner & Stockhausen, 1988), cholesterol levels in adulthood could be expected to be higher in breastfed individuals. The reverse, however, may well be true: exposure to cholesterol in breastmilk may be an advantage later in life. At least one study (Osborn, 1968) reported that coronary artery disease in persons up to 20 years of age is seen less frequently in individuals who were breastfed. A "cholesterol-challenge" hypothesis proposes that exposure to cholesterol early in life may contribute to a more efficient cholesterol metabolism in adulthood and thus greater protection against heart disease. This hypothesis has been criticized on two counts. First,

human milk is not high in cholesterol–10 to 15 mg/dl versus none in formula. Second, the validity of a complex study that tries to measure the long-term effect of intake of different fats early in life is questionable (Jensen et al., 1988).

Fat content of milk changes throughout a breastfeeding and, generally speaking, increases more steeply as more milk is taken. Daly et al. (1993) argued that the long-established observation that fat concentration is always higher at the end of the feeding is not accurate. Instead, they claimed that the fat content varies according to the degree to which the breast is emptied at that breastfeeding and that fat content increases markedly after *most of the milk in the breast has been taken*. Moreover, they claimed that the amount of milk consumed at a breastfeeding does not necessarily correlate with fat intake but rather with the interval between feedings. The longer the time interval between two breastfeedings, the less likely is the infant to empty the breast and thus the lower the fat concentration in the subsequent feeding. Although the work of Daly et al. (1993) indicated that the pattern of feedings dictates the infant's fat intake, this is not necessarily the case. Woolridge (1990) studied mothers who fed in two patterns—either feeding at one breast or at two breasts during a feeding. The infants thus fed were able to regulate their fat intake and to achieve stable fat intakes in spite of disparate patterns of feedings. His findings support flexible "baby-led" feedings.

Lactose

Lactose, a disaccharide, accounts for most of the carbohydrates in human milk, although small quantities of oligosaccharides, galactose, and fructose are also present. Although lactose concentration is relatively constant (7 gm/dl) in mature milk, it is affected by maternal diet. In his longitudinal study of breastfeeding women in the Gambia, Prentice (1980) found that the milk-lactose concentration of these women was higher during the wet season (hungry period), when energy intakes were very low, than it was during the dry season (when food was more plentiful).

Lactose enhances calcium absorption and metabolizes readily to galactose and glucose, which supply energy to the rapidly growing brain of the infant. Some oligosaccharides promote the growth of *Lactobacillus bifidus,* thus increasing intestinal acidity and stemming the growth of pathogens.

The enzyme lactase is necessary to convert lactose into simple sugars that can be easily assimilated by the infant. The enzyme is present in the infant's intestinal mucosa from birth. Congenital, or primary, lactase deficiency is exceedingly rare; some authorities question its existence. Lactose intolerance, however, is common in many mammals as they grow older and is the result of diminishing activity of intestinal lactase after weaning. In humans, lactose intolerance is more prevalent in adults of Asian and African heritage.

Protein

Protein content of mature human milk from well-nourished mothers is about 0.8 to 0.9 gm protein per deciliter (Butte et al., 1984). Some of the protein in human milk is probably not nutritionally available to the infant; it serves immunological purposes instead. The high quality of protein in human milk and its precisely balanced quantity meet the energy needs of both term and preterm infants (Gaull, 1985; Raiha, 1985).

Human milk contains casein and whey protein. Casein accounts for 40 percent of the total protein, about one-half that in bovine milk; 60 percent is whey protein. Whey proteins, which predominate in human milk, are acidified in the stomach, forming soft flocculant curds. These digest quickly, supplying a continuous flow of nutrients to the baby. By contrast, caseins (the primary protein in untreated bovine milk) form a tough, less digestible curd that requires high expenditure of energy for an incomplete digestive process.

Whey protein is composed of five major components: alpha-lactalbumin, serum albumin, lactoferrin, immunoglobulins, and lysozyme. The latter three elements play important roles in immunological defense. Lactoferrin concentration of milk is higher in iron-deficient women as compared with well-nourished mothers; therefore milk lactoferrin may also help protect the infant against iron deficiency (Raiha, 1985). A large number of other proteins (enzymes, growth modulators, and hormones) are present in low concentrations.

Nonprotein Nitrogen of Breastmilk. Milk proteins are synthesized from amino acids derived from the bloodstream. Nonprotein nitrogen contains a number of free amino acids, including glutamic acid, glycine, alanine, valine, leucine, aspartic acid, serine, threonine, proline, and taurine. When amino acids exist singly or in free form, they are known as *free amino acids.* Of these, leucine, valine, and threonine are essential amino acids; they must be consumed in the diet because the body does not manufacture them.

The percentage of protein in human colostrum is much greater than that in mature breastmilk. This high level is due to the presence of several additional amino acids and antibody-rich proteins, especially secretory IgA and lactoferrin. All 10 essential amino acids are present in colostrum and account for approximately 45 percent of its total nitrogen content.

Nucleotides. Nucleotides are low-molecular-weight compounds with a nitrogenous base. Necessary for energy metabolism, enzymatic reactions, and growth and maturation of the developing gastrointestinal tract, they also play several roles in immune function, including enhanced lymphocytic proliferation, stimulation of immunoglobulin production in lymphocytes, and increased natural killer-cell activity. Clinical research on nucleotides in human milk attempts to emulate the amount of nucleotides as much as possible in infant formula (Leach et al., 1995). At this writing (1997), at least one formula company is marketing an "advance" formula that contains nucleotides.

The importance to the baby of available nitrogen cannot be overstated. Atkinson, Anderson, and Bryan (1980) have shown that the concentration of nitrogen in the milk of women who deliver preterm infants is 20 percent greater than that in milk of women delivering at term. The higher levels of available protein and fat in preterm mother's milk underscore the importance of using the milk of the preterm infant's mother rather than pooled milk from women in other stages of lactation (Table 5–1). Donated milk, however, can be modified with components from other human milk to make a preterm human milk formula with none of the dangers of commerical bovine-based preterm formulas.

Table 5-1

COMPOSITION OF TERM AND PRETERM MILK DURING THE FIRST MONTH OF LACTATION

Nutrients	3–5 Days		8–11 Days		15–18 Days		26–29 Days	
	Full-Term	Preterm	Full-Term	Preterm	Full-Term	Preterm	Full-Term	Preterm
Energy (kcal/dl)	48	58	59	71	62	71	62	70
Lipid (gm/dl)	1.85	3.00	2.9	4.14	3.06	4.33	3.05	4.09
Protein (gm/dl)	1.87	2.10	1.7	1.86	1.52	1.71	1.29	1.41
Lactose (gm/dl)	5.14	5.04	5.98	5.55	6.00	5.63	6.51	5.97

Source: Adapted from CH Anderson: Human milk feeding. Pediatr Clin North Am *32:335–52, 1985.*

Vitamins and Micronutrients

The amounts of vitamins and micronutrients in human milk vary from one person to another because of diet and genetic differences. However, it is generally true that human milk will satisfy the micronutrient requirements of a full-term healthy infant and thus can be taken as the primary yardstick of dietary recommendations, or reference values. Generally, as lactation progresses, the level of water-soluble vitamins in breastmilk increases, and the level of fat-soluble vitamins declines. Fat-soluble vitamin (A, D, K, E) levels in human milk are minimally influenced by recent maternal diet, as these vitamins can be drawn from storage in the body. Although several micronutrients can produce toxic effects when given in large doses to adults or infants, the only recorded case of toxicity to breastfed infants through excessive accumulation in breastmilk was due to excessive vitamin D (Greer et al., 1984).

Fat Solubility. Human milk is a good source of vitamin A (200 IU/dl), which is present mainly as retinol (40–53 ng/dl). Required for vision and maintenance of epithelial structures, vitamin A is at highest levels in the first week after birth and then gradually declines. Deficiency of vitamin A is a serious health problem for young children in many developing countries, leading to blindess through damage to the corneal epithelium (xerophthalmia) and to increased morbidity from infectious dis-

eases. The prolongation of even partial breastfeeding provides an important source of vitamin A to children in developing countries (Bates & Prentice, 1994; West et al., 1986).

Human milk has very little fat-soluble vitamin D. Concentrations in human milk range between 5 IU and 20 IU per liter. A water-soluble variant of vitamin D has been found (Lakdawala & Widdowson, 1977), but further study has not supported a major role for this compound (Reeve, Chesney, & De Luca, 1982). Increased vitamin D intake results in increased levels in human milk (Specker et al., 1985). Ingestion of oral vitamin D supplements (60 ug/day) for two weeks raised the level of vitamin D in the milk of a lactating woman 40 times (Hollis, 1983). Vitamin D may constitute an exception to the general rule that breastmilk micronutrient levels are protected from the effect of maternal deficiency (Bates & Prentice, 1994). Although rickets is rarely seen in breastfed children, especially if their mothers are well nourished, scattered reports of rickets have led the American Academy of Pediatrics to recommend vitamin D supplements (400 IU/day) for children subject to certain conditions (AAP, 1980). The risk of rickets is greatest for dark-skinned children living in inner-city areas, children whose clothing lowers skin exposure to the sun, and children of mothers eating vegetarian diets that exclude meat, fish, and dairy products. The child who is adequately exposed to the sun (and thus to radiation-formed precursors of vitamin D) and whose mother consumes adequate nutrients does not need routine vitamin D supplements (Greer & Marshall, 1989; Roberts, 1981).

Human colostrum is particularly rich in vitamin E (tocopherol). Milk of mothers with preterm and term infants have similar levels of vitamin E (3 IU/100 kcal) and beta-carotene levels, which are higher than those in bovine milk levels (Ostrea, 1986; Jansson, Akesson, & Holmberg, 1981). A deficiency of vitamin E in infancy can result in hemolytic anemia, especially in the premature infant. Because it is an antioxidant, vitamin E protects cell membranes in the retina and lungs against oxidant-induced injury. The requirement for vitamin E increases with intake of polyunsaturated fatty acids in breastmilk. Mothers who eat foods high in polyunsaturated fats and "fast foods" add to oxidant stress (Guthrie et al., 1977).

Vitamin K, which is required for the synthesis of blood-clotting factors, is present in human milk in small amounts. Within a few days after the baby's birth, vitamin K is normally produced in sufficient quantities by enteric bacteria. However, neonates are susceptible to vitamin K deficiency until ingestion of copious amounts of breastmilk can promote gastrointestinal bacterial colonization, which enhances their low levels of vitamin K.

Insufficient vitamin K in neonates can lead to vitamin K-responsive hemorrhagic disease. To prevent hemorrhage and to raise prothrombin levels, 1 mg vitamin K is routinely given intramuscularly. Alternatively, an equal oral dose of vitamin K may be absorbed in the intestinal tract in amounts sufficient to prevent bleeding (Haroon et al., 1982), and the infant is spared the pain of an injection and the risk of nerve damage always possible with any intramuscular injection. However, because of the difficulty of measuring the low levels of vitamin K in milk and other body fluids, this subject is still at an early stage of investigation (Bates & Prentice, 1994; Canfield & Hopkinson, 1989).

Water Solubility. Water-soluble vitamins—ascorbic acid, nicotinic acid, B_{12} (thiamine), riboflavin, and B_6 (pyridoxine)—are readily influenced by the maternal diet. If maternal supplements are present, the vitamin levels in the milk increase and then plateau. Although supplementation may be beneficial for undernourished women, it is not necessary if the mother is well nourished and eating a diet

that contains foods close to their natural state. (See Chapter 16 for a detailed discussion of maternal diet and lactation.)

Vitamin B_{12} is needed for early development of the baby's central nervous system, and its presence in human milk is critical. A mother eating a vegan diet (i.e., without meat or dairy products) may produce milk deficient in B_{12}. This was demonstrated by a breastfed infant who developed severe hematological and neurological problems that resolved rapidly with B_{12} supplementation (Higginbottom et al., 1978). The literature contains several reports of megaloblastic anemia in breastfeeding infants of mothers with this deficiency (Worthington-Roberts & Williams, 1993). Unlike other micronutrients, folate (which is bound to a folate-binding protein) remains at the same level throughout all stages of lactation. This consistent, adequate level of folate reduces the risks of folate deficiency and megaloblastic anemia in breastfed infants (Ek & Magnus, 1979). It should be noted that a deficiency of B-vitamin folate during pregnancy is associated with neural-tube defects.

High pharmacological doses of vitamin B_6 have been reported to suppress prolactin and thus lactation. However, low nutritionally relevant doses have no effect on plasma prolactin or on breastmilk volume. Doses as high as 4.0 mg of vitamin B_6 taken as part of a vitamin B complex supplement are considered safe for both the lactating mother and the infant (Andon et al., 1985).

Minerals

The total mineral content in human milk is fairly constant. Except for magnesium, minerals tend to be highest in human milk in the first few days after birth and decrease slightly in a consistent pattern throughout lactation, with little diurnal or within-feeding variation. Maternal age, parity, and diet, even when supplemented, usually have minimal influence on mineral concentrations in milk, probably because of their regulation from maternal body stores (Butte et al., 1987; Casey et al., 1989; Freely et al., 1983; Karra et al., 1986).

Sodium. Breastmilk sodium is elevated in early colostrum but falls dramatically by the third day postpartum and declines at a slower rate for six months. Elevated human-milk sodium levels occur during weaning, in women with mastitis, and during the first months of gestation. A high concentration of sodium has also been found in the milk of mothers whose infants develop malnutrition, dehydration, and hypernatremia. Persistent high levels may also be a marker for impaired lactation (Morton, 1994).

Zinc. Zinc is actively transported into the mammary gland. Zinc levels rise to a peak on the second day postpartum and then decline for the duration of lactation (Casey et al., 1989). Zinc is eight times more abundant in human colostrum than in mature milk. Krebs and Hambidge (1986) suggested that zinc requirements are based on growth velocity; therefore, requirements are relatively high in the very young infant and decrease with increasing age of the infant. For fully breastfed infants, a combination of high absorption and efficient conservation of intestinal endogenous zinc allows them to retain enough zinc to meet the demands of infant growth even in the face of modest intake (Abrams et al., 1996; Krebs et al., 1996).

Zinc is known to dramatically alleviate the symptoms of acrodermatitis enteropathica, a rare but serious congenital metabolic disorder that manifests itself in part in severe dermatitis (Evans & Johnson, 1980). While an infant with this disorder continues to receive human milk, he has no symptoms. The high bioavailability of zinc in human milk is brought about by a low-molecular-weight zinc-binding ligand that facilitates zinc absorption (Sandstrom et al., 1983). Abnormally low zinc levels in breastmilk are rare but apparently can sometimes occur in mothers of infants with low birth weight. A slowing growth rate and persistent perioral or perianal rash (with or without diarrhea) in infants fed solely breastmilk may be due to zinc depletion (Atkinson et al., 1989). These infants should continue to breastfeed but they may require zinc supplementation. Maternal supplementation of zinc will also raise the level in breastmilk (see Chapter 16).

Iron. Although human milk has only a small amount of iron (0.5–1.0 mg/liter), breastfed babies rarely are iron deficient. They maintain their iron status at the same level as that of formula-fed infants receiving iron supplements for up to nine months (Duncan et al., 1985; McMillan et al., 1976; Salmenpera et al., 1986; Siimes et al., 1984).

Breastfed infants are sustained by sufficient iron stores laid down in utero and by the high lactose and vitamin C levels in human milk, which facilitate iron absorption. Also, breastfed infants do not risk loss of iron as do infants fed cow's milk; the latter may experience microhemorrhages of the bowel as a result of mucosal damage by nonhuman milk (Woodruff et al., 1977).

During the first few months of life, healthy, full-term infants draw on extensive iron reserves generally present at birth. Normally, an infant's hemoglobin level is high (16–22 gm/dl) at birth and decreases rapidly as physiological adjustment is made to extrauterine life. At four months of age, normal hemoglobin ranges between 10.2 and 15 gm/dl. Iron is well absorbed by older infants and is not affected by mineral intake from solid foods in the diet (Abrams, Wen, & Stuff, 1996). Iron supplementation is not usually needed and may, in fact, be detrimental to the breastfeeding baby during the first half-year after birth. Excess iron tends to saturate lactoferrin and thereby diminish its anti-infective properties (Bullen et al., 1972). Iron supplements taken by the mother will not increase iron levels in her milk, but they may produce constipation in the infant.

Calcium. Like iron, calcium appears in only small quantities in human milk (20–34 mg/dl). Yet babies absorb 67 percent of the calcium in human milk as compared to only 25 percent of that in cow's milk. Neonatal hypocalcemia and tetany are more commonly seen in the formula-fed infant, because cow's milk has a much higher concentration of phosphorus (calcium-phosphorus ratio of 1.2 : 1.0 versus 2 : 1 in human milk), which leads to decreased absorption and increased excretion of calcium. Calcium and phosphorus supplements are sometimes given to breastfed infants with low birth weight who should be monitored for hypercalcemia (calcium >11 mg/dl) (Steichen et al., 1987).

Other Minerals. Copper levels are highest during the first few days postpartum, decrease for about five to six months, and then tend to remain stable. Magnesium, on the other hand, gradually increases after four to six months postpartum or remains constant (Butte et al., 1987). Selenium is usually higher in human milk than in formula (Kumpulain et al., 1987; Smith et al., 1982). Minute amounts of aluminum, iodine, chromium, and fluorine are also found in breastmilk. Very little is known about the mechanisms or control of the secretion of trace elements into human milk.

Renal Solute Load

Human milk produces a small renal solute load, thus aiding the infant's kidney function and general state of hydration. Human milk has significantly lower levels of calcium, phosphorus, sodium, and potassium than does bovine milk. Formula-fed infants also have higher urinary oxalate excretion than do those fed human milk (Campfield et al., 1994). Oxalate is an insoluble end product of metabolism. Because of these factors and the low protein content of human milk, the solute load on the immature kidney of the breastfed infant is approximately one-third that of the infant fed bovine milk. Because excess salts require additional water for excretion, greater obligatory water loss occurs when the infant is not fed human milk. Improvements in formula composition have reduced the renal solute load produced by artificial foods, but there is always the possibility of error in preparing formulas (e.g., using excessive amounts of powder, which results in a high-protein concentration) (Miller & Chopra, 1984). Table 5–2 lists the major components of human milk and their functions.

Antiinfective Properties

Breastmilk offers the newborn protection against disease. This benefit has been recognized for hundreds of years; however, only in the last few decades have investigators begun to identify the specific antiinfective components of human milk that make it a peerless substance for feeding the human infant. Breastmilk has been viewed from ancient times as living tissue and rightly so. This "white blood" contains enzymes, immunoglobulins, and leukocytes in abundance. These components, one frequently enhancing the efficacy of another, account for most of the unique antiinfective properties of human milk. In some cultures, fresh breastmilk is used as eyedrops to treat conjunctivitis; elsewhere, it is common practice to apply breastmilk on the skin to heal cracked nipples.

Many studies that measured the protectiveness of human milk reaffirm its significance in prevent-

ing infections (Cunningham, 1977, 1979; Dewey et al., 1995; Frank et al., 1982; Gulick, 1986; Kovar et al., 1984; Pullan et al., 1980; Rosenberg, 1989; Victora et al., 1987; Watkins et al., 1979). The evidence is strongest for bacterial infections, gastroenteritis, and necrotizing enterocolitis but is likewise convincing for respiratory infections. This protective effect is most striking in communities with poor sewage systems, poverty, and malnutrition. According to the WHO (Snyder & Merson, 1982), more than 5 million children under the age of five years die annually from gastrointestinally related disease, and many more suffer from gastrointestinal illness.

Wherever infant morbidity and mortality are high, breastfeeding conclusively helps to prevent infantile diarrhea and gastrointestinal infections (Almroth & Latham, 1982; Brown et al., 1989; Clavano, 1982; Granthan-McGregor & Back, 1972; Habicht et al., 1988; Jason et al., 1984; Kanaaneh, 1972; Koopman et al., 1985; Kovar et al., 1984; Mata, 1979; Mitra & Rabbani, 1995; Ravelomanana et al., 1995; Shoub, 1977). Breastfeeding minimizes diarrhea both by providing protective factors and by reducing exposure to other foods or water that may contain enteropathogens (Van Derslice et al., 1994). In a review of field studies conducted to identify the effect of breastfeeding on childhood diarrhea in Bangladesh, Glass and Stoll (1989) found that during the first six months of life, breastfeeding protected children against diarrhea. Those children partially breastfed had a greater risk of diarrhea than had those who were exclusively breastfed. Although breastmilk's protective effect is most easily demonstrated in areas of poverty and malnutrition, worldwide data consistently indicate protective effects. In China, Chen et al. (1988) showed that compared with breastfed infants, artificially fed infants are more likely to be admitted to the hospital for gastroenteritis and other conditions. In the Cebu region of the Philippines, giving water, teas, and other liquids to breastfed babies doubles or triples the likelihood of diarrhea (Popkin et al., 1990).

Cunningham (1977, 1979) reviewed hospital and clinical records of children hospitalized in Cooperstown, NY, during the mid-1970s. During their first year, breastfed infants had significantly fewer episodes of illness than did those not breast-

Table 5-2

MAJOR COMPONENTS OF HUMAN MILK AND THEIR FUNCTIONS

Component	Function
Ascorbic acid	Antioxidant
Epidermal growth factor	Stimulates epithelial proliferation
Enzymes	
Amylase	Facilitates infant digestion of polysaccharides
Lipase	Hydrolizes fat in infant intestine; bactericidal activity
Lactose	Major carbohydrate; breaks down into galactose and glucose; enhances absorption of Ca, Mg, and Mn
Lipids (fat)	Major source of calories
Long-chain polyunsaturated fatty acids	Docosahexanoic acid may enhance visual and neural development
Short-chain fatty acids	Antiinfective effects
Minerals	Regulates normal body functions; minimal influence by maternal diet
Nonprotein nitrogen	Contains free amino acids necessary for growth
Oligosaccharides	Contribute to bifidus activity and prevent adhesion of microbes to tissue walls
Protein	
Whey	Contains lactalbumin, lactoferrin, lysozyme, albumin, and immunoglobulins
Nonprotein nitrogen	Frees amino acids for infant growth
Taurine	Possible function in brain development and maturation
Thyroxine	Regulates basal metabolic rate
Triglycerides	Largest source of calories for infant; broken down to free fatty acids and glycerol by lipase; types of fat depend on maternal diet
Water	Constitutes 87.5 percent of human milk volume; provides adequate hydration to infant

fed. The differences remained statistically significant even after controlling for paternal education, maternal age, presence of older siblings, exposure to day-care centers, and parental smoking.

Chandra (1979) prospectively studied 30 breastfed and 30 bottle-fed Canadian babies for two years. Infants exclusively breastfed for the first two months had significantly fewer episodes of diarrhea than did infants bottle-fed from birth. Khin-Maung et al. (1985) compared clinical outcomes in two groups of children younger than two years with acute diarrhea: one group received oral rehydration solution alone, and the other group breastfed in addition to receiving oral rehydration solution. The breastfed children passed 250 ml less of diarrheal stools and recovered from diarrhea more quickly than did children who were not breastfed. The breastfed children also required less oral rehydration solution than did those who were not breastfed during the early acute phase of diarrhea.

Epidemiological evidence indicates that human milk continues to confer protection even with supplementation. Partial breastfeeding is better than no breastfeeding at all. This protection is specific mainly to pathogens in the mother's and infant's environment. Thus the infant receives protection against the pathogens it is most likely to encounter. Table 5–3 summarizes the ameliorating and protective effects of human milk. The authors assume that breastfeeding is the norm and that artificial feeding is a deviation from the norm that brings about hazards to infant health. Two infant health problems exacerbated by lack of breastfeeding—respiratory illness and otitis media—are discussed here. Others are discussed throughout this text, especially in Chapters 19 and 20.

Respiratory Illness

Studies of the protective effects of breastfeeding against respiratory tract infections are conflicting (Adebonojo, 1972; Cunningham, 1979; Paine & Coble, 1982; Watkins et al., 1979). Several studies suggest that breastfeeding helps to prevent respiratory infections (Lopez-Alarcon et al., 1997). When Chen et al. (1988) looked for an association between type of feeding and hospitalization of infants in Shanghai, People's Republic of China, they found that artificial feeding was associated with more frequent hospitalizations for respiratory infections during the first 18 months of life. The effect of artificial feeding was independent of demographic characteristics and socioeducational status. In a careful review of Chen's study, Kramer (1988) concluded that the findings "are convincing and add to the accumulating and now overwhelming evidence that breast-feeding protects against infant and early childhood infection, particularly in non-Western, less industrialized countries."

There is mounting evidence that breastmilk protects against respiratory syncytial virus (RSV) infection (Bell, 1988; Downham et al., 1976; Duffy et al., 1986; Holberg et al., 1991; Rahman et al., 1987). Duffy et al. (1986) prospectively studied 197 infants to examine the relationship between mode of feeding and risk of rotavirus infection. Infants

exclusively breastfed for at least four months had the lowest attack rates (5 percent) for rotavirus-related gastroenteritis, as compared to infants fed formula or a combination of breastmilk and formula. Similar protection has been established for *Haemophilus influenzae* bacteremia and meningitis (Cochi et al., 1986; Istre et al., 1985; Silfverdal et al., 1997; Takala et al., 1989). Downham et al. (1976) compared 115 infants hospitalized with RSV who were younger than 12 months with 162 control infants. Only 7 percent of the hospitalized infants were breastfed, compared with 27.5 percent of the control infants, a statistically significant difference.

Otitis Media

Breastfeeding protects against ear infections (otitis media) for reasons that are not completely clear. However, immunological factors, feeding position, and lack of irritation from bovine-based formula may explain it. Saarinen et al. (1982) followed healthy, full-term infants through their first three years of life. Up to six months of age, no infant had otitis during the period of exclusive breastfeeding, whereas 10 percent of the babies who were given any cow's milk did. These significant differences persisted up to three years of age. Other studies (Aniansson et al., 1994; Chandra, 1979; Cunningham, 1979; Dewey et al., 1995; Schaefer, 1971) support an inverse relationship between ear infections and breastfeeding.

In contrast to global evidence that breastfeeding helps to protect infants against health problems, Bauchner, Levanthal, and Shapiro (1986), Leventhal et al. (1986), and Sauls (1979) have challenged the claim that breastfeeding protects infants in developed countries, citing lack of control for potentially confounding factors, such as low birth weight, parental smoking, crowding, sanitation, and other characteristics of socioeconomic status.

Howie et al. (1990) settled this controversy by examining the effect of breastfeeding on childhood illness in Scotland in a study using an adequate sample that met the methodological criteria set by Bauchner et al. (1986). Howie concluded that breastfeeding during the first 13 weeks of life confers protection against gastrointestinal illness beyond the period of breastfeeding itself. A few years later, Fuchs et al. (1996) questioned this long-

Table 5-3

AMELIORATION BY HUMAN MILK OF DISEASE IN INFANTS AND CHILDREN

Disease in Child	Ameliorating Properties of Human Milk
Acrodermatitis enteropathica	More efficient zinc absorption (Evans & Johnson, 1980)
Appendicitis	Antiinflammatory properties (Pisacane et al., 1995b)
Atopic disease (allergies, asthma)	Inhibits potential antigen molecules from entering neonate by providing passive barrier (numerous studies found throughout text)
Bacterial infections, neonatal sepsis	Leukocytes, lactoferrin, immune properties (Ashraf et al., 1991; Fallot et al., 1980; Levanthal et al., 1986)
Celiac disease	Protects against development of villous atrophy in intestinal mucosa (Auricchio, 1983; Greco et al., 1983; Kelly et al., 1989; Logan, 1990)
Childhood lymphoma	Increases resistance and immunity; strengthens defenses (Davis, Savitz, & Graubard, 1988; Mathur et al., 1993; Shu et al., 1995; Swartzbaum et al., 1991)
Chronic constipation	Stools soft
Colitis	Less exposure to cow's milk proteins (Anveden-Hertzberg, 1996; Jenkins et al., 1984; Rigas et al., 1993)
Crohn's disease	Uncertain but possibly reduced exposure to foreigh proteins (Bergstrand & Hellers, 1983; Koletzko et al., 1989; Rigas et al., 1993)
Diabetes, type 1	Lack of antigenic peptides helps protect against autoimmune disease (Borch-Johnson et al., 1984; Kostraba et al., 1993; Mayer et al., 1988; Perez-Bravolt et al., 1996)
Gastrointestinal infection	Humoral and cellular antiinfectious factors (Dewey et al., 1995; Howie et al., 1990; numerous other studies discussed throughout this text)
Gastroesophageal reflux	More rapid gastric emptying; lower esophageal pH (Heacock et al., 1992)
Hypernatremic dehydration	Low mineral and sodium content
Hypertrophic pyloric stenosis	Uncertain; breastfeeding may prevent pyloric spasm and edema (Habbick et al., 1989)
Infantile eczema	No species-nonspecific proteins (Blair, 1977)
Inguinal hernia	Hormones in breastmilk might stimulate neonatal testicular function to close inguinal canal and promote descent of testes (Pisacane et al., 1995a)
Iron-deficiency anemia	Better iron resorption, no blood loss from intestines (Woodruff et al., 1977)

Table 5-3 (cont.)

Juvenile rheumatoid arthritis	Antiinflammatory properties protect against autoimmune disease (Mason et al., 1995)
Liver disease	Protease inhibitors (including antitrypsin) protect children with ∂_1-AT (alpha-antitrypsin) deficiency (Udall et al., 1985)
Malocclusion	Physiological suckling patterns (Labbok & Hendershot, 1987)
Multiple sclerosis	Protects against autoimmune disease (Pisacane et al., 1994)
Necrotizing enterocolitis	Immunological factors, macrophages, osmolarity of human milk (Lucas & Cole, 1990)
Otitis media	Antibody, T- and B-cell protection; lack of irritation from cow's milk; upright feeding position (Aniansson et al., 1994; Duncan et al., 1993; Saarinen et al., 1982; Sassen et al., 1994)
Respiratory syncytial virus	IgA, IgG antibody transmitted to breastmilk and infant through gut-associated or bronchus-associated lymphoid tissue (GALT and BALT) (Bell, 1988; Downham et al., 1976; Duffy et al., 1986; Holberg et al., 1991; Pullan et al., 1980; Rahman et al., 1987)
Sudden infant death syndrome	Uncertain; possibly antiinfectious, antiallergic (Ford et al., 1993; Gilbert et al., 1995; Mosko et al., 1997) Mitchell, 1990)
Tonsillitis	Antibacterial properties (Pisacane et al., 1996)
Urinary tract infections	Antibacterial properties (Marild et al., 1990; Pisacane et al., 1996)
Vitamin E–deficiency anemia	Sufficient vitamin E in human milk

term protection for diarrhea. They found that children who stopped breastfeeding in the previous two months were vulnerable to developing dehydrating diarrhea.

In a prospective multicenter study on the effect of breastmilk in preventing necrotizing enterocolitis in premature infants, Lucas and Cole (1990) found that the disease was 6 to 10 times more common in exclusively formula-fed babies than in exclusively breastmilk-fed babies. This held true even though the human milk received was often pooled, deriving from mothers other than the babies'. These findings support our contention that breastfeeding is more than a lifestyle choice; it has profound implications for the health of the child.

The Immune System

The body's overall immune system is known as the *systemic immune system*. Another immune system, the *secretory immune system,* invokes surfaces of the body (such as the breast) and acts locally. Lymphocytes in the secretory immune system are different from other lymphocytes. Sensitized to antigens found in the gastrointestinal or the respiratory tracts, these lymphocytes travel through mucosal lymphoid tissues (e.g., breasts, salivary glands, bronchi, intestines, and genitourinary tract) where they secrete antibodies.

Most antigens to which a mother has been exposed sensitize lymphocytes migrating to the breast. There they secrete immunoglobulins into the milk, hence the term *secretory IgA* or *sIgA*. These components are further described later under Immunoglobulins.

Immunity occurs actively and passively. Maternal antibodies passed to the fetus through the placenta before birth present an example of passive immunity. Passive immunological protection is only temporary, because the infant's immune system has not itself responded.

Breastfeeding can also confer long-term protection by stimulating an active immune response. Active immunity is a specific immunity by which the immune system formulates a long-term memory of exposure to a certain antigen. Later exposure to the same antigen will produce an immune response. Poliovirus or rubella immunization of women or any attenuated virus immunization of the mother provides active immunity to the infant, because the virus will likely appear in her milk and thus immunize the infant. Another example of active immunity is the breastfed infant's immune reponse to cytomegalovirus in human milk.

Protective factors in human milk discussed in this chapter are grouped under specific headings: cells (macrophages and lymphocytes), antibodies and immunoglobulins, non–antibody factors, and antiinflammatory components.

Cells

Human milk contains two main types of white cells: phagocytes and lymphocytes (Figs. 5–5, 5–6). Although phagocytes (mostly macrophages) are most abundant (90 percent), the lymphocyte population (10 percent) provides significant protective effects to the recipient infant. The concentration of these cells and the predominant cell type vary with the duration of lactation. After birth, the number of these cells is higher than at any other time; they decline progessively thereafter.

Phagocytes. Macrophages, a type of leukocyte, are the dominant phagocyte in human milk. They engulf and absorb pathogens. Macrophages release IgA, although they probably do not synthesize it. Macrophages are both polymorphonuclear (PMN) and mononuclear. Because PMN numbers increase dramatically during inflammation of the breast, they may function to protect the mammary tissue

per se rather than to impart protection to the newborn (Buescher & Pickering, 1986). Macrophages also produce complement, lactoferrin, and lysozymes, which are discussed later in this section. Neutrophils are yet another phagocytic leukocyte. Short-lived but effective, they are first to arrive at an inflamed site, such as that which may occur during mastitis.

Lymphocytes. Lymphocytes are also leukocytes and include T cells, B cells, and assorted T-cell subsets. Lymphocytes compose about 4 percent of the total leukocytes in early lactation; about 83 percent of the lymphocytes are T cells that appear to transfer through human milk to infants (Wirt et al., 1992). The several ways in which lymphocytes recognize and help to destroy antigens are called *cell-mediated immunity*. Cell-mediated immunity is important in the destruction of viruses because the cells within which viruses live shield them from the action of antibodies.

T cells decrease rapidly in the first week after birth and continue to decline steadily. T cells are a special and separate immune component that can be activated into memory T cells (Wirt et al., 1992). These memory cells are the key to active immunity. Antibodies persist for only a few weeks before breaking down; however, memory cells can live for years, providing long-lasting protection. It is not clear whether T cells are activated in human milk or whether there is a specific homing of activated and memory T lymphocytes to the breast. B cells have functional capabilities similar to those of T cells. They mature into plasmalike cells that travel to epithelial tissues in the breast and release antibodies (Bellig, 1995; Newman, 1995).

Antibodies and Other Immunoglobulins

Immunoglobulins are proteins produced by plasma cells in response to an immunogen. Antibodies are immunoglobulins that recognize and act on a particular antigen. There are five types of immunoglobulins: IgG, IgA, IgM, IgE, and IgD. Both IgA and IgE play a critical role in biological specificity of human milk on the recipient infant.

Secretory IgA (sIgA) is the major immunoglobulin in all human secretions. SIgA provides the initial bolus that supplements immunoglobulins

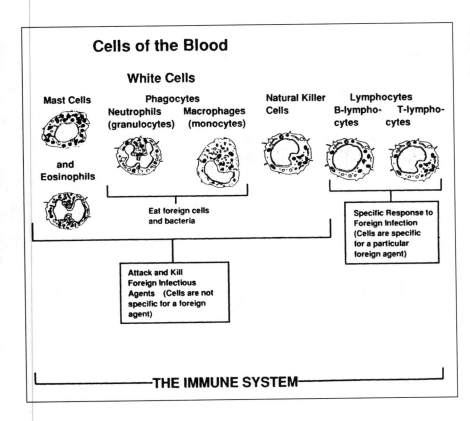

Cells of the Blood

White Cells

Mast Cells and **Eosinophils**

Phagocytes
Neutrophils (granulocytes) Macrophages (monocytes)

Natural Killer Cells

Lymphocytes
B-lympho-cytes T-lympho-cytes

Eat foreign cells and bacteria

Specific Response to Foreign Infection (Cells are specific for a particular foreign agent)

Attack and Kill Foreign Infectious Agents (Cells are not specific for a foreign agent)

THE IMMUNE SYSTEM

FIGURE 5–5. White cells of the blood. *(From H Fan, R Conner, L Villarreal:* The Biology of AIDS. *Boston: Jones and Bartlett, 1989:28.)*

transferred earlier across the placenta to the fetus. It is the immunoglobulin most frequently noted in medical literature as having immense immunological value to the neonate. SIgA, which is both synthesized and stored in the breast, reaches levels up to 5 mg/ml in colostrum, then decreases to 1 mg/ml in mature milk. Interleukin-6 in human milk may be partly responsible for the genesis of IgA- and IgM-producing cells in the mammary gland (Rudloff et al., 1993). As the mother yields more milk, the infant receives more sIgA so that the total dose of sIgA the baby receives throughout lactation is constant or even increases (depending on the milk intake). For unknown reasons, mothers of infants with poor suckling have higher IgA levels in their breastmilk (Groer et al., 1994).

SIgA synthesis via the secretory immune system described is an elegant lymphocyte traffic pathway called *gut-associated lymphoid tissue* (GALT) or *bronchus-associated lymphoid tissue* (BALT). This pathway leads to the development of lymphoid cells in the mammary gland, which produce IgA antibodies after exposure to specific microbial or environmental antigens on the intestinal or the respiratory mucosa (Goldman et al., 1983; Okamoto & Ogra, 1989). This migration of immunological responsiveness from both BALT and GALT to the mammary glands supports the unique concept of a common mucosal immune system. (See Fig. 5–8.)

Because the infant's own IgA is deficient and only slowly increases during the first several months after birth, sIgA in human milk provides important passive immunological protection to the digestive tract of newborn infants. SIgA is only minimally absorbed from the intestine: sIgA levels in the feces of breastfed infants are significantly higher than in those of formula-fed infants at the same age (Garza et al., 1987; Jatsyk et al., 1985).

A number of IgA antibodies in human milk which act upon viruses or bacteria that cause respiratory and gastrointestinal tract infections have been reported. These infecting agents include *E. coli, V. cholerae, Clostridium difficile, Salmonella,* rotavirus, poliovirus, *G. lamblia, E. histolytica,* and *Camplylobacter* (Pickering & Kohl, 1986; Ruiz-Palacios et al., 1990). As stated earlier, immunizing

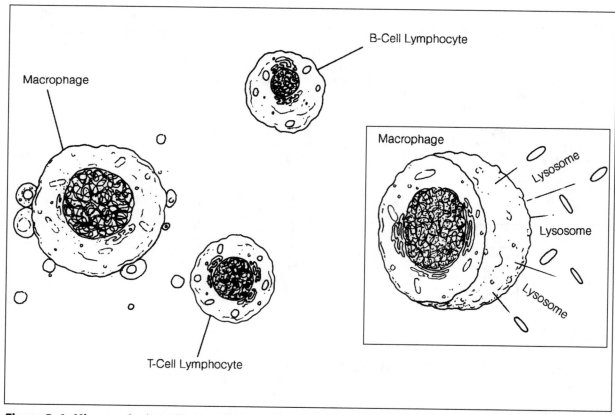

Figure 5–6. Microscopic view of living cells in human milk. *The 4,000 cells per centimeter of human milk consist mainly of macrophages and T-cell and B-cell lymphocytes. Macrophages secrete lysozyme, which helps destroy the cell walls of bacteria. (Drawing by Ka Botzis.)*

breastfeeding women with poliovirus or rubella creates IgA antibodies in milk that specifically target these agents. IgA_4 may also play a role in host defense of mucosal surfaces; in some women IgA_4 is produced locally in the mammary gland (Keller, et al., 1988). In addition to IgA, other Ig classes, including IgD, may be involved in local immunity of the breast. Several investigators (Bahna et al., 1982; Litwin et al., 1990; Steel & Leslie, 1985) have demonstrated high levels of locally produced IgD in breast tissues and breastmilk.

As shown in Figure 5–6, clear biological rhythms of protective factors predictably rise and fall as lactation progresses. The reasons for waxing and waning of various antiinfective components are not always clear but are assumed to be adapted to the needs of the infant (Figs. 5–7, 5–8).

Nonantibody Antibacterial Protection

Nonantibody factors in human milk, an elegant and intricate system, protect the infant against bacterial infection. These factors include lactoferrin, the bifidus factor, lactoperoxidase, oligosaccharides, and complement.

Lactoferrin. Lactoferrin, a potent bacteriostatic iron-binding protein, is abundant in human milk (1–6 mg/ml) but is not present in bovine milk. In the presence of IgA antibody and bicarbonate, lactoferrin readily absorbs enteric iron and thus prevents pathogenic organisms, particularly *Escherichia coli* and *Candida albicans* (Borgnolo et al., 1996; Kirkpatrick et al., 1971), from obtaining the iron needed for survival. Because exogenous iron may well interfere with the protective effects of

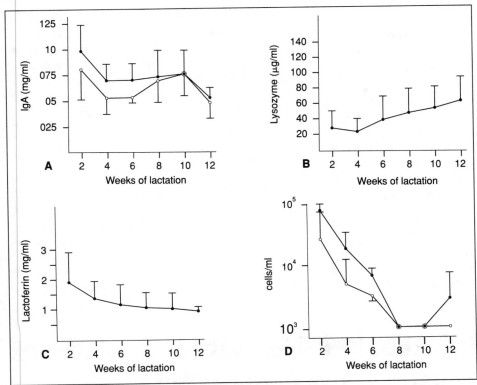

FIGURE 5–7. A longitudinal study of selected resistance factors in human milk.
(A) Total (•) and secretory (°) IgA. (B) Lysozyme. (C) Lactoferrin. (D) Macrophages-neutrophils (•–•) and lymphocytes (°–°). (Modified from AS Goldman et al: Immunological factors in human milk during the first year of lactation. J Pediatr *100:663, 1982.)*

lactoferrin, giving iron supplements to the healthy breastfed infant must be carefully weighed. Lactoferrin also has been shown to be an essential growth factor for human B and T lymphocytes (Hashizume et al., 1983).

The Bifidus Factor. The intestinal flora of breast-fed infants is dominated by gram-positive lactobacilli, especially *Lactobacillus bifidus*. This bifidus factor in human milk, first recognized by György (1953), promotes the growth of these beneficial bacteria. Together with the low protein, phosphate, and buffering capacities of milk, the bifidus factor contributes to the low pH (5–6) of stools. This acid environment discourages replication of enteropathogens such as *Shigella*, *Salmonella*, and some *E. coli*.

Lactoperoxidase. Although levels of the enzyme lactoperoxidase are low, substantial amounts are present in the newborn's saliva. It is thought that IgA in milk enhances the ability of lactoperoxidase to kill streptococci.

Oligosaccharides. Oligosaccharides (carbohydrates composed of a few monosaccharides) in human milk help to block antigens from attaching to the epithelium of the gastrointestinal tract. This blocking mechanism prevents the attachment of *Pneumococcus*, which is particularly adhesive (Goldman et al., 1986). Human milk contains about 10 times the amount of oligosaccharides that are found in bovine milk.

Complement. The complement system is a non-specific body defense system against inflammation. Although the major component of the complement system, C3, is biologically active in human milk, there is little evidence that it has a significant protective effect.

Fecal Flora

Fecal flora of breastmilk-fed infants differs strikingly from that of formula-fed infants. Among breastfed infants, bifidobacteria, lactobacilli, and staphylococci are the predominant organisms. In formula-fed infants, by contrast, the predominant organisms are enterococci, coliforms, and bacterioids similar to those of adults. Even when bovine lactoferrin is added to an infant formula, it has little effect on the fecal flora.

Antiinflammatory Components

Human milk, rich in antiinflammatory agents, supplies key protection during the vulnerable period of infancy. Major biochemical pathways of inflammations are either absent or poorly represented in breastmilk. Goldman (1993) has identified several antiinflammatory factors in breastmilk, such as antioxidants, alpha$_1$-antitrypsin, cortisol, epidermal growth factor, IgA, lysozyme, and prostaglandins. The antiinflammatory effects of these components have not as yet been directly demonstrated in the nursing infant. The specific properties of breastmilk shown to be active against bacteria, viruses, and parasites are listed in Tables 5–4 through 5–6.

Bioactive Components

Hamosh (1985) designated a special group of substances in human milk as *bioactive components*. These substances promote growth and development of the newborn by special activities that continue after the infant ingests breastmilk. Most are not available to the infant in commercial infant formula. Research on bioactive components is a

---

Table 5-4

ANTIBACTERIAL FACTORS FOUND IN HUMAN MILK

Factor	Shown in vitro to Be Active Against:	Effect of Heat
Secretory IgA	*E. coli* (also pili and capsular antigens), *C. tetani, C. diphtheriae, K. pneumoniae, Salmonella* (6 groups), *Shigella* (2 groups), *Streptococcus, S. mutans, S. sanguis, S. mitis, S. salivarius, S. pneumoniae, C. burnetti, H. influenzae* *E. coli* enterotoxin, *V. cholerae* enterotoxin, *C. difficile* toxins, *H. influenzae* capsule	Stable at 56°C for 30 min; some loss (0–30 percent) at 62.5°C for 30 min; destroyed by boiling
IgM, IgG	*V. cholerae* lipopolysaccharide; *E. coli*	IgM destroyed and IgG decreased by a third at 62.5°C for 30 min
IgD	*E. coli*	
Bifidobacterium bifidum growth z factor	Enterobacteriacea, enteric pathogens	Stable to boiling
Factor binding proteins (zinc, vitamin B$_{12}$, folate)	Dependent *E. coli*	Destroyed by boiling
Complement C1–C9 (mainly C3 and C4)	Effect not known	Destroyed by heating at 56°C for 30 min
Lactoferrin	*E. coli*	Two-thirds destroyed at 62.5°C for 30 min

Table 5-4 (cont.)

Lactoperoxidase	*Streptococcus, Pseudomonas, E. coli, S. typhimurium*	Destroyed by boiling
Lysozyme	*E. coli, Salmonella, Micrococcus lysodeikticus*	Some loss (0–23 percent) at 62.5°C for 30 min; essentially destroyed by boiling for 15 min
Unidentified factors	*S. aureus, C. difficile* toxin B	Stable at autoclaving; stable at 56°C for 30 min
Carbohydrate	*E. coli* enterotoxin	Stable at 85°C for 30 min
Lipid	*S. aureus*	Stable to boiling
Ganglioside (GMI-like)	*E. coli* enterotoxin, *V. cholerae* enterotoxin	Stable to boiling
Glycoproteins (receptor-like) + oligosaccharides	*V. cholerae*	Stable to boiling for 15 min
Analogues of epithelial cell receptors (oligosaccharides)	*S. pneumoniae, H. influenzae*	Stable to boiling
Milk cells (macrophages, neutrophils, B and T lymphocytes)	By phagocytosis and killing: *E. coli, S. aureus, S. enteritidis* By sensitized lymphocytes: *E. coli* By phagocytosis: *C. albicans, E. coli* Lymphocyte stimulation: *E. coli* K antigen, tuberculin purified protein derivative (PPD). Monocyte chemotactic factor production: PPD	Destroyed at 62.5°C for 30 min

Source: JT May: Microbial contaminants and antimicrobial properties of human milk. Microbiol Sci 5:42–46, 1988.

rapidly growing area of investigation. These bioactive components may play a significant role in child health.

Enzymes

Mammalian milk contains a large number of enzymes, some of which appear to have a beneficial effect on the development of the newborn. The enzyme content of human milk and bovine milk differ substantially (Hamosh, 1985). For example, lysozyme activity is several thousand times greater in human milk than in bovine milk. The alkaline pH of the human infant's stomach has a limited effect on the antitrypsin activity of breastmilk, thereby protecting children with alpha$_1$-antitrypsin deficiency against severe liver disease and early death (Udall et al., 1985). Most mammal milks

contain many enzymes that appear to be species-specific because of their varying level of activity in different species. A few enzymes (discussed further on) serve a digestive function in the infant or may be important to neonatal development.

Lysozyme. Lysozyme, a major component of human milk whey fraction, produces both bactericidal and antiinflammatory action. It acts with peroxide and ascorbate to destroy *E. coli* and some *Salmonella* strains (Pickering & Kohl, 1986). Lysozyme is much more abundant in human milk (400 ug/ml) than in bovine milk. Rather than slowly declining as lactation progresses, lysozyme activity increases progressively, beginning about six months after delivery (Goldman et al., 1982; Prentice et al., 1984). The lysozyme differs from other protective factors in this respect because

Table 5-5

ANTIVIRAL FACTORS FOUND IN HUMAN MILK

Factor	Shown in vitro to Be Active Against:	Effect of Heat
Secretory IgA	Poliovirus types 1, 2, 3; coxsackievirus types A9, B3, B5; echovirus types 6, 9; Semliki Forest virus, Ross River virus, rotavirus, cytomegalovirus, retrovirus type 3, rubella virus, herpes simplex virus, mumps virus, influenza virus, respiratory syncytial virus	Stable at 56°C for 30 min; some loss (0–30 percent) at 62.5°C for 30 min; destroyed by boiling
IgM, IgG	Rubella virus, cytomegalovirus, respiratory syncytial virus	IgM destroyed and IgG decreased by one-third at 62.5°C for 30 min
Lipid (unsaturated fatty acids and monoglycerides)	Herpes simplex virus, Semliki Forest virus, influenza virus, dengue, Ross River virus, Japanese B encephalitis virus, Sindbis virus, West Nile virus	Stable to boiling for 30 min
Nonimmunoglobulin macromolecules	Herpes simplex virus, vesicular stomatitis virus, coxsackievirus B4, Semliki Forest virus, retrovirus 3, poliotype 2, cytomegalovirus, respiratory syncytial virus, rotavirus	Most stable at 56°C for 30 min and destroyed by boiling
Alpha$_2$-macroglobulin (like)	Influenza virus hemagglutinin, parainfluenza virus hemagglutin	Stable to boiling for 15 min
Ribonuclease	Murine leukemia virus	Stable at 62.5°C for 30 min
Hemagglutinin inhibitors	Influenza and mumps viruses	Destroyed by boiling
Milk cells	Induced interferon: virus or phytohemagglutinin Induced lymphokine (LDCF): phytohemagglutinin Induced cytokine: by herpes simplex virus Lymphocyte stimulation: cytomegalovirus, rubella, herpes, measles, mumps, respiratory syncytial viruses	Destroyed at 62.5°C for 30 min

Source: JT May: Microbial contaminants and antimicrobial properties of human milk. Microbiol Sci *5:42–46, 1988.*

many babies begin receiving solid foods around six months, and high levels of lysozyme may be a teleological, practical safeguard against the greater risk from pathogens and diarrheal disease at this time.

Lipase. For human infants to digest fat, adequate lipase activity and bile salt levels must be present. Bile-salt–stimulated lipase and lipoprotein lipase present in human milk compensate for immature pancreatic function and for the absence of amylaze in neonates, especially in the premature infant. When human milk is frozen or refrigerated (Hamosh et al., 1997), lipase is not affected; however, heating severely reduces lipase activity.

Table 5-6

ANTIPARASITE FACTORS FOUND IN HUMAN MILK

Factor	Shown in vitro to Be Active Against:	Effect of Heat
Secretory IgA	*G. lamblia* *E. histolytica* *S. mansoni* *Cryptosporidium*	Stable at 56°C for 30 min, some loss (0–30 percent) at 62.5°C for 30 min, destroyed by boiling
Lipid (free)	*G. lamblia* *E. histolytica* *T. vaginalis*	Stable to boiling
Unidentified	*T. rhodesiense*	

Source: JT May: Microbial contaminants and antimicrobial properties of human milk. Microbiol Sci *5:42–46, 1988.*

Several protozoa—*Giardia lamblia, Entamoeba histolytica,* and *Trichomonas vaginalis*—have been shown in vitro to be killed rapidly by exposure to salt-stimulated lipase, which is found only in the milk of humans and mountain gorillas (Blackberg et al., 1980).

Amylase. Amylase is necessary for the digestion of starch. Although amylase is synthesized and stored in the pancreas of the newborn, the infant is around six months old before amylase is released into the duodenum. Human milk contains about 10 to 60 times as much alpha-amylase as does normal human serum, thus providing an alternate source of this starch-digestive substance. No alpha-amylase is present in bovine, goat, or swine milk, suggesting that this enzyme appeared late in the evolutionary continuum. Hamosh (1985) observed that breastfed infants have fewer problems digesting solid foods than do formula-fed infants, even if these foods are introduced early. Breastfed infants may tolerate the early introduction of solids because of the alpha-amylase provided by breastmilk. Amylase is stable when refrigerated (95–100 percent activity after 24 hours storage at 15–25°C) (Hamosh et al., 1997).

Biotinidase. The enzyme biotinidase regulates the metabolism of biotin. Biotinidase activity in colostrum is about five times higher than that in human milk. Although the role of biotinidase is not yet known, its high levels in colostrum suggest that it might have a special nutritional role in neonates (Oizumi & Hayakawa, 1988).

Growth Factors

Human milk contains growth-promoting components also known as *growth modulators*. As with its antiinfective properties, these substances are more pronounced in colostrum than in mature milk. Neither their biological significance nor their method of action is yet clear. It is not certain, for instance, whether growth factors influence growth and repair of mammary tissue or promote growth and repair cells within the intestines of the neonate, are absorbed from the neonatal gastrointestinal tract, enter the circulation of the neonate, and exert an effect on enteric or target organs or whether some combination of these possible actions occurs (Morriss et al., 1986).

Epidermal Growth Factor. Epidermal growth factor (EGF) is a major growth-promoting agent in breastmilk, which stimulates proliferation of intestinal mucosa and epithelium and strengthens the mucosal barrier to antigens (Carpenter, 1980; Petschow et al., 1993). A polypeptide that contains 53 amino acids, EGF is highest in human milk after delivery (15 µg/dl) and decreases rapidly thereafter (Matsuoka & Idota, 1995). There is no diurnal variation or variation between preterm and term milk. EGF is also present in plasma, saliva, and amniotic fluid, but human milk contains a higher concentration. EGF may also be involved in the development of low-density lipoprotein receptors and in cholesterol metabolism.

Human Growth Factors I, II, and III. Three polypeptides, called *human-milk growth factors* (HMGF) *I, II, and III,* have been isolated (Shing & Klagsburn, 1984). HMGF III stimulates DNA synthesis and cellular proliferation, suggesting that it is an epidermal growth factor. Several in vivo studies (Heird et al., 1984; Widdowson et al., 1976) on growth factors in animal milk have shown striking increases in the mass of intestinal mucosa. Morriss et al. (1986) point out that "the presence of growth factors in human milk may influence the growth of target tissues in the suckled infant by provoking an *endogenous hormonal response* that is different from that provoked by ingestion of a proprietary formula." Different growth factors may have overlapping functions, both stimulating cell growth and indirectly affecting the infant's defense mechanisms against disease.

Hormones

Insulinlike Growth Factor. An insulinlike growth factor (IGF-I) in human milk is thought to have a growth-promoting role. The concentration of this factor in colostrum is about 30 times that in human serum. These high levels (4.1 nmol/liter) decrease rapidly (to 1.3 nmol/liter) as colostrum alters to transitional milk (Read et al., 1984) but do not decline further. In fact, Corps et al. (1988) found that the concentration of an insulinlike growth factor in human milk increased (2.5 nmol/liter) by the sixth week postpartum.

Thyroxine and Thyrotropin-Releasing Hormone. Thyroxine is present in human milk in small quantities but is not found in commercial formulas. The concentration in colostrum is low, increases by the first week postpartum, and gradually declines thereafter. It has been suggested that thyroxine may stimulate the maturation of the infant's intestine (Morriss, 1985).

Although the thyroxine level is significantly higher in breastfed children than in formula-fed children at one and two months of age (Rovet, 1990), it is unclear whether breastfeeding protects breastfed infants against clinical evidence of congenital hypothyroidism (Bode, Vanjonack, & Crawford, 1978; Latarte et al., 1980; Rovet, 1990). Some infants receive sufficient thyroxine in their mother's milk to compensate for hypothyroidism; thus the symptoms may be masked for several months. Although this does not appear to be true for all infants, the results of thyroid studies after the first week of life should be interpreted with caution in breastfed infants and should include measurements of both thyroxine and thyroid-stimulating hormone (TSH) concentrations.

Cortisol. Cortisol is present in relatively high concentrations in colostrum, declines rapidly by the second day, and remains low thereafter. Its role in infant physiology is not clear. Three theories have been presented concerning the function of cortisol in the infant:

1. It may control the transport of fluids and salts in the infant's gastrointestinal tract (Kulski & Hartmann, 1981).

2. It may play a role in the growth of the infant's pancreas (Morisset & Jolicoeur, 1980).

3. Cortisol may serve as a hormone released during chronic stress. Mothers' higher level of satisfaction with breastfeeding is associated with lower levels of cortisol in their milk. The amount of cortisol in milk is inversely related to sIgA, suggesting that cortisol may suppress the function of immunoglobulin-producing cells in milk (Groer et al., 1994).

Cholecystokinin (CCK). CCK is a gastrointestinal hormone that enhances digestion, sedation, and a feeling of satiation and well-being. During suckling, vagal stimulation causes CCK release in both mother and infant, producing a sleepy feeling. The infant's CCK level peaks twice after suckling. The first peak occurs immediately after the feeding. It peaks again 30 to 60 minutes later. The first CCK rise is probably induced by suckling; the second by the presence of milk in the gastrointestional tract (Marchini & Linden, 1992; Uvnas-Moberg et al., 1993).

Prostaglandins. Prostaglandins, a special group of lipids, are present in most mammal cells and tissues and affect almost every biological system.

Prostaglandins are formed by numerous body tissues and affect many physiological functions, including local circulation, gastric and mucous secretion, electrolyte balance, zinc absorption, and the release of brush border enzymes. The protective activity of milk lipids is thought to be due to the presence of prostaglandins PGE_2 and PGF_{2a} present in both colostrum and mature milk. Concentrations there are about 100 times greater than their levels in adult plasma (Lucas & Mitchell, 1980). PGE_2 particularly is thought to exert a cytoprotective action (protection against inflammation and necrosis) on the gastric mucosa by promoting the accumulation of phospholipids in the neonatal stomach (Reid, Smith, & Friedman, 1980). The full extent of the beneficial effects of prostaglandins in human milk awaits future scientific investigation.

Taurine

Taurine, absent in bovine milk, is the second most abundant amino acid in human milk (Raiha, 1985). This unusual amino acid, which may function as a neurotransmitter, plays an important role in early brain maturation (Gaull, 1985). Before 1983, taurine was thought to act only in the conjugation of bile acids. Infants who do not receive taurine in their diet conjugate bile acids with glycine, which less effectively assists in absorbing dietary fats. Although deleterious effects of low taurine levels are not known in humans, deficiencies have caused retinal problems in cats and monkeys (Jensen et al., 1988). Taurine was added to most commercial formulas when formula-fed infants were found to have plasma taurine levels only half as high as those of breastfed infants.

Antiallergenic Properties

In 1936, Grulee and Sanford published a classic study demonstrating for the first time that breastfeeding, compared to cow's-milk feeding, reduced the incidence of eczema sevenfold. There is general agreement that allergies are less common in completely breastfed babies, because foreign food intake is limited to those eaten by the mother and secreted into her breastmilk. At the same time, this topic is controversial and engenders considerable debate in published literature and in discussions.

The incidence of food-induced allergic disease in children has been estimated to be between 0.3 to 7.5 percent (Metcalfe, 1984). Heredity is a significant predictor of allergic disease (Savilahti et al., 1987), even when the mother is on a milk-free diet during late pregnancy and lactation (Lovegrove et al., 1994). Sixty percent of all those who will develop atopic eczema do so within the first year of life, and 90 percent do so within the first five years (Hanifin, 1984). Before six to nine months of age, the infant's intestinal mucosa is permeable to proteins; moreover, his secretory IgA, which later will "paint" the mucosa and bind sensitizing proteins to itself, is not yet functioning effectively.

Bovine milk is the most common single allergen affecting infants. Proteins in bovine milk known to act as allergens include lactoglobulin, casein, bovine serum albumin, and lactalbumin. Modern heat treatment of formula may have reduced—but has certainly not eliminated—the allergic potential of these proteins. The problem is probably increased by the sizable dose of allergens in formula and by the large volume of formula ingested. At two to four months of age, for example, a baby consumes his body weight in milk each week. This is the equivalent of nearly seven quarts per day for an adult—truly a macrodose!

Symptoms of allergy to cow's milk commonly appear during the first few months of life. Cow's milk most frequently affects the gastrointestinal tract. Vomiting, diarrhea, colic, and occult bleeding are symptoms. It also affects the respiratory tract (runny nose, cough, asthma) and the skin (dermatitis, urticaria). Because the symptoms are varied and nonspecific, the diagnosis is often mistaken or missed (Bahna, 1987).

At birth, the IgE system is defective in the potentially allergic infant, and problems arise if this system is activated by allergens. When the introduction of foreign proteins is delayed for four to six months, the baby's own IgA system is permitted to become more fully functional; thus allergic responses may be minimized or entirely avoided. Exclusive consumption of breastmilk facilitates the early maturation of the intestinal barrier and provides an exogenous passive barrier; it also provides an exogenous passive barrier to potentially antigenic molecules until the baby's own natural barriers develop. The rationale for delay of solids for the first half year after birth is thus reinforced.

High levels of neonatal blood IgE are thought to predict later development of atopic symptoms. When the relationship between fecal IgE levels, a reliable indicator of serum IgE levels, was compared in one-month-old infants, formula-fed babies showed a higher incidence of high fecal IgE levels than did the breastfed infants (Furukawa et al., 1994).

Studies of the effect of breastfeeding on allergic disease are conflicting, and some are seriously flawed (Kovar et al., 1984; Kramer, 1988). The majority of studies, however, show that breastmilk has a protective effect against allergies. The longest prospective study, by Saarinen and Kajosaari (1995), followed breastfed Finnish infants of atopic parents for 17 years. The prevalence of atopy was highest in the group of children who were not breastfed at all or were breastfed for less than one month. Hide and Guyer (1981) conducted a large cohort study of atopic disease in infants and found a small, statistically nonsignificant difference of eczema between breastfed and bottle-fed infants. Jenkins et al. (1984) looked at 46 children with colitis and identified food allergy as a major cause of colitis. In eight children in the study, the onset of colitis occurred soon after starting foods other than breastmilk. Prolonged breastfeeding has been reported to reduce the severity of diarrhea in atopic infants aged 7 to 12 months, although not in older infants (Ruuska, 1992).

Taylor et al. (1982) reported that increased duration of breastfeeding, both exclusive and nonexclusive, was associated with decreasing likelihood of eczema at any time during a child's life. Blair (1977) followed children in his private London practice for five years to determine whether asthma was affected by infant feeding. More children who had not been breastfed had severe asthma than did those who had been breastfed. Twenty years later, the differences were still statistically significant: some 64 percent who had not been breastfed had chronic or recurrent asthma, contrasted with 46 percent who had been breastfed for one week or less and 35 percent who had been breastfed for eight weeks or more. Another study (Wright et al., 1995) found that breastfeeding was associated with lower rates of recurrent wheezing at age six years but only in nonatopic children; this relationship was not significant for atopic children. When 83 mother-and-infant pairs were followed in a pediatric clinic for routine care for 12 months, infants who were nursed for 6 months or more had significantly fewer allergies than did those who were on formula or were nursed for less than 6 months (Strimas & Chi, 1988). Conversely, the Italian Collaborative Study (1988), a multisite study of allergies in 303 infants less than one year old, showed that breastfeeding was not more common and did not last longer in controls (those without allergies) as compared to cases (those with allergies).

As a result of this conflicting information, not everyone agrees that breastfeeding reduces food allergies. After conducting a meta-analysis of 22 original research reports on infant feeding and atopic disease, Kramer (1988) decided that errors in research methods preclude definitive conclusions.

Problems in this type of research are manifold. Because it is not possible to classify mothers randomly into breastfeeding and nonbreastfeeding groups, are those infants with a family history of atopic eczema more likely to be breastfed because the parents are aware that it has a protective effect? When the infant is identified as *breastfed,* does that mean that the baby received no other nutriments? If so, for how long was exclusive breastfeeding continued?

A few breastfed infants develop atopic eczema. Of those who do, according to several well-documented studies, the culprit is often foods ingested by the mother, especially cow's milk (Gerrard et al., 1973; Jakobsson et al., 1985). Chandra et al. (1986) completed a prospective study of 109 women who had a previous child with atopic disease. By almost completely excluding milk, other dairy products, egg, fish, beef, and peanuts throughout pregnancy and lactation, these authors documented a significant reduction in the incidence and severity of atopic eczema among breastfed infants of these mothers. Several studies have reported the detection of cow's-milk antigen in breastmilk (Axelsson et al., 1986; Cavagni et al., 1988; Jakobsson et al., 1985; Odze et al., 1995; Paganelli et al., 1986; Stuart et al., 1984). Early and occasional exposure to cow's-milk protein sensitizes neonates so that even minute amounts of bovine milk protein in human milk may later act as booster doses that elict allergic reactions (Host et al., 1988).

Others disagree that symptoms of allergy in a breastfed infant may be due to the passage of a food antigen into the mother's milk (Herrmann et al., 1996). A Swedish study (Lilja et al., 1989) found no preventive effect on the development of atopic disease in infants up to 18 months of age when their mothers avoided chicken's eggs and cow's milk during late pregnancy and the first two months of lactation. Because immune responses are present in the fetus before the end of the first trimester and because many other potential allergens were neither assessed nor controlled in this study, such a finding is hardly surprising.

Implications for Clinical Practice

Human milk is a species-specific fluid of diverse composition that includes nonnutrient substances, all of which protect the infant. Although the significance of these nonnutrient components is well known, their influence on the growth and development and subsequent health of infants is a new field that is just beginning to be explored.

With the advent of managed care that rewards prevention of health problems and avoidance of health services, health care corporations look for cost-effective ways to keep their insured clients healthy. Although it is difficult to calculate the actual costs of the widespread use of artificial, commercial baby milks, one study showed that the cost of not breastfeeding for four medical diagnoses (gastroenteritis, RSV, insulin-dependent diabetes mellitus, and otitis media) alone results in an estimated extra $1.9 billion annual health care costs (Riordan, 1997).

A thorough understanding of the biological components of human and bovine milks and of manufactured formulas is essential for the health care specialist who is providing lactation assistance. Parents have a right to make an informed decision about how they will feed their infant. When prenatal discussion with the parents and prenatal classes include information about the advantages of immunological protection and its absence from not breastfeeding, the parents can make a truly informed choice.

Very little research has been done on the perceptions of mothers about breastmilk. In a qualitative study, Bottorff and Morse (1990) revealed that mothers clearly recognize the difference between colostrum and mature breastmilk. Because of the relative thickness of colostrum, some mothers believe it is the "strongest" milk, significant for its "rich" supply of antibodies rather than for its nutritional properties. Breastmilk was frequently "described by using fat-related terms (e.g., lean, creamy, rich) and evaluated by drawing comparisons to cow's milk and infant formula, as if some similarities should exist between the two [p. 520]."

Given the differences between the growth patterns of breastfed infants and infants fed human-milk substitutes, practitioners need to question the use of standardized growth charts (developed primarily on the basis of results from bottle-fed infants) to evaluate breastfed infants. Otherwise, breastfeeding mothers might be told that their babies are gaining too slowly and that their milk production must be insufficient, when obviously their babies are healthy in all respects. The WHO has recently developed growth guidelines based on results from studies of breastfed infants (WHO, 1994). (See Chapter 11 on slow weight gain for a more detailed discussion of this issue.)

Knowledge of physiology provides us direction for lactation practice and advice to mothers. For example, the high fat (and thus calories) in hindmilk, when the breast has less milk, imply caution in routinely recommending "switch" nursing (repeatedly switching feedings from breast to breast during a breastfeeding) (Woolridge & Fisher, 1988). On the other hand, infants whose requirements may fluctuate with time are amazingly adept at self-regulating their nutrient intake (Woolridge et al., 1990). Thus we can encourage women to be flexible about breastfeedings and to be led by infants' cues that tell mothers when the baby wants to be fed and when to stop the feeding. Also it would be helpful to have a way to identify mothers who might be at risk for delay in lactogenesis. Humenick's (1987) MICAM method, which uses filter papers, appears to be an inexpensive and easy way to do this.

The drop of infant CCK levels 10 minutes after the feeding implies a "window" within which the infant can be awakened to feed from the second breast or to reattach to the first side for additional fat-rich milk. Waiting 30 minutes after the feeding before laying the baby down takes advantage of the second CCK peak to help the infant to stay asleep.

Given the high water content coupled with the low solute load and mineral content in human milk, the breastfed infant with free access to this mother's breast needs no additional water. Healthy infants who consume enough breastmilk to satisfy their energy needs receive, with a considerable margin of safety, enough fluid to satisfy their requirements even in hot and dry environments (Almroth & Bidinger, 1978; Brown et al., 1986b). Water and teas given in addition to breastmilk for hydration in hot weather produce the opposite effect by increasing the risk of diarrhea. If a breastfeeding infant does develop diarrhea, the low mineral level in human milk prevents a rapid osmotic shift of free (extracellular) water so that dehydration is less severe and recovery is more rapid than in the artificially fed infant (Khin-Maung-U, 1985).

The studies cited here support giving fresh, rather than heat-treated or frozen, human milk whenever possible. Some living cells are killed by both of these treatments. Also, due to the action of the bile-salt–stimulated lipase, fat in fresh human milk is absorbed more completely than that in pasteurized milk.

During the assessment phase of working with a breastfeeding family, the practitioner needs to ask if there is a family history of allergies. If so, the mother should be encouraged to breastfeed for a minimum of nine months and to delay feeding the infant solid foods until the baby shows signs of readiness. Because of risk of sensitization to allergenic proteins, particularly in babies who have a family history of allergies, even occasional formula supplements can trigger an allergic reaction and should be avoided as long as possible. In addition to preventing allergies, infant malabsorption problems, such as celiac disease, are lessened when the baby is breastfed and solid foods are delayed (Auricchio et al., 1983; Logan, 1990). Solid foods are usually started around six months of age as babies' intestinal enzymes mature and they become increasingly capable of digesting complex proteins and starches. After six months, babies can generally eat whatever they like (with few exceptions) and in any order they want.

In the maternal diet, dairy products particularly are potential allergens to the breastfeeding baby. If the mother notices that a particular food seems to cause an allergic response in her infant, she needs to consider eliminating it from her diet. A case report (Wilson, Self, & Hamburger, 1990) describes rectal bleeding in a four-day-old infant who was exclusively breastfed: her mother was drinking four to five glasses of cow's milk per day. Although this case is extreme and rare, it demonstrates the potential for problems when a breastfeeding mother drinks large quantities of cow's milk. Discussion of diet and appropriate substitution should be part of the care provided the mother by the health care worker offering lactation consultation and support.

SUMMARY

The nutritional components of human milk, combined with its immune and antiallergic properties, make it the ideal foundation for optimal infant health. Immunological and allergy protection are obvious, but more difficult is substantiating the protection by breastfeeding against inflammatory and immunologically determined disorders that emerge later in life. Allowed to breastfeed at will in response to their own needs, infants generally obtain milk in amounts that satisfy their energy needs and maintain normal patterns of growth.

Practical experience clearly supports the benefits of breastfeeding. In recent years, scientific data from all parts of the world confirm what the practitioner has long observed. It is ironic that many of the complex properties of human milk described in this chapter have been identified through research funded by formula companies, which stand to make large sums of money if they can develop products for which they can claim a close resemblance to human milk.

Commenting on its unique adaptability, Ratner (1981) noted, "Human milk has a remarkable fitness in terms of the demands and needs of the infant. . . . The configuration of elements in breastmilk are like computer information with a reciprocal fitness between the mother and the infant." Moreover, even in special cases, such as the accelerated energy needs of the premature infant, this adaptability is seen in the greater availability of energy in preterm milk. Jensen et al. (1988) poetically describes this reciprocity as "human milk as a carrier of important physiological messages" to the recipient infant.

REFERENCES

Abrams SA, Wen H, Stuff JE: Absorption of calcium, zinc, and iron from breast milk by five- to seven-month-old infants. *Pediatr Res* 39:384–90, 1996.

Adebonojo FO: Artificial vs breast-feeding: relation to infant health in a middle-class American community. *Clin Pediatr* 11:25–9, 1972.

Almroth SG, Bidinger PD: No need for water supplementation for exclusively breast-fed infants under hot and arid conditions. *Trans Roy Soc Trop Med Hygiene* 84:602–4, 1990.

Almroth SG, Latham MC: Breast feeding practices in rural Jamaica. *J Trop Pediatr* 28:103–9, 1982.

American Academy of Pediatrics, Committee on Nutrition. Commentary on breastfeeding and infant formulas, including standards for formulas. *Pediatrics* 57:278–85, 1976.

American Academy of Pediatrics, Committee on Nutrition: vitamin and mineral supplement needs in normal children in the United States. *Pediatrics* 66:1015–21, 1980.

Anderson CH: Human milk feeding. *Pediatr Clin North Am* 32:338–52, 1985.

Andon MB, et al: Nutritionally relevant supplementation of vitamin B_6 in lactating women: effect on plasma prolactin. *Pediatrics* 76:769–73, 1985.

Aniansson G, et al: A prospective cohort study on breast-feeding and otitis media in Swedish infants. *Pediatr Infect Dis J* 13:183–8, 1994.

Anveden-Hertzberg L: Proctocolitis in exclusively breast-fed infants. *Eur J Pediatr* 155:464–7, 1996.

Arthur PG, et al: Measuring short-term rates of milk synthesis in breast-feeding mothers. *Q J Exp Physiol* 47:419–28, 1989.

Arthur PG, Smith M, Hartmann PE: Milk lactose, citrate, and glucose as markers of lactogenesis in normal and diabetic women. *J Pediatr Gastroenterol Nutr* 9:488–96, 1989.

Ashraf RN, et al: Breast feeding and protection against neonatal sepsis in a high risk population. *Arch Dis Child* 66:488–90, 1991.

Atkinson SA, Anderson G, Bryan MH: Human milk: comparison of the nitrogen composition of milk from mothers of premature infants. *Am J Clin Nutr* 33:811–5, 1980.

Atkinson SA, et al: Abnormal zinc content in human milk: risk for development of nutritional zinc deficiency in infants. *Am J Dis Child* 143:608–11, 1989.

Auricchio S, et al: Does breast feeding protect against the development of clinical symptoms of celiac disease in children? *J Pediatr Gastroenterol Nutr* 2:428–33, 1983.

Axelsson I, et al: Bovine beta-lactoglobulin in the human milk. *Acta Pediatr Scand* 75:702, 1986.

Bahna SL: Milk allergy in infancy. *Ann Allergy* 59:131–6, 1987.

Bates CJ, Prentice A: Breast milk as a source of vitamins, essential minerals and trace elements. *Pharmacol Ther* 62:193–220, 1994.

Bauchner J, Levanthal JM, Shapiro ED: Studies of breastfeeding and infections: how good is the evidence? *JAMA* 256:887–92, 1986.

Beijers RJW, Schaafsma A: Long-chain polyunsaturated fatty acid content in Dutch preterm breast milk: differences in the concentrations of docosahexaenoic acid and arachidonic acid due to length of gestation. *Early Hum Dev* 44:215–23, 1996.

Bell LM, et al: Rotavirus serotype-specific neutralizing activity in human milk. *Am J Dis Child* 142:275–8, 1988.

Bellig LL: Immunization and the prevention of childhood diseases. *JOGNN* 24:469-77, 1995.

Bergstrand O, Hellers G: Breast-feeding during infancy in patients who develop Crohn's Disease. *Scand J Gastroenterol* 18:903–6, 1983.

Birch DG, et al: Retinal development in very-low-birth-weight infants fed diets differing in omega-3 fatty acids. *Invest Ophthalmol Vis Sci* 33:2365–76, 1992.

Birch E, et al: Breast-feeding and optimal visual development. *J Pediatr Ophthalmol Strabismus* 30: 30–8, 1993.

Blackberg LD, et al: The bile salt stimulated lipase in human milk is an evolutionary newcomer derived from a non-milk protein. *FEBS Lett* 112:51, 1980.

Blair H: Natural history of childhood asthma: a twenty-year follow-up. *Arch Dis Child* 52:613–9, 1977.

Bode HH, Vanjonack WJ, Crawford JD: Mitigation of cretinism by breast feeding. *Pediatrics* 62:13, 1978.

Borch-Johnson K, et al: Relation between breast-feeding and incidence rates of insulin-dependent diabetes mellitus. *Lancet* 2:1083–6, 1984.

Borgnolo G, et al: A case-control study of *Salmonella* gastrointestinal infection in Italian children. *Acta Paediatr* 85:804–8, 1996.

Bottorff JL, Morse JM: Mother's perceptions of breast milk. *JOGNN* 19:518–27, 1990.

Brown KH, et al: Infant-feeding practices and their relationship with diarrheal and other diseases in Huascar (Lima), Peru. *Pediatrics* 83:31–40, 1989.

Brown KH, et al: Lactational capacity of marginally nourished mothers: relationships between maternal nutritional status and quantity and proximate composition of milk. *Pediatrics* 78:909–19, 1986a.

Brown KH, et al: Milk consumption and hydration status of exclusively breast-fed infants in a warm climate. *J Pediatr* 108:677–80, 1986b.

Buescher ES, Pickering LK: Polymorphonuclear leukocytes in human colostrum and milk. In: Howell RR, Morriss FH, Pickering LK, eds. *Human milk in infant nutrition and health*. Springfield, IL: Thomas, 1986: 160–73.

Bullen JJ, Rogers HJ, Leigh L: Iron-binding proteins in milk and resistance to *Escherichia coli* infection in infants. *Br Med J* 1:69–75, 1972.

Butte NF, et al: Human milk intake and growth in exclusively breast-fed infants. *J Pediatr* 104:187–95, 1984.

Butte NF, et al: Influence of early feeding mode on body composition of infants. *Biol Neonate* 67: 414–24, 1995.

Butte NF, et al: Macro- and trace-mineral intakes of exclusively breast-fed infants. *Am J Clin Nutr* 45:42–7, 1987.

Butte NF, Smith EO, Garza C: Energy utilization of breast-fed and formula-fed infants. *Am J Clin Nutr* 51:350–8, 1990.

Campfield T, et al: Urinary oxalate excretion in premature infants: effect of human milk versus formula feeding. *Pediatrics* 94:674–8, 1994.

Canfield LM, Hopkinson JM: State of the art of vitamin K in human milk. *J Pediatr Gastroenterol Nutr* 8:430–41, 1989.

Carlson SE, et al: Visual-acuity development in healthy preterm infants: effect of marine-oil supplementation. *Am J Clin Nutr* 57:35–41, 1993.

Carpenter G: Epidermal growth factor is a major growth-promoting agent in human milk. *Science* 210:198–9, 1980.

Casey CE, Hambidge KM, Neville MC: Studies in human lactation: zinc, copper, manganese and chromium in human milk in the first month of lactation. *Am J Clin Nutr* 41:1193–200, 1985.

Casey CE, Neville MC, Hambidge KM: Studies in human lactation: secretion of zinc, copper, and manganese in human milk. *Am J Clin Nutr* 49:773–85, 1989.

Cavagni G, et al: Passage of food antigens into circulation of breast-fed infants with atopic dermatitis. *Ann Allergy* 61:361–5, 1988.

Cavell B: Gastric emptying in infants fed human or infant formula. *Acta Paediatr Scand* 70:639–41, 1981.

Chandra RK: Prospective studies of the effect of breast-feeding on incidence of infection and allergy. *Acta Paediatr Scand* 68:691–4, 1979.

Chandra RK, et al: Influence of maternal food antigen avoidance during pregnancy and lactation on incidence of atopic eczema in infants. *Clin Allergy* 16:563–9, 1986.

Chen Y, Yu S, Li W: Artificial feeding and hospitalization in the first 18 months of life. *Pediatrics* 81:58–62, 1988.

Clavano NR: Mode of feeding and its effect on infant mortality and morbidity. *J Trop Pediatr* 28:287–93, 1982.

Cochi SL, et al: Primary invasive *Haemophilus influenzae* type b disease: a population-based assessment of risk factors. *J Pediatr* 108:8-87-96, 1986.

Committee on Dietary Allowances: *Recommended Dietary Allowances*. Washington, DC: National Academy of Sciences, 1980: 46–7.

Corps et al: The insulin-like growth factor I content in human milk increases between early and full lactation. *J Clin Endocrinol Metab* 67(1): 25–9, 1988.

Cox DB, Owens RA, Hartmann PE: Blood and milk prolactin and the rate of milk synthesis in women. *Exp Physiol* 81:1007–20, 1996.

Cunningham AS: Morbidity in breast-fed and artificially fed infants: I. *J Pediatr* 90:726–9, 1977.

Cunningham AS: Morbidity in breast-fed and artificially fed infants: II. *J Pediatr* 95:685–9, 1979.

Daly SE, et al: Degree of breast emptying explains changes in the fat content, but not fatty acid compositon of human milk. *Exp Physiol* 78:741–55, 1993.

Daly SE, et al: The determination of short-term breast volume changes and the rate of synthesis of human milk using computerized breast measurement. *Exp Physiol* 77:79–87, 1992.

Daly SE, Owens RA, Hartmann PE: The short-term synthesis and infant-regulated removal of milk in lactating women. *Exp Physiol* 78: 209–20, 1993.

Davis MK, Savitz DA, Graubard B: Infant feeding and childhood cancer. *Lancet* 2(8607):365–8, 1988.

Dewey KG, et al: Growth of breast-fed infants deviates from current reference data: a pooled analysis of US, Canadian, and European data sets. *Pediatrics* 96:495–503, 1995.

Dewey KG, et al: Breast-fed infants are leaner than formula-fed infants at 1 year of age: the DARLING study. *Am J Clin Nutr* 57:140–5, 1993.

Dewey KG, Heinig J, Nommsen-Rivers LA: Differences in morbidity between breast-fed and formula-fed infants. *J Pediatr* 126:697–702, 1995.

Dewey KG, Lönnerdal B: Milk and nutrient intake of breast-fed infants from 1 to 6 months: relation to growth and fatness. *J Pediatr Gastroenterol Nutr* 2:497–506, 1983.

Downham MA, et al: Breast-feeding protects against respiratory syncytial virus infection. *Br Med J* 2:274–6, 1976.

Duffy LC, et al: The effects of infant feeding on rotavirus-induced gastroenteritis: a prospective study. *Am J Public Health* 76:259–63, 1986.

Duncan B, et al: Iron and the exclusively breast-fed infant from birth to six months. *J Pediatr Gastroenterol Nutr* 4:412–25, 1985.

Duncan J, et al: Exclusive breast-feeding for at least 4 months protects against otitis media. *Pediatrics* 91:867–72, 1993.

Ek J, Magnus EM: Plasma and red cell folate in beast-fed infants. *Acta Paediatr Scand* 68:239–43, 1979.

Evans GS, Johnson PE: Characterization and quantitation of a zinc-binding ligand and human milk. *Pediatr Res* 14:876–80, 1980.

Fallot MB, et al: Breast-feeding reduces incidence of hospital admissions for infections in infants. *Pediatrics* 65:1121–24, 1980.

Fan H, Conner R, Villareal L: *The biology of AIDS.* Boston: Jones and Bartlett, 1989: 28.

Fawzi WW, et al: Maternal anthropometry and infant feeding practices in Israel in relation to growth in infancy: the North African Infant Feeding Study. *Am J Clin Nutr* 65:1731–7, 1997.

Ford RPK, et al: Breastfeeding and the risk of sudden infant death syndrome. *Int J Epidemiol* 22:885–90, 1993.

Forman MR, et al: Undernutrition among Bedouin Arab infants: the Bedouin Infant Feeding Study. *Am J Clin Nutr* 51:339–43, 1990.

Frank AL, et al: Breast-feeding and respiratory virus infection. *Pediatrics* 70:239–45, 1982.

Freely RM, et al: Calcium, phosphorus, and magnesium contents of human milk during early lactation. *J Pediatr Gastroenterol Nutr* 2:262–7, 1983.

Fuchs SC, Victor CG, Martines J: Case-control study of risk of dehydrating diarrhoea in infants in vulnerable period after full weaning. *Br Med J* 313:391–4, 1996.

Furukawa SK, et al: Fecal IgE in infants at 1 month of age as indicator of atopic disease. *Allergy* 49:791–4, 1994.

Gale CR, Martyn CN: Breastfeeding, dummy use, and adult intelligence. *Lancet* 347(9009):1072–5, 1996.

Garza C, et al: Changes in the nutrient compositon of human milk during gradual weaning. *Am J Clin Nutr* 37:61–5, 1983.

Garza C, et al: Special properties of human milk. *Clin Perinatol* 14:11–31, 1987.

Garza C, Stuff J, Butte N: Growth of the breast-fed infant. In: Goldman AS, Atkinson SA, Hanson LA, eds. *Human lactation: the effects of human milk on the recipient infant.* New York: Plenum, 1986:109–21.

Gaull GE: Significance of growth modulators in human milk. *Pediatrics* 75(suppl):142–5, 1985.

Gerrard JW, et al: Cow's milk allergy: prevalence and manifestations in an unselected series of newborns. *Acta Paediatr Scand* 234(suppl):1–21, 1973.

Gilbert RE, et al: Bottle-feeding and the sudden infant death syndrome. *Br Med J* 310:88–90, 1995.

Glass RI, Stoll BJ: The protective effect of human milk against diarrhea: a review of studies from Bangladesh. *Acta Paediatr Scand* 351(suppl):131–6, 1989.

Goldman AS: The immune system of human milk: antimicrobial, antiinflammatory and immunomodulating properties. *Pediatr Infect Dis J* 12:664–71, 1993.

Goldman AS, et al: Antiinflammatory properties of human milk. *Acta Paediatr Scand* 75:689–95, 1986.

Goldman AS, et al: Immunologic factors in human milk during the first year of lactation. *J Pediatr* 100:563–67, 1982.

Goldman AS, et al: Immunologic components in human milk during gradual weaning. *Acta Paediatr Scand* 72:133–4, 1983.

Grantham-McGregor SM, Back EH: Breast feeding in Kingston, Jamaica. *Arch Dis Child* 45:404–9, 1972.

Greco L, et al: Case control study on nutritional risk factors in celiac disease. *J Pediar Gastroenterol Nutr* 7:395–99, 1983.

Greer FR, Hollis BW, Napoli JL: High concentrations of vitamin D_2 in human milk associated with pharmacological doses of vitamin D_2. *J Pediatr* 105:61–4, 1984.

Greer FR, Marshall S: Bone mineral content, serum vitamin D metabolite concentrations and ultraviolet B light exposure in infants fed human milk with and without vitamin D_2 supplements. *J Pediatr* 114:204–12, 1989.

Groer MW, Humenick S, Hill P: Characterizations and psychoneuroimmunolgic implications of secretory immunoglobulin A and cortisol in preterm and term breast milk. *J Perinat Neonatal Nurse* 7:42–51, 1994.

Grulee CG, Sanford HN: The influence of breast and artificial feeding on infantile eczema. *J Pediatr* 9:223–5, 1936.

Gulick EE: The effect of breast-feeding on toddler health. *Pediatr Nurs* 12:51–4, 1986.

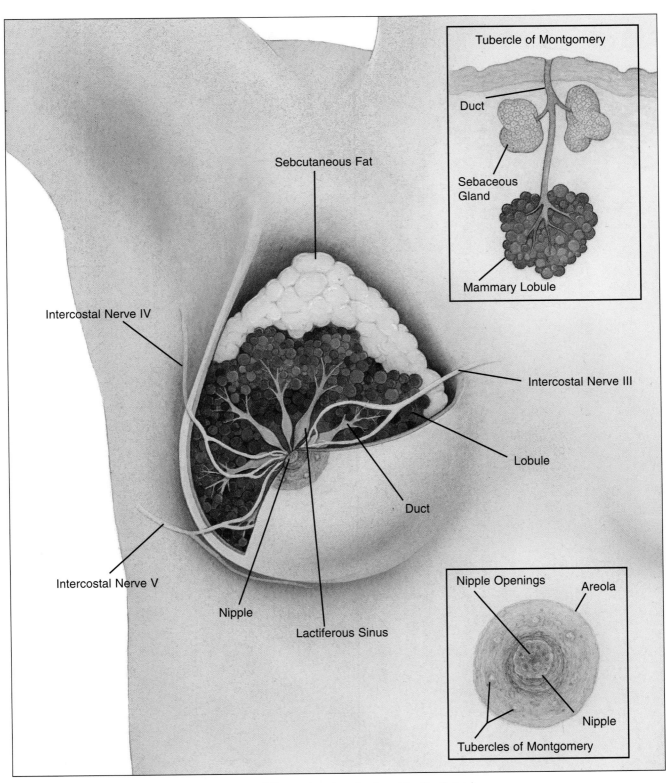

FIGURE 4–5. Frontal view of lactating breast. *(Illustrations in color insert by Ka Botzis)*

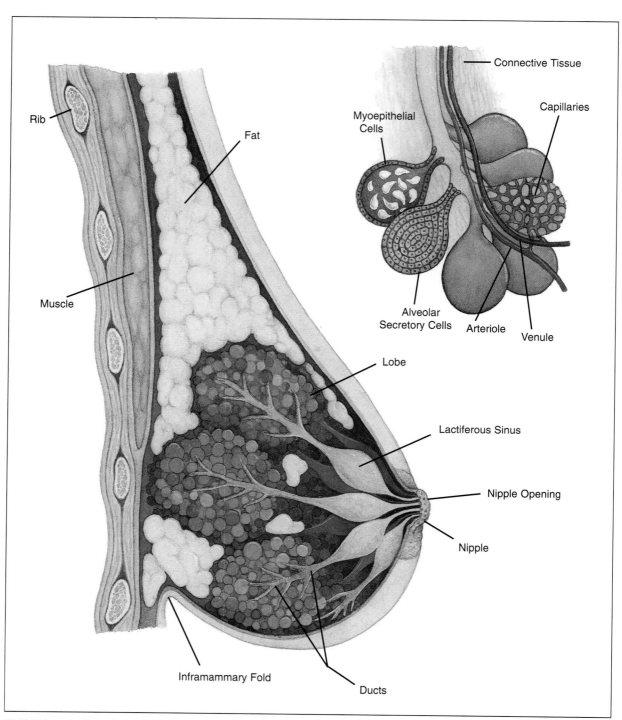

FIGURE 4–6. Side view of lactating breast.

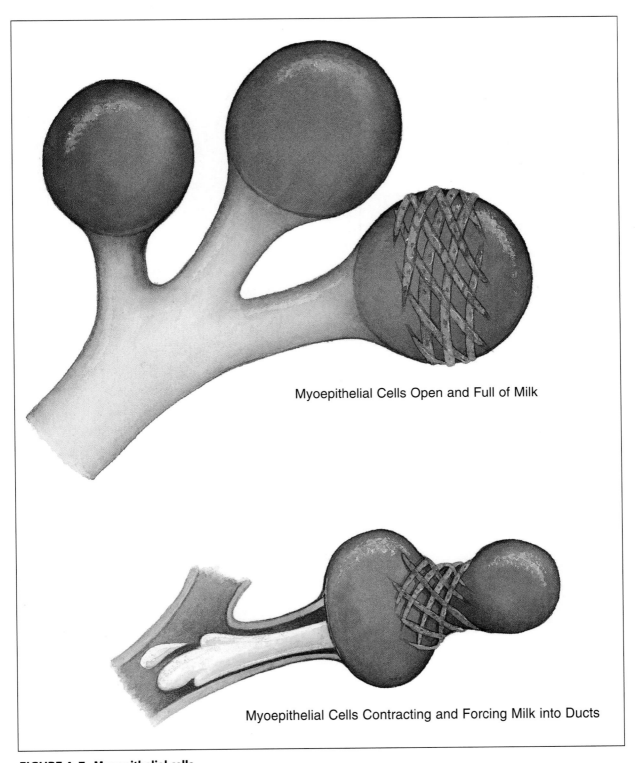

Myoepithelial Cells Open and Full of Milk

Myoepithelial Cells Contracting and Forcing Milk into Ducts

FIGURE 4–7. Myoepithelial cells.

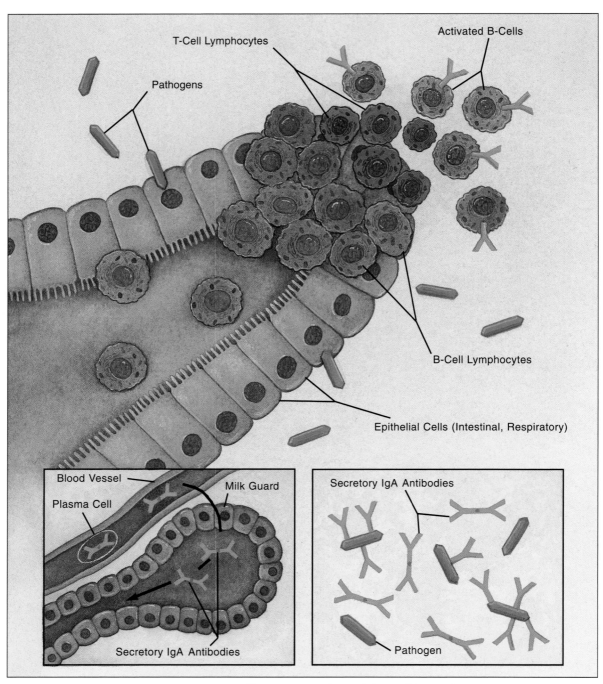

FIGURE 5–8. BALT and GALT migration. *B cells originate in the epithelium of the mother's intestinal tract or respiratory tract. These B-cell lymphocytes are sensitized by microbial antigens from bacteria in the mother's intestines and activated by a chemical from T-cell lymphocytes. The sensitized B cells migrate to the mother's breast by a special "homing" system (GALT or BALT) described in the text. Once there, they can secrete IgA that enters into breastmilk. When the infant consumes the milk, it coats his intestinal walls, providing protection. The B-cell lymphocytes can also travel in milk to the baby and secrete IgA antibodies in the infant's own intestinal tract. Either way, the infant has secretory IgA antibodies against the specific bacteria he will most likely encounter in his environment.*

COLOR PLATE 1. Nipple bruised and cracked from poor positioning. This trauma occurred on postpartum day 1. It was corrected by lifting the baby out of the mother's lap and into her arms and turning the baby so that his entire body faced the mother.

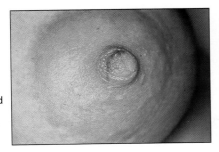

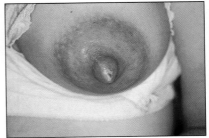

COLOR PLATE 2. Sore nipple with trauma from poor positioning. The white streak across the face of the nipple is a sign that the baby's lower jaw was too close to the tip of the nipple. Positioning the baby centrally across the mother's torso resulted in the baby driving his chin in closer to the breast rather than to the nipple. (Photo with permission from Barbara Wilson-Clay.)

COLOR PLATE 3. Nipple fissure that resulted from use of a poorly designed breast pump for three days. Even short-term use of a poorly designed pump can cause significant nipple damage. (Photo with permission of Catherine Watson Genna.)

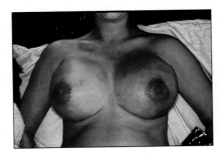

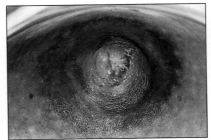

COLOR PLATE 4. Badly cracked nipple with possible bacterial infection. Such trauma can become an entry point for bacterial invasion and subsequent inflammation or infection. (Photo with permission of Kay Hoover.)

COLOR PLATE 5. Extreme engorgement. Engorgement occurred 30 to 36 hours postpartum, secondary to ineffective and infrequent breastfeeding and no expression or pumping when the infant did not obtain milk. (With permission from Chele Marmet/ Lactation Institute.)

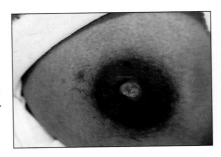

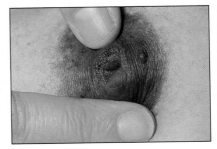

COLOR PLATE 6. Abraded folded nipple. The abrasion occurred when the nipple tissue remained wet between feedings; air-drying after each breastfeeding resolved the problem.

COLOR PLATE 7. Milk plugs at nipple pores, often characterized by acute pain. When milk is released from the duct, relief is immediate.

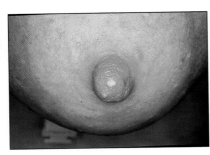

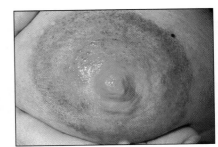

COLOR PLATE 8. Candidiasis (thrush) of the breast. This mother experienced four separate episodes in which her breasts, but not the baby's mouth, were treated. Within one week of simultaneous treatment of mother and baby, neither the baby's mouth nor the mother's breasts were infected.

COLOR PLATE 9. Breast abscess prior to excision. A breast abscess will often present with generalized redness. When the affected area is palpated, it is hot and hard to the touch. (Photo with permission from Barbara Wilson-Clay.)

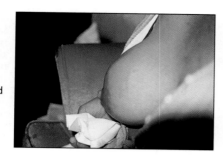

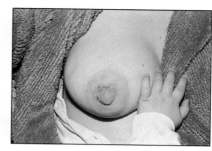

COLOR PLATE 10. Herpes on the areola. A thirteen-month-old nursing toddler contracted oral herpes by using a playmate's contaminated rattle; the mother was then infected. The breast lesion appeared soon after the baby's infection was identified. (With permission from Chele Marmet/Lactation Institute.)

COLOR PLATE 11. Psoriasis of the nipples. Although previous lesions had occurred on her breasts (but never on her nipples or areolae), this mother developed psoriasis on her nipples within a week of her baby's birth. When the baby latched on at the beginning of each breastfeeding session, she felt pain, which gradually subsided as the feeding progressed. (Photo with permission of Karen Foard.)

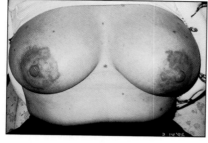

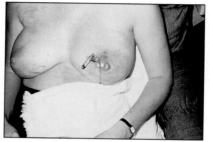

COLOR PLATE 12. Breast abscess with iodoform gauze drain in place; the safety pin is not holding the drain in place. (Photo with permission of Donna Corrieri.)

COLOR PLATE 13. Pumping the breast following abscess drainage. When a mother cannot put a baby to breast following treatment for a breast abscess, pumping may be necessary. The LC's gloved hand is placing gentle, even pressure over the area of the abscess drain to create a seal, in order to pump both breasts simultaneously and comfortably. (Photo with permission from Donna Corrieri.)

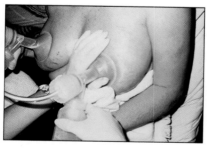

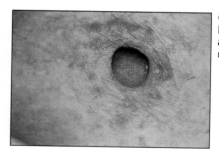

COLOR PLATE 14. Poison ivy on the areola. (Photo with permission of Kay Hoover.)

COLOR PLATE 15. Mastitis involving the lower outer quadrant of the breast. The mother was placed on intravenous antibiotics in the hospital, and lactation continued throughout the IV therapy. Her baby was housed with her during her hospitalization.

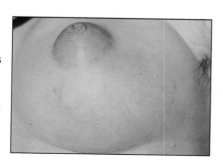

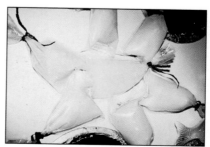

COLOR PLATE 16. Green (fresh) milk and white, creamy frozen milk, all from the same mother. When a mother expresses her milk, she may be surprised that it is not always white or creamy in color. In this case, the fresh milk had a greenish tint; when frozen, the previously green milk became creamy white. (Photo with permission from Jane Bradshaw.)

COLOR PLATE 17. Auxiliary breast and nipple tissue. A common site for additional breast or nipple tissue. In the absence of stimulation, milk production and tissue swelling ceases.

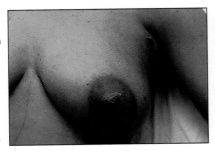

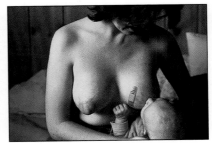

COLOR PLATE 18. Breastfeeding following biopsy for a benign tumor. The mother, with a totally breastfed infant, is shown four months post-partum. The tumor was discovered during lactation two weeks prior to biopsy. The baby is breastfeeding four hours after biopsy, the mother keeping the baby's hand away from the biopsy incision area. (With permission from Chele Marmet/Lactation Institute.)

COLOR PLATE 19. Nipple inversion. The mother had successfully breastfed her previous baby using both breasts.

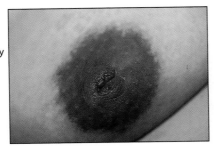

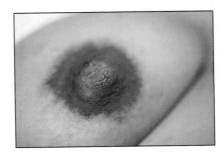

COLOR PLATE 20. Nipple eversion. Following gentle suction with a hand breast pump, the nipple completely everted.

COLOR PLATE 21. Burn scars on breast. This mother sustained third-degree burns as a child and experienced numerous subsequent reconstructive surgeries, including one to reconstruct her nipples. Although the breast tissue was difficult to compress because of extensive scar tissue, the baby was able to breastfeed.

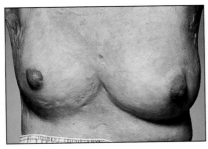

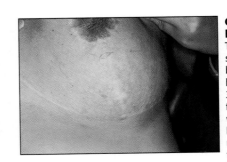

COLOR PLATE 22. Breast-reduction scars. This mother had breast surgery at age 28, two years before her first pregnancy; her bra size changed from a 32HH to a 36B prior to her first pregnancy. The nipples were not entirely detached, but both areolae were reduced in size and repositioned on the breast. Following surgery, the left breast had heightened sensation; the right nipple had no sensation at all. Some milk was obtained from each breast. (With permission from Chele Marmet/Lactation Institute.)

COLOR PLATE 23. Significantly different breast size and shape, suggestive of primary breast insufficiency; this mother was referred for a lactation consultation for her inadequate milk supply. (Photo with permission from Kay Hoover.)

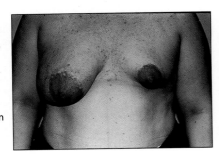

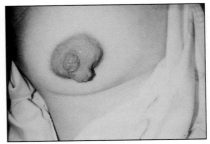

COLOR PLATE 24. Double nipple on the same breast. This mother's baby needed to gape widely enough to take both nipples into his mouth. (Photo with permission of Linda Stewart.)

COLOR PLATE 25. Oral Candidiasis (thrush). When first seen, the baby was fifteen days old; the gums and inner cheeks were as involved as his tongue. The mother's nipples were also inflamed. After four weeks of intermittent treatment, neither the baby's mouth nor the mother's breasts were infected. (With permission from Chele Marmet/Lactation Institute.)

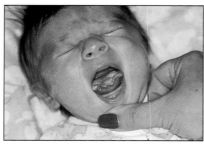

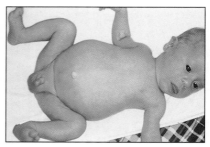

COLOR PLATE 26. Baby with Down syndrome. Note the small genitalia characteristic of a child with Down syndrome. Poor head and neck control, weak jaw and other motor abilities, and a poor suck often require special assistance while the baby is learning how to suckle the breast. (With permission from Chele Marmet/Lactation Institute.)

COLOR PLATE 27. Baby with FTT. At birth, this baby weighed 8 lbs 12 oz. When referred to the LC at 4½ months, he still weighed only 10 lbs 11 oz. He avidly sucked his own fingers and slept for long periods; when put to breast, he was extremely lethargic. In addition, he sucked in his cheeks, generating no effective negative pressure on the breast. (Photo with permission from Jane Bradshaw.)

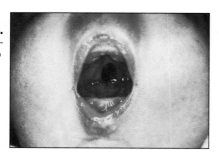

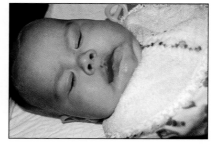

COLOR PLATE 28. Hemangioma of the infant's lip. Although it may appear to be troublesome, this condition did not cause feeding problems for the baby. (Photo with permission of Barbara Wilson-Clay.)

COLOR PLATE 29. Cleft of the soft palate. Such a cleft can occur without a cleft of the lip. (Photo with permission from Jane Bradshaw.)

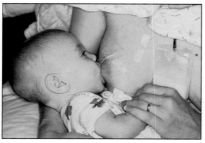

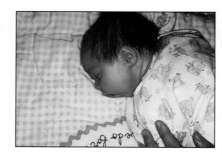

COLOR PLATE 30. Baby with Pierre Robin syndrome. This syndrome is characterized by a severely receded chin, which can often require special assistance and creative positioning to help the baby latch on. Other characteristics of this syndrome, such as cleft palate, may also render breastfeeding difficult or impossible to achieve for varying lengths of time. (Photo with permission from Jane Bradshaw.)

COLOR PLATE 31. Baby being fed by NG tube while at breast. Sometimes a baby unable to feed directly can be fed with a nasogastric tube. Doing so while holding her baby next to her breast and allowing the baby to suck on a finger or thumb can help the mother to normalize this feeding situation. (Photo with permission of Jane Bradshaw.)

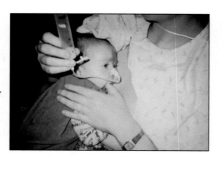

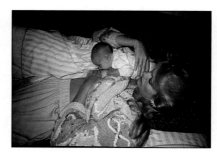

COLOR PLATE 32. Over-the-shoulder positioning of baby. This mother with extremely sore nipples was referred to a lactation consultant. The position shown here was taught as an alternative, to move the baby's mouth away from very tender areas and allow breastfeeding to continue during the healing period. The mother was placed on the LC's couch on her back, with the baby approaching the breast from over her shoulder. (Photo with permission from Jane Bradshaw.)

Guthrie HA, Picciano MF, Sheehe D: Fatty acid patterns of human milk. *J Pediatr* 90:39–41, 1977.

György P: A hitherto unrecognized biochemical difference between human milk and cow's milk. *Pediatrics* 11:98–104, 1953.

Habbick BF, Kahnna C, To T: Infantile hypertropic pyloric stenosis: a study of feeding practices and other possible causes. *Can Med Assoc J* 140:401–4, 1989.

Habicht JP, DaVanso J, Butz WP: Mother's milk and sewage: their interactive effects on infant mortality. *Pediatrics* 81:456–60, 1988.

Hamosh M: Human milk. In: Colon AR, Mohsen Z, eds. *Pediatric pathophysiology*. Boston: Little, Brown, 1985:69–85.

Hamosh M, et al: Digestive enzymes in human milk: stability at suboptimal storage temperatures. *J Pediatr Gastroenterol Nutr* 24:38–43, 1997.

Hanifin JM: Atopic dermatitis. *J Allergy Clin Immunol* 73:211–22, 1984.

Haroon Y, et al: The content of phylloquinone (vitamin K_1) in human milk, cow's milk and infant formula foods determined by high performance liquid chromatography. *J Nutr* 112:1105–17, 1982.

Hartmann PE: Lactation and reproduction in Western Australian women. *J Reprod Med* 32:543–7, 1987.

Hartmann PE, Prosser CG: Physiological basis of longitudinal changes in human milk yield and composition. *Fed Proc* 43:2448–53, 1984.

Hashizume S, Kuroda K, Murakami H: Identification of lactoferrin as an essential growth factor for human lymphocytic cell lines in serum-free medium. *Biochem Biophys Acta* 763:377, 1983.

Hasselbalch H, et al: Decreased thymus size in formula-fed infants compared with breastfed infants. *Acta Paediatr* 85:1029–32, 1996.

Heacock H, et al: Influence of breast versus formula milk on physiological gastroesophageal reflux in healthy, newborn infants. *J Pediatr Gastroenterol* 14:41–6, 1992.

Heird WC, Schward SM, Hansen IH: Colostrum-induced enteric mucosal growth in beagle puppies. *Pediatr Res* 18:512, 1984.

Herrmann ME, et al: Prospective study on the atopy preventive effect of maternal avoidance of milk and eggs during pregnancy and lactation. *Eur J Pediatr* 155:770–4, 1996.

Hide DW, Guyer BM: Clinical manifestations of allergy related to breast and cows' milk feeding. *Arch Dis Child* 56:172–5, 1981.

Higginbottom MD, Sweetman L, Hyhan WL: A syndrome of methylmalonic aciduria, homocystinuria, megaloblastic anemia, and neurologic abnormalities in a vitamin B_{12} deficient breast-fed infant of a strict vegetarian. *N Engl J Med* 299:317, 1978.

Holberg CJ, et al: Risk factors for respiratory syncytial virus-associated lower respiratory illnesses in the first year of life. *Am J Epidemiol* 133:1135–51, 1991.

Hollis BW: Individual quantitation of vitamin D_2, vitamin D_3, 25-hydroxyvitamin D_2, and 25-hydroxyvitamin D_3 in human milk. *Anal Biochem* 131:211–9, 1983.

Host A, Husby S, Österballe O: A prospective study of cow's milk allergy in exclusively breast-fed infants. *Acta Paediatr Scand* 77:663–70, 1988.

Houston MJ, Howie PW, McNeilly AS: Factors affecting the duration of breast feeding: 1. Measurement of breast milk intake in the first week of life. *Early Hum Dev* 8:49–54, 1983.

Howie PW, et al: Protective effect of breast feeding against infection. *Br Med J* 300:11–16, 1990.

Humenick SS: The clinical significance of breastmilk maturation rates. *Birth* 14(4):174–9, 1987.

Humenick SS, et al: The maturation index of colostrum and milk (MICAM): a measurement of breast milk maturation. *J Nurs Measurement* 2:169–86, 1994.

Inch S, Renfrew M: Common breastfeeding problems. In: Chalmers I, Enkin M, Keirse MJNC, eds. *Effective care in pregnancy and childbirth*. Oxford: Oxford University Press, 1989:1375–89.

Innis SM, et al: Feeding formula without arachidonic acid and docosahexanoic acid has no effect on preferential looking acuity or recognition memory in healthy full-term infants at 9 mo of age. *Am J Clin Nutr* 64:40–6, 1996.

Istre GR, et al: Risk factors for primary *Haemophilus influenzae* disease: increased risk from day care attendance and school-aged household members. *J Pediatr* 106:190–5, 1985.

Italian Collaborative Study: Cow's milk allergy in the first year of life. *Acta Paediatr Scand* Suppl 348 (entire issue), 1988.

Jackson RL, et al: Growth of "well-born" American infants fed human and cow's milk. *Pediatrics* 33:642, 1964.

Jakobsson I, et al: Dietary bovine beta-lactoglobulin is transferred to human milk. *Acta Paediatr Scand* 74:342, 1985.

Jansson L, Akesson B, Holmberg L: Vitamin E and fatty acid composition of human milk. *Am J Clin Nutr* 34:8–13, 1981.

Jason JM, Niebury P, Marks JS: Mortality and infectious disease associated with infant-feeding practices in developing countries. *Pediatrics* 74(suppl):702–27, 1984.

Jatsyk GV, Kuvaeva IB, Gribakin SG: Immunological protection for the neonatal gastrointestinal tract: the importance of breast feeding. *Acta Paediatr Scan* 74:246–9.

Jenkins HR, et al: Food allergy: the major cause of infantile colitis. *Arch Dis Child* 59:326–9, 1984.

Jensen RG, et al: Human milk as a carrier of messages to the nursing infant. *Nutr Today* 23:20–5, 1988.

Johnson DL, et al: Breastfeeding and children's intelligence. Psych Rep 79:1179–85.

Juex G, et al: Growth pattern of selected urban Chilean infants during exclusive breast feeding. *Am J Clin Nutr* 38:462–8, 1983.

Kanaaneh H: The relationship of bottle feeding to malnutrition and gastroenteritis in a pre-industrial setting. *J Trop Pediatr Environ Child Health* 18:302–6, 1972.

Karra MV, et al: Changes in specific nutrients in breast milk during extended lactation. *Am J Clin Nutr* 43:495–503, 1986.

Keller MA, et al: $IgAG_4$ in human colostrum and human milk: continued local production or selective transport from serum. *Acta Paediatr Scand* 77:24–9, 1988.

Kelly DW, et al: Rise and fall of coeliac disease 1960–1985. *Arch Dis Child* 64:1157–60, 1989.

Khin-Maung-U J, et al: Effect of clinical outcome of breastfeeding during acute diarrhea. *Br Med J* 290:587–9, 1985.

Kirkpatrick CH, et al: Inhibition of growth of *Candida albicans* by iron-unsaturated lactoferrin: relation to host defense mechanisms in chronic mucocutaneous candidiasis. *J Infect Dis* 124:539, 1971.

Kohn G, et al: Diet and the essential fatty acid status of term infants. *Acta Paediatr* Suppl 402: 69–74, 1994.

Koletzko S, et al: Role of infant feeding practices in development of Crohn's disease in childhood. *Br Med J* 298:1617–8, 1989.

Koopman JS, et al: Infant formulas and gastrointestinal illness. *Am J Public Health* 75:477–80, 1985.

Kostraba JN, et al: Early exposure to cow's milk and solid foods in infancy, genetic predisposition and risk of IDDM. *Diabetes* 42:288–95, 1993.

Kovar MG, et al: Review of the epidemiologic evidence for an association between infant feeding and infant health. *Pediatrics* 74(suppl):615–38, 1984.

Kramer MS: Infant feeding, infection, and public health. *Pediatrics* 81:164–6, 1988.

Krebs NF, et al: Zinc homeostasis in breast-fed infant. *Pediatr Res* 39:661–5, 1996.

Krebs NF, Hambidge KM: Zinc requirements and zinc intakes of breast-fed infants. *Am J Clin Nutr* 43:288–92, 1986.

Kulski JK, Hartmann PE: Changes in the concentration of cortisol in milk during different stages of human lactation. *Aust J Exp Biol Med Sci* 59:769, 1981.

Kumpulain et al: Formula feeding results in lower selenium status than breast-feeding or selenium-supplemented formula feeding: a longitudinal study. *Am J Clin Nutr* 45:49–53, 1987.

Labbok M, Hendershot GE: Does breast-feeding protect against malocclusion? An analysis of the 1981 Child Health Supplement to the National Health Interview survey. *Am J Prev Med* 3:227–32, 1987.

Lakdawala DR, Widdowson EM: Vitamin D in human milk. *Lancet* 1:167–8, 1977.

Latarte J, et al: Lack of protective effect of breast-feeding in congenital hypothyroidism: report of 12 cases. *Pediatrics* 65:703–5, 1980.

Leach JL, et al: Total potentially available nucleotides of human milk by stage of lactation. *Am J Clin Nutr* 61:1224–30, 1995.

Lemons JA, et al: Differences in the composition of preterm and term human milk during early lactation. *Pediatr Res* 16:113–7, 1982.

Lepage G, et al: The composition of preterm milk in relation to the degree of prematurity. *Am J Clin Nutr* 40:1042–9, 1984.

Leventhal JM, et al: Does breastfeeding protect against infection in infants less than 3 months of age? *Pediatrics* 78:896–903, 1986.

Lilja G, et al: Effects of maternal diet during late pregnancy and lactation on the development of atopic diseases in infants up to 18 months of age—*in-vivo* results. *Clin Exp Allergy* 19:473–9, 1989.

Litwin SD, Zehr BD, Insel RA: Selective concentration of IgD class-specific antibodies in human milk. *Clin Exp Immunol* 80:262–7, 1990.

Logan RF: Coeliac disease [letter]. *Lancet* 336:633, 1990.

Lopez-Alarcon M, Villalpando S, Fajardo A: Breast-feeding lowers the frequency and duration of acute respiratory infection and diarrhea in infants under six months of age. *J Nutr* 127:436–443, 1997.

Lovegrove JA, Hampton SM, Morgan JB: The immunological and long-term atopic outcome of infants born to women following a milk-free diet during late pregnancy and lactation: a pilot study. *Br J Nutr* 71:223–38, 1994.

Lucas A, Cole TJ: Breast milk and neonatal necrotizing enterocolitis. *Lancet* 336:1519–23, 1990.

Lucas A, et al: Breast milk and subsequent intelligence quotient in children born preterm. *Lancet* 339:261–4, 1992.

Lucas A, Mitchell MD: Prostaglandins in human milk. *Arch Dis Child* 55:950, 1980.

McMillan JA, Landaw SA, Oski FA: Iron sufficiency in breast-fed infants and the availability of iron from human milk. *Pediatrics* 58:686–91, 1976.

Makrides M, et al: Are long-chain polyunsaturated fatty acids essential nutrients in infancy? *Lancet* 345:1463–8, 1995.

Makrides M, et al: Erythrocyte docosahexaenoic acid correlates with the visual response of healthy term infants. *Pediatr Res* 33:425–7, 1993.

Marchini G, Linden A: Cholecystokinin, a satiety signal in newborn infants? *J Dev Physiol* 17:215–9, 1992.

Marild S, et al: Breastfeeding and urinary tract infection [letter]. *Lancet* 336(8720):942, 1990.

Mason T, et al: Breast feeding and the development of juvenile rheumatoid arthritis. *J Rheumatol* 22:1166–70, 1995.

Mata L: The malnutrition-infection complex and and its environment factors. *Proc Nutr Soc* 38:29–40, 1979.

Mathur GP, et al: Breastfeeding and childhood cancer. *Ind Pediatr* 30:651–7, 1993.

Matsuoka Y, Idota T: The concentration of epidermal growth factor in Japanese mother's milk. *J Nutr Sci Vitaminol* 41:24–51, 1995.

May JT: Microbial contaminants and antimicrobial properties of human milk. *Microbiol Sci* 5:42–6, 1988.

Mayer EJ, et al: Reduced risk of IDDM among breast-fed children. *Diabetes* 37:1625–32, 1988.

Metcalfe DD: Food hypersensitivity. *J Allergy Clin Immunol* 73:749–62, 1984.

Miller SA, Chopra JG: Problems with human milk and infant formulas. *Pediatrics* 74(suppl):639–47, 1984.

Mitchell EA, et al: Results from the first year of the New Zealand cot death study. *NZ Med J* 10:71–76, 1991.

Mitra AK, Rabbani F: The importance of breast-feeding in minimizing mortality and morbidity from diarrhoeal diseases: the Bangladesh perspective. *J Diarrhoeal Dis Res* 13(1):1–7, 1995.

Morriss FH: Method for investigating the presence and physiologic role of growth factors in milk. In: Jensen RG, Neville MC, eds. *Human lactation: milk components and methodologies*. New York: Plenum, 1985:193–200.

Morriss FH, et al: Relationship of human milk pH during course of lactation to concentrations of citrate and fatty acids. *Pediatrics* 78:458–64, 1986.

Morrisset J, Jolicoeur L: Effect of hydrocortisone on pancreatic growth in rats. *Am J Physiol* 239:295, 1980.

Morton JA: The clinical usefulness of breast milk sodium in the assessment of lactogenesis. *Pediatrics* 93:802–6, 1994.

Mosko S, et al: Maternal proximity and infant CO_2 environment during bedsharing and possible implications for SIDS research. *Am J Phys Anthrop* 103:315–28, 1997.

Motil KJ, et al: Human milk protein does not limit growth of breast-fed infants. *J Pediatr Gastroenterol Nutr* 24:10–7, 1997.

Neville MC, et al: Studies in human lactation: milk volumes in lactating women during the onset of lactation and full lactation. *Am J Clin Nutr* 48:1375–86, 1988.

Neville MC, Oliva-Rasbach J: Is maternal milk production limiting for infant growth during the first year of life in breast-fed infants? In: Goldman AS, Atkinson SA, Hanson LA, eds. *Human lactation 3: the effects of human milk on the recipient infant*. New York: Plenum, 1987:123–33.

Newman J: How breast milk protects newborns. *Sci Am* 372(b):76–9.

Odze RD, et al: Allergic colitis in infants. *J Pediatr* 126:163–70, 1995.

Oizumi J, Hayakawa K: Biotinidase in human breast milk. *Am J Clin Nutr* 48:295–7, 1988.

Okamoto Y, Ogra P: Antiviral factors in human milk: implications in respiratory syncytial virus infection. *Acta Paediatr Scand* Suppl 351:137–43, 1989.

Osborn FR: Relationship of hypotension and infant feeding to the aetiology of coronary disease. *Colleques Int Cont Natl Res Sci* 169:93, 1968.

Ostrea EM, et al: Influence of breast-feeding on the restoration of the low serum concentration of vitamin E and beta-carotene in the newborn infant. *Am J Obstet Gynecol* 154:1014–7, 1986.

Paganelli R, Cavagni G, Pallone F: The role of antigenic absorption and circulating immune complexes in food allergy. *Ann Allergy* 57:330–6, 1986.

Paine F, Coble RJ: Breast-feeding and infant health in a rural U.S. community. *Am J Dis Child* 136:36–8, 1982.

Perez-Bravolt F, et al: Genetic predisposition and environmental factors leading to the development of insulin-dependent diabetes mellitus in Chilean children. *J Mol Med* 74:105–9, 1996.

Petschow B, et al: Influence of orally administered epidermal growth factor on normal and damaged intestinal mucosa in rats. *J Pediatr Gastroenterol Nutr* 17:49–57, 1993.

Pickering LK, Kohl S: Human milk humoral immunity and infant defense mechanisms. In: Howell RR, Morriss FH, Pickering LK, eds. *Human milk in infant nutrition and health*. Springfield, IL: Thomas, 1986:123–40.

Pisacane A, et al: Breast-feeding and inguinal hernia. *J Pediatr* 127:109–11, 1995a.

Pisacane A, et al: Breast feeding and acute appendicitis. *Br Med J* 310:836–7, 1995b.

Pisacane A, et al: Breast feeding and multiple sclerosis. *Br Med J* 308:1411–2, 1994.

Pisacane A, et al: Breast feeding and tonsillectomy. *Br Med J* 312:746–7, 1996.

Pisacane A, et al: Breast feeding and urinary tract infection. *Lancet* 336:50, 1990.

Popkin BM, et al: Breast-feeding and diarrheal morbidity. *Pediatrics* 86:874–82, 1990.

Prentice AM: Variations in maternal dietary intake, birthweight and breastmilk output in the Gambia. In: Aebi H, Whitehead R, eds. *Maternal nutrition during pregnancy and lactation.* Bern: Hans Huber, 1980:167–83.

Prentice AM, et al: Breast-milk antimicrobial factors of rural Gambian mothers. *Acta Paediatr Scand* 73:796–812, 1984.

Prosser CG, Saint L, Hartmann PE: Mammary gland function during gradual weaning and early gestation in women. *Aust J Exp Biol Med Sci* 62:215–28, 1984.

Pullan CR, et al: Breast-feeding and respiratory syncytial virus infection. *Br Med J* 281(6247): 1034–6, 1980.

Quinlan PT, et al: The relationship between stool hardness and stool composition in breast- and formula-fed infants. *J Pediatr Gastroenterol Nutr* 20:81–90, 1995.

Rahman MM, et al: Local production of rotavirus specific IgA in breast tissue and transfer to neonates. *Arch Dis Child* 62:401–5, 1987.

Raiha NCR: Nutritional proteins in milk and the protein requirement of normal infants. *Pediatrics* 75(suppl):136–41, 1985.

Ratner H: Presentation at La Leche League International, Ninth Annual Seminar on Breast-feeding for Physicians, Chicago, July 1981.

Ravelomanana N, et al: Risk factors for fatal diarrhoea among dehydrated malnourished children in a Madagascar hospital. *Eur J Clin Nutr* 49:91–7, 1995.

Read L, et al: Changes in the growth-promoting activity of human milk during lactation. *Pediatr Res* 18:133–8, 1984.

Reeve LE, Chesney RW, DeLuca HF: Vitamin D of human milk: identification of biologically active forms. *Am J Clin Nutr* 36:122–6, 1982.

Reid B, Smith H, Friedman Z: Prostaglandins in human milk. *Pediatrics* 66:870–2, 1980.

Rigas A, et al: Breast-feeding and maternal smoking in the etiology of Crohn's disease and ulcerative colitis in childhood. *Ann Epidemiol* 3:387–92, 1993.

Riordan J: The cost of not breastfeeding. *J Hum Lact* 13:93–7, 1997.

Roberts CC, et al: Adequate bone mineralization in breast-fed infants. *J Pediatr* 99:192–6, 1981.

Rosenberg M: Breast-feeding and infant mortality in Norway 1860–1930. *J Biosoc Sci* 21:335–48, 1989.

Rovet JF: Does breast-feeding protect the hypothyroid infant whose condition is diagnosed by newborn screening? *Am J Dis Child* 144:319–23, 1990.

Rudloff EH, et al: Interleukin-6 in human milk. *J Reprod Immunol* 23:13–20, 1993.

Ruiz-Palacios GM, et al: Protection of breast-fed infants against *Campylobacter* diarrhea by antibodies in human milk. *J Pediatr* 116:707–13, 1990.

Ruuska R: Occurrence of acute diarrhea in atopic and nonatopic infant: the role of prolonged breast-feeding. *J Pediatr Gastroenterol Nutr* 14:27–33, 1992.

Saarinen JM, et al: Prolonged breast feeding as prophylaxis for recurrent otitis media. *Acta Paediatr Scand* 71:567–71, 1982.

Saarinen I, Kajosaari M: Breastfeeding as prophylaxis against atopic disease: prospective follow-up study until 17 years old. *Lancet* 346:1065–9, 1995.

Saint L, Smith M, Hartmann PE: The yield and nutrient content of colostrum and milk of women giving birth to 1 month postpartum. *Br J Nutr* 52:87–95, 1984.

Salmenpera L, et al: Folate nutrition is optimal in exclusively breast-fed infants but inadequate in some of their mothers and in formula-fed infants. *J Pediatr Gastroenterol Nutr* 5:283–9, 1986.

Sandstrom BA, et al: Zinc absorption from human milk, cow's milk, and infant formulas. *Am J Dis Child* 137:726–9, 1983.

Sanjurjo P, et al: Plasma fatty acid composition during the first week of life following feeding with human milk or formula. *Acta Paediatr Scand* 77:202–6, 1988.

Sassen ML, Brand R, Grote JJ: Breast-feeding and acute otitis media. *Am J Otolaryngol* 15:351–7, 1994.

Sauls JS: Potential effect of demographic and other variables in studies comparing morbidity of breast-fed and bottle-fed infants. *Pediatrics* 64:523–7, 1979.

Savilahti E, et al: Prolonged exclusive breast feeding and heredity as determinants in infantile atopy. *Arch Dis Child* 62:269–73, 1987.

Schaefer O: Otitis media and bottle-feeding: an epidemiological study of infant feeding habits and incidence of recurrent and chronic middle ear diseases in Canadian Eskimos. *Can J Public Health* 62:478–89, 1971.

Serdula MK, Seward J, Marks JS: Seasonal differences in breast-feeding in rural Egypt. *Am J Clin Nutr* 44:405–9, 1986.

Shing YW, Klagsburn M: Human and bovine milk contain different sets of growth factors. *Endocrinology* 115:273, 1984.

Shoub BD: A microbiological investigation of acute summer gastroenteritis in Black South African infants. *J Hygiene* 78:377–80, 1977.

Shu XO, et al: Infant breastfeeding and the risk of childhood lymphoma and leukaemia. *Int J Epidemiol* 24:27–34, 1995.

Siigur U, Ormission A, Tamm A: Faecal short-chain fatty acids in breast-fed and bottle-fed infants. *Acta Paediatr* 82:536–8, 1993.

Siimes MA, et al: Exclusive breast-feeding for nine months: risk of iron deficiency. *J Pediatr* 104:196–9, 1984.

Silfverdal SA, et al: Protective effect of breastfeeding on invasive *Haemophilus influenzae* infection: a case-control study in Swedish preschool children. *Int J Epidemiol* 26:443–50, 1997.

Smith AM, Picciano MF, Milner JA: Selenium intakes and status of human milk and formula fed infants. *Am J Clin Nutr* 35:521, 1982.

Snyder JD, Merson MH: The magnitude of the global problem of acute diarrhoeal disease: a review of active surveillance data. Bull WHO 60:605–13, 1982.

Specker BL, et al: Sunshine exposure and serum 25-hydroxyvitamin D concentrations in exclusively breast-fed infant. *J Pediatr* 107:372–6, 1985.

Steel MG, Leslie GA: Immunoglobulin D in rat serum, saliva and milk. *Immunology* 55:571–77, 1985.

Steichen JJ, Krug-Wispe SK, Tsang RC: Breast-feeding the low birth weight preterm infant. *Clin Perinatol* 14:131–71, 1987.

Strimas JH, Chi DS: Significance of IgE level in amniotic fluid and cord blood for the prediction of allergy. *Ann Allergy* 61:133–6, 1988.

Stuart CA, et al: Passage of cow's milk protein into breast milk. *Clin Allergy* 14:533–5, 1984.

Stuff JE, Nichols GL: Nutrient intake and growth performance of older infants fed human milk. *J Pediatr* 115:959–68, 1989.

Swartzbaum JA, et al: An exploratory study of environmental and medical factors potentially related to childhood cancer. *Med Pediatr Oncol* 19:115–21, 1991.

Takala AK, et al: Risk factors of invasive *Haemophilus influenzae* type b disease among children in Finland. *J Pediatr* 115:694–701, 1989.

Taylor B, et al: Breast-feeding, bronchitis and admissions for lower-respiratory illness and gastroenteritis during the first five years. *Lancet* 1:1227–9, 1982.

Uauy RD, et al: Effect of dietary omega-3 fatty acids on retinal function of very-low-birth-eight neonates. *Pediatr Res* 28:485–92, 1990.

Udall JN, et al: Liver disease in a_1-antitrypsin deficiency. *JAMA* 253:2679–82, 1985.

Uvnas-Moberg K, Marchini G, Windberg J: Plasma cholecystokinin concentrations after breast-feeding in healthy 4 day old infants. *Arch Dis Child* 68:46–8, 1993.

Van Derslice J, Popkin B, Briscoe J: Drinking-water quality, sanitation, and breast-feeding: their interactive effects on infant health. *Bull WHO* 72:589–601, 1994.

van der Westhuyzen, Chetty M, Atkinson PM: Fatty acid composition of human milk from South African black mother consuming a traditional maize diet. *Eur J Clin Nutr* 42:213–20, 1988.

van Steenbergen WM, et al: Energy supplementation in the last trimester of pregnancy in East Java, Indonesia: effect on breast-milk output. *Am J Clin Nutr* 50:274–9, 1989.

Victora CG, et al: Evidence for protection by breastfeeding against infant deaths from infectious diseases in Brazil. *Lancet* 2(8554):319–21, 1987.

Wagner V, Stockhausen JG: The effect of feeding human milk and adapted milk formulae on serum lipid and lipoprotein levels in young infants. *Eur J Pediatr* 147:292–5, 1988.

Watkins CJ, Leeker SR, Corkhill RT: The relationship between breast and bottle feeding and respiratory illness in the first year of life. *J Epidemiol Commun Health* 33:180–2, 1979.

West KP, et al: Breast-feeding, weaning patterns, and the risk of xerophthalmia in Southern Malawi. *Am J Clin Nutr* 44:690–7, 1986.

Whitehead RG, et al: Factors influencing lactation performance in rural Gambian mothers. *Lancet* 2:178–81, 1978.

Whitehead RG, Paul AA: Infant growth and human milk requirement, a fresh approach. *Lancet* 2:161–3, 1981.

Widdowson EM, Colombo VE, Artavanis CA: Changes in the organs of pigs in response to feeding for the first 24 hours after birth: II. The digestive tract. *Biol Neonate* 28:272, 1976.

Wilson JV, Self TW, Hamburger R: Severe cow's milk induced colitis in an exclusively breast-fed neonate. *Clin Pediatr* 29:77–80, 1990.

Wirt DP, et al: Activated and memory T lymphocytes in human milk. *Cytometry* 13:282–90, 1992.

Wood CS, et al: Exclusively breast-fed infants: growth and caloric intake. *Pediatr Nurs* 14(2): 117–24, 1988.

Woodruff CW, Latham E, McDavid S: Iron nutrition in the breast-fed infant. *J Pediatr* 90:36–8, 1977.

Woolridge MW, Fisher C: Colic, "overfeeding," and symptoms of lactose malabsorption in the breast-fed baby: a possible artifact of feed management? *Lancet* 2:382–4, 1988.

Woolridge MW, Ingram JC, Baum JD: Do changes in pattern of breast usage alter the baby's nutrient intake? *Lancet* 336:395–7, 1990.

World Health Organization Working Group on Infant Growth, Nutrition unit: *an evaluation of infant growth*. Geneva: WHO, 1994.

World Health Organization and Agricultural Organization of the United States (WHO/FAO): Report of a joint FAO/WHO ad hoc expert committee, Rome, 1980, National Academy of Science on Dietary Allowances, 1980.

Worthington-Roberts B, Williams SR: *Nutrition in pregnancy and lactation,* (5th ed). St Louis: Mosby, 1993: 24.

Wright AL, et al: Relationship of infant feeding to recurrent wheezing at age 6 years. *Arch Pediatr Adolesc Med* 149:758–63, 1995.

Yamauchi Y, Yamanouchi I: Breast-feeding frequency during the first 24 hours after birth in full-term neonates. *Pediatrics* 86:171–5, 1990.

Yoneyama K, Nagata H, Asano H: Growth of Japanese breast-fed and bottle-fed infants from birth to 20 months. *Annu Hum Biol* 21:597–608, 1994.

DRUGS AND BREASTFEEDING

Jan Riordan

The current rise in the popularity of breastfeeding parallels the rise in the use of drugs, both therapeutic and illegal; therefore, health professionals often are asked by lactating mothers about the safety of taking a certain medication. There are three "knowns" about drugs and human milk: *1. Most drugs pass into breastmilk. 2. Almost all medication appears in only small amounts in human milk, usually less than 1 percent of the maternal dosage. 3. Very few drugs are contraindicated for breastfeeding women.*

The methods used to measure chemicals in breastmilk have changed remarkably in the last two decades. Gas-liquid chromatography, atomic absorption spectrophotometry, and radioimmunoassay have vastly improved our ability to measure drugs in milk; thus even microscopic amounts can be detected.

As a result, more is known now about the effect of maternal drugs on the breastfeeding baby than ever before. At the same time, our improved ability to measure drugs in human milk far exceeds our ability to make clinical judgments about their presence (Roberts, 1984). This easy detection of drugs in human milk, even in minute amounts, is a double-edged sword. On the positive side, it facilitates close monitoring of drug levels in the mother and the infant. Even microscopic amounts of a drug in milk may be clinically significant in the case of a premature infant who is ill or in the instance of a mother who must take a medication for a long time or in combination with other medications.

On the negative side, authorities often recommend that a mother not breastfeed when she must use a medication known to pass into milk. There are other problems. Many research reports on lactation and drugs are single-case reports that lack the validity of reports based on the experiences of many women. Milk sampling is often not done when the drug is at a steady-state plasma concentration. The daily variability of milk fat is not considered, nor are infant plasma drug concentrations measured (Giacoia & Catz, 1988). A drug can be relegated to the contraindicated list for years on the basis of a single, often faulty, case report.

Despite the availability of information about medication during lactation, too few physicians know much about the effect on the nursling of drugs in breastmilk. Such doctors are unduly influenced by the well-known teratogenic effects of drugs taken during pregnancy. This awareness makes them fear the potential of similar toxic effects of drugs in breastmilk. However, the analogy is unwarranted. Whereas the placenta permits drugs to cross over to the fetus, the breast serves as a nearly impermeable barrier. At the same time, too many physicians are concerned about legal repercussions when they order medication for a nursing woman. Because the health of the vulnerable infant is so important, the value of breastfeeding is so poorly appreciated, and the climate (in the United States) is so litigious, most tend to err on the side of caution (Riordan, 1987). The net result is that it is easier and less threatening to recommend weaning than it is to look into the matter and be reassured that medication poses no danger to the baby (Tyree, 1992). The victim of such caution is the breastfeeding woman who, lacking time, energy, and wherewithal to sift through the research literature, succumbs to her physician's advice and weans her infant.

Roberts (1984) warned that a physician should recommend weaning only when scientific documentation indicates that a drug will be harmful to the infant. It is no longer acceptable for the physician to intervene arbitrarily in the mother's wish to breastfeed her infant merely because maternal drug therapy is indicated (Dillon et al., 1997). Also, it does not seem reasonable to discontinue breastfeeding solely because the drug in question has been implicated in one or two case reports of toxic side effects in primary recipients.

The Passage of Maternal Drugs into Breastfeeding Infants

Several authors (Atkinson & Begg, 1990; Wilson, 1981) have developed equation models that permit prediction of the concentration of a drug in breastmilk; however, the concentration in breastmilk may be of limited clinical use, because so many other maternal and infant factors are involved. For example, a drug present in breastmilk may be destroyed in the infant's gastrointestinal (GI) tract before it is absorbed. Because the drug levels in the nursing baby are usually not measured, we have little information about the actual dose that the infant receives from the milk.

Drug Factors

The amount of drug transported into breastmilk partially depends on the drug's characteristics. These characteristics include the drug's molecular weight, the degree to which the drug is bound to

plasma and milk proteins, its solubility in lipids and in water, the proportion of the drug that is ionized (i.e., carries a positive or negative charge), its pH factor, its half-life, and its milk/plasma ratio. Simplified, general guidelines apply to drug factors:

1. *The lower the drug's molecular weight, the more easily it passes through to a mother's milk.* Drugs with a high molecular weight (>200) (heparin, insulin, warfarin) are restricted from passing into human milk. Because of their high molecular weight, they are also not absorbed in the GI tract.

2. *The more a drug binds to plasma proteins (is protein-bound), the less likely it freely diffuses through the alveolar membranes into breastmilk.* Conversely, if a drug binds readily to milk proteins in the mother's milk, the drug tends to accumulate in the milk. Proteins are found in smaller proportions (0.8–0.9 percent) in human milk than in other elements (e.g., lipids), so even if it does bind to protein, it may not represent a substantial burden.

3. *The more lipid-soluble a medication or substance, the greater the quantity of medication transferred and the greater the speed of transfer into breastmilk. Medications with a low lipid solubility diffuse slowly into milk.* Lipid-soluble drugs more readily cross cell membranes by dissolving in the lipid layer, whereas water-soluble drugs must cross cell membranes through pores or openings. Because of the greater amount of lipids in breastmilk as compared to protein, for example, binding to lipid by itself may enable a larger proportion of the drug to transfer into the infant.

4. *The greater the proportion of a drug in a nonionized form, the more readily it diffuses across the lipid cellular membrane and into breastmilk.* When a nonionized molecule enters the milk compartment, it is quickly ionized, and back-diffusion is prevented; it becomes "trapped" in this form and accumulates in the milk. This accumulation is reflected in a high milk/plasma (M/P) ratio.

5. *Drugs that are weak bases (more alkaline) tend to concentrate more in breastmilk. Conversely, drugs*

that are weak acids do not readily transfer (Feldman & Pickering, 1986). This is because acids tend to attract bases. Because human milk is usually more acid (7.0–7.4) than is plasma (7.4), drugs that are weak bases (lincomycin, erythromycin, antihistamines, alkaloids, and isoniazid) would theoretically be more likely to cross the membranes from plasma into milk than would drugs that are weak acids (barbiturates, sulfonamides, penicillins, and diuretics).

6. *The longer the half-life of the drug, the greater the risk of accumulation in the mother and in the infant.* The rate of removal of a drug from the body is known as *clearance*. Half-life ($t^{1}/_{2}$) is another term frequently used to estimate how fast a drug leaves the body. Half-life is the time necessary for the drug serum concentration to decrease by one-half. Half-life is determined by the drug's rates of absorption, metabolism, and excretion from the body. Half-life varies considerably from one drug to another. For instance, penicillin has a serum half-life of less than one hour, whereas that of digitoxin is about one week. A drug with a short half-life is taken more frequently than is one with a long half-life. When a drug is given at a fixed dose, about four or five half-lives are required to achieve *steady-state* serum concentration in which plasma drug levels remain fairly steady.

7. *The higher the M/P ratio, the greater the amount of the drug found in milk. The M/P ratio refers to the concentration of the protein-free fractions in milk and in plasma.* For example, the M/P ratio of a particular sulfonamide is 0.08. This means that the level of the medication in the milk is 8 percent of the level of the medication in the plasma. An M/P ratio of 4.0 means that the level of the medication in milk is four times higher than the level in plasma. A medication with an M/P ratio of 1.0 has the same concentration in milk as that in plasma (Lipkin, 1989). M/P ratios are only estimations, but special concern should be given to drugs that have an M/P greater than 1.0 (Wilson, 1981).

Maternal Factors

The amount of medication the mother takes, how often she takes it, and the route of administration affect the magnitude and duration of drug passage into breastmilk. As expected, the higher the dosage, the more the drug transfers into the milk. If the medication is taken right after breastfeeding, the drug has the maximum time to clear the maternal blood. Drugs taken 30 to 60 minutes before a feeding are likely to be at maximum serum levels when the infant breastfeeds. On the other hand, when feedings are frequent (up to 16 times per day in some cultures), timing the dose would make little difference.

The level of a drug in the breastmilk and how soon it appears also depends on where the drug enters the mother's system. Whereas the infant's exposure to the substance is always through the gastrointestinal (GI) tract, the drug can enter the mother through one of several routes: orally, intravenously, intramuscularly, topically, or through inhalation. Oral medications have a slower drug action and take longer to reach breastmilk. The intravenous route, which bypasses GI barriers to absorption, allows a drug to enter the milk quickly and at higher levels than if the drug were given orally. The intramuscular route also allows quick transfer of drugs, because muscles have an abundant blood supply. Generally, topical medications (e.g., skin creams) reach breastmilk more slowly and in lesser amounts than do medications administered in other ways.

The mother's and the infant's genetic makeup and health play a role in their response to certain drugs. For instance, some breastfed infants are sensitive to certain drugs, such as caffeine from coffee drunk by the mother, whereas others feel no effect from it (Ryu, 1985; Yurchak & Jusko, 1976). Finally, if the mother's kidney or liver functions are impaired, normal metabolic pathways that excrete the drug are less effective, and there is greater or more prolonged presence of the drug in breastmilk.

Infant Factors

The age and maturity of the breastfeeding infant are important in light of the risks and benefits of maternal ingestion of a drug. Because infants are dynamic, changing organisms, what adversely affects them at one point may not be an issue a week or a month later. Premature infants have immature renal and hepatic systems and are at risk for developing high plasma drug concentrations. Premature infants' livers may be overwhelmed by breakdown products from hemoglobin or from medications administered directly to them. As their renal and liver systems develop, they may then be able to handle medication that previously might have triggered harmful consequences.

The full-term newborn's developing enzyme systems, lipid-brain barrier, and renal function are not yet fully developed. Thus, during the first week or so of life for the healthy neonate, and much later for the premature infant, detoxification of chemicals in the milk by either acetylation or oxidation is hampered. A healthy, three-month-old baby whose liver and renal systems have matured is much better equipped to metabolize a drug and has far fewer problems. Moreover, babies tolerate maternal drugs more easily as they get older because they are larger; therefore, the drug is distributed over a larger volume. For example, a male baby in the 50th percentile almost doubles his birth weight by three months.

The frequency of feedings and volume of breastmilk the infant takes must be considered. The child who is feeding only once or twice a day and taking other nourishment consumes considerably less drug than does a baby who breastfeeds 10 times daily and receives no other form of nourishment. Calculations of infant dose are often made on the assumption of exclusive breastfeeding. Such calculations are helpful because they give the maximum drug transfer. At the same time, they exaggerate the hazard in the case of an infant who takes other nutriments. Also, the presence of a substance in milk does not necessarily mean that it is absorbed in the infant's GI tract. Some drugs, such as gentamicin, kanamycin, tetracycline, and insulin, are absorbed very poorly in the GI tract of infants (and of adults as well).

Breast and Milk Factors

Most breastmilk is manufactured during feedings; the breast "stores" only a minimal quantity of milk. Therefore, the timing of a drug dose relative to breastfeeding influences how much of the drug will appear in breastmilk. If the infant feeds when the mother's drug serum levels are at a peak (highest) level, the amount of the drug that transfers into her milk (while it is being manufactured) is also higher than if her drug serum levels are at a trough (lowest) level. This is true in part because changes in mammary blood flow alter the amount of drug transported to the breast. The blood flow in the breast increases many times over when the breast begins to lactate; high mammary blood flow at the time the drug peaks—or any other time—delivers an even greater quantity of drug to milk (Vorherr, 1978; Wilson, 1981).

Breastmilk composition also affects the ability of the drug to cross the plasma into milk. Colostrum is high in protein and low in lactose, the reverse of mature milk. As milk composition changes, especially its fluctuations in fat content, drug-transport mechanisms also change. In addition, mammary blood pH, permeability of cellular and extracellular membranes within the secretory unit, cellular transport mechanisms in the alveoli, drug metabolism by breast tissue, and a drug's characteristics (such as pH and protein-binding ability) affect the passage of drugs into human milk.

Routes of Transport

Nature provides a series of barriers that help to prevent drugs from getting into human milk. A drug in a mother's bloodstream first passes out of the blood capillary lumen into the mammary interstitium, the connective tissue space surrounding the secretory lobules. To pass into the alveolar lumen, the drug must first penetrate the membranes of the myoepithelial cells and walls of the secretory cells lining the alveolus. It does this either by diffusion through the lipid portion of the membranes or through protein channels in the membranes. There are two main types of diffusion: passive (movement from higher concentration to lower concentration) and active (movement from lower concentration to higher concentration). Passive diffusion is the more common mechanism. In an alternate route, a drug molecule may travel from the interstitium to the alveolar lumen via small intercellular clefts, bypassing the secretory and myoepithelial cells. Table 6–1 lists the approximate percentage of maternal drugs that pass into milk, each drug's half-life, and safety-of-use ratings by the American Academy of Pediatrics.

Drugs That Affect Milk Volume

A number of drugs inhibit or enhance milk secretion. This effect is achieved by stimulating or suppressing prolactin or by steroidlike activity (Table 6–2). Thyrotropin-releasing hormone (TRH or protirelin) increases serum prolactin and has been used investigationally as a nasal spray to increase milk yield in mothers with insufficient milk supply at five days postpartum. It increased milk volume by 78 percent (Peters et al., 1991). Human growth hormone was shown to increase milk yield by 18.5 percent (Milsom et al., 1992). According to Anderson and Valdes (1993), both TRH and human growth hormone have been insufficiently studied and are too expensive to be recommended for routine use.

Some medications used in the treatment of psychiatric disorders cause an increase in breastmilk production (galactorrhea) by interfering with dopamine release. Because dopamine inhibits prolactin, a decrease in dopamine stimulates lactation. Drugs that interfere with dopamine release include reserpines (Serpasil), rauwolfia derivatives (Raudixin), and phenothiazines (Thorazine, Stelazine, Mellaril).

Metoclopramide (Reglan) is commonly used to treat gastroesophageal reflux and other gastric problems in infants and is routinely ordered for preventing nausea after a cesarean birth. It also increases breastmilk volume by inducing prolactin release and by blocking dopamine (Ehrenkranz & Ackerman, 1986; Guzman et al., 1979; Kauppila et al., 1983). Metoclopramide appears to be effective for women who are having problems maintaining an adequate milk supply, and it has few side effects (Gupta & Gupta, 1985; Kauppila et al., 1983; Sousa, 1975). Metoclopramide is usually taken as a 10-mg tablet orally three or four times per day. Cost for 30 tablets is about $33 for the trade product and $15 for the generic brand, which is just as effective (Wright, 1995). The average interval between the first dose of metoclopramide and improvement in lactation is about three days. In a case report, because of lack of breastmilk, a moth-

er received metoclopramide, 10 mg three times per day, along with breast stimulation using an electric pump. Within 48 hours of the first dose, the mother pumped 45 to 60 ml per breast every four hours, and her serum prolactin concentration increased from 125 ng/ml to 172 ng/ml (Budd et al., 1993). Domperidone (Motilium), a dopamine antagonist that increases breastmilk volume, is a popular galactologue in Canada. Like metoclopramide, it is an antiemetic. Unlike metoclopramide, it appears to act primarily in the periphery, with minimal access across the blood-brain barrier (Maddern, 1983).

Ergot alkaloids, such as bromocriptine, inhibit prolactin secretion. Bromocriptine (Parlodel) was extensively used to suppress lactation postpartum. However, after reports of serious adverse cardiovascular effects (Canterbury et al., 1987; U.S. Food and Drug Administration, 1982; Hopp et al., 1996; Watson et al., 1989), it is rarely used to reduce engorgement. Treating postpartum engorgement in mothers who do not intend to breastfeed once again relies on "old-fashioned" methods: ice, breast binders, analgesics, and sympathy. Other ergot derivatives, such as ergonovine maleate (Ergotrate) and methylergonovine maleate (Methergine), may be given once or twice to control postpartum bleeding and do not significantly affect milk yields (Bowes, 1980; Jolivet et al., 1978).

Alcohol ingestion by the mother results in the infant consuming significantly less breastmilk (Mennella & Beauchamp, 1991); however, it is not clear whether alcohol also reduces breastmilk production. Combined (estrogen and progestogen) oral contraceptives may inhibit milk production if estrogen dosage is high (Koetsawang et al., 1972; Miller & Hughes, 1970). There is also some evidence that oral contraceptives can slightly lower protein, fat, and minerals in breastmilk (Kader et al., 1969).

Drug Safety

The following brief discussion of the safety of drugs for breastfeeding mothers and infants is organized by pharmaceutical classifications. This information is derived from the references cited at the end of the chapter.

Table 6-1

MATERNAL DRUGS APPEARING IN BREASTMILK

Drug	Percentage (Approx.)	Half-Life (Hours)	AAP Review
Acebutolol	3.5	3–4	A[a]
Acetaminophen	0.04–0.23	1–3	A
Amitriptyline	< 1.0	31–46	B
Amoxicillin	< 0.07	4	A
Aspirin	0.5	0.25	C
Atenolol	5.7–19.2	6.4[b]	A[a]
Azactam	0.03	1.7	A
Baclofen	< 0.1	3–4	A
Caffeine	0.06–0.15	80–97[b]	A
Carbamazepine	3–5	8–28[b]	A
Carbenicillin	0.001	3.4–5.7	NR
Cefoperazone sodium	< 0.9	6–10 (neonatal)	NR
Cefpodoxine proxetil	0–6	2–3	NR
Cefprozil	< 0.03	1.3	A
Ceftriaxone	3–4	7.3	A
Chloramphenicol	1.3	22[b]	B
Cetirizine	3.0	6.2[b]	NR
Chlorpromazien	0.07	12	B
Clomipramine	trace	92.8[b]	A[a]
Clonazepam	4.8	23	NR
Codeine	0.1	2.9	A
Corticosteroids	< 0.01	24+	NR
Diazepam	0.7–7.8	20–50[b]	B
Digoxin	0.07–0.14	20–180[b]	A
Erythromycin	< 1.0	1.5–2	A
Fluoxetine	5–9	48–72	B
Ibuprofen	0.6	2	A
Imipramine	0.1	18	B
Indocin	0.07–0.98	4.5	A
Isoniazid	0.75	8–20[b] (neonatal)	A
Kanamycin	0.05	4–18[b]	A

Table 6-1 (cont.)

Ketorolac	< 0.4	2–8	A
Labetalol	0.07	6–8	A
Lincomycin	0.025	4.4–6.4	NR
Lithium	0.12	22	D
Methotrexate	0.01	7.2	D
Methlydopa	0.02	1.5	A
Methylergonovine	0.003	0.5	NR
Nadolol	5.1	20–24	A
Nalidixic acid	0.05	2	A
Naproxen	1.1	12–15[b]	A
Nortriptyline	2.3	16–90	NR
Paroxetine	0.002	21	NR
Phenobarbital	1.5	99	C
Phenytoin	< 5.0	20–160 (premature)	A
Prednisolone	0.12	8.2	A
Prednisone	0.04	3	A
Propranolol	< 0.1	3–5	A
Rifampin	0.05	2.9[b]	A
Rocephin	3–4	7.3	A
Sotalol	22.0	12	A
Spironolactone	0.2	10–35	A
Streptomycin	0.5	4–10[b] (neonates)	A
Sulfisoxazole	< 1.0	4.6–7.8	A
Sumatriptan succinate	0.2–0.5	1.3	NR
Terbutaline	0.2–0.7	14	A
Terfenadine	0.45	11.7	NR
Tetracycline	0.03	6–11	A
Theophylline	< 1.0	30[b]	A
Tramadol HCL	0.1	7	NR
Valproic acid	< 3.0	6–10 (neonates)	NR

AAP = American Academy of Pediatrics; A = approved by the American Academy of Pediatrics for use in breastfeeding mothers; B = drug whose effect on nursing infants is unknown but may be of concern; C = drugs associated with significant side effects, should be given with caution; D = contraindicated by the American Academy of Pediatrics for use by breastfeeding mothers; NR = not reviewed.
[a] Under consideration for removal from A list.
[b] Pediatric elimination half-life (no asterisk indicates adult-elimination half-life).

Table 6-1 (cont.)

Source: From American Academy of Pediatrics, Committee on Drugs: Transfer of drugs and other chemicals into human milk, *American Academy of Pediatrics, 1994; T Hale: Medications and mothers' milk (6th ed). 1997; G Pon, E Rey, I Matheson: Excretion of psychoactive drugs into breast milk.* Clin Pharmacol Ther *27:270–89, 1994; H Vorherr: Human lactation and breastfeeding. In: BL Larson, ed.* Lactation: a comprehensive treatise, *vol 4. New York: Academic, 1978; 181–279; CM Berlin: The excretion of drugs and chemicals in human milk. In: SJ Yaffe,* Pediatric pharmacology. *New York: Grune & Stratton, 1980; 137–47; R Lawrence:* Breastfeeding: a guide for the medical profession. *St Louis: Mosby, 1994; L Rivera-Calimlim: The significance of drugs in breast milk.* Clin Perinat *14(1):51–70, 1987.*

Nonsteroidal Antiinflammatory Drugs

Nonsteroidal antiinflammatory drugs (NSAIDs) act as analgesics to relieve pain by interfering with the release of prostaglandins and the antiinflammatory process. Ibuprofen (Motrin), commonly used for postpartum analgesia and as an antiinflammatory drug for breastfeeding mothers, crosses into breastmilk in trivial amounts and does not appear to have adverse effects on infants (Ito, 1993; Townsend et al., 1984). Acetaminophen (Tylenol) alone or with codeine is another common postpartum pain medication. Acetaminophen enters the maternal milk rapidly but is only 0.52 percent of the lowest recommended infant single dose. It is given directly to infants as the drug of choice for reducing fever. Ketorolac (Toradol), a popular NSAID, is contraindicated in labor and delivery because, through its prostaglandin synthesis inhibitory effect, it may adversely affect fetal circulation and inhibit uterine contractions, thus increasing the risk of uterine hemorrhage. During breastfeeding, an infant would receive less than 0.4 percent of the daily maternal dose (Hale, 1997; Wischnik, Manth, & Lloyd, 1989). Although aspirin is still the antiarthritic drug of choice for the breastfeeding mother, her infant should be monitored for increased prothrombin time and signs of bleeding.

Analgesics and Narcotics

If the mother needs narcotic analgesia postpartum, short-term use probably does not adversely affect the infant (Findlay, 1981). When narcotics are used repeatedly, the infant should be monitored for drowsiness, poor breastfeeding, and weight loss. Narcotics frequently used postpartum are oxycodone and aspirin (Percodan), propoxyphene (Darvon), codeine, and meperidine (Demerol).

Anesthetics

A breastfeeding mother who must undergo a surgical procedure is more likely to be treated as an outpatient than to be hospitalized. As a result, separation because of hospitalization is not as frequent a problem for breastfeeding as it was a few years ago. Most concerns center around the transfer of anesthesia and analgesia into breastmilk. See Table 6–3 for information on common anesthetics. A discussion of breastfeeding for the mother facing surgery appears in Chapter 17.

Anticoagulants

Previously, all anticoagulants were contraindicated for nursing mothers. Newer research indicates that some anticoagulants are not a problem. Warfarin (Coumadin) is present in breastmilk but only in very small amounts. The prothrombin time is usually normal in infants whose mothers are taking warfarin and dicumarol. Heparin does not appear in breastmilk. To be on the safe side, monitoring of the infant's prothrombin time is recommended. The baby is given vitamin K (Mephyton) if needed. Phenindione (Hedulin, Dindevan) is contraindicated when the mother is breastfeeding because it has been reported to cause bleeding in breastfed infants.

Anticonvulsants

Most anticonvulsant drugs are generally considered to be compatible with breastfeeding. Common medications used to treat seizure disorders are phenytoin (Dilantin), carbamazepine (Tegretol, Primidone, Mysoline), valproic acid (Depakene), ethosuximide (Zarontin) and phenobarbital. Given a maximum dose of carbamazepine, the breastfed infant would ingest in breastmilk only 3 to 5 per-

Table 6–2

Drugs That Affect Milk Production

Generic Name	Trade Name	Generic Name	Trade Name
Inhibitors of Milk Production			
Levodopa	Dopar, Larodopa	Pyridoxine	Vitamin B_6
Phenelzine	Nardil	Prostaglandin E_2	–
Tranylcypromine EE	Parnate	Estrogens	(numerous)
Ergocryptine	Ergocryptine	Androgens	(numerous)
Barbiturates	(numerous)	Bromocriptine	Parlodel
Apomorphine	Apomorphine	Alcohol (excessive)	–
Antihistamines	(numerous)		
Enhancers of Milk Production			
Rauwolfia	Roudisin, Rauval	Metoclopramide	Reglan
Reserpine	Serpasil	Thiothixene	Navrane
Chlorpromazine	Thorazine	Amitriptyline	Elavil
Perphenazine	Trilafon, Triavil	Imipramine	Trofranil
Prochlorperazine	Compazine	Methyldopa	Aldomet
Promazine	Sparine	Thyroid-releasing hormone	Thyroid-releasing hormone
Thioridazine	Mellaril	Insulin	insulin
Trifluoperazine	Stelazine	Oxytocin (nasally)	Syntocinon
Chlorprothixene	Taractan	Sulpiride	
Haloperidol	Haldol		

Source: Derived from Dickey RP, Stone SC: Drugs that affect the breast and lactation. Clin Obstet Gynecol *18:95–111, 1975; Peterson RG, Bowes WA: Drugs, toxins and environmental agents in breast milk. In: Neville MC, Neifert M, eds.,* Physiology, nutrition and breast-feeding. *New York: Plenum, 1983, 367–403.*

cent of the infant's therapeutic exposure (Ito et al., 1995)–not a significant level of exposure in breast-fed infants (Bailey & Ito, 1997). Similar results are reported for phenytoin and valproic acid. Phenobarbital and phenytoin transfer into milk in insignificant amounts and are generally considered safe for the breastfeeding mother to use. If the mother takes high doses of phenobarbital, however, her baby may become drowsy. Short-acting phenobarbiturates (secobarbital, pentobarbital) are preferred to the long-acting agents, because they appear in lower concentrations in milk. Despite consensus among neurologists that breastfeeding is safe for a mother taking antiepileptic drugs (especially carbamazepine, valproic acid, and phenytoin), many physicians recommend against breastfeeding in this situation (Ito et al, 1995). When a mother receives magnesium sulfate for pregnancy-induced hypertension or seizures, lactogenesis and engorgement may be delayed for several days (Halderman, 1993).

Table 6–3

COMMON ANESTHETICS USED FOR MATERNAL SURGERY

Drug	Peak Milk Concentration	Comments
Thiopental	At 2 hr = 0.9 μg/ml	Used to induce general anesthesia; transfer to infant inconsequential
Propofol	0.7 μg/ml	Used to induce general anesthesia; rapid clearance
Fentanyl	Within 1 hr = 0.4 ng/ml; adult half-life: 3–4 hr; newborn half-life: 3–13 hr	Rapid clearance; not detectable in breastmilk 4–7 hr after administration
Meperidine (Demerol)	500 ng/ml	Infant neurobehavioral depression possible
Morphine	60 ng/ml	Multiple doses may cause infant sedation and ineffective suckling
Midazolam (Versed)	9 ng/ml	Low passage rate into breastmilk; not detected at 7 hr; no apparent effect on breastfed infants

Source: Derived from C Biddle: When the breast-feeding mother faces surgery. Contemp Nurse Pract *July/August 15–20, 1995.*

Antidepressants

Medications given for depression are usually given over a long period; therefore, they have a greater potential for accumulating than do other medications. At the same time, drug levels are easily monitored by measuring serum drug levels (peak and trough) in both the mother and the infant.

Fluoxetine (Prozac), paroxetine (Paxil), and sertraline (Zoloft), drugs of choice for first-line treatment of depression, belong to a class of drugs known as *selected serotinin re-uptake inhibitors* (SSRIs). SSRIs have minimal anticholinergic effects (dry mouth, blurred vision, constipation, urinary retention), are safer in overdose situations, and need to be taken only once daily. The most common side effect is nausea. When mothers take standard doses, the amount of SSRIs found in human milk and in infant serum levels is very small. According to estimates, a breastfeeding infant would receive 5 to 9 percent of the maternal dose of fluoxetine and 0.34 percent of paroxetine (Hale, 1997). Probably the preferred SSRI for breastfeeding women is sertraline, as serum levels in a three-week-old infant were not detectable, and no abnormal occurrences have been noted in the development of the infant (Altshuler, 1995). One case study reports colic in a six-week-old infant whose mother was taking fluoxetine while breastfeeding (Lester et al., 1993).

The tricyclic antidepressants (TCAs) desipramine (Norpramine) and imipramine (Trofanil) are widely used to treat postpartum depression. Clomipramine (Anafranil), used to treat obsessive-compulsive disorder in the postpartum period, is either undetectable or below the quantifiable limit in infant serums (Wisner, Perel, & Folgia, 1995). In one study (Misri & Sivertz, 1991), no adverse effects were noted in breastfed infants of 20 breastfeeding women taking TCAs. Although negligible amounts of TCAs pass into breastmilk, anticholinergic effects are common. Doxepin is the least favorable choice of this group of compounds, as several reports suggest problems with this medication in the infant (Hale, 1997). Amitriptyline, nortriptyline, desipramine, clomipramine, or sertraline are favored to treat breastfeeding women, according to one study (Wisner, Perel, & Findling, 1996).

Lithium is listed as contraindicated on the most recently published Drug List from the American Academy of Pediatrics Committee on Drugs (AAP, 1994). (See Appendix 6–1 at the end of this chapter.) However, breastfeeding mothers should be able to take lithium with careful monitoring (Roberts, 1990). In discussing lithium and breastfeeding, Schou (1990) states:

Accumulating evidence points strongly to the beneficial effects of breastfeeding for both child and mother, mentally and physically, and it is an open question whether the gain outweighs the losses when breastfeeding is avoided. Supported by husband and physician, the mother must make her own choice.

Diazepam (Valium), a tranquilizer, is a commonly prescribed psychotherapeutic agent. High doses have been associated with infant lethargy, drowsiness, and jaundice. Ayd (1973) warned that competition for glucuronic acid by diazepam may result in hyperbilirubinemia in breastfed infants of Valium-treated mothers. As discussed, some psychotherapeutic medications increase the mother's milk supply. A mother should be forewarned that she may have more milk as a result of taking such a medication.

Antihistamines

Antihistamines specifically compete with histamine, a naturally occurring amine that causes allergy symptoms. Many lactating women have taken terfenadine (Seldane), a second-generation antihistamine, for seasonal allergic rhinitis, because it is nonsedating compared with such first-generation antihistamines as diphenhydramine (Benadryl) and brompheniramine (Dimetane). Terfenadine is undetected in breastmilk; its metabolite passes into breastmilk in small amounts (Lucas et al., 1995). However, the FDA has proposed a ban of Seldane because it has been associated with potentially fatal heart-rhythm disturbances. Seldane must *not* be taken in conjunction with such antifungal drugs as ketoconazole or itraconazole or with the antibiotic erythromycin, as dangerous cardiac arrhythmias have occurred (Hale, 1997). If a nonsedating antihistamine is needed, Claritin (loratidine), Hismanal (astemizole), or Allegra (hexofenadine) are recommended instead.

Antimicrobials

According to a rule of thumb, if an antibiotic can be given directly to an infant, it can also be taken by the nursing mother. With the exception of cephalexin (Keflex), cephalothin (Keflin), oxacillin (Prostaphlin), and nystatin (Mycostatin), antibiotics transfer into milk. Because any oral antibiotic changes the GI flora and mucosa, the infant's stools may loosen and change in color. Because antibiotics predispose the mother and the infant to candidiasis, monitoring for this problem is advised.

The breastfeeding baby may develop sensitization to the antibiotics the mother is taking. A strong family history of drug sensitization should be considered in deciding whether a mother should take antibiotics and related drugs (Roberts, 1984). Allergies may be a problem. The author saw a case in which the mother, who was highly allergic to penicillin, developed a rash and hives on her breasts from nursing her baby, who was on ampicillin. The mother resolved her allergic response by giving her baby the ampicillin immediately after nursing instead of before the feeding. Chloramphenicol has relatively high concentration in milk. Most physicians avoid using tetracycline because it can discolor teeth during the formative years. The infant receives such a minute amount through breastmilk, however, that the possibility of this happening is remote. Maternal use of minocycline, a derivative of tetracyline used to treat acne, may result in a black discoloration of breastmilk (Hunt et al., 1996).

Quinolones are synthetics that differ chemically from other antibiotics. Ofloxacin (Floxin) and ciprofloxacin (Cipro) are quinolones effective in treating a wide variety of infections. A week-long exposure of this drug is probably not detrimental to nursing infants as long as the dose is modest. Many current studies do not support the contention that fluoroquinolones induce arthropathy in pediatric patients (Hale, 1997). The mother should be encouraged to avoid breastfeeding at the time of peak levels.

Metronidazole (Flagyl) should be given in a single 2-gm dose, and breastfeeding should be interrupted for 12 hours after the dose. Such a plan interrupts breastfeeding for only 12 hours rather than for a week (Erickson, Oppenheim, & Smith, 1981). Sulfa drugs should not be taken by the mother during the first month of the infant's life because of the risk of neonatal jaundice. Sulfa drugs may be used after the first month of life; short-acting sulfonamides are preferred to the long-acting agents.

Antifungals

Nystatin (Mycostatin), miconazole (Monistat), clotrimazole (Lotrimin, Mycelex), and fluconaxole (Diflucan) are antifungals used in the treatment of candidiasis. They are used topically and orally for treating fungal infections of the breastfeeding woman and her infant. Nystatin is the main therapeutic agent to control overgrowth of *Candida albicans,* including thrush and diaper rash in infants; it is poorly absorbed in the GI tract, skin, or mucous membranes and is used for a local effect to reduce the total load of candida in the woman's body. Nystatin can be given directly to the infant; it is safe, without serious side effects, and very reasonably priced.

Miconazole (Monistat) is a relatively new synthetic antifungal agent. About 50 percent of miconazole is absorbed from the GI tract and is widely distributed into body tissues and fluids. Clotrimazole (Gyne-Lotrimin) has been used safely for more than a decade to treat vaginal yeast infection or candidiasis and is highly effective, with minimum risk. Only small amounts of clotrimazole are absorbed systemically. The FDA approved clotrimazole as an over-the-counter (OTC) drug.

Fluconazole (Diflucan), a newer and more expensive preparation, is used to treat oral-pharyngeal candidiasis. It is available in pill form and in an orange-flavored suspension for children. The initial dose is usually 200 mg followed by 100 mg daily. Two weeks of therapy are recommended. An infant taking 450 ml of milk daily would receive about 5 to 10 percent of a recommended therapeutic dose for candidiasis from breastmilk and thus would need separate therapy (Hale, 1997). The recommended pediatric dosage is an initial dose of 6 mg/kg followed by 3 mg/kg/day. There are conflicting anecdotal reports about the effectiveness of fluconazole in treating candidiasis in breastfeeding women and infants and about its overuse.

Bronchodilators

Ephedrine, epinephrine, and cromolyn (Intal) are destroyed in the infant's GI tract. Although relatively safe for breastfeeding infants, theophylline tends to accumulate in infants, who should be monitored for irritability and insomnia. Nursing women who take theophylline should avoid eating chocolate, another source of theophylline. Use of an inhaler minimizes the amount of theophylline passed into breastmilk.

Beta-Blockers and Antihypertensives

In this group of medications, the amount of drug transferred through breastmilk varies considerably from drug to drug. Ellsworth (1994) reviewed the literature and advised that atenolol (Tenormin), acebutolol (Sectral), nadolol (Corgard), soltalol (Betapace), and timolol (Blocadren) should be avoided in breastfeeding women with younger infants and when high doses are required. Propranolol, metoprolol, and labetolol are excreted in milk in low quantities to allow breastfeeding even by the compromised infant. A mother using propranolol as prophylaxis against migraine, for example, would expose her infant to 2 percent of the therapeutic dose. Such a small dose is unlikely to cause clinical effects (Bailey & Ito, 1997). Digoxin is considered safe during lactation if maternal serum levels are carefully monitored. Methyldopa increases milk volume, but no adverse effects have been reported. Maternal use of oral sumatriptan, a relatively new drug to treat migraine headaches, results in the breastfed infant's absorption of only 0.2 to 0.5 percent of his mother's dose (Bailey & Ito, 1997; Wojnar-Horton et al., 1996).

Calcium Channel Blockers

Verapamil and nifedipine are used to treat hypertension. Both have relatively short half-lives, and both appear in generally low levels in breastmilk. Less than .01 percent of verapamil and 5 percent of nifedipine is transferred daily to the breastfeeding infant (Ehrenkranz, 1989); no drug could be detected in the plasma of breastfeeding infants according to one study (Miller et al., 1986). Both drugs are given in release formulations; therefore, it makes no sense to try to breastfeed around peak serum levels. Low doses (5–10 mg, two to three times per day) of nifedipine are used to treat vasospasm in lactating breasts, sometimes termed *Raynaud's syndrome of the nipple.* Overdoses of calcium channel blockers can be lethal, so they should be kept out children's reach.

Contraceptives

Combined (estrogen and progestin) oral contraceptives (OCs), especially those with more than 50 µg estrogen, significantly decrease milk output and are contraindicated during lactation (Croxato et al., 1983; Peralta et al., 1983). Anecdotal reports also suggest that combined OCs may cause malodorous stools and GI distress in some infants. Alternatively, Progestin-only OCs and methods (DMPA, Norplant) appear to have no effect on breastmilk and are not contraindicated during lactation, particularly if they are started when lactation is well established and the lowest effective dose is used (McCann & Potter, 1994; Visness & Rivera, 1995; WHO Task Force, 1994b). Depomedroxy-progesterone (DMPA or Depo-Provera) is a pregnancy prevention method of choice to 9 million women worldwide (Kaunitz, 1993). The amount of steroids absorbed by the breastfeeding infant of a mother using OCs is small and appears to have no long-term effects on children (Nilsson et al., 1986).

Ideally, the use of progestin-only contraceptive methods should be delayed until at least six weeks postpartum, as it may suppress lactation if it is given in the early weeks after birth. Moreover, most fully breastfeeding women are not at risk of ovulating during this time, and delaying the medication avoids exposing newborns to exogenous steroids during the more vulnerable early weeks of life. (See Chapter 21 for additional discussion of contraceptive use during lactation.)

Diuretics

Large doses of short-acting thiazide-type diuretics, usual doses of loop diuretics (furosemide [Lasix]) or long-acting thiazide diuretics (bendroflumethiazide [Corzide], chlorthalidone [Hygroton]) can reduce milk production and potentially cause dehydration in the infant (Ellsworth, 1994). The infant should be weighed regularly, and the number of wet diapers should be noted. Low doses of thiazide diuretics (Hydro-Diuril, Esidrix, Oretic) are considered by the American Academy of Pediatrics (1994) to be compatible with breastfeeding.

Laxatives

Laxatives are given routinely postpartum. Such bulk-forming laxatives as Metamucil are considered a natural laxative; they are preferable to irritant cathartics (Peri-Colace, Dulcolax), which stimulate intestinal peristalsis and inhibit the reabsorption of water in the large intestine. Although there may be some concern about the possibility of dehydration, Peri-Colace and Dulcolax are frequently taken by breastfeeding mothers, apparently without ill effects. Mothers should be taught that use of a stimulant cathartic for more than one week may cause the large intestine to lose its tone.

Herbs

Herbs, especially herbal teas, are currently very popular. Herbs and related compounds have been used since antiquity for a variety of purposes, especially for medicinal purposes and the restoration of health. Some herbal remedies do work, are safe when used as directed, are less expensive than are drugs, and have their place as partners with pharmaceuticals. On the other hand, some herbals do not work, are poisonous, and have unknown potency and efficacy (Ehudin-Pagano et al., 1987).

More than 30 herbs are considered to be powerful galactagogues (Fleiss, 1988). Perhaps the most widely known is fennel or fenugreek, the principal ingredient in the legendary Lydia Pinkham's Vegetable Compound. Prior to the dubious use of bovine growth hormone, dairy farmers used to increase milk production from their dairy cows by adding fennel to the animals' fodder (Miczak, 1996). Ixbut, an herb from Guatemala, is used to help women to increase their breastmilk.

Cascara and senna are two herbal remedies not recommended for the breastfeeding woman because they can cause diarrhea in the baby (Thorley, 1996). Sage acts like estrogen; therefore, it can reduce milk production. In South India, jasmine flowers suppress lactation when fashioned into a bralike "wreath" over engorged breasts (Shrivastav et al., 1988). Similarly, in Australia, raw cabbage leaves placed on the breasts are routine treatment for engorgement (Rosier, 1988; Roberts, 1995).

Herbs contain active ingredients that, when purified and standardized as a chemical isolate (e.g., digitoxin from the foxglove plant), are marketed and sold as drugs. The plant's other constituents, which together form the complete picture of the plant's medicinal worth, are discarded (Miczak, 1996). Only a few research-based articles on herbs and breastfeeding have been published in the Western world. Most of them are case reports, such as those discussed later, of adverse outcomes from breastfeeding mothers who consistently ingested large quantities of herbs, a result similar to overdosing from a commercial drug.

Only one report (Sharma et al., 1996) looked prospectively at outcomes in lactating women who used herbs in moderation. In this randomized clinical trial of lactating women in New Delhi diagnosed as having insufficient milk supply, each mother was randomly assigned to receive either a placebo or a galactagogue (*Asparagus racemosus*) twice daily for four weeks. At the end of four weeks, prolactin levels were somewhat higher in the placebo group; however, infants whose mothers took the galactagogue fed their babies 44 percent less supplemental milk, and their infants had gained slightly more weight than those of the placebo group. There were no biochemical liver cell dysfunction or other significant side effects in any of the women in either group.

Several case reports on breastfeeding and herbs have appeared in the literature. A Canadian report (Koren et al., 1990) cited a mother who took ginseng in high doses during her pregnancy and while breastfeeding. Her full-term baby boy was noted to have thick black pubic hair, hair over his forehead, and swollen red nipples. Although this case cannot establish ginseng as the cause of neonatal hirsutism, reversal of hair growth after the mother discontinued taking ginseng suggested a cause-and-effect relationship. Another report from Italy (Rosti et al., 1994) concerned two ill neonates whose mothers had taken teas containing licorice, fennel, anise, and French lilac. When the teas were stopped, the infants' symptoms of lethargy and hypotonia ceased. The authors identified licorice as the harmful ingredient, claiming it to be unsafe if taken in large doses.

Countless numbers of breastfeeding women around the globe daily take herbal compounds without adverse effects. Although herbs can have strong pharmocological properties, their effect when taken during lactation is wrongly perceived as being the same as the effect of herbs taken during pregnancy. This is clearly *not* the case (as is noted elsewhere in the chapter). Health care providers, including lactation consultants (LCs), are not generally knowledgeable in the usage of herbs and should be cautious. Box 6–1 lists some of the herbs used by lactating women around the world.

Scabicides and Pediculicides

Infestation with mites or lice continues to be a problem throughout the world; yet there is very little information on the use of medications for this condition during lactation. Lindane (gamma benzine hexachloride) is used for treatment of pediculosis or scabies. Lindane is absorbed through the skin after topical use as a shampoo or lotion, but its drug levels in human milk are not known (Morin & Stoukides, 1994). Until toxicological data are available, the Centers for Disease Control (CDC, 1985) does not recommend its use. Pyrethrins with piperonyl butoxide are OTC products effective topically for treating pediculoses but not scabies in breastfeeding women. For scabies, the CDC recommends crotamiton, 10 percent, or sulfur, 6 percent in petrolatum.

Steroids

Prednisone passes into human milk in small amounts and, in small doses over a short period, is not contraindicated in nursing mothers. Hale (1997) estimated that an infant consuming a liter of milk per day from a mother taking a 10-mg/day oral dose would consume 28.3 μg of prednisone, an insignificant dose. A dose of 80 mg/day would result in the infant's receiving <.1 percent mg of the dose. Women taking prednisone for multiple sclerosis report a significant decrease in milk supply with doses of prednisone greater than 20 to 30 mg/day, a process that reverses when the dose is lowered or discontinued. Nursing children report that prednisone can cause breastmilk to taste bitter.

Clinical Implications

Pharmaceuticals commonly taken by childbearing women include antibiotics, antidepressants, thyroid preparations, OCs, and OTC medications for colds and minor respiratory problems. Ito et al. (1993) followed a cohort of 838 infants breastfed by women taking medications. By identifying the 31 most frequently used drugs in their cohort, they provided the first prospective information on safety of breastfeeding during maternal therapy with many commonly taken drugs. They found no major adverse reactions necessitating medical attention, and only 94 women (11.2 percent) reported infants' minor adverse reactions (those not requiring medical attention):

- antibiotics, 19.2 percent (32 of 166)
- analgesics or narcotics, 11.2 percent (22 of 196)
- antihistamines, 9.4 percent (8 of 85)
- sedatives, antidepressants, or antiepileptics, 7.1 percent (3 of 42)
- others, 9.9 percent (42 out of 435)

When a mother calls and asks whether she can continue to breastfeed while she takes a certain drug, the LC faces the dilemma (as well as the legal implications) of being asked a "medical" question. Although the final decision must be made by the woman and her physician, the LC can be an invaluable source of information and can provide up-to-date information about studies done on the safety of a particular drug during breastfeeding (Box 6–2). Many available drug lists provide the needed information. The most current recommendations regarding drugs and breastmilk from the Committee on Drugs of the American Academy of Pediatrics are presented at the end of this chapter.

When using such literature provided by drug manufacturers as the information sheets in the medication packet, the following should be kept in mind: pharmaceutical houses protect themselves legally by taking the "guilty-unless-proved-innocent" approach. Unless documentation proves otherwise, many medications are "not recommended for breastfeeding." General pharmacology textbooks take a similar conservative stance, warning readers that nursing mothers should not take any medications.

The first task is to find a discussion of the drug in question in current drug literature. Identifying the *generic* name of the drug will simplify the search. The generic name is the drug's chemical or official name as opposed to its *trade,* or *brand,* name. For example, ampicillin is the generic name of an antibiotic. Ampicillin is manufactured by

---

BOX 6–1

Herbs Used for Health and Breastfeeding-Related Conditions

Condition	Herbs[a]
Anemia	Nettle, yellow dock root (*Rumex* species)
Galactagogues	*Asparagus racemosus* (Shatavari)[b]
	Ginseng[b]
	Fennel
	Fennugreek
	Red raspberry
	Red clover blossoms (*Trifolium pratense*)
Postpartum "blues"	St. John's wort (*Hypericum perfora tum*)
Fatigue and tension	Borage (*Borago officinalis*)
	Chamomille (catnip tea)
	Mint
Mastitis	Dandelion tea
	Compresses of raw scraped carrot
	Comfrey root
	Yarrow juice, parsley leaves
Weaning or reducing	Periwinkle
	Sage (*Saliva officinalis*)
milk supply	Sassafras
	Yarrow (*Achillea milleolium*)[b]

[a] *All herbs should be taken only in* low to moderate doses.
[b] *Reports of adverse consequences to the infants' health with high doses.*

BOX 6–2

Questions to Be Asked of Breastfeeding Mothers Needing Medications

---

• *What did your physician tell you in ordering this medication for you?*

Identify the medical reason for taking the medication and the doctor's opinion about whether the mother should continue breastfeeding. Phrased this way, the question captures the mother's reaction and her feelings about what she has been told.

• *What is the drug's name, what is the prescribed dosage, and what is the time scheduled for taking the drug?*

This query should yield basic information for evaluating the drug's action, its excretion rate, and possible effects on the infant or on the mother's milk supply.

• *How old is your baby, and how often are you breastfeeding?*

The infant's maturity makes a difference in its ability to metabolize drugs; the

older the baby, the better. It may be possible to schedule ingestion of the drug at certain times during the day that avoid peak plasma and milk drug levels, minimizing the amount of drug the baby receives through the milk. Usually, the best time to take the medication is right after feeding.

• *Do you know how to hand-express or use a breast pump?*

If the mother must interrupt breastfeeding, these activities provide options. Sometimes feedings need to be interrupted for only a few hours or for a day or two; hand expression avoids the expense and bother of renting or purchasing a pump. Reassure her that her milk production will continue if she expresses her milk regularly.

---

several pharmaceutical companies and is sold under a trade name, such as Amoxil, Omnipen, or Amcill. Trade names are capitalized; generic names appear in lower case. Most drug lists use the generic name followed by its popular trade names. Generic names of drugs are given with their common trade names in the American Academy of Pediatrics Committee on Drugs appendix at the end of this chapter.

Nonprescription, OTC drug sales rise each year. The drugs sold are frequently combination drugs. Popular OTC drugs include analgesics (ibuprofen, acetaminophen, and aspirin), antihistamines (diphenhydramine and chlopheniramine) for colds and sinus conditions, bronchodilators (ephedrine), antacids, and cathartics. Generally, OTC drugs are compatible with lactation.

The many OTC cold preparations that produce long-acting or sustained action are advertised to "last" 12 hours. Fillers are added to the drug to produce a timed release so that the mother cannot excrete it all within a 12-hour period. Such drugs will be long acting for the infant as well; these preparations increase the potential for accumulation in both the mother and the infant.

Scheduling the best time of day for a mother to take medication minimizes the amount of drug the infant receives. If a mother is taking penicillin with a known half-life of one hour, the infant theoretically receives the least amount of penicillin through her milk if she nurses her baby just before taking the medication, when serum levels are likely to be at their lowest. Whenever the mother takes a medication over a long period, the timing of the

BOX 6–3

General Guidelines for Combined Breastfeeding and Medication Use

- Use a medication only if it is absolutely necessary. Consider alternative nondrug therapies.

- Delay starting the medication (if there is a choice) until the infant is more mature and better able to detoxify and metabolize drugs that might be transported through the breastmilk.

- Take the lowest dose possible for the shortest time possible.

- Choose a drug that transfers the least amount into breastmilk, using its reported M/P ratio as a guide. Avoid drugs with an M/P greater than or equal to 1.

- Avoid a drug with a long half-life, if possible.

- Avoid sustained-release preparations.

- Schedule taking the medication so that the lowest amount gets into the milk (usually immediately after a feeding or before the infant has a long sleep period).

- Watch for any untoward reaction, such as fussiness, rash, colic, or change in feeding or sleeping habits. If any of these occur, notify the physician and provide needed information about all of the drugs used by the mother.

- Teach hand-expression or provide a breast pump and instructions for its use if the mother must take a contraindicated drug for a short time.

medication in relation to feeding her baby is less important, because the concentration of the drug in her serum remains relatively stable.

At least one drug appears to make breastmilk taste bitter. In one case (Smolek-Houghton, 1984), after a nursing mother took an OTC antihistamine, her toddler refused to breastfeed, spitting out her milk. The mother stopped taking the drug, and the toddler promptly resumed breastfeeding.

Health professionals have a formidable responsibility when it comes to making decisions about drugs and breastfeeding (Box 6–3). On the one hand, physicians are anxious (and rightly so) about their legal risk if something adverse happens. On the other hand, if the doctor recommends weaning, the result can be disastrous. Abrupt weaning can be so traumatic that many women painfully recall the experience in vivid detail decades later—sometimes with hostility toward the

physician if they realize that weaning was not necessary. The infant who is weaned even temporarily is at greater risk of infection and may develop allergies or other severe health problems. The following example illustrates, in the extreme, what may happen when breastfeeding is interrupted because of maternal medication.

Diagnosed as having a urinary-tract infection and started on a sulfonamide medication, a breastfeeding mother was told to discontinue breastfeeding for the duration of the therapy (10 days). Already discouraged because she had to pump her breasts earlier when her infant was jaundiced, the mother felt overwhelmed and decided to give up breastfeeding. Later the physician's office called to say that her urine culture was negative, but that she should continue the drug as a precautionary measure. Shortly after discontinuing breastfeeding, her infant developed vomiting, diarrhea, and later eczema. The parents and physician desperately switched from one formula to another to find one that the infant could tolerate. The infant developed periods of apnea and was placed on a home apnea monitor between hospitalizations. Ultimately, more complications developed, and an ileostomy was performed. Desperate, the mother began relactating while she collected fresh breastmilk donated by other women; eventually she was able to sustain the infant on her milk (Riordan & Riordan, 1984).

Finally, the LC may find herself in a tug-of-war between the mother and the physician about the safety of taking a medication. The author found herself in this situation when a breastfeeding mother called for help. She was ordered by her psychiatrist to take an antidepressant and to wean her baby immediately. Several drug lists showed the drug in question to be considered safe for breastfeeding. The author relayed this information to the family. The psychiatrist held firm. After several heated discussions between the mother and her psychiatrist, the mother relented and weaned.

Although there are no easy answers to resolve this kind of problem, the LC, acting as a client advocate and using reliable information, can only advise or recommend but cannot force a decision.

Maternal Substance Abuse and Addiction

According to a 1985 survey by the U.S. National Institute on Drug Abuse, about 70 million Americans have used an illegal substance, such as cocaine, marijuana, or heroin, on at least one occasion (National Institute on Drug Abuse, 1986). Persons with the highest rate of use are those between 18 and 25 years old. Most breastfeeding women do not use illegal drugs, but some do. Although there are many illegal drugs, this discussion is limited to those most commonly used.

Marijuana

Marijuana is so widely used today that it is probably the most commonly used illegal drug among breastfeeding women. In a 1985 survey (Johnson, 1987), 21 percent of women 18 to 25 years old reported use within the last month. Braude et al. (1987) estimated that 5 to 15 percent of pregnant

women use or have used marijuana. Marijuana purportedly impairs DNA and RNA formation in laboratory animals (Nahas & Panon, 1976), but there have been no reports of infant health problems solely from maternal use of marijuana during lactation or pregnancy. However, anecdotal reports have cited marijuana-induced drowsiness in breastfeeding infants. Tetrahydrocannabinol, the active ingredient in marijuana, is readily absorbed from the GI tract and is metabolized by the baby (Perez & Wall, 1982). Marijuana cigarette sidestream smoke inhaled by the infant increases his exposure to the drug.

Thus the dilemma arises: should a woman be advised not to breastfeed if she refuses to give up her recreational use of marijuana? Obviously, smoking marijuana is not wise; the optimal situation is for the mother to be free of all drugs while breastfeeding. However, because there is little evidence that marijuana causes serious harm, it is probably better for the occasional marijuana user to continue to breastfeed rather than wean her baby. On the other hand, no infant should ever have to inhale passive smoke from marijuana or any cigarette, cigar, or pipe.

Cocaine

Cocaine use in the United States has dramatically increased in the last several years. More recently, a cheaper and more popular form of cocaine known as crack has emerged. Cocaine harms the fetus and the nursing infant. Because it is highly lipid-soluble and readily crosses biological membranes, its use by a breastfeeding mother can have serious effects.

Chasnoff, Lewis, and Squires (1987) reported a case in which a mother who was a cocaine user brought her two-week-old infant girl to a hospital emergency room. The baby was extremely irritable and was frequently startled by minimal stimulation. She also exhibited dilated pupils, vomiting, and tachycardia, all symptoms of cocaine intoxication. Intravenous fluids were started and breastfeeding was discontinued. Milk samples were negative for cocaine and its metabolites by 36 hours after the mother's last cocaine use. The infant's urine was negative by 60 hours after the last breastfeeding. The baby fully recovered and was discharged home with the parent under court supervision. Another infant reportedly developed apnea and seizures from direct ingestion of cocaine that her mother had used as a topical anesthetic for sore nipples (Chaney, Franke, & Wadlington, 1988). These reports are the basis for legal action on charges of child abuse against breastfeeding women who use cocaine.

The recommendation is clear: cocaine should never be used by the breastfeeding mother. Those who do so risk not only the health of their child but also legal action, which may result in the removal of the child from their custody.

Amphetamines

Amphetamines readily transfer into breastmilk; levels are three times higher than those in the mother's plasma. Despite these high levels, a case report (Steiner et al., 1984) of a mother taking high doses of amphetamines recounts that a nursing infant had no adverse effects and developed normally. A large study of more than 100 breastfeeding women taking amphetamines failed to detect any adverse changes in the behavior of their infants (Ayd, 1973).

Alcohol

Alcohol affects the central nervous system of both the breastfeeding mother and the infant. When taken in sufficient quantity it can inhibit milk ejection. Although "social" drinking is usually not considered a problem for breastfeeding women, a troubling study (Little et al., 1989) showed that the motor development of breastfed infants may be slower if their mothers frequently or regularly drink alcohol. Mennella and Beauchamp (1991) found that alcohol ingestion changed the flavor of the mother's milk in direct proportion to the timing of alcohol ingestion and the consequent breastfeeding episode. Additionally, they found that the baby's suck behavior changed, sucking more but obtaining less milk. In a later article, Mennella and Beauchamp (1993; see also Mennella, 1997) reported that milk odor was different when mothers ingested alcohol and that their babies ingested less milk, although they suckled for periods similar to those infants not exposed to alcohol through their mother's milk. They suggest that the babies may be reacting to the odor of the milk in addition to being directly affected by the alcohol they receive.

Lawton (1985) contended that alcohol, which appears quickly in both hindmilk and foremilk at levels equivalent to maternal serum levels, is quickly diluted by the baby's own body water. Thus occasional alcohol consumption by the mother may not represent a serious risk for her breastfeeding baby (Jason, 1991).

It is clear that alcohol ingestion decreases prolactin yield, blocks release of oxytocin and can result in a reduction in milk yield (Anderson, 1995). Unanswered is whether the infant sucks less effectively as well, thus contributing yet another reason for reduced maternal milk yield. The timing of alcohol ingestion also makes a difference, in that peak levels are reached within 30 to 60 minutes if the woman is drinking on an empty stomach and 60 to 90 minutes if she is drinking while also eating. Other factors such as maternal weight, menstrual cycle, and the age of the baby, will influence the potential effects of alcohol on the mother and her baby (Schulte, 1995). It is best if the breastfeeding woman avoids all alcohol ingestion during breastfeeding; Schulte recommends that if the breastfeeding mother insists on drinking, she should wait at least two hours for every drink consumed before putting the baby to breast.

Clinical Implications

Generally, if the mother has been detoxified and is narcotic-free, she should be encouraged to breastfeed. A woman on an average methadone maintenance dose will theoretically excrete only about 57 µg/day in her first five weeks, which is considered a trace amount not harmful to her infant (Beeley, 1986; Ostrea et al., 1978) and may minimize withdrawal symptoms to the infant.

According to Ostrea et al. (1978) when these mothers were under care and supervision, their children's mental and psychomotor development was within normal limits up to two years of age. Although the drug-dependent mother needs support and guidance, fears of the addicted mother's unstable lifestyle, potential for child abuse, and neglect have been overrated. Others disagree about this mother's ability to function and provide adequate care for her infant. Kantor (1978) considered the addicted mother a poor risk for parenting, even though she is receiving help. In the United States, it is becoming more common for grandmothers and others to take over parental care when addicted women voluntarily relinquish their children or are required by the court to do so.

The desire to mother and to breastfeed can be a powerful motivator to stay off drugs, at least for a while. It is not at all uncommon for a drug user to give up her drug habit during pregnancy and lactation; the experience of childbearing is a "high" in itself. For some, this is their one opportunity to "be normal," even if temporarily, and to give something of themselves. Williams (1990) interviewed women who had been addicted to heroin for more than 15 years. Children were central to the lives of these women. Several described how they had stopped drug use when they were pregnant but then resumed their habits after their children were born.

Environmental Contaminants

The great concern—perhaps the tragedy of our age—is the ever-increasing contamination of our planet. A global problem shared by all countries, industrial pollution of air and water respects no boundaries. The threat that a mother's milk may no longer be safe causes justifiable public alarm and outcry. The degree of environmental contamination has no feasible solution, even if unlimited funds were available.

Generally, older women, primiparas, and cigarette smokers have higher level of contaminants in their first lactation. The levels decline both with duration of breastfeeding and with the number of children breastfed (Hong et al., 1994). Although human milk appears to be a useful medium for monitoring organochlorine pesticides (Niessen et al., 1984; Stacey et al., 1985), there is little evidence that contaminants in human milk cause harm to the nursling. Further, although numerous toxins can enter breastmilk, the major contaminants are pesticides (DDT, DDE, chlordane, heptachlor), other organohalogen compounds (PCBs, PBBs, dioxin, benzofurans, benzene hexachloride), and radioactivity. Polybrominated biphenyls (PBBs) are chemical compounds similar to PCBs and DDT. Although PCBs are banned in the U.S., they will remain a problem for decades.

Laug, Kunze, and Prickett (1951) published a report on DDT levels in human milk exceeding that permitted by the WHO and the U.S. Code of Federal Regulations. The widespread use of DDT was halted in 1972 when its FDA registration was withdrawn. The first widespread alarm over breastmilk contamination occurred in 1973, when Michigan farm animals were contaminated with PBBs that were accidentally mixed with their feed. Breastfeeding mothers living on the contaminated Michigan farms were advised to wean their infants. Later, Rogan (1983) found no difference in the levels of PCBs in the milk of women exposed to PCBs and those not exposed to a given spill.

Dioxin is another name for a series of chemicals called *polychlorinated dibenzodioxins* (or PCDDs). Women exposed to these herbicides have high levels of the toxin during their first lactation but have lower levels with subsequent lactation. Overweight women have somewhat lower PCDD levels, whereas underweight women have slightly higher levels (Ahlborg et al., 1987).

Many women are exposed to mercury from food, amalgam fillings in their teeth, and other sources. Breastfed Swedish infants have one-half the tolerable daily intake for adults recommended by the WHO (Oskarsson et al., 1996). Yet this exposure does not appear to be harmful to breastfeeding babies. Mothers eating food contaminated with mercury have not been associated with toxicity in their breastfeeding infants, even though the infants had high serum levels of mercury (Amin-Zaki et al., 1974). A study of children in the Faeroe Islands of Denmark showed that breastfed children who were breastfed for a longer time reached developmental milestones earlier than did children who were breastfed for a shorter period, even though their mercury exposure was slightly higher (Grandjean et al., 1995).

The effect of nuclear pollution on breastmilk has been studied after the massive release of radioactivity at the Chernobyl nuclear power plant. Following the 1986 explosion at Chernobyl, radioactive fallout occurred throughout many areas of western Europe. Radioactive levels in cow's milk and in leafy vegetables were sufficiently high that these foods were banned for consumption by pregnant women and children. DeLallo et al. (1987) measured the [131]I (radioactive iodine) concentrations in human milk from women in two hospitals in Rome and from a milk bank in Rome for the first seven months after the explosion. Gori et al. (1988) examined samples of human placenta and human milk in Italy for one year after the accident to determine radioactive levels. Placental levels climbed rapidly. Although levels in human milk increased, the increase was much lower from the start, and it continued at a substantially slower rate. Radioactivity in human milk was about one-third the level found in placentas.

Shortly after the DeLallo report, Lindemann and Christensen (1987) reported their findings from Norway, Sweden, and Austria. In Sweden, identical amounts of [137]I were found in both cow's milk and human milk. In Austria, the amount in human milk was only one-tenth that found in cow's milk. In Norway, the total amount of radioactive cesium in cow's milk never exceeded 60 Bq/liter. The accepted upper limit of radioactive cesium in milk or baby food is 370 Bq/kg. Radioactive cesium has a biological half-life of 70 to 110 days. Because the amount in human milk was negligible, these investigators also concluded that "there was never any danger for the breast-fed infants. . . . If a similar accident should occur, the infants may safely be nursed but the mothers should take care and be advised when using local vegetables, meat, fish, and milk products" (Lindemann & Christensen, 1987). All of these reports document that radioactive levels rose much higher in cow's milk than in human milk, probably because of the bovine diet of plant foods. These authors concluded that the concentrations in human milk were low enough that they did not present a threat to the breastfeeding infant.

A massive release of radioactivity occurred in the United States during the mid-1940s. A nuclear weapons plant in Hanford, Washington, poured so much radioactive iodine into the air that children living nearby were exposed to massive and cumulative doses (Church, 1990). Presumably, infants in the area were being breastfed. No known studies were done on the milk of mothers in the area or on the breastfed children who are now adults; consequently, long-term outcomes related to breastfeeding are unknown. Table 6-4 lists the half-life of selected chemicals.

Although environmental pollution is of tremendous concern, there are few reports of either

Table 6–4	
HALF-LIFE OF CHEMICALS IN BREASTMILK	
Substance	**Half-Life**
Lead	13 weeks
Iodine	20 weeks
Nicotine	1.5 hours
PCBs	5–8 hours
Ethanol	3 hours

PCB = polychlorinated biphenyl.
Source: Adapted from M Wolff: Lactation. In: M Paul, ed., Occupational and environmental reproductive hazards: a guide for clinicians. *Baltimore: Williams & Wilkins, 1993:6.*

short- or long-term adverse effects on infants from pollutants in mother's milk. Is it possible, for instance, that higher levels of DDE are associated with shorter length of breastfeeding as Gladen and Rogan (1995) suggested? Earlier, Rogan (1990) projected that even under the worst conditions, breastfed children would lose only two days of life from exposure to such pollutants in human milk if they lived a normal life span. Moreover, even though they have received higher contaminant lead levels through human milk than have children who had been formula-fed, breastfed children score significantly high on mental and development tests over several time points (Rogan & Gladen, 1993).

The lead in breastmilk in the general population has declined, probably because less leaded gasoline is used (Wolff, 1993). The amount of lead in breastmilk is relatively stable over the breastfeeding period. If the infant consumes 700 ml of breastmilk per day, the result is a daily dose of 0.7 μg of lead, a low level of dietary lead intake as compared to the average total dietary lead intake of 5 μg/day (Wolff, 1983).

If the baby is weaned to formula or cow's milk, these foods also carry the risk of toxicity from lead or other contaminants. For example, concentrated formula that requires dilution reflects the lead or nitrate content of the water used. Formula mixed with water from a contaminated private well can cause severe illness (and perhaps death) in an infant. Eventually, the child eats the same foods as the rest of the family and is equally exposed to any contaminants. The risk of pollution exists for everyone, not just breastfeeding babies. Routine blood lead screening of breastfeeding mothers to determine infant risk is not necessary (Tellier & Aronson, 1994). The benefits of breastfeeding outweigh concerns about infant exposure to lead from breastmilk.

Although most lactating women are at minimal risk for contamination of their milk, there are exceptions, depending on where one lives and works. The risk is greater in an agricultural area where chemicals are sprayed, particularly by aerial spraying; in an industrial area where chemicals are used; or near contaminated water (e.g., the Great Lakes). German women living in both rural and urban areas have about the same dioxin residues in breastmilk, even though rural women are presumably exposed to higher levels of pesticides (Schlaud et al., 1995). Women can minimize their risk for pollutant contamination (Bartmess, 1988; Drijver et al., 1988; Stacey et al., 1985). Lactating women should take care to follow certain safeguards:

- Avoid freshwater fish from waters known to be contaminated.

- Wash and peel nonorganically grown vegetables and fruits thoroughly before eating.

- Eat low-fat foods and cut fat from meats.

- Avoid using pesticides in the home or on the lawn.

- Avoid a "crash" diet, thereby preventing the sudden release of toxins from body fat into breastmilk.

- Avoid contact with wood preservatives containing pentachlorophenol.

- Avoid fatty meat and fatty fish in the diet to minimize the amount of animal fat.

- Avoid buildings or homes treated with dieldrin for termites.

Even using lanolin as a nipple ointment is suspect, and only a medical grade of lanolin should be used, because pesticide residues in lanolin have been found in Australia and the United States (Copeland et al., 1989). A mother who is concerned about environmental contamination can contact the local Department of Health and the Environmental Protection Agency, Human Effects Monitoring Branch in the Office of Pesticide Programs, for information about a milk analysis (Lauwers & Woessner, 1990). Although analysis of the level of contaminants in breastmilk may be helpful, the results are of limited value unless the clinical history (including exposure events and chronic illness) justifies them. Another problem is unreliability of one-time results. A Norwegian study (Bakken & Seip, 1976) showed a dramatic variance of insecticide levels in the same mother's milk at different times. Although breastfeeding is still considered "safe," active efforts to diminish contaminants in our environment, and subsequently in human milk, must continue.

SUMMARY

The issue that pervades this chapter is the effect of drugs and contaminants on a mother's milk and on her baby. More drugs are used in the management of human illness and for recreational purposes than ever before. There is a dangerous tendency to believe that drugs are the answer to any problem. Perhaps this is a notion left over from times when infectious diseases were the major health problem—even though infectious diseases are reduced pri-

marily through public health measures such as improved sanitation. Many illnesses are self-limiting, causing only minor discomforts that subside with or without drugs. For example, a tense new mother taught to use progressive relaxation techniques or meditation avoids exposing her infant to a chemical tranquilizer. In some cases, maternal drug treatment can be delayed until after infants have weaned on their own. In essence, the question should not be, "Can this medicated mother be allowed to breastfeed?" but rather, "Does this mother really need to be medicated?"

The question of drugs and breastfeeding also depends on belief systems. If involved health professionals believe that breastfeeding is important, they will make every effort to find a safe way for a mother to continue breastfeeding. If they do not value it, they probably will not make the effort and will recommend that the mother wean. The same is true for breastfeeding during recreational drug use: some people believe that the lactating woman must make a clear choice between taking drugs or breastfeeding her baby; others prefer to weigh the risks and benefits of each situation.

More and more foreign substances in milk will continue to be found as analytical tools are improved. The problem now lies in evaluating this information and translating it into practical and safe action while respecting the wishes (and rights) of women who bear children and desire to breastfeed. Better surveillance systems are needed to alert us to potential problems before the child is exposed to drug or environmental toxins. Health care providers can help to reduce these risks by awareness that commercially prepared formula may contain similar amounts of contaminants, by staying current with new findings and by teaching parents methods for avoiding unnecessary exposure.

REFERENCES

Ahlborg GG, Waern F, Hakansson H: Interactive effects of PCDDs and PCDFs occurring in human mother's milk. *Chemosphere* 16:1701–6, 1987.

Altshuler LL: Breastfeeding and sertraline: a 24 hours analysis. *J Clin Psychiatry* 56:6, 1995.

Anderson PO: Alcohol and breastfeeding. *J Hum Lact* 11:321–3, 1995.

Anderson PO, Valdes V: Therapy consultation: increasing breast milk supply. *Clin Pharm* 12:479–50, 1993.

American Academy of Pediatrics, Committee on Drugs: The transfer of drugs and other chemicals into human milk. *Pediatrics* 84:924–36, 1994.

Amin-Zaki L, et al: Studies of infants postnatally exposed to methylmercury. *J Pediatr* 85:81–4, 1974.

Atkinson JC, Begg EJ: Prediction of drug distribution into human milk from physicochemical characteristics. *Clin Pharmacokin* 18:151–67, 1990.

Ayd FJ: Excretion of psychotropic drugs in human breast milk. *Int Drug Ther Newsl* 8:33–5, 1973.

Bailey B, Ito S: Breast-feeding and maternal drug use. *Pediat Clin North Am* 44:41–55, 1997.

Bakken AR, Seip M: Insecticides in human breast milk. *Acta Paediatr Scand* 65:535–9, 1976.

Bartmess JE: The risk of polychlorinated dibenzodioxins in human milk. *J Hum Lact* 4:105–7, 1988.

Beeley L: Drugs and breastfeeding. *Clin Obstet Gynecol* 13:24–51, 1986.

Berlin CM: The excretion of drugs and chemicals in human milk. In: SJ Yaffe: *Pediatric Pharmacology.* New York Grune & Stratton, 1980; 137–47.

Biddle C: When the breast-feeding mother faces surgery. *Contemp Nurse Pract.* (July/August), 15–20, 1995.

Bowes WA: The effect of medications on the lactating mother and her infant. *Clin Obstet Gynecol* 23:1073–9, 1980.

Braude MC, et al: Perinatal effects of drugs of abuse. *Fed Proc* 46:2446–53, 1987.

Budd SC, et al: Improved lactation with metoclopramide. *Clin Pediatr* 32:53–7, 1993.

Canterbury RJ, et al: Postpartum psychosis induced by bromocriptine. *South Med J* 80:1463–4, 1987.

Centers for Disease Control Guidelines: Parasitic skin infections. *MMWR* 34:915, 1985.

Chaney NE, Franke J, Wadlington WB: Cocaine convulsions in a breast-feeding baby. *J Pediatr* 112:134–5, 1988.

Chasnoff IJ, Lewis DE, Squires L: Cocaine intoxication in a breast-fed infant. *Pediatrics* 80:836–8, 1987.

Church GJ: There was death in the milk. *Time,* July 23, 1990, p 28.

Copeland C, Raebel MA, Wagner SL: Pesticide residue in lanolin [letter]. *JAMA* 261:242, 1989.

Croxato HB, et al: Fertility regulation in nursing women: IV. Long-term influence of a low-dose combined oral contraceptive initiated at day 30 postpartum upon lactation and infant growth. *Contraception* 27:27–37, 1983.

DeLallo E, et al: Radioactivity in breast milk in central Italy in the aftermath of Chernobyl [letter]. *Acta Paediatr Scand* 76:530–1, 1987.

Dickey RP, Stone SC: Drugs that affect the breast and lactation. *Clin Obstet Gynecol* 18:95–111, 1975.

Dillon AE, et al: Drug therapy in the nursing mother. *Obstet Gynecol Clin North Am* 24:675–96, 1997.

Drijver M, et al: Determinants of polychlorinated biphenyls (PCBs) in human milk. *Acta Paediatr Scand* 77:30–6, 1988.

Ehrenkranz TA, Ackerman BA: Metoclopramide effect on faltering milk production by mothers of premature infants. *Pediatrics* 78:614–20, 1986.

Ehrenkranz TA, et al: Nifedipine transfer into human milk. *J Pediatr* 114:478–80, 1989.

Ehudin-Pagano E, et al: The use of herbs in nurse-midwifery practice. *J Nurse Midwifery* 32:260–2, 1987.

Ellsworth A: Pharmacotherapy of hypertension while breastfeeding. *J Hum Lact* 10:121–4, 1994.

Erickson SH, Oppenheim GL, Smith GH: Metronidazole in breast milk. *Obstet Gynecol* 57:48–50, 1981.

Feldman S, Pickering LK: Pharmacokinetics of drugs in human milk. In: Howell RR, Morriss FH, Pickering LK, eds. *Human milk in infant nutrition and health.* Springfield, IL: Charles C. Thomas, 1986; 256–78.

Findlay JW, et al: Analgesic drugs in breast milk and plasma. *Clin Pharmacol Ther* 29:625–33, 1981.

Fleiss P: Herbal remedies for the breastfeeding mother. *Mothering* 48:68–70, 1988.

Giacoia GP, Catz CS: Drug therapy in the lactating mother. *Postgrad Med* 83:211–8, 1988.

Gladen BC, Rogan WJ: DDE and shortened duration of lactation in a northern Mexican town. *Am J Public Health* 85:504–8, 1995.

Gori G, et al: Radioactivity in breast milk and placentas during the year after Chernobyl. *Am J Obstet Gynecol* 159:1232–4, 1988.

Grandjean P, Weihe P, While RF: Milestone development in infants exposed to methylmercury from human milk. *Neurotoxicology* 16:27–34, 1995.

Gupta AP, Gupta PK: Metoclopramide as a lactogogue. *Clin Pediatr* 24:269–72, 1985.

Guzman V, et al: Improvement of defective lactation by using oral metoclopramide. *Acta Obstet Gynecol Scand* 58:53–5, 1979.

Halderman W: Can magnesium sulfate therapy impact lactogenesis? *J Hum Lact* 9:249–52, 1993.

Hale T: *Medications and mothers' milk.* Amarillo, TX: Pharmasoft Medical Publishing, 1997.

Hong CS, et al: Mono-Ortho- and non-ortho-substituted ploychlorinated biphenyls in human milk from Mohawk and control women: effects of maternal factors and previous lactation. *Arch Environ Contam Toxicol* 27:431–7, 1994.

Hopp L, Weiss AB, Iffy L: Acute myocardial infarction in a healthy mother using bromocriptine for milk suppression. *Can J Cardiol* 12:415–8, 1996.

Hunt MJ, et al: Black breast milk due to minocycline therapy. *Br J Dermatol* 134:943–4, 1996.

Ito S, et al: Initiation and duration of breast-feeding in women receiving antiepileptics. *Obstet Gynecol* 172:881–6, 1995.

Ito S, et al: Prospective follow-up of adverse reactions in breast-fed infants exposed to maternal medication. *Am J Obstet Gynecol* 168:1293–9, 1993.

Jason J: Breast-feeding in 1991 [editorial]. *N Engl J Med* 325:1036–7, 1991.

Johnson EM: Substance abuse and women's health. *Public Health Rep* (suppl) 101:42–48, 1987.

Jolivet A, et al: Effect of ergot alkaloid derivatives on milk secretion in the immediate postpartum period. *J Gynecol Obstet Biol Reprod* (Paris) 1:129–34, 1978.

Kader A, et al: Biochemical and experimental studies on lactation: III. Clinical changes induced in human milk by gestagens. *Am J Obstet Gynecol* 105:978–85, 1969.

Kantor GK: Addicted mother, addicted baby: a challenge to health care providers. *MCN* 3:281–4, 1978.

Kaunitz AM: A new contraception option. *Contemp Obstet Gynecol* 38:19–34, 1993.

Kauppila A, et al: A dose response relation between improved lactation and metoclopramide. *Lancet* 1(8231):1175–7, 1983.

Koetsawang S, Bhiraleus P, Chiemprajert T: Effects of oral contraceptives on lactation. *Fertil Steril* 23:24–8, 1972.

Koren G, et al: Maternal ginseng use associated with neonatal androgenization [letter]. *JAMA* 264:1866, 1990.

Laug EP, Kunze FMN, Prickett CS: Occurrence of DDT in human fat and milk. *Arch Ind Hyg* 3:245–6, 1951.

Lauwers J, Woessner C: *Chemical agents and breast milk.* Garden City Park, NY: Avery Publishing Group, 1990: 3–6.

Lawrence R: *Breastfeeding: a guide for the medical profession.* St. Louis: Mosby, 1994.

Lawton ME: Alcohol in breast milk. *Aust NZ J Obstet Gynecol* 25:71–3, 1985.

Lester BM, et al: Possible association between fluoxetine hydrochloride and colic in an infant.. *J Am Acad Child Adolesc Psychiatry* 32:1253–5, 1993.

Lindemann R, Christensen. GC: Radioactivity in breastmilk after the Chernobyl accident [letter]. *Acta Paediatr Scand* 76:981–2, 1987.

Lipkin GB: Drug therapy in maternal care. In: Spencer RT, et al, eds. *Clinical pharmacology and nursing management.* (3rd ed.). Philadelphia: Lippincott, 1989: 1132–70.

Little RE, et al: Maternal alcohol use during breastfeeding and infant mental and motor development at one year. *N Engl J Med* 321:425–30, 1989.

Lucas BD, et al: Terfenadine pharmacokinetics in breast milk in lactating women. *Clin Pharmacol Ther* 57:398–402, 1995.

Maddern G: Galactorhoea due to domperidone. *Med J Aust* 2:539–40, 1983.

McCann MF, Potter LS: Progestin-only oral contraception: a comprehensive review. *Contraception* 50(suppl 1):S140–8, 1994.

Mennella, JA: Infants' suckling responses to the flavor of alcohol in mothers' milk. *Alcohol Clin Exp Res* 21:581–55, 1997.

Mennella JA, Beauchamp GK: The transfer of alcohol to human milk: effects on flavor and the infant's behavior. *N Engl J Med* 325:981–5, 1991.

Mennella JA, Beauchamp GK: Beer, breast feeding and folklore. *Dev Psychobiol* 26:459–66, 1993.

Miczak M: Herbs and healthy lactation. *Mothering* 78:60–3, 1996.

Miller MR, et al: Verapamil and breast-feeding. *Eur J Clin Pharmacol* 30:125–6, 1986.

Miller GH, Hughes LR: Lactation and genital involution effects of a new low-dose oral contraceptive on breastfeeding mothers and their infants. *Obstet Gynecol* 35:44–50, 1970.

Milsom SR, et al: Growth hormone stimulates galactopoiesis in healthy lactating women. *Acta Endocrinol* 127:337–43, 1992.

Misri S, Sivertz K: Tricyclic drugs in pregnancy and lactation: a preliminary report. *Int J Psychiatry Med* 21:157–71, 1991.

Morin AK, Stoukides CA: Scabicides and pediculocides and breastfeeding. *J Hum Lact* 10:267–68, 1994.

Nahas G, Panon W, eds: *Marihuana: chemistry, biochemistry, and cellular effect.* New York: Springer-Verlag, 1976.

National Institute on Drug Abuse: *Drug abuse statistics 1985 population estimates.* Washington DC: Alcohol, Drug Abuse, and Mental Health, United States Public Health Service, 1986.

Niessen KH, et al: Chlorinated hydrocarbons in adipose tissue of infants and toddlers: inventory and studies on their association with intake of mothers' milk. *Eur J Pediatr* 142:238–43, 1984.

Nilsson S, et al: Long-term follow-up of children breast-fed by mothers using oral contraceptives. *Contraception* 34:443–57, 1986.

Oskarsson A, et al: Total and inorganic mercury in breast milk and blood in relation to fish consumption and amalgam fillings in lactating women. *Arch Environ Health* 51:234–41, 1996

Ostrea EM, Chavez DJ, Stryker JC: *The care of the drug dependent woman and her infant.* Lansing, MI: Michigan Department of Public Health, 1978.

Peralta O, et al: Fertility regulation in nursing women: V. Long-term influence of a low-dose combined oral contraceptive initiated at day 90 postpartum upon lactation and infant growth. *Contraception* 27:27–37, 1983.

Perez RM, Wall ME: Presence of D-9-tetrahydrocannabinol in human milk. *N Engl J Med* 307:819–20, 1982.

Peters F, Schulze-Tollert J, Schuth W: Thyrotropin-releasing hormone–a lactation-promoting agent? *Br J Obstet Gynaecol* 98:880–5, 1991.

Peterson RG, Bowes WA: Drugs, toxins and environmental agents in breast milk. In: Neville MC, and Neifert M, eds. *Physiology, nutrition and breastfeeding.* New York: Plenum, 1983, 367–403.

Pon G, Ray E, Matheson I: Excretion of psychoactive drugs into breast milk. *Clin Pharmacol Ther* 27:270–89, 1994.

Postpartum hypertension, seizures, strokes reported with bromocriptime. *FDA Bull* 14:3, 1982.

Riordan J: Drugs in breastmilk. In: Pagliaro LA, Pagliaro AM, eds: *Problems in pediatric drug therapy.* Hamilton, IL: Drug Intelligence Publishers, 1987: 194–258.

Riordan J, Riordan M: Drugs in breastmilk: Is the risk exaggerated? *Am J Nurs* 84:328–32, 1984.

Rivera-Calimlim L: The significance of drugs in breast milk. *Clin Perinatal* 14:51–70, 1987.

Roberts KL: A comparison of chilled cabbage leaves and chilled gelpaks in reducing breast engorgement. *J Hum Lact* 11:17–20, 1995.

Roberts RJ: *Drug therapy in infants.* Philadelphia: Saunders, 1984: 346–83.

Roberts RJ: Drugs and breastfeeding: an overview. Presentation at La Leche League International, Seminar for Physicians, Boston, July 12–13, 1990.

Rogan W: Should the presence of carcinogens in breastmilk discourage breastfeeding? Presentation at International Society for Research on Human Milk and Lactation. 1990, Ambulatory Pediatric Association Annual Meeting, Anaheim, CA, 1990.

Rogan WJ: Chromatographic evidence of polychlorinated biphenyl exposure from a spill. *JAMA* 249:1057–8, 1983.

Rogan WJ, Gladen BC: Breast-feeding and cognitive development. *Early Hum Dev* 31:181–93, 1993.

Rosier W: Cool cabbage compresses. *Breastfeed Rev* 11:28–31, 1988.

Rosti L, et al: Toxic effects of a herbal tea mixture in two newborns. *Acta Paediat* 83:683–5, 1994.

Ryu JE: Effect of maternal caffeine consumption on heart rate and sleep time of breast-fed infants. *Dev Pharmacol Ther* 8:355–63, 1985.

Schlaud M, et al: Organochlorine residues in human breast mik: analysis through a sentinel practice network. *J Epidemiol Comm Health* 49(suppl 1):17–21, 1995.

Schou M: Lithium treatment during pregnancy, delivery, and lactation: an update. *J Clin Psychiatry* 51(10):410–3, 1990.

Schulte P: Minimizing alcohol exposure to the breastfeeding infant. *J Hum Lact* 11:317–9, 1995.

Sharma S, et al: Randomized controlled trial of *Asparagus racemosus* (Shatavari) as a lactogogue in lactational inadequacy. *Ind Pediatr* 33:675–7, 1996.

Shrivastav P, et al: Suppression of puerperal lactation using jasmine flowers. *Aust NZ Obstet Gynaecol* 28:68–71, 1988.

Smolek-Houghton M: My milk connoisseur. *La Leche League News* 26:50, 1984.

Sousa PLR: Metoclopramide and breast-feeding. *Br Med J* 1:512, 1975.

Stacey CI, Perriman WS, and Whitney S: Organochlorine pesticide residue levels in human milk, Western Australia, 1979–1980. *Arch Environ Health* 40:102–8, 1985.

Steiner E, et al: Amphetamine secretion in breast milk. *Eur J Clin Pharmacol* 27:123–4, 1984.

Tellier L, Aronson RA: Lead in breast milk: should mothers be routinely screened? *Wisc Med J* 93: 257–8, 1994.

Thorley V: Letter to the editor. *Breastfeed Rev* 4:82, 1996.

Townsend RJ, et al: Excretion of ibuprofen into breast milk. *Am J Obstet Gynecol* 149:184–6, 1984.

Tyree DJ: Perinatal medications and breastfeeding. *J Hum Lact* 8:87–90, 1992.

Visness CM, Rivera R: Progestin-only pill use and pill switching during breastfeeding. *Contraception* 51:279–81, 1995.

Vorherr H: Human lactation and breastfeeding. In: Larson BL, ed. *Lactation: a comprehensive treatise.* vol 4. New York: Academic, 1978:181–279.

Watson DL, et al: Bromocriptine mesylate for lactation suppression: a risk for postpartum hypertension? *Obstet Gynecol* 74:573–6, 1989.

Williams AB: Reproductive concerns of women at risk for HIV infection. *J Nurse Midwifery* 35:292–8, 1990.

Wilson J: Drugs in breast milk. Balgowlah, South Australia: ADIS Press, 1981.

Wischnik A, Manth SM, Lloyd J: The excretion of ketorolac tromethamine into breastmilk after multiple oral dosing. *Eur J Clin Pharmacol* 36:521–4, 1989.

Wisner KL, Perel JM, Findling RL: Antidepressant treatment during breast-feeding. *Am J Psychiatry* 153:1132–6, 1996.

Wisner KL, Perel JM, Folgia JP: Serum clomipramine and metabolite levels in four nursing mother-infant pairs. *J Clin Psychiatry* 56:17–20, 1995.

Wojnar-Horton RE, et al: Distribution and excretion of sumatriptan in human milk. *Br J Clin Pharmacol* 41:217, 1996.

Wolff M: Lactation. In: Paul M, ed. *Occupational and environmental reproductive hazards: a guide for clinicians.* Baltimore: Williams & Wilkins, 1993: 60–75.

Wolff M: Occupationally derived chemicals in breast milk. *Am J Industr Med* 4:259–81, 1983.

World Health Organization Task Force for Epidemiological Research on Reproductive Health. Progestogen-only contraceptives during lactation: I. Infant growth. *Contraception* 50:35–53, 1994a.

World Health Organization Task Force for Epidemiological Research on Reproductive Health. Progestogen-only contraceptives during lactation: II. Infant development. *Contraception* 50:55–68, 1994b.

Wright NE: Use of Reglan (metoclopramide) to increase maternal milk supply. *Med Assoc Newsl* 10:2–7, 1995.

Yurchak AM, Jusko WJ: Theophylline secretion into breast milk. *Pediatrics* 57:518–20, 1976.

APPENDIX 6-A

The Transfer of Drugs and Other Chemicals into Human Milk

American Academy of Pediatrics
Committee on Drugs

This statement was first published in 1983,[1] with a revision published in 1989.[2] Information about the transfer of drugs and chemicals into human milk continues to become available. This current statement is intended to revise the lists of agents transferred into human milk and describe their possible effects on the infant or on lactation, if known (Tables 6A–1 through 6A–7). The fact that a pharmacologic or chemical agent does not appear on the lists is not meant to imply that it is not transferred into human milk or that it does not have an effect on the infant; it only indicates that there were no reports found in the literature. These tables should assist the physician in counseling a nursing mother regarding breast-feeding when the mother has a condition for which a drug is medically indicated.

The following question and options should be considered when prescribing drug therapy to lactating women. (1) Is the drug therapy really necessary? Consultation between the pediatrician and the mother's physician can be most useful. (2) Use the safest drug, for example, acetaminophen rather than aspirin for analgesia. (3) If there is a possibility that a drug may present a risk to the infant, consideration should be given to measurement of blood concentrations in the nursing infant. (4) Drug exposure to the nursing infant may be minimized by having the mother take the medication just after she has breast-fed the infant and/or just

before the infant is due to have a lengthy sleep period.

Data have been obtained from a search of the medical literature. Because methodologies used to quantitate drugs in milk continue to improve, this current information will require continuous updating. Drugs cited in Tables 6A–1 through 6A–7 are listed in alphabetical order by generic name; brand names are listed in Tables 6A–8 and 6A–9 in accordance with the current *Physicians Desk Reference, AMA Drug Evaluation,* and the *USAN and the USP Dictionary of Drug Names.* The reference list is not inclusive of all articles published.

Physicians who encounter adverse effects in infants fed drug-contaminated human milk are urged to document these effects in a communication to the American Academy of Pediatrics Committee on Drugs and to the Food and Drug Administration. This communication should include the generic and brand name of the drug, the maternal dose and mode of administration, the concentration of the drug in milk and maternal and infant blood in relation to the time of ingestion, the method used for laboratory identification, the age of the infant, and the adverse effect. Such reports may significantly increase the pediatric community's fund of knowledge regarding drug transfer into human milk and the potential or actual risk to the infant.

Acknowledgment

The Committee would like to thank Linda Watson for her work in reference identification, document retrieval, and manuscript preparation.

COMMITTEE ON DRUGS, 1992 TO 1993
Ralph E. Kauffman, MD, PhD, Chairperson
William Banner, Jr, MD, PhD
Cheston M. Berlin, Jr, MD
Jeffrey L. Blumer, MD, PhD
Richard L. Gorman, MD
George H. Lambert, MD
Geraldine S. Wilson, MD

LIAISON REPRESENTATIVES
Donald R. Bennett, MD, PhD, American Medical
    Association

Jose F. Cordero, MD, MPH, Centers for Disease
Control and Prevention
Paul Kaufman, MD, Pharmaceutical
Manufacturers' Association
Sam A. Licata, MD, National Health and Welfare,
Health Protection Branch, Canada
Paul Tomich, MD, American College of
Obstetricians and Gynecologists
Gloria Troendle, MD, Food and Drug
Administration

Sumner J. Yaffe, MD, National Institute of Child
Health and Human Development, National
Institutes of Health
AAP Section Liaison
Charles J. Coté, MD, Section on Anesthesiology

CONSULTANT
Anthony R. Temple, MD

Table 6A-1

DRUGS THAT ARE CONTRAINDICATED DURING BREAST-FEEDING

Drug	Reason for Concern, Reported Sign or Symptom in Infant, or Effect on Lactation	Reference No.
Bromocriptine	Suppresses lactation; may be hazardous to the mother	3, 4
Cocaine	Cocaine intoxication	5
Cyclophosphamide	Possible immune suppression; unknown effect on growth or association with carcinogenesis; neutropenia	6, 7
Cyclosporine	Possible immune suppression; unknown effect on growth or association with carcinogenesis	8
Doxorubicin*	Possible immune suppression; unknown effect on growth or association with carcinogenesis	9
Ergotamine	Vomiting, diarrhea, convulsions (doses used in migraine medications)	10
Lithium	One-third to one-half therapeutic blood concentration in infants	11–13
Methotrexate	Possible immune suppression; unknown effect on growth or association with carcinogenesis; neutropenia	14
Phencyclidine (PCP)	Potent hallucinogen	15
Phenindione	Anticoagulant; increased prothrombin and partial thromboplastin time in one infant; not used in United States	16

Drug is concentrated in human milk.

Table 6A-2

DRUGS OF ABUSE: CONTRAINDICATED DURING BREAST-FEEDING*

Drug Reference	Reported Effect or Reasons for Concern	Reference No.
Amphetamine[†]	Irritability, poor sleeping pattern	17
Cocaine	Cocaine intoxication	5
Heroin	Tremors, restlessness, vomiting, poor feeding	18
Marijuana	Only one report in literature; no effect mentioned	19
Nicotine (smoking)	Shock, vomiting, diarrhea, rapid heart rate, restlessness; decreased milk production	20–26
Phencyclidine	Potent hallucination	15

* The Committee on Drugs strongly believes that nursing mothers should not ingest any compounds listed in Table 6A–2. Not only are they hazardous to the nursing infant, but they are also detrimental to the physical and emotional health of the mother. This list is obviously not complete; no drug of abuse should be ingested by nursing mothers even though adverse reports are not in the literature.
† Drug is concentrated in human milk.

Table 6A-3

RADIOACTIVE COMPOUNDS THAT REQUIRE TEMPORARY CESSATION OF BREAST-FEEDING*

Drug	Recommended Time for Cessation of Breast-Feeding	Reference No.
Copper 64 (^{64}Cu)	Radioactivity in milk present at 50 h	27
Gallium 67 (^{67}GA)	Radioactivity in milk present for 2 wk	28
Indium 111 (^{111}In)	Very small amount present at 20 h	29
Iodine 123 (^{123}I)	Radioactivity in milk present up to 36 h	30
Iodine 125 (^{125}I)	Radioactivity in milk present for 12 d	31
Iodine 131 (^{131}I)	Radioactivity in milk present 2–14 d, depending on study	32–35
Radioactive sodium	Radioactivity in milk present 96 h	36
Technetium-99m (^{99m}Tc), ^{99m}Rc macroaggregates, ^{99m}TC O4	Radioactivity in milk present 15 h to 3 d	37–42

*Consult nuclear medicine physician before performing diagnostic study so that radionuclide that has shortest excretion time in breast milk can be used. Before study, the mother should pump her breast and store enough milk in freezer for feeding the infant; after study, the mother should pump her breast to maintain milk production but discard all milk pumped for the required time that radioactivity is present in milk. Milk samples can be screened by radiology departments for radioactivity before resumption of nursing.

Table 6A-4

Drugs Whose Effect on Nursing Infants Is Unknown but May Be of Concern

Psychotropic drugs, the compounds listed under antianxiety, antidepressant, and antipsychotic categories, are of special concern when given to nursing mothers for long periods. Although there are no case reports of adverse effects in breast-feeding infants, these drugs do appear in human milk and thus could conceivably alter short-term and long-term central nervous system function.[43]

Drug	Reported or Possible Effect	Reference No.
Antianxiety		
Diazepam	None	44–46
Lorazepam	None	47
Midazolam	. . .	48
Perphenazine	None	49
Prazepam*	None	50
Quazepam	None	51
Temazepam	. . .	52
Antidepressants		
Amitriptyline	None	53, 54
Amoxapine	None	55
Desipramine	None	56, 57
Dothiepin	None	58, 59
Doxepin	None	60
Fluoxetine	. . .	61
Fluvoxamine	. . .	62
Imipramine	None	56
Trazodone	None	63
Antipsychotic		
Chlorpromazine	Galactorrhea in adult; drowsiness and lethargy in infant	64, 65
Chlorprothixene	None	66
Haloperidol	None	67, 68
Mesoridazine	None	69
Chloramphenicol	Possible idiosyncratic bone marrow suppression	70, 71
Metoclopramide*	None described; dopaminergic blocking agent	72, 73
Metronidazole	In vitro mutagen; may discontinue breast-feeding 12–24 h to allow excretion of dose when single-dose therapy given to mother	74, 75
Tinidazole	See metronidazole	76

* Drug is concentrated in human milk.

Table 6A-5

DRUGS THAT HAVE BEEN ASSOCIATED WITH SIGNIFICANT EFFECTS ON SOME NURSING INFANTS AND SHOULD BE GIVEN TO NURSING MOTHERS WITH CAUTION*

Drug	Reported Effect	Reference No.
5-Aminosalicylic acid	Diarrhea (1 case)	77, 78
Aspirin (salicylates)	Metabolic acidosis (1 case)	79–81
Clemastine	Drowsiness, irritability, refusal to feed, high-pitched cry, neck stiffness (1 case)	82
Phenobarbital	Sedation; infantile spasms after weaning from milk containing phenobarbital, methemoglobinemia (1 case)	83–87
Primidone	Sedation, feeding problems	83, 84
Sulfasalazine (salicylazosulfapyridine)	Bloody diarrhea (1 case)	88

Measure blood concentration in the infant when possible.

Table 6A-6

MATERNAL MEDICATIONS USUALLY COMPATIBLE WITH BREAST-FEEDING*

Drug	Reported Sign or Symptom in Infant or Effect on Lactation	Reference No.
Acebutolol	None	89
Acetaminophen	None	90–92
Acetazolamide	None	93
Acitretin	. . .	94
Acyclovir†	None	95, 96
Alcohol (ethanol)	With large amounts drowsiness, diaphoresis, deep sleep, weakness, decrease in linear growth, abnormal weight gain; maternal ingestion of 1 g/kg daily decreases milk ejection reflex	20, 97–100
Allopurinol	. . .	101

Table 6A-6

Amoxicillin	None	102
Antimony	. . .	103
Atenolol	None	104–106
Atropine	None	107
Azapropazone (apazone)	. . .	108
Aztreonam	None	109
B_1 (thiamin)	None	110
B_6 (pyridoxine)	None	111–113
B_{12}	None	114
Baclofen	None	115
Barbiturate	See Table 6A–5	
Bendroflumethiazide	Suppresses lactation	116
Bishydroxycoumarin (dicumarol)	None	117
Bromide	Rash, weakness, absence of cry with maternal intake of 5.4 g/d	118
Butorphanol	None	119
Caffeine	Irritability, poor sleeping pattern, excreted slowly; no effect with usual amount of caffeine beverages	120–125
Captopril	None	126
Carbamazepine	None	127, 128
Carbimazole	Goiter	129, 130
Cascara	None	131
Cefadroxil	None	102
Cefazolin	None	132
Cefotaxime	None	133
Cefoxitin	None	133
Cefprozil	. . .	134
Ceftazidime	None	135
Ceftriaxone	None	136
Chloral hydrate	Sleepiness	137
Chloroform	None	138
Chloroquine	None	139–141
Chlorothiazide	None	142–143
Chlorthalidone	Excreted slowly	144
Cimetidine[†]	None	145

Table 6A-6 (cont.)

Agent	Reported Sign or Symptom in Infant or Effect on Lactation	Reference No.
Cisapride	None	146
Cisplatin	Not found in milk	9
Clindamycin	None	147
Clogestone	None	148
Clomipramine	. . .	149
Codeine	None	92, 107
Colchicine	. . .	15
Contraceptive pill with estrogen/progesterone	Rare breast enlargement; decrease in milk production and protein content (not confirmed in several studies)	151–158
Cycloserine	None	159
D (vitamin)	None; follow up infant's serum calcium level if mother receives pharmacological doses	160–162
Danthron	Increased bowel activity	163
Dapsone	None; sulfonamide detected in infant's urine	141, 164
Dexbrompheniramine maleate with *d*-isoephedrine	Crying, poor sleeping patterns, irritability	165
Digoxin	None	166, 167
Diltiazem	None	168
Dipyrone	None	169
Disopyramide	None	170–171
Domperidone	None	172
Dyphylline†	None	173
Enalapril	. . .	174
Erythromycin†	None	175
Estradiol	Withdrawal, vaginal bleeding	176
Ethambutol	None	159
Ethanol (cf. alcohol)	. . .	
Ethosuximide	None, drug appears in infant serum	127, 177
Fentanyl	. . .	178
Flecainide	. . .	179, 180
Flufenamic acid	None	181
Fluorescein	. . .	182
Folic acid	None	183

Table 6A-6

Gold salts	None	184–188
Halothane	None	189
Hydralazine	None	190
Hydrochlorothiazide	. . .	142, 143
Hydroxychloroquine[†]	None	191, 192
Ibuprofen	None	193, 194
Indomethacin	Seizure (1 case)	195–197
Iodides	May affect thyroid activity; see miscellaneous iodine	198
Iodine (providone-iodine/ vaginal douche)	Elevated iodine levels in breast milk, odor of iodine on infant's skin	198
Iodine	Goiter; see miscellaneous, iodine	198
Iopanoic acid	None	199
Isoniazid	None; acetyl metabolite also secreted; hepatotoxic	159, 200
K_1 (vitamin)	None	201, 202
Kanamycin	None	159
Ketorolac	. . .	203
Labetalol	None	204, 205
Levonorgestrel	. . .	206–209
Lidocaine	None	210
Loperamide	. . .	211
Magnesium sulfate	None	212
Medroxyprogesterone	None	148
Mefenamic acid	None	213
Methadone	None if mother receiving ≤ 20 mg/24 h	214, 215
Methimazole (active metabolite of carbimazole)	None	216
Methocarbamol	None	217
Methyldopa	None	218
Methyprylon	Drowsiness	219
Metoprolol[†]	None	104
Metrizamide	None	220
Mexiletine	None	221
Minoxidil	None	222
Morphine	None; infant may have significant blood concentration	223, 224
Moxalactam	None	225

Table 6A-6 *(cont.)*

Agent	Reported Sign or Symptom in Infant or Effect on Lactation	Reference No.
Nadolol [†]	None	226
Nalidixic acid	Hemolysis in infant with glucose-6-phosphate dehydrogenase (G-6-PD) deficiency	227
Naproxen	. . .	228
Nefopam	None	229
Nifedipine	. . .	230
Nitrofurantoin	Hemolysis in infant with G-6-PD deficiency	231
Norethynodrel	None	232
Norsteroids	None	233
Noscapine	None	234
Oxprenolol	None	235, 236
Phenylbutazone	None	237
Phenytoin	Methemoglobinemia (1 case)	85, 127, 238
Piroxicam	None	239
Prednisone	None	241
Procainamide	None	242
Progesterone	None	243
Propoxyphene	None	244
Propranolol	None	245–247
Propylthiouracil	None	248
Pseudoephedrine [†]	None	249
Pyridostigmine	None	250
Pyrimethamine	None	141, 251
Quinidine	None	252
Quinine	None	223
Riboflavin	None	110
Rifampin	None	159
Scopolamine	. . .	107
Secobarbital	None	253
Senna	None	254
Sotalol	. . .	180, 255
Spironolactone	None	256
Streptomycin	None	159
Sulbactam	None	257

Table 6A-6

Sulfapyridine	Caution in infant with jaundice or G-6-PD deficiency, and ill, stressed, or premature infant; appears in infant's milk	258, 259
Sulfisoxazole	Caution in infant with jaundice or G-6-PD deficiency, and ill, stressed, or premature infant; appears in infant's milk	260
Suprofen	None	261
Terbutaline	None	262
Tetracycline	None; negligible absorption by infant	263, 264
Theophylline	Irritability	120, 265
Thiopental	None	86, 266
Thiouracil	None mentioned; drug not used in United States	267
Ticarcillin	None	268
Timolol	None	236
Tolbutamide	Possible jaundice	269
Tolmetin	None	270
Trimethoprim/sulfamethoxazole	None	271, 272
Triprolidine	None	249
Valproic acid	None	127, 273, 274
Verapamil	None	275
Warfarin	None	276
Zolpidem	None	277

*Drugs listed have been reported in the literature as having the effects listed or no effect. The word "none" means that no observable change was seen in the nursing infant while the mother was ingesting the compound. It is emphasized that most of the literature citations concern single case reports or small series of infants.

†Drug is concentrated in human milk.

Table 6A-7

FOOD AND ENVIRONMENTAL AGENTS: EFFECTS ON BREAST-FEEDING

Agent	Reported Sign or Symptom in Infant or Effect on Lactation	Reference No.
Aflatoxin	None	278–280
Aspartame	Caution if mother or infant has phenylketonuria	281
Bromide (photographic laboratory)	Potential absorption and bromide transfer into milk; see Table 6A–6	282
Cadmium	None reported	283
Chlordane	None reported	284
Chocolate (theobromine)	Irritability or increased bowel activity if excess amounts (16 oz/d) consumed by mother	120, 285
DDT, benzenehexachlorides, dieldrin, aldrin, hepatachlorepoxide	None	286–293
Fava beans	Hemolysis in patient with glucose-6-phosphate dehydrogenase (G-6-PD) deficiency	294
Fluorides	None	295, 296
Hexachlorobenzene	Skin rash, diarrhea, vomiting, dark urine, neurotoxicity, death	297, 298
Hexachlorophene	None, possible contamination of milk from nipple washing	299
Lead	Possible neurotoxicity	300–301
Methyl mercury, mercury	May affect neurodevelopment	302–304
Monosodium glutamate	None	305
Polychlorinated biphenyls and polybrominated biphenyls	Lack of endurance, hypotonia, sullen expressionless facies	306–310
Tetrachlorethylene-cleaning fluid (perchloroethylene)	Obstructive jaundice, dark urine	311
Vegetarian diet	Signs of B_{12} deficiency	312

Table 6A-8

GENERIC DRUGS AND CORRESPONDING TRADE NAMES*†

Generic	Trade	Generic	Trade
acebutolol	Sectral	cefazolin	Ancef, Kefzol
acetaminophen	Tylenol, Anacin-3, Panadol, Tempra, Phenaphen	cefotaxime	Claforan
		cefprozil	Cefzil
		ceftazidime	Fortaz
acetazolamide	Diamox	ceftriaxone	Rocephin
acitretin	Soriatane	chloramphenicol	Chloromycetin
acyclovir	Zovirax	chloroquine	Aralen
allopurinol	Zyloprim	chlorothiazide	Diuril, Chlotride (foreign)
aminosalicylic acid	Rowasa	chlorpromazine	Thorazine
amitriptyline	Elavil, Endep	chlorprothixene	Taractan
amoxapine	Asendin	chlorthalidone	Hygroton, as Combipres
amoxicillin	Amoxil	cimetidine	Tagamet
amphetamine (dextroamphetamine)	Dexedrine	cisapride	Benzamide (foreign)
		cisplatin	Platinol
aspartame	NutraSweet	clemastine	Tavegil (foreign), Tavist
atenolol	Tenormin	clindamycin	Cleocin
azapropazone (apazone)	Not available in United States	clomipramine	Anafranil
		colchicine	(generic only)
aztreonam	Azactam	cyclophosphamide	Cytoxan
baclofen	Lioresal	cycloserine	Seromycin
bendroflumethiazide	Naturetin	danthron	Dorbane, Istizin
bishydroxycoumarin	Dicumarol	dapsone	(generic only)
bromocriptine	Parlodel	desipramine	Norpramin, Pertofrane
butorphanol	Stadol	dexbrompheniramine maleate with *d*-isoephedrine	as Disophrol, as Drixoral
captopril	Capoten		
carbamazepine	Tegretol		
carbimazole	Neo-mercazole (foreign)	dextroamphetamine	Dexedrine
cefadroxil	Duricef	diazepam	Valium

* *For convenience, one or more examples of the trade name are given.*

† *Inclusion of drug names in Table 6A–8 does not constitute an endorsement by the American Academy of Pediatrics of the products listed. Names are included for informational purposes only.*

Table 6A-8 *(cont.)*

Generic	Trade	Generic	Trade
digoxin	Lanoxin, Lanoxicaps	ketorolac	Toradol
diltiazem	Cardizem	labetalol	Normodyne, Trandate
dipyrone	Diprofarn, Novaldin (unavailable in United States)	levonorgestrel	as Levlen, as Nordette, as Norplant, as Tri-Levlen, as Triphasil
disopyramide	Norpace	lidocaine	Xylocaine
domperidone	Motilium (unavailable in United States)	loperamide	Imodium
		lorazepam	Ativan
dothiepin	Prothiaden (unavailable in United States)	medroxyprogesterone	Provera, Depo-Provera
		mefenamic acid	Ponstel
doxepin	Sinequan	mesoridazine	Serentil
doxorubicin	Adriamycin	methadone	Dolophine
dyphylline	Dilor	methimazole	Tapazole
enalapril	Vasotec	methocarbamol	Robaxin
ergotamine tartrate with caffeine	as Cafergot	methotrexate (amethopterin)	Folex, Rheumatrex
estradiol	Estrace	methyprylon	Noludar
ethambutol	Myambutol	metoclopramide	Reglan
ethosuximide	Zarontin	metoprolol	Lopressor
fentanyl	Sublimaze	metrizamide	Amipaque
flecainide	Tambocor	metronidazole	Flagyl, Protostat
flufenamic acid	Arlef (foreign)	mexiletine	Mexitil
fluoxetine	Prozac	midazolam	Versed
fluvoxamine	. . .	minoxidil	Loniten, Rogaine
gold sodium thiomalate	Myochrysine	monosodium glutamate	MSG, Accent
haloperidol	Haldol	moxalactam	Moxam
hydralazine	Apresoline	nadolol	Corgard
hydrochlorothiazide	HydroDIURIL	nalidixic acid	NegGram
hydroxychloroquine	Plaquenil	naproxen	Naprosyn
ibuprofen	Advil, Motrin	nefopam	Acupan (unavailable in the United States)
imipramine	Tofranil, Janimine		
indomethacin	Indocin	nifedipine	Procardia
iopanoic acid	Telepaque	nitrofurantoin	Furadantin, Macrodantin
isoniazid	INH		
kanamycin	Kantrex	[3H]norethynodrel	as Enovid

Table 6A-8

Generic	Trade	Generic	Trade
noscapine	Tusscapine	sulbactam	as Unasyn
oxprenolol	Trasicor (foreign)	sulfasalazine (salicylazo-sulfapyridine)	Azulfidine
perphenazine	Trilafon, as Etrafon, as Triavil	sulfisoxazole	Gantrisin
phenindione	Hedulin, Indon (unavailable in United States)	suprofen	Suprol
		temazepam	Restoril
		terbutaline	Bricanyl, Brethine
phenylbutazone	Azolid, Butazolidin	tetracycline	Achromycin
phenytoin	Dilantin	theophylline	Bronkodyl, Elixophyllin, Slo-Phyllin, Theo-Dur
piroxicam	Feldene		
prazepam	Centrax		
prednisolone	Delta-Cortef, Meti-Derm, Prelone	thiopental	Pentothal
		thiouracil	Thiouracil (no longer marketed in United States)
prednisone	Deltasone, Meticorten, Sterapred		
primidone	Mysoline	ticarcillin	as Timentin
procainamide	Pronestyl	timolol	Blocadren, Timoptic
propoxyphene	Darvon, Dolene, SK65	tinidazole	Fasigyn, Simplotan (unavailable in United States)
propranolol	Inderal		
propylthiouracil	(generic only)		
pseudoephedrine	as Actifed, Novafed, as Sudafed	tolbutamide	Orinase
		tolmetin	Tolectin
pyridostigmin	Mestinon	trazodone	Desyrel
pyrimethamine	Daraprim	trimethoprim with sulfamethoxazole	Bactrim, Septra
quazepam	Dormalin		
quinine	as Quinamm	triprolidine	Actidil, as Actifed
rifampin	Rifadin, Rimactane	valproic acid	Depakene
secobarbital	Seconal	verapamil	Calan
senna	Senokot	warfarin	Coumadin, Panwarfin
sotalol	(investigational)	zolpidem	Ambien
spironolactone	Aldactone		

Table 6A-9

TRADE NAMES AND GENERIC EQUIVALENTS*

Trade	Generic	Trade	Generic
Accent	monosodium glutamate	Bronkodyl	theophylline
Achromycin	tetracycline	Butazolidin	phenylbutazone
Actidil	triprolidine	as Cafergot	ergotamine tartrate with caffeine
as Actifed	triprolidine		
as Actifed	pseudoephedrine	Calan	verapamil
Acupan (unavailable in United States)	nefopam	Capoten	captopril
		Cardizem	dilitiazem
Adriamycin	doxorubicin	Cefzil	cefprozil
Advil	ibuprofen	Centrax	prazepam
Aldactone	spironolactone	Chloromycetin	chloramphenicol
Ambien	zolpidem	Chlotride (foreign)	cholothiazide
Amipaque	metrizamide	Claforan	cefotaxime
Amoxil	amoxicillin	Cleocin	clindamycin
Anacin-3	acetamethophan	as Combipres	chlorthalidone
Anafranil	clomipramine	Corgard	nadolol
Ancef	cefazolin	Coumadin	warfarin
Apresoline	hydralazine	Cytoxan	cyclophosphamide
Aralen	chloroquine	Daraprim	pyrimethamine
Arlef (foreign)	flufenamic acid	Darvon	propoxyphene
Asendin	amoxapine	Delta-Cortef	prednisolone
Ativan	lorazepam	Deltasone	prednisone
Azactam	aztreonam	Depakene	valproic acid
Azolid	phenylbutazone	Depo-Provera	medroxyprogesterone
Azulfidine	sulfasalazine	Desyrel	trazodone
Bactrim	trimethoprim with sulfamethoxazole	Dexedrine	dextroamphetamine
		Diamox	acetazolamide
Benzamide (foreign)	cisapride	Dicumarol	bishydroxycoumarin
Blocadren	timolol	Dilantin	phenytoin
Brethine	terbutaline	Dilor	dyphylline
Bricanyl	terbutaline	Diprofarn (foreign)	dipyrone

Inclusion of drug names in Table 6A-9 does not constitute an endorsement by the American Academy of Pediatrics of the products listed. Names are included for informational purposes only.

Table 6A-9

Trade	Generic	Trade	Generic
as Disophrol	dexbrompheniramine maleate	Kantrex	kanamycin
		Kefzol	cefazolin
Diuril	chlorothiazide	Lanoxicaps	digoxin
Dolene	propoxyphene	Lanoxin	digoxin
Dolophine	methadone	as Levlen	levonorgestrel
Dorbane	danthron	Lioresal	baclofen
Dormalin	quazepam	Loniten	minoxidil
as Drixoral	dexbrompheniramine maleate	Lopressor	metoprolol
		Macrodantin	nitrofurantoin
Duricef	cefadroxil	Mestinon	pyridostigmine
Elavil	amitriptyline	Meticorten	prednisone
Elixophyllin	theophylline	Meti-Derm	prednisolone
Endep	amitriptyline	Mexitil	mexiletine
Enovid	[³H]norethynodrel	Motilium	domperidone
Estrace	estradiol	Motrin	Ibuprofen
as Etrafon	perphenazine	Moxam	moxalactam
Fasigyn	tinidazole	MSG	monosodium glutamate
Feldene	piroxicam	Myambutol	ethambutol
Flagyl	metronidazole	Myochrysine	gold sodium thiomalate
Folex	methotrexate (amethopterin)	Mysoline	primidone
		Naprosyn	naproxen
Fortaz	ceftazidime	Naturetin	bendroflumethiazide
Furadantin	nitrofurantoin	NegGram	nalidixic acid
Gantrisin	sulfisoxazole	Neo-mercazole (foreign)	carbimazole
Haldol	haloperidol	Noludar	methyprylon
Hedulin	phenindione	as Nordette	levonorgestrel
HydroDIURIL	hydrochlorothiazide	Normodyne	labetalol
Hygroton	chlorthalidone	Norpace	disopyramide
Imodium	loperamide	as Norplant	levonorgestrel
Inderal	propranolol	Norpramin	desipramine
Indocin	indomethacin	Novafed	pseudoephedrine
Indon	phenindione	Novaldin (unavailable in United States)	dipyrone
INH	isoniazid		
Istizin	danthron	NutraSweet	aspartame
Janimine	imipramine	Orinase	tolbutamide

Table 6A-9 (cont.)

Trade	Generic	Trade	Generic
Parlodel	bromocriptine	Serentil	mesoridazine
Panadol	acetomethophan	Seromycin	cycloserine
Panwarfin	warfarin	Simplotan (unavailable in United States)	tinidazole
Pentothal	thiopental		
Pertofrane	desipramine	Sinequan	doxepin
Phenaphen	acetomethophan	SK65	propoxyphene
Plaquenil	hydroxychloroquine	Slo-Phyllin	theophylline
Platinol	cisplatin	Soriatane	acitretin
Ponstel	mefenamic acid	Sotalol	sotalol
Prelone	prednisolone	Stadol	butorphanol
Procardia	nifedipine	Sterapred	prednisone
Pronestyl	procainamide	Sublimaze	fentanyl
Propacil	propylthiouracil	as Sudafed	pseudoephridine
Prothiaden (unavailable in United States)	dothiepin	Suprol	suprofen
		Tagamet	cimetidine
Protostat	metronidazole	Tambocor	flecainide
Provera	medroxyprogesterone	Tapazole	methimazole
Prozac	fluoxetine	Taractan	chlorprothixene
as Quinamm	quinine	Tavegil (foreign)	clemastine
Quine	quinine	Tavist	clemastine
Reglan	metoclopramide	Tegretol	carbamazepine
Restoril	temazepam	Telepaque	iopanoic acid
Rheumatrex	methotrexate	Tempra	acetomethophan
Rifadin	rifampin	Tenormin	atenolol
Rifamycin	rifampin	Theo-Dur	theophylline
Rimactane	rifampin	Thiouracil (no longer marketed in United States)	thiouracil
Robaxin	methocarbamal		
Rocephin	ceftriaxone		
Rogaine	minoxidil	Thorazine	chlorpromazine
Rowasa	mesalamine	as Timentin	ticarcillin
Seconal	secobarbital	Timoptic	timolol
Sectral	acebutolol	Tofranil	imipramine
Senokot	senna	Tolectin	tolmetin
Septra	trimethoprim with sulfamethoxazole	Toradol	ketorolac
		Trandate	labetalol

Table 6A-9

Trade	Generic	Trade	Generic
Trasicor (foreign)	oxprenolol	Valium	diazepam
Triavil	perphenazine	Vasotec	enalapril
Trilafon	perphenazine	Versed	midazolam
as Tri-Levlen	levonorgestrel	Xylocaine	lidocaine
as Triphasil	levonorgestrel	Zarontin	ethosuximide
Tusscapine (foreign)	noscapine	Zovirax	acyclovir
Tylenol	acetaminophen	Zyloprim	allopurinol
as Unazyn	sulbactam		

APPENDIX 6-A TABLE REFERENCES

1. American Academy of Pediatrics, Committee on Drugs. The transfer of drugs and other chemicals into human breast milk. *Pediatrics.* 1983;72:375–383

2. American Academy of Pediatrics, Committee on Drugs. Transfer of drugs and other chemicals into human milk. *Pediatrics.* 1989; 84:924–936

3. Kulski JK, Hartmann PE, Martin JD, et al. Effects of bromocriptine mesylate on the composition of the mammary secretion in non-breast-feeding women. *Obstet Gynecol.* 1978; 52:38

4. Katz M, Kroll D, Pak I, et al. Puerperal hypertension, stroke, and seizures after suppression of lactation with bromocriptine. *Obstet Gynecol.* 1985;66:822–824

5. Chasnoff IJ, Lewis DE, Squires L. Cocaine intoxication in a breast-fed infant. *Pediatrics.* 1987;80:836–838

6. Wiernik PH, Duncan JH. Cyclophosphamide in human milk. *Lancet.* 1971;1:912

7. Amato D, Niblett JS. Neutropenia from cyclophosphamide in breast milk. *Med J Aust.* 1977;1:383

8. Fletcher SM, Katz AR, Rogers AJ, et al. The presence of cyclosporine in body tissue and fluids during pregnancy. *Am J Kidney Dis.* 1985;5:60

9. Egan PC, Costanza ME, Dodion P, et al. Doxorubicin and cisplatin excretion into human milk. *Cancer Treat Rep.* 1985;69:1387

10. Fomina PI. Untersuchungen uber den Ubergang des aktiven agens des Mutterkorns in die milch stillender Mutter. *Arch Gynecol.* 1934;157:275

11. Schou M, Amdisen A. Lithium and pregnancy, III: lithium ingestion by children breast-fed by women on lithium treatment. *Br Med J.* 1973;2:138

12. Tunnessen WW Jr, Hertz C. Toxic effects of lithium in newborn infants: a commentary. *J Pediatr.* 1972;81:804

13. Sykes PA, Quarrie J, Alexander FW. Lithium carbonate and breast-feeding. *Br Med J.* 1976;2:1299

14. Johns DG, Rutherford LD, Leighton PC, et al. Secretion of methotrexate into human milk. *Am J Obstet Gynecol.* 1972;12:978

15. Kaufman KR, Petrucha RA, Pitts Jr FN, et al. PCP in amniotic fluid breast milk: case report. *J Clin Psychiatry.* 1983;44:269

16. Eckstein HB, Jack B. Breast-feeding anticoagulant therapy. *Lancet.* 1970;1:672

17. Steiner E, Villen T, Hallberg M, et al. Amphetamine secretion in breast milk. *Eur J Clin Pharmacol.* 1984;27:123

18. Cobrinik RW, Hood RT Jr, Chusid E. The effect of maternal narcotic addiction on the newborn infant: review of literature and report of 22 cases. *Pediatrics.* 1959;24:288

19. Perez-Reyes M, Wall ME. Presence of tetrahydrocannabinol in human milk. *N Engl J Med.* 1982;307:819

20. Bisdom W. Alcohol and nicotine poisoning in nurslings. *JAMA.* 1937;109:178

21. Ferguson BB, Wilson DJ, Schaffner W. Determination of nicotine concentrations in human milk. *AJDC.* 1976;130:837

22. Luck W, Nau H. Nicotine and cotinine concentrations in the milk of smoking mothers: influence of cigarette consumption and diurnal variation. *Eur J Pediatr.* 1987;146:21–26

23. Luck W, Nau H. Nicotine and cotinine concentrations in serum and milk of nursing mothers. *Br J Clin Pharmacol.* 1984;18:9–15

24. Luck W, Nau H. Nicotine and cotinine concentrations in serum and urine of infants exposed via passive smoking or milk from smoking mothers. *J Pediatr.* 1985;107;816–820

25. Labrecque M, Marcoux S, Weber J-P, et al. Feeding and urine cotinine values in babies whose mothers smoke. *Pediatrics.* 1989;83:93–97

26. Schwartz-Bickenbach D, Schulte-Hobein B, Abt S, et al. Smoking and passive smoking during pregnancy and early infancy: effects on birth weight, lactation period, and cotinine concentrations in mother's milk and infant's urine. *Toxicol Lett.* 1987;35:73–81

27. McArdle HJ, Danks DM. Secretion of copper 64 into breast milk following intravenous injection in a human subject. *J Trace Elem Exp Med.* 1991;4:81–84

28. Tobin RE, Schneider PB. Uptake of ^{67}Ga in the lactating breast and its persistence in milk: case report. *J Nucl Med* 1976;17:1055

29. Butt D, Szaz KF. Indium-111 radioactivity in breast milk. *Br J Radiol.* 1986;59:80

30. Hedrick WR, Di Simone RN, Keen RL. Radiation dosimetry from breast milk excretion of radioiodine and pertechnetate. *J Nucl Med.* 1986;27:1569–1571

31. Palmer KE. Excretion of ^{125}I in breast milk following administration labelled fibrinogen. *Br J Radiol.* 1979;52:672

32. Honour AJ, Myant NB, Rowlands EN. Secretion of radioiodine in digestive juices and milk in man. *Clin Sci.* 1952;11:447

33. Karjalainen P, Penttila IM, Pystynen P. The amount and form of radioactivity in human milk after lung scanning, renography and placental localization by ^{131}I labelled tracers. *Acta Obstet Gynecol Scand.* 1971;50:357

34. Bland EP, Crawford JS, Docker MF, et al. Radioactive iodine uptake by thyroid of breastfed infants after maternal blood-volume measurements. *Lancet.* 1969;2:1039

35. Nurnberger CE, Lipscomb A. Transmission of radioiodine (I^{131}) to infants through human maternal milk. *JAMA.* 1952;150:1398

36. Pommerenke WT, Hahn PF. Secretion of radioactive sodium in human milk. *Proc Soc Exp Biol Med.* 1943;52:223

37. O'Connell MEA, Sutton H. Excretion of radioactivity in breast milk following ^{99}Tcm-Sn polyphosphate. *Br J Radiol.* 1976;49:377

38. Berke RA, Hoops EC, Kereiakes JC, et al. Radiation dose to breast-feeding child after mother has ^{99m}Tc-MAA lung scan. *J Nucl Med* 1973;14:51

39. Vagenakis AG, Abreau CM, Braverman LE. Duration of radioactivity in the milk of a nursing mother following ^{99m}Tc administration. *J Nucl Med.* 1971;12:188

40. Wyburn JR. Human breast milk excretion of radionuclides following administration of radiopharmaceuticals. *J Nucl Med.* 1973;14:115

41. Pittard WB III, Merkatz R, Fletcher BD. Radioactive excretion in human milk following administration of technetium Tc 99 m macroaggregated albumin. *Pediatrics.* 1982; 70:231

42. Maisels MJ, Gilcher RO. Excretion of technetium in human milk. *Pediatrics.* 1983;71:841

43. American Academy of Pediatrics, Committee on Drugs. Psychotropic drugs in pregnancy and lactation. *Pediatrics.* 1982;69:241–244

44. Patrick MJ, Tilstone WJH, Reavey P. Diazepam and breast-feeding. *Lancet.* 1972;1:542

45. Cole AP, Hailey DM. Diazepam and active metabolite in breast milk and their transfer to the neonate. *Arch Dis Child.* 1975;50:741

46. Dusci LJ, Goods M, Hall RW, et al. Excretion of diazepam and its metabolites in human milk during withdrawal from combination high dose diazepam and oxazepam. *Br J Clin Pharmacol.* 1990;29:123–126

47. Summerfield RJ, Nielson MS. Excretion of lorazepam into breast milk. *Br J Anaesth.* 1985;57:1042

48. Matheson I, Lunde PK, Bredesen JE. Midazolam and nitrazepam in the maternity ward: milk concentrations and clinical effects. *Br J Clin Pharmacol.* 1990;30:787–793

49. Olesen OV, Bartels U, Poulsen JH. Perphenazine in breast milk and serum. *Am J Psychiatry.* 1990;147:1378–1379

50. Brodie RR, Chasseaud LF, Taylor T. Concentrations of N-descyclopropylmethyl-prazepam in whole-blood, plasma, and milk after administration of prazepam to humans. *Biopharm Drug Dispos.* 1981;2:59

51. Hilbert JM, Gural RP, Symchowicz S, et al. Excretion of quazepam into human breast milk. *J Clin Pharmacol.* 1984;24:457

52. Lebedevs TH, Wojnar-Horton RE, Yapp P, et al. Excretion of temazepam in breast milk. *Br J Clin Pharmacol.* 1992;33:204–206

53. Bader TF, Newman K. Amitriptyline in human breast milk and the nursing infant's serum. *Am J Psychiatry.* 1980;137:855

54. Erickson SH, Smith GH, Heidrich T. Tricyclics and breast feeding. *Am J Psychiatry.* 1979;136:1483

55. Gelenberg AJ. Amoxapine: a new antidepressant appears in human milk. *J Nerv Ment Dis.* 1979;167:635

56. Sovner R, Orsulak PJ. Excretion of imipramine and desipramine in human breast milk. *Am J Psychiatry.* 1979;136:451

57. Stancer HC, Reed KL. Desipramine and 2-hydroxydesipramine in human breast milk and the nursery infant's serum. *Am J Psychiatry.* 1986;143:1597

58. Rees JA, Glass RC, Sporne GA. Serum and breast milk concentrations of dothiepin. *Practitioner.* 1976;217:686

59. Ilett KF, Lebedevs TH, Wojnar-Horton RE, et al. The excretion of dothiepin and its primary metabolites in breast milk. *Br J Clin Pharmacol.* 1992;33:635–639

60. Kemp J, Ilett KF, Booth J, et al. Excretion of doxepin and N-desmethyldoxepin in human milk. *Br J Clin Pharmacol.* 1985;20:497

61. Burch KJ, Wells BG. Fluoxetine/norfluoxetine concentrations in human milk. *Pediatrics.* 1992;33:676–7

62. Wright S, Dawling S, Ashford JJ. Excretion of fluvoxamine in breast milk. *Br J Clin Pharmacol.* 1993;31:209

63. Verbeeck RK, Ross SG, McKenna EA. Excretion of trazodone in breast milk. *Br J Clin Pharmacol.* 1986;22:367

64. Polishuk WZ, Kulcsar SA. Effects of chlorpromazine on pituitary function. *J Clin Endocrinol Metab.* 1956;16:292

65. Wiles DH, Orr MW, Kolakowska T. Chlorpromazine levels in plasma and milk of nursing mothers. *Br J Clin Pharmacol.* 1978;5:272

66. Matheson I, Evang A, Fredricson Overo K, et al. Presence of chlorprothixene and its metabolites in breast milk. *Eur J Clin Pharmacol.* 1984;27:611

67. Stewart RB, Karas B, Springer PK. Haloperidol excretion in human milk. *Am J Psychiatry.* 1980;137:859

68. Whalley LJ, Blain PG, Prime JK. Haloperidol secreted in breast milk. *Br Med J.* 1981;282:1746

69. Ananth J. Side effects in the neonate from psychotropic agents excreted through breast-feeding. *Am J Psychiatry.* 1978;135:801

70. Havelka J, Hejzlar M. Popov V. Excretion of chloramphenicol in human milk. *Chemotherapy.* 1968.13:204

71. Smadel JE, Woodward TE, Ley HL Jr, et al. Chloramphenicol (Chloromycetin) in the treatment of tsutsugamushi disease (scrub typhus). *J Clin Invest.* 1949;28:1196

72. Gupta AP, Gupta PK. Metaclopramide as a lactogogue. *Clin Pediatr.* 1985;24:269

73. Kauppela A, Arvela P, Koivisto M, et al. Metaclopramide and breast-feeding: transfer into milk and the newborn. *Eur J Clin Pharmacol.* 1983;25:819

74. Erickson SH, Oppenheim GL, Smith GH. Metronidazole in breast milk. *Obstet Gynecol.* 1981;57:48

75. Heisterberg L, Branebjerg PE. Blood and milk concentrations of metronidazole in mothers and infants. *J Perinat Med.* 1983;11:114

76. Evaldson GR, Lindgren S, Nord CE, et al. Tinidazole milk excretion and pharmacokinetics in lactating women. *Br J Clin Pharmacol.* 1985;19:503

77. Nelis GF. Diarrhoea due to 5-aminosalicylic acid in breast milk. *Lancet.* 1989;383

78. Jenss H, Weber P, Hartmann F. 5-Aminosalicylic acid its metabolite in breast milk during lactation. *Am J Gastroenterol.* 1990;85:331

79. Clark JH, Wilson WG. A 16-day-old breast-fed infant with metabolic acidosis caused by salicylate. *Clin Pediatr.* 1981;20:53

80. Levy G. Salicylate pharmacokinetics in the human neonate. In: Marselli PL, ed. *Basic and Therapeutic Aspects of Perinatal Pharmacology.* New York, NY: Raven Press; 1975:319

81. Fakhredding J, Keshavarz E. Salicylate excretion in breast milk. *Int J Pharm* 1981;8:285

82. Kok THHG, Taitz LS, Bennett MJ. Drowsiness due to clemastine transmitted in breast milk. *Lancet.* 1982;1:914

83. Nau H, Rating D, Hauser I, et al. Placental transfer and pharmacokinetics of primidone and its metabolites phenobarbital, PEMA and hydroxyphenobarbital in neonates and infants of epileptic mothers. *Eur J Clin Pharmacol.* 1980;18:31

84. Kuhnz W, Koch S, Helge H, et al. Primidone and phenobarbital during lactation period in epileptic women: total and free drug serum levels in the nursed infants and their effects on neonatal behavior. *Dev Pharmacol Ther.* 1988;11:147

85. Finch E, Lorber J. Methaemoglobinaemia in the newborn: probably due to phenytoin excreted in human milk. *J Obstet Gynaecol Br Emp.* 1954;61:833

86. Tyson RM, Shrader EA, Perlman HH. Drugs transmitted through breast milk, II: barbiturates. *J Pediatr.* 1938;13:86

87. Knott C, Reynolds F, Clayden G. Infantile spasms on weaning from breast milk containing anticonvulsants. *Lancet.* 1987;2:272

88. Branski D, Kerem E, Gross-Kieselstein E, et al. Bloody diarrhea—a possible complication of sulfasalazine transferred through human breast milk. *J Pediatr Gastroenterol Nutr.* 1986;5:316

89. Boutroy MJ, Bianchetti G, Dubruc C, et al. To nurse when receiving acebutolol: is it dangerous for the neonate? *Eur J Clin Pharmacol.* 1986;30:737

90. Berlin CM Jr, Yaffe SJ, Ragni M. Disposition of acetaminophen in milk, saliva, and plasma of lactating women. *Pediatr Pharmacol.* 1980;1:135

91. Bitzen PO, Gustafsson B, Jostell KG, et al. Excretion of paracetamol in human breast milk. *Eur J Clin Pharmacol.* 1981;20:123

92. Findlay JWA, DeAngelis RL, Kearney MF, et al. Analgesic drugs in breast milk and plasma. *Clin Pharmacol Ther.* 1981;20:123

93. Soderman P, Hartvig P, Fagerlund C. Acetazolamide excretion into human breast milk. *Br J Clin Pharmacol.* 1984;17:599

94. Rollman O, Pihl-Lundin I. Acitretin excretion into human breast milk. *Acta Derm Venereol (Stockh).* 1990;70:487–490

95. Lau RJ, Emery MG, Galinsky RE. Unexpected accumulation of acyclovir in breast milk with estimation of infant exposure. *Obstet Gynecol.* 1987;69:468

96. Meyer LJ, de Miranda P, Sheth N, et al. Acyclovir in human breast milk. *Am J Obstet Gynecol.* 1988;158:586–588

97. Binkiewicz A, Robinson MJ, Senior B. Pseudo-cushing syndrome caused by alcohol in breast milk. *J Pediatr.* 1978;93:965

98. Cobo E. Effect of different dose of ethanol on the milk-ejecting reflex in lactating women. *Am J Obstet Gynecol.* 1973;115:817

99. Kesaniemi YA. Ethanol and acetaldehyde in the milk and peripheral blood of lactating women after ethanol administration. *J Obstet Gynaecol Br Commonw.* 1974;81:84

100. Little RE, Anderson KW, Ervin CH, et al. Maternal alcohol use during breast-feeding and infant mental and motor development at one year. *N Engl J Med.* 1989;321:425–430

101. Kamilli I, Gresser U, Schaefer C, et al. Allopurinol in breast milk. *Adv Exp Med Biol.* 1991;309A:143–145

102. Kafetzis DA, Siafas CA, Georgakopoulos PA, et al. Passage of cephalosporins and amoxicillin into the breast milk. *Acta Paediatr Scand.* 1981;70:285

103. Berman JD, Melby PC, Neva FA. Concentration of Pentosam in human breast milk. *Trans R Soc Trop Med Hyg.* 1989;83:784–785

104. Liedholm H, Melander A, Bitzen P-O, et al. Accumulation of atenolol and metoprolol in human breast milk. *Eur J Clin Pharmacol.* 1981;20:229

105. Schimmel MS, Edelman AI, Wilschanski MA, et al. Toxic effects of atenolol consumed during breast feeding. *J Pediatr.* 1989;114:476–478

106. Thorley KJ, McAinsh J. Levels of the beta-blockers atenolol and propanolol in the breast milk of women treated for hypertension in pregnancy. *Biopharm Drug Dispos.* 1983;4:299–301

107. Sapeika N. The excretion of drugs in human milk—a review. *J Obstet Gynaecol Br Commonw.* 1947;54:426

108. Bald R, Bernbeck-Betthauser E-M, Spahn H, et al. Excretion of azpropazone in human breast milk. *Eur J Clin Pharmacol.* 1990;39:271–273

109. Fleiss PM, Richwald GA, Gordon J, et al. Aztreonam in human serum and breast milk. *Br J Clin Pharmacol.* 1985;19:509

110. Nail PA, Thomas MR, Eakin R. The effect of thiamin and riboflavin supplementation on the level of those vitamins in human breast milk and urine. *Am J Clin Nutr.* 1980;33:198

111. Roepke JLB, Kirksey A. Vitamin B_6 nutrature during pregnancy lactation: I. vitamin B_6 intake, levels of the vitamin in biological fluids, condition of the infant at birth. *Am J Clin Nutr.* 1979;32:2249

112. West KD, Kirksey A. Influence of vitamin B_6 intake on the content of the vitamin in human milk. *Am J Clin Nutr.* 1976;29:961

113. Greentree LB. Dangers of vitamin B_6 in nursing mothers. *N Engl J Med.* 1979;300:141

114. Samson RR, McClelland DBL. Vitamin B_{12} in human colostrum milk: quantitation of the vitamin its binder the uptake of bound vitamin B_{12} by intestinal bacteria. *Acta Paediatr Scand.* 1980;69:93

115. Eriksson G, Swahn CG. Concentrations of baclofen in serum and breast milk from a lactating woman. *Scand J Clin Lab Invest.* 1981;41:185

116. Healy M. Suppressing lactation with oral diuretics. *Lancet.* 1961;1:1353

117. Brambel CE, Hunter RE. Effect of dicumarol on the nursing infant. *Am J Obstet Gynecol.* 1950;59:1153

118. Tyson RM, Shrader EA, Perlman HH. Drugs transmitted through breast milk, III: bromides. *J Pediatr.* 1938;13:91

119. Pittman KA, Smyth RD, Losada M, et al. Human perinatal distribution of butorphanol. *Am J Obstet Gynecol.* 1980;138:797

120. Berlin CM Jr. Excretion of the methylxanthines in human milk. *Semin Perinatol.* 1981;5:389

121. Tyrala EE, Dodson WE. Caffeine secretion into breast milk. *Arch Dis Child.* 1979;54:787

122. Hildebrandt R, Gundert-Remy V. Lack of pharmacological active saliva levels of caffeine in breast-fed infants. *Pediatr Pharmacol.* 1983;3:237

123. Berlin CM Jr, Denson HM, Daniel CH, Ward RM. Disposition of dietary caffeine in milk, saliva and plasma of lactating women. *Pediatrics.* 1984;73:59–63

124. Ryu JE. Caffeine in human milk and in serum of breast-fed infants. *Dev Pharmacol Ther.* 1985;8:329

125. Ryu JE. Effect of maternal caffeine consumption on heart rate and sleep time of breast-fed infants. *Dev Pharmacol Ther.* 1985;8:355

126. Devlin RG, Fleiss PM. Captopril in human blood and breast milk. *J Clin Pharmacol.* 1981;21:110

127. Nau H, Kuhnz W, Egger JH, et al. Anticonvulsants during pregnancy and lactation. *Clin Pharmacokinet.* 1982;7:508

128. Pynnonen S, Kanto J, Sillanpaa M, et al. Carbamazepine: placental transport, tissue concentrations in foetus newborn, level in milk. *Acta Pharmacol Toxicol.* 1977;41:244

129. Cooper DS, Antithyroid drugs: to breast-feed or not to breast-feed. *Am J Obstet Gynecol.* 1987;157:234

130. Lamberg B-A, Ikonen E, Österlund K, et al. Antithyroid treatment of maternal hyperthy-roidism during lactation. *Clin Endocrinol.* 1984;21:81–87

131. Tyson RM, Shrader EA, Perlman HH. Drugs transmitted through breast milk, I: laxatives. *J Pediatr.* 1937;11:824

132. Yoshioka H, Cho K, Takimoto M, et al. Transfer of cefazolin into human milk. *J Pediatr.* 1979;94:151

133. Dresse A, Lambotte R, Dubois M, et al. Transmammary passage of cefoxitin: additional results. *J Clin Pharmacol.* 1983;23:438

134. Shyu WC, Shah Vr, Campbell DA, et al. Excretion of cefprozil into human breast milk. *Antimicrob Agents Chemother.* 1992;36:938–941

135. Blanco JD, Jorgensen JH, Castaneda YS, et al. Ceftazidine levels in human breast milk. *Antimicrob Agents Chemother.* 1983;23:479

136. Kafetzis DA, Brater DC, Fanourgakis JE, et al. Ceftriaxone distribution between maternal blood and fetal blood and tissues at parturition and between blood and milk postpartum. *Antimicrob Agents Chemother.* 1983;23:870

137. Lacey JH. Dichloralphenazone breast milk. *Br Med J.* 1971;4:684

138. Reed CB. A study of the conditions that require the removal of the child from the breast. *Surg Gynecol Obstet.* 1908;6:514

139. Soares R, Paulini E, Pereira JP. Da concentra-cao e eliminacao da cloroquina atraves da cir-culacao placentaria e do leite materno, de pacientes sob regime do sal loroquinado. *Rev Bras Malariol Doencas Trop.* 1957;9:19

140. Ogunbona FA, Onyizi CO, Bolaji OO, et al. Excretion of chloroquine and desethylchloro-quin in human milk. *Br J Clin Pharmacol.* 1987;23:476

141. Edstein MD, Veenendaal JR, Newman K, et al. Excretion of chloroquine, dapsone and pyrimethamine in human milk. *Br J Clin Pharmacol.* 1986;22:733

142. Werthmann MW Jr, Krees SV, Excretion of chlorothiazide in human breast milk. *J Pediatr.* 1972;81:781

143. Miller EM, Cohn RD, Burghart PH. Hydrochlorothiazide disposition in a mother her breast-fed infant. *J Pediatr.* 1982;101:789

144. Mulley BA, Parr GD, Pau WK, et al. Placental transfer of chlorthalidone and its elimination in maternal milk. *Eur J Clin Pharmacol.* 1978; 13:129

145. Somogyi A, Gugler R. Cimetidine excretion into breast milk. *Br J Clin Pharmacol.* 1979; 7:627

146. Hofmeyr GJ, Sonnendecker EWW. Secretion of the gastrokinetic agent cisapride in human milk. *Eur J Clin Pharmacol.* 1986;30:735

147. Smith JA, Morgan JR, Rachlis AR, et al. Clindamycin in human breast milk. *Can Med Assoc J.* 1975;112:806

148. Zacharias S, Aguillern E, Assenzo Jr, et al. Effects of hormonal and nonhormonal contraceptives on lactation and incidence of pregnancy. *Contraception.* 1986;33:203

149. Schimmell MS, Katz EZ, Shaag Y, et al. Toxic neonatal effects following maternal clomipramine therapy. *J Toxicol Clin Toxicol.* 1991;29:479–484

150. Milunsky JM. Breast-feeding during colchicine therapy for familial Mediterranean fever. *J Pediatr.* 1991;119:164

151. Nilsson S, Mellbin T, Hofvander Y, et al. Long-term followup of children breast-fed by mothers using oral contraceptives. *Contraception.* 1986;34:443

152. Nilsson S, Nygren KG. Transfer of contraceptives steroids to human milk. *Res Reprod.* 1979;11:1

153. American Academy of Pediatrics, Committee on Drugs. Breast-feeding and contraception. *Pediatrics.* 1981;68:138–140.

154. Barsivala VM, Virkar KD. The effect of oral contraceptives on concentration of various components of human milk. *Contraception.* 1973;7:307

155. Borglin NE, Sandholm LE. Effect of oral contraceptives on lactation. *Fertil. Steril.* 1971; 22:39

156. Curtis EM. Oral-contraceptive feminization of a normal male infant: report of a case. *Obstet Gynecol.* 1964;23:295

157. Kora SJ. Effect of oral contraceptives on lactation. *Fertil Steril.* 1969;20:419

158. Toaff R, Ashkenazi H, Schwartz A, et al. Effects of oestrogen and progestagen on the composition of human milk. *J Reprod Fertil.* 1969;19:475

159. Snyder DR Jr, Powell KE. Should women taking antituberculosis drugs breast-feed? *Arch Intern Med.* 1984;144:589

160. Cancela L, LeBoulch N, Miravet L. Relationship between the vitamin D content of maternal milk and the vitamin D status of nursing women and breast-fed infants. *J Endrocinol.* 1986;110:43

161. Rothberg AD, Pettifor JM, Cohen DF, et al. Maternal-infant vitamin D relationships during breast-feeding. *J Pediatr.* 1982;101:500

162. Greer FR, Hollis BW, Napoli JL. High concentrations of vitamin D_2 in human milk associated with pharmacologic doses of vitamin D_2. *J Pediatr.* 1984;105:61

163. Greenhalf JO, Leonard HSD. Laxatives in the treatment of constipation in pregnant and breast-feeding mothers. *Practitioner.* 1973; 210:259

164. Dreisbach JA. Sulphone levels in breast milk of mothers on sulphone therapy. *Lepr Rev.* 1952;23:101

165. Mortimer EA Jr. Drug toxicity from breast milk? *Pediatrics.* 1977;60:780

166. Loughnan PM. Digoxin excretion in human breast milk. *J Pediatr.* 1978;92:1019

167. Levy M, Granit L, Laufer N. Excretion of drugs in human milk. *N Engl J Med.* 1977;297:789

168. Okada M, Inoue H, Nakamura Y, et al. Excretion of diltiazem in human milk. *N Engl J Med.* 1985;312:992

169. Zylber-Katz E, Linder N, Granit L, et al. Excretion of dipyrone metabolites in human breast milk. *Eur J Clin Pharmacol.* 1986;30:359

170. MacKintosh D, Buchanan N. Excretion of disopyramide in human breast milk. *Br J Clin Pharmacol.* 1985;19:856

171. Hoppu K, Neuvonen PJ, Korte T. Disopyramide and breast feeding. *Br J Clin Pharmacol.* 1986;21:553

172. Hofmeyr GJ, van Idlekinge B. Domperidone and lactation. *Lancet.* 1983;1:647

173. Jorboe CH, Cook LN, Malesic I, et al. Dyphylline elimination kinetics in lactating women: blood milk transfer. *J Clin Pharmacol.* 1981;21:405

174. Redman CW, Kelly JG, Cooper WD. The excretion of enalapril and enalaprilat in human breast milk. *Eur J Clin Pharmacol.* 1990;38:99

175. Matsuda S. Transfer of antibiotics into maternal milk. *Biol Res Pregnancy.* 1984;5:57

176. Nilsson S, Nygren KG, Johansson EDB. Transfer of estradiol to human milk. *Am J Obstet Gynecol.* 1978;132:653

177. Koup JR, Rose JQ, Cohen ME. Ethosuximide pharmacokinetics in a pregnant patient and her newborn. *Epilepsia.* 1978;19:535

178. Steer PL, Biddle CJ, Marley WS, et al. Concentration of fentanyl in colostrum after an analgesic dose. *Can J Anaesth.* 1992; 39:231–235

179. McQuinn RL, Pisani A, Wafa S, et al. Flecainide excretion in human breast milk. *Clin Pharmacol Ther.* 1990;48:262–267

180. Wagner X, Jouglard J, Moulin M, et al. Coadministration of flecainide acetate and sotalol during pregnancy: lack of teratogenic effects, passage across the placenta, and excretion in human breast milk. *Am Heart J.* 1990;119:700–702

181. Buchanan RA, Eaton CJ, Koeff ST, et al. The breast milk excretion of flufenamic acid. *Curr Ther Res.* 1969;11:533

182. Mattern J, Mayer PR. Excretion of fluorescein into breast milk. *Am J Ophthalmol.* 1990; 109:598–599

183. Retief EF, Heyns ADuP, Oosthuizen M, et al. Aspects of folate metabolism in lactating women studied after ingestion of ^{14}C-methylfolate. *Am J Med Sci.* 1979;277:281

184. Bell RAF, Dale IM. Gold secretion in maternal milk. *Arthritis Rheum.* 1976;19:1374

185. Blau SP. Metabolism of gold during lactation. *Arthritis Rheum.* 1973;16:777

186. Gottlieb NL. Suggested errata. *Arthritis Rheum.* 1974;17:1057

187. Ostensen M, Skavdal K, Myklebust G, et al. Excretion of gold into human breast milk. *Eur J Clin Pharmacol.* 1986;31:251

188. Bennett PN, Humphries SJ, Osborne JP, et al. Use of sodium aurothiomalate during lactation. *Br J Clin Pharmacol.* 1990;29:777–779

189. Cote CJ, Kenepp NB, Reed SB, et al. Trace concentrations of halothane in human breast milk. *Br J Anaesth.* 1976;48:541

190. Liedholm H, Wahlin-Boll E, Hanson A, et al. Transplacental passage and breast milk concentrations of hydralazine. *Eur J Clin Pharmacol.* 1982;21:417

191. Ostensen M, Brown ND, Chiang PK, et al. Hydroxychoroquine in human breast milk. *Eur J Clin Pharmacol.* 1985;28:357

192. Nation RL, Hackett LP, Dusci LJ, et al. Excretion of hydroxychloroquine in human milk. *Br J Clin Pharmacol.* 1984;17:368

193. Townsend RJ, Benedetti T, Erickson SH, et al. A study to evaluate the passage of ibuprofen into breast milk. *Drug Intell Clin Pharm.* 1982;16:482

194. Townsend RJ, Benedetti T, Erickson SH, et al. Excretion of ibuprofen into breast milk. *Am J Obstet Gynecol.* 1984;149:184

195. Eeg-Olofsson O, Malmros I, Elwin CE, et al. Convulsions in a breast-fed infant after maternal indomethacin. *Lancet.* 1978;2:215

196. Fairhead FW. Convulsions in a breast-fed infant after maternal indomethacin. *Lancet.* 1978;2:576

197. Lebedevs TH, Wojnar-Horton RE, Yapp P, et al. Excretion of indomethacin in breast milk. *Br J Clin Pharmacol.* 1991;32:751–754

198. Postellon DC, Aronow R. Iodine in mother's milk. *JAMA.* 1982;247:463

199. Holmdahl KH. Cholecystography during lactation. *Acta Radiol.* 1955;45:305

200. Berlin CM Jr, Lee C. Isoniazid and acetylisoniazid disposition in human milk, saliva and plasma. *Fed Proc.* 1979;38:426

201. Dyggve HV, Dam H, Sondergaard E. Influence on the prothrombin time of breast-fed newborn babies of one single dose of vitamin K_1, or synkavit given to the mother within 2 hours after birth. *Acta Obstet Gynecol Scand.* 1956;35:440

202. Kries RV, Shearer M, McCarthy PT, et al. Vitamin K_1 content of maternal milk: Influence of the stage of lactation, lipid composition, vitamin K_1 supplements given to the mother. *Pediatr Res.* 1987;22:513

203. Wischnik A, Manth SM, Lloyd J, et al. The excretion of ketorolac tromethamine into breast milk after multiple oral dosing. *Eur J Clin Pharmacol.* 1989;36:521–524

204. Lunell HO, Kulas J, Rane A. Transfer of labetalol into amniotic fluid and breast milk in lactating women. *Eur J Clin Pharmacol.* 1985;28:597

205. Atkinson H, Begg EJ. Concentration of beta-blocking drugs in human milk. *J Pediatr.* 1990;116:156

206. Díaz S, Herreros C, Juez G, et al. Fertility regulation in nursing women, VII: influence of Norplant levonorgestrel implants upon lactation and infant growth. *Contraception.* 1985;32:53–74

207. Shaaban MM, Odlind V, Salem HT, et al. Levonorgestrel concentrations in maternal and infant serum during use of subdermal levonorgestrel contraceptive implants, Norplant by nursing mothers. *Contraception.* 1986;33:357–363

208. Shikary ZK, Betrabet SS, Patel ZM, et al. Transfer of levonorgestrel (LNG) administered through different drug delivery systems from the maternal circulation into the newborn infant's circulation via breast milk. *Contraception.* 1987;35:477–486

209. McCann MF, Moggia AV, Higgins JE, et al. The effects of a progestin-only oral contraceptive (levonorgestrel 0.03 mg) on breast-feeding. *Contraception.* 1987;40:635–648

210. Zeisler JA, Gaarder TD, DeMesquita SA. Lidocaine excretion in breast milk. *Drug Intell Clin Pharm.* 1986;20:691

211. Nikodem VC, Hofmeyr GJ. Secretion of the antidiarrhoel agent loperamide oxide in breast milk. *Eur J Clin Pharmacol.* 1992;42:695–696

212. Cruikshank DP, Varner MW, Pitkin RM. Breast milk magnesium and calcium concentrations following magnesium sulfate treatment. *Am J Obstet Gynecol.* 1982;143:685

213. Buchanan RA, Eaton CJ, Koeff ST, et al. The breast milk excretion of mefenamic acid. *Curr Ther Res Clin Exp.* 1968;10:592

214. Blinick G, Inturrisi CE, Jerez E, et al. Methadone assays in pregnant women and pregnancy. *Am J Obstet Gynecol.* 1975;121:617

215. Blinick G, Wallach RC, Jerez E, et al. Drug addiction in pregnancy and the neonate. *Am J Obstet Gynecol.* 1976;125:135

216. Cooper DS, Bode HH, Nath B, et al. Methimazole pharmacology in man: studies using or newly developed radioimmunoassay for methimazole. *J Clin Endocrinol Metab.* 1984;58:473

217. Campbell AD, Coles FK, Eubank LLK, et al. Distribution and metabolism of methocarbamol. *J Pharmacol Exp Ther.* 1961;131:18

218. White WB, Andreoli JW, Cohn RD. Alpha-methyldopa disposition in mothers with hypertension in their breast-fed infants. *Clin Pharmacol Ther.* 1985;37:387

219. Shore MF. Drugs can be dangerous during pregnancy and lactations. *Can Pharm J.* 1970; 103:358

220. Ilett KF, Hackett LP, Paterson JW. Excretion of metrizamide in milk. *Br J Radiol.* 1981; 54:537

221. Lownes HE, Ives TJ. Mexiletine use in pregnancy and lactation. *Am J Obstet Gynecol.* 1987;157:446

222. Valdivieso A, Valdes G, Spiro TE, et al. Minoxidil in breast milk. *Ann Intern Med.* 1985;102:135

223. Terwilliger WG, Hatcher RA. The elimination of morphine and quinine in human milk. *Surg Gynecol Obstet.* 1934;58:823

224. Robieux I, Koren G, Vandenbergh H, et al. Morphine excretion in breast milk and resultant exposure of a nursing infant. *J Toxicol Clin Toxicol.* 1990;28:365–370

225. Miller RD, Keegan KA, Thrupp LD, et al. Human breast milk concentration of moxalactam. *Am J Obstet Gynecol.* 1984;148:348

226. Devlin RG, Duchin KL, Fleiss PM. Nadolol in human serum and breast milk. *Br J Clin Pharmacol.* 1981;12:393

227. Belton EM, Jones RV. Haemolytic anaemia due to nalidixic acid. *Lancet.* 1965;2:691

228. Jamali F, Tam YK, Stevens RD. Naproxen excretion in breast milk and its uptake by suckling infant. *Drug Intell Clin Pharm.* 1982;16

229. Liu DTY, Savage JM, Donnell D. Nefopam excretion in human milk. *Br J Clin Pharmacol.* 1987;23:99

230. Ehrenkranz RA, Ackerman BA, Hulse JD. Nifedipine transfer into human milk. *J Pediatr.* 1989;114:478–480

231. Varsano I, Fischl J, Tikvah P, et al. The excretion of orally ingested nitrofurantoin in human milk. *J Pediatr.* 1973;82:886

232. Laumas KR, Malkani PK, Bhatnagar S, et al. Radioactivity in the breast milk of lactating women after oral administration of ³H-norethynodrel. *Am J Obstet Gynecol.* 1967; 98:411

233. Pincus G, Bialy G, Layne DS, et al. Radioactivity in the milk of subjects receiving radioactive 19-norsteroids. *Nature.* 1966; 212:924

234. Olsson B, Bolme P, Dahlstrom B, et al. Excretion of noscapine in human breast milk. *Eur J Clin Pharmacol.* 1986;30:213

235. Sioufi A, Hillion D, Lumbroso P, et al. Oxprenolol placental transfer plasma concentrations in newborns and passage into breast milk. *Br J Clin Pharmacol.* 1984;18:453

236. Fidler J, Smith V, DeSwiet M. Excretion of oxprenolol and timolol in breast milk. *Br J Obstet Gynaecol.* 1983;90:961

237. Leuxner E, Pulver R. Verabreichung von irgapyrin bei Schwangeren und Wocherinnen. *MMW.* 1956;98:84

238. Mirkin B. Diphenylhydantoin: placental transport, fetal localization, neonatal metabolism, possible teratogenic effects. *J Pediatr.* 1971;78:329

239. Ostensen M. Piroxicam in human breast milk. *Eur J Clin Pharmacol.* 1983;25:829

240. McKenzie SA, Selley JA, Agnew JE. Secretion of predisolone into breast milk. *Arch Dis Child.* 1975;50:894

241. Katz FH, Duncan BR. Entry of prednisone into human milk. *N Engl J Med.* 1975;293:1154

242. Pittard WB III, Glazier H. Procainamide excretion in human milk. *J Pediatr.* 1983; 102:631

243. Díaz S, Jackanicz TM, Herreros C, et al. Fertility regulation in nursing women, VIII: progesterone plasma levels and contraceptive efficacy of a progesterone-releasing vaginal ring. *Contraception.* 1985;32:603

244. Kunka RL, Venkataramanan R, Stern RM, et al. Excretion of propoxyphene and norpropoxyphene in breast milk. *Clin Pharmacol Ther.* 1984;35:675

245. Levitan AA, Manion JC. Propranolol therapy during pregnancy and lactation. *Am J Cardiol.* 1973;32:247

246. Karlberg B, Lundberg D, Aberg H. Excretion of propranolol in human breast milk. *Acta Pharmacol Toxicol.* 1974;34:222

247. Bauer JH, Pape B, Zajicek J, et al. Propranolol in human plasma and breast milk. *Am J Cardiol.* 1979;43:860

248. Kampmann JP, Johansen K, Hansen JM, et al. Propylthiouracil in human milk. revision of a dogma. *Lancet.* 1980;1:736

249. Findlay JWA, Butz RF, Sailstad JM, et al. Pseudoephedrine and triprolidine in plasma and breast milk of nursing mothers. *Br J Clin Pharmacol.* 1984;18:901

250. Hardell L-I, Lindstrom B, Lonnerholm G, et al. Pyridostigmine in human breast milk. *Br J Clin Pharmacol.* 1982;14:656

251. Clyde DF, Shute GT, Press J. Transfer of pyrimethamine in human milk. *J Trop Med Hyg.* 1956;59:277

252. Hill LM, Malkasian GD Jr. The use of quinidine sulfate throughout pregnancy. *Obstet Gynecol.* 1979;54:366

253. Horning MG, Stillwell WG, Nowlin J, et al. Identification and quantification of drugs and drug metabolites in human breast milk using GC-MS-COM methods. *Mod Probl Paediatr.* 1975;15:73

254. Werthmann MW, Krees SV. Quantitative excretion of senokot in human breast milk. *Med Ann DC.* 1973;42:4

255. Hackett LP, Wojnar-Horton RE, Dusci LJ, et al. Excretion of sotalol in breast milk. *Br J Clin Pharmacol.* 1990;29:277–278

256. Phelps DL, Karim A. Spironolactone: relationship between concentrations of dethioacetylated metabolite in human serum milk. *J Pharm Sci.* 1977;66:1203

257. Foulds G, Miller RD, Knirsch AK, et al. Sulbactam kinetics and excretion into breast milk in postpartum women. *Clin Pharmacol Ther.* 1985;38:692

258. Jarnerot G, Into-Malmberg MB. Sulphasalazine treatment during breast feeding. *Scand J Gastroenterol.* 1979;14:869

259. Berlin CM Jr, Yaffe SJ. Disposition of salicylazosufapyridine (Axulfidine) and metabolites in human breast milk. *Dev Pharmacol Ther.* 1980;1:31

260. Kauffman RE, O'Brien C, Gilford P. Sulfisoxazole secretion into human milk. *J Pediatr.* 1980;97:839

261. Chaiken P, Chasin M, Kennedy B, et al. Suprafen concentrations in human breast milk. *J Clin Pharmacol.* 1983;23:385

262. Lindberberg C, Boreus LO, DeChateau P, et al. Transfer of terbutaline into breast milk. *Eur J Respir Dis.* 1984;65:87

263. Tetracycline in breast milk. *Br Med J.* 1969; 4:791.

264. Posner AC, Prigot A, Konicoff NG. Further observations on the use of tetracycline hydrochloride in prophylaxis and treatment of obstetric infections. In: Welch H, Marti-Ibanez F, eds. *Antibiotics Annual* 1954–1955. New York, NY: Medical Encyclopedia Inc; 1955:594

265. Yurchak AM, Jusko WJ. Theophylline secretion into breast milk. *Pediatrics.* 1976;57:518

266. Anderson LW, Qvist T, Hertz J, et al. Concentrations of thiopentone in mature breast milk and colostrum following an induction dose. *Acta Anaesthesiol Scand.* 1987;31:30

267. Williams RH, Kay GA, Jandorf BJ. Thiouracil: its absorption, distribution, excretion. *J Clin Invest.* 1944;23:613

268. Von Kobyletzki D, Dalhoff A, Lindemeyer H, et al. Ticarcillin serum and tissue concentrations in gynecology and obstetrics. *Infection.* 1983;11:144

269. Moiel RH, Ryan JR. Tolbutamide (Orinase) in human breast milk. *Clin Pediatr.* 1967;6:480

270. Sagranes R, Waller ES, Goehrs HR. Tolmetin in breast milk. *Drug Intell Clin Pharm.* 1985; 19:55

271. Arnauld R. Etude du passage de la trimetho-prime dans le lait maternel. *Ouest Med.* 1972; 25:959

272. Miller RD, Salter AJ. The passage of trimetho-prim/sulpha-methoxazole into breast milk and its significance. Proceedings of the 8th International Conference of Chemotherapy, Athens. *Hellenic Soc Chemother.* 1974;1:687

273. Alexander FW. Sodium valproate and pregnancy. *Arch Dis Child.* 1979;54:240

274. Von Unruh GE, Froescher W, Hoffman F, et al. Valproic acid in breast milk: how much is real there? *Ther Drug Monit.* 1984;6:272

275. Anderson P, Bondesson U, Mattiasson I, et al. Verapamil and norverapamil in plasma and breast milk during breast feeding. *Eur J Clin Pharmacol.* 1987;31:625

276. Orme ML'E, Lewis PJ, deSwiet M, et al. May mothers given warfarin breast-feed their infant? *Br Med J.* 1977;1:1564

277. Pons G, Francoual C, Guillet P, et al. Zolpidem excretion in breast milk. *Eur J Clin Pharmacol.* 1989;37:245–248

278. Wild CP, Pionneau FA, Montesano R, et al. Aflatoxin detected in human breast milk by immunoassay. *Int. J Cancer.* 1987;40:328

279. Maxwell SM, Apeagyei F, de Vries HR, et al. Aflatoxins in breast milk, neonatal cord blood and sera of pregnant women. *J Toxicol Toxin Rev.* 1989;8:19–29

280. Zarba A, Wild CP, Hall AJ, et al. Aflatoxin M_1 in human breast milk from The Gambia, West Africa, quantified by combined monoclonal antibody immunoaffinity chromatography HPLC. *Carcinogenesis.* 1992;13:891–894

281. Steglink LD, Filer LJ Jr, Baker BL. Plasma, erythrocyte human milk levels of free amino acids in lactating women administered aspartame or lactose. *J Nutr.* 1979;109:2173

282. Mangurten HH, Kaye CI. Neonatal bromism secondary to maternal exposure to a photographic laboratory. *J Pediatr.* 1982;100:596

283. Radisch B, Luck W, Nau H. Cadmium concentrations in milk and blood of smoking mothers. *Toxicol Lett.* 1987;36:147

284. Miyazaki T, Akiyama K, Kaneko S, et al. Chlordane residues in human milk. *Bull Environ Contam Toxicol.* 1980;25:518

285. Resman BH, Blumenthal HP, Jusko WJ. Breast milk distribution of theobromine from chocolate. *J Pediatr.* 1977;91:477

286. Wolff MS. Occupationally derived chemicals in breast milk. *Am J Ind Med.* 1983;4:259

287. Egan H, Goulding R, Roburn J, et al. Organochlorine pesticide residues in human fat human milk. *Br Med J.* 1965;2:66

288. Quinby GE, Armstrong JF, Durham WF. DDT in human milk. *Nature.* 1965;207:726

289. Bakken AF, Seip M. Insecticides in human breast milk. *Acta Paediatr Scand.* 1976;65:535

290. Adamovic VM, Sokic B, Smiljanski MJ. Some observations concerning the ratio of the intake of organochlorine insecticides through food and amounts excreted in the milk of breast-feeding mothers. *Bull Environ Contam Toxicol.* 1978;20:280

291. Savage EP, Keefe TJ, Tessari JD, et al. National study of chlorinated hydrocarbon insecticide residues in human milk, USA. *Am J Epidemiol.* 1981;113.413

292. Wilson DJ, Locker DG, Ritzen CA, et al. DDT concentrations in human milk. *AJDC.* 1973;125:814

293. Bouwman H, Becker PJ, Cooppan RM, et al. Transfer of DDT used in malaria control to infants via breast milk. *Bull World Health Organ.* 1992;70:241–250

294. Emanuel B, Schoenfeld A. Favism in a nursing infant. *J Pediatr.* 1961;58:263

295. Simpson WJ, Tuba J. An investigation of fluoride concentration in the milk of nursing mothers. *J Oral Med.* 1968;23:104

296. Esala S, Vuori E, Helle A. Effect of maternal fluorine intake on breast milk fluorine content. *Br J Nutr.* 1982;48:201

297. Dreyfus-See G. Le passage dans le lait des aliments ou medicaments absorbes par denourrices. *Rev Med Interne.* 1934;51:198

298. Ando M, Hirano S, Itoh Y. Transfer of hexachlorobenzene from mother to newborn baby through placenta and milk. *Arch Toxicol.* 1985; 56:195

299. West RW, Wilson DJ, Schaffner W. Hexachlorophene concentrations in human milk. *Bull Environ. Contam Toxicol.* 1975;13:167

300. Rabinowitz M, Leviton A, Needelman H. Lead in milk and infant blood: a dose-response model. *Arch Environ Health.* 1985;40:283

301. Sternowsky JH, Wessolowski R. Lead and cadmium in breast milk. *Arch Toxicol.* 1985;57:41

302. Koos BJ, Longo LD. Mercury toxicity in the pregnant woman, fetus, and newborn infant: a review. *Am J Obstet Gynecol.* 1976;126:390

303. Amin-Zaki L, Elhassani S, Majeed MA, et al. Studies of infants post-natally exposed to methylmercury. *J Pediatr.* 1974;85:81

304. Pitkin RM, Bahns JA, Filer LA Jr, et al. Mercury in human maternal and cord blood, placenta, and milk. *Proc Soc Exp Biol Med.* 1976;151:565

305. Stegink LD, Filer LJ Jr, Baker GL. Monosodium glutamate: effect on plasma and breast milk amino acid levels in lactating women. *Proc Soc Exp Biol Med.* 1972;140:836

306. Miller RW. Pollutants in breast milk. *J Pediatr.* 1977;90:510

307. Rogan WJ, Bagniewska A, Damstra T. Pollutants in breast milk. *N Engl J Med.* 1980;302:1450

308. Wickizer TM, Brilliant LB, Copeland R, et al. Polychlorinated biphenyl contamination of nursing mothers in Michigan. *Am J Public Health.* 1981;71:132

309. Brilliant LB, Van Amburg G, Isbister J, et al. Breast milk monitoring to measure Michigan's contamination with polybrominated biphenyls. *Lancet.* 1978;2:643

310. Wickizer TM, Brilliant LB. Testing for polychlorinated biphenyls in human milk. *Pediatrics.* 1981;68:411–415

311. Bagnell PC, Ellenberg HA. Obstructive jaundice due to a chlorinated hydrocarbon in breast milk. *Can Med Assoc J.* 1977;117:1047

312. Higginbottom MC, Sweetman L, Nyhan WL. A syndrome of methylmalonic aciduria, homocystinuria, megaloblastic anemia neurologic abnormalities in a vitamin B_{12}-deficient breast-fed infant of a strict vegetarian. *N Engl J Med.* 1978;299:317

Viruses in Human Milk

Jan Riordan

Mother-to-infant transmission, a passage of infection known as *vertical transmission,* can occur during pregnancy, birthing, and the postpartum period through breastfeeding. Specific concerns about viral diseases and possible transmission through breastfeeding include the risks from mothers who acquire an infection while breastfeeding and the risks from mothers who acquired an infection during or before pregnancy. Questions abound: Which viruses are found in the milk of infected or seropositive women? What is the risk of transmission of such viruses by breastfeeding? What effect does the infection have on the child? Do protective maternal antibodies in the milk limit transmission or reduce the severity of viral infection in the child? Is there an effective treatment for the mother or the baby? This chapter seeks to answer these questions, although we recognize that there are no simple answers to the complex puzzle of viral transmission from mother to infant.

Antibodies, interferon, and white blood cells in human milk, nature's most perfect vaccine model, play a vital role in protecting the suckling young from viral infections. At the same time, a variety of animal and human viruses can be transmitted through mothers' milk (Ruff, 1994). Because breastmilk is a highly cellular fluid and viruses are intracellular (i.e., live within the cell), the passage of viruses through milk is possible. The transmission of cytomegalovirus (CMV) through breastmilk, for instance, which occurs frequently, provides a natural vaccine that confers active immunity to the infant against infection. In contrast, hepatitis B virus and rubella virus appear in human milk, but breastfeeding does not appear to be a common mode of transmission for either. The opposite is true of human immunodeficiency virus (HIV) and human T-cell lymphotropic virus type I (HTLV-1). Both are transmitted by breastmilk, with potentially adverse effects on the child.

Human Immunodeficiency Virus

Transmission of HIV to a fetus during pregnancy can occur as early as the eighth week. About one-half of perinatally transmitted infection from non-breastfeeding women occurs shortly before or during delivery. Breastfeeding may increase the rate of transmission above that related to fetal exposure by 8 to 18 percent. Public health policy on mother-to-child HIV transmission is being largely reevaluated, because it was found that anti-retroviral therapy is profoundly effective in preventing perinatal transmission. The results from a placebo-controlled clinical trial indicated that administration of zidovudine (AZT) to HIV-infected pregnant women and their newborns reduced the risk for perinatal transmission of HIV by approximately two-thirds (Connor et al., 1994). Routine HIV testing and counseling to all pregnant women, and AZT administration to those who are HIV positive is now considered the standard of care in the United States. The goal is to reduce perinatal transmission to less than 2 percent.

Laboratory Tests

HIV is one of the envelope viruses known as *retroviruses*. Standard tests for HIV that detect anti-HIV immunoglobulin A (IgA) antibody (enzyme immunoassay or Western blot) are of little use in diagnosing HIV infection in children younger than 18 months as *all* babies born to infected mothers have high HIV antibody levels. Tests that can detect HIV or part of its genetic material are HIV culture, polymerase chain reaction (PCR), and the p24 antigen test. All three tests have a high specificity for HIV, with few false-positive results (Benson, 1994). PCR is now considered the standard of care, along with HIV culture, for HIV detection in young infants; however, such testing is expensive, so few developing countries offer testing to the general population.

What We Know in the Late 1990s

HIV infection and acquired immune deficiency syndrome (AIDS) are the most serious threat to worldwide public health since the poliomyelitis epidemics earlier in the twentieth century. More than one-half of the estimated 8 million virus carriers worldwide live on the African continent. The number of AIDS cases in the developed world began to explode sometime in the late 1970s, particularly among the U.S. male homosexual population. Formerly considered a "gay" or drug abusers' disease in the developed world, AIDS is also a woman's disease, as evidenced by the annual increase in the number of HIV-infected women. More than 4 in 10 HIV-infected people are women, and this number is rising at a faster rate than that of men. An estimated 1,000 to 2,000 HIV-infected infants are born annually in the United States (Centers for Disease Control [CDC], 1995).

Early concerns about the safety of breastfeeding by HIV-positive women were modulated by evidence that anti-HIV properties in human milk may diminish transmission (Belec et al., 1990; Malaviya et al., 1992). A study in Zaire, for example, found no difference in HIV transmission between infants of seropositive mothers who had breastfed and those who had not (Ryder, 1989, 1991). Also, transmission rates in developing countries (25–48 percent) and in poor communities were higher than those in more industrialized, affluent areas (13–32 percent) (Newell & Peckham, 1994).

As more controlled studies were published, investigators reported that breastfeeding is associated with an increased risk of HIV transmission. In women who were already infected before they became pregnant, an additional risk of 8 to 18 percent was attributed to breastfeeding. If a mother became infected postnatally while breastfeeding, the risk of transmission rose to 26 to 29 percent (Dunn et al., 1992; Van de Perre, 1995).

Mother-to-infant HIV transmission rates vary depending on the number of risk factors involved. Factors associated with an increased risk of transmission are the presence of cells infected by HIV, low CD4+ T-lymphocyte counts, low vitamin A levels, premature rupture of the membranes, and an immunodeficiency in the mother (Boyer et al., 1994; Ryder et al., 1989; Van de Perre et al., 1995).

A vast amount of AIDS research is being conducted, especially in the United States, where millions of dollars have been allocated to researchers. Some investigations are promising. Newburg et al. (1992) identified a possible "blocking" factor in human milk that inhibits the binding of HIV on the CD4 receptor and thus impairs viral entry into the cells. More studies are needed to evaluate transmission rates according to type of feeding. Human milk lipids appear to inactivate enveloped viruses, and some fatty acids found in human milk are efficient antiviral agents (Begin, 1989; Isaacs & Thormar, 1990; McDougal, 1991). In testing antiviral activity of human milk, Isaacs and Thormar (1990) showed that all enveloped viruses exposed to antiviral milk lipids or milk stomach contents were inactivated, including herpes simplex virus type 1 (HSV-1), CMV, and HIV-1. These perplexing areas of study beg additional examination.

The World Health Organization (WHO)/ United Nations Childrens' Fund (UNICEF) consultants acknowledged in 1992 that breastfeeding was associated with HIV transmission (WHO, 1992). They advised that where infectious disease was not a primary cause of infant death, women known to be HIV-1 infected should be advised not to breastfeed (AAP, 1992). Where the primary causes of infant death were infections and malnutrition, breastfeeding should continue to be protected, promoted, and supported. These recommendations are similar to those of the WHO published in 1987 (WHO, 1987) and of the CDC in 1985. See Box 7–1.

Several mathematical models have been presented that estimate infant mortality in developing countries in the presence and in the absence of breastfeeding (Del Fante et al., 1992; Heymann, 1990; Hu et al., 1992; Kennedy et al., 1990; Lederman, 1992). Kennedy et al. (1990) estimate that deaths from HIV infection through breastfeeding could number between 1,000 and 19,000 annually. By contrast, deaths due to diseases of infancy that occur in the absence of breastfeeding range from 10,000 to 75,000 in a year's time. Another decision-analysis model demonstrated that in communities in which the HIV prevalence rate among mothers reaches 40 percent, breastfeeding should still be recommended in the absence of HIV screening unless HIV transmission via breastmilk surpasses 30 percent (Heymann, 1990). Nagelkerke et al. (1995; see also Kuhn & Stein, 1997) calculated that, in *developing countries,* the duration of breastfeeding that minimizes mortality is between three and seven months. These researchers suggest that HIV-1 mothers discontinue breastfeeding between three and seven months to preserve the benefits of breastfeeding but to reduce future HIV-1 transmission.

It is important to bear in mind that these models apply consistently in circumstances in which infant mortality and risks from artificial feeding are high. In more affluent, industrialized environments in which infant mortality is low, AZT therapy is available, and manufactured baby milk can be supplied cleanly, bottle-feeding by known HIV-infected mothers would increase child survival. In environments with moderate HIV-1 prevalence, moderately high risks from artificial feeding, and limited availability of antiretroviral therapy, the effects of feeding policies for HIV-infected mothers are more difficult to predict (Nicoll et al., 1994). In every setting, the final decision rests with the mother.

Clinical Implications

The most important medications for treating HIV are AZT and protease inhibitors, which block one step of HIV's reproductive cycle. Both medications sharply reduce the risk of transmission from mother to infant. AZT given in a combined regimen to the mother during pregnancy and during labor and to the infant after birth reduces the transmission rate of HIV by two-thirds (AAP, 1997; Bryson, 1996; Cotton, 1994; Fiscus et al., 1996; Matheson et al., 1995). The following factors, other than AZT treatment, may affect transmission of HIV through breastfeeding:

- *Maternal virus load:* The higher the virus load, the greater the risk of transmission; therefore, transmission of HIV-1 to children through breastfeeding is more likely for mothers who seroconvert while breastfeeding (Bryson, 1996; Mulder et al., 1996).

- *Duration of breastfeeding:* Duration of breastfeeding may be related to rate of transmission, but these data are not consistent. According to two studies (Datta et al., 1992; de Martino et al., 1994), children who breastfed for longer than 15 months were at increased risk for developing HIV-1 infection, presumably from continuing postnatal exposure through breastfeeding. Ekpini et al. (1997) found that babies breastfed longer than 6 months were at greater risk of seroconverting than those children who breastfed less than 6 months. However, a study by Guay et al. (1996) found that the duration of breastfeeding (>15 months) and the transmission rate of HIV were not associated.

- *Prenatal maternal infection:* Transmission of HIV is more likely if the mother was infected before the baby's birth; most postnatal transmission through breastfeeding occurs early in lactation.

- *Cesarean birth:* HIV transmission in children delivered by cesarean birth may be lower as compared with those delivered vaginally (Villari et al., 1993).

- *Maternal seropositivity:* The seropositive mother may, as her condition deteriorates, increase the risk of transmission through her milk (Van de Perre, 1991).

BOX 7–1

Joint United Nations Programme on HIV-AIDS (UNAIDS): HIV and Infant Feeding–An Interim Statement

The number of infants born with HIV infection is growing every day. The AIDS pandemic represents a tragic setback in the progress made on child welfare and survival. Given the vital importance of breast milk and breast-feeding for child health, the increasing prevalence of HIV infection around the world, and the evidence of a risk of HIV transmission through breast-feeding, it is now crucial that policies be developed on HIV infection and infant feeding.

The following statement provides policymakers with a number of key elements for the formulation of such policies.

THE HUMAN RIGHTS PERSPECTIVE

All women and men, irrespective of the HIV status, have the right to determine the course of their reproductive life and health, and to have access to information and services that allow them to protect their own and their family's health. Where the welfare of children is concerned, decisions should be made that are in keeping with children's best interests.

These principles are derived from international human rights instruments, including the Declaration of Human Rights (1948), the Convention on the Elimination of All Forms of Discrimination Against Women (1979), and the Convention on the Rights of the Child (1989), and they are consistent with the Cairo Declaration (1994) and the Beijing Platform for Action (1995).

PREVENTING HIV INFECTION IN WOMEN

The vast majority of HIV-infected children have been infected through their mothers, most of whom have been infected through unprotected heterosexual intercourse. High priority, therefore, now and in the long term, should be given to policies and programmes aimed at reducing women's vulnerability to HIV infection, especially their social and economic vulnerability–through improving their status in society. Immediate practical measures should include ensuring access to information about HIV/AIDS and its prevention, promotion of safer sex including the use of condoms, and adequate treatment of sexually transmitted diseases which significantly increase the risk of HIV transmission.

THE HEALTH OF MOTHERS AND CHILDREN

Overall, breast-feeding provides substantial benefits to both children and mothers. It significantly improves child survival by protecting against diarrhoeal diseases, pneumonia and other potentially fatal infections, while it enhances quality of life through its nutritional and psychosocial benefits. In contrast, artificial feeding increases risks to child health and contributes to child mortality. Breast-feeding contributes to maternal health in various ways including prolonging the interval between births and helping to protect against ovarian and breast cancers.

However, there is evidence that HIV–the virus that causes AIDS–can be transmitted through breast-feeding. Various studies conducted to date indicate that between one-quarter and one-third of infants born worldwide to women infected with HIV become infected with the virus themselves. While in most cases transmission occurs during late pregnancy and delivery, preliminary studies indicate that more than one-third of these infected infants are infected through breast-feeding. These studies suggest an average risk for HIV transmission through breast-feeding of 1 in 7 children born to, and breast-fed by, a woman living with HIV (i.e., infected with HIV).

Additional data are needed to identify precisely the timing of transmission through breast-feeding (in order to provide mothers living with HIV with better information about the risks and benefits of early weaning), to quantify the risk attributable to breast-feeding, and to determine the associated risk factors. Studies are also needed to assess other interventions for reducing mother-to-child transmission of HIV infection.

ELEMENTS FOR ESTABLISHING A POLICY ON HIV AND INFANT FEEDING

1. Supporting breast-feeding

As a general principle, in all populations, irrespective of HIV infection rates, breast-feeding should continue to be protected, promoted and supported.

2. Improving access to HIV counseling and testing

Access to voluntary and confidential HIV counseling and testing should be facilitated for women and men of reproductive age, in part by ensuring a supportive environment that encourages individuals to be informed and counseled about their HIV status rather than one that discourages them out of fear of discrimination or stigmatization.

As part of the counseling process, women and men of reproductive age should be informed of the implications of their HIV status for the health and welfare of their children.

Counseling for women who are aware of their HIV status should include the best available information on the benefits of breast-feeding, on the risk of HIV transmission through breast-feeding, and on the risks and possible advantages associated with other methods of infant feeding.

3. Ensuring informed choice

Because both parents have a responsibility for the health and welfare of their children, and because the infant feeding method chosen has health and financial implications for the entire family, mothers and fathers should be encouraged to reach a decision together on this matter. However, it is mothers who are in the best position to decide whether to breast-feed, particularly when they alone may know their HIV status and wish to exercise their right to keep that information confidential. It is therefore important that women be empowered to make fully informed decisions about infant feeding and that they be suitably supported in carrying them out. This should include efforts to promote a hygienic environment, essentially clean water and sanitation, that will minimize health risks when a breast-milk substitute is used.

When children born to women living with HIV can be ensured uninterrupted access to nutritionally adequate breast-milk substitutes that are safely prepared and fed to them, they are at less risk of illness and death if they are not breast-fed. However, when these conditions are not fulfilled, in particular in an environment where infectious diseases and malnutrition are the primary causes of death during infancy, artificial feeding substantially increases children's risk of illness and death.

4. Preventing commercial pressures for artificial feeding

Manufacturers and distributors of products which fall within the scope of the

| **BOX 7-1** | **(cont.)** |

International Code of Marketing of Breast-milk Substitutes (1981) should be reminded of their responsibilities under the Code and continue to take the necessary action to

ensure that their conduct at every level conforms to the principles and aim of the Code.

Source: Weekly Epidemiological Record, 71(Sept 27):289–91, 1996.

- *High-risk practices that might increase exposure to HIV:* Uninfected mothers who are breastfeeding should be especially careful to avoid high-risk practices (e.g., drug abuse or a sexual partner who is bisexual or has engaged in practices linked to HIV transmission) that might expose them to a primary HIV infection (Dunn et al., 1992; Van de Perre, 1991).

Practitioners who work with human milk or with breastfeeding women are rightly concerned about their own protection. In 1987, the CDC published a document that recommended precautions to be used when handling blood and body fluid of all patients regardless of their infection status. These universal precautions apply to blood and other body fluids that contain visible blood (e.g., semen and vaginal secretions). Universal precautions *do not apply* to human milk unless it contains visible blood (CDC, June 24, 1988). Occupational exposure to human milk has not been implicated in the transmission of HIV. Gloves are not needed when touching the breasts (e.g., in breast assessment), and they usually are not necessary for handling breastmilk, either. However, if the health care worker comes into frequent contact with human milk, (e.g., while working in human milk banking), he or she may choose to wear gloves (CDC, 1987). Also, if the mother has an open wound on her breast, glove wearing is warranted for the protection of both the mother and her care provider.

Gloves are routinely worn by staff during delivery, for newborn care until the infant has been washed and dried, and for a suckling assessment. Vigorous hand washing by the care provider—both before and after any physical contact with a client or with any body fluid—is standard practice for

infection control and should be performed consistently to prevent transmission of *any* infection in the mother, the child, and the health care worker. As discussed in Chapter 24, pasteurization is now advised for all pooled breastmilk and should eliminate any risk of transmission of HIV, making unnecessary HIV antibody screening of donors.

U.S. Public Health Service Recommendations

With proven reduction of HIV infection from AZT treatment, the U.S. Public Health Service (USPHS) now recommends routine HIV counseling and voluntary testing for all pregnant women (CDC, 1995). HIV counseling and testing offers prevention to both uninfected and infected women and their infants. Diagnosis of HIV infection before or during pregnancy allows women to make informed decisions regarding prevention of perinatal transmission. Knowledge of HIV serostatus allows early identification of the HIV-exposed infant. Prompt identification is essential for optimal treatment. About 10 to 20 percent of perinatally infected children develop rapidly progressive disease and die by 24 months. USPHS recommendations issued in 1995 include the following (CDC, 1995):

- *Voluntary testing:* Health providers should ensure that all pregnant women are counseled and encouraged to be tested for HIV infection to allow women to know their infection status both for their own health and to reduce the risk for perinatal HIV transmission.

- *Counseling regarding the risk for HIV infection,* the risk for transmission to the woman's infant if she is infected, and the availability of therapy to reduce this risk.

- *Providing information concerning AZT therapy* to reduce the risk for perinatal HIV transmission. This information should address the potential benefit and short-term and long-term safety of AZT therapy.

- *Advising HIV-infected women in developed countries not to breastfeed* to reduce the risk for HIV transmission to their infants.

To optimize medical management, the USPHS also recommends that HIV test results be made available to a woman's health care provider and be included on both her and her infant's confidential medical records. After consent has been obtained, the USPHS recommends that the provider notify the pediatric care provider. Identification of newborn babies who test positively for HIV is a controversial topic that has triggered vigorous debate. In New York, for example, testing is performed on all newborn babies, but the tests are anonymous, and mothers and their doctors do not know the results. Such a policy of nondisclosure could prevent early identification and treatment that might significantly prolong children's lives. However, identification might jeopardize the privacy rights of the mother and her child. These ethical and legal issues must continue to be addressed.

Counseling

Voluntary testing implies that women will know their infection status and receive counseling if they are found to be HIV-1 infected. Care must be taken, however, to ensure that all women tested for HIV-1 are given sufficient information to make informed decisions regarding continuation of their pregnancies and the mode of feeding they intend to use (Nicoll et al., 1994).

All women who are seropositive for HIV are advised to defer pregnancy. Pregnant women who are HIV positive will most likely begin the pregnancy as asymptomatic carriers and develop additional symptoms as the pregnancy progresses. Although the recommendation for women who are seropositive is to defer pregnancy, Fekety (1989, p. 255) reports three realities in practice:

Clients who have tested positive prior to the pregnancy fail to effectively contracept; clients whose sero status is unknown until early pregnancy testing is performed do not elect, for a host of reasons, to terminate the pregnancy; or prenatal testing may be delayed to a point in gestation where termination, even if desired, is not possible.

A primary concern of women at risk for AIDS relates to infecting their unborn children. Most at-risk women interviewed by Williams (1990) were sure they would transmit AIDS to their unborn children. They greatly feared the results of antibody testing. One woman in the study was so afraid of being told her test results that she continued her pregnancy without that information.

HIV-infected women come from all walks of life; some are not drug abusers or prostitutes and are victims themselves. Whatever the direct cause of their illness, their lives are shattered by the knowledge that they are HIV positive, which may be disclosed when their babies are born or when their spouses become ill or die. Often they feel dirty, useless, unwanted, and unlovable (Wofsy, 1987). Although they desperately need help from family, friends, and other support groups, they may be isolated because HIV is a "secret" disease. They suffer profound grief over the loss of their health, their sexuality, their chance to have more children, and their ability to breastfeed safely. Their counseling needs are necessarily complex, because these women must make difficult decisions while trying to cope with the implications of HIV for themselves and their families. When offering counseling, the care provider must recognize that children are central to many of these women's lives and they are reluctant to forgo childbearing (Lindberg, 1995; Williams, 1990).

Herpes Simplex

HSV-1, caused by *Herpesvirus hominus,* is a common viral infection in humans. HSV-1 is most serious during pregnancy and in the neonate. Herpetic lesions can erupt anywhere in the body, including the breast or the genital area, usually as a result of direct contact. The infection may be either primary or recurrent. Diagnosis is made either by culturing the lesion or by drawing serum-antibody titers.

The painful mucocutaneous blisterlike vesicles of herpes can appear within a few hours or up to 20 days after exposure. After the lesions heal, the virus enters a dormant phase and resides in the nerve ganglia in the affected area. Usually the primary infection is the most severe. Neonatal HSV-1 infection is usually acquired when the newborn passes through an infected genital tract; congenital infection is responsible for the most serious illness in neonates. Vaginal delivery is safe in most women with a history of recurrent genital herpes unless active lesions are present at term. As an indiscriminate preventive strategy, cesarean section is ineffective and expensive and exposes the mother and fetus to unjustifiable risks (Brown, 1995).

The seriousness of HSV-1 infection appears to be age-related. Neonates may become seriously ill; beyond the first few weeks of the neonate's life, however, there are few adverse consequences. Despite the high prevalence of genital herpes in the general population, the incidence of neonatal herpes is low and ranges from 1 in 2,000 to about 1 in 10,000 births (Brown, 1995). It is doubtful that neonatal herpes is transmitted through human milk. Transmission during breastfeeding, if it occurs, is most likely from direct contact with the herpes vesicle on the breast (Oxtoby, 1988; Quinn & Lofberg, 1978; Sealander & Kerr, 1989; Sullivan-Bolyai et al., 1983).

Sealander and Kerr (1989) report a case of a nursing toddler transmitting HSV to the mother through breastfeeding. In this case, the child's oral lesions (on the inner aspect of the lower lip) caused painful blisters on the mother's nipples. Culture of the child's oral lesions and the mother's nipple lesions were positive for HSV-1. After one week's cessation of breastfeeding, during which the mother was given oral acylclovir–200 mg five times daily for five days–the mother resumed breastfeeding. The authors recommended that whenever a young child develops oral HSV lesions, the mother should be asked whether she is breastfeeding this child, in order that the risk of contracting HSV from her child can be explained and appropriate intervention offered.

Sullivan-Bolyai et al. (1983) reported a case of a mother with a maternal breast lesion identified as HSV-1. Although her infant experienced an uneventful nursery course and was discharged from the hospital at two days of age, the mother reported developing a "skin sore" on the areola of her left breast during her postpartum stay. On the fourth day of life, the baby appeared to have pustules in the corner of his mouth and on his chin. On days six and seven, HSV was isolated from the mouth of the infant; on day seven, the virus was isolated from the mother's breast lesions also. The infant died at 11 days of age. This case points out the need to avoid direct infant contact with an HSV-1 lesion. Although the mother's milk may be free of the virus, the lesion itself is not. In another case, the milk from the mother of an infected infant was found to contain HSV; however, it appeared that the transmission had probably occurred at delivery, and it was unknown whether the infant became infected by the mother or the mother became infected by the infant (Duckle, Schmidt, & O'Connor, 1979).

Although HSV-1 can occasionally be cultured from breastmilk, this appears to be rare (Oxtoby, 1988). HSV-1 has not been isolated in any of the CMV studies that used culture techniques appropriate for HSV-1 (Pass, 1986a), and no role in transmitting infection in the absence of a local HSV-1 lesion has been demonstrated. Breast lesions are seldom the first clinical evidence of herpes in the family (Sullivan-Bolyai et al., 1983). The primary herpetic lesion can be manifested in other family members who then pass it on (e.g., the father while making love with the mother, or a sibling who kisses a baby brother or sister). Therefore, transmission can be from mother to infant or from infant to mother; or some other family member can infect the infant, who then passes the virus on to the mother during feedings.

Women with herpetic lesions on their breasts should refrain from breastfeeding; active lesions should be covered (AAP, 1997). In the absence of breast lesions, the newborn of a mother with HSV-1, if the baby is well, may breastfeed and be with the mother in her room; however, scrupulous hand washing, gowning, and covering of any lesions must be practiced to prevent possible cross-contamination. The mother does not need to wear rubber gloves while breastfeeding.

Treatment is usually directed toward symptomatic relief and prevention of a secondary infection, because there is no known cure for HSV (Table 7–1). Two antiviral drugs, acyclovir (Zovirax) and vidarabine, are specifically indicated for HSV infections. Aggressive and early use of intravenous acyclovir results in apparent improvement for the mother and infant. Acyclovir can be given orally (Sealander & Kerr, 1989), applied topically, or given intravenously (usually for treating neonatal HSV). Vidarabine is given by intravenous infusion as an alternative to acyclovir treatment (Spencer et al., 1989). Cleaning affected areas with povidone-iodine (Betadine) solution is thought to help prevent a secondary infection, and applying Burrow's solution (aluminum acetate) may relieve some of the discomfort. Vitamin C or lysine and lysine supplements are frequently suggested to prevent recurrence, although their efficacy is unknown (Olds et al., 1988).

Chickenpox

Most people have had chickenpox (varicella-zoster virus) and have lifelong immunity. The incubation period is usually 14 to 16 days. Lesions begin on the neck or trunk and spread to the face, scalp, mucous membranes, and extremities. Lesions first appear as small, flat, red blotches and progress to raised vesicles that form crusts over a period from two to four days. A varicella vaccine was licensed for use in the United States in early 1985. The varicella-zoster DNA has been detected in breastmilk, suggesting the possibility of mother-to-infant transmission (Yoshida et al., 1992).

Because chickenpox can occur during the reproductive years, a woman may develop this infection while she is breastfeeding. If a mother contracts chickenpox while breastfeeding, she should continue to breastfeed, because the antibodies in her milk confer immunity against chickenpox to her baby. This passive immunization may even spare the breastfed baby symptoms of chickenpox; if the disease is contracted, the course of the infant's disease is usually mild (Berman, 1982).

If the mother has never had chickenpox, she will have no antibodies in her breastmilk to protect the baby against chickenpox. A mother who develops chickenpox several days before she delivers her baby presents a special, complex medical case that can be potentially life-threatening. In this case,

the mother and baby should be isolated separately if the neonate does not develop lesions. Only about 50 percent of exposed infants will develop the disease. The mother should express breastmilk if the baby is housed elsewhere. If the baby has lesions, the baby can be isolated with the mother, and breastfeeding may occur uninterruptedly.

Two cases of varicella-zoster are described by Frederick, White, and Braddock (1986). In the first case, a 33-year-old mother developed classic herpetiform lesions on her left back and side. The breast was not involved. Expressed milk obtained within 24 hours of the appearance of the lesions revealed no varicella-zoster virus. Breastfeeding continued from both breasts, with slight position changes to avoid direct infant contact with the lesions. The infant remained healthy throughout the course of the mother's illness. The second case involved a mother who developed chickenpox at 40 weeks' gestation after contracting the virus from her older child. No history of chickenpox was noted, and she developed severe pulmonary problems due to varicella pneumonia. After an emergency cesarean section, this mother's healthy infant was treated prophylactically with varicella-zoster immune globulin and parenteral acyclovir. The mother was isolated, and her infant was not put to breast because of the mother's extensive cutaneous lesions and the danger of neonatal varicella infection from contact with the mother. During the mother's isolation, the baby remained healthy, and lactation was sustained through breast pumping.

According to Mohrbacher and Stock (1997), there is no benefit of delaying breastfeeding after the mother is no longer contagious. If the mother develops lesions four days before birth, the mother and baby can breastfeed on the child's second day with no risk of contagion if the mother's lesions have crusted.

Cytomegalovirus

Cytomegalovirus (CMV), another herpesvirus, is probably the most prevalent infection in the TORCH group. Almost half of all adults have antibodies for CMV, which provide evidence of an infection at some point in their lives. The incidence of CMV antibody in young children is highest in developing countries and in countries in which

Table 7–1

CLINICAL CARE PLAN FOR BREASTFEEDING MOTHER WITH HERPES SIMPLEX VIRUS (HSV) INFECTION

Problem	Intervention	Rationale
Seropositive for HSV	Encourage continued breastfeeding unless breast lesions are present.	Provides protective antibodies to infant
Herpes	Instruct mother to wash hands thoroughly with soap before breastfeeding.	Helps prevent spreading infection
No breast lesion	Caution mother against touching baby or breast after touching lesion from any site.	Avoid risks of shedding
	Caution mother to avoid tub bath with infant; use universal precautions (hospital staff).	Avoid risks of shedding
Breast lesion present	Discourage breastfeeding from affected breast; encourage use of breast pump to maintain comfort and milk supply; after each use, sterilize pump part that comes in contact with breast lesion.	Prevents infant's direct contact with lesion
Pain	Administer acetaminophen.	Analgesia
	Apply Burrow's solution topically.	Soothing effect
	Employ imagery.	Distraction by focusing
Feelings of shame	Reassure mother that HSV occurs frequently.	Mothers tend to blame themselves
Secondary infection	Cleanse lesion with Betadine.	Antibacterial
Recurrence	Recommend vitamin C supplements.	Possibly prevents recurrence
	Ensure that antiviral medication is taken as prescribed.	

communal child care and breastfeeding are common (Yow et al., 1987). The virus can be found in the breast, genital tract, urine, and pharynx and is transmitted by any close contact. As with other herpesviruses, it remains in host cells indefinitely. CMV can be transmitted through human milk; in fact, breastfeeding has proven to be an important means of conveying passive immunity to CMV, a so-called natural immunization.

In Japanese children whose mothers were seropositive, mother-to-child CMV transmission was 64.7 percent if the child was breastfed, as compared to 27.6 percent if bottle-fed (Minamishima et al., 1994). Breastfed children thus immunized to CMV by breastfeeding are protected later in life from symptomatic infection and from primary infection during pregnancy, which can cause intrauterine tissue damage (Pass, 1986b). Other studies (Dworsky et al., 1983; Peckham et al., 1987) show a mother-to-infant transmission of CMV in the majority of infants. Premature infants, particularly if they are seronegative, are at risk for serious illness if they acquire CMV. Pasteurization of milk appears to inactivate CMV; freezing milk at −20°C (−4°F) will decrease vital titers but does not reliably eliminate CMV; therefore, premature infants should receive only banked human milk from seronegative donors.

It is relevant that primates delivered by cesarean birth and bottle-fed are free of antibodies for simian CMV, thereby eliminating natural protection to the next generation, whereas primates captured in the wild are seropositive for their own CMV (Minamishima, Graham, & Melnick, 1971). Extrapolating this simian model to the human, a combination of a cesarean birth and artificial feeding may bypass the natural protection of mother-to-infant transmission of antibodies.

Rubella

Because rubella in the first trimester of pregnancy causes serious birth defects, the uninformed person might be unduly concerned that rubella in human milk is likewise deleterious. Although the rubella virus can be passed through maternal milk lymphocytes to the infant, there is no evidence that the baby who acquires rubella in this manner becomes ill (Losonsky et al., 1982). As with CMV, transmission of maternal antibodies against rubella, though at lower levels, is beneficial to the infant by serving as a natural vaccine (Adu & Adeniji, 1995).

If the mother is immunized to rubella postpartum, the breastfeeding infant will develop antibodies to rubella but will not show symptoms of the disease. Buimovici-Klein et al. (1977) describe a case in which the mother developed a rash, glandular swelling, and fever 12 days after postpartum vaccination. The infant had no clear antibody response; however, one year later when the child was immunized, his antibody response suggested that he had sometime earlier acquired the virus. In another case (Klein, Byrne, & Cooper, 1980), a breastfeeding mother developed a rubellalike rash 8 days after a normal birth; 18 days before the onset of the rash, she had been in close contact with a person with a clinically diagnosed case of

rubella. Her newborn daughter was followed for signs of rubella. The mother stopped breastfeeding for the first 2 days of her rash but resumed without incident on the third day. Her daughter remained clinically well, without sign of infection. The American Academy of Pediatrics (1997, p. 75) states, "Women with rubella, or those who have just been immunized with rubella live-attenuated virus vaccine need not refrain from breastfeeding."

Hepatitis B

Hepatitis B virus (HBV) causes a systemic illness that involves the liver. The patient may be asymptomatic or may experience anything from mild flu-like symptoms to a fulminating illness. HBV is usually transmitted by contact with infected blood or body secretions or through transfusion of contaminated blood. Contamination of the mucous membranes during the birth or during sexual intercourse is another method of transmission. Approximately 5 to 15 percent of pregnant women with HBV will infect their babies before labor begins. The vast majority of exposure occurs during or immediately preceding labor, so that immunoprophylaxis and vaccination in the early postnatal period have an excellent chance of preventing infection. Medical and birthing centers routinely screen for HBV from umbilical-cord blood. Indicators of HBV are the presence of hepatitis B_e antigen (HB_eAg) in the blood, serological testing for antibody to the hepatitis B surface antigen (HB_sAg), and the hepatitis B virus DNA probe (HBV DNA). Hepatitis B vaccination is recommended for all infants as part of the routine childhood immunization schedule.

Infants born to an HBV-positive mother, already exposed to maternal blood, amniotic fluid, and vaginal secretions during delivery, may breastfeed (Krugman, 1985; Peter et al., 1994). The neonate should receive hepatitis B immunoglobulin (HBIG) within 12 hours after birth, followed by a series of injections of HBV vaccine: the first during the first week, the second at one month, and the third at six months. All infants should undergo pediatric follow-up including repeated screening for HB_sAg to rule out chronic carriers. Most untreated infants of HB_sAg- and HB_eAg-positive mothers will develop active hepatitis and become chronic carriers.

Several investigators have examined the risk to the breastfeeding infant if the mother is infected. Lee, Ip, and Wong (1978) found that after immunization of 447 infants born to mothers who were positive for the hepatitis B antigen, infection was somewhat higher in the infants born vaginally as compared with those delivered by cesarean section (24.9 percent versus less than 10 percent). At birth, none of the newborns delivered by cesarean, compared with 13 of the 67 infants born vaginally, were positive for HBV DNA. The investigators concluded that the risk of infection to the infants was diminished if cesarean section was performed. Follow-up with administration of passive antibodies from HBIG vaccine further reduces the risk of infants born to infected mothers.

Tseng, Lam, and Tam (1988) report that there is no evidence that breastfeeding will increase the risk of HBV infection in infants, regardless of their immunization status. There were no differences in the rate of development of antigenemia or immunity against hepatitis B between the breastfed and bottle-fed babies during the first year of life, and almost all infants were HB_sAg-positive at one year of age, regardless of how they were fed. These researchers concluded that there was "no valid contraindication for breastfeeding in infants born to HB_sAg-positive mothers," especially if the infants were immunized soon after birth.

De Martino et al. (1987) followed 47 breastfed and 112 formula-fed infants born to mothers who were positive for HB_sAg. No difference was observed between the groups regarding the percentage of infants who seroconverted. Seven months after birth, the formula-fed infants developed transient but significantly higher anti-HB_sAg levels, as compared with the breastfeeding infants. The authors speculate that suppressive factors in human milk and orally induced tolerance (55 percent of the milk samples were found to have detectable HB_sAg) may contribute to this suppression.

Breastfeeding does not appear to increase the rate of infection among infants. Moreover, in areas of high prevalence of HBV and environmental exposure, lack of breastfeeding places the infant at greater risk of contracting the disease.

Hepatitis C

Hepatitis C (HCV), a viral infection of the liver, accounts for about 80 percent of cases of non-A, non-B posttransfusion hepatitis. HCV is associated with a high risk for developing chronic liver disease and is spread through blood-to-blood contact. Vertical transmission is believed to be less than 10 percent and depends on the viral load level during the pregnancy. The interval from the onset of hepatitis to seroconversion to anti-HCV antibody is 4 to 32 weeks (Alter et al., 1994).

Breastfeeding in the presence of HCV is a controversial topic; however, the benefits to the infant's health relative to the potential for HCV infection favor continued breastfeeding (AAP, 1997; Mohrbacher & Stock, 1997). In many countries, including Australia, health authorities do not recommend avoidance of breastfeeding for women who are HCV-positive, especially if the titer levels are not high (Grayson et al., 1995).

Several studies support continued breastfeeding. Although HCV can be found in breastmilk, infection through breastfeeding appears to be infrequent. Kage et al. (1997) identified hepatitis C virus in saliva but not in the breastmilk of the 11 HCV carrier mothers they followed. These investigators found no evidence of viral transmission through breastfeeding. In a study of 40 breastfeeding mothers who were HCV-positive, all infants were HCV RNA-negative according to the PCR test, and maternally acquired anti-HCV antibodies disappeared by 9 months in 78 percent of the infants (Fischler et al., 1996). Ho-Hsiung et al. (1995) found that none of 15 infants of HCV-infected mothers who were fed human milk for up to 4 months had HCV infection by one year of age, probably because of one or more of the following:

- The amount of HCV in the colostrum may be so low as to be unable to infect the newborn infant.

- The amount of HCV in the colostrum may be easily inactivated in the gastrointestinal tract.

- The integrity of the oral and gastrointestinal mucosa may effectively preclude HCV infection via the oral route.

Table 7–2

Viruses in Milk

Virus	Transmission Through Milk	Associated Disease	Breastfeeding
Chickenpox	Probably not	None apparent	Permitted unless mother develops chickenpox several days before delivering baby
Cytomegalovirus	Proven	None	Permitted; protective effect
Hepatitis B	Unknown	Hepatitis	Permitted if infant and mother have HBIG and HB_sAg
Hepatitis C	Proven	Unknown	Permitted if titers are not high
Herpes simplex	Probably not	Disseminated herpes possible in neonate	Permitted if no lesions on the breast
HIV	Possibly	AIDS	Not in developed countries
HTLV-1	Probably	Leukemia or lymphoma	Not permitted
Rubella	Proven	None	Encouraged; protective effect

HIV, human immunodeficiency virus; HTLV-1, human T-lymphotropic virus type 1; AIDS, acquired immunodeficiency syndrome; HBIG, hepatitis B immunoglobulin; HB_sAg, hepatitis B surface antigen.

Source: Derived from Mohrbacher N, Stock J: The breastfeeding answer book *(rev ed.). Schaumburg, IL: La Leche League International, 1997; RF Pass, Viral contamination of milk. In: Goldman AS, Atkinson SA, Hanson A, eds.* Human lactation 3: the effects of milk on recipient infant. *New York: Plenum, 1986:279–87; and AJ Ruff: Breastmilk, breastfeeding, and transmission of viruses to the neonate.* Semin Perinatol *18:510–6, 1994.*

Human T-Lymphotropic Virus

HTLV-1, endemic in the Caribbean Islands and certain parts of Japan and Africa, is linked with adult T-cell leukemia and lymphoma. This virus is rare in the United States, but American women who are seropositive should not breastfeed (AAP, 1997).

Although breastfed babies of HTLV-1-infected mothers are more likely to become infected (20–25 percent) than are artificially fed infants (3 percent) (Kinoshita et al., 1987; Lal et al., 1993), the duration of breastfeeding appears to be critical to the child's development of the disease. Children who are breastfed for a long period (more than seven months) are more likely to develop HTLV-1 infection than are those breastfed for a shorter period (CDC, 1985). Several Japanese studies substantiate this finding. The seroconversion rate of infants

breastfed short-term (fewer than seven months) was nearly equal to that of bottle-feeders: 4.4 percent (4 of 90 cases) versus 5.7 percent (9 of 158 cases) (Takahashi et al., 1991). Similarly, Oki et al. (1992) established that the seroconversion rate of short-term breastfeeders was nearly equal to that of bottle-feeders: 3.8 percent to 5.6 percent in 885 HTLV-1-seropositive pregnant women. Hino et al. (1995; see also Takezaki et al., 1997) also found that antibody titers in short-term breastfeeders were about the same as those in bottle-feeders.

Thus breastfeeding that extends after disappearance of the maternal antibody appears to be an important risk factor for mother-to-child transmission of HTLV-1. Children born to seropositive carrier mothers passively acquire maternal antibodies prenatally that gradually disappear by nine months of age. Thus babies who breastfeed for a long time would still be exposed to HTLV-1-infected lymphocytes from breastmilk after the passively acquired high-titer antibodies disappear from their circulation.

Implications for Practice

Breastfeeding infants do develop viral infections, but their illnesses are usually less serious than similar infections in nonbreastfed infants. Acquisition of their own antibodies via breastmilk is critical to an infant's survival after his or her level of protective maternal antibodies begins to decrease. A viral infection in the mother rarely requires terminating breastfeeding (Table 7–2). From a practical standpoint, the infant has already been exposed to the virus, usually transplacentally and during the birth process. The only antibody protection that is available to the infant is from the mother's milk as a result of her infection. If the mother is well enough to care for her baby and the infant does not require special care, mother and baby should stay in the same hospital room. The concern of health care providers should be directed not at mothers known to have an infection but at those with an unidentified infection.

For the breastfeeding mother with a viral disease, isolation precautions should be used while she is hospitalized. If the infant's mother tests positively for HBV or other viruses, scrupulous hand washing and gowning are routinely practiced to prevent possible cross-contamination. Although antiseptic soaps for hand washing will more effectively kill organisms, no data prove that infection rates vary depending on whether plain or antiseptic soap is used. The mother does not need to wear rubber gloves while breastfeeding. The most effective ways to prevent the spread of infections among neonates, parents, and staff is for staff to maintain body-substance precautions and to teach others to do so also (Larson, 1987).

A new mother is already under stress. The news that she has a viral infection, which may or may not be considered a sexually transmitted disease, may cause her to feel pain, anger, and guilt. These feelings can be compounded by a fear that she should not breastfeed her baby. Encouraging the mother to express her fears, answering her questions, and then supporting her desires is a vital contribution that the nurse or lactation consultant can make to her care and well-being.

SUMMARY

Toward the end of pregnancy, the fetus receives passive immunity from the mother; the baby is, therefore, born with the mother's immunities. Breastfed infants acquire additional antibodies to influenza, mumps, chickenpox, and other viruses, either through the mother's clinical exposure or through immunization. This passive immunity lasts from three to six months and protects the infant from childhood diseases. Concern about the risk of viral transmission through breastmilk appears to be limited to HIV and HTLV-1. Thus, for all other viral infections, breastfeeding should continue except in the case of a mother who has a herpetic lesion on her breast.

The possibility of HIV transmission by human milk has had a negative effect on breastfeeding that is as yet unmeasured. In developing countries, where artificial feeding is often lethal, this effect is a major concern (Cutting, 1994). Even if antiretroviral treatment is available, such medications and artificial feeding are expensive. On the basis of realistic costs, decisions must be made as to whether individual families' incomes and countries' scarce foreign currency can support these high costs (Nicoll et al., 1994). Before large-scale testing is initiated or required, the rights of women and the care of HIV-infected women must be considered.

REFERENCES

Adu FD, Adeniji JA: Measles antibodies in the breast milk of nursing mothers. *Afr J Med Sci* 24:385–8, 1995.

Alter HJ: Transmission of hepatitis C virus—route, dose and titer. *N Engl J Med* 330:784–6, 1994.

American Academy of Pediatrics. *1997 Red book: report of the Committee on Infectious Diseases,* 24th ed. Elk Grove Village, IL: American Academy of Pediatrics, 1997:73–9.

American Academy of Pediatrics, Committee on Pediatric AIDS: Human milk, breastfeeding, and transmission of human immunodeficiency virus in the United States. *Pediatrics* 96:977–9, 1992.

Begin M: Possible role of polyunsaturated fatty acids in the pathogenesis of AIDS. *Arch AIDS Res* 4:93–104, 1989.

Belec L, et al: Antibodies to human immunodeficiency virus in the breast milk of healthy, seropositive women. *Pediatrics* 85:1022–6, 1990.

Benson MS: Management of infants born to women infected with the human immunodeficiency virus. *J Perin Neon Nurs* 7:79–89, 1994.

Berman A: Varicella and breast feeding [letter]. *J Fam Pract* 15:617–20, 1982.

Boyer PJ, et al: Factors predictive of maternal-fetal transmission of HIV-1: preliminary analysis of zidovudine given during pregnancy and/or delivery. *JAMA* 271:1925–30, 1994.

Brown ZA: Preventing transmission of herpes simplex to newborns. *Contemp Nurse Pract* Sept–Oct: 29–35, 1995.

Bryson YJ: Perinatal HIV-1 transmission; recent advances and therapeutic interventions. *AIDS* 10(suppl 3):S33–42, 1996.

Buimovici-Klein E, et al: Isolation of rubella virus in milk after postpartum immunization. *J Pediatr* 6:939–41, 1977.

Centers for Disease Control: Recommendations for assisting in the prevention of perinatal transmission of human T-lymphotrophic virus type III

lymphadenopathy–associated virus and acquired immunodeficiency virus. *MMWR* 34:721–26, 1985.

Centers for Disease Control: Recommendations for prevention of HIV transmission in health care settings. *MMWR* 36(suppl 25), 1987.

Centers for Disease Control: Update: universal precautions for prevention of transmission of human immune deficiency virus, hepatitis B virus, and other bloodborne pathogens in health-care settings. *MMWR* 37:378–87, 1988.

Centers for Disease Control: U.S. Public Health recommendations for human immunodeficiency virus counseling and voluntary testing for pregnant women. *MMWR* 44(RR-7):81–84, 1995.

Connor EM, et al: Reduction of maternal-infant transmission of human immunodeficiency virus type 1 with zidovudine treatment. *N Engl J Med* 331:1173–80, 1994.

Cotton P: Trial halted after drug cuts maternal HIV transmission rate by two thirds. *JAMA* 271:807, 1994.

Cutting WA: Breast-feeding and HIV—a balance of risks. *J Trop Pediatr* 40:6–11, 1994.

Datta P, et al: Resumption of breast-feeding in later childhood: a risk factor for mother to child human immunodeficiency virus type 1 transmission. *Pediatr Infect Dis* 11:974–6, 1992.

Del Fante P, et al: HIV, breast-feeding and under-5 mortality: modelling the impact of policy decisions for or against breast-feeding. *J Trop Med Hyg* 96:203–11, 1993.

de Martino M, et al: Different degree of antibody response to hepatitis B virus vaccine in breast- and formula-fed infants born to HB$_S$Ag-positive mothers. *J Pediatr Gastroenterol Nutr* 6:208–11, 1987.

de Martino M, et al: HIV-1 transmission of human immunodeficiency virus type 1: report from the Nairobi study. *J Infect Dis* 170:134–40, 1994.

Duckle LM, Schmidt R, O'Connor DM: Neonatal herpes simplex infection possibly acquired via maternal breast milk. *Pediatrics* 63:250–1, 1979.

Dunn DT, et al: Risk of human immunodeficiency virus, type 1, transmission through breastfeeding. *Lancet* 340:585–8, 1992.

Dworsky M, Yow MY, Stagno S, et al: Cytomegalovirus infection of breast milk and transmission in infancy. *Pediatrics* 72:295–9, 1983.

Ekpini ER, et al: Late postnatal mother-to-child transmission of HIV-1 in Abidjan, Cote d'Ivoire. *Lancet* 349(9058):1054–59, 1997.

Fekety SE: Managing the HIV-positive patient and her newborn in a CNM service. *J Nurse Midwifery* 34:253–8, 1989.

Fischler B, et al: Vertical transmission of hepatitis C virus infection. *Scand J Infect Dis* 28:353–6, 1996.

Fiscus SA, et al: Perinatal HIV infection and the effect of zidovudine therapy on transmission in rural and urban counties. *JAMA* 275:1504–6, 1996.

Frederick IB, White RJ, Braddock SW: Excretion of varicella-herpes zoster virus in breast milk. *Am J Obstet Gynecol* 154:1116–7, 1986.

Grayson M, et al: Breastfeeding and the risk of vertical transmission of hepatitis C virus. *Med J Aust* 163:107–9, 1995.

Guay LA, et al: Detection of human immunodeficiency virus type 1 (HIV-1) DNA and p24 antigen in breast milk of HIV-1 infected Ugandan women and vertical transmission. *Pediatrics* 98:438–44, 1996.

Heymann SJ: Modeling the impact of breast-feeding by HIV-infected women on child survival. *Am J Public Health* 80:1305–9, 1990.

Hino S, et al: Association between maternal antibodies to the external envelope glycoprotein and vertical transmission of human T-lymphotropic virus type 1. *J Clin Invest* 95:2920–5, 1995.

Ho-Hsiung L, et al: Absence of infection in breast-fed infants born to hepatitis C virus-infected mothers. *J Pediatr* 126:589–91, 1995.

Hu DJ, et al: HIV infection and breast-feeding: policy implication through a decision analysis model. *AIDS* 6:1505–13, 1992.

Isaacs CE, Thormar H: Human milk lipids inactivate enveloped viruses. In: Atkinson SA, Hanson

LA, Chandra RK, eds. *Breastfeeding, nutrition, infection and infant growth in developed and emerging countries.* St. John's, Newfoundland: ARTS Biomedical Publishing, 1990: 161–74.

Kage M, et al: Hepatitis C virus RNA present in saliva but absent in breast-milk of the hepatitis C carrier mother. *J Gastroenterol Hepatol* 12:518–21, 1997.

Kennedy KI, et al: Do the benefits of breastfeeding outweigh the risk of postnatal transmission of HIV via breastmilk? *Trop Doct* 20:25–9, 1990.

Kinoshita K, et al: Milk-borne transmission of HTLV-I from carrier mothers to their children. *Jpn J Cancer Res* 78:674–80, 1987.

Klein EB, Byrne T, Cooper LZ: Neonatal rubella in a breast-fed infant after postpartum maternal infection. *J Pediatr* 97:774–5, 1980.

Krugman S: Viral hepatitis: 1985 update. *Pediatr Rev* 7(1): 3–10, 1985.

Kuhn L, Stein Z: Infant survival, HIV infection, and feeding alternatives in less-developed countries. *Am J Public Health* 87:926–31, 1997.

Lal RB, et al: Evidence for mother-to-child transmission of human T-lymphotropic virus type II. *J Infect Dis* 168:586–91, 1993.

Larson E: Trends in neonatal infections. *JOGNN* 16:404–9, 1987.

Lederman SA: Estimating infant mortality from human immunodeficiency virus and other causes in breast-feeding and bottle-feeding populations. *Pediatrics* 89:290–6, 1992.

Lee AK, Ip HM, Wong VC: Mechanisms of maternal-fetal transmission of hepatitis B virus. *J Infect Dis* 138:668–71, 1978.

Lindberg CE: Perinatal transmission of HIV: how to counsel women. *Matern Child Nurs J* 20:207–12, 1995.

Losonsky GA, et al: Effect of immunization against rubella on lactation products: I. Development and characterization of specific immunologic reactivity in breast milk. *J Infect Dis* 145:661–6, 1982.

Malaviya AN, et al: Circumstantial evidence of HIV transmission via breastmilk [letter]. *J Acq Immune Defic Synd* 5:102, 1992.

Matheson PB et al: Efficacy of antenatal zidovudine in reducing perinatal transmission of human immunodeficiency virus type 1. *J Infect Dis* 172:353–8, 1995.

McDougal JS: Pasteurization of human breast milk and its effect on HIV infectivity. *AMBANA Newsl* 7, Winter 1991.

Minamishima I, et al: Role of breast milk in acquisition of cytomegalovirus infection. *Microbiol Immunol* 38:549–52, 1994.

Minamishima Y, Graham BJ, Melnick MB: Neutralizing antibodies to cytomegaloviruses in normal simian and human sera. *Infect Immun* 4:368–73, 1971.

Mohrbacher N, Stock J: *The breastfeeding answer book* (rev ed.). Schaumburg, IL: La Leche League International, 1997.

Mulder DQ, et al: Post-natal incidence of HIV-1 infection among children in a rural Ugandan population: no evidence for transmission other than mother to child. *Trop Med Int Health* 1:81–5, 1996.

Nagelkerke JD, et al: The duration of breastfeeding by HIV-1 infected mothers in developing countries: balancing benefits and risks. *J Acq Immune Defic Synd Hum Retrovirol* 8:176–81, 1995.

Newburg DS, et al: A human milk factor inhibits binding of human immunodeficiency virus to the CD4 receptor. *Pediatr Res* 31:22–8, 1992.

Newell ML, Peckham C: Vertical transmission of HIV infection. *Acta Paediatr Suppl* 400:43–5, 1994.

Nicoll A, Newell ML, Praag EV: Infant feeding policy and practice in the presence of HIV-1 infection. *AIDS* 9:107–19, 1994.

Oki T, et al: A sero-epidemiological study on mother-to-child transmission of HTLV-1 in Southern Kyushu, Japan. *Asia Oceania J Obstet Gynaecol* 44:371–7, 1992.

Olds S, London ML, Ladewig PA: *Maternal-newborn nursing,* 3rd ed. Menlo Park, CA: Addison-Wesley, 1988:237–8.

Oxtoby MJ: Human immunodeficiency virus and other viruses in human milk: placing the issues in broader perspective. *Pediatr Infect Dis* 7:825–35, 1988.

Pass RF: Transmission of viruses through human milk. In: Howell RR, Morriss FG, Pickering LK, eds. *Human milk in infant nutrition and health.* Springfield, IL: Thomas, 1986a:205–23.

Pass RF: Viral contamination of milk. In: Goldman AS, Atkinson SA, Hanson A, eds. *Human lactation 3: the effects of milk on recipient infant.* New York: Plenum, 1986b:279–87.

Peckham CS, et al: Early acquisition of cytomegalovirus infection. *Arch Dis Child* 62:780–5, 1987.

Peter G, et al, eds: *1994 Red Book: American Academy of Pediatrics: Report of the Committee on Infectious Diseases,* 23rd ed. Elk Grove Village, IL: American Academy of Pediatrics, 1994.

Quinn PT, Lofberg JV: Maternal herpetic breast infection: another hazard of neonatal herpes simplex. *Med J Aust* 2:411–2, 1978.

Ruff AJ: Breastmilk, breastfeeding, and transmission of viruses to the neonate. *Sem Perinatol* 18:510–6, 1994.

Ryder RW, et al: Evidence from Zaire that breast-feeding by HIV-1 seropositive mothers is not a major route for perinatal HIV-1 transmission but does decrease morbidity. *AIDS* 5:709–14, 1991.

Ryder RW, Nsa W, Hassig SE: Perinatal transmission of the human immunodeficiency virus type 1 to infants of seropositive women in Zaire. *N Engl J Med* 320:1637–42, 1989.

Sealander JY, Kerr CP: Herpes simplex of the nipple: infant-to-mother transmission. *Am Fam Pract* 39:111–3, 1989.

Spencer RT, et al: *Clinical pharmacology and nursing management,* 3rd ed. Philadelphia: Lippincott, 1989:252–5.

Sullivan-Bolyai JS, et al: Disseminated neonatal herpes simplex virus type 1 from a maternal breast lesion. *Pediatrics* 71:455–7, 1983.

Takahashi K, et al: Inhibitory effect of maternal antibody on mother-to-child transmission of human T-lymphotrophic virus, type 1. *Int J Cancer* 49:673–7, 1991.

Takezaki T, et al: Short-term breast-feeding may reduce the risk of vertical transmission of HTLV-1. The Tsushima ATL Study Group. *Leukemia* 11(suppl 3):60–62, 1997.

Tseng RYM, Lam CWK, Tam J: Breastfeeding babies of HB$_S$Ag-positive mothers. *Lancet* 2(8618): 1032, 1988.

Van de Perre P: Postnatal transmission of human immunodeficiency virus type 1: the breast-feeding dilemma. *Am J Obstet Gynecol* 173:483–7, 1995.

Van de Perre P: Postnatal transmission of human immunodeficiency virus type 1 from mother to infant: a prospective cohort study in Kigali, Rwanda. *N Engl J Med* 325:593–8, 1991.

Villari P, et al: Cesarean section to reduce perinatal transmission of human immunodeficiency virus. A meta analysis. *Online J Curr Clin Trials* 74, 1993.

WHO. *Consensus statement from the WHO/ UNICEF consultation on HIV transmission and breastfeeding.* Geneva: Global Programme on AIDS (WHO/GPA/INF/92.1), 1992.

Williams AB: Reproductive concerns of women at risk for HIV infection. *J Nurse Midwif* 35:292–8, 1990.

Wofsy CB: Intravenous drug abuse and women's medical issues. *Report of the Surgeon General's Workshop on children with HIV infection and their families.* [USDHHS publ. no. HRS-D-MC 87–1]. 1987:32–3.

Yoshida M, et al: Case report: detection of varicella-zoster virus DNA in maternal breast milk. *J Med Virol* 38:108–19, 1992.

Yow MD, et al: Acquisition of cytomegalovirus infection from birth to 10 years: a longitudinal serologic study. *J Pediatr* 110:37–42, 1987.

Prenatal, Perinatal, and Postnatal Periods

Educating parents and professionals about breastfeeding leads to better care and a more satisfying experience. Clinical care during pregnancy, the interpartum and the immediate postpartum, the imprimatur of lactation consulting, is best when caring, knowledge, and clinical skills merge. Most breastfeeding infants are born at or near term and are healthy.

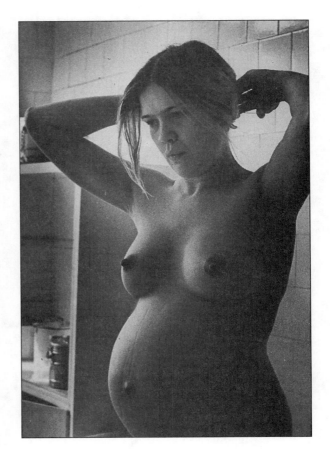

Some babies grow poorly when breastfed. Is this a problem deriving from the mother, the baby, or both? How can it be resolved without compromising the breastfeeding relationship? Although not premature, some breastfeeding babies become ill. Jaundice is an outcome of early extrauterine life. How it is managed can influence the breastfeeding course, often negatively and unnecessarily. Too often, breastfeeding succumbs to technologically based decisions designed to help the baby survive in the short term without also considering his needs or those of his mother in the long term. Those who are born early or at risk represent a small percentage of the total, yet they require major caretaking by their mothers and the caregivers assisting them. When mothers encounter difficulties while breastfeeding, more than the infants' opportunity to receive breastmilk can be affected. These chapters highlight the breastfeeding baby's needs and how they can be met—even in situations that do not at first appear to be conducive to continued breastfeeding.

CHAPTER 8

Breastfeeding Education

Debi Leslie Bocar and Jan Riordan

Education is the cornerstone supporting the framework of lactation and breastfeeding. This chapter provides the health care provider with tools to fashion meaningful educational experiences for breastfeeding families and colleagues. Two types of programs are addressed: those aimed at assisting families in having a positive breastfeeding experience and those designed to increase the knowledge base of the health care providers so that they can effectively assist with breastfeeding. Because education permeates all activities in the field of breastfeeding, isolating the educational component is an enormous challenge. This chapter addresses a broad range of educational issues, from theory to practical application. An overview of research related to breastfeeding education is provided, along with strategies for teaching adult learners.

In traditional societies, an inexperienced woman turns to her mother, aunts, or grandmothers for emotional support during childbearing and breastfeeding. Breastfeeding "education" involves lifelong immersion in a culture in which seeing a baby at breast is a normal, welcome sight. Even though formal breastfeeding and parent education is common in many parts of the world, it is still only a replacement for a time-honored family function.

The dramatic decrease in breastfeeding in industrialized societies during the first half of the twentieth century reduced the number of mothers who could share their breastfeeding experiences.

Over time, expectant mothers were less likely to see an infant breastfeed or to know someone who could provide practical assistance. Geographical mobility further isolated young families from traditional support networks. Into the vacuum came alternative support systems for the few women who chose to breastfeed. Self-help groups such as La Leche League International, Nursing Mothers Association of Australia, and childbirth education groups began to organize. They flourished worldwide, providing accurate information, practical assistance, and emotional support for breastfeeding families using a mother-to-mother approach.

As breastfeeding rates increased, health care systems began to offer formal breastfeeding assistance. Hospitals, clinics, health maintenance organizations, and medical practice groups increasingly offer classes of all types to parents, siblings, and grandparents. Although the primary purpose of these programs is educational, they are also effective public relations techniques for attracting families to those institutions. In an era in which health care agencies are increasingly competitive, patient-client education can be an effective marketing strategy. Shifts in the U.S. health care industry affect breastfeeding education of parents. Third-party reimbursement rewards birth settings from which patients are discharged quickly. When families leave the hospital or birthing center within hours or days after birth, teaching opportunities shift to prenatal education or postdischarge follow-up.

Educational programs for health professionals and lactation consultants have proliferated along with parent education. Several medical centers and academic institutions regularly offer systematic training in lactation management to health professionals. Some programs offer completion certificates or titles, such as breastfeeding educator. These programs, as well as many high-quality, one-day and two-day seminars offered throughout the world, are useful preparation for individuals seeking to improve their knowledge of breastfeeding. Many individuals also seek certification by the International Board of Lactation Consultant Examiners (IBLCE), Inc.

Lactation training through distance learning is a growing area. Distance learning enjoys a rich heritage, beginning when the printing press met the pony express. Because breastfeeding courses have limited audiences, distance education offers a way for people to "attend" a course without leaving their home area. Breastfeeding Support-Consultants of Philadelphia has offered long-distance education since the mid-1980s. The first Internet course on breastfeeding came on-line in 1997 from Wichita State University School of Nursing. Modeled after the long-distance CNEP (Community-Based Nurse-Midwifery Education Program) Midwifery program, it is taught entirely through the Internet. As of this writing, nearly 2,000 lactation consultants take part in an Internet discussion group called LACTNET. In daily posts, LACTNET participants seek and receive help with difficult clinical cases and discuss current issues that relate to breastfeeding. LACTNET is a cross between having a daily coffee klatch with friends and attending a leading-edge clinical seminar on breastfeeding.

Learning Principles

Learning is most effective when individuals are ready to learn (i.e., when they feel a need to know something) (Redman, 1988). "Teachable moments" refer to those periods when learners perceive the need for information and skills. Motivation is further enhanced when the material to be learned is organized in a manner that makes it meaningful to the learner. Activities that are novel and interesting encourage learning. Active, rather than passive, participation is associated with more meaningful and permanent learning (Brillinger, 1990; Darkenwald & Merriam, 1982). Learning is divided into three domains, and breastfeeding education incorporates all three (Bloom, 1956):

- Cognitive skills (gathering information, linking concepts, problem solving)
- Psychomotor skills (listening to instructions, observing skills, repetitive practice, mastery of skill performance)
- Affective learning (modifying attitudes, values, and preferences)

Individual learning styles should also be considered when planning teaching strategies (Dunn, 1979). Some participants learn primarily through auditory perceptions; they listen intently and remember what they hear. Others learn best visually and retain information about what they see. These learners benefit from visual aids and printed materials (Fig. 8–1). A third mode of learning is kinesthetic or psychomotor learning. Kinesthetic learners benefit from touching and handling equipment and models. Most learners use all three modalities. Therefore, in teaching about breast pumps, learning is strengthened by discussion coupled with the showing of slides that demonstrate how pumps work and by having the learners manipulate the equipment themselves.

Because success is predictably more motivating than is failure, dividing tasks and information into easily mastered segments keeps the adult learners motivated to continue the program. Learners respond to specific descriptions of their positive performance. Praise enhances feelings of self-confidence and conveys respect for the learner.

Adult Education

Adult learners differ widely from children in their learning styles. Unlike children, who are required to attend school, adults are self-directed when they choose to attend educational activities (Knowles, 1980). Adults perceive time as one of their most valued and scarce assets, and they are not willing to

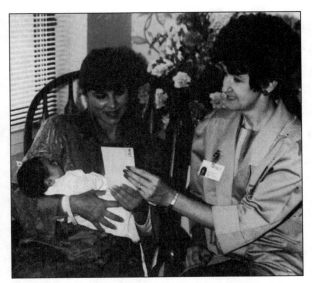

FIGURE 8–1. *Pamphlets and other written materials reinforce one-to-one teaching. (Courtesy Debi Leslie Bocar.)*

spend it in meaningless activity. Education programs must, therefore, demonstrate a clear applicability to the adult's everyday life. For example, discussion of the anatomy of the breast and the physiology of breastfeeding is more meaningful when related directly to practical skills, such as latch-on techniques and how often to feed the baby.

Adult learners have a rich variety of backgrounds and motivations for participating in educational programs. They appreciate and expect respect as unique individuals. Adults know what they want to learn. If the instructor identifies what these personal learning needs are and fulfills them, learning occurs quickly and easily. Adult learning should be self-directed and provide feedback about the learner's progress toward achieving these goals. Parents should be considered "co-learners" in that they teach each other as well as the instructor, who will invariably learn at least one new piece of information at every class. Principles of adult education are easily applied to breastfeeding education using these approaches:

- Ensure that content and timing of teaching coincides with parents' "readiness" to learn (prior to conception, during pregnancy, immediately postbirth, later postpartum).

- Prioritize and present information in easily understood and easily mastered segments.

- Organize activities in increments to increase the likelihood of success.

- Give explicit instructions so that participants clearly understand what they are being asked to do.

- Provide specific, immediate feedback following each activity.

- Respect participants who do not perceive a topic as meaningful.

- Recognize the importance of body language and nonverbal communication.

- Recognize the social and recreational aspect of adult learning by providing refreshments and a relaxed atmosphere during breaks.

- Assist participants in focusing on their own activities, resourcefulness, and increased self-sufficiency.

- Use handouts and other media to reinforce and augment rather than to replace individualized assessment and teaching.

- Identify breastfeeding support resources, including telephone numbers of local resources.

There are several factors that enhance a positive learning climate for adult learners. Lighting, temperature, seating, the availability of writing surfaces furnished with paper and pencils, and the ability to view learning materials comfortably have a tremendous impact on learning (Darkenwald & Merriam, 1982). Adults appreciate physical comfort and knowing where drinks, food, and restroom facilities are located.

Adult education programs tend to be a social as well as a learning activity, because they afford opportunities to become acquainted with other adults. Greet each person warmly; demonstrate genuine concern for each one as an individual. Use first names if it seems appropriate. It is a good idea to structure break periods with refreshments to encourage socializing. Adults enjoy sharing informal learning activities with others, and successful programs encourage adults to have fun as they learn. Adults also expect teachers to value student opinions about the usefulness of learning activities. One way to find out what areas of the program were helpful is to request informal verbal feedback or formal written evaluations. Evaluations are important data to modify and improve programs.

Curriculum Development

Assessing learning needs is mandatory in working with adult learners. There must be a "match" between what the learner needs to know and what the teacher presents. If the teacher assumes that learners already possess a high level of knowledge, learners can be frustrated because the information is too complex. Conversely, learners may be offended if the instructor assumes they have minimal knowledge. Accurate assessment is essential in providing relevant information.

To assess levels of knowledge when working with small groups, the facilitator can ask non-threatening questions, such as, "What have you heard about breastfeeding?" In larger class settings, the content cannot be customized to each participant. Asking participants at the beginning of class what specific topics they would like to discuss helps to assess their learning needs and involves them in establishing the curriculum. If the topics are written on the blackboard as they are suggested, and each topic is crossed off as it is addressed, the participants are more likely to feel that their learning needs are respected.

In addition to the participants' perceived learning needs, critical breastfeeding knowledge and skills must be identified and included in the curriculum. Several organizational models can be used to organize curriculum (Posner & Rudnitsky, 1982):

- The *chronological model* presents information in the order of its usual occurrence. Thus prenatal nipple assessment precedes a discussion of the importance of early breastfeeding opportunities, which in turn precedes an explanation of positioning and latch-on techniques.
- The *utilization model* presents information when participants are likely to need it. Therefore, information on breastmilk expres-

sion techniques precedes discussion of the storage of breastmilk.

- Organizing content *from simple to complex* is also a helpful strategy. A lecture on simple infant cueing and latch-on techniques precedes one on difficult latch-on management. Preventive strategies for avoiding problems are covered before moving on to the management of existing problems. Thus a discussion on preventing nipple trauma precedes one on the treatment of sore nipples.
- *Moving from the general to the specific* places information in perspective. Discussing the concept of nutritional supplementation precedes an explanation of specific techniques for supplementation.
- *Proceeding from the known to the unknown* is helpful in relating new tasks to those already known, making the new task seem less difficult. For example, when teaching an alternative breastfeeding position, explain that cueing and latch-on are completed in the same manner as with a previous position.

The importance of a topic should be reflected in the time given to it, taking into consideration how frequently the information will be used. For example, positioning and latch-on are fundamental to breastfeeding and so deserve a more thorough discussion than does adoptive nursing, which is relevant to a much smaller group of learners.

Too much information at one time is overwhelming and prioritizing teaching is critical. Basic physiological requirements (e.g., adequacy of the infant's nutrient intake) help to guide prioritization. Health care providers also must be aware of additional family resources and defer some teaching for later health visits. Thus, when a family is in the birth setting, the health care provider may share with the mother that breastfeeding can continue when she is employed outside the home. However, specific techniques for doing so will be taught after breastfeeding is established.

The Change Process

Educating expectant families and breastfeeding mothers is a good beginning point for breastfeeding support. However, for mothers to have positive breastfeeding experiences, it is also necessary that practices in the birth setting assist, rather than hinder, early breastfeeding. Covey (1989) points out that common sense is not always common practice. Specific hospital practices are detrimental to the establishment of lactation. These include mother-infant separation, delay in initial breastfeeding, prelacteal feeds, complementary or supplementary bottle-feeding, prolonged intervals between feedings, and failure to give individual breastfeeding assistance. Changing such practices is essential to achieving goals of maximizing breastfeeding outcomes.

An understanding of the change process can help to accomplish a complex change that, though desirable, may nevertheless be resisted. According to Nyberg (1980), "planned change is a conscious, deliberate attempt to apply new knowledge in order to modify behavior or practices." The change agent must not only identify the desired outcome but also consider *how* to make the change.

Change is inevitable. Planned, rather than haphazard, change is characteristic of a professional approach. Planned change is characterized by a clearly defined goal (vision) and a systematic problem-solving approach (Galpin, 1996). Breaking the change process into small, attainable steps increases confidence and maintains enthusiasm in the team directing the change. Organizations and people are motivated to change when the dissatisfaction and frustration associated with the current situation (status quo) is greater than the resistance and discomfort associated with change. The change process can be thought of as a mathematical equation:

Dissatisfaction (with the status quo) + Vision (for change) + Small Steps = Change

Lewin (1951) noted that unfreezing the old status quo is necessary to initiate change. After change occurs, a new status quo develops that will be thawed during the next change process. Changes in the health care industry are unfreezing the status quo. The present is an opportune time to initiate change related to prenatal education, specialized assistance in the birth setting, follow-up telephone calls, home health care visits, and outpatient services for breastfeeding families.

Establishing a sense of urgency for the change by identifying crises, potential crises, or major opportunities helps to propel the change process (Kotter, 1996). Developing time lines for specific steps in the change process can provide short-term evaluation points. Deadlines create momentum. Time frames, however, must be realistic to avoid discouragement; change activities tend to take longer than expected. Celebrating small increments of change as steps toward the envisioned goal helps to maintain enthusiasm.

Assessing and planning for change are the most critical and the most time-consuming components of the change process. However, implementation is often the most challenging aspect because of the human tendency to resist change. Resistance to change is not inherently bad. It enables individuals and society to avoid destabilization and inefficiency, which could result from trivial or nonbeneficial change. Resistance also stimulates the change agent to convincingly support and modify, if necessary, the recommended innovation. Resistance to change can stem from threatened self-interest, inaccurate perceptions of the intended change, objective disagreement with the change, psychological reaction, or low tolerance for change (New & Couillard, 1981). Strategies frequently used to avoid change include: minimizing the problem ("It's not that bad"), focusing on distractions ("We have enough changes going on now"), and delaying action ("We'll address that later").

Numerous techniques are available for dealing with resistance to change. These include participation, coercion, manipulation, education, use of an external agent, incentives, supportive behavior, and gradual introduction (New & Couillard, 1981). The broken-record strategy, calmly repeating perceptions and desires ("I continue to see this problem . . . ," "It is significant because . . . ," "I think we should address it now") serves to make the issue visible to others and thus more likely to be addressed. Strategies, either singly or in combination, must be individualized to each situation. Common mistakes in attempting to implement change include ambiguous objectives, poorly defined strategies, and the use of a limited number of change agents and techniques.

An important strategy for change is to recruit the support of formal and informal leaders within the organization. The primary change agent should not "own the project." Rather, the change agent should involve a variety of participants in the change process–from initial assessment through planning, implementation, and evaluation (Garcia, 1996). People are more likely to support, rather than sabotage, a project that they helped to create. Planning should involve both supportive participants, who provide enthusiasm for the project, and nonsupportive participants, whose concerns should be considered early in the project.

The change process can be broken down into specific steps. The identification of these steps can help to accomplish desired change and includes the following steps in the process:

1. Assess the current situation, program, or practice.

2. Identify a focus of dissatisfaction with the current situation (unfreezing the status quo).

3. Recruit a wide base of support to form a task force or change group.

4. Establish a sense of urgency for change.

5. Develop a vision of change outcome, communicate the vision to all people involved, and ask for suggestions.

6. Identify small steps in the process (starting with challenges big enough to make a difference, small enough to be successful).

7. Select criteria to measure outcomes.

8. Develop a flow chart with a sequence of actions and target the time frame necessary to move the system from the present state to the desired state.

9. Assign specific individuals to lead each step.

10. Create support for the change agents, including self-renewal and activities that build enthusiasm.

11. Provide support, coordination, supervision, and resources to ensure performance of assignments.

12. Reinforce desired behaviors and directly address undesired behaviors (Carr et al., 1996).

13. Evaluate the process and outcomes.

14. Recognize accomplishments and celebrate achievements.

15. Revise the plan as necessary.

How professionals approach colleagues with proposed changes can affect how new ideas are received. One nonthreatening approach is to focus on improving patient care. It is helpful to point out the vulnerability of new parents. They become frustrated when encountering inconsistent recommendations from health care providers whom they regard as knowledgeable authorities. That frustration negatively influences parents' perceptions of the institution.

To facilitate change in presenting new ideas, credibility is important. This requires preparation involving thorough review and sharing of relevant literature, such as references, articles, and texts. It is best to identify specific recommendations rather than to present vague goals. Role playing with a supportive person can help to identify possible responses and barriers that the change agent may encounter and offers an opportunity for brainstorming and experimentation in a nonthreatening setting.

"Constructive confrontation" of colleagues is an approach in which one shares information and seeks input from another person in a way that respects that person's expertise. It helps to create a conducive time and private place for discussion; it is essential to be thoroughly prepared. Body language should reflect confidence rather than defensiveness or aggressiveness. The presenter should describe the problem situation with a patient-centered focus and avoid casting blame. The person or group addressed by the change agent should be asked to consider reference materials as they apply to the identified problem. A time is then set to meet again for further discussion. With the patient's optimal care as a shared goal, there need be no winner or loser among professional colleagues. Sharing, discussing, and asking for feedback demonstrate a belief in the abilities of one's colleagues and help to elicit mutual respect.

Parent Education

Facilitating the learning experience for parents requires an understanding of the tasks of adulthood

(Darkenwald & Merriam, 1982). People seeking breastfeeding assistance are couples involved in a major life change: acquisition of the parental role. There are four stages of transition into parenthood: anticipatory, formal, informal, and personal (Bocar & Moore, 1987). During the *anticipatory stage,* before the birth of the infant, expectant parents benefit from realistic information about infant care. It is important for parents to understand that, in the first weeks after the baby is born, they will experience loss of sleep, fatigue, and episodes of crying (by baby, mom, and possibly dad). In this phase, parents should be encouraged to perform in certain ways:

- Form realistic expectations of infant care.
- Identify responsibilities that they can relinquish to devote time and energy to infant care.
- Learn practical aspects of infant care (including psychomotor experiences with dolls or infants).
- Begin to identify philosophical approaches to child care (such as how they will respond to a crying infant).
- Learn about typical emotional responses to new parenthood so that their experiences can be placed in perspective.
- Review previous personal successful experiences to support self-confidence.
- Socialize with other new families to increase opportunities for incidental learning and for developing a support network.
- Identify community resources that can facilitate the transition into parenthood.

The *formal stage* begins with the birth of the infant. Parents are often surprised at their intense feelings about the responsibilities of parenthood. Although forming attachment bonds with their infant, they are simultaneously achieving parental roles. Attachment is enhanced if parents room in, which enables them to get acquainted with their baby (Anderson, 1989). Health care providers can also use the infant's given name frequently to personalize the infant.

Parental caretaking behavior is often characterized by rigidity as parents seek to perform psychomotor tasks "the one best way." They are often overwhelmed if given too many equally attractive alternatives in child care. They may become noticeably frustrated if they receive conflicting information during this phase of role acquisition. New parents often feel awkward and inadequate because they lack experience and confidence in caretaking skills. They often equate their performance of infant care with their ability to parent effectively. During this stage, new parents are extremely vulnerable to implied judgment of their caretaking abilities. They are quite sensitive to nonverbal communication regarding their performance. Health care providers and experienced parents are particularly powerful role models as the self-image of the new parents emerges. The most persistent feelings during such role transition are those of inadequacy and lack of self-confidence.

During this time, mothers are fatigued and feel overwhelmed. In the days immediately after giving birth, women have impaired cognitive function, particularly in memory function (Eidelman et al., 1993). Therefore, new parents benefit from simple, concrete instructions divided into easily mastered segments. Specific, positive feedback about their performance, coupled with an expression of confidence by someone whose opinion is important to them, can greatly enhance their self-confidence. They need frequent assistance in placing their experiences in perspective.

The *informal stage* begins when parents feel that they have mastered child-care tasks. Self-confidence increases as a person accrues successful experiences (Coopersmith, 1967). Several weeks or months are required by most parents to amass adequate positive experiences so that they can proceed to the informal stage of role acquisition. Health care providers are in a unique position to enhance parental self-confidence by providing enthusiastic praise of performance and reviewing positive experiences. The relatively restrictive behavior of the formal stage is replaced by a willingness to consider options. Behavior becomes more spontaneous and there is less fear of imperfection. A reassuring environment that supports experimentation and provides stimulation through a variety of role models enables parents to progress to the final stage of parental role acquisition.

During the *personal stage,* behaviors are further modified, so that a parental role style evolves that is consistent with the parents' personalities. Relinquishing the fantasy of being the "perfect parent" frees parents to develop a unique set of behaviors with which they are comfortable. Support groups and classes provide ideal social settings in which parents can share their personal child-care techniques and approaches with other parents, thus integrating their new parental role into their personalities (Fig. 8–2).

Because breastfeeding is considered instinctive by many mothers and health care providers, the need for knowledge about the process often remains unrecognized. Yet, as mothers encounter difficulties and abandon breastfeeding for readily available alternatives, the need for knowledge and expert assistance becomes more obvious. It is not enough to promote breastfeeding. Health care providers need to empower mothers to have positive breastfeeding experiences by increasing their knowledge of the practical aspects of the management of breastfeeding (Locklin & Naber, 1993; Shelton, 1994). Because a large volume of information is needed by mothers who have had little or no experience with breastfeeding, it is appropriate to present content in small segments over time. Breastfeeding education programs usually have three purposes:

1. to influence or to support prenatal decision making regarding infant feeding choice,

2. to provide practical information on management of lactation at the onset of the breastfeeding experience, and

3. to provide ongoing support after the initiation of breastfeeding.

Modifying attitudes, sharing knowledge, and teaching specific skills are essential components of breastfeeding education (Hanson, 1996).

Prenatal Education

Most mothers make decisions about how they will feed their baby before they become pregnant or during pregnancy. Pregnancy is an appropriate time to support a mother's decision to breastfeed, to correct inaccurate information, to add to the information she already has about breastfeeding, and to encourage undecided expectant mothers to

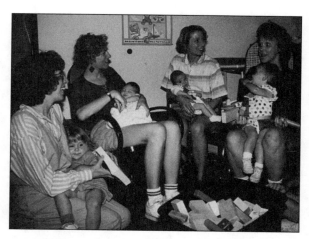

FIGURE 8–2. La Leche League meeting: *adult learning in action. (Courtesy Debi Leslie Bocar.)*

consider breastfeeding. Infant feeding should be discussed before mothers start feeling the baby's movements. (Quickening usually occurs around the fifth month of pregnancy.) When mothers begin to perceive their babies as separate beings, they start making concrete plans for care, including how they will feed their babies. Mothers need information about infant feeding before being asked, "How are you going to feed your baby?" Because of the influence of the baby's father or the mother's partner and other family members, breastfeeding education programs should include support persons by encouraging their attendance at classes and group meetings and by providing educational materials specifically directed to them (Freed et al., 1993b; Giugliani et al., 1994; Littman et al., 1994; Matich & Sims, 1992; Sciacca et al., 1995a).

Breastfeeding education programs during early pregnancy must describe the benefits of breastfeeding to both mothers and to infants. An awareness of the values in a particular culture is essential (Libbus, 1992). For instance, the primary reason given by women for selecting breastfeeding in certain cultures is its contraceptive effect. In other cultures, breastfeeding is selected primarily for the protective health benefits it affords the infant (Kocturk, 1988).

Breastfeeding programs designed to influence the decision to breastfeed must address maternal concerns, including those related to convenience, modesty, participation of the father in infant care and to incorporating breastfeeding into the mother's lifestyle, her return to employment, any previous negative experiences with breastfeeding by the mother or her peers, and contraceptive considerations (Grassley & Davis, 1978; Jones, 1987; Young & Kaufman, 1988). Educational programs instigated early in pregnancy must provide adequate information, so that expectant parents can make an informed choice regarding infant feeding. In addition, these programs should address specific maternal concerns, include support persons, and identify additional resources for information.

Early Breastfeeding Education

Toward the end of pregnancy, breastfeeding education appropriately focuses on the basics of breastfeeding initiation and management during the early days and weeks following the baby's birth. The site where mothers receive prenatal care is optimal for access to expectant mothers and their support people. Classes can be offered at times convenient to these families. Pamphlets and videos can be used by patients while they are waiting for appointments. Health care providers can also assess and add to the patients' knowledge during appointments. It is generally better to have frequent, short discussions about breastfeeding throughout the course of prenatal care rather than to attempt to say everything a mother may need to know in one breastfeeding talk. Free-standing classes can be provided by institutions and health care professionals in the community: hospitals, clinics, libraries, childbirth education programs, breastfeeding support groups, and lactation consultants.

The content of breastfeeding classes offered during pregnancy should include information necessary to initiate breastfeeding (e.g., timing of the first breastfeeding, positioning and assisting the infant to latch onto the breast, prevention of nipple trauma, management of engorgement, assessment adequate milk intake, and establishing, maintaining, and increasing milk supply [Box 8–1]). A variety of techniques can be used, including formal or informal classes, videos, and printed materials. Educational programs, however well developed, augment rather than replace the responsibility of the health care professional for individualized

assessment and one-to-one teaching specific to each breastfeeding family.

Supplying information about breastfeeding management is insufficient to ensure continual breastfeeding. Mothers still need expert assistance during the hours and days immediately after birth to acquire experiential skills. Dr. Audrey Naylor, Director of Wellstart in San Diego, CA, says, "Successful breastfeeding requires more than words of encouragement. It requires a continuum of skilled services designed to enhance the synchronous breastfeeding duet learned by the mother-infant couple" (Riordan, 1983).

Although mothers can have a positive breastfeeding experience at the birth setting, breastfeeding continuance is influenced by situations she encounters after she returns home. Given the mother's limited stamina and inability to retain large quantities of new information, care should be taken not to overwhelm families with the sheer volume of material. Prioritize the content of classes in the birth setting, from most important to least important. For example, information that relates to continuing breastfeeding and insuring infant well-being is most important, whereas information that pertains to returning to employment and weaning can be covered later.

Individualize the content based on the mother's concerns (Box 8–2). For example, if a pregnant mother wants to select a pump to prepare for going back to work, the lactation consultant provides this information. Families do not attend to information that health care providers *think* they should have until their own concerns have been addressed.

When special circumstances, such as prematurity, multiple births, congenital anomalies, or infant neurological impairment, affect the initiation of breastfeeding, the learning needs of the parents are complicated by the emotional ramifications of the experience. Families with special needs benefit from individualized teaching and assistance and from specific educational materials and ongoing group support that addresses their unique needs.

Continuing Support for Breastfeeding Families

The sharp decline in breastfeeding in the early weeks postpartum (see Chapter 1) demonstrates

BOX 8–1

Recommended Topics for Prenatal Breastfeeding Classes

EARLY PREGNANCY

"How do you plan to feed your baby?"
Importance of decision about feeding choice

Assess knowledge and perceptions regarding breastfeeding
Reasons mothers choose (breastfeeding, bottle-feeding, combined feeding)

Explore and identify concerns
Personal feelings and perceptions regarding breastfeeding

Families' feelings (including partner, significant other)

Dealing with disapproval

Acknowledge and validate feelings

Educate using carefully targeted messages to address individual concerns
Benefits of breastfeeding (infant, mother, community)

Risks of formula feeding

Doctors' recommendations

Issues to address
Ease of breastfeeding
Breastfeeding with modesty
Family involvement

Lack of dietary restrictions and lifestyle changes
Feasibility with employment or school
Availability of people to assist

Identify breastfeeding resource network
Family and friends who enjoyed breastfeeding

Health care providers who are knowledgeable

Mother-to-mother support group

Enthusiastically support any interest in breastfeeding
Encourage ambivalent mothers to breastfeed

LATER PREGNANCY

Nipple and breast preparation *not* necessary (breastfeeding is easy)

Assess nipple eversion (treat with shells if necessary)

Discuss nursing bras, clothes for discrete nursing

No need for nipple creams, ointments, and the like

---

the need that mothers have for assistance and follow-up. A systematic program to ensure contact with the new breastfeeding mother can be a powerful influence on breastfeeding duration. Where feasible, telephone contact is ideal. Home care or early return visits to a clinic are also helpful. Each mother should be able to identify at least one resource person for information, support, and assistance.

In addition to needing information and assistance with solving breastfeeding challenges, mothers need support and encouragement to continue breastfeeding. Family, peers, and community resources are often her primary sources of support.

BOX 8–2

Sample Content for "How-To" Breastfeeding Class

Based on three common concerns of mothers:
- Will I have enough milk?
- Will breastfeeding hurt?
- Where can I get help?

I. WILL I HAVE ENOUGH MILK?

How milk is made (milk removal, milk production)

Getting off to a good start

Best time for breastfeeding: within first hour after birth (importance of colostrum)

Rooming-in

What if separation is medically necessary?

How often to breastfeed
- Baby-led feedings
- Identify early hunger cues (crying is a *late* cue)
- Guidelines
  - Feed at least every 3 hours during day (8–12 feedings each 24 hours)
  - Feed at least 5–10 minutes each side
  - Listen for swallowing
  - Watch infant for satiety cues (identify satiety cues)
  - Avoid intense clock watching

What causes decreased milk production?
- Long intervals between feedings
- Formula or water supplements
- Smoking

Do I have to change my lifestyle?

Nutrition, fluids, rest
- Listen to your body: eat when hungry, drink when thirsty, rest when tired

Medications: over-the-counter drugs, prescription drugs, recreational drugs, alcohol, nicotine

If mother gets a cold

II. WILL BREASTFEEDING HURT?

Making breastfeeding comfortable

Do I have to prepare my nipples?
- Check for nipple protrusion (treat with breast shells)

Do I need any special supplies or equipment?

Positioning and latch-on
- Alerting infants: techniques
- Avoid overuse of swaddling
- Impact of pacifiers on breastfeeding
- Mother's position and breast support
- Infant's position (cradle hold, football hold, side-lying)
- Discuss with visual aids, video demonstration
- Demonstrate with doll, mother to return demonstrate

What is a good latch?
- Wide-open mouth
- Lips flanged
- Nose and chin to breast
- No sharp pain

Can I prevent sore nipples?
- Break latch if it hurts, breastfeed frequently, start on less sore side
- Creams and ointments (not always helpful)

BOX 8–2　*(cont.)*

What is engorgement? How do I manage engorgement?

 Breastfeed frequently

 Cold packs to breasts

 Use breast pump if necessary

 Softer, smaller breasts (after engorgement) does not mean lost milk supply

III. WHERE CAN I GET HELP?

Dad's special role (special role of primary support person)

Types of help (practical help, emotional help, skilled assistance)

Dealing with advice and opinions

Sources for expert help with breastfeeding

 Lactation consultants, breastfeeding and lactation educators, peer counselors (provide local telephone numbers)

 Baby's doctor, nurse

 La Leche League, local mothering groups (provide local telephone numbers)

How do I know if baby is getting enough?

 Swallowing

 Bowel movements (at least four per 24 hours)

 Satisfied between feedings

 Feeding at least eight times each 24 hours

Family life with baby: enjoying baby, consoling baby, fear of "spoiling"

When to call for help

 Baby feeding every hour

 Feedings lasting > 1 hour

 Baby sleeping for > 4–5 hours more than once each 24 hours

 Baby feeds fewer than 7 times in 24 hours

 Baby has fewer than 4 bowel movements in 24 Hours

 Severe nipple pain

 Tender, swollen area in breast

Important things to remember

 Early, frequent feedings are important

  Know if baby is getting milk

   Correct latch-on (that is comfortable), swallowing, frequent bowel movements (more than four in 24 hours)

 Learn baby's cues

 Use expert resources

 No supplements unless medical doctor recommends

  (Find out why supplementation is medically necessary and what can be done to increase milk supply)

Realistic expectations

 What to expect during first weeks; withhold judgment about breastfeeding for two weeks

Source: Adapted from a presentation by Linda J. Smith, International Lactation Consultant Association Conference, Arlington Heights, IL, 1992.

However, health care professionals have a role to play in assessing and augmenting or creating support systems.

 Fathers are often the most influential support persons in the early breastfeeding period (Bar-Yam & Darby, 1997; Beske & Garvis, 1982; Freed, 1993b; Gorman et al., 1995). Fathers benefit from suggestions of specific ways by which they can support their partners. They can help the mother to achieve a comfortable breastfeeding position, provide nutritional support and household assistance, burp and console the infant, monitor the mother's fatigue level, limit visitors, and show delight in the decision to breastfeed.

As breastfeeding continues, the baby is a powerful source of positive feedback for the mother (Beske & Garvis, 1982). The baby who thrives on mother's milk and who is healthy and contented offers obvious validation of the unique nourishment the mother provides.

However, even the evidence of a healthy infant and the encouragement of health care providers may be insufficient to overcome lack of support among peers and the community. In industrialized cultures in particular, where artificial feeding has been viewed as the cultural norm, breastfeeding support may be inversely related to the age of the infant. Assisting mothers to become a part of formal or informal support systems, or even creating an ongoing support system, is an appropriate focus for the health care professional who wishes to encourage continued breastfeeding (Box 8–3). Ideally, mothers are able to identify at least one mother whom they know who enjoyed breastfeeding and who can give them practical assistance.

How Effective Is Breastfeeding Education?

With short hospital stays and tight hospital budgets, we need to know what strategies work most effectively. Because education can change only those elements that are modifiable, we first need to identify what *can* be changed. When Janke (1993) extensively reviewed the research literature a few years ago, she found only six modifiable variables that predict breastfeeding outcomes:

- Mother intends to breastfeed a long time.

- Mother is strongly committed to breastfeeding.

- Mother and family have a strong support system.

- Mother expresses a positive attitude toward breastfeeding.

- Baby has an early first feeding.

- Mother avoids supplemental feedings of water or formula.

Note that the effect of health professionals was not on this list. Although a few studies (Balcazar et al., 1995; Wiles, 1984) indicate that health care providers are an important factor in mothers' decision to breastfeed, most controlled studies indicate that professionals have little influence on the feeding decisions made by expectant mothers (Aberman & Kirchoff, 1985; Auerbach, 1984; Baranowski et al., 1983; Beske & Garvis, 1982; Bryant, 1982; Gulick, 1982; Lawrence, 1982; Sullivan & Jones, 1986). More influential are the baby's father, peers, and maternal grandmother (Aberman & Kirchhoff, 1985; Baranowski et al., 1983; Beske & Garvis, 1982; Bryant, 1982; Freed, 1993a; Littman et al., 1994; Sullivan & Jones, 1986).

The influence of health care professionals may be minimized by the timing of their contact with expectant parents, which usually occurs only during pregnancy. How the mother will feed her baby is a decision that often is made prior to conception (Birenbaum, Fuchs, & Reichman, 1989; Ekwo, Dusdieker, & Booth, 1983; Kaplowitz & Olson, 1983) or very early in pregnancy (Beske & Garvis, 1982). Therefore, educational efforts may have to target future parents prior to conception through the elementary and secondary school systems, the mass media, churches, community organizations, and other influential institutions.

The lack of influence of health care providers on breastfeeding decisions also may reflect the fact that in many cases infant feeding is not discussed with patients. Health care providers may be reluctant to encourage breastfeeding. They may assume they will contribute to feelings of guilt a mother may experience if she chooses not to breastfeed. However, such concerns do not negate the responsibility to provide families with accurate and complete information so that they can make an informed choice.

Health care professionals have a responsibility to provide accurate information and to actively encourage the decision to breastfeed, just as they encourage other health-optimizing choices, such as early prenatal care, appropriate nutrition, use of car restraint systems, immunizations, and avoidance of smoking, drinking alcohol, and using drugs

BOX 8–3

Recommended Topics for an Ongoing Breastfeeding Support Class

NEWBORN ADJUSTMENT

Parental fatigue, time management

Physical changes during postpartum

Maternal mood changes

Management of fussiness, crying

   Concerns about "spoiling" infants

   Consoling techniques

Infant sleeping issues, nighttime parenting

Transition from two to three (feeling left out)

   Being a person and partner as well as a parent

   Sexuality and contraception

Dealing with unsolicited advice

Blended families, sibling or pet adjustments

BREASTFEEDING CONCERNS

Milk supply concerns

Assessing adequacy of infant intake

Strategies to increase milk supply

Appetite and growth spurts

Frequency of breastfeeding as baby gets older

Involving family members

Obstructed ducts and mastitis

Weaning

RETURNING TO AN EMPLOYMENT SETTING

Feasibility of combining breastfeeding and employment outside the home

Feeding options

Child-care considerations

Time management

Selecting a breastmilk expression technique (hand expression and breast pump options)

Expressing and storing breastmilk

Maintaining milk supply; maintaining baby's interest in breastfeeding

Keeping breastfeeding in perspective

---

of abuse. A neutral attitude toward feeding choice is inappropriate, as it implies an equivalence of breastmilk and its substitutes. Hewat and Ellis (1986) suggest that mothers benefit from realistic guidance about breastfeeding, not just information that stresses its positive aspects.

The effect of breastfeeding education on WIC participants is mixed. A lack of effect is usually found in older studies before 1988, when WIC began receiving federal funding for breastfeeding education and promotion. In fact, the recent increases in U.S. rates of breastfeeding are mostly due to more mothers on WIC choosing to breastfeed. State WIC promotion efforts are spotty, how-

ever, with only a few states developing what could be considered model programs for breastfeeding education.

Young and Kaufman (1988) reported an increase in breastfeeding initiation among a low-income group of expectant mothers who attended prenatal education classes. Auerbach (1985) also found that mothers breastfed longer when WIC staff members were educated in breastfeeding management and when a lactation consultant saw mothers at least once.

Although professional influence may be minimal in influencing the mother's decision to breastfeed, it is invaluable during the perinatal and postnatal periods. Numerous studies show that education and professional interventions make a difference in the birth setting and postpartum by extending breastfeeding continuation (Cohen, 1980; Hall, 1978; Palti et al., 1988; Wiles, 1984; Young & Kaufman, 1988). More recent educational programs designed to promote the decision to breastfeed and to influence its continuance are summarized in Table 8–1.

Teaching Strategies

Good teaching involves organizing learning experiences that keep the participant's interest and use the facilitator's time efficiently. The lecture format yields an efficient use of the instructor's time; however, it requires that participants remain passive, and it is associated with decreased retention. An effective strategy is to vary the teaching format. Team presentations, small group discussions, demonstrations, role playing, question-and-answer sessions with teacher-led or student-led questioning, observations and comments by participants, group projects, and individualized instruction modules are effective ways to break the monotony of lecture presentations.

Each teaching session should include an introduction, learning experience, and conclusion or summary. A fundamental axiom is to "explain what you're going to teach, teach, and then describe what you have taught." When using the lecture format, remember certain essential guidelines:

- Use a conversational tone (avoid reading notes word for word).
- Vary speech (inflection, speed, and tone).
- Wear bright, interesting clothing.
- Move around while lecturing and use gestures for emphasis.
- Use visual aids liberally (slides, charts, models, portions of videotapes and films).
- Use humor.
- Demonstrate psychomotor tasks.
- Encourage the audience to participate by practicing psychomotor skills and with questions, comments, and small group discussion.

- Schedule breaks every 50 minutes for maximum retention.

Charts, slides, line drawings, and role playing are useful in dividing a psychomotor skill, such as positioning and latch-on, into understandable steps. Follow this with a videotape presentation of the skill. The facilitator must always preview audiovisual materials and be knowledgeable about equipment operation so that each learner's time is used efficiently.

Therapeutic Communication

Communication is a process by which we transmit information, thoughts, ideas, and feelings. It is often categorized into two types: verbal (spoken or written) and nonverbal. Although both types of communication may occur concurrently, experts estimate that between 65 percent (Haber & Hoskins, 1987) and 90 percent (Kozier & Erb, 1987) of messages received are nonverbal.

Nonverbal communications not only portray a person's feelings but also indicate how people are coping with their feelings. How words are spoken (i.e., the rate of speech, tone of voice, pitch, inflection, volume, rhythm, pauses and silence) conveys more reliable information than do actual words. Nonlanguage vocalizations, such as sighing, gasping, sobbing, moaning, grunting, and laughing, also communicate significant messages.

Body motion and posture along with facial expressions are important sources of nonverbal messages (Haber & Hoskins, 1987) and communicate self-image, mood, and state of health. The face discloses specific emotions, and intensity can telegraph the importance of a topic. Eye contact can communicate the amount of trust and acceptance between people and level of interest and involvement. In Western societies, direct eye contact usually communicates a high level of interest and implies positive regard for another person. Mutual eye contact conveys a willingness to maintain communication. Eye contact is often averted or avoided when a person feels weak, defenseless, or embarrassed. Hand movement and gestures convey such messages as anxiety, impatience, avoidance, indifference, relaxation, and confidence.

Table 8–1

EFFECTIVENESS OF BREASTFEEDING EDUCATION

Reference	Findings and Conclusions
Prenatal Education	
Pugin et al., 1996	A control-intervention study in Chile found a statistically significant increase in full breastfeeding at six months among women who attended a prenatal breastfeeding group.
In-Hospital Education	
Schy et al., 1996	U.S. in-hospital education was not associated with increased satisfaction with breastfeeding or duration. Duration was associated with satisfaction, maternal education level, and expected length of breastfeeding. Need for follow-up telephone calls was identified.
Postpartum Education	
Grossman et al., 1990	Ninety-seven low-income women were randomized to receive intensive postpartum breastfeeding education or routine assistance. There was no statistically significant difference between groups at six weeks postpartum. Participation in prenatal classes predicted breastfeeding duration by logistic regression.
Peer Counselors	
Kistin et al., 1994	Low-income U.S. women who received support from peer counselors had significantly greater breastfeeding initiation, exclusivity, and duration than those who did not.
Social and Informational Support	
Buckner & Matsubara, 1993	At two weeks postpartum, U.S. breastfeeding mothers had statistically significantly higher support scores than mothers who discontinued breastfeeding. At four weeks, this difference was no longer statistically significant.
McNatt & Freston, 1992	There was no statistically significant difference between perceived support scores of women who considered themselves successful with breastfeeding and those who did not. There was a positive correlation between health care provider support, informational support, and perception of successful lactation.
Education of Professionals	
Valdes et al., 1995	Pretest and posttest revealed increased knowledge in all areas after attending a three-day course on breastfeeding in Chile. A survey completed two years after the course showed 69 percent of respondents had changed their clinical practice after attending the course.
Westphal et al., 1995	Pretest and posttest revealed improved knowledge of health care providers and improved institutional scores related to the WHO/UNICEF "Ten Steps to Successful Breast-Feeding" after a Brazilian training course.

Body movement changes as we continue to interact with each other. Initially, participants in a class maintain physical distance. As the working phase begins, they move more loosely and even lean toward each other. Empathy and understanding are conveyed by mirroring another person's posture or body position. Desire to terminate an interaction is indicated by stretching, averting eye contact, straightening papers, closing a purse, or standing in preparation for leaving.

Touch is another powerful way we communicate. A hand placed on the shoulder conveys compassion and support. In Western cultures, touch validates the spoken message. As with all nonverbal communication, it must be used with sensitivity, always considering how it can affect an individual and always using it within a cultural context. Appearance, including physical characteristics and manner of dress, acts as a nonverbal message that confirms or contradicts verbal messages. Choice of clothing, adornments, and grooming practices are highly personal and convey social and financial status, religion, and group association.

There are two types of therapeutic communication skills: attending skills and responding skills. Attending skills include active listening, which uses all of the senses. Therapeutic listening is an active process that requires energy and concentration. Egan (1982) identified four ways to convey physical attending skills: facing the other person squarely, maintaining comfortable eye contact, leaning toward the other person to convey interest and involvement, and maintaining an open posture in which neither arms nor legs are crossed.

Sitting with a family, rather than standing above them, decreases the listener's feelings of condescension. People often perceive that more time is spent with them when the health care provider sits rather than stands. Focusing complete attention on the speaker and identifying themes and patterns in the family's message provides the basis for responding effectively. Responding skills include reflecting, restating, and paraphrasing; clarifying and validating; asking open-ended questions; stating observations and sharing interpretations; identifying strengths and building hope; and summarizing.

Reflecting, restating, and paraphrasing help the listener to convey understanding of the initial message. Reflecting the feelings implied in a message helps families to identify underlying themes in the primary message. Clarifying identifies areas of confusion and enables the listener to request more information. Validating confirms that the restated message is what the person meant to communicate.

Questions or statements that are open-ended often yield significant information by encouraging parents to express themselves fully. Open-ended questions typically start with *how* or *tell me about.* For example, if a mother is asked where she is having breast tenderness, the answer will probably relate only to the site. However, if she is asked to talk about the tenderness, she may give information about its location, intensity, and duration. As more specific information is needed, questions begin with *who, what, when, where, how much,* and *how often.* Closed-ended questions usually start with *are, is, do,* and *does.* Such questions can also be answered with a *yes* or *no* and yield the least amount of information. (e.g., "Is your breast tender?") (Lauwers & Woessner, 1989).

Asking too many questions in sequence or in an interrogating manner (such as *why* questions) is threatening. Balancing questioning with other therapeutic skills promotes the family's problem-solving abilities by involving the family in clarifying the problem, generating resolution strategies, and evaluating the outcome. Focusing on central issues and returning to the main topic keeps the interaction purposeful and goal-directed rather than rambling.

Stating observations and sharing interpretations provides constructive feedback to families about how their messages are perceived. Identifying strengths helps families to focus on their positive qualities. Indicating that a family's specific concerns are common experiences helps to place the concern in perspective and builds hope that there is a solution. It is extremely important not to discount or trivialize a family's concerns in an attempt to decrease their anxiety. Personal concerns are valid and must be treated with respect. The intent is to offer empathy, genuine concern, and assistance in problem solving. Summarizing unifies pieces of information into themes of content and feeling. By highlighting the most significant information they have shared, families are more easily able to participate in the problem-solving process. Effective communication between health care providers and parents is *disconnected* by assuming, ordering, blaming, generalizing, trivializing and discounting, negative prognosticating, and providing conflicting information (Driscoll, 1992).

Learners retain information and psychomotor skills more effectively if they incorporate the information they have received and practice their new skills (Kozier & Erb, 1987). Return demonstrations in which learners repeat the teacher's demonstration provide opportunities for reinforcing correct execution. This increases learner confidence. Clarifying suggested actions facilitates appropriate performance of a skill.

Evaluation of the learning experience should be a joint effort by both learner and instructor. Attainment of goals and enjoyment of the learning process are important criteria for evaluating success. Adults want recognition for their efforts and appreciate awards of completion (e.g., certificates, ceremonies, public listings).

Small-Group Dynamics

Formal classes and educational media might provide information to large numbers of people, but small-group teaching is a much more powerful method for behavior change. Group discussions enhance peer support and decision making, and decrease dependence on health care professionals. A group is two or more people who interact and influence each other, accomplish common goals, and derive satisfaction from maintaining membership in the group. The ideal group size ranges from 8 to 12 people. More than 10 people in a subgroup decreases productivity (Tubbs, 1984).

Small-group interaction has the advantage of stimulating a free flow of information and encouragement among participants as different questions are asked and new topics are raised. Small groups meet human needs for companionship, knowledge, and identity. Discussion in a small group is more likely to answer participants' information needs, because they usually feel more comfortable asking questions and changing the topic than when they are in a large group.

An informal, relaxed setting encourages participation. The group leader needs to be expert in the subject content area and skilled in group dynamics. Familiarity with the different roles played by group members (initiator, elaborator, evaluator, coordinator, encourager, harmonizer, compromiser, aggressor, recognition-seeker, confessor, dominator) enhances the group leader's effectiveness in moving the group in a fruitful direction (Sampson & Marthas, 1981).

Although the group leader may have to actively guide the discussion initially, the goal is to act as a resource for information, encouraging participants to develop their own creative and problem-solving abilities (Nichols & Edwards, 1988). When participants share their personal experiences, it enhances learning and increases self-worth as individuals' efforts are reinforced and supported by the group. A variety of techniques can be used by a group leader or facilitator to enhance the group process. These include supporting, clarifying, probing, summarizing, paraphrasing, reflecting, confronting, highlighting, suggesting, questioning, repeating, interpreting and analyzing, and listening (Sampson & Marthas, 1981).

Multimedia Presentations

Education programs must compete with television, videotapes, CD ROMs, and the Internet. Audio or visual enhancements are almost mandatory for educational programs. In an age of television and computers, people expect visual and auditory stimulation. Some say our current expectations harken back to the way humankind has communicated during most of our existence on earth, before written language and the printing press. The following items offer ways to present breastfeeding information visually:

- Use computer technology, such as PowerPoint software and LCDs (computerized slides that reside on a computer diskette). PowerPoint presentations are becoming the norm for slide presentations. It is easy to print professional-looking outlines of your talk for handouts and to make speaker's notes for each slide.

- Arrange for all necessary equipment (projectors, screens, videotape equipment, tape recorder, pointer, light stick, podium light, chart stands) well in advance of the presentation. If using the Internet on the LCD, ensure that the hotel or speaking facility has a telephone line to access the Net.

- Identify light switches and sound control panels; make certain that a responsible person is available to operate them.

- Set up and test all equipment. Have a back-up plan for all equipment. Always have a spare projector bulb in the room.

- Adjust the volume of the microphone so that persons in the back of the room can hear easily. Make adjustments before beginning the presentation.

- Tape extension cords and cables to the floor to reduce the likelihood of an accident.

- Adjust the location of the slide projector so that images fill the entire screen and can be seen clearly by all participants.

- Adjust the position of the television monitor(s) so that videotapes can be seen by all participants.

- Adjust the lighting in the room to enhance the visual presentation and still allow for taking notes.

- Arrange equipment so that it does not block the view of the screen(s).

- When showing part of a videotape, preset the tape to the place where it is to begin.

- Meet with the equipment operator, review the audiovisual component of the presentation, and explain what the operator will need to do during the presentation (e.g., change slide trays, press "play" on the videotape player).

- Avoid using supercapability (140-slot) slide trays; they often jam when slides are warped or slightly frayed.

- Always screen visual aids before the presentation (unmarked slides are especially prone to being placed backward or upside down).

- Avoid facing the audiovisual aids when speaking or standing between them and the audience. Audiovisual aids that are presented effectively greatly enhance teaching. Learners are frustrated when such aids are poorly pre-

sented or the instructor talks about a wonderful component that is not available. Adequate planning and preparation are the best insurance for an effective presentation.

Slides

Slides are easily stored and transported and are flexible; there is wide variety in how they can be sequenced. Slides might be "worth a thousand words," but they can be expensive to make. Some lactation consultants working in hospitals and health care agencies have access to audiovisual staff whose sole job is to produce audiovisual aids.

Computer-generated slides are fast becoming the standard for presentations. As mentioned, some software programs create slides that can be easily modified, so there is little or no expense in revising and updating slides.

Transparencies

Transparencies or overhead projections are easy to make and the least expensive of all the media options. Almost every classroom has an overhead projector. However, transparencies are easily damaged, are difficult to combine with slide presentations, and may require a second person at the overhead projector. Transparencies are generally limited to charts and words (photographs do not reproduce well) and appear to be less "professional" than do other formats.

Videotapes

Videotapes are excellent for demonstrating live-action psychomotor skills (e.g., positioning mother and baby for breastfeeding) and are easily transported and stored. Many households in the United States now have videotape players. For these families, videotapes are a natural way to reinforce teaching after early hospital discharge. However, videotapes are usually expensive to purchase, and equipment to present them (especially in hotel conferences) is also expensive. Because people are so accustomed to the high visual quality they see on television, a teaching videotape must be sophisticated; lesser-quality videotape productions are rarely appreciated.

CD ROMs

CD ROMS are one of the newest technologies in education. Several CD ROMS on breastfeeding have been developed. Advantages are that they are individually paced and everyone receives consistent information. Because they are not usable without computers and they are expensive, CD ROMS are mainly used in tertiary health centers and colleges and universities. At the University of Kansas School of Medicine, pediatric residents, medical students, and nurse practitioners review a CD ROM on breastfeeding and complete a posttest as part of their ambulatory pediatric rotation.

When developing a presentation using a visual format, first apply these general principles:

- Identify key concepts to be emphasized. Write them out on a "story board" before developing slides or transparencies. A story board is a sequence of the presentation's main points. Drawing boxes on a paper pad and filling them in with the secondary points works just fine for a story board.

- Keep the content simple: one idea per slide.

- Ensure that all lettering is large enough to be read in the back of the room.

- Insist that all lettering, artwork, and photography be of professional quality. Use multiple colors to maintain interest.

- Avoid overuse of clip art. It can distract learners.

- Use simple, clearly labeled graphs and drawings.

- Avoid complicated, detailed artwork that is more suitable for print publications.

- Choose photographs that are sharp, clear, visually appealing, uncluttered, and convey a single key point. Well-selected photographs help viewers to see how information can be used in their lives. A presentation on breastfeeding that uses attractive photos of breastfeeding mothers and infants is rated higher by participants than is one in which no such photos are used.

- Include photographs that are several feet away from the subject, within a few feet of the subject, and very close to the subject.

Educational Materials

Retention of new information is always shorter under stress. After the physical and emotional stress of childbirth, families benefit from educational materials that reinforce verbal teaching; therefore, educational materials should be used throughout pregnancy and after childbirth to reinforce, but not replace, individualized teaching. If the educator uses audiovisual aids in addition to printed matter, retention is usually improved. Adult learners retain only about 30 percent of the information they hear. A multimodal approach (seeing and hearing) increases retention to 50 percent (Becton & Dickenson, 1981).

Materials must be scrutinized closely for their accuracy to determine that no outdated information is included. Information must be consistent. New parents are frustrated by conflicting recommendations. Because nonverbal messages have a more profound impact on behavior than do verbal instructions (Pease, 1984), materials must be carefully evaluated for correctness of maternal-infant positioning and latch-on (Shrago & Bocar, 1990). Use only those visuals that show discreet breastfeeding where public exposure of the breasts is discouraged or considered taboo.

Educational materials aimed at promoting breastfeeding should include practical tips for breastfeeding and resources for additional information. It is a disservice to enthusiastically expound the benefits of breastfeeding without providing practical assistance to help families to meet their breastfeeding goals. Mothers need to make informed decisions about how they will feed their babies. Mothers, however, do not need to know how to manage every potential breastfeeding difficulty. Materials that dwell on the management of complications (i.e., breast abscess) may be frightening to mothers still considering how they will feed their baby. Materials should indicate when a mother should seek assistance and should always include a local resource telephone number. The telephone number can be printed or written on the materials, or a business card can be attached to the materials.

Printed matter should be attractively packaged. Families from a variety of socioeconomic backgrounds have access to sophisticated printed materials and commercial television programs; they expect similar quality in materials about breastfeeding. Pamphlets must be inviting, easy to read, and organized for scanning (with bold headings and generous amounts of white space). Too many words on a page can overwhelm a reader. Pictorial learning is superior to verbal learning for recognition and recall (Redman, 1988). Pictures and drawings make materials more interesting. Although books on breastfeeding are welcomed by some mothers, women who have not read a book since they completed their formal education may think that if they have to read a comprehensive book, breastfeeding may be too difficult for them. Interest in reading should always be individually assessed before making recommendations about written materials. Written materials are not helpful for the 27 million functionally illiterate people in the United States. Riordan (1985) identifies readability, relevancy, and reliability as important components in evaluating breastfeeding literature.

More printed materials are not always better. If families are bombarded with thick stacks of pamphlets and materials, the likelihood of their use is decreased. A few carefully selected pamphlets can convey the idea that breastfeeding is uncomplicated and enjoyable. Pamphlets and short audiovisual programs are preferable to lengthy materials that attempt to cover the gamut of breastfeeding experiences. Brief, focused materials should address the issues that the family perceives as meaningful and that they are motivated to learn. This concept applies especially to mothers and families in special circumstances (such as prematurity, birth anomalies, and relactation). Books that are divided into small segments and have detailed indexes help families to locate needed information. Visual materials are more effective if they depict parents with ethnic, socioeconomic, and cultural backgrounds that are similar to the target audience. For example, teenage mothers respond most favorably to visual representations of adolescent mothers. A lending library of books and videotapes conveys a commitment to empowering families.

The source of materials must be considered in evaluating educational materials. Organizations whose purpose is to promote human milk substitutes cannot be expected to genuinely promote breastfeeding (Valaitis & Shay, 1993). Underlying messages may communicate that bottle-feeding is the cultural norm and that breastfeeding is difficult, complicated, uncomfortable, immodest, and inconvenient (Auerbach, 1988; see also Curro et al., 1997). There is often an explicit message that when families begin using formula, the product of that company is optimal. Smith (1995) has developed a score sheet for evaluating breastfeeding educational materials.

Because it is an established fact that mothers who receive samples of commercial formula in health care settings discontinue breastfeeding sooner than do mothers who do not receive samples (Adair et al., 1993; Auerbach, 1993a, b, 1997; Howard et al., 1993, 1994; Hunt, 1994; Janke, 1995; Owen, 1994; Snell et al., 1992), educational materials should comply with the International Code of Marketing of Breast-Milk Substitutes (WHO 34.22, 1981), often called the WHO Code. The Code was designed to apply to all countries and restricts advertising and promotion of products through health care facilities. No words or pictures idealizing artificial feeding should be included in materials given to childbearing families. Giving families written materials that contain incorrect or misleading information, conflicting messages, and subtle themes that undermine breastfeeding may be more detrimental than giving them nothing. Riordan (1985) notes in her review of breastfeeding pamphlets that the price of some "free" pamphlets is one's credibility. Individual health care providers can make a personal commitment to abide by the Code provisions by not providing materials produced by infant-formula companies. The WHO Code provisions are discussed in Chapter 1.

Parents are not the only audience for breastfeeding education. One of the concerns of LCs working in clinical agencies is conveying current breastfeeding information about breastfeeding to the staff. This problem was creatively solved by a lactation consultant in Washington State (Aken, 1993, p. 183):

When I became a lactation consultant I was very concerned about how to reach this large number of staff. My thought was to post basic as well as new breastfeeding information on the bulletin board that everyone would see—and I hoped, take the time to read. I was unable to find a bulletin board that all three Birth Center departments would read. The only place that everyone frequented was the staff bathroom. I had my captive audience. So I created a newsletter, "Milkline," that can be read easily in a couple of minutes. I post a new sheet every other week. My audience is so captive that one Friday when I hung a new sheet, I noticed that someone had moved the sheet closer to the stool. It now hung directly above the toilet paper dispenser. I was told later that it had been too far away to sit and read.

The target audience should be considered in evaluating educational information. Materials must be written at a reading level that the reader can understand. For materials developed on a desktop computer, most word-processing programs have the ability to calculate the reading level of the material being created by a simple push of a button. The FOG index is a useful tool for assessing reading levels for materials that are already printed (Gunning, 1968). A simple method to calculate reading level is to count the number of multisyllabic words in a sample of 100 words. Less than 4 multisyllabic words is equal to less than a high school level; 16 multisyllabic words is equivalent to a high school level; and more than 16 multisyllabic words is equal to a college level. Box 8–4 lists the criteria for evaluating educational material.

Education for At-Risk Populations

In the United States, women who have low incomes, who are minimally educated, or who are members of particular ethnic groups initiate and sustain breastfeeding at rates lower than those of the national average. Although mothers with limited formal education are likely to be economically disadvantaged, their breastfeeding concerns are similar to those of more affluent mothers: modesty, partner participation, lifestyle changes, contraception, and fear of difficulty or pain.

In addition, they are influenced by the relative absence of peer models and social support. Women with minimal formal education may be more influenced by advertisements and media portrayal of artificial feeding as the cultural norm. They may also lack self-confidence, a sense of control over

their lives, and assertiveness skills that are likely to enhance their experience with breastfeeding. Thus mothers with limited formal education should receive informational support and follow-up to enhance their breastfeeding experiences. Because partners, family members, and social-support people exert considerable influence on mothers with limited formal education, they should be included in breastfeeding education (Buckner & Matsubara, 1993; Gielen et al., 1992; Libbus, 1992; McClurg-Hitt & Olsen, 1994; McNatt & Freston, 1992).

U.S. families who do not speak English create challenges regarding health education. Ideally, an interpreter will be available to assist in providing critical information if the educator or care provider is not fluent in the patient's language. If a facility serves a large population that speaks English as a second language, the agency should consider translating educational materials. Also, they can purchase translated breastfeeding materials. La Leche League International sells pamphlets in many different languages. Pictures are an excellent way to teach the basics of breastfeeding. The *Illustrated Multi-Language Pocket Glossary* has line drawings and breastfeeding phrases translated into seven languages. The *Pocket Guide to Breastfeeding* has pictures of breastfeeding positions and latch-on techniques. Both resources are published by and available through Childbirth Graphics, a division of WRS Group.

If the teacher or leader of a breastfeeding class comes from a different socioeconomic or ethnic group than do the mothers she is teaching, she may have a difficult time being accepted as a peer in whom the mothers can confide and trust. An example is a white, highly educated, articulate, and well-dressed woman leading an inner-city group of African-American or Hispanic mothers in a WIC program. On the other hand, peers who are especially trained to help other women in their community with breastfeeding (peer counselors) have a positive effect on initiation and continuation of breastfeeding among low-income urban women (Kistin et al., 1994; Lapierre, Perrault, & Goulet, 1995; Locklin, 1995; Long et al., 1995; Naber & Locklin, 1994; Sciacca et al., 1995b; Turner, 1995). Locklin (1993, p. 181) described peer counselors trained by members of the Chicago Breastfeeding Task Force, a grass-roots organization consisting of

BOX 8–4

Criteria for Evaluating Educational Materials

CONTENT

- Specific to family's needs?
- Accurate, reliable information based on valid research reports?
- Accepted principles of anatomy and physiology?
- Up-to-date recommendations?
- Consistency between narrative and visual aids?
- Simple, uncomplicated approach? Avoids dwelling on difficulties or potential complications?

PRESENTATION

- Attractive, inviting?
- Organized for easy scanning: bold headings, short paragraphs, ample amounts of white space?
- Appropriate reading level? Less than high school education (grade 3). Need more visuals, less narrative. High school graduate (grades 5–7). Newspapers are written at this level. College graduate (grades 12–13). Professional journals are written at this level.

- Generous use of appropriate pictures, drawings, and graphs that are consistent with the narrative?
- Visual aids depict families from similar backgrounds of audience?
- Appropriate length to maintain interest?

PROMOTIONAL MATERIALS

- Enthusiastically discusses benefits of breastfeeding?
- Includes risks of bottle-feeding?
- Culturally appropriate breastfeeding is modeled?
- Includes practical tips for successful breastfeeding?
- Provides information for additional resources?

SOURCE OF MATERIALS

- No underlying or hidden messages about the use of formula?
- Breastfeeding presented as complicated, uncomfortable, immodest, inconvenient?
- Complies with WHO Code, which precludes health care providers from distributing materials provided by formula and baby-food companies?

committed professionals whose mission is to train peer counselors:

The peer counselors who are passionate about their mission have certain characteristics in common. They frequently call their clients, they make themselves available at all hours of the day and night within the early postpartum weeks, and they use assertive language in their encounters. I often hear

mothers say in the same breath, "She cares for me, she's there for me, she wants me to keep it up, she won't let me stop." The counselors provide ego strength and integrity and a sense of purpose in the lives of these women.

Adolescents' concerns regarding breastfeeding are influenced by their developmental stage (Flanagan et al., 1995; Yoos, 1985). The primary focus of the young adolescent is the self. In discussing the advantages of breastfeeding with an adolescent, it is important to emphasize the advantages of breastfeeding for mothers. Self-consciousness and modesty may be so pronounced that the young mother may be reluctant to consider breastfeeding. Typical concerns of North American adolescent mothers include issues of modesty, sexuality, mobility, lifestyle, peer approval, the wish to return to school, and the attitude of the baby's father (Alexy & Martin, 1994; Freed, 1993a; Marchand & Morrow, 1994; Peterson & DaVanzo, 1992; Purtell, 1994; Robinson et al., 1993). A focus group of U.S. teens identified fears related to breastfeeding, which included lack of confidence, dietary concerns, loss of freedom, pain and discomfort, and disfigurement (Bryant, 1992; Motil et al., 1997).

Peer role models exert a strong influence in favor of breastfeeding (Radius & Joffe, 1988). Teen mothers who have enjoyed breastfeeding should be encouraged to discuss their experiences among pregnant peers. Adolescents are typically interested in having new experiences; some teenage mothers show interest in breastfeeding because they do not want to miss the "novel" experience of breastfeeding. Some teens find that breastfeeding is a source of pride; they gain positive attention from health care providers, family members, and peers. Choosing to breastfeed can demonstrate their maturity and show that they are individualists. Because adolescents want to be loved and to give love, it can be effective to emphasize that breastfed babies and mothers feel a special closeness and love for each other.

"Whose baby is this?" is sometimes an issue between the adolescent mother and her baby's grandmother. Breastfeeding can be attractive, because only the mother can breastfeed. It is important to emphasize flexibility in feeding plans with teen mothers. Although there are numerous advantages to exclusive breastfeeding, an all-or-none approach will usually result in teens declining to breastfeed. It is more appealing for teens to discuss feeding plans in which the teen mother decides what the baby will be fed and by whom. Remembering that partial breastfeeding provides more advantages to mothers and babies than no breastfeeding helps health care providers to place their recommendations in perspective. Teens are

especially sensitive to others' opinions. Conveying confidence in the adolescent mother's ability to care for her baby validates her role as a mother.

When working with adolescent mothers, avoid rigid rules about positioning, dietary intake, and exclusive breastfeeding. As they complete their developmental tasks of adolescence, teenagers tend to distance themselves from (and sometimes actively rebel against) rules and regulations. It is more effective to suggest ideas that have worked for other young mothers. It is also important to emphasize the ease of breastfeeding (after the first weeks), because teens may lack self-confidence (Benson, 1996). Teenagers tend to think more concretely than abstractly and thus benefit from hands-on activities, such as positioning dolls in prenatal classes. Learning activities should be fun, geared to what the mothers believe is important, and quickly paced, remembering that adolescents are used to being entertained with television and videotapes. Enthusiastic praise for any interest in breastfeeding, practical assistance in the birth setting, supportive social networks, and close follow-up during the week after birth are critical factors in facilitating successful breastfeeding among teenage mothers (Benson, 1996; Maehr et al., 1993).

Parents who have delayed childbearing, whether by choice or as a result of infertility, have unique concerns. Incorporating an infant and breastfeeding into their established lifestyles is not easy, and they may require frequent reassurance. On the positive side, older parents have the advantages of varied life experiences and perhaps wisdom and patience that enhance parenting skills. They may need assistance to locate peers with whom they can relate. The older mother may need reassurance that the ability to breastfeed does not decrease with increasing maternal age.

Educational Needs and Early Discharge

As families are discharged from the birth setting more quickly, educational opportunities are abbreviated. There are fewer hours to discuss educational needs, there are more visitors, and mother's retention of information is affected by her need for physical recovery. More medical and birthing centers are finding that prenatal classes and outpatient follow-up, including home care, result in positive outcomes, including saving health care dollars (Braveman et al, 1995; Britton, Britton, & Beebe, 1994; Lawrence, 1995; Neyzi et al., 1991; Rouke, 1995; Weinberg, 1994).

In the birth setting, it is critical that health care providers prioritize discharge teaching so that parents have information that is critical. *Infant hydration and nourishment is top priority.* Teaching latch-on and assessment of milk intake is far more important than is teaching bathing, which can be reviewed by other resource persons (family members, friends, or health care providers) following discharge. Special concerns identified by the family and when and from whom to get help are other areas that should be covered before the family leaves the birth setting. To avoid problems with infant dehydration and to heighten parent awareness, a feeding log and questionnaire used at Mercy Health Center in Oklahoma City helps parents to assess whether breastfeeding is going well and whether they need to contact a health care provider (Box 8–5). Early self-referrals increase when parents use this tool.

When teaching for discharge, be optimistic yet realistic. The maxim "Expect the best and prepare for the worst" is appropriate. Using a chronological approach, discussing what parents should expect in the first few days, is helpful. Subsequent visits with a physician or nurse practitioner (ideally within a few days after discharge) provide opportunities to discuss ensuing concerns. Concrete time frames (i.e., "You will probably begin to notice that your breasts are fuller on Tuesday") is easier for a postpartum mother to comprehend than is using phrases that include professional "jargon" (i.e., "You'll probably notice that your breasts are fuller four to five days postpartum"). Written information regarding engorgement, nipple tenderness, and the like (ideally in separate pamphlets or fliers) can reinforce earlier teaching if the mother is experiencing these situations.

Health Care Provider Education

Basic educational programs in medicine, nursing, and nutrition prepare students to be generalists (Crowder, 1981; Hayes, 1981). Additional study and clinical experience are necessary to develop expertise in the speciality of lactation consulting (Bagwell et al., 1993; Freed, 1995; Lewinski, 1992). Recognition of the need for additional education is demonstrated by the emergence of programs that prepare health providers to assist breastfeeding families (Davies-Adetugbo & Adebawa, 1997; Naylor et al., 1990, 1994; Newton, 1992; Valdes, 1995; Westphal, 1995).

It is necessary to distinguish between programs that prepare participants to be peer counselors, breastfeeding educators, and lactation consultants. In all categories, there is a wide range of knowledge and expertise. In general, peer counselors and breastfeeding educators are prepared to provide education and assistance relating to the management of normal lactation. They are also prepared to identify and to refer more complicated breastfeeding situations. Lactation consultants have more extensive education than peer counselors and breastfeeding educators, in both lactation and basic educational preparation and are prepared to assist breastfeeding families in complex situations. Lactation consultants are discussed in greater detail in Chapter 22.

Although, at present, there is no national accreditation system with established criteria for professional lactation education programs, various educational programs are available to prepare practitioners in lactation management. Each program has a slightly different focus and requirements. A few offer academic credit; most award continuing education credits only. The International Lactation Consultant Association (4101 Lake Boone Trail, Suite 201, Raleigh NC) has a listing of educational preparation programs for lactation consultants.

Continuing Education

Almost all large medical centers now offer at least some staff or continuing education related to breastfeeding. Some of these programs are highly successful and bring in welcome revenue (Box 8–6). Others less financially successful are considered "loss leaders." The strategy is to attract young families to a particular health care system that employs nurses and other providers who are knowledgeable in and supportive of breastfeeding.

BOX 8–5

Breastfeeding Log and Questionnaire

BREASTFEEDING LOG

INSTRUCTIONS: Each day, circle the approximate time to the nearest hour that you **start** breastfeeding. Mark off the first four bowel movements that your baby has during each 24-hour period.

If you are breastfeeding AT LEAST **8 times** daily, you hear your baby **swallowing,** and your baby is having AT LEAST **3–4 bowel movements** daily (more than 4 is great), you can be assured that your baby is doing well with breastfeeding.

Breastfeeding Start Time   Date _____

Midnight   Noon

12 1 2 3 4 5 6 7 8 9 10 11 12 1 2 3 4 5 6 7 8 9 10 11

Bowel Movements 1 2 3 4+   Total number of feedings in 24 hours _____

Breastfeeding Start Time   Date _____

Midnight   Noon

12 1 2 3 4 5 6 7 8 9 10 11 12 1 2 3 4 5 6 7 8 9 10 11

Bowel Movements 1 2 3 4+   Total number of feedings in 24 hours _____

Breastfeeding Start Time   Date _____

Midnight   Noon

12 1 2 3 4 5 6 7 8 9 10 11 12 1 2 3 4 5 6 7 8 9 10 11

Bowel Movements 1 2 3 4+   Total number of feedings in 24 hours _____

Breastfeeding Start Time   Date _____

Midnight   Noon

12 1 2 3 4 5 6 7 8 9 10 11 12 1 2 3 4 5 6 7 8 9 10 11

Bowel Movements 1 2 3 4+   Total number of feedings in 24 hours _____

Breastfeeding Start Time   Date _____

Midnight   Noon

12 1 2 3 4 5 6 7 8 9 10 11 12 1 2 3 4 5 6 7 8 9 10 11

Bowel Movements 1 2 3 4+   Total number of feedings in 24 hours _____

Breastfeeding Start Time   Date _____

Midnight   Noon

12   1   2   3   4   5   6   7   8   9   10   11   12   1   2   3   4   5   6   7   8   9   10   11

Bowel Movements   1 2 3 4+   Total number of feedings in 24 hours _____

Breastfeeding Start Time   Date _____

Midnight   Noon

12   1   2   3   4   5   6   7   8   9   10   11   12   1   2   3   4   5   6   7   8   9   10   11

Bowel Movements   1 2 3 4+   Total number of feedings in 24 hours _____

IF YOU HAVE ANY CONCERNS OR QUESTIONS ABOUT BREASTFEEDING, CALL

Local Breastfeeding Resource Name Here
Telephone Number Here

HOW DO I KNOW IF BREASTFEEDING IS GOING WELL?

The following questions will help you know whether you and your baby are off to a good start with breastfeeding.

Directions: Answer these questions when your baby is **5 to 7 days old.** If you circle an answer in the right-hand column, call your breastfeeding resource person at (**Local Telephone Number Here**).

1. Do you feel breastfeeding is going well for you now?	Yes	No
2. Have you noticed an increase in your milk supply?	Yes	No
3. Is your baby able to latch onto your breasts with her mouth covering all of your nipple and some of the dark area?	Yes	No
4. Does your baby swallow at least 5 minutes at each breast?	Yes	No
5. Does your baby let you know when he/she is hungry? (Answer no if you have to wake your baby up for most feedings.)	Yes	No
6. Does your baby usually nurse at both breasts each feeding?	Yes	No
7. Does your baby nurse about every 2 to 3 hours, with no more than one long sleep interval of up to 5 hours (at least 8 nursings each 24 hours)?	Yes	No
8. Do your breasts feel full before feedings?	Yes	No
9. Do your breasts feel soft after feedings?	Yes	No
10. Are your nipples so sore that you dread breastfeeding?	No	Yes

---

BOX 8–5   *(cont.)*

11. Is your baby having bowel movements that are soft and
    mustard-yellow with small curds?   Yes   No

12. Is your baby having at least 4 bowel movements each day
    that are more than a "stain" on the diaper?   Yes   No

13. When you notice a wet diaper, is it pale yellow or clear?   Yes   No

14. Does your baby seem to be hungry after most feedings
    (is he/she fussy, sucking his/her hands, or vigorously sucking
    a pacifier after most feedings)?   No   Yes

15. Do you have any sore, tender areas in your breast that are
    firm and red?   No   Yes

Local Breastfeeding Resource Name Here
Telephone Number Here

Source: Adapted by the Breastfeeding Resource Center, Mercy Health Center, Oklahoma City, OK, from materials originally developed by the Lactation Program, Presbyterian/St. Luke's Medical Center, Denver, CO.

As birth settings that support breastfeeding are recognized and rewarded by the community, families will, in turn, become lifelong paying "customers" of the health care system offering them. Core components of developing and presenting continuing education programs follow these sequential steps:

1. Assess the learning needs of the participants.

2. Assess participants' motivation and readiness to learn.

3. Plan and develop learning objectives, curriculum content, and teaching methods.

4. Implement teaching strategies and assist participants in focusing attention on learning tasks.

5. Evaluate the outcome of teaching activities.

Managers become aware of learning needs and deficits in the clinical staff through feedback from families and from other health care providers. In addition to gaining administrative input regarding learning needs, potential participants of the educational program should be involved in assessing their own learning needs. Their involvement in the planning stage will enhance their belief that the program will benefit them in their clinical practice. Staff members may attend educational programs either because their employer requires attendance or because they need to attend a certain number of continuing-education offerings to maintain their professional registration or certification (extrinsic motivation). However, if participants are there because they want to be (intrinsic motivation), they are self-directed learners who have identified their learning goals and are enthusiastic about learning. Relating the curriculum content directly to a clinician's practice is a key strategy for arousing and maintaining interest in the program.

Teaching strategies for staff or continuing professional education are similar to those used with breastfeeding families. Health care providers are generally action-oriented; they do not enjoy being passive participants. They also appreciate frequent breaks, because they are rarely sedentary in their employment settings.

Evaluating professional educational programs includes the staff's own assessment of the useful-

BOX 8–6

Sample Continuing-Education Program

Program title: Insufficient Lactation and Infant Weight Gain

Description: This two-hour course reviews the characteristics and interventions of a situation where infant is gaining weight at below acceptable levels owing to apparent maternal lactation insufficiency.

Objectives:

1. Correlate normal growth with expected nutritional intake.

2. Assess the mother-infant to determine probable causes of insufficient milk supply.

3. Identify variation in the lactating breast that may potentially impact a mother's milk supply.

4. Distinguish between primary and secondary lactation insufficiency.

5. Describe effective interventions, including supplementation of the infant while maintaining lactation and feedings at the breast.

(Three objectives can usually be adequately covered in one hour.)

Teaching Methodology: Lecture, slides, videotape, case study for discussion

Instructor: Jane Smith, PhD, IBCLC

References:

Hillervik-Lindquist C: Studies on perceived breastmilk insufficiency. A prospective study in a group of Swedish women. *Acta Paediatr Scand Suppl* 376:1–27, 1991.

Livingstone V: Problem-solving formula for failure-to-thrive infants. *Can Fam Phys* 36:1541-5, 1990.

Neifert M, Seacat J, Jobe W: Lactation failure due to insufficient glandular development of the breasts. *Pediatrics* 76:823-8, 1985.

Willis DE, Livingstone V: Infant insufficient milk syndrome associated with maternal postpartum hemorrhage. *J Hum Lact* 11:123–6, 1995.

Evaluation: Program will be evaluated by participants using the standardized Comprehensive Evaluation Tool for Continuing Health Education Programs (CETCHEP). Faculty/presenter will receive evaluation results and participant comments.

---

ness of the program to their clinical practices and an appraisal of the speaker and the content. This information is invaluable in modifying future programs; it also helps to convey the goal of clinical applicability and communicates respect for participants as valuable individuals.

Objectives and Outcomes

In developing education programs for health care professionals, it is useful to clearly identify what the learner is expected to master. Writing behavioral objectives is one concrete way of identifying learning goals. A behavioral objective states what the student will be able to do at the end of the session. See Table 8–2 for examples of the correct way and the incorrect way to write behavioral objectives.

Program outcomes are different from objectives. Objectives have to do with what a learner is able to do as a result of an education program, whereas outcomes are the *results* of clinical practice

Table 8–2

EXAMPLES OF BEHAVIORAL OBJECTIVES

Incorrect

The participant will understand the relationship between breastfeeding and jaundice.
(Note: the student's "understanding" is not observable.)

Not Observable

Understand, know, appreciate, learn, perceive, recognize, be aware of, comprehend, grasp the significance of, gain a working knowledge of

Correct

The learner will list three types of neonatal jaundice and will describe the relationship of each type to breastfeeding.

Observable

State, list, define, identify, describe, compare, critique, rate, demonstrate, plan, design, choose, discuss, match, relate, categorize, distinguish between, select, locate

---

that may be an indirect result of educational programs. An example is staff nurses who become more knowledgeable about breastfeeding after attending a series of continuing-education programs, and this new knowledge ultimately results in fewer mothers weaning early. Outcomes must be relevant and measurable and a logical result of clinical practices or of institutional effort. Examples of breastfeeding outcomes are

- the number of mothers who initiate breastfeeding,

- length of time the mothers breastfed,

- rate of ER visits for breastfeeding infants with dehydration, and

- cost savings to the managed care organization due to the better health of infants because they were breastfed (Riordan, 1997).

All of these outcomes are relevant, and measurable and reflect staff and institutional knowledge and effort. Managed-care organizations now require not only clinical-outcomes data periodically but in "real time" (i.e., weekly or monthly). As hospital information systems are developed, it is important that outcome parameters relevant to breastfeeding are incorporated into databases. A breastfeeding promotion program in Santiago,

Chile, is a model for describing the impact of education on breastfeeding outcomes and the measurement of those outcomes. As a result of this hospital's breastfeeding promotion program that included training a health team at the Wellstart San Diego Lactation Program, the number of women delivering at the hospital who fully breastfed and experienced lactational amenorrhea doubled. Costs saved by the hospital were estimated to be 14 percent (Valdes et al., 1995).

The Team Approach

A team approach to breastfeeding education enhances the learning experiences of childbearing families. Health care providers cannot simply promote breastfeeding; they must provide specific information to enhance breastfeeding success. It is crucial that each team member present consistent information. Acquisition of the parental role is enhanced when new parents are given specific, concrete recommendations (Bocar & Moore, 1987). Conflicting information frustrates the patient and erodes new parents' trust in the health care system.

The health care team is responsible for a comprehensive approach. The fragmented care that often typifies women's health care today is not conducive to effective breastfeeding education. Families need a thorough understanding of the dynamics of breastfeeding. Consistent information shared by a variety of providers on multiple occasions strengthens the impact of each breastfeeding education encounter. Each family has varying breastfeeding goals. Health care providers can assist families to meet their goals on the basis of informed decisions.

Each member of the team must be aware of the content discussed by other members, to avoid unintentional contradiction. Documenting what has been discussed with teaching checklists and care maps allows the educator to build on that foundation and to reinforce key points. Networking among local and regional colleagues provides many opportunities to improve educational programs and to avoid the omission of key topics. Each health care provider develops a unique relationship with a breastfeeding family and can make unique contributions to the family's education (Bocar, 1992).

Childbirth Educators. Childbirth educators develop rapport with breastfeeding families during their multisession classes. They provide invaluable anticipatory guidance by including breastfeeding information in general childbirth education programs. Following childbirth, families frequently seek breastfeeding assistance from childbirth instructors.

Perinatal Nurses and Health Care Providers. Perinatal nurses and health care providers possess basic competencies related to breastfeeding education and provide breastfeeding education along with many other types of health education that communicate the normalcy of breastfeeding. Perinatal nurses often provide assistance with early breastfeeding and refer more complex cases to lactation consultants. They may be certified as breastfeeding educators, lactation educators, or lactation counselors or may possess other titles that indicate completion of a study of breastfeeding basics (Fig. 8–3).

Lactation Consultants

Lactation consultants are health care providers whose primary focus is providing breastfeeding assistance. Lactation consultants provide a variety of specialized services, including individual consultations for unusual breastfeeding situations, care plans developed in collaboration with other health

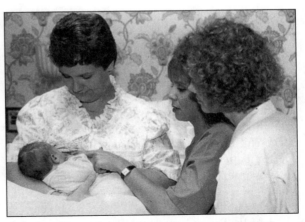

FIGURE 8–3. Perinatal nurse learning new skills from lactation consultant. *(Courtesy Debi Leslie Bocar.)*

care providers, breastfeeding class sessions, and instruction in the use of specific breastfeeding products. They also serve as a resource for information and data, develop special programs or projects related to breastfeeding, provide continuing education programs for health care providers, and conduct research (see Chapter 22).

Physicians. Physicians can serve as powerful breastfeeding promoters. Their support of breastfeeding can be a potent force in a family's decision to begin and continue breastfeeding (Graffy, 1992). Physicians often refer families to lactation consultants for time-intensive treatment of breastfeeding difficulties or follow-up.

Dietitians. Dietitians' responsibilities include nutritional counseling for childbearing families. They can describe the influence of breastfeeding on maternal and infant nutrition needs. Many dietitians working with breastfeeding families are employed by WIC programs and in other community health settings.

Community Support Groups. Mother-to-mother support groups create an invaluable social support network for breastfeeding families. Practical tips and much incidental learning about parenting are derived from these important support groups. The largest and most effective self-care group for breastfeeding support is La Leche League International (LLLI). Founded in 1956, LLLI's core service is mother-to-mother support and information provided through small neighborhood-based groups. Four monthly topics are provided throughout the year on a rotating basis.

Leaders are available between meetings for individual assistance and problem solving. The relaxed, friendly interchange between women with common interests in breastfeeding, childbearing, and childrearing is a basic strength of this highly successful organization. LLLI is effective in meeting the educational and support needs of middle-class women in 46 countries. More than 9,000 volunteer leaders are estimated to serve more than 100,000 families in the United States each year.

LLLI's Peer Counseling Program was developed in 1986 to meet the needs of socioeconomically disadvantaged families in the United States. The program educates mothers from low-income areas and provides up-to-date information and assistance to their peers. Instructors are LLL leaders with additional training in working in this program. LLLI requires that peer counselor candidates have three to six months of breastfeeding experience. Other programs are generally modeled on LLLI's program but may lack the "buddy" concept. All require close coordination with professionals in the sponsoring agency. Several training manuals have been developed. Some childbirth-education groups in the United States have developed additional mother-to-mother breastfeeding support groups. Peer-support programs are often sponsored by state WIC agencies. Peer-support groups have also been developed in other countries.

SUMMARY

Breastfeeding families are empowered for self-sufficiency when health care providers furnish information in an accurate, well-organized manner. When good information is coupled with identification of the family's goals and with problem solving, parents have greater self-confidence and self-reliance.

Although providing information to families and assisting with problem solving are components of empowerment, removing specific barriers to breastfeeding also is essential. Strategies that promote breastfeeding include facilitating early, frequent breastfeeding; encouraging rooming-in; avoiding routine formula supplementation; providing early assistance and follow-up; teaching families the signs of adequate nutritional intake by the infant; and instructing families about the relationship between milk removal from the breast and continued milk production. Applying principles of the change process can assist health care providers in promoting practices that improve breastfeeding success.

Underestimating a family's desire to breastfeed may be an unrecognized barrier to its continuance. This is particularly true with adolescent mothers, single mothers, immigrant women, mothers from ethnic minority populations, or mothers who are employed outside the home. Health care providers tend to underestimate a family's interest in such information (Waitzkin, 1985).

Developing and presenting educational programs for health care providers who assist breastfeeding families requires significant time and energy. One needs to remember the ripple effect related to education; enormous numbers of breastfeeding families benefit from the enhanced knowledge of health care providers. A successful education program—regardless of its subject matter—entails positive experiences for learners and educators. Identifying the components of effective breastfeeding education programs can assist health care providers who are involved in planning, implementing, and evaluating breastfeeding services.

REFERENCES

Aberman S, Kirchoff KT: Infant-feeding practices: mothers' decision-making. *JOGN Nurs* 14:394–8, 1985.

Adair LS, Popkin BM, Guilday DK: The duration of breast-feeding: how it is affected by biological, sociodemographic, health sector, and food industry factors. *Demography* 30:63–80, 1993.

Aken J: A captive audience for breastfeeding information. *J Hum Lact* 9(3):183, 1993.

Alexy B, Martin CA: Breastfeeding: perceived barriers and benefits/enhancers in a rural and urban setting. *Public Health Nurs* 11:214–18, 1994.

Anderson GC: Risk in mother-infant separation postbirth. *Image* 21:196–9, 1989.

Auerbach KG: Beyond the issue of accuracy: evaluating patient education materials for breastfeeding mothers. *J Hum Lact* 4:108–10, 1988.

Auerbach KG: Discharge milk samples. (letter) *Pediatrics* 91:518–19, 1993a.

Auerbach KG: Employed breastfeeding mothers: problems they encounter. *Birth* 11:17–20, 1984.

Auerbach, KG: Hospital discharge formula packs: do they really hinder breastfeeding? *Mo Baby J* 2:41–46, 1997.

Auerbach KG: One result of marketing: breastfeeding is the exception in infant feeding. (editorial) *J Trop Pediatr* 38:210–13, 1993b.

Auerbach, KG: The influence of lactation consultant contact on breastfeeding duration in a low-income population. *Neb Med J* 70:341–6, 1985.

Bagwell JE, et al: Knowledge and attitudes toward breast-feeding among dietitians, nurses, and physicians working with WIC clients. *J Am Diet Assoc* 93:801–4, 1993.

Balcazar H, Trier C, Coba J: What predicts breast-feeding intention in Mexican-American and non-Hispanic white women? Evidence from a national survey. *Birth* 22:74–80, 1995.

Baranowski T, et al: Social support, social influence, ethnicity and the breastfeeding decision. *Soc Sci Med* 17:1599–1611, 1983.

Becton LG, Dickenson CC: Patient comprehension profiles: recent findings and strategies. *Pat Counsel Health Educ* 2:101–6, 1981.

Bar-Yam NB, Darby L: Fathers and breastfeeding: a review of the literature. *J Hum Lact* 13:45–50, 1997.

Benson S: Adolescent mothers experience of parenting and breastfeeding—a descriptive study. *Breastfeed Rev* 5:19–26, 1996.

Beske EJ, Garvis MS: Important factors in breastfeeding success. *MCN* 7:174–9, 1982.

Birenbaum E, Fuchs C, Reichman B: Demographic factors influencing the initiation of breast-feeding in an Israeli urban population. *Pediatrics* 83:519–23, 1989.

Bloom BS: *Taxonomy of educational objectives.* New York: David McKay Co., 1956:7–8.

Bocar DL: The lactation consultant: part of the health care team. *Clin Iss Perinat Wom Health Nurs* 3:731–7, 1992.

Bocar DL, Moore K: *Acquiring the parental role: a theoretical perspective* (Unit 16, Lactation Consultant Series). Garden City Park, NY: Avery Publishing Group, 1987:2–11.

Braveman P, et al: Early discharge of newborns and mothers: a critical review of the literature. *Pediatrics* 96:716–26, 1995.

Brillinger MF: Helping adults learn. *J Hum Lact* 6:171–5, 1990.

Britton JR, Britton HL, Beebe SA: Early discharge of the term newborn: a continued dilemma. *Pediatrics* 94:291–5, 1994.

Bryant CA: The impact of kin, friend, and neighbor networks on infant feeding practices. *Soc Sci Med* 16:1757–65, 1982.

Bryant CA: Promoting breastfeeding among economically disadvantaged women and adolescents. *Clin Iss Perinat Wom Health Nurs* 3:723–30, 1992.

Buckner E, Matsubara M: Support network by breastfeeding mothers. *J Hum Lact* 9:231–5, 1993.

Carr DK, Hard KJ, Trahant WJ: *Managing the change process*. New York: McGraw-Hill, 1996: 115–31.

Cohen SA: Postpartum teaching and the subsequent use of milk supplements. *Birth Fam J* 7:163–7, 1980.

Coopersmith S: *The antecedents of self-esteem*. San Francisco: W.H. Freeman, 1967:37–8.

Covey S: *Seven habits of highly effective people*. New York: Simon and Shuster, 1989: 287–307.

Crowder DS: Maternity nurses' knowledge of factors promoting successful breastfeeding: a survey of two hospitals. *JOGN Nurs* 10:28–30, 1981.

Curro V, et al: Randomized controlled trial assessing the effectiveness of a booklet on the duration of breast feeding. *Arch Dis Child* 76:500–4, 1997.

Darkenwald GG, Merriam SB: *Adult education: foundations of practice*. New York: Harper & Row, 1982.

Davies-Adetugbo AA, Adebawa AA: The Ife South Breastfeeding Project: training community health extension workers to promote and manage breastfeeding in rural communities. *Bull WHO* 75:323–32, 1997.

Driscoll JW: Breastfeeding success and failure: implications for nurses. *Clin Iss Perinat Wom Health Nurs* 3:565–9, 1992.

Dunn R: Learning–a matter of style. *Educ Lead* 36:430–2, 1979.

Egan G: *The skilled helper: model skills and methods of effective helping*. 2nd ed. Monterey, CA: Brooks-Cole, 1982, 60–1.

Eidelman A, Hoffmann NW, Kaitz M: Cognitive deficits in women after childbirth. *Obstet Gynecol* 81:764–7, 1993.

Ekwo EE, Dusdieker LB, Booth BM: Factors influencing initiation of breast-feeding. *Am J Dis Child* 137:375–77.

Flanagan PJ, et al: Adolescent development and transitions to motherhood. *Pediatrics* 96:273–7, 1995.

Freed GL, et al: Pediatrician involvement in breast-feeding promotion: a national study of residents and practitioners. *Pediatrics* 96:490–4, 1995.

Freed GL, Fraley JK, Schanler RJ: Accuracy of expectant mothers' predictions of fathers' attitudes regarding breast-feeding. *J Fam Pract* 37:148–52, 1993a.

Freed GL, Fraley JK, Schanler RJ: Effect of expectant mothers' feeding plan on prediction of fathers' attitudes regarding breast-feeding. *Am J Perinatol* 10:300–3, 1993b.

Galpin TJ: *The human side of change*. San Francisco: Josey-Bass, 1996:123–33.

Garcia E: Moving change through the system: a model for staff involvement. *MCN* 21:219–21, 1996.

Gielen AC, et al: Determinates of breastfeeding in a rural WIC population. *J Hum Lact* 8:11–15, 1992.

Giugliani ERJ, et al: Effect of breastfeeding support from different sources on mothers' decisions to breastfeed. *J Hum Lact* 10:157–61, 1994.

Gorman T, Byrd TL, VanDerslice J: Breast-feeding practices, attitudes, and beliefs among Hispanic women and men in a border community. *Fam Commun Health* 18:17–27, 1995.

Graffy J: Breastfeeding: the GD's role. *Practitioner* 236:322–4, 1992.

Grassley J, Davis K: Common concerns of mothers who breast-feed. *MCN* 6:347–51, 1978.

Grossman LK, et al: The effect of postpartum lactation counseling on the duration of breastfeeding in low-income women. *Am J Dis Child* 144:471–74, 1990.

Gulick E: Informational correlates of successful breastfeeding. *MCN* 7:370–5, 1982.

Gunning R: *The technique of clear writing* (rev ed). New York: McGraw-Hill, 1968:38–40.

Haber J, Hoskins PP: *Comprehensive psychiatric nursing* (3rd ed). New York: McGraw-Hill, 1987.

Hall JM: Influencing breastfeeding success. *JOGN Nurs* 7:28–32, 1978.

Hanson J: Breastfeeding education: meeting the needs of the expectant parent. *Breastfeed Rev* 4(2):65–8, 1996.

Hayes B: Inconsistencies among nurses in breastfeeding knowledge and counselling. *JOGN Nurs* 10:430–3, 1981.

Hewat RJ, Ellis DJ: Similarities and differences between women who breastfeed for short and long duration. *Midwifery* 2:37–43, 1986.

Howard FM, Howard CR, Weitzman M: Infant formula distribution and advertising in pregnancy: a hospital survey. *Birth* 21:14–19, 1994.

Howard FM, Howard CR, Weitzman M: The physician as advertiser: the unintentional discouragement of breastfeeding. *Obstet Gynecol* 81:1048–51, 1993.

Hunt CE: Antenatal formula advertising: another potential threat to breastfeeding. *Pediatrics* 94:102–7, 1994.

Janke S: Free formula samples for all. *Child Instruct Magazine* 5:32–5, 1995.

Janke JR: The incidence, benefits, and variables associated with breastfeeding: implications for practice. *Nurse Pract* 18:22–32, 1993.

Jones DA: The choice to breast feed or bottle feed and influences upon that choice: a survey of 1525 mothers. *Child Care Health Dev* 13:75–85, 1987.

Kaplowitz DD, Olson CM: The effect of an education program on the decision to breastfeed. *J Nutr Educ* 15:61–5, 1983.

Kistin N, Abramson R, Dublin P: Effect of peer counselors on breastfeeding initiation, exclusivity, and duration among low-income urban women. *J Hum Lact* 10:11–15, 1994.

Knowles M: *The modern practice of adult education*. New York: Cambridge University, 1980.

Kocturk T: Advantages of breastfeeding according to Turkish mothers living in Istanbul and Stockholm. *Soc Sci Med* 27:405–10, 1988.

Kotter JP: *Leading change*. Boston: Harvard Business School Press, 1996:20–1.

Kozier B, Erb G: *Fundamentals of nursing: concepts and procedures* (3rd ed). Menlo Park, CA: Addison-Wesley, 1987.

Lapierre J, Perrault M, Goulet C: Prenatal peer counseling: an answer to the persistent difficulties with prenatal care for low-income women. *J Public Health Nurs* 12:53, 1995.

Lauwers J, Woessner C: *Counseling the nursing mother* (2nd ed). Garden City Park, NY: Avery Publishing Group, 1989:13.

Lawrence RA: Early discharge alert. *Pediatrics* 96:966–7, 1995.

Lawrence RA: Practices and attitudes toward breastfeeding among medical professionals. *Pediatrics* 70:912–20, 1982.

Lewin K: *Field theory in social science*. New York: Harper & Row, 1951.

Lewinski CA: Nurse's knowledge of breastfeeding in a clinical setting. *J Hum Lact* 8:143–6, 1992.

Libbus MK: Perspectives of common breastfeeding situations: a known group comparison. *J Hum Lact* 8:199–203, 1992.

Littman H, et al: The decision to breastfeed: the importance of fathers' approval. *Clin Pediatr* 33:214–19, 1994.

Locklin MP: Passionate advocacy: a look back, a look forward. *J Hum Lact* 9:181, 1993.

Locklin MP: Telling the world: low income women and their breastfeeding experiences. *J Hum Lact* 285–91, 1995.

Locklin MP, Naber SJ: Does breastfeeding empower women? Insights from a select group of educated, low-income, minority women. *Birth* 20:30–5, 1993.

Long DG, et al: Peer counselor program increases breastfeeding rates in Utah Native American WIC population. *J Hum Lact* 11:279–84, 1995.

Maehr JC, et al: A comparative study of adolescent and adult mothers who intend to breastfeed. *J Adolesc Health* 14:453–7, 1993.

Marchand L, Morrow MH: Infant feeding practices: understanding the decision-making process. *Fam Med* 26:319–24, 1994.

Matich J, Sims LS: A comparison of social support variables between women who intend to breast or bottlefeed. *Soc Sci Med* 34:919–27, 1992.

McClurg–Hitt D, Olsen J: Infant feeding decisions in the Missouri WIC program. *J Hum Lact* 10:253–6, 1994.

McNatt MH, Freston MS: Social support and lactation outcomes in postpartum women. *J Hum Lact* 8:73–7, 1992.

Motil KJ, Kertz B, Thotathuckery M: Lactational performance of adolescent mothers shows preliminary differences from that of adult women. *J Adolesc Health* 20:442–49, 1997.

Nabor SJ, Locklin MP: Are peer counselors the key to achieving breastfeeding success with low income women? *Breastfeed Abstr* 13:19–20, 1994.

Naylor AJ, et al: Lactation management education for physicians. *Semin Perinatol* 18:525–31, 1994.

Naylor A: Professional education and training for trainers. *Int J Gynecol Obstet* 31(suppl1):25–7, 1990.

New JR, Couillard NA: Guidelines for introducing change. *J Nurs Admin* 11:17–21, 1981.

Newton E: Breastfeeding/lactation and the medical school curriculum. *J Hum Lact* 8:122–4, 1992.

Neyzi O, et al: An educational intervention on promotion of breastfeeding complemented by continuing support. *Paediatr Perinat Epidemiol* 5:299–303, 1991.

Nichols FH, Edwards MR: Are your group process skills up to par? *Nurs Health Care* 9:205–8, 1988.

Nyberg J: Probing the change process. *Superv Nurs* 11:31–3, 1980.

Owen AM: Impediments to breast-feeding in hospitals. *World Health Forum* 15:373–4, 1994.

Palti H, et al: Evaluation of the effectiveness of a structured breast-feeding promotion program integrated into a maternal and child health service in Jerusalem. *Isr J Med Sci* 24:342–8, 1988.

Pease A: *Signals*. New York: Bantam 1984:6–7.

Peterson CE, DaVanzo J: Why are teenagers in the United States less likely to breast-feed than older women? *Demography* 29:431–50, 1992.

Posner GJ, Rudnitsky AN: *Course design: a guide to curriculum development for teachers* (2nd ed). New York: Longman Publishing Group, 1982:108–17.

Pugin E, et al: Does prenatal breastfeeding skills group education increase the effectiveness of a comprehensive breastfeeding promotion program? *J Hum Lact* 12:15–19, 1996.

Purtell M: Teenage girls' attitudes to breastfeeding. *Health Vis* 67:156–7, 1994.

Radius SM, Joffe A: Understanding adolescent mothers' feelings about breastfeeding: a study of perceived benefits and barriers. *J Adolesc Health Care* 9:156–60, 1988.

Redman BK: *The process of patient education* (6th ed). St Louis: Mosby, 1988.

Riordan J: *A practical guide to breastfeeding*. St Louis: Mosby, 1983.

Riordan J: Readable, relevant, reliable: the three "R's" of breastfeeding pamphlets. *Breastfeed Abstr* 5:5–6, 1985.

Riordan JM: the cost of not breastfeeding: a commentary. *J Hum Lact* 13:93–97, 1997.

Robinson JB, et al: Attitudes toward infant feeding among adolescent mothers from a WIC population in northern Louisiana. *J Am Diet Assoc* 93:1311–13, 1993.

Rouke L: Earlier postdischarge visits promote breastfeeding. *Can Fam Phys* 41:374, 1995.

Sampson EE, Marthas M: *Group process for the health professions*. New York: Wiley, 1981.

Schy DS, et al: The effects of in-hospital lactation education on breastfeeding practice. *J Hum Lact* 12:117–22, 1996.

Sciacca JP, et al: A breast feeding education and promotion program: effects on knowledge, attitudes and support for breast feeding. *J Commun Health* 20:473–90, 1995a.

Sciacca JP, et al: Influences on breast-feeding by lower-income women: an incentive-based, partner supported educational program. *J Am Diet Assoc* 95:323–8, 1995b.

Shelton K: Empowering women to breastfeed successfully. *Breastfeed Rev* 2:455–8, 1994.

Shrago LC, Bocar DL: The infant's contribution to breastfeeding. *JOGNN* 19:209–15, 1990.

Smith LJ: A score sheet for evaluating breastfeeding educational materials. *J Hum Lact* 11:307–11, 1995.

Snell BJ, et al: The association of formula samples given at hospital discharge with the duration of breastfeeding. *J Hum Lact* 8:67–72, 1992.

Sullivan J, Jones LC: Breastfeeding adoption by low-income black women. *Health Care Wom Int* 7:295–309, 1986.

Tubbs SL: *A systems approach to small group interaction*. Reading, MA: Addison-Wesley, 1984.

Turner GM: Peer counseling. *Pediatr Ann* 24:330, 1995.

Valaitis RK, Shea E: An evaluation of breastfeeding promotion literature: does it really promote breastfeeding? *Can J Public Health* 84:24–7, 1993.

Valdes V, Pugin E, Labbok MH: The effects of professional practice of a three-day course on breastfeeding. *J Hum Lact* 11:185–90, 1995.

Waitzkin H: Information giving in medical care. *J Health Soc Behav* 26:81–101, 1985.

Weinberg SH: An alternative to meet the needs of early discharge: the tender beginnings postpartum visit. *MCN* 19:339–42, 1994.

Westphal MF, et al: Breast-feeding training for health professionals and resultant institutional changes. *Bull WHO* 73:461–8, 1995.

Wiles LS: The effect of prenatal breastfeeding education on breastfeeding success and maternal perception of the infant. *JOGN Nurs* 13:253–7, 1984.

Yoos L: Developmental issues and the choice of feeding method of adolescent mothers. *JOGN Nurs* 14:68–72, 1985.

Young SA, Kaufman M: Promoting breastfeeding at a migrant health center. *Am J Public Health* 78:523–5, 1988.

The Breastfeeding Process: The Perinatal and Intrapartum Period

Kathleen G. Auerbach and Jan Riordan

Helping new mothers during the lactation process is a rewarding experience for the nurse or lactation consultant. With a basic understanding of the anatomy and physiology of the breast and of the nutritional and immunological properties of breastmilk, the health care worker can contribute greatly to a mother's breastfeeding experience. However, the care provider must be prepared to offer practical assistance supported by relevant research findings and to meet the urgent needs of mothers with little or no breastfeeding experience. The provider must also be able to assist new mothers who, despite previous breastfeeding experience, are still anxious about doing it. Emphasis on confident self-care is a major goal.

What the mother learns about breastfeeding and caring for herself and her baby in the medical office, the hospital, or the clinic will affect her breastfeeding relationship for a long time and may influence how she feeds not one but all of her children. Many women who initiate breastfeeding wean after two months or even sooner. Thus we emphasize the necessity for self-care skills. *Self-care,* the guiding framework for this book, can be defined as "the practice of activities that individuals person-

ally initiate and perform on their own behalf in maintaining life, health, and well-being" (Orem, 1980). In the self-care approach to breastfeeding, each care provider educates, assists, encourages, and nurtures the mother and her family toward effective use of each member's resources for achieving an optimal breastfeeding experience. As Rubin (1961, 1967a, b) so clearly demonstrated, the maternal role, far from being intuitive, is learned.

The self-care orientation is congruent with the current recognition of consumer participation and partnership in health care. Self-care education is based on the parent's perceived needs rather than needs identified by the health care provider. It is especially appropriate for maternal infant-care nursing, a field in which, unlike other areas of nursing, clients are usually healthy. In no other area of health care is the consumer's involvement in her own care more rewarding to assist and to observe.

Breastfeeding Preparation

Although preparation for breastfeeding is often given a great deal of importance, the best preparation for breastfeeding is for the mother to learn as much as possible before she embarks on her own lactation adventure. Gaining this knowledge can be accomplished in any number of ways. She may choose to take a prenatal breastfeeding class. Classes are offered by health care organizations, independent lactation consultants, or by community-based breastfeeding support groups, such as La Leche League International (LLLI) or the Nursing Mothers Associations (NMA). Both LLLI and NMA groups offer ongoing support and are not dependent on a single institution. Thus they are less likely to include questionable recommendations that stem from the practices or routines of a particular hospital or clinic.

Some physicians in pediatrics or family practice also offer breastfeeding classes in their offices. These classes usually are part of these doctors' regular services, which cover the prenatal through the immediate postbirth periods. Breastfeeding classes are also offered by hospitals as a way of encouraging parents to use their facility. In still other cases, breastfeeding is the topic for one or two sessions of a childbirth preparation or parenting class.

In addition to attending a class, mothers can prepare by reading books about breastfeeding. Learning about breastfeeding through reading requires proper choice of the reading material. Information by reputable authors is best; the recommendations of knowledgeable reviewers may be quite valuable. Although many brochures and book-length materials are available, not all are accurate or up-to-date. Reading material prepared by proprietary formula companies or companies that make infant-feeding equipment, for example, often leave the impression that breastfeeding is difficult and requires the use of supplemental infant formula and a variety of other equipment. Such material may also imply that weaning from the breast occurs early.

Discussing breastfeeding with one or more women who have experienced it is another way to learn. If they also share the same career or live in the same neighborhood, they may become a mutual resource for finding a pediatrician or a reputable babysitting service and for comparing breastfeeding experiences. The experienced breastfeeding mother who acts as a mentor to the less knowledgeable woman can teach her much how-to information. She also can respond to the new mother's concerns and feelings and advise her on aspects of breastfeeding that are more difficult to address in written form or in a less personal setting.

Breast and Nipple Preparation

Prenatal preparation of nipple tissue, a frequent recommendation, is unnecessary and is based on a faulty assumption: that the nipple and breast tissue require treatment in preparing for breastfeeding. On the contrary, the mother who makes no such efforts will be just as ready to breastfeed as the mother who spends time and effort attempting to condition her breasts (Brown & Hurlock, 1975; Whitley, 1974).

Some mothers are told to attempt to express colostrum, to roll their nipples, or to condition the nipple through the use of friction. There is no need to express colostrum prior to the birth of the baby. The mother with a history of preterm labor should avoid stimulating her breasts through expression or nipple rolling. The latter technique—especially if practiced frequently by women with a history of preterm labor—may stimulate labor contractions (Capeless & Mann, 1984; Elliot & Flaherty, 1983; Oki et al., 1987). Colostrum is produced throughout the pregnancy and need not be expressed to determine its presence. In some mothers, colostrum spontaneously leaks during sexual intercourse and late in pregnancy when nipples rub against clothing. Nipple rolling, too, is unnecessary to prepare the breasts for breastfeeding, although women learn how quickly the nipples respond to stimulation when they do so. During pregnancy, the breasts begin making milk, and the nipples become more elastic, which may explain why many women characterize their nipples as "flat" or "inverted" at the beginning, but not at the end, of pregnancy.

If the nipple remains flat or retracted, nipple rolling may stimulate a greater degree of eversion than might otherwise be observed; however, the negative pressure exerted by the baby in the act of suckling will have the same effect. How the nipple looks when the baby is not suckling bears little resemblance to its appearance in the baby's mouth, nor is it necessary for the nipple to be everted when not in the baby's mouth. Hoffmann's exercises for nipple inversion or flatness have no noticeable impact on the appearance of the nipple (Hoffmann, 1953) or on the degree of inversion or protractility (MAIN Collaborative Group Preparing for Breast Feeding, 1994). For women who have never handled their breasts except in a sexual context, occasional nipple rolling, Hoffmann's exercises and other manipulations may help them to view their breasts in a more matter-of-fact manner. For that reason, such preparation may be helpful.

It is a fallacy to assume that nipple tissue, with stimulation (or use by the baby) will become "toughened" (Auerbach, 1990). Such a term implies a reduction in sensitivity, but the nipple, which is highly ennervated, must remain sensitive to the baby's stimulation if it is to send to the brain the messages that trigger milk production and milk ejection.

If the nipples appear functional and are not inverted, the best preparation is to do as little as possible. Involving the breasts and nipples in lovemaking (except when the mother has a history of preterm labor; Salmon et al., 1986), washing without soap, and providing occasional brief exposure to sun and air are sufficient to prepare the nipples for breastfeeding (Riordan & Countryman, 1980).

The most important organ for breastfeeding is the mother's brain. When it receives signals from the nipple and breast, milk production and ejection will occur. Mothering is more learned than instinctive (Rubin, 1967a, b), and a mother's best "teacher" is her own baby. When reaffirmed as a person and supported in her early efforts to breastfeed, a mother will have most of what she needs to assume her new role and relish the unique joys it will provide her.

The Birth Plan and Feeding Plan

The prospective mother in the United States must purchase her health care; thus it is her right to get what she pays for. This right may seem most obvious when relating to childbirth, but it also applies to her feeding plan and to how and when she intends to act on that plan. Frequently, expectant parents identify issues of importance to them, develop a birth plan, and use this plan to discuss with their midwife or physician their goals for the birth of their baby.

Using the same principles, parents may devise a feeding plan. Breastfeeding is the means by which the infant receives optimal nutrition. The infant's right to this milk must be preserved and protected, even if the baby is not immediately able to receive this milk. The family's wishes as they relate to breastfeeding must be understood by health care workers at the outset of their contact with the pregnant woman, particularly when the mother gives birth in a setting away from her own home. The feeding plan in Box 9–1 addresses issues to be included in an infant-feeding plan in a hospital setting.

In some institutions, specific elements in the feeding plan may be more difficult to implement than in other settings. For example, where glucose and artificial formula feedings are considered routine and where parental consent is not usually obtained prior to their use, provisions that restrict feeding at the breast alone will require that hospital caregivers furnish a kind of care that they may be unaccustomed to giving. It is the responsibility of the parents to speak for the infant, who is unable to voice his preference.

Early Feedings

Following birth, continuing assessment of the mother's physical condition and psychosocial status is essential. The optimal time for initiating breastfeeding depends on these factors and on the mother's informed choice and will not be the same for all individuals. If the birth process has been relatively uncomplicated, the mother should be encouraged to breastfeed immediately after birth and regularly thereafter.

The study by Crowell, Hill, and Humenick (1994) highlights the potential interaction effect of two background (nonchangeable) and two care-related variables. In their study, 48 healthy infants were followed. A key question was, at what time will the neonate exhibit effective breastfeeding? Four factors influenced that time: maternal parity, neonatal gender, timing of the baby's first feeding at the breast, and exposure to maternal labor analgesia.

How those four variables interacted made a difference. Specifically, the babies who took the longest time to demonstrate effective breastfeeding

BOX 9–1

Feeding Plan

- The mother's chart will indicate that she plans to breastfeed her baby.
- The baby's chart will be similarly marked to indicate that the baby is to be breastfed.
- The mother indicates the degree to which she expects to receive assistance with breastfeedings during her stay in the hospital and from whom she expects to receive such assistance. If her doctor employs a lactation consultant, that person needs to have hospital privileges to see the physician's patients while they are in the hospital. It is appropriate to ask whether the physician's LC can see patients in the hospital.
- The mother indicates whether she is willing to allow the baby to be fed by someone other than herself at any time during the hospital stay and whether she will provide her own milk for someone else to feed. She also specifies how her milk is to be given and under what conditions this may occur.
- The mother indicates what fluids, other than human milk, she will allow her baby to receive during the hospital stay, how such fluids are to be given, and under what conditions this may occur.
- If a family history of allergies has been identified (in a sibling of the new baby, his mother, his father, or other relative), that fact should be noted on both the mother's and the baby's charts; recommendations relating to the risks of using

fluids other than human milk should be noted accordingly (Heacock et al., 1992; Lifschitz et al., 1988).
- The mother indicates whether she expects the baby to be housed exclusively with her in her room and under what conditions, if any, the baby may be housed elsewhere.
- The mother indicates the frequency with which she expects to breastfeed her baby and under what circumstances, if any, she will not breastfeed the baby.
- The mother indicates whether she will provide her own milk to her baby in the event the baby is unable to suckle directly and whether she will arrange to provide fresh unrefrigerated, fresh refrigerated, fresh-frozen, or deep-frozen human milk in containers acceptable to the hospital in which her newborn is receiving care.

Each of the preceding points should be stated in writing, thereby providing a record of parental expectations about optimal care. A written feeding plan protects the parents, the outpatient caregivers, and all hospital staff members who work with the family by providing a clear understanding of the preferences and expectations of the parents with regard to the care and feeding of their child. It also serves to generate discussions between the caregivers and the parents about how their baby will be fed, and about the advantages and disadvantages of each chosen element in the plan.

(as independently measured by an observer trained to use the Matthews IBFAT scale and blind to when the mother first breastfed and whether she

received labor analgesia) were those males (presumably because most male babies were circumcised) born to primiparous women who had received labor analgesia and whose first breast-feeding encounter occurred more than one hour after birth. By contrast, those babies who demonstrated effective breastfeeding most rapidly were more likely to be females born to multiparous women who put the baby to breast within the first hour postbirth and who received less than one hour (or no) labor analgesia.

Although the health care provider has no control over the parity of the mother or the gender of the baby she will birth, the time at which she chooses (or is urged) to accept medication may be related to how much assistance she receives during her labor. Furthermore, when she puts her baby to breast for the first time is often related to the interest of the care provider in encouraging her to do so. Knowing how these variables interrelate may have not only short-term but long-term effects on the mother's breastfeeding course and the ease with which her baby learns to breastfeed in the first several days postbirth.

Several reasons support early and frequent breastfeeding for optimal functioning for both the infant and the mother:

- Suckling stimulates uterine contractions, aids in expulsion of the placenta, and helps to control maternal blood loss.

- The infant's suckling reflex is usually most intense 45 minutes through the second hour after birth. Delaying gratification of this reflex can make it more difficult for the baby to learn to suckle later on (Anderson et al., 1982; Eppink, 1969).

- The infant promptly begins to receive the immunological advantages of colostrum (Shortridge, 1990; Silva & Giampaglia, 1992).

- The infant's digestive peristalsis is stimulated, thereby promoting elimination of the by-products of hemoglobin breakdown. Jaundice is more likely to occur when feeding and peristalsis are delayed (Buescher & McIlheran, 1992).

- Breast engorgement is minimized or prevented by the early and frequent removal of milk from the ducts and sinuses of the breast (Moon & Humenick, 1989; Newton, 1961).

- Lactation is accelerated, and early and frequent intake of breastmilk lessens infant weight loss after birth (de Carvalho et al., 1983).

- Attachment and bonding are enhanced at a time when both the mother and the infant are in a heightened state of readiness (Hewat & Ellis, 1984).

When access to the mother is not restricted after birth, the breastfeeding neonate exhibits a pattern similar to that illustrated in Table 9–1. The initial alertness and eagerness of the baby to suckle (Anderson et al., 1982) is followed by progressively deeper sleep and then increased wakefulness and interest in nursing. During this period of increased wakefulness, the baby may want to feed frequently, alternating between relatively short periods of light sleep and quiet wakefulness (Williams & Mueller, 1989). Mothers may interpret these "cluster feedings" as indicators that the baby is not getting any milk or is getting an insufficient amount. However, they actually constitute a series of minifeedings, snacks, or courses in a larger banquet that is part of a single breastfeeding episode. A cluster of minifeedings by the baby is usually followed by a period of deep sleep, during which time the mother should be encouraged to catch up on her own sleep.

This period of deep sleep following cluster feedings is particularly important to the infant. Babies whose mothers have received medication in labor may engage in their first cluster of minifeedings 20 to 24 hours after birth. This time lag may reflect the effect of the mother's medication on the neonate. Often this phenomenon occurs late at night or in the very early morning hours when the mother may be urged to sleep or to let others take care of the baby. If a baby is born at home or in an institutional setting where he is not removed from the mother's room, cluster feedings usually occur much earlier, often within one or two hours after birth, thereby "cementing" suckling behavior sooner. These feedings are followed by a period of deep sleep, after which the infant breastfeeds frequently but with more regular spacing between suckling episodes.

If the baby is denied access to the mother when the cluster feedings are most likely to occur,

Table 9-1

First-Day Sleep Patterns of Neonates Born in Hospital

Infant State	Time Period
Alert and eager	Birth–2 hours
Light and deep sleep	2–20+ hours
Increasing wakefulness*	20–24 hours

Often includes a cluster of 5–10 feeding episodes over 2–3 hours followed by a 4–5-hour deep sleep.

this behavior may not occur until after the mother is home. If she is not told to expect it, she may be concerned that her milk production is not meeting the baby's needs and may think that she should supplement. In truth, what both mother and baby need is time to get to know one another and to practice their new skills.

The pattern of normal infant suckling was discussed earlier in this book. Neonates housed with their mothers immediately after birth quickly learn how to suckle effectively and show increasing facility with each subsequent feeding. In general, full-term infants demonstrate a well-organized sequence of suckling behaviors, including bringing the hand to the mouth, rooting and suckling within the first hour after birth (Klaus, 1987; Widström et al., 1987). Delays in getting the baby to breast (Taylor, Maloni, & Brown, 1986) as a result of maternal labor analgesia (Matthews, 1989) or routine suctioning of gastric fluids (Widström et al., 1987) can disrupt this pattern of behavior. Another potential disruption is suctioning the infant's nares with a bulb syringe or a DeLee mucus trap after birth. The suction tends to cause the infant to have nasal edema and "stuffiness." Because the baby's airway is somewhat obstructed, the baby does not feed well (breast or bottle) until the swelling subsides.

If there are no intervening complications, the first breastfeeding will take place immediately after the infant's birth. After his airway has been cleared, the infant can be placed in the mother's arms to breastfeed. Mother-infant body contact is as effec-

tive as supplemental heat in maintaining the healthy newborn's temperature (Johanson et al., 1992). The placenta is normally expelled soon after birth, often before the infant is put to breast for the first time, but if a delay occurs, breastfeeding may hasten detachment and expulsion.

With the mother propped on her side and a pillow at her back for support, the baby may suckle in the delivery room. If the mother delivers in a birthing suite, so much the better. The ambience and homey comforts of the setting encourage early breastfeeding. When the father is present, he can share the enjoyment of these first moments together and can help to position the mother and infant in a comfortable chair or in the birthing bed.

Newborns often suckle minimally at this time; frequently they only lick or nuzzle the nipple. Given ample opportunity, however, they will attempt to move up the mother's trunk and suckle strongly and at length (Righard, 1995; Widström et al., 1987). Regardless of the baby's initial suckling behavior, this interaction is advantageous, because it stimulates uterine contractions, promotes colonization of harmless bacteria on the nipple, and helps to protect the infant from pathogenic bacteria—a very pleasant method of infection control. Explaining to the mother that "nuzzling" is normal behavior will help her to see this activity as a positive response rather than as disinterest or "rejection" of the breast.

Sometimes, the first breastfeeding takes place after the mother and her newborn are transferred from the delivery area to their room. Wherever it may be, if the mother is awake and oriented, it is best that she put her baby to breast as soon as possible, because during this period the baby is usually in an alert state and later falls asleep (Fig. 9–1).

Women breastfeed for a longer duration if feedings are initiated early (Endresen & Helsing, 1995; Lawson & Tulloch, 1995; Lothian, 1995; Wright et al., 1996). The first several feedings have an imprinting effect. A positive, satisfying experience gets breastfeeding off to a good start, and parents often recall this experience in great detail many years later. The caregiver's unhurried nurturing approach helps to establish rapport with the mother. It is important to explain to the first-time mother that breastfeeding is not as automatic for her as the suckling and rooting reflexes are for her

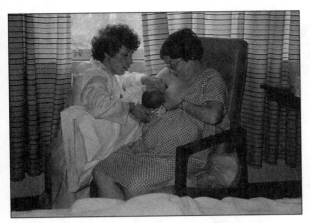

FIGURE 9–1. Lactation consultant assisting mother at eye level during first breastfeeding.

baby. Yet the experience is new to the baby too, and the first few times at breast offer opportunities for each to learn from the other. Early breastfeedings may be optimized in the following ways:

1. *Arrange for privacy.* Concentrating on learning a new skill is easier when it is not attempted in public. Shut the door of the mother's room or pull the curtains around her bed if she wishes. Suggest that she wash her hands with soap and rinse them.

2. *Help the mother to find the most comfortable position* and ensure that there are several pillows available. Women who have had a cesarean birth often find it more comfortable to breastfeed while sitting in a chair with low arms. Almost always, the least comfortable position is leaning back in the bed, as if in a lounge chair. At the first feeding, arrange pillows on her lap, behind her back, and under her arm and shoulder on the side on which the baby is to nurse. If the mother is in bed, raise the back of the bed to high Fowler's position with plenty of pillows for additional support. The experienced breastfeeder or the mother who must remain flat because regional anesthesia has been administered during labor or birth may lie on her side with pillows at her back and between her knees.

3. *Work with the mother at her eye level.* If she is in a chair, kneel down; if she is in bed, pull up a chair; if the bed is electronically operated, raise the bed to bring her to your eye level. When an individual is engaging in a new activity, anyone standing higher than the learner provokes anxiety in the learner.

4. *Help the mother to position the baby's head.* It should be snuggled securely in the mother's arms and rotated toward her. This permits the mother to easily maintain eye contact with her baby. By cradling the infant's thigh or the buttock of his lower leg with her arm, the mother can change the baby's position with ease.

5. *Ask the mother to support her breast with her hand.* Advise her to keep her thumb well above the areola and the rest of her fingers below and under the breast. This is sometimes called the *C-hold* (Fig. 9–2). In this position, the mother is able to lift the breast and guide her nipple in any direction as she assists the baby in taking more of the areola in his mouth. By lifting her breast slightly, she can easily maintain the infant's airway.

6. *Help the mother to position her baby so that his mouth is at the level of the mother's nipple.* Ask the mother to brush her nipple lightly against the baby's lower lip. When the infant opens his mouth wide (rooting reflex) in response to this stimulus, signal the mother to bring him to her breast in one quick movement of her hand or forearm, slipping the nipple in toward the upper part of his wide open mouth. Bringing the baby to the breast at the exact moment that his mouth is at its widest gape is desirable

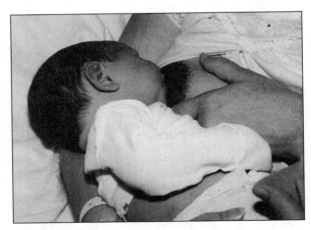

FIGURE 9–2. The C-hold.

because it maximizes the amount of breast tissue he grasps. The baby's lower lip should be flanged outward and his nose resting against the surface of the breast so that he can easily breathe (Fig. 9–3).

7. Explain that for these early feedings, *her infant should be offered both breasts at each feeding.* This will stimulate the need-supply response. In some cases, the neonate will suckle only one breast well before falling asleep. As long as each breast is offered frequently (at least every two hours), single-breast feedings of whatever duration the baby wishes are an appropriate option until the baby shows a desire for both breasts (Woolridge & Fisher, 1988; Woolridge, Ingram, & Baum, 1990). "Finishing the first breast first" is an easy rule of thumb to suggest to the mother if she is concerned about when to move her baby from the first to the second breast (Righard et al., 1993). Suggest that the mother feed until she becomes relaxed to the point of sleepiness–a delightful side effect of oxytocin secretion (Mulford, 1990)–or until she notes cues from the infant suggesting satiety (suckling activity ceases or he falls asleep). The length of the feedings is up to her. The rule here is, "Watch the baby, not the clock." If the mother is breastfeeding for the first time and feels more comfortable with knowing an approximate length of time to feed, suggest that she feed 20 to 30 minutes on the first side or until infant satiety, and that she then offer the other side.

8. If the mother elects to end a feeding before her baby has slipped off the breast or pushed the nipple out of his mouth, *teach her how to break the infant's suction on the breast* by placing her finger in the corner of his mouth between his gums.

Occasionally, an otherwise healthy newborn will not latch onto his mother's breast or suckle even after several attempts. Most nurses and lactation consultants have witnessed the frustrating situation in which a distraught mother repeatedly tries to breastfeed her neonate. The baby's lack of interest may be due to labor-related or postbirth narcotics, to the infant's neurological immaturity, to inappropriate timing by those who attempt to pro-

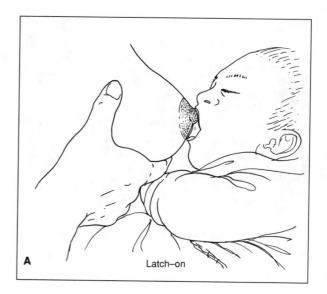

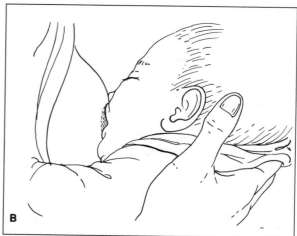

FIGURE 9–3. Latch-on. *A. Mouth gaped open. B. Grasping breast.*

mote suckling before the baby is rousable and shows active interest, or to "forcing" the baby onto the breast, an action that may result in an aversive reaction (Widström & Thingström-Paulsson, 1993).

Although epidural anesthesia or analgesia during labor is common in some areas (the U.S. rate is about 80 percent at this writing) and allow the mother to be awake during cesarean birth, studies implicate its use with a three- to fourfold increase in prolonged labor and cesarean sections (Goer, 1995; Newton et al., 1994; Nissen et. al., 1997) and a variety of adverse consequences for both mother and infant (Thorp & Breedlove, 1996). Prolonged labor and increased likelihood of an operative delivery are more likely if the epidural anesthesia is administered when the mother's cervix is dilated less than 5 cm. In addition, epidural anesthetics, primarily because of their deleterious impact on labor, delay or disrupt neonatal suckling (Loftus et al., 1995; Murray et al., 1981; Sepkoski et al., 1992). Pregnant women are seldom informed of the risks of such anesthetics. Some childbirth educators report that they have been told not to mention these risk factors in hospital-sponsored childbirth classes. Thus discussions of epidural anesthesia in prenatal classes tend to center around *when,* rather than *whether,* they should be given.

Most maternal and infant problems resolve with time; meanwhile, the infant should not go without nourishment or fluids for a long period. Figure 9–4 is a flowchart that can be used as an algorithm indicating appropriate actions for early feedings or lack of feedings. The full-term infant is born with additional extracellular fluid; however, after one to two days without receiving fluid nutriment, the neonate is at risk for rapid dehydration. We recommend the guidelines in Box 9–2 for intervention when the infant does not latch onto the breast 12 to 24 hours after birth.

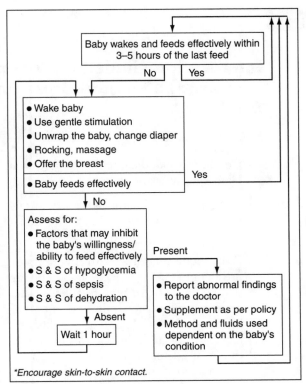

FIGURE 9–4. Breastfeeding flowchart.
(Source: Reprinted with permission from Plenum Publishing Corp. and J Glover: Supplementation of breastfeeding newborns: a flowchart for decision-making. J Hum Lact *11:127–131, 1995.)*

Cup-Feeding the Neonate

Babies can be fed by cup from birth. For this purpose, a small cup with stiff sides and a rounded edge is preferred. Paper cups generally do not work well, nor is a sipper edge necessary. Medicine cups are readily available in hospitals and do not hold large quantities; they are thus appropriate for early feedings when volume will rarely exceed one to two ounces. The baby should be placed in an upright, sitting position. As the cup is brought to a position resting just below his lower lip, he may smell the milk it contains and move his tongue forward in a lapping action. Tipping the cup slightly to allow access to the fluid allows the baby to be fed without the risk of developing a preference for rubber teats or nipple sets. As long as the caregiver does not attempt to pour too much milk into the baby's mouth, risk of aspiration is minimal, and the feeding can be accomplished quickly (Davis et al., 1949; Lang et al., 1994) (Fig. 9–5).

Nipple Shields

Nipple shields have a controversial history, largely because they have been overused or were given to more mothers than needed them, often with minimal instruction in their appropriate application. As a result, they came to be viewed as interfering with, rather than assisting, the new mother's attempts at breastfeeding. More recently, experienced lactation consultants have described how they might be used to appropriate advantage, particularly in the case of the baby who has developed a preference for the more obvious cue of a rubber teat on a bottle and thus refuses to suckle when put back to breast. In many cases, the short-term use of a nipple shield will preserve the breastfeeding relationship while the baby learns to suckle at the breast, thus relieving the mother of concerns she has about being able to induce her baby to breastfeed

BOX 9–2

Intervention Guidelines When Neonate Does Not Latch onto Breast by 12–24 Hours After Birth

1. Continue to put the infant to the breast at least eight times per day.

2. Ask the mother to express her breastmilk to stimulate her supply after each feeding attempt.

3. If the mother has flat or inverted nipples, use a pump to evert the nipples just before putting the baby to breast. If the mother received intravenous fluid during her labor or immediately postpartum, her nipples may appear to be flat; this is an indication of edema and may resolve on its own over the first few days postpartum. In the meantime, if the baby is unable or unwilling to latch, nipple shields can be used for short-term assistance.

4. Give the infant expressed breastmilk using a cup, regular syringe, peridontal syringe, or other feeding-tube device, or by finger-feeding. (See Box 9–3, Instructions for Finger-Feeding a Neonate.)

5. Alternate cup or syringe feedings with putting the infant on the breast while continuing feedings using a No. 5 French gavage tube attached to the syringe or a feeding-tube device, if necessary.

6. Continue to alternate cup or syringe feedings with regular breastfeedings for 48 hours.

7. To ensure adequate calorie intake, supplements should be human milk or formula, not glucose or sterile water.

(Nicholson, 1993; Wilson-Clay, 1996). For additional discussion of these devices, see Chapter 13.

Hypoglycemia

Hypoglycemia, a deficiency of blood glucose, is partially a matter of definition. Whether a baby is considered to have a low blood-glucose level depends on the laboratory values used as criteria for hypoglycemia and the reliability of the methods used to measure blood glucose. Before deciding what is abnormal, one must first establish what is *normal*.

On the basis of research findings from a large sample of well, full-term infants, Heck and Erenberg (1987) recommend that hypoglycemia in full-term infants be defined as serum glucose concentration of less than 30 mg/dl in the first day of life or less than 40 mg/dl in the second day of life. According to another study (Sexson, 1984), if the higher level of 40 mg/dl is used, 20.6 percent of well, full-term infants would be considered hypoglycemic and unnecessarily would receive glucose water. Intrapartum management plays a role in the neonate's glucose level. The routine use of hypertonic glucose infusions during labor can lead to elevation in maternal blood glucose, which can in turn result in fetal hyperglycemia and hyperinsulinemia and eventually neonatal hypoglycemia (Keppler, 1988; Newton, Newton, & Broach, 1988). Moreover, the amount of intravenous fluid given during the intrapartum period is often more than that ordered (Cotton, 1984).

The most common method used in the birth setting to assess neonates' blood-glucose levels is a heel stick to obtain blood, then use of Dextrostix

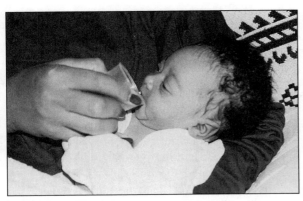

FIGURE 9–5. Baby cup-feeding. *(Courtesy of Kay Hoover, M Ed, IBCLC.)*

with the glucometer or Chemstrips with an Accu-Check 11 reflectance meter. Dextrostix and Chemstrips are easily used and inexpensive; however, they have been shown to record levels at considerable variance from true blood-glucose levels and, as such, are considered unreliable (Cornblath et al., 1990; Hawdon et al., 1993).

According to the American Academy on Pediatrics, Committee on Fetus and Newborn (AAP, 1993), there is no evidence that asymptomatic hypoglycemic infants benefit from treatment or that glucose administration has a better short-term or long-term outcome. The AAP also recommended that routine neonatal screening of blood glucose is not warranted in most nurseries.

Hawdon et al. (1993) noted that breastfed babies are more likely than are bottle-fed neonates to stay in glucose balance when they are fed frequently. Furthermore, these authors recommended against measuring blood-glucose concentrations in asymptomatic babies in the first two postnatal hours, on the grounds that it is unnecessary, potentially harmful to parental well-being, and interferes with establishing breastfeeding (Hawdon et al., 1994). Wang et al. (1994) agreed. In their study of 30 newborns who were exclusively breastfed and 30 newborns who received mixed foods or were exclusively formula-fed, an incidence of only 2.5 percent of the babies in each group were found to have low blood-glucose levels. However, no clinical symptoms or signs of hypoglycemia were observed in any of these babies. These authors

noted that newborns experience a physiological decrease in blood-glucose levels after birth, that they soon adapt to the extrauterine environment and regain normal blood-glucose levels rapidly. Transient asymptomatic low blood-glucose levels (< 30 mg/dl) are not evidence of pathology but rather an expression of individual differences. Furthermore, Yamauchi (1997) found that hypoglycemia seldom occurred in the healthy full-term neonates who roomed in with their mothers and who suckled frequently after birth.

Hypoglycemia is most often a concern for the infant of a mother with diabetes, a postmature neonate, or an infant who is small for gestational age. The infant of a mother with diabetes is most apt to experience hypoglycemia shortly after birth, because he continues to produce a high level of insulin, which depletes the blood glucose within hours after birth. The degree of infant hypoglycemia is usually in proportion to the success achieved in controlling the mother's blood glucose during her pregnancy. Symptomatic neonates are given 10 to 15 percent glucose intravenously immediately after birth until they stabilize.

Postmature infants also need early frequent breastfeedings to normalize their glucose levels. Lethargy and poor feeding in these babies may contribute to hypoglycemia; thus any interest shown in feeding should be followed by immediate, unrestricted access to the breast as often and as long as the baby wishes. Most postmature neonates, after a first breastfeeding, show increased interest in subsequent breastfeeding, thus reducing the risk of continued hypoglycemia.

The newborn who is small for his gestational age is also at risk for hypoglycemia. A prompt first breastfeeding followed by very frequent nursing thereafter is usually sufficient to bring the baby's blood-glucose level to normal. In some cases, continued poor feeding may require a supplement, but this practice need not be repeated once the baby is nursing well.

Whenever glucose feeds are offered to the neonate, whether routinely or in an attempt to resolve a problem, such as hypoglycemia, the health care worker needs to be mindful of the negative effects such feedings have on infant interest in breastfeeding and effective suckling at the breast. Unless nonhuman milk is used, any fluid

BOX 9–3

Instructions for Finger-Feeding a Neonate

• Ensure that your hands are clean and your nails are short before you begin finger-feeding. In some institutions, wearing a rubber glove or finger cott is required when the baby is finger-fed by someone other than the mother or father. Babies do not always respond well to the feel or taste of rubber in their mouths. If the baby refuses to suck when finger-feeding is attempted and the person finger-feeding is wearing a glove or a finger cott, assume that the baby is rejecting the glove or cott, not the attempt at finger-feeding.

• Place the baby in the football or cradle position or prop him high in your lap. This may require the use of a pillow in your lap while your legs are elevated on a footstool to keep the baby comfortably in place. If you are using a dropper or syringe, both hands will be needed.

• When using a dropper, avoid squeezing the milk into the baby's mouth. This can cause gagging, aspiration, and other problems, particularly if the baby is not ready to suck when the milk is squeezed into his mouth. A more appropriate approach is to drip a drop or two into the baby's mouth so that the taste of the milk coaxes the baby to suck.

• When using a feeding-tube device that can be worn around the neck, the tube can be held or taped to the finger. If tape is used, it should be placed back far enough on the finger and tube so that the tape is not drawn into the baby's mouth. Fluid can loosen the tape.

• Use a medium tube in most cases involving a normal full-term neonate.

However, small or large tubing may be necessary, depending on the baby's sucking response and his overall condition. In cases in which the baby's suck is very poor and the goal is to present as much milk with as little effort by the baby as possible, both tubes of the same size (e.g., the smallest tubing) can be used at the same time.

• Select a finger that is about the same size as the breadth of the mother's nipple.

• Slide the finger in so that the pad side touches the baby's hard palate and nail bed rests on his tongue. The tube should be taped to the pad side of the provider's finger and placed in the baby's mouth past the alveolar ridge (gum line) but not so deep in his mouth that you trigger the gag reflex. In most instances, the baby will begin suckling as soon as he feels the finger pad on the hard palate (Fig. 9–6).

• If the baby is suckling effectively, the person who is finger-feeding the baby will feel a pulling sensation along the nail bed with each exertion of negative pressure (suckle), as if the nail is being pulled deeper into the baby's mouth, and will feel a reduction of such pressure when the baby swallows. The suck-swallow pattern will be rhythmic.

• Record the amount of human milk (or formula) that the baby takes with each finger-feeding. Neonates should be offered one to two ounces with each such feeding. Many times, the baby will take some but not all of this amount. By offering a bit more than you expect the baby will take, you prevent him from sucking air through the tube if he drains all of the milk from the container.

- Record the baby's response to finger-feeding, including his willingness to do so, his suck pattern, the duration of rhythmic suckling, the presence (if any) of nonrhythmic suckling, and any difficulties the baby exhibited.

- After showing the mother how to finger-feed, help her to learn how to do so, particularly if you anticipate that the baby may need more finger-feedings or that they are likely to occur when you are not available to assist.

Source: Derived from M Walker: Breastfeeding premature babies *(Unit 14, Lactation Consultant Series). Garden City Park, NY: Avery Publishing Group, 1991:23.*

(e.g., sterile water or glucose) that is substituted for breastfeedings will result in a lower-calorie feeding and subsequent greater early weight loss than is likely to occur from colostrum-to-mature-milk feedings (Glover & Sandilands, 1990). Such a reduction in caloric intake must be considered a risk to avoid if possible. If they are deemed essential, limit such feedings to as few as possible.

Problems that are most likely to be of concern in the early days of breastfeeding relate to method of birth, breast engorgement, sore nipples, and other perceived problems that usually disappear quickly. Chapter 10 focuses on breastfeeding events during the early postpartum period.

Cesarean Births

The impact of cesarean birth on breastfeeding has been extensively studied, and the results are mixed. Cesarean birth appears to be a risk factor, in several studies, for failure to breastfeed (Ford & Labbok, 1990; Perez-Escamilla et al., 1996; Procianoy et al., 1984; Rush et al., 1988; Samuels et al., 1985; Whichelow, 1982; Wittels et al., 1997). In other studies (Ellis, 1984; Gulick, 1982; Janke, 1988; Kearney et al., 1990; Kulski et al., 1981; Loughlin et al., 1985; Padawer et al., 1988; Tamminen et al., 1983; Victora et al., 1990; Wright & Walker, 1983), researchers report no such risk. The impact on breastfeeding may be culture bound, in that in regions in which cesarean births

are common, the impact on breastfeeding would be expected to be less. Also, reviewing these studies indicates that it is likely cesarean births affect breastfeeding primarily by delaying the initiation and establishment of lactation but not the continuance of breastfeeding.

An unexpected cesarean delivery may be a major disappointment for the mother and may require more time from the community-based nurse (Brooten et al., 1996) to resolve issues relating to the unplanned operative birth and subsequent experiences, including feeding. In addition,

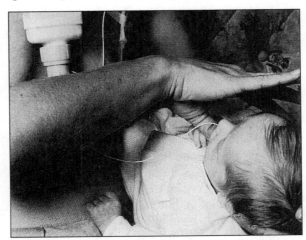

FIGURE 9–6. Finger-feeding. *A technique to feed the infant breastmilk and avoid rubber nipple preference when the infant is not latching onto the breast. (Courtesy of Pat Bull, RN, IBCLC.)*

recovery from major surgery takes more time, is more painful, and represents additional risks compared to an uneventful vaginal birth, which explains why breastfeeding occurs later following cesarean birth (Kearney et al., 1990). A woman may interpret such a birth as a reflection on her adequacy and may be more fearful that she will fail at breastfeeding because she perceives that she failed with birthing (Pietz, 1989). To the degree that she feels violated, the shock of the cesarean birth may also reflect on her self-esteem. "From the waist up, I felt like a success; from the waist down, a failure!" In these few words, one mother summed up the feelings of guilt, frustration, and loss of self-esteem that a mother may experience following a cesarean. Some Asian women consider a cesarean birth to be a form of mutilation (Taylor, 1985). The sensitive caregiver can assist the mother to see that breastfeeding is not another proving ground but rather an affirmation of her femininity, a experience that she need not forgo because she had an operative delivery.

This view is balanced by the findings of a study on mothers' adaptation to cesarean birth, which found a normalizing effect of the high cesarean birth rate (Fawcett et al., 1993). New parents tended to view cesarean birth as a normal or alternative mode of delivery. Childbirth educators and others have effectively conveyed the message that cesarean birth does not have to be a threat. Moreover, the parents' concerns may be reduced by the knowledge that regional anesthesia is available and that the baby's father can be present at the birth.

The type of labor and birth medication influences how soon mother and baby begin breastfeeding (Rajan, 1994). The attachment process is often delayed for mothers who have delivered by cesarean section, because they need extra time to recover before they can move into mothering and breastfeeding. Lie and Juul (1988) found that mothers who had epidural, rather than general, anesthesia for such surgery not only held and breastfed their babies sooner but nursed longer than did women who had general anesthesia. This finding held with elective versus emergency cesarean section. Another study (Nissen et al., 1996) found that mothers who had an emergency cesarean birth did not breastfeed until an average of six hours postdelivery, whereas mothers who had a vaginal delivery breastfed an average of 75 minutes after giving birth. Compared with the vaginal delivery group, the women who had a cesarean birth in this study lacked a significant rise in prolactin levels at 20 to 30 minutes after starting to breastfeed and had fewer pulsations of prolactin. Despite these differences, neither the duration of breastfeeding nor the duration of exclusive or total breastfeeding differed between the groups. The mother's commitment to breastfeeding plays a substantial role despite unexpected birth outcomes. A greater commitment to breastfeeding, regardless of the manner of birth, results in longer duration of breastfeeding (Janke, 1988).

When mothers give birth to premature infants and the birth is by cesarean section, they are significantly more likely to provide milk for the preterm baby than are women who have given birth vaginally. Difficulties may strengthen a committed mother's resolve to breastfeed. Kearney, Cronenwett, and Reinhardt (1990) reported that mothers giving birth by cesarean section had a later first breastfeeding and expressed less satisfaction with the birth experience than did those who delivered vaginally. The delayed first breastfeeding, however, did not affect breastfeeding duration.

In working with a mother who has had a cesarean birth, the nurse or the lactation consultant needs to assess the mother's degree of physical comfort and awareness. If she is not fully conscious, she is not ready to put her baby to breast. Once the mother is alert and able to hold her baby, however, she can begin breastfeeding. The mother should be asked how she wants to hold her infant. Some mothers, particularly those still receiving intravenous pain medication or those who have had an epidural narcotic, are quite comfortable holding their babies in the cradle position. Others are hesitant to hold the baby at all until they have been reassured that they can do so without touching or placing any pressure near their abdominal incision. If the mother holds her baby in a football (clutch) position, she will avoid the sensitive incision area. As the pain of her incision decreases, the mother can be instructed and assisted in the use of positions other than the football hold, as discussed later in this chapter. By the second or third day postpartum, side-lying is generally comfortable, especially if the mother is adequately supported

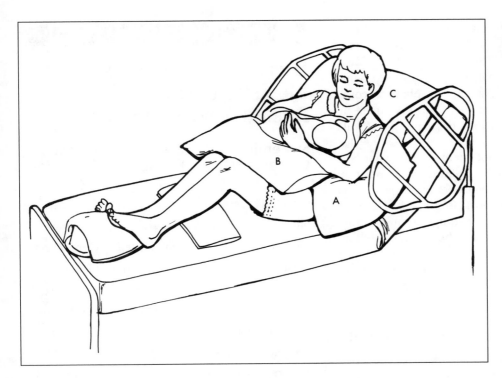

FIGURE 9–7.
Comfortable position for breastfeeding, *especially for women who have delivered by cesarean.*

with pillows at her back and beneath her abdomen or can sit supine with her knees supported, as in Figure 9–7.

The baby born by cesarean section may be lethargic, particularly if the birth followed a long period of exposure to analgesia or anesthesia in labor. If so, explain to the mother that a delay in feeding will not deter breastfeeding; rather, her milk supply may be established slightly later than it would following a vaginal birth (Moon & Humenick, 1989). If, as a result of early bottle-feedings, the mother is concerned about infant nipple preference, reassure her that some babies are affected by this to a greater degree than others but that it can be overcome. Observing the baby at the breast will enable the lactation consultant or nurse to evaluate the extent to which the baby has been affected by bottle-feedings and to offer appropriate help to restore suckling at breast during subsequent feedings (Neifert et al., 1995).

As the mother progresses through her post-partum course, breastfeeding will sometimes be satisfying, at other times not. When she is very tired, for example, she may be easily frustrated if the baby does not readily take the breast or suckle enthusiastically. At other feedings, the new mother will be gratified to find that she and her baby need little or no assistance—proof that each is learning to work with the other. The mother may need an occasional reminder that both she and her baby are learning a new skill; she should expect that some feedings will go better than others. The goal is not to have a perfect breastfeeding each time but rather many opportunities for each to practice and to learn about—and from—the other. This uneven pattern from one feeding to another characterizes early feeding behavior following both vaginal and cesarean births.

Epidural morphine and other narcotics given following cesarean birth relieve pain so effectively that many women are up and about within hours of delivery (Rimar, 1986). If a longer postpartum hospital stay following a cesarean birth is available, the new mother may benefit from direct assistance for a somewhat longer period.

An unknown element is the effect of antihistamines, which are used to relieve generalized itching, a common reaction in a mother who has had epidural morphine following a cesarean birth or a birth in which she has sustained a severe tear. Trimeprazine tartrate (Temaril) is a phenothiazine. Because phenothiazines usually increase milk supply, theoretically this class of medications should not affect breastfeeding. Furthermore, they are not considered harmful to the infant. Diphenhydramine (Benadryl) is also used; sometimes it is mixed with Narcan or Nubain to counteract pruritis in the mother. At this time, no studies report that Benadryl decreases breastmilk production.

Encouraging the mother to decide when she would like to nurse the baby in the cradle position will help her to see herself as being in charge of at least this aspect of her own progress. Just as with a vaginal birth, frequent feedings stimulate milk production after a cesarean. The mother will benefit from encouragement that she now shares yet another similarity with women whose births were what she expected but did not experience.

Breast Fullness Versus Engorgement

Breast engorgement is a major issue in most discussions of early breastfeeding. Such preoccupation stems from many factors, not the least of which is the assumption that the condition is normal (i.e., that it occurs in all breastfeeding women). Most published materials continue to present the condition as a norm or an indication of early lactation. This assumption is, in part, incorrect. Although the gradual buildup of fluid in the breasts following parturition is a welcome sign of breastmilk, breast engorgement and breast fullness are two different matters. The nearly universal experience of transient breast fullness does not prevent the infant from feeding; however, clinical engorgement usually precludes breastfeeding. The distinction between breast fullness and breast engorgement may be seen in Newton and Newton's (1948) operational definitions of these two conditions, from which many later discussions derive. However, often such discussions do not note that the Newtons' definitions provide a four-step progression, beginning with mild fullness that, if mishandled, can result in severe breast engorgement. (Table 9–2).

As noted in Table 9–2, with breast fullness the mother's breast tissue remains compressible, thus enabling the infant to suckle comfortably and efficiently, without risk of trauma to the breast or

Table 9-2		

DIFFERENCES BETWEEN BREAST FULLNESS AND BREAST ENGORGEMENT

Systemic Characteristics	Breast Fullness	Breast Engorgement
Onset of symptoms	2–4 days	2–10 days
Site	Bilateral	Bilateral
Swelling	Generalized	Generalized
Heat	Occasional	Generalized
Pain	None-rare	Generalized
Palpation of breast	Soft	Hard
Breast tenderness	None	Generalized
Body temperature	< 38°C	> 38.4°C
Maternal symptoms	Feels well	Breast tightness, discomfort

Source: Derived in part from RA Lawrence: Breastfeeding: a guide for the medical profession. *St Louis: Mosby, 1989:209.*

nipple tissue. Breast fullness rarely lasts more than 24 hours, during which time breastfeeding can continue without discomfort. The mother with breast fullness should be encouraged to view this state as an increase in fluid in the breast tissue that will subside on its own simultaneously with an increase in milk production that will begin to regulate to meet the baby's needs as the infant suckles. She should be encouraged to offer the breast frequently to reduce the likelihood that breast fullness will become breast engorgement.

Breast engorgement, by contrast, is often the consequence of mismanagement of the normal state of transient breast fullness caused by the delay or restriction in duration and frequency of breastfeeding. Such delay or restriction allows milk stasis to occur. The infant then finds it difficult or impossible to grasp the severely engorged breast. When the baby is unable to suckle, the mother's discomfort mounts, and her breast and nipple tissue may be so significantly stretched that even leaking cannot occur. Under such conditions, further trauma to the tissue is apt to occur when a vigorous baby attempts unsuccessfully to grasp and draw the nipple and areola into his mouth. Numbness and tingling of the mother's hand and arm may occur with severe engorgement because of pressure on brachial-plexus nerves in the axilla (Simkin, 1988).

In their study of postpartum women, Humenick et al. (1994) identified four distinct patterns of breast engorgement, only one of which is similar to the usual expectation of a gradual increase to a single peak on day three or day four followed by a gradual cessation of engorgement. Other patterns noted included a multimodel form that included a decline in a "saw-tooth" pattern lasting over several days, an intense pattern with a single peak and a gradual decline lasting as long as two weeks, and a minimal engorgement pattern characterized by few changes in intensity. They also found that multiparous women were more likely to report more intense engorgement than were primiparous women (Hill & Humenick, 1994). This landmark work requires that the clinician remain sensitive to the potential for variation in the kind of engorgement a mother may report, particularly because this is likely to occur *after* the mother's very short hospital stay if she was discharged within the first two days postpartum.

Techniques for reducing engorgement vary and have included cold packs and both room-temperature and cold cabbage compresses (Roberts, 1995; Roberts, Reiter, & Schuster, 1995; Rosier, 1988). Whatever technique is used, mothers report feeling better after having taken some kind of action in addition to increasing the frequency of breastfeeding. This finding suggests that any method that reduces the sensation of tightness in the breast tissue is likely to help the mother to see that this aspect of the early breastfeeding process is transitory and can be managed with minimal difficulty.

A fever of unknown origin in a mother during the first week postpartum may be another sign of breast engorgement. Epidural anesthesia also has been implicated in increased likelihood of maternal fever (and an unnecessary subsequent workup for sepsis in her infant). Because most women who receive labor medication have intravenous fluids throughout labor, they are more likely to experience engorgement as a function of supersaturation of their body tissues, including the breasts. Severe engorgement has been noted in women who receive excessive intravenous infusions during the intrapartum period. One LC described such a mother's breasts as being "hard as rocks"; as a result, her neonate was unable to latch onto her breasts for several days, until the edema subsided. Mothers can be spared this discomfort, and breastfeeding need not be jeopardized if the intrapartum intravenous line is maintained by a heparin lock and intravenous fluids are given only if they are needed.

Management during the intrapartum period itself may contribute to later difficulties that impinge on the postpartum and breastfeeding course. It is not known to what extent the use of vacuum extractors during birthing and suctioning of the neonate has on breastfeeding. Anecdotal reports indicate that neonates who have ungone these procedures have difficulty with suckling and appear to be in pain when they attempt to feed.

If the mother is breastfeeding, how often and how long her infant is suckling should be assessed. If the baby is being offered the breast fewer than eight times in 24 hours or is feeding infrequently and for less than an average of 15 minutes per feeding, it may not be enough. If the mother is unable to increase the number of feedings, she may obtain relief with the judicious use of hand expression or a fully automatic intermittent electric breast pump. Under no circumstances should a mother whose breasts are engorged be allowed to use an electric breast pump that does not provide intermittent minimum pressure. Pumping should also be limited to a maximum duration of 10 minutes to avoid traumatizing the distended breast tissues.

Hand Expression

Although many women in the United States think first of using a breast pump to obtain milk when the baby cannot breastfeed, expressing milk by hand is a skill that has been used by many mothers for millennia. The mother's own hands represent several advantages over breast pumps:

- their presence costs her nothing,
- she may trigger a more effective milk-ejection reflex with her own hands, and
- they are always available.

After the mother has practiced this skill, she may find she can obtain more milk more quickly than her neighbor who is using an electric device for the same purpose! Techniques vary across cultures and are most effective when the tissue behind the milk sinuses is compressed, thus moving the milk out of the nipple pores and into the collection container (Fig. 9–8). The most effective teaching is often accomplished by a mother experienced in the technique who can demonstrate to the novice. Rolling the fingers is recommended rather than sliding the fingers down the breast, to avoid inadvertently bruising or abrading the tissue. The mother should be cautioned that she may have greater difficulty with expression if she is attempting to relieve engorgement or her breasts are very tender. She should be encouraged to be patient, to shower or use warm compresses, and to stimulate milk ejection with gentle breast massage in advance of attempting to express her milk.

If breast massage is practiced with each expression, encourage the mother to avoid creating a ritual that becomes so time consuming that it interferes with the process. This is particularly relevant if the mother is expressing her milk at work or some other site where she has limited time in which to accomplish it. Some mothers have used Syntocinon (synthetic oxytocin) for short-term assistance; however, it is no longer on the market unless it is formulated by the pharmacist on prescription.

If the woman is not breastfeeding and her breasts are engorged, she needs instruction in gentle breast massage and the use of warm showers to reduce her discomfort while her body is ceasing to produce milk. Cold reduces fluid filtration into the interstitium, owing to vasoconstriction. As in other areas of the body, tissue edema in the breast is reduced by cold and is increased by heat (Michlovitz & Wolf, 1986; Shrago, 1991). Washcloths or small towels, wrung out in water and folded, serve as inexpensive, moist compresses and are less time consuming than are showers. Immersing her breasts in a basin of tepid water also may work well if the mother takes care to avoid a backache. Wearing a tight-fitting breast binder is unnecessary and should be avoided in the interests of reducing the risks of iatrogenically induced mastitis.

In a press release of September 1989, the U.S. Food and Drug Administration recommended against the use of bromocriptine and related dopamine-receptor antagonists when the need for medication is minimal. Fewer than 10 percent of women have been found to need drug therapy to control symptoms of breast engorgement when they do not breastfeed. The serious side effects of bromocriptine–including stroke (Watson et al., 1989), myocardial infarction (Ruch & Duhring, 1989), puerperal seizures (Rothman et al., 1990), and postpartum psychosis (Canterbury et al., 1987)–support its avoidance. In addition, women who have received lactation suppressants often report significant rebound engorgement after withdrawal of the medication. Usually, rebound engorgement occurs after the mother has left the hospital, so the likelihood that she will be seen by a knowledgeable health care worker is reduced.

A nipple shield is sometimes offered in an attempt to reduce engorgement. However, a nipple shield does not reduce engorgement unless it encourages a previously reluctant neonate to suckle effectively. If the mother's excess breast fullness is related to the infant's infrequent suckling and use of a nipple shield increases the baby's willingness to stay on the breast and actively feed, the shield may assist the process. However, other methods should be attempted first.

Moon and Humenick (1989) identified several factors that increase the risk of breast engorgement. They and others (Stamp & Crowther, 1995; Wright et al., 1996) found that supplementing the breastfeeding infant with other feeds contributes to breast engorgement, whereas allowing breastfeedings to last as long as the mother and baby wish decreases breast engorgement. For example, Lawson & Tulloch (1995) reported that mothers whose babies fed on only one breast (adhering to

FIGURE 9–8. Hand expression.

A. Wash hands and any collection equipment to be used. Sit or stand comfortably and place the collection cup near breast. Apply warm, moist towel to enhance milk flow. Massage breasts and nipples to stimulate milk-ejection reflex. Use gentle pressure in a circular motion and move around the breast.

B. Squeeze the breast gently, rolling the hands forward from the chest toward the nipple.

C. Place thumb and forefingers approximately two to three cm (one to one and a half inches) behind the nipple and press into the breast.

D. Press inward toward the chest wall, squeezing gently with a slight rolling action toward the chest wall. Release pressure and repeat as needed to obtain milk. If pain results, something is wrong, and the mother should be observed to identify what may be causing her discomfort.

E. Change position of the fingers around the areola to express milk from as many sinuses as possible. Within three to five minutes, the milk flow may slow; this is a signal to express milk from the other breast. Both sides may be expressed as often as the mother wishes in a given session or until she tires. Particularly in the beginning, the mother should expect to spend 20–30 minutes in expressing milk. As she becomes more adept at it, the time will decrease even as the amount of milk obtained increases.

Derived from S Jolley: Breastfeeding triage tool *(3rd ed). Seattle, WA: Seattle-King County Department of Public Health, 1996:83; FS King:* Helping mothers to breastfeed *(rev ed). Nairobi: African Medical and Research Foundation, 1992:119–20; and K Frantz:* Hand expression *(videotape presentation). (Drawing by Ruth Linstromberg.)*

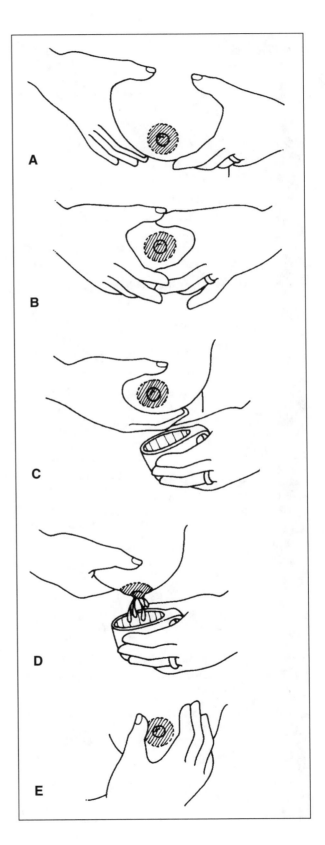

BOX 9–4

Post on Baby's Crib in Hospital

Dear Nurse:

IF I AM A HEALTHY, FULL-TERM BABY,

1. Please don't give me any water bottles, formula, or pacifiers.

2. I eat "on demand" or q2–3hr., whichever comes first, AM & PM.

3. I may be allowed to sleep one 4–5 hr. period at night—if I have already had 8 feedings that day.

4. My mom allows "bunching" (i.e., frequent feedings) whenever I want it.

5. My mom feeds me from both breasts at each feeding for as long as I want it.

6. My mom wants to feed me 8–12 times in 24 hrs.

7. Thank you for helping me get off to a good start!

Mother's signature_____

Reprinted with permission from and credit to
Lactation Consultants
of Cincinnati
Jo Williams (513) 251-3176
Susan Mueller (513) 542-2576
©1988

Source: From J Williams, and S Mueller: A message to the nurse from the baby. J Hum Lact 5:19, 1989. Reprinted with permission.

the policy of finishing the first breast first) were less likely to experience engorgement in the first week postpartum and to report less infant colic in the baby's first six months of life.

There is wide variation in the length of a feeding. Between the fifth and seventh day postpartum, a baby may spend from 7 to 30 minutes at the breast; the mean is about 17 minutes (Howie, Houston, & Cook, 1981). Breast changes are also related to the timing of the first feed; mothers feeding soon after birth are more likely to have full breasts sooner than are mothers whose first feeding is delayed. Mothers have fewer breast changes following a cesarean birth than after a vaginal birth because of the usual pattern of delayed breastfeeding among women who have experienced a cesarean birth.

The notice shown in Box 9–4 can be posted on the baby's crib in the hospital as a reminder to staff not to feed supplements to the infant.

Clinical Implications

Assessment is a critical first step in working with a client. LCs often find that identifying problems that a client had with a previous infant may be helpful. Reviewing the risk factors or red flags will often identify issues to pay particular attention to as the mother begins her breastfeeding career (Box 9–5). For example, if the mother had maternal analgesia and her baby is sleepy and nursing infrequently, the hospital caregiver can

- reassure the mother that the baby's sleepiness may be the result of the analgesia to which he was exposed prior to his birth,

- encourage the mother to take every opportunity when the baby is awake to offer the breast,

- suggest that the mother let the baby stay on the first breast until he has completed a feeding when he does begin suckling well, and

- provide specific suggestions regarding home visitation and follow-up with a lactation consultant in private practice and a community-based breastfeeding support group.

BOX 9–5

Risk Factors or Red Flags Indicating a Need for Skilled Assessment and Follow-Up

If at least two starred items (*) or four or more nonstarred items are checked prior to the mother's and baby's discharge from the hospital, a referral for postpartum follow-up is recommended.

MOTHER

____ Gained less than 18 lb during her full-term pregnancy
____ History of breast surgery or breast trauma*
____ Reports few or no breast changes (such as size, shape, color) throughout her pregnancy*
____ History of hormone-related infertility
____ History of low or no milk production for one or more previous infants or reports breastfeeding "failure" with a previous baby
____ Flat or inverted nipples or taut, tight breast tissue[†]
____ First baby (primipara)
____ Received medications during her labor or delivery*[‡]
____ Epidural analgesia or anesthesia was in place more than three hours before birth
____ Mother received more than one bolus of analgesia/anesthesia[†]
____ Mother received continuous intravenous fluids
____ Labor was induced or augmented with pitocin*
____ Received pain medication more than one hour before baby's birth*
____ Had unplanned cesarean section*[†]
____ Birth was assisted with vacuum extraction or forceps delivery
____ Ankles or other tissues are edematous postbirth but were not edematous before the mother went into labor[†]
____ First breastfeeding occurred more than one hour after the baby's birth*
____ First breast pumping (if baby is not breastfeeding) was begun more than one day after the baby's birth*
____ Sore nipples throughout feedings prior to hospital discharge*

INFANT

____ Younger than 37 weeks' gestational age
____ History of fetal distress or meconium staining during delivery
____ Considered SGA or LGA[§]
____ Weighs less than seven pounds at birth
____ History of insult to the oral cavity (laryngoscope and deep suctioning)
____ Is male

[†] *Verify whether mother had intravenous fluids during labor and, if so, for how long.*
[‡] *Verify the duration of labor or delivery medications, type, and dosage(s).*
[§] *SGA: small for gestational age; LGA: large for gestational age.*

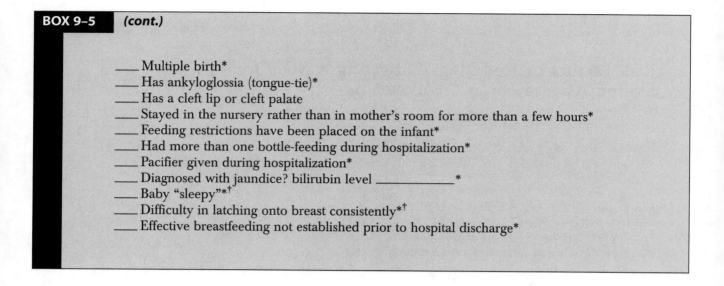

____ Multiple birth*
____ Has ankyloglossia (tongue-tie)*
____ Has a cleft lip or cleft palate
____ Stayed in the nursery rather than in mother's room for more than a few hours*
____ Feeding restrictions have been placed on the infant*
____ Had more than one bottle-feeding during hospitalization*
____ Pacifier given during hospitalization*
____ Diagnosed with jaundice? bilirubin level _____ *
____ Baby "sleepy"*[†]
____ Difficulty in latching onto breast consistently*[†]
____ Effective breastfeeding not established prior to hospital discharge*

If the mother experienced difficulty in breastfeeding with an earlier baby, the caregiver may need to reassure the concerned or anxious mother that a similar condition need not recur.

Several assessment tools specific to feedings at the breast are now available. These tools are presented and discussed in Chapter 21. They can also be found in the *Resource Guide to Accompany Breastfeeding and Human Lactation* (1996). Assessment tools are useful for evaluating infant suckling over several feedings to show mothers that their babies are learning with each feeding and are becoming more efficient at obtaining milk. They also can be used to alert the caregiver to specific "red flags." If the mother-baby dyad is not feeding effectively, they may need special attention to prevent a problem with dehydration and weight loss. Breastfeeding assessment tools also remind the mother that what her baby does is both complex and predictable and that he needs lots of opportunities to practice, just as she needs many opportunities to learn how to hold and position him for optimal breastfeeding. The ease of using these tools means that the mother can evaluate for herself what occurs at each feeding. Despite the usefulness of these tools, reliability and validity testing indicate that they need further development (Riordan & Koehn, 1997).

Discharge Planning

Early discharge from the hospital, a fact of life today for most new mothers and their neonates, has had a major impact on postpartum care. Mothers and infants often return home in the first 24 to 48 hours after a vaginal birth and two to four days after a cesarean birth. It is the responsibility of the hospital caregiver to highlight particular elements to which the mother needs to pay attention when she returns home with her new baby. Foremost among these concerns is seeing to it that the baby feeds often and effectively. The mother needs guidelines that will help her to assess whether this is occurring and what to do and whom to contact for assistance if this is not occurring (Hall & Carty, 1993).

Early discharge from the hospital may negatively influence the mother's feeling of competence in her mothering (Waldenstrom, Sundelin, & Lindmark, 1987), particularly if she is unprepared or unsure of how to care for her newborn. Contact with mother-to-mother organizations can help the mother to place her experiences in the context of other women's comments about their breastfeeding course. In addition, home health care opportunities are now being developed to provide the care that used to be provided in longer-term hospitalization (Brucker & MacMullen, 1985; Jansson, 1985; Page-Goertz, 1989).

The goal of discharge planning is twofold: to prevent common problems and to provide emotional support (Page-Goertz, 1989). With such a brief time in the hospital, the mother needs a caregiver who imparts as much basic information as possible without overwhelming her. She also needs reinforcement of her self-confidence in her role as a new mother. These two goals are mutually reinforcing, and as the caregiver instructs the mother in the prevention of problems, she is in a position to simultaneously enhance the new mother's self-esteem and self-confidence; in short, the mother is able to "take control" of her experience (Hall & Carty, 1993). The mother's perceptions of her infant not only reflect how she and the baby will interact but can also influence how long she breastfeeds (Vandiver, 1997).

In endeavoring to prevent the most common problems that may arise, three priorities need to be addressed: positioning the baby at the breast, understanding basic feeding techniques, and recognizing signs of the need for additional help or intervention.

Feeding Positions

Prior to hospital discharge, the new mother needs to know ways to position her neonate. The three most frequently taught techniques are the Madonna (cradle or cross-chest, Fig. 9–9), the football (or clutch, Fig. 9–10), and the side-lying positions (Fig. 9–11), or variations on these general themes. Although there is nothing magical about a particular position, the mother may feel uncomfortable in experimenting with more than three different positions prior to her discharge from the hospital. However, she needs to be encouraged to experiment and to use whatever position works best for her and her nursling. Mothers who had vaginal deliveries report less fatigue if they breastfeed in the side-lying rather than the sitting position (Milligan, Flenniken, & Pugh, 1996). Before discharge, the mother should have more than one opportunity to practice each position with assistance and to demonstrate that she can place her baby in each position without assistance.

Each position has its positive and negative elements. The mother who is informed about each

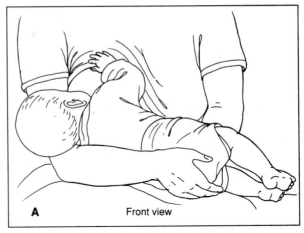

A   Front view

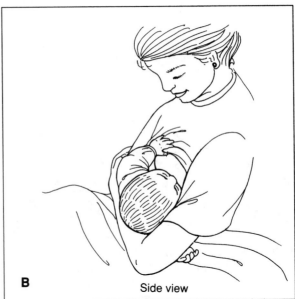

B   Side view

FIGURE 9–9. Madonna (cradle) position. *A. Front view. B. Side view.*

position and has practiced each prior to discharge will be more likely to select the position that works best for her at different times (Table 9–3).

Basic Feeding Techniques

In teaching basic feeding techniques, priority must be given to certain guidelines:

- *Feed the baby frequently* (eight or more feedings in a 24-hour period). Using a visual aid to demonstrate the size of the newborn's stomach

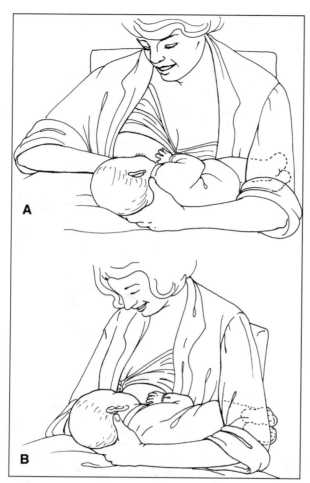

FIGURE 9–10. Football position. *A. Modified clutch position. B. Clutch hold.*

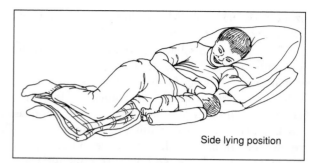

Side lying position

FIGURE 9–11. Side-lying position.

is an excellent way to illustrate why the neonate needs frequent feedings: his stomach is simply too small to hold large quantities at a time! Additionally, the small curd formed by human milk is more easily digested than is the large curd formed by artificial baby milks. The breastfeeding infant, therefore, is less likely to experience a sense of fullness for an extended period.

• *Offer (and keep the baby on) the first breast until he has completed the feeding.* If he wants more, offer the second breast, and as many others as the baby asks to take! Some babies will be satiated with one breast; others prefer two, and still others may have some early marathon feed-

ings in which they move from one to the other four or more times!

• *Avoid watching the clock;* the best timer of the feeding is the baby. After breastfeeding is established, the mother may identify cues that the baby is happy with one breast or wants more than one.

• *Avoid the use of artificial teats, pacifiers (dummies), supplemental infant formula, water, or glucose feeds* for the first two to four weeks. The infant may substitute nonnutritive suckling for milk intake at the breast, resulting in poor weight gain. The pacifier can also become a source of nipple confusion (Powers & Slusser, 1997) and a possible marker for other difficulties that can result in shorter breastfeeding duration (Victora et al., 1993, 1997). Telling the mother why these practices can interfere with early, effective breastfeeding will give her the ammunition she may need to fend off well-meaning but uninformed attempts to "assist" her with unnecessary, potentially interfering practices. The exception is preterm infants, who may benefit from nonnutritive suckling during the period that they are unable to take oral feedings (see Chapter 14).

• *Identify various ways in which the mother can recognize that her infant is getting sufficient milk.* These include listening for and identifying the infant's swallows (Lau & Henning, 1989). Another way, particularly in the early days, is noting the number of stools (the number of which should increase each day past the birth day) and the changes in their color and consistency that occur with the increase in the num-

Table 9–3

POSITIVE AND NEGATIVE ELEMENTS OF INFANT FEEDING POSITIONS

Infant Positioning Options	Positive Elements	Negative Elements
Madonna (cross-chest or cradle) position	Most frequently pictured. Most often used by experienced mothers.	Often most difficult to master. Baby's head tends to wobble around on the mother's arm. Mother may feel she has minimal control over baby's head. Sometimes difficult to keep baby's head close to the breast or appropriately high on mother's chest wall.
Football (clutch) position	Provides most complete control of the baby's head. An excellent option following cesarean birth or tubal ligation. Easily accomplished with a small baby [SGA or preterm].	Least frequently pictured in books. Least familiar to caregivers. Some mothers are not comfortable holding their babies in this manner.
Side-lying position	Often expected to be used before breastfeeding in a chair. Enables the mother to rest more completely than is possible if she is sitting up.	Not always taught in hospital. Mothers often fear smothering baby in this position. Rarely practiced as often as the Madonna position.

SGA: small-for-gestational-age.

ber of feedings and the volume of milk transferred. The mother should also note an increase in the frequency of wet diapers as well. A good rule of thumb is that the baby should produce at least as many wet diapers as his age in days.

Signs That Intervention Is Needed

Seven signs indicate a need for health care intervention:

1. The infant is producing scant, often highly concentrated urine or no urine at all.

2. The infant has infrequent stools (fewer than four per day by the end of the first week of life).

3. The baby is lethargic (difficult or impossible to waken for feedings).

4. The baby is extremely fretful (never contented after any feedings).

5. No swallowing is felt or heard during feedings; when a feeding is evaluated, the clinician does not observe an "open-pause-close" pattern of suckling (Newman, 1996).

6. The mother is experiencing nipple soreness that is more intense if it existed earlier, or that suddenly develops if it was previously absent.

7. The mother's breasts are clinically engorged and very painful, making it difficult or impossible for the baby to breastfeed.

At discharge, the parents need clear, simply written materials that provide step-by-step information and are individualized as much as possible. Walker (1989) suggested that Polaroid photographs of positioning and other techniques might be helpful, depending on the situation. The hospital caregiver should establish a definite plan for follow-up: making a phone call to the mother at a specific time postdischarge or providing her with the phone numbers of the hospital "warm milk" line and of lactation consultants or LLLI leaders in the area. A referral to an LC made from the mother's room prior to her discharge from the hospital is appropriate, particularly if the baby has not been observed to have had at least two effective feedings per day. Public health, home health, or nurse case-manager follow-ups are other options in some communities.

In many countries other than the United States, new mothers are routinely visited by midwives and home health visitors. The optimal time for a follow-up visit or call is no later than two to four days after discharge from the hospital. This is an especially crucial period, because enough time has passed to make an accurate evaluation of the mother's milk supply and the infant's intake. By this time, too, the mother has probably passed the peak of transient sore nipples and, if things are progressing normally, is beginning to feel comfortable with breastfeeding. Three to five days after hospital discharge is also about the midpoint between discharge and the baby's first scheduled visit to the physician. This is a critical period that is underserved by the U.S. health care system in most communities.

SUMMARY

Consumer advocacy, the expectations of parents, childbirth education, early hospital discharge, frequent cesarean births, and technologies all affect birthing and early breastfeeding. In recent years, the emphasis has changed from a management approach to support and education of childbearing families for their own self-care. No longer do we view the mother and her infant as separate entities; rather we care for them as a natural single unit. Many hospitals now boast a family-centered birthing unit or labor-delivery room postpartum (also called *family birthplace, single-room maternity care,* or *new-life center*) where the mother and infant are cared for together in one room. Birthing rooms today look much like a bedroom, with a comfortable recliner chair for the mother's support person; hookups for medical equipment are concealed behind wall prints and other decorations. A major benefit of this kind of mother-baby care is that families receive more comprehensive, coordinated care, which facilitates breastfeeding.

At the same time that we are seeing improvements in mother-baby care, the use of medical interventions, particularly epidural analgesia and anesthesia, has skyrocketed. Two opposing forces appear to be battling each other for control of childbirth: on one side, childbirth education, midwifery, doula services, and free-standing birthing centers; on the other, hospitals with routine epidural injections, high rates of cesarean births, and other technologies that medicalize the intrapartum experience.

Until recently, the transition process after discharge was a neglected element in the prospective payment system; this situation is changing. Follow-up care in the home is beginning to be regarded as a necessity rather than a luxury. Nevertheless, it is a minority of mothers in the United States who will be seen by a visiting nurse or in-home care program that is designed to ensure that she and her baby are healthy and doing well together.

Too few mothers learn enough about breastfeeding in the hospital before being asked to assume full responsibility for themselves and their babies. Rarely are they informed of the red flags that indicate that they should seek expert help and when to do so. Thus what should be a natural function is perceived as complicated. New mothers need reassurance that they can enjoy an uncomplicated breastfeeding experience and that common concerns can be easily managed.

As public awareness grows that breastfeeding sustains the baby's health, and government and insurance companies become more aware of cost savings, breastfeeding will be promoted as the feeding of choice. Insurance companies will provide household help and visiting nurses to assess breastfeeding mothers and infants, in addition to giving substantial rebates to mothers who breastfeed. Breastfeeding will be not only socially acceptable but socially responsible.

REFERENCES

American Academy of Pediatrics Committee on the Fetus and the Newborn: Routine evaluation of blood pressure hematocrit and glucose in newborns. *Pediatrics* 92:474–6, 1993.

Anderson GC, et al: Development of sucking in term infants from birth to four hours postbirth. *Res Nurs Health* 5:21–7, 1982.

Auerbach KG: Breastfeeding fallacies: their relationship to understanding lactation. *Birth* 17:44–9, 1990.

Brooten D, et al: Early discharge and home care after unplanned cesarean birth: nursing care time. *JOGNN* 25:595–600, 1996.

Brown MS, Hurlock JT: Preparation of the breast for breastfeeding. *Nurs Res* 24:448–51, 1975.

Brucker MC, MacMullen NJ: Bridging the gap between hospital and home. *Child Today* 14:19–22, 1985.

Buescher ES, McIlheran SM: Colostral antioxidants: separation and characterization of two activities in human colostrum. *J Pediatr Gastroenterol Nutr* 14:47–56, 1992.

Canterbury RJ, et al: Postpartum psychosis induced by bromocriptine. *South Med J* 80:1463–4, 1987.

Capeless EL, Mann LI: Use of breast stimulation for antepartum stress testing. *Obstet Gynecol* 64:641–5, 1984.

de Carvalho M, et al: Effect of frequent breast-feeding on early milk production and infant weight gain. *Pediatrics* 72:307–11, 1983.

Cornblath M, et al: Hypoglycemia in infancy: the need for a rational definition. *Pediatrics* 85:834–7, 1990.

Cotton DB, et al: L Intrapartum to postpartum changes in colloid osmotic pressure. *Am J Obstet Gynecol* 149:174–7, 1984.

Crowell MK, Hill PD, Humenick SS: Relationship between obstetric analgesia and time of effective breastfeeding. *J Nurse Midwif* 39:150–6, 1994.

Davis HV, et al: Effects of cup, bottle and breast feeding on oral activities of newborn infants. *Pediatrics* 23:549–58, 1949.

Elliott JP, Flaherty JF: The use of breast stimulation to ripen the cervix in term pregnancies. *Am J Obstet Gynecol* 145:553–6, 1983.

Ellis DJ, Hewat RJ: Factors related to breastfeeding duration. *Can Fam Phys* 30:1479–85, 1984.

Endresen EH, Helsing E: Changes in breastfeeding practices in Norwegian maternity wards: national surveys 1973, 1982 and 1991. *Acta Paediatr* 84:719–24, 1995.

Eppink H: Experiment to determine a basis for nursing decisions in regard to initiation of breastfeeding. *Nurs Res* 18:292, 1969.

Fawcett, et al: Effects of information on adaptation to cesarean birth. *Nurs Res* 42:49–53, 1993.

Ford K, Labbok M: Who is breast-feeding? Implications of associated social and biomedical variables for research on the consequences of methods of infant feeding. *Am J Clin Nutr* 52:451–6, 1990.

Glover J, Sandilands M: Supplementation of breastfeeding infants and weight loss in hospital. *J Hum Lact* 6:163–6, 1990.

Goer H. *Obstetric myths versus research realities: a guide to the medical literature.* Westport, CT: Bergin & Garvey, 1995:21–39.

Gulick E: Informational correlates of successful breastfeeding. *MCN* 7:37–75, 1982.

Hall WA, Carty EM: Managing the early discharge experience: taking control. *J Adv Nurs* 18:574–82, 1993.

Hawdon JM, Ward-Platt MPW, Aynsley-Green A: Neonatal hypoglycaemia–blood glucose monitoring and baby feeding. *Midwifery* 9:3–6, 1993.

Hawdon JM, Platt MPW, Aynsley-Green A: Prevention and management of neonatal hypoglycaemia. *Arch Dis Child* 70:F65–F70, 1994.

Heacock HJ, et al: Influence of breast versus formula milk on physiological gastroesophageal reflux in healthy, newborn infants. *J Pediatr Gastroenterol Nutr* 14:41–6, 1992.

Heck LJ, Erenberg A: Serum glucose levels in term neonates during the first 48 hours of life. *J Pediatr* 110: 119–22, 1987.

Hewat RJ, Ellis DJ: Breastfeeding as a maternal-child team effort: women's perceptions. *Health Care Women Int* 5:437–52, 1984.

Hill PD, Humenick SS: The occurrence of breast engorgement. *J Hum Lact* 10:79–86, 1994.

Hoffmann JB: A suggested treatment for inverted nipples. *Am J Obstet Gynecol* 66:346, 1953.

Howie PW, Houston MJ, Cook A: How long should a breast feed last? *Early Hum Dev* 5:71–7, 1981.

Humenick SS, Hill PD, Anderson MA: Breast engorgement: patterns and selected outcomes. *J Hum Lact* 10:87–93, 1994.

Janke JR: Breastfeeding duration following cesarean and vaginal births. *J Nurse Midwif* 33:159–64, 1988.

Jansson P: Early postpartum discharge. *Am J Nurs* 85:547–50, 1985.

Johanson RB, et al: Effect of post-delivery care on neonatal body temperature. *Acta Paediatr* 81:859–62, 1992.

Jolley S: *Breastfeeding Triage Tool,* 3rd ed. Seattle: Seattle–King County Department of Public Health, 1996:83.

Kearney MH, Cronenwett LR, Barrett JA: Breastfeeding problems in the first week postpartum. *Nurs Res* 39:90–5, 1990.

Kearney MH, Cronenwett LR, Reinhardt R: Cesarean delivery and breastfeeding outcomes. *Birth* 17:97–103, 1990.

Keppler AB: The use of intravenous fluids during labor. *Birth* 15:75–79, 1988.

King FS: *Helping Mothers to Breastfeed* (rev. ed.) Nairobi: Aftican Medical and Research Foundation, 1992:119–20.

Klaus MH: The frequency of suckling: a neglected but essential ingredient of breast-feeding. *Obstet Gynecol Clin North Am* 14:623–33, 1987.

Kulski JK, Smith M, Hartman PE: Normal and cesarean section delivery and the initiation of lactation in women. *Aust J Exp Biol Med Sci* 59:405–12, 1981.

Lang S, Lawrence CJ, Orme RLE: Cup feeding: an alternative method of infant feeding. *Arch Dis Child* 71:365–9, 1994.

Lau C, Henning SJ: Noninvasive method for determining patterns of milk intake in the breast-fed infant. *J Pediatr Gastroenterol Nutr* 9:481–7, 1989.

Lawrence RA: *Breastfeeding: a guide for the medical profession.* St Louis: Mosby, 1989.

Lawson T, Tulloch MI: Breastfeeding duration: prenatal intentions and postnatal practices. *J Adv Nurs* 22:841–9, 1995.

Lie B, Juul J: Effect of epidural vs. general anesthesia on breastfeeding. *Acta Obstet Gynecol Scand* 67:207–9, 1988.

Lifschitz CH, et al: Anaphylactic shock due to cow's milk protein hypersensitivity in a breast-fed infant. *J Pediatr Gastroenterol Nutr* 7:141–4, 1988.

Loftus JR, et al: Placental transfer and neonatal effects of epidural sufentanil and fentanyl administered with bupivacaine during labor. *Anesthesiology* 83:300–8, 1995.

Lothian JA: It takes two to breastfeed: the baby's role in successful breastfeeding. *J Nurs Midwif* 40:328–34, 1995.

Loughlin H et al: Early termination of breastfeeding: identifying those at risk. *Pediatrics* 75:508–13, 1985.

MAIN Collaborative Group Preparing for Breast Feeding: Treatment of inverted and non-protractile nipples in pregnancy. *Midwif* 10:200–14, 1994.

Matthews MK: The relationship between maternal labour analgesia and delay in the initiation of breastfeeding in healthy neonates in the early neonatal period. *Midwif* 5:3–10, 1989.

Michlovitz SL, Wolf SL: *Thermal agents in rehabilitation.* Philadelphia: Davis, 1986.

Milligan RA, Flenniken PM, Pugh LC: Positioning intervention to minimize fatigue in breastfeeding women. *Appl Nurs Res* 9:67–70, 1996.

Moon JL, Humenick SS: Breast engorgement: contributing variables and variables amenable to nursing intervention. *JOGNN* 18:309–15, 1989.

Mulford C: Subtle signs and symptoms of the milk ejection reflex. *J Hum Lact* 6:177–8, 1990.

Murray AD, et al: Effects of epidural anesthesia on newborns and their mothers. *Child Dev* 52:71–82, 1981.

Neifert M, Lawrence R, Seacat J: Nipple confusion: toward a formal definition. *J Pediatr* 126:s125–s129, 1995.

Newman J: Decision tree and postpartum management for preventing dehydration in the "breastfed" baby. *J Hum Lact* 12:129–35, 1996.

Newton E, et al: Epidural analgesia and uterine function. *Obstet Gynecol* 85:749–55, 1994.

Newton M: Human lactation. In: Kon SK, Cowie AT, eds. *Milk, the mammary gland and its secretion,* vol 1. New York: Academic, 1961.

Newton M, Newton N: The let-down reflex in human lactation. *J Pediatr* 33:698–704, 1948.

Newton N, Newton M, Broach J: Psychologic, physical, nutritional and technologic aspects of intravenous infusion during labor. *Birth* 15:67–72, 1988.

Nicholson WL: The use of nipple shields by breastfeeding women. *Aust Coll Midwives J* 6:18–24, 1993.

Nissen, et al: Different patterns of oxytocin, prolactin but not cortisol release during breastfeeding in women delivered by Cesarean section or by the vaginal route. *Early Hum Dev* 45:103–8, 1996.

Nissen E, et al: Effects of routinely given pethidine during labour on infants' developing breastfeeding behaviour: effects of dose-delivery time interval and various concentrations of pethidine/norpethidine in cord plasma. *Acta Paediatr* 86:201–8, 1997.

Oki EY, et al: The breast-stimulated contraction stress test. *J Reprod Med* 32:919–23, 1987.

Orem DE: *Nursing: concepts of practice* (2nd ed). New York: McGraw-Hill, 1980.

Padawer JA, et al: Women's psychological adjustment following emergency Cesarean versus vaginal delivery. *Psychol Women Q* 12:25–34, 1988.

Page-Goertz S: Discharge planning for the breastfeeding dyad. *Pediatr Nurs* 15:543–4, 1989.

Perez-Escamilla R, Maulen-Radovan I, Dewey KG: Association between cesarean delivery and breastfeeding outcomes among Mexican women. *Am J Public Health* 86:832–6, 1996.

Pietz CL: The emotional impact of breastfeeding after a cesarean. *Int J Child Educ* 4:20–1, 1989.

Powers NG, Slusser W: Breastfeeding update 2: clinical lactation management. *Pediatr Rev* 18:147–61, 1997.

Procianoy R, et al: Factors affecting breastfeeding: the influence of cesarean section. *J Trop Pediatr* 30:39–42, 1984.

Rajan L: The impact of obstetric procedures and analgesia/anesthesia during labour and delivery on breastfeeding. *Midwif* 10:87–103, 1994.

Righard L: How do newborns find their mother's breast? *Birth* 22:174–5, 1995.

Righard L, et al: Breastfeeding patterns: comparing the effects on infant behavior and maternal satisfaction of using one or two breasts. *Birth* 20:182–5, 1993.

Rimar JM: Epidural morphine for analgesia following a cesarean. *MCN* 11:345, 1986.

Riordan J, Countryman BA: Basics of breastfeeding: IV: Preparation of breastfeeding and early optimal functioning. *JOGN Nurs* 9:273–83, 1980.

Riordan J, Koehn M: Reliability and validity testing of three breastfeeding assessment tools. *JOGNN* 26:181–87, 1997.

Roberts KL: A comparison of chilled cabbage leaves and chilled gelpaks in reducing breast engorgement. *J Hum Lact* 11:17–20, 1995.

Roberts KL, Reiter M, Schuster D: A comparison of chilled and room temperature cabbage leaves in treating breast engorgement. *J Hum Lact* 11:191–4, 1995.

Rosier W: Cool cabbage compresses. *Breastfeed Rev* 11:28–31, 1988.

Rothman KJ, Runch DP, Dreyer NA: Bromocriptine and puerperal seizures. *Epidemiology* 1:232–8, 1990.

Rubin R: Attainment of the maternal role: I. Processes. *Nurs Res* 16:237–41, 1967a.

Rubin R: Attainment of the maternal role: II. Models and referrants. *Nurs Res* 16:342–6, 1967b.

Rubin R: Basic maternal behavior. *Nurs Outlook* 9:683–6, 1961.

Ruch A, Duhring JL: Postpartum myocardial infarction in a patient receiving bromocriptine. *Obstet Gynecol* 74:448–51, 1989.

Rush D, et al: Longitudinal study of pregnant women. *Am J Clin Nutr* 48:439–83, 1988.

Salmon YM, et al: Cervical ripening by breast stimulation. *Obstet Gynecol* 67:21–4, 1986.

Samuels S, Margen S, Schoen E: Incidence and duration of breastfeeding in a health maintenance organization population. *Am J Clin Nutr* 42:504–10, 1985.

Sepkoski CM, et al: The effects of maternal epidural anesthesia on neonatal behavior during the first month. *Dev Med Child Neurol* 34:1072–80, 1992.

Sexson WR: Incidence of neonatal hypoglycemia: a matter of definition. *J Pediatr* 105:149–50, 1984.

Shortridge KF, et al: Protective potential of colostrum and early milk against prospective influenzae viruses. *J Trop Pediatr* 36:94–5, 1990.

Shrago LC: Engorgement reconsidered. *Breastfeeding Abstr* 11(1):1–2, 1991.

Silva MLM, Giampaglia CMS: Colostrum and human milk inhibit localized adherence of enteropathogenic *Escherichia coli* to HeLa cells. *Acta Paediatr* 81:266–7, 1992.

Simkin P: Intermittent brachial plexus neuropathy secondary to breast engorgement. *Birth* 15:102–4, 1988.

Stamp GE, Crowther CA: Breastfeeding—why start? why stop? A prospective survey of South Australian women. *Breastfeed Rev* 3:15–9, 1995.

Tamminen T, et al: The influence of perinatal factors on breastfeeding. *Acta Paediatr Scand* 72:9–12, 1983.

Taylor MM: *Transcultural aspects of breastfeeding–USA* (Unit 2). Lactation Consultant Series, Garden City Park, NY: Avery Publishing Group, 1985: 18–19.

Taylor PM, Maloni JA, Brown DR: Early suckling and prolonged breast-feeding. *Am J Dis Child* 140:151–4, 1986.

Thorp JA, Breedlove G: Epidural analgesia in labor: an evaluation of risks and benefits. *Birth* 23:63–83, 1996.

Vandiver TA: Relationship of mothers' perceptions and behaviors to the duration of breastfeeding. *Psychol Rep* 80(3 Pt 2):1375–84, 1997.

Victora CG, et al: Caesarean section and duration of breast feeding among Brazilians. *Arch Dis Child* 65:632–4, 1990.

Victora CG, et al: Pacifier use and short breast-feeding duration: cause, consequence, or coincidence? *Pediatrics* 99:445–53, 1997.

Waldenstrom U, Sundelin C, Lindmark G: Early and late discharge after hospital birth: breastfeeding. *Acta Paediatr Scand* 76:727–32, 1987.

Walker M: *Breastfeeding premature babies* (Unit 14, Lactation Consultant Series). Garden City Park, NY: Avery Publishing Group, 1991.

Wang YS, et al: Preliminary study on the blood glucose level in the exclusively breastfeeding newborn. *J Trop Pediatr* 40:187–8, 1994.

Watson DL, et al: Bromocriptine mesylate for lactation suppression: a risk for postpartum hypertension? *Obstet Gynecol* 74:573–6, 1989.

Whitley N: Preparation for breastfeeding: a one-year follow-up of 34 nursing mothers. *JOGN Nurs* 7:44–8, 1974.

Whichelow M: Factors associated with the duration of breastfeeding in a privileged society. *Early Hum Dev* 7:273–80, 1982.

Widström A-M, et al: Gastric suction in healthy newborn infants. *Acta Paediatr Scand* 76:566–72, 1987.

Widström A-M, Thingström-Paulsson J: The position of the tongue during rooting reflexes elicited in newborn infants before the first suckle. *Acta Paediatr* 82:281–3, 1993.

Williams J, Mueller S: A message to the nurse from the baby. *J Hum Lact* 5:19, 1989.

Wilson-Clay B: Clinical use of silicone nipple shields. *J Hum Lact* 12:279–85, 1996.

Wittels B, et al: Postcesarean analgesia with both epidural morphine and intravenous patient-controlled analgesia: neurobehavioral outcomes among nursing neonates. *Anesth Analg* 85:600–6, 1997.

Woolridge MW, Fisher C: Colic, "overfeeding," and symptoms of lactose malabsorption in the breast-fed baby: a possible artifact of feed management? *Lancet* 2:382–4, 1988.

Woolridge MW, Ingram JC, Baum JD: Do changes in pattern of breast usage alter the baby's nutrient intake? *Lancet* 336(8712):395–7, 1990.

Wright A, et al: Changing hospital practices to increase the duration of breastfeeding. *Pediatrics* 97:669–75, 1996.

Wright H, Walker P: Prediction of duration of breastfeeding in primiparas. *J Epidemiol Commun Health* 37:89–94, 1983.

Yamauchi Y: Hypoglycemia in health, full-term, breast-fed neonates during the early days of life: preliminary observation. *Acta Paediatr Japon* 39 Suppl 1:544–47, 1997.

THE BREASTFEEDING PROCESS: THE POSTPARTUM PERIOD

Jan Riordan and Kathleen G. Auerbach

This chapter follows the mother-infant dyad as they rejoin the family at home after birth in the early postpartum period. Most hospitals in the United States and Canada now discharge mothers who have given birth vaginally within 24 to 48 hours postpartum and mothers whose infants are born by cesarean section within four days. In birthing centers, the mother and infant may return home within hours after birth. The intent of health maintenance organizations (HMOs) and insurers in encouraging early postpartum discharge is greater corporate profits. With about 4 million births annually (United States) and maternity beds averaging $1,000 per day, insurers save $4 billion annually for every day they shorten the hospital stay (_onLine Birth Wars, AP US & World, Sun, July 16, 1995).

Early discharge offers advantages to the family as well. For instance, there is less time for hospital routines to interfere with early lactation and less opportunity for cross-infection. Alternatively, the disadvantages of early discharge include less time for health care workers to assess, teach, and refer patients. In response to national concerns about early discharge, the Newborns' and Mothers' Health Protection Act (1997) requires insurers to pay for at least two days in a hospital after a vaginal birth.

Early discharge may increase feeding-related readmissions to the hospital but research findings on this topic conflict, probably because of a lack of consensus about case definition. At least three studies (Lee et al., 1995; Soskolne et al., 1996; Pascale et al., 1996) showed that early postpartum discharge is linked with increasing hospital readmission for both jaundice and dehydration. In their study, Pascale et al. (1996) asked whether reduced staffing (LC services and birthing-center staffing over the weekend) contributed to a reduced likelihood of teaching and breastfeeding assessment, especially for primiparous mothers. Results of others failed to demonstrate a significant, independent effect (Braverman et al., 1995). Edmonson et al. (1997), conducted a case-control analysis of 210 normal Wisconsin newborns who were readmitted to the hospital. Early discharges increased threefold during the study period, but feeding-related admissions remained stable. Readmitted newborns were significantly ($p < .05$) more likely to have been breastfed, first-born, or preterm, or to have mothers who were poorly educated (less than a twelfth-grade education), unmarried, or receiving Medicaid. Readmission was not associated with early discharge (adjusted odds ratio, 1.05; 95 percent confidence interval, 0.71–1.53). Early discharge does not appear to result in earlier weaning, especially if postpartum follow-up is integrated into care (Quinn et al., 1997).

The first challenge for health professionals is to identify and prioritize major concerns of the breast-feeding mother and family in the first few weeks. These major issues, in order of priority, include

- adequate hydration and nutrition of the neonate
- the mother's concern over whether she has enough milk (perceived or actual)
- sore nipples

The chapter addresses each of these critical topics, and then discusses other common issues during the "fourth trimester" for the mother, baby, and family (Basire et al., 1997).

Adequate Hydration and Nutrition of the Neonate

The priority for follow-up care of the mother-infant pair following birthing center discharge is the determination that the baby is receiving sufficient breastmilk to maintain hydration and calories for growth. The neonate is much more likely to develop fluid and electrolyte disturbances within a shorter period of time than would an older infant, with a small margin between homeostasis and overload or underload (Blackburn & Loper, 1992). Although the American Academy of Pediatrics (AAP, 1995) lists among its guidelines for early discharge the recommendation that the baby have at least two effective feedings before discharge, mothers are still leaving the hospital with a breast pump, a hope, and a prayer but without having engaged in an adequate feeding in the hospital. An early post-discharge appointment with the pediatrician or primary practitioner during the first week should be routine so that mothers and infants do not "fall through the cracks" of health care. Those families who lack a private health care provider should be scheduled for a postdischarge clinic visit or a home visit by a visiting nurse or other care provider.

To grow and thrive, the baby must receive milk. When milk transfer occurs frequently and in sufficient volume, several indicators will be present

that will reassure the parents and the professionals with whom they have contact that all is well (Box 10–1). Once at home, the mother, especially if she is a first-time mother, needs to know which signs indicate that her infant is taking adequate amounts of breastmilk. Ideally, these indicators are shared with the parents before discharge so that they understand what to do if these indicators are not present.

Ideally, within two to four days of her return home, the mother should be seen by a health professional who observes a feeding, weighs the baby using an electronic scale (Meier et al., 1994), and evaluates how mother and baby are progressing toward the indicators listed in Box 10–1. The infant regains his birth weight no later than the end of two weeks postpartum and, after that time, gains at least four to seven ounces (113–219 gm) per week or at least a pound a month. If 7 percent weight loss from birth weight has occurred, the health care provider should assess the factors that might be contributing to this situation and should take steps to reduce the likelihood that additional weight loss will occur. If 10 percent weight loss has occurred, supplementary milk should be offered to the baby to ensure that milk transfer is occurring with sufficient frequency and volume to rehydrate the neonate. An additional clinic appointment or home visit is needed within seven days of the first visit if any of the indicators in Box 10–1 are present. This visit should also include a weight check using an electronic scale.

Insufficient Milk Supply (IMS)
Perceived Insufficient Milk Supply

A major worry of many new mothers during the first few weeks postpartum is that their milk supply might not be enough for their baby. This is the almost universal reason given by mothers for early weaning and for supplementation (Hill & Humenick, 1989; Hillervick-Lindquist et al., 1991). Although many women fear that they will not be able to produce enough milk to feed their babies, the conclusion that many women have an insufficient milk supply is unsubstantiated. Some argue that mammalian survival has depended on sufficient milk production to enable the young of the

BOX 10–1

Indicators of sufficient milk intake

INDICATORS

By the end of the first week, 5 to 10 mostly yellow milk stools per day should be seen.

The infant should wet at least six to eight cloth diapers (three to five paper diapers) daily by the end of the first week; the urine should look clear, not dark or concentrated.

The baby is alert, acts hungry at times, is fussy at certain times of the day, and acts satiated after each feeding.

The baby's mucous membranes are wet and, when pinched, the skin does not remain above the normal surface (tenting).

RATIONALE

Frequent stool output is usually the most reliable indicator of adequate nutrient intake.

After the first few days, urine output is an indicator of hydration.

An alert baby is giving appropriate cues to indicate that he is hungry and then satisfied.

These are physiological signs that the infant is sufficiently hydrated.

---

species to survive beyond the period when they are completely dependent on mother's milk. If real milk insufficiency occurred frequently, the species' survival would be in jeopardy.

Breastmilk insufficiency may often be a perceived problem rather than an actual one, generated in part by societal ignorance of normal breastfeeding and in part by iatrogenic elements that make breastfeeding difficult to accomplish or sustain (Beeken & Waterston, 1992; Newman, 1986). This claim is buttressed by the knowledge that the problem of insufficient milk appears to be culture-bound: for example, it is milk *oversupply,* not undersupply, that has been observed in breastfeeding women in Australia and New Zealand and elsewhere (Livingstone, 1996), suggesting that appropriate assistance may enable more women to have more milk than their babies need. Over many years of practice, the authors note the frequency of conversations they have had with mothers who expressed concerns that they did not have enough milk; on assessing the situation, they found that the

infant was thriving, but the mother misunderstood infant cues or other indications that breastfeeding was going well. Such misunderstanding of the baby's cues can result in unnecessary supplementation, which may then result in a reduction in milk production from reduced stimulation. One frequent outcome of such early supplementation is early weaning (Hill et al., 1997).

Before insufficient milk supply can be assumed to exist, a wide variety of factors that the mother may accept as evidence of insufficient milk must be ruled out. For example, if the mother does not know that breastfed infants need to feed frequently, she may conclude that her baby's behavior suggests that she has insufficient milk. The reality is that the baby is not being offered the breast frequently enough. In reviewing the data on newborns readmitted to the hospital within the first month to rule out sepsis, most had negative cultures but were dehydrated. The babies responded well to rehydration; however, McGregor (1996) found that the mothers believed that their infants were "nursing a lot," when in fact the babies were not being fed frequently *enough*. McGregor concluded that the mothers who were discharged early did not know how often their babies should have been feeding.

In addition, breastfed infants typically have a sleep/wake cycle that includes a tendency for wakefulness and frequent ("cluster") feedings in the late afternoon and evening–an ancient pattern emanating from hunter-gatherer tribes of the past, according to anthropologists. This wakeful, sometimes fussy, period at the end of the day may be particularly trying for the inexperienced mother who is unsure of her ability to breastfeed and unaware that wakefulness and frequent feedings at these times are entirely normal and do not reflect poor mothering skills. Lactation consultants can expect that many of the distress calls from mothers during the second and third week after delivery stem from a lack of knowledge of this common pattern.

The mother may complain about any of the following concerns:

The baby

- is restless or irritable during or between feedings.
- acts "hungry all the time," sucks his fists or blanket, moves his head rapidly from side to side at the breast.
- comes off the breast frequently.
- cries or is fussy constantly, is difficult to console, is fussy right after a feeding.
- has feedings that seem longer than the mother may have been told (or may have read) to expect.
- takes formula from a bottle right after a feeding.
- falls asleep at the breast.
- nurses less than 15 to 20 minutes on either or both breasts, leading the mother to believe she does not have enough milk.

The mother

- does not feel the milk-ejection reflex as she thinks she should.
- reports that her breasts feel soft before each feeding, not just afterward.
- cannot express much milk (or expresses less than previously).

- has been told that frequent feedings indicate a decreased milk supply.
- was told not to put baby to breast because of cracked nipples.
- reports that her breasts did not enlarge or become tender during pregnancy; that she did not become engorged; or that she is concerned about the possible effects of previous breast surgery.

Others have noted that a low milk supply can occur after a mother has experienced significant stress (Ruvalcaba, 1987), as following the 1985 Mexican earthquake; after breast biopsy (Day, 1986) or other breast surgery (Hughes & Owen, 1993; Hurst, 1996); and when the mother is a smoker (Hill & Aldag, 1996). These reports emphasize the need to rule out as many factors as possible that could have a direct or indirect influence on milk production before one assumes that primary breast insufficiency exists.

Actual or Primary Insufficient Milk Supply

Very few women may have a true low milk supply caused by (1) congenital insufficient glandular tissue, (2) breast surgery, (3) postpartum hemorrhage, or (4) anemia. Neifert, Seacat, and Jobe (1985) described three cases of congenital insufficient glandular tissue. In all of these women, marked size or shape differences (or both) were noted from one breast to the other. Women who have had breast surgery, especially one involving the periareolar region in which the nerves surrounding the areola are severed, are at risk for a low milk supply (Neifert et al., 1990; Widdice, 1993). See Chapter 15 for a detailed discussion of this topic.

Perinatal nurses have long noted that women who have suffered postpartum hemorrhage experience difficulty producing breastmilk. Willis and Livingstone (1995) studied 10 mothers who experienced normal mammogenesis and then suffered a large obstetrical hemorrhage, which was followed by failure to lactate adequately. Estimated blood loss ranged from 500 to 1,500 ml (average blood loss during delivery, 500 ml). Five of seven infants had hypernatremic dehydration, with serum sodium levels ranging from 148 to 166 mmol/L. Sodium levels in the breastmilk of five of the six mothers were elevated. None of the mothers were diagnosed with Sheehan's syndrome. With health care support, most of these mothers were producing sufficient breastmilk a month later. Because lactation failure reversed over time in two mothers, the disruption of pituitary function was likely due to ischemia rather than infarction, as it is in Sheehan's syndrome. Another study also noted reduced or absent lactation in 6 of 20 women who had experienced a postpartum hemorrhage and otherwise had no signs of hypopituitarism (Schneeberg et al., 1960). Concomitantly, new mothers with anemia are also more likely to produce less breastmilk (Henly et al., 1995).

If such problems are encountered, there is no need to discontinue breastfeeding. Rather, the mother can use a tube-feeding device to deliver additional nutrition to the infant while he is at the breast. In some cases, metoclopramide (Reglan) given to the mother orally for several days is an option for treating a low milk supply. For example, clinicians have found that metoclopramide is very helpful for mothers of premature babies in enhancing milk ejection (and the mother's confidence). To date, no adverse effects have been observed with short-term use of the drug; however, long-term use may be associated with maternal depression.

Hill and Humenick (1989) have proposed a conceptual model describing insufficient milk supply as well as some potential antecedents and indicators (Fig. 10–1). With early discharge, close follow-up of mothers–especially those who are breastfeeding for the first time–can prevent many problems and subsequent unintended weaning. It is helpful to provide each breastfeeding family with a written list of "red flags" that signal underfeeding and other guidelines.

Breast Massage

Massage has been used extensively and effectively during the childbearing period. It relieves the discomforts of labor and is often used for infant stimulation. Massage of the lactating breasts is common in many parts of the world and is often used to stimulate milk production, to promote drainage, and to relieve engorged breasts.

A special technique, Alternate Breast Massage, in which the mother alternately massages each breast, was developed by Iffrig (1968) and later tested by Bowles et al. (1988). The mother massages the base of her breast when she observes the infant begin rapid, shallow suckling movements. She then alternates massage with the infant's suckling. Infants of mothers who use such breast massage have been reported to gain more weight than do other infants whose mothers did not practice this technique.

In Japan, breast massage is popular. Many people in that country, including physicians, are convinced that it effectively increases the milk supply and relieves plugged ducts (Riordan, 1990). In fact, some Japanese hospitals offer both mothers (and fathers) breast massage classes that confer certification. Figure 10–2 shows the Japanese technique for breast massage.

Massaging the mother's back to relieve discomfort from engorgement or to relax her if she has difficulty letting down her milk is an acupressure technique recommended for years by La Leche League leaders. While the mother sits in a chair, someone stands behind her and briskly rubs the knuckles of a fist from the base of the mother's neck to the bottom of her shoulder blades on both sides of her spine.

Sore Nipples

Sore nipples (of two types) are a common, early postpartum concern and a frequent reason that mothers stop breastfeeding before they intended to do so. *Transient soreness* can occur during the first week postpartum, usually peaking between the third and sixth days. *Prolonged, abnormal soreness* lasts beyond the first week. Most women develop some nipple tenderness as they begin to feed their new baby (Chapman et al., 1985; de Carvalho et al., 1984; Foxman et al., 1994; Gunther, 1945; Hewat & Ellis, 1987; Riordan, 1985; Walker & Driscoll, 1989; Woolridge, 1986; Ziemer et al., 1990). Skin color, hair color, and prenatal nipple preparation all appear to be unrelated to nipple pain (de Carvalho et al., 1984; Hewat & Ellis, 1987; Ziemer et al., 1990). This transient tenderness usually resolves after about one week.

Unfortunately, hospital personnel often advise that, to prevent sore nipples, mothers should limit the duration of feedings. Hospital staff rarely see

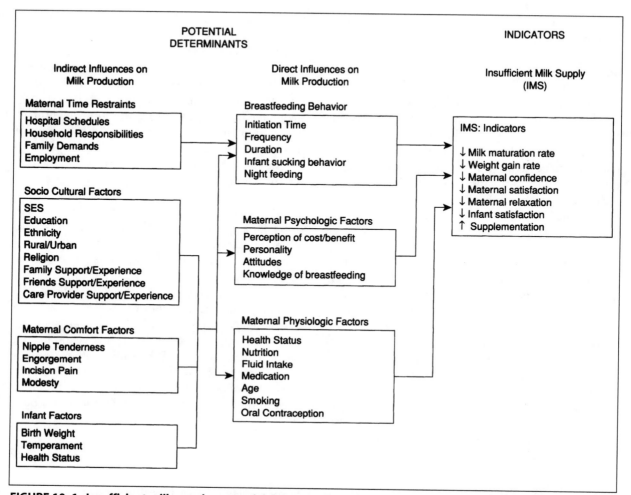

FIGURE 10–1. Insufficient milk supply: potential determinants and indicators. *(From Hill, PD, and Humenick, SS: Nurs Res 21:145, 1989.)*

the mother after discharge and, given today's brief hospital stay, they may continue to hold the erroneous belief that restricting time at the breast is a good preventive measure. In reality, placing a time limit on the length of each feeding has several negative effects:

- It simply delays nipple soreness.

- Short feedings prevent the baby from receiving the creamier hindmilk.

- Short feedings may necessitate that the mother remove the baby from the breast; if this is not done carefully, repeated attempts to break the baby's suction can result in unnecessary pain and trauma.

Nipple soreness that increases or lasts beyond the first week is abnormal. Chronic pain is a warning that something is wrong. Because breastfeeding is a two-person activity, it is imperative that both partners be considered during assessment of possible causes of protracted nipple pain and trauma (Amir, 1993; Huggins & Billon, 1993; Pugh et al., 1996; Walker & Driscoll, 1989). A number of factors may be responsible:

Ankyloglossia (tongue-tie)
Impetigo
Disorganized or dysfunctional infant suckling engorgement
Eczema
Flat or retracted nipples

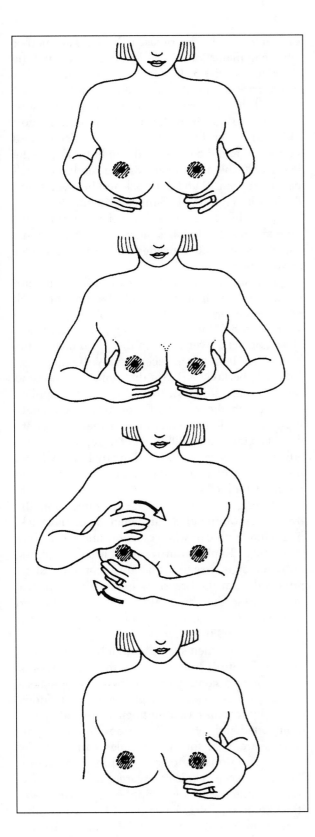

FIGURE 10–2. Japanese breast massage. *A. Improve breastfeeding by massaging the base of the breast. B. Place the thumbs of both hands in armpits. The rest of the fingers support the breast from the side. Thrust the chest forward by moving the elbows back as far as possible ("chicken-wing position"). Push the breasts toward the center as if trying to press the nipples together. This will improve the milk flow from the base of the breast. C. Cup the breast with both hands and gently rotate, as if making a rice bowl or shaping bread dough, for one to two minutes Repeat the first two steps two or three times. D. Hold one breast at a time and squeeze before putting the baby to breast. (Drawing by Ruth Linstromberg.)*

> Herpes simplex
> Improper breaking of suction
> Improper infant positioning at breast
> Improper or excessive use of breast pumps
> Nipple shields
> Presence of *Staphylococcus aureus*
> Prolonged exposure to wet nursing pads or to moisture buildup in poorly vented breast shells
> Sensitivity to nipple creams, lotions, or oils
> Severe breast engorgement
> Thrush
> Unrelieved negative pressure

Infant suckling patterns can contribute to nipple tenderness in the mother, particularly if the baby's first suckling has been conditioned by a rubber teat from bottle-feeding or a pacifier (Newman, 1990). In mothers with moderate to severe nipple pain, *S. aureus* was more likely to be found on the nipples, possibly contributing to prolonged soreness (Livingstone et al., 1996). Another recently "rediscovered" factor is a frenulum attached too near the tip of the tongue, which might cause nipple or areolar abrasions (Berg, 1990; Marmet et al., 1990; Notestine, 1990; Wiessinger & Miller, 1995; Wilton, 1990).

Evaluation. Careful evaluation of the infant at the breast must include asking the mother how the breast feels when the baby is suckling and examining the frenulum. The following assessments also should be made:

- *What do the baby's cheeks look like?* The baby's cheeks should round outward if he is suckling effectively. Cheeks that are drawn inward, causing "dimpling," are an indication that the baby may be tongue-sucking rather than stimulating the maternal milk-ejection response. Thus the baby is not receiving milk. When this occurs, the mother will feel minimal negative pressure or sensation, indicating that the baby is suckling. It is appropriate to verify this by asking the mother what she feels when dimpling of the cheeks is observed.

- *Where is the baby's tongue?* If the corner of the baby's mouth is pulled slightly away from the breast while the baby is suckling, the tongue should be visible under the areolar tissue and nipple and forward over the baby's gumline. If the tongue is not visible, it may be curled backward. If the tongue does not extend over the gumline, if it assumes a heart shape if the baby cries and attempts to lift the tongue, or if the mother complains of pain when the baby is nursing, the health care provider should check the frenulum for shortness or for attachment that prevents the tongue from extending forward sufficiently to allow effective suckling.

- *What is heard when the baby is suckling?* The health care provider should listen to the baby. A baby who is breastfeeding effectively will make a swallowing sound that is sometimes very quiet but will occur after one to three sucks. Additionally, no slurping sounds should be heard, as this is usually an indication that the baby is sucking his own tongue or is not creating a complete seal around the areola.

- *How tight is the baby's seal on the breast?* The suction of the baby on the breast should be checked. If a good seal is formed, the mother may need to insert her finger into the side of the baby's mouth to effect removal without causing pain. If the baby easily falls from the breast when he appears to be suckling actively, the seal is inadequate (Escott, 1989).

The baby is only one member of the breastfeeding partnership. The mother's breasts also need to be inspected. The position of bruises on the breast may indicate the cause of the problem. For example, if too much of the top of the areola and too little of the bottom is drawn into the baby's mouth, stretching and cracking of nipple tissue on the underside of the breast is likely. The mother who complains of nipple tenderness should be asked to visualize a clock face superimposed on her breast and to indicate where there is a bruise or a crack. If the baby suckles too low on the breast or too close to the tip of the nipple, trauma is most likely to occur between 10 and 12 o'clock and between 4 and 6 o'clock on the right breast; on the left breast, the areas of maximum tenderness will occur between 12 and 2 o'clock and between 6 and 8 o'clock (Fig. 10–3). Simply bringing the baby closer to the mother's body so that the tip of his nose and his chin brushes the mother's breast tissue usually is all that is needed to allow the tender areas to heal.

In cases in which both a crack and a bruise are evident on the nipple and areola, bathing the crack with fresh expressed milk will aid healing and prevent bacterial infection. Usually, the crack will close and scab over prior to disappearance of the bruise. In light of a recent study (Livingstone, Willis, & Berkowitz, 1996) that links *S. aureus* and severe nipple soreness, topical antibiotics applied to breaks in the skin and, possibly, low-strength topical steroids for inflammation may be beneficial. Huggins and Billon (1993) report that no adverse effects were observed in any infant when a thin coating of these preparations applied to the mother's nipples.

Resting the nipple by not feeding from the breast is recommended only when the pain of suckling is intolerable or when bleeding and erosion are worsening. Rapid improvement usually follows; however, it is essential that milk continue to be removed from the breast by expressing or pumping. During this time, the infant may be fed expressed breastmilk by spoon, cup, or dropper (Ellis et al., 1993).

Nipple ointments are commonly used for sore nipples. There is little evidence that ointments or creams have a salutary effect either on nipple healing or on soreness, although such preparations, especially lanolin-based ointments, are widely recommended and sold. A discussion of which nipple creams are best for sore nipples can engender strong emotions among lactation consultants. Based on recent clinical research, the most effective treatment for sore nipples is warm water (Buchko et al., 1993; Lavergne, 1997), confirming what Niles Newton's study (1952) found to be true

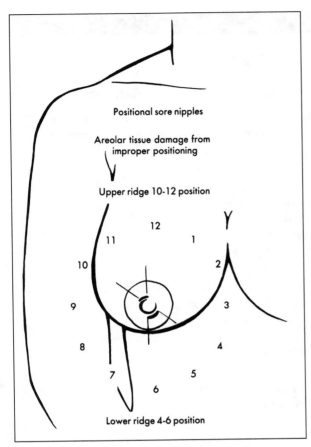

Positional sore nipples

Areolar tissue damage from
improper positioning

Upper ridge 10-12 position

Lower ridge 4-6 position

FIGURE 10–3. Area of breast soreness and trauma, as related to a clock face. *Imagine the face of a clock superimposed on right breast. Soreness usually develops in the crescent around the perimeter of the nipple at 10 to 12 o'clock position and below the perimeter of the nipple at 4 to 6 o'clock position. With the left breast, maximal potential for soreness is, similarly, at 12 to 2 o'clock and 6 to 8 o'clock positions.*

more than 40 years ago. Treatments for sore nipples—including the use of Massé cream (Brown & Hurlock, 1975), tea bags (Lavergne, 1997; Riordan, 1985), or lanolin (Brown & Hurlock, 1975; Newton, 1952)—appear to neither prevent nor reduce nipple soreness. Mothers who used a purified lanolin product, reported reduced nipple pain during days 6 through 10 of breastfeeding (Spangler & Hildebrandt, 1993). Purified lanolin is purported to promote "moist healing," which is considered to occur when the nipple is covered by a moisture barrier that helps prevent evaporation and drying

(Mohrbacher & Stock, 1997, p. 394). See the clinical care plan for sore nipples in Table 10–1.

Nonetheless, in most cases, nipple treatments are relatively harmless. They are a form of nurturing the mother, and new mothers like to use them; it makes the mothers feel as if something is being done for them. Given the low cost of such products, it seems harsh to deny mothers ointment and creams for sore nipples unless some harm results. For instance, some institutions discontinued using unpurified lanolin for breastfeeding mothers when pesticides were found (Copeland et al., 1989; Rosanove, 1987). Marx et al. (1985) reported increased serum concentrations of vitamin E in breastfeeding babies after six days of ingesting milk from their mothers who were applying vitamin E to their nipples. Belief in a certain type of cream as the "magic cure-all" caused an outbreak of breast infections when an Australian nurse, carrying her own container of pawpaw ointment, gave a little dab to all mothers who complained of sore or cracked nipples. The ointment was found to be contaminated (Lesley McBurney, personal communication, 1997). Gribetz (1974) described an infant who developed an intestinal obstruction thought to be caused by bismuth subnitrate (40 percent of constituents) in Mammol ointment.

Table 10–2 contains some of the products used for nipple soreness. There are dozens more—for example, aloe vera, olive oil, pawpaw cream (Australia), Bepanthen (Australia), maize oil (Kamillsoan) (Africa), Coopers Milking Salve (Africa), Rose Calendar Cream (New Zealand), Rectinol, and chapstick. As discussed in Chapter 15, warm water and purified lanolin (if used in later weeks) are the only products that have been studied and found to actually reduce soreness. Medicated creams such as neosporin, bacitracin and clotrimazole, and hydrocortisone are also used for *Candida* infections and other nipple conditions. In considering each item's use, the care provider should keep in mind that two people are exposed to the product in question whenever it is used on the mother's nipples. What may be appropriate to use for the mother may expose the infant to unnecessary risk. If the product must be removed completely from the nipple to avoid infant exposure, the care provider should consider whether such action is self-defeating for the mother and whether some other element might be more appropriate.

Table 10-1

CLINICAL CARE PLAN FOR SORE NIPPLES

Assessment	Interventions	Rationale
Nipples appear slightly red and chapped in white mother; appear shiny in very dark-skinned mother.	Reassure mother that discomfort is temporary and condition will improve.	Breast is sensitive at start of breastfeeding. Many mothers experience some early nipple soreness.
Mother complains of soreness at latch-on or at start of pumping. Soreness subsides when milk-ejection reflex occurs.	Encourage mother to discontinue use of soap or antiseptic to clean breasts; apply purified lanolin or warm water to promote moist healing; and air-dry the nipples by leaving bra flaps down.	Maintains natural skin oils and moisture.
Wincing as infant grasps breast (or draws nipple into mouth).	Encourage mother to massage breast to milk-ejection reflex to stimulate flow; wear an all-cotton bra; and apply crushed ice in plastic bag (covered by washcloth) to nipples.	Softens nipple and breast before latch-on. Cold relieves discomfort.
Nipple sticks to bra or breast pad.	Encourage mother to moisten bra or breast pads before removing and to change pads more frequently.	Avoids removing keratin layer of skin.
Mother using breast cream.	Instruct mother to discontinue using cream and note any change.	Mother may be allergic, especially if cream contains unpurified lanolin.
Crescent-shaped abrasions above or below the nipple. Nipple tip is blanched after suckling episode. Discomfort and pain throughout feeding.	Review feeding position, making sure infant's mouth is open wide before latching on and baby is held high on mother's chest wall with entire body facing mother. Reposition as necessary.	Infant is gumming and pinching nipple or sliding up and down because of poor positioning.
Baby's tongue is retracted behind lower gum.	Draw infant in closely enough that breast is positioned deep in baby's mouth. Bring baby's tongue forward. Pull baby's lower lip out if it is drawn inward while feeding. Mother should be shown alternative nursing positions.	Tongue retraction prevents normal perfusion to nipple. Pressure on other areas of nipple allows healing of abraded areas.

Table 10-1

Bright, pinkish red area extending beyond nipple and areola. Mother complains of pain that extends throughout feeding.	Apply antifungal medication to nipples. Treat infant for thrush. Treat family for candidiasis.	Prompt treatment alleviates problem. Candidiasis spreads with warm, moist contact among family members.
Reddish lesions on breast that do not appear to be candidiasis.	Refer to health care provider for possible treatment with antibiotic cream for bacterial infection.	Topical antibiotics are effective for treating bacterial infection of nipple areas.

Nicholson (1986) investigated three separate treatments for cracked nipples: expressing milk and not breastfeeding while the cracked nipple was healing; using a nipple shield during breastfeeding; and continuing breastfeeding and receiving assistance designed to improve the baby's position on the breast. She found no significant differences in outcome. Gosha and Tichy (1988) provided new mothers with a breast shell designed with multiple air-holes and found that postpartum nipple pain was unaffected by its use.

Neonatal Physiological Jaundice

Typically, most infants will be jaundiced to some extent between the third and sixth days after birth. This means that jaundice will be most evident after the baby and mother are at home. Jaundice is normal in healthy full-term babies and is more exaggerated in those who are breastfed, which can concern parents (Brown, 1992). Sometimes this concern results in an unnecessary trip to the emergency room or clinic. Part of the postdischarge visit will include assessing the infant for hyperbilirubinemia. Asking the parents the questions listed in Box 12–2 will help to determine whether the baby is taking sufficient nutriment.

If it is determined that the infant is not feeding frequently or is not latching on effectively, a complete feeding assessment and review of the breastfeeding basics is necessary. The breastfeeding behavior found to correlate most highly with milk intake is audible swallowing while the baby is feeding. If the baby has prolonged, exaggerated jaundice, a bilirubin level should be drawn and plans made for close monitoring and follow-up.

Hyperbilirubinemia and treatment guidelines are discussed in detail in Chapter 12. Because interruption of breastfeeding may lead to early, unintended weaning, the focus of care should be on maintaining lactation while temporarily supplementing the baby's intake (if necessary) to reduce bilirubin levels (Auerbach, 1992; James et al., 1993).

Crying and Colic

An infant cries to signal a need. That need may be for comfort, a diaper change, a change of position, or suckling. Most parents go to their infant when they hear the baby cry, and they make every possible effort to comfort the child. The baby whose cries are responded to quickly soon learns to trust his parents (or caregivers). The baby who is responded to quickly generally stops crying sooner than the infant whose cry does not promptly receive a response. (Barr & Elias, 1988). Prompt response reduces the baby's stress level and enhances the parents' enjoyment of the baby and of their new role as parents. The hospital-based caregiver who assists new parents has a unique opportunity to help them interpret their baby's cry—and other earlier cues—and to learn the importance of meeting the baby's needs promptly. In time, as the baby learns to distinguish between stresses and the parents learn to interpret the baby's signals, the specific cause of the baby's distress will be more easily recognized and dealt with.

Unlike other cries, colic usually is characterized by a high-pitched wail or scream, a sign that the baby is in pain. Colic is the result of sudden, spasmodic abdominal cramping. Often the baby

Table 10–2

Products Used for Nipple Soreness

Name	Description and Ingredients	Comments
A&D Ointment	Ointment in tube. Contains anhydrous lanolin, petrolatum, fragrance, mineral oil, fish liver oil, and cholecalciferol	For *external use* only. In case of ingestion, contact a poison control center. There are no vitamins in this ointment.
Bag Balm	Stiff yellow ointment. Contains petrolatum, lanolin, 8-hydroxyquinoline sulfate, sanitas, and water.	A fungistat and bactericide for farm use. *Not for internal use* since 1969, because it causes cancer in laboratory animals.
Eucerin Cream	Cream in a jar. Contains petrolatum, mineral oil, mineral wax, lanolin wax, lanolin alcohol, methylchloroisothiazolinone, methylisothiazolinone.	For *external use* only.
Mammol Ointment	Contains bismuth subnitrate, castor oil, anhydrous lanolin, ceresin wax.	Advertised as a dressing for nipples of nursing mothers. However, instructions advise washing and drying nipples before and after use. *Warning:* Case report exists of bismuth subnitrate causing intestinal obstruction in infant.
Massé Cream	Contains glyceryl stearate, glycerin, cetyl alcohol, stearate, stearic acid, polysorbate 60, propylparaben, methylparaben, potassium hydroxide.	Advised for prenatal and postnatal nipple care. However, instructions advise to cleanse the breasts before and after each nursing with a clean cloth and water. Contraindicated in mastitis and breast abscess. Although most of the ingredients are innocuous, the glycerin is rapidly metabolized and can cause hyperglycemia. The cetyl alcohol is a laxative, and aspiration of peanut oil can cause severe and fatal bronchitis in small children.

Source: Derived from Drug evaluations *(6th ed). Chicago: American Medical Association Department of Drugs, Division of Drugs and Technology, in cooperation with the American Society for Clinical Pharmacology and Therapeutics, 1986; RE Gosselin, RP Simth, HC Hodge:* Clinical toxicology of commercial products *(5th ed). Baltimore, MD: Williams & Wilkins, 1984;* Handbook of nonprescription drugs *(7th ed). Washington, DC: American Pharmaceutical Association, 1982; D Grilbetz:* Ingestion of bismuth-containing ointment by a breast-fed infant. Mt Sinai J Med *41:498–510, 1974; CM Marx, et al: Vitamin E concentrations in serum of newborn infants after topical use of vitamin E by nursing mothers.* Am J Obstet Gynecol *152:668–70, 1985; BM Monheit, BG Luke: Pesticides in breastmilk—a public health perspective.* Commun Health Stud *14:269–73, 1990; J Morse: The hazards of lanolin.* MCN *14:204, 1989; Physicians' desk reference for non-prescription drugs (11th ed). Oradell, NJ: Medical Economics, 1990; ALW Po: Non-prescription drugs, London: Blackwell Scientific, 1982; R Rosanove: Dangers of the application of lanolin [letter].* Med J Aust *146:232, 1987; E Spannraft: A hidden source of vitamin E.* MCN *14:204, 1989; Springhouse drug reference: Springhouse, PA: Springhouse Corporation, 1988. Compiled by Angela Jacobi, RN, MN, IBCLC, Rush-Presbyterian-St. Luke's Medical Center, Chicago, IL.*

Table 10-2

USP Modified Lanolin (Lansinoh, Purelan, Marcalan)	Contains 100% anhydrous, modified lanolin.	Hypoallergenic. Estimated to contain fewer than 1.5 ppm of combined impurities. No caution required for use on open wounds or where ingestion may occur. Used in moist healing.
USP Lanolin ("Lanum")	Tube or cream. Contains hydrous lanolin.	Highly allergenic wool derivative. Analysis of a range of lanolin creams revealed that all contained organophosphorous pesticide residue, including Diazinon.
Vaseline Petroleum Jelly	Gel in a jar. Contains white petrolatum.	Not recommended for sore nipples.
Vitamin E (generic)	Vitamin capsules, oil, gelatin, or cream. Contains vitamin E in suspension. Capsules = 400 IU each.	U.S. recommended daily allowance for vitamin E in infants is 5 IU/day. Effect of increased serum concentrations of vitamin E is unknown.

draws up his knees and, in some cases, his abdomen will be distended. Some infants experience colic only once or twice daily, at about the same time each day. In others, the colic occurs after nearly every feeding and gradually disappears in about three to four months.

Reasons for colic abound. Explanations, many of which relate to feeding, include the following:

- Infant's allergies to cow's milk–based formula (Bishop et al., 1990; Clyne & Kulczycki, 1991; Jakobsson & Lindberg, 1983; Lifschitz et al., 1988; Lothe et al., 1982) or to some other element in the lactating mother's diet

- Overfeeding of infant, especially if bottle-feeding, although this can occur in some infants who are breastfeeding (Evans et al., 1995; Woolridge and Fisher, 1988)

- Underfeeding of infant, especially if the baby is not offered feedings frequently and is allowed to cry until it is "time" to feed

- "Too rich" or "too weak" milk

- Too much fat, sugar, or protein (especially if the baby receives artificial milk)

- Too large or too small holes in the bottle teat

- Excessive swallowing of air by infant, especially if bottle-fed, if given a pacifier frequently or for long periods, or if poorly positioned at the breast

- Temperament of the baby (Barr et al., 1989)

- Smoke inhalation by infant, particularly if the mother smokes (Matheson, 1989; Said et al., 1984)

- Anxious mother or a mother who interprets all crying as a sign of hunger (an interpretation that often leads a mother to stop breastfeeding in the mistaken belief that her emotional state has somehow affected her milk and her baby's ability to digest it) (Taubman, 1988)

Bottle-feedings of artificial bovine- or vegetable-based baby milk may at times be responsible for colic (Chandra et al., 1989; Høst et al., 1988; Working Group on Cow's Milk Protein Allergy, 1988). Sometimes breastfeeding techniques may be the culprit. For example, correcting poor positioning will reduce the likelihood that the baby will swallow air while suckling, if this is the problem. Forcing the baby to feed from both breasts can cause distress and colic (Evans et al., 1995).

If the colicky baby is fully breastfed, the mother's diet should be reviewed. If she drinks large quantities of cow's milk, a diet from which all dairy products are eliminated for at least one week is indicated (Clyne & Kulczycki, 1991; Jakobsson et al., 1985). The mother begins by eliminating all dairy products and foods containing dairy products from her diet. If this is the cause of the baby's distress after feedings, the mother will note a marked change in the baby's behavior within three to eight days. Without the offending bovine milk proteins in the mother's milk, the baby remains comfortable after each breastfeeding. At the end of the first week of dairy food elimination, if the mother confirms that the baby is better, she can begin to reintroduce dairy products slowly into her diet. She might be encouraged to try the following approach:

First week: eliminate all dairy products. Calcium is available in foods other than those in the dairy group. (If the mother is concerned about her calcium intake, she may use calcium tablets.)

Second week: reintroduce only hard cheeses (e.g., cheddar, Swiss) or yogurt in small quantities.

Third week: reintroduce soft cheeses (e.g., Gouda, Brie, cottage, American, cream) in small quantities.

Fourth week: reintroduce butter, ice cream, and milk in cooked form.

Fifth week: reintroduce cow's milk in small quantities.

Usually, while reintroducing dairy products into her diet, the mother will discover how much and in what form the baby can tolerate her intake of these foods. She should be encouraged to ingest only those dairy products to which the baby does not react. Waiting several weeks or months—depending on the baby's reactivity—before challenging the baby with an increase of dairy products in the mother's diet is essential.

Occasionally, a week of elimination may not be sufficient to eliminate the offending proteins. Clyne and Kulcyzcki (1991) note that bovine IgG levels were markedly higher in the milk of mothers of colicky babies than in the milk of mothers whose babies were not colicky. Bovine IgG has a prolonged half-life, and its presence in high levels may require a longer period of elimination than is usually suggested for short dietary trials. Particularly if a mother is sensitive to cow's milk, the lactation consultant may ask the mother to extend her dairy elimination somewhat longer if her baby's colic is believed to reflect the mother's dietary intake.

Although cow's milk appears to be the single most frequent offender in a mother's diet, other foods also have been implicated (Cant et al., 1985; Cavagni et al., 1988; Chandra et al., 1986). They include beef, eggs, peanut butter, wheat (and related glutens such as nuts), and high-acid fruits and vegetables (Chandra et al., 1986). Lactation consultants have also observed that mothers taking additional iron tablets report that their babies are colicky. This distress may relate to the effect of iron on neonatal gastrointestinal flora (Jackson & Lee, 1990; Mevissen-Verhage et al., 1985). Elimination of the extra iron readily solves the problem, often within a few days. Often babies who develop colic in response to foods in the breastfeeding mother's diet exhibit allergic symptoms when exposed to the same foods later in life. (Kajosaari & Saarinen, 1983; Pittschieler, 1990). The "colic hold" (La Leche League International, 1997, p. 99) provides relief, particularly during the period when the effects of elimination of the offending foods is not yet fully realized.

Stooling Patterns
Changes Over Time

As discussed earlier, the stools of the breastfed newborn go through several changes and can be used as an indicator of milk intake. These changes are easily observed and occur at predictable intervals (Table 10–3). Black, tarry stools (meconium) are passed in the first several days. With each succeeding milk feeding, the (transitional) stool gradually lightens and becomes less sticky and more liquid. The totally breastmilk stool is yellow and generally very soft or liquid. Breastfed infants have an average of 4.2 daily stools, twice as many as those fed a cow's milk or soy preparation (Hyams et al., 1995). At times, the stool may contain small curds, whereas at other times, it has a mushy consistency and is greenish yellow to mustard yellow. As the color changes, an odor develops that is sweeter and not as strong as the stool of artificially fed infants. It has been likened to a "yeasty" odor rather than the bile-predominant odor of the formula-fed infant. In contrast, the stools of non-breastfed infants are darker and firmer and have an unpleasant odor. By 14 days of age, formula-fed babies have a fecal flora that is very similar to that of

Table 10–3

CHARACTERISTIC STOOL CHANGES OVER TIME

Time Period	Type of Stool	Number per Day	Amount
0–6 days	Meconium, transitional, milk stool	2+	Scant to copious
7–28 days	Milk stool	5–10+	Scant
29+ days	Milk stool	1 every 4–12 days*	Copious

* Occasionally infants may go as long as 3–4 weeks between copious stools.

adults with predominance of coliforms and enterocci, whereas the flora of the breastfed baby is dominated by lactobacilli and bifidobacteria (Quinlan et al., 1995; Wharton et al., 1994).

As does color, the frequency of the stool changes. Stooling usually begins shortly after birth and continues two or more times daily during the first week of life. Often these relatively infrequent, mostly meconium stools are copious and explosive. As the frequency of stools increases, the amount of stool passed each time declines. After the first week, when the infant passes some stool during or immediately after nearly every breastfeeding, the amount of liquid yellow stool may be no more than a stain on the diaper rather than a gush that leaks out. The greater frequency and liquid nature of the totally breastfed infant's stool is neither a cause for concern nor an indication of diarrhea. Grandmothers and other helpers whose experience has been with artificially fed infants need to be reassured that these are normal stool patterns for the breastfed infant and are not a cause for concern.

After the first month to six weeks of life, however, the totally breastfed baby's stool pattern changes again. The frequency of stooling gradually declines, and the volume of stool passed each time increases. The color of the stool remains the characteristic mustard yellow, and the odor remains the same as well. Many infants stool only once every 4 to 12 days on average, although longer periods also have been noted (Weaver et al., 1988). The long period between stools in the second and later months after birth in a baby who is obviously thriving is not a cause for concern if his abdomen remains soft and he seems content and alert (Riordan, 1990).

Whenever artificial formula is offered, the stools change. The stool becomes darker, more formed, and more odorous. Curds are usually larger than in the stool of the totally breastfed baby, and the frequency of the stool varies. Whereas the totally breastfed infant passes very frequent, scanty stools during the first month of life, the bottle-fed infant tends to pass larger, more copious, more odorous, but less frequent stools (Quinlan et al., 1995). Whereas the totally breastfed infant passes copious stools very infrequently after the fourth week of life, the bottle-fed infant tends to pass larger and more odorous stools more frequently. As the volume of artificial formula increases in the diet of the breastfeeding baby, the stools reflect this intake.

This is also true when solid foods are added. Generally, the odor of the breastfed baby's stool becomes more noticeable as solid food is added to the baby's diet. Early occasional meals of solid foods that represent only a small proportion of the infant's total daily intake will not cause a marked change in the stool pattern. As the proportion of solid foods increases, however, the stooling occurs two or three times per day and the odor, color, and consistency reflect the food that the baby has ingested. In some cases, portions of undigested food may be visible in the stool. An example is peas, the casing of which may appear virtually unchanged in the stool. If the infant is growing well, the appearance of such food particles in the stool is not a cause for concern.

Stooling as an Indication of a Problem

The newborn who does not pass stool may have an organic problem that needs to be addressed. Hirschsprung's disease and cystic fibrosis are two such entities. The newborn who does not pass stool frequently in the first month of life but who is growing well in all parameters (head circumference, height, and weight) may be one of those relatively rare individuals who adopts an infrequent stool pattern earlier than usual. Occasionally, some element in the mother's diet may contribute to an unexpected stool pattern. The authors are aware of one infant whose stools were hard and occurred only every five to six days until his mother stopped taking prenatal multivitamins that contained extra iron.

Generally, an infant who is stooling fewer than four times daily *and* who is not gaining weight appropriately must be evaluated; infrequent stooling in such cases may be an early sign of inadequate milk intake (Auerbach & Eggert, 1987; Livingstone, 1990) or inadequate intake of the hindmilk, which tends to stimulate stooling (Woodward et al., 1989, Woolridge et al., 1990; see also Chapter 11).

Multiple Infants

The use of hormones for infertility has spawned an increase in the number of multiple births over the past several years. Lactation consultants are likely to work with these families, for many parents who undergo fertility treatment tend to breastfeed. Parents of multiple infants can be reassured that breastfeeding more than one infant at a time not only is possible but is done frequently (Gromada, 1991) (Fig. 10–4).

The needs of term or near-term multiples are the same as those of full-term singletons; the mother's needs, however, are likely to be greater. The mother of multiples is more likely to have had a difficult and complicated pregnancy and childbirth, and she may need more time to recover physically. She and her partner, if they live in a region where sonography is commonly used during pregnancy, are usually aware of the impending multiple birth. Because many parents are uncertain whether breastfeeding is possible after a multiple birth, the decision about infant feeding will be heavily influenced by the information the parents receive from their health care providers.

In addition to conferring superior nutrition and protection to the infants, breastfeeding helps to ensure frequent mother-infant interaction with each baby. Although the frequency of feedings can seem overwhelming to new mothers, they soon find that feedings give them many daily opportunities to rest and relax (Gromada, 1992). At the same time, the caloric needs of the mother of multiple infants are greater than those of the mother of a single breastfeeding infant, and the physical demands leave a mother little time to eat. Well-wishers who want to assist the new parents of multiples should be encouraged to bring over a meal to the family or to send food as a gift. "Fast" whole foods that are nutritious yet require little or no preparation are preferred.

Mothers need help and support with the early feedings, as they can easily feel overwhelmed. The lactation consultant should show the mother various positions for feedings so that she realizes she has many choices for comfortable breastfeeding. Simultaneous feedings save time and effort and can be easily accomplished with twins during the first few weeks postpartum. After that time, each infant starts to develop his own wake/sleep pattern, and often one baby is ready to go to the breast before his sibling(s). LaFleur and Niesen (1996) describe one mother's experience with breastfeeding conjoined twins. Single feedings give the mother an opportunity to learn to nurse one baby and can be a private time for each child. When breastfeeding is begun after days or weeks of pumping, the mother may need to be reminded that she might not be able to breastfeed fully for some time. Storr (1989; see also Duggin, 1994; Mead et al., 1992) describes the approach of one mother of triplets who used interim bottle-feedings with each baby as she gradually increased her milk supply. Milk production *will* increase to meet the needs of multiple infants (Saint et al., 1986).

Gromada (1992) contends that household help is not a luxury for mothers recuperating from a multiple pregnancy and birth, who must care for and form attachments with more than one neonate simultaneously. The mother of multiples needs the assistance of at least one other pair of hands and additional ongoing assistance with household chores as she spends more time and energy meeting the needs of her babies. This helper is expected to assume household tasks and to provide physical support to the mother.

Mothering and nursing multiples requires greater organization by the mother than does caring for a single baby or two babies of different ages

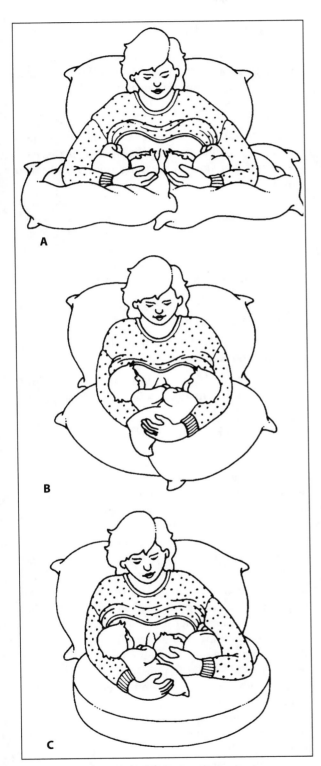

FIGURE 10–4. Feeding positions for twins.
A. Football. B. Cross. C. Mixed. (Drawing by Ruth Linstromberg.)

(Sollid et al., 1989). The mother of twins may wish to keep a chart of daily activities, especially those related to the babies' feedings (e.g., which breast each baby used at the most recent feeding, as a reminder to switch the babies so that each uses both breasts at subsequent feedings. This will avoid stimulation of only one breast by the more vigorous twin. A record of wet diapers and stools reassures the mother that the babies are receiving sufficient nutriments (Driscoll & Walker, 1985).

When twins, triplets, or quadruplets are born prematurely or have other medical complications, the mother can begin to provide breastmilk for her babies with the assistance of hand expression or a breast pump. Feedings at the breast may be delayed for weeks but need not imply that the babies will not go to breast or will not breastfeed exclusively (Liang et al., 1997). Simultaneous pumping from a hospital-grade electric pump is the most effective strategy for obtaining maximum amounts of milk and for maintaining lactation (see Chapter 13). Most hospitals with neonatal intensive care units make these pumps available for mothers to use.

Needs, problems, and solutions vary with each situation. One lactation consultant has assisted several mothers who had quadruplets and pumped for many weeks before all the babies were on the breast. Representative of the situation of many, mother A gave birth to her quads at 34 weeks. She took the first baby home one week after birth, feeding from a bottle; direct nursing did not occur until almost five weeks later. The second and third babies went home at 5 weeks postpartum; one was a good nurser from the start, the other a very poor nurser. The fourth baby went home after 8 weeks of hospitalization for respiratory distress; however, within one week, he was breastfeeding. Mother B nursed and pumped and fed one or more babies with a bottle for at least 8 weeks. Her youngest quad never breastfed well, requiring both breastfeedings and bottle-feedings for most of the breastfeeding course. The mother weaned all four babies at around seven months of age.

The caregiver can employ practical strategies that promote rest, diet, and bonding for mothers of multiples when breastfeeding:

- Emphasize the need for housekeeping help for several months at least. This person should be supportive of breastfeeding.

- Link the mother with other women who have breastfed multiples.

- Provide several pillows to position and stabilize the infants during the early weeks. The mother needs help to support each infant's head as he latches on. The mother in Figure 10–4C is using a special pillow, especially designed for feeding multiples. This pillow stabilizes the babies for feedings and is invaluable during the early weeks postpartum.

- Review the basics of breastfeeding and maintenance of milk production and the advantages of breastfeeding, including the fast return of the uterus to its original size.

- Help to develop a plan for alternating infants and breasts, to rotate breastfeeding positions. Rotation provides equal stimulation both for the mother's breasts and for the babies' eyes.

- Suggest that the mother create a "breastfeeding station" where she keeps nutritious liquids and foods to supplement her diet, breast pads, infant-care items such as diapers and wipes, and, if available, a portable telephone.

An important consideration for the caregiver is to remain sensitive to the need of the mother to attach or bond to each baby individually (Ander-son & Anderson, 1990). The attachment process is more likely to be disrupted when more than one infant is born, particularly if the twin or triplet birth was a surprise or was not discovered until very shortly before the babies' birth. Assisting the mother to see and relate to each baby as an individual rather than as part of a multiple unit is important. It can begin with the caregiver pointing out unique qualities in each baby as she helps the mother to get to know her offspring. Multiples wean as individuals; they may stop breastfeeding at about the same time, or one may wean long before the other infant(s).

Despite concerns about the difficulty that the mother might have in bonding with two or more babies, Abbink et al. (1982) found that only 25 percent of mothers, when asked to describe differences in their feelings toward one or the other baby during the early newborn period, identified any difference in their early bonding feeling. These differences were primarily related to one of the babies being less healthy than the other.

Refusing the Breast

Although it may occur throughout the breastfeeding course, some infants suddenly refuse to breastfeed at seven to nine months of age. The mother may think that the infant has weaned himself, but this is not necessarily so. The abruptness of the infant's refusal to breastfeed usually is the mother's best clue that what is occurring is a so-called breastfeeding strike; normal weaning seldom occurs as rapidly.

Most mothers whose infants have refused to breastfeed believe the strike is a signal of the baby's distress, dissatisfaction, or confusion associated with feedings, over which the baby attempts to exert some control. The older breastfeeding infant might suddenly refuse to nurse when the mother

- begins a new feeding schedule (e.g., when the mother returns to work),

- leaves the infant with a bottle (even breastmilk) when he is unaccustomed to it,

- rebukes the baby (understandably) for biting her breast, usually early in the teething period, or

- leaves the baby for several days.

When the baby refuses the breast, efforts to encourage resumption of breastfeeding may take several days or longer. During this period, the mother needs to spend more time with the baby, carrying him more, and offering a great deal of skin-to-skin contact. It is generally useless to attempt to put the baby to breast while he is awake; mothers often are more successful offering the breast to the baby while he is dropping off to sleep or just waking. Using the feeding-tube device and finger-feeding are other techniques that have been successful for overcoming breast refusal (Newman, 1990). Finger-feeding calms the baby so he will be less hungry when he is put to breast. The health care provider or family member can support the mother by helping her to sort out the circumstances surrounding the baby's refusal, by encouraging her to maintain her milk supply, and by assuring her that the problem does not lie with her.

Every so often an infant will refuse to feed from one breast. This sometimes occurs after mastitis if an infant discovers that the milk from the previously infected breast tastes salty, and so "boy-cotts" that breast. At other times, no reason for the refusal is apparent.

One-sided breastfeeding provides adequate nourishment for the baby. Infants who prefer to breastfeed from the same breast tend to refuse the right rather than the left breast. This may relate to mothers' tendency to hold and feed their babies more often on the left side (Nakamichi & Takeda, 1995). The opposite also appears to be true: babies who favor the right breast are usually cradled in their mother's right arm (Chapman et al., 1985).

Too Much Milk

In the United States, until recently, little attention was paid to those women who made more milk than their babies needed. Women who breastfeed their infants at will, without concern for frequency and duration of feedings, have noted that milk production may exceed the baby's need (Daly et al., 1992; Daly & Hartmann, 1995; Rattigan et al., 1981). Feeding technique may account for oversupply. Switching the baby from the first breast before he has shown that he wishes to go to the other has been offered by some investigators as an explanation for overfeeding (Woolridge & Fisher, 1988). The subsequent colicky behavior in the baby has often been characterized as "overactive letdown reflex" (Andrusiak & Larose-Kuzenko, 1987). The infant may have frequent watery stools and may develop a sore perianal area as a result.

A more recent examination (Woolridge et al., 1990) of the nutrient intake from feedings in which only one breast was used as compared with two found that babies received slightly less milk when breastfed from only one breast per feeding but that total fat intake was slightly higher with one-breast feedings. The authors urged mothers to allow their babies to set the breastfeeding pattern, which will vary throughout the course of breastfeeding. Based on a description of "overactive letdown reflex" by Andrusiak and Larose-Kuzenko (1987), the clinician should be aware that this "embarrassment of riches" can cause the baby to wean early. Choking and having to struggle with a fast, abundant flow of milk at each feeding is simply too difficult for some babies to handle.

Women with overabundant milk supplies often have a moment of intense pain as the milk-ejection reflex occurs. The following step-by-step approach, used by one of the authors of this chapter, has been found to be effective in reducing the mother's milk supply sufficiently to make the mother more comfortable and to enable the baby to suckle more comfortably:

1. Encourage the mother to offer *only one breast* at each feeding; if the second breast becomes uncomfortably full, the mother should express just enough milk to reduce ductal pressure. (Vigorous pumping should be avoided.) Remind the mother that her baby is not in danger of weight loss. Often these infants are well above the average weight at the time that the mother seeks help.

2. Position the baby so that he is straddling the mother's leg, directly facing the breast, with his head slightly above the mother's nipple. Ask the mother to lean back slightly, as in a lounge chair, and to support the baby at the breast. The mother may wish to slip a towel under the breast to catch any dripping or leaking milk. Because the mother is leaning back, excess milk is more likely to drip out of the baby's mouth rather than to make him choke. Some women find that lying on their side to nurse also is helpful, using a diaper or towel to catch the excess. Phillips (1991) recommends "posture feeding," which simply means that the mother lies down with baby on top of her, so that he is feeding "uphill." If the baby is small, an underarm (football) position may be used, but the baby's head should be higher than the rest of his body.

3. If the baby stops nursing and wants to return to the breast in less than an hour, encourage the mother to offer the same breast that was used at the previous feeding.

4. Ask the mother to take a deep breath, count to 10, breathe deeply, and make a conscious effort to relax during the first milk-ejection reflex. In many cases, the first ejection consists exclusively of forceful sprays; thereafter, sprays appear to be less forceful. Some mothers have found that the initial sprays of milk

are so overwhelming that they should be allowed to escape into a towel. The baby is then put to breast after the first spray has subsided to drips.

5. Advise the mother to burp the baby frequently, particularly if she hears continuing loud gulping throughout the feeding. In the upright position, the baby is less likely to have to struggle to stay ahead of the milk flow.

6. Encourage the mother to avoid expressing or pumping milk unless this is absolutely necessary for comfort.

Within a week, the mother's milk supply will generally diminish sufficiently so that the baby can breastfeed comfortably with a minimum of burping, little or no choking, and a resumption of comfort suckling. In some cases, babies of mothers with too much milk are not able to engage in comfort suckling until the milk supply has been reduced. Such babies may be offered the comfort of a pacifier. Once the milk supply has been reduced, the baby may again suckle at both breasts without subsequent difficulties. As always, the mother should be encouraged to follow the baby's lead.

Leaking and Breast Pads

Most breastfeeding women experience leaking milk in the early weeks of lactation when infant needs and maternal responses are not yet well attuned to one another and when daily variability of feeding frequency and duration is greatest. The amount of leaking usually declines over time. A variety of stimuli may cause the mother's breasts to leak milk. The sound of her own or another baby's stirring or crying is a common stimulus. The scent of her baby's clothes, thinking about her baby, the sound of a breast pump (if she has been using one regularly), listening to music she has heard while breastfeeding, or seeing or sitting in the chair she has used while breastfeeding often stimulates a mother's milk let-down or leaking.

Leaking varies among mothers with respect to stimuli, amount of leaked milk, and the length of time the leaking continues. Most mothers leak enough milk in the early weeks to soak their clothing (Morse & Bottorff, 1989). Many are embarrassed and concerned at the unpredictability and inability to control leaking, especially if it continues beyond the first several months. Mothers report leaking for a long period or leaking milk in quantities sufficient to soak a cloth diaper. These mothers need to be instructed in ways to reduce spontaneous milk release. Gentle pressure for a few seconds on a leaking breast is usually sufficient to cue it to retain milk until an "official" feeding. When modesty is not an issue, pressure can be applied to the breast with fingers or the palm of the hand. In a public setting, pressing the upper arm or elbow against the breast while touching one's earlobe will usually be interpreted by others as an attempt to scratch one's ear or adjust an earring. When the mother feels her milk letting down, crossing both arms over her chest and pressing gently for 5 to 10 seconds usually stops the leaking. Only another breastfeeding mother is likely to recognize the maneuver as a means of halting inadvertent leaking.

Breast pads are often worn by lactating women. Although many commercial brands of breast pads are available, inexpensive homemade pads can be fashioned from folded men's handerchiefs, nappy or diaper liners wrapped around paper tissue, or folded clean cotton or toweling. In order of preference, women want breast pads that are disposable, comfortable, re-usable, affordable, and absorbent (Griffiths, 1993). They also want the protection against leaking in public that is afforded by plastic-lined pads. Traditional advice is to avoid using these pads because they prevent air circulation and so are thought to contribute to nipple soreness; however, in a study of several hundred South African women, Griffiths (1993) found that plastic-backed pads did not increase nipple soreness. Based on Griffiths' work, the most efficient breast pad is one made of a diaper liner encasing toilet paper. This type of pad keeps the breast surface driest, offers good protection against leaking to the clothing, and is economical and easy to make.

Clothing

Clothing needs in the puerperium are simple. Mothers are concerned with ease of laundering as well as comfort and convenience for breastfeeding. A dress that closes in the back has no place in the breastfeeding mother's wardrobe—unless she can guarantee that she will not need to feed the baby and will not experience any leaking while she is wearing it!

Increasingly, clothing stores and catalogues carry attractive garments designed for the breast-feeding mother. Designs today include hidden zippers, snaps, Velcro closures, and buttons that cleverly hide the openings incorporated into darts, seams, pockets, or other fashion details.

Cotton tends to be cooler in warm months and warmer in cool months than are other fabrics; in addition, it allows greater flow of air to the skin. Wrinkles are less likely with some of the cotton-synthetic blends. Two-piece outfits that allow the blouse to be pulled up from the waist offer easy access to the breasts while maintaining modesty. Many experienced mothers are well aware that breastfeeding "from the waist up" rather than "from the neck down" enables them to feed their babies in virtually any setting. Light-colored, patterned clothes (rather than dark solid colors) camouflage tell-tale leaking (Phillips, 1991).

Cotton bras—100 percent cotton, if possible—tend to be more comfortable than those made of synthetic materials. Bras with plastic liners or so-called moisture barriers should be avoided, because they keep the skin damp, potentially creating an ideal environment for candidiasis. Cup closures should be easy to manage with one hand. In most stores, the pregnant mother not only can obtain a personalized fitting but can test whether the openings are easy to manage prior to purchasing a bra. Some bras have front openings that enable the mother to remove the bra from both breasts, if she prefers the greater freedom this affords. Small-breasted women unused to wearing a bra often find that the lightweight bras made of multistretch material provide adequate support. Lactating women should be cautioned against wearing underwire bras during the course of breastfeeding. Underwires tend to constrict and compress the milk ducts and predispose to recurrent plugged ducts or mastitis.

Breastfeeding During Pregnancy

Population studies of the likelihood of becoming pregnant while fully breastfeeding reveals that this risk is extremely small. However, when it does occur, the mother may feel betrayed by her body,

particularly if she was told that breastfeeding women cannot become pregnant.

Women who continue breastfeeding past the child's first year may become pregnant. When asked, many of these mothers report that the emotional needs of the child is their principal motivation for continued breastfeeding, followed by their belief in child-led weaning. Some common outcomes when breastfeeding continues through a pregnancy are listed here: (Gopalan, 1958; Mohrbacher & Stock, 1997; Moscone & Moore, 1993; Newton & Theotokatos, 1979).

- *Nipples and breast soreness:* One of the first signs of pregnancy in a lactating woman is the sudden onset of sore nipples and pain during breastfeeding. Breast pain involves the whole breast and may be intense. It is likely related to hormonal changes rather than to difficulties with positioning.

- *Maternal fatigue:* The hormones of early pregnancy that often impel women to want to sleep are implicated here as well. However, most mothers with an active toddler or young child often feel they cannot lie down and rest if their child is not also willing to do so. This sensation of fatigue is not a result of breastfeeding while pregnant but rather of the mother's bodily reaction to early pregnancy. As the pregnancy progresses, this complaint tends to subside. However, the pregnant mother of a young child should be encouraged to nap when her child naps, so that she will feel able to keep up with her active soon-to-be-older child.

- *Decline in milk supply and number of feedings:* About 70 percent of mothers who become pregnant while breastfeeding report a decrease in their milk production; most nursing children breastfeed less often than they have before. As the pregnancy progresses, the milk volume appears to decline. Sometimes the child will wean during this period. If already talking, the child may complain that the milk is "all gone" or that it takes "too long to get it."

- *Change in taste of milk:* The milk may taste bitter or different from the way it tasted before the pregnancy. The nursing child may even ask to drink juice or some other liquid after nursing, as if washing his mouth out. The talking nursling may state quite clearly how the milk tastes or may simply indicate by his actions that it is not the same. This taste change is likely related to the increase in sodium and total protein and the decrease in concentrations of glucose and lactose resulting from the pregnancy (Prosser et al., 1984).

- *Uterine contractions:* A small percentage of women experience uterine contractions during breastfeeding. One woman reported that her fetus responded by "kicking violently." In most cases, breastfeeding will not affect the fetus in any way, and there is no evidence that uterine contractions are associated with fetal loss.

- *Weaning:* Many nursing children wean before their sibling is born, presumably because of the decline of milk available, its change in taste, or their mother's urging to wean. Another factor is the gradual disappearance of the mother's lap as her pregnancy becomes noticeable. A change in the way the child is held for breastfeeding may make such interaction less desirable. As feeding sessions decline in frequency, weaning may occur without the mother having to do anything other than to breastfeed when asked but not to offer as she might have in the past.

There is no documented danger to the mother or fetus when mothers breastfeed through a healthy pregnancy (La Leche League International, 1997). This mother will need to eat a nutritious diet; she may choose to take supplemental vitamins as a precaution. In the study by Moscone and Moore (1993), most mothers reported continued good general health throughout their pregnancy as well as healthy outcomes in the new baby. However, the mother who breastfeeds during pregnancy faces potential criticism from her family, friends, and health care provider. The lactation consultant may be asked for her opinion after the mother has been told by her physician that she must wean her child, even in the absence of indicators that continuing to breastfeed is in any way a risk for the mother or her developing fetus. This is especially true in developed, industrialized countries, and it is not uncommon for these mothers to "hide" their nursing. In developing countries too, traditional beliefs about weaning when the mother's pregnancy is confirmed may reduce the frequency with which such a combination occurs. The lactation consultant or nurse who openly accepts individual choices of breastfeeding women can be helpful in providing information and guidance that supports a mother's choice.

Clinical Implications

Medical centers report increased readmissions of neonates after discharge from the hospital. Factors other than early discharge may precipitate these readmissions. According to one study of readmissions of neonates (Pascale et al., 1996), none of the mothers had attended prenatal breastfeeding classes; moreover, the number of lactation consultant hours had been cut in half in order to "cut costs," and so these women had not been seen by the lactation consultant prior to their discharge from the hospital.

These experiences need not have occurred. Preparing the mother to go home after a birth confident in her ability to meet her own and her baby's needs should be the goal of every hospital or birthing center professional. Reaching this goal requires that the new mother be provided with appropriate anticipatory guidance, including behaviors that she should expect from her baby in the first few days at home, the first week, and the first month, of breastfeeding. Figure 10–5 shows a time line of potential events that commonly occur in the postpartum period. This time line can be used to teach anticipatory guidance for both mothers and for health care personnel.

If a home visit is scheduled within the first week, the mother needs to know when it will occur and who will be providing that home visit (a staff nurse or case manager, a community health nurse, a lactation consultant in private practice, etc.). Ideally, the information she learned prenatally about the infant's need for frequent feedings and ways to determine whether the baby is breastfeeding well will be reemphasized by the discharge planner. The mother will go home knowing the importance of assessing milk transfer by noting the baby's output (wet and soiled diapers). She will know whom to contact (1) when she has questions; (2) if the baby is not following expected patterns of feeding, voiding, or stooling; and (3) if the baby has a fever or appears to be dehydrated.

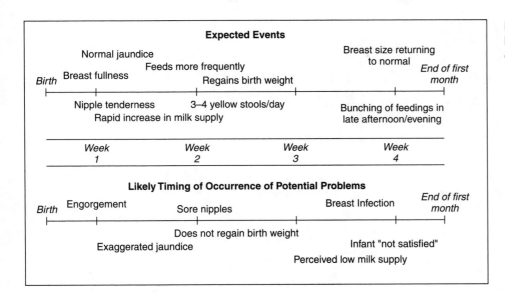

FIGURE 10–5. Time line of postpartum events.

Many health care organizations pay for an early office visit with the family physician or a home visit by a nurse or lactation consultant. This visitor may be a member of the nursing staff from the hospital or birthing center, may be employed by a home health agency, or may be in private practice and contracted to provide these services. In some cases, referrals are made directly to a private lactation consultant in the community. Commonly, professionals who spot early breastfeeding difficulties at these postdischarge visits then refer the mother to a La Leche League leader or similar mother-to-mother support group. During the home visit, mother's knowledge should be reinforced through review of basic breastfeeding techniques. According to adult education principles (described in Chapter 8), this is the "teachable moment" in which the parents are highly receptive to information that helps them to deal with practical life dilemmas. Priority information includes the following:

- *Feeding the baby often.*
- *Watching for early cues that the baby wants to feed, such as rooting and fussing* (crying is a very late cue).
- *Allowing the baby to finish the first breast before offering the second,* so that the baby will receive the creamier milk as the feeding progresses, and watching the baby for cues that he is finished with the feeding. Limiting the duration of the feeds can interfere with adequate milk transfer. The mother should be reminded to watch the clock only when she is timing the food that is cooking on the stove or in the oven!

- *Reinforcing the mother's confidence in her ability to produce milk.* Because the mother's breasts will be filling at about the time of the usual postpartum arrangement, this visit provides an ideal opportunity to build the mother's confidence in her milk supply by making positive comments: "You have lots of good milk for your baby." "What a lot of milk you have!" "Your leaking means you have lots of milk for the baby." "It looks like you could feed twins."

Assessment is a critical first step in working with a client. Lactation consultants find that identifying problems that a client had with a previous infant often may be helpful in identifying her unspoken fears or anticipated problems with the new baby. For instance, if the mother suffered sore nipples with an earlier baby, the caregiver may need to reassure the concerned or anxious mother that a similar condition need not recur. Dodgson (1989) urges that risk assessment be used to identify women for whom the anticipated course of lactation may hold special worries (Box 10–2). Unfortunately, not all health care organizations realize the benefits of breastfeeding and are committed to early postpartum support for breastfeeding families.

BOX 10–2

Lactation History and Risk Assessment

G _____ P _____ EDC _____ Age _____

FEEDING CHOICE:

Breast _____   Breast/Formula _____   Undecided _____

PHYSICAL EXAM:

Nipples: Flat _____   Breasts: Size increase during pregnancy?
          Inverted _____   Yes _____ No _____
          Other _____   Other _____
          WNL _____

HISTORY:

Previous breastfeeding experience?   Yes _____ No _____
How long? _____
Did you want to breastfeed but were unable to for some reason?   Yes _____ No _____
Why? _____

Did you have any of the following (check all that apply)?
_____ Sore nipples   _____ Not enough milk
_____ Cracked or bleeding nipples   _____ Breast infection
_____ Baby did not gain weight well

Did you stop nursing before you really wanted to?   Yes _____ No _____
Why? _____

RISK FACTORS (check all that apply):

_____ Multiple gestation   _____ Breast surgery
_____ History of preterm infant   _____ Diabetes

Medications (prescription and nonprescription) taken:
_____
_____

Medical condition: _____
_____

Source: Derived from J Dodgson: Early identification of potential breastfeeding problems. J Hum Lact *5:80–81, 1989.*

SUMMARY

Chapters 9 and 10 are the key twin chapters on the breastfeeding process. In each, we have presented the most current, research-based clinical knowledge and techniques.

In writing these chapters, the authors were reminded that clinical research on breastfeeding and lactation is sadly lacking. For example, we still know little about the causes of nipple pain and trauma. Clinicians have long observed that the positon of the infant at breast improves maternal comfort and infant suckling, yet no studies carefully substantiate the role of optimal positioning. The same deficit exists in our knowledge about the effectiveness of nipple creams: myriad proprietary and "natural" products are used, but few studies on them are available. We have no information regarding why some women leak and others do not, or why some women appear to produce small quantities of colostrum whereas others seem to have copious amounts and why some women seem to have colostrum for a considerably longer period than others, even in the face of similar breastfeeding episodes. We remain poorly informed about the effect on breastfeeding of intrapartum interventions such as epidural analgesia or anesthesia, suctioning of the infant, and vacuum extraction. In this dynamic, rapidly growing field, the clinical questions that remain to be answered far outnumber those for which we have definitive answers.

Finally, national news stories about breastfed babies with dehydration and hyperbilirubinemia (Seidman et al., 1995) are reminders that breastfeeding cannot be assumed to occur easily for all women. As lactation consultants know from clinical experience, a mother needs time to learn how to breastfeed, and the health care provider needs time to assist—more time than is needed if the mother bottle-feeds her infant. An early visit with the health care provider is an opportunity to intervene when it is likely to have the greatest preventive pay-off for mother and baby. Guidance given by the knowledgeable health care provider not only helps to assure the infant a healthy start in life but also provides valuable lifelong health education for the family. The effort expended may be great, but the rewards are greater still.

REFERENCES

Abbink C, et al: Bonding as perceived by mothers of twins. *Pediatr Nurs* 8:411–3, 1982.

American Academy of Pediatrics, Committee on Fetus and Newborn: Hospital stay for healthy newborns. *Pediatrics* 96:716–23, 1995.

Amir L: Eczema of the nipple and breast: a case report. *J Hum Lact* 9:173–5, 1993.

Anderson A, Anderson B: Toward a substantive theory of mother-twin attachment. *MCN* 15:373–7, 1990.

Andrusiak F, Larose-Kuzenko M: *The effects of an overactive let-down reflex* (Unit 13, Lactation Consultant Series). Garden City Park, NY: Avery Publishing, 1987.

Auerbach KG: When treatment for jaundice undermines breastfeeding. *Contemp Pediatr* 9:105–6, 1992.

Auerbach KG, Eggert LD: The importance of infant suckling patterns when a breast-fed baby fails to thrive [letter]. *J Trop Pediatr* 33:156–7, 1987.

Barr RG, Elias MF: Nursing interval and maternal responsivity: effect on early infant crying. *Pediatrics* 81:529–36, 1988.

Barr RG, et al: Feeding and temperament as determinants of early infant crying/fussing. *Pediatrics* 84:514–21, 1989.

Basire K, Pullon S, McLeod D: Baby feeding: the thoughts behind the statistics. *NZ Med J* 110(1044):184–7, 1997.

Beeken S, Waterston T: Health service support of breast feeding–are we practising what we preach? *Br Med J* 305(6848):285–7, 1992.

Berg KL: Two cases of tongue-tie and breastfeeding. *J Hum Lact* 6:124–26, 1990.

Bishop JM, Hill DJ, Hosking CS: Natural history of cow milk allergy: clinical outcome. *J Pediatr* 116:862–7, 1990.

Blackburn ST, Loper DL: *Maternal, fetal, and neonatal physiology*. Philadelphia: Saunders, 1992.

Bowles BC, Stutte PC, Hensley J: Alternate massage in breastfeeding. *Genesis* 9:5–9, 1988.

Bravermen P, et al: Early discharge of newborn and mothers: a critical review of the literature. *Pediatrics* 96:716–26, 1995.

Brown LP: Breastfeeding and jaundice: cause for concern? *Clin Iss Perin Wom Health Nurs* 3:613–9, 1992.

Brown MS, Hurlock JT: Preparation of the breast for breastfeeding. *Nurs Res* 24:448–51, 1975.

Buchko BL, et al: Comfort measures in breastfeeding, primiparous women. *JOGNN* 23:46–52, 1993.

Cant A, Marsden RA, Kilshaw PJ: Egg and cow's milk hypersensitivity in exclusively breast fed infants with eczema. *Br Med J* 291:932–5, 1985.

Cavagni G, et al: Passage of food antigens into circulation of breast-fed infants with atopic dermatitis. *Ann Allergy* 61:361–5, 1988.

Chandra RK, et al: Influence of maternal food antigen avoidance during pregnancy and lactation on incidence of atopic eczema in infants. *Clin Allergy* 16:563–9, 1986.

Chandra RK, Puri S, Hamed A: Influence of maternal diet during lactation and use of formula feeds on development of atopic eczema in high risk infants. *Br Med J* 299:228–30, 1989.

Chapman J, et al: Concerns of breast-feeding mothers from birth to 4 months. *Nurs Res* 34:374–7, 1985.

Clyne PS Kulczycki A: Human breast milk contains bovine IgG. Relationship to infant colic? *Pediatrics* 87:439–44, 1991.

Copeland CA, Raebel MA, Wagner SL: Pesticide residue in lanolin [letter]. *JAMA* 261:242, 1989

Daly SEJ, et al: The determination of short-term breast volume changes and the rate of synthesis of human milk using computerized breast measurement. *Exp Physiol* 77:79–87, 1992.

Daly SEJ, Hartmann PE: Infant demand and milk supply: Part 1. Infant demand and milk production in lactating women. *J Hum Lact* 11:21–6, 1995.

Day TW: Unilateral failure of lactation after breast biopsy. *J Fam Pract* 23:161–2, 1986.

de Carvalho M, Robertson S, Klaus MH: Does the duration and frequency of early breastfeeding affect nipple pain? *Birth* 11:81–4, 1984.

Dodgson J: Early identification of potential breast-feeding problems. *J Hum Lact* 5:80–1, 1989.

Driscoll JW, Walker M: *Breastfeeding your twins.* Weston, MA: Lactation Associates, 1985.

Duggin J: Breastfeeding triplets—it can be done! *Breastfeed Rev* 2(10):469–70, 1994.

Edmonson MB, Stoddard JJ, Owens LM: Hospital readmission with feeding-related problems after early postpartum discharge of normal newborns. *JAMA* 278:299–303, 1997.

Ellis DJ, Livingstone VH, Hewat RJ: Assisting the breastfeeding mother: a problem-solving process. *J Hum Lact* 9:89–93, 1993.

Escott R: Positioning, attachment and milk transfer. *Breastfeed Rev* 14:31–7, 1989.

Evans K, et al: Effects of the method of breastfeeding on breast engorgement, mastitis, and infantile colic. *Acta Paediatr* 84:849–52, 1995.

Foxman B, Schwartz K, Looman SJ: Breastfeeding practices and lactation mastitis. *Soc Sci Med* 38:75–61, 1994.

Gopalan C: Studies on lactation in poor communities. *J Trop Pediatr Environ Health* 4:87–97, 1958.

Gosha JL, Tichy AM: Effect of a breast shell on postpartum nipple pain: an exploratory study. *J Nurse Midwifery* 33:74–7, 1988.

Griffiths RJ: Breast pads: their effectiveness and use by lactating women. *J Hum Lact* 9:19–26, 1993.

Gribetz D: Ingestion of bismuth-containing ointment by a breast-fed infant. *Mt Sinai J Med* 41:498–510, 1974.

Gromada KK: Breastfeeding more than one: multiples and tandem breastfeeding. *Clin Iss Perin Wom Health Nurs* 3:656–66.

Gromada KK: *Mothering multiples.* Schaumberg, IL: La Leche League International, 1991.

Gunther M: Sore nipples: causes and prevention. *Lancet* 2:347–51, 1945.

Henly SJ, et al: Anemia and insufficient milk in first-time mothers. *Birth* 22:87–92, 1995.

Hewat RJ, Ellis DJ: Comparison of the effectiveness of two methods of nipple care. *Birth* 14:41–5, 1987.

Hill PD, Aldag JC: Smoking and breastfeeding status. *Res Nurs Health* 19:125–32, 1996.

Hill PD, et al: Does early supplementation affect long-term breastfeeding? *Clin Pediatr* 36:345–50, 1997.

Hill PD, Humenick SS: Insufficient milk supply. *Image* 21:145–8, 1989.

Hillervik-Lindquist C, Hofvander Y, Sjölin S: Studies on perceived milk insufficiency III. Consequences of breast milk consumption and growth. *Acta Paediatr Scand* 80:297–303, 1991.

Høst A, Husby S, Osterballe O: A prospective study of cow's milk allergy in exclusively breast-fed infants. *Acta Paediatr Scand* 77:663–70, 1988.

Huggins K, Billon SF: Twenty cases of persistent sore nipples: collaboration between lactation consultant and dermatologist. *J Hum Lact* 9:155–60, 1993.

Hughes V, Owen J: Is breast-feeding possible after breast surgery? *MCN* 18:213–7, 1993.

Hurst NM: Lactation after augmentation mammoplasty. *Obstet Gynecol* 87:30–4, 1996.

Hyams JS, et al: Effect of infant formula on stool characteristics of young infants. *Pediatrics* 95:50–4, 1995.

Iffrig MC: Nursing care and success in breastfeeding. *Nurs Clin North Am* 3:347–9, 1968.

Jackson LS, Lee K: The effect of dairy products on iron availability. *Crit Rev Food Sci Nutr* 31:259–70, 1990.

Jakobsson I, et al: Dietary bovine beta-lactoglobulin is transferred to human milk. *Acta Paediatr Scand* 74:342–5, 1985.

Jakobsson I, Lindberg T: Cow's milk proteins cause infantile colic in breast-fed infants: a double-blind crossover study. *Pediatrics* 71:268–71, 1983.

James JM, et al: Discontinuation of breast-feeding infrequent among jaundiced neonates treated at home. *Pediatrics* 92:153–5, 1993.

Kajosaari M, Saarinen UM: Prophylaxis of atopic disease by six months' total solid food elimination. *Acta Paediatr Scand* 72:411–4, 1983.

LaFleur EA, Niesen KM: Breastfeeding conjoined twins. *JOGNN* 25:241–4, 1996.

La Leche League International: *The womanly art of breastfeeding* (6th ed). Franklin Park, IL: La Leche League International, 1997:98–9.

Lavergne NA: Does application of tea bags to sore nipples while breastfeeding provide effective relief? *JOGNN* 26:53–8, 1997.

Lee KS, et al: Association between duration of neonatal hospital stay and readmission rate. *J Pediatr* 127: 758–66, 1995.

Liang R, Gunn AJ, Gunn TR: Can preterm twins breast feed successfully? *NZ Med J* 110(1045): 209–12, 1997.

Lifschitz CH, et al: Anaphylactic shock due to cow's milk protein hypersensitivity in a breast-fed infant. *J Pediatr Gastroenterol Nutr* 7:141–4, 1988.

Livingstone VH: Problem-solving formula for failure to thrive in breast-fed infants. *Can Fam Phys* 36:1541–5, 1990.

Livingstone VH: Too much of a good thing: maternal and infant hyperlactation syndromes. *Can Fam Phys* 42:89–99, 1996.

Livingstone VH, Willis CE, Berkowitz J: *Staphylococcus aureus* and sore nipples. *Can Fam Phys* 42:654–9, 1996.

Lothe L, Lindberg T, Jakobsson I: Cow's milk formula as a cause of infantile colic: a double-blind study. *Pediatrics* 70:7–10, 1982.

Marmet C, Shell E, Marmet R: Neonatal frenotomy may be necessary to correct breastfeeding problems. *J Hum Lact* 6:117–21, 1990.

Marx CM, et al: Vitamin E concentrations in serum of newborn infants after topical use of vitamin E in nursing mothers. *Am J Obstet Gynecol* 152:668–70, 1985.

Matheson I: The effect of smoking on lactation and infantile colic. *JAMA* 261:42–3, 1989.

McGregor LA: Short, shorter, shortest: continuing to improve the hospital stay for mothers and newborns. *MCN* 21:191–6, 1996.

Mead LJ, et al: Breastfeeding success with preterm quadruplets. *JOGNN* 21:221–7, 1992.

Meier P, et al: A new scale for in-home test weighing for mothers of preterm and high risk infants. *J Hum Lact* 10:163–8, 1994.

Mevissen-Verhage EAE, et al: Effect of iron on neonatal gut flora during the first three months of life. *Eur J Clin Microbiol* 4:273–8, 1985.

Mohrbacher N, and Stock J: *The breastfeeding answer book* (rev ed). Schaumburg, IL: La Leche League International, 1997.

Morse JM, Bottorff JL: Leaking: a problem of lactation. *J Nurse Midwif* 34:15–20, 1989.

Moscone SR, Moore MJ: Breastfeeding during pregnancy. *J Hum Lact* 9:83–8, 1993.

Nakamichi M, Takeda S: A child-holding thought experiment: students prefer to imagine holding an infant on the left side of the body. *Percept Mot Skills* 80:687–90, 1995.

Neifert M, et al: The influence of breast surgery, breast appearance and pregnancy-induced changes on lactation sufficiency as measured by weight gain. *Birth* 17:31–8, 1990.

Neifert MR, Seacat JM, Jobe WE: Lactation failure due to insufficient glandular development of the breast. *Pediatrics* 76:823–8, 1985.

Newborns' and Mothers' Health Protection Act of 1996. Public Law 104–204, September 26, 1996. Enacted as Title VI of the Departments of Veterans Affairs and Housing Urban Development, and Independent Agencies Appropriations Act, 1997.

Newman J: Breast-feeding: the problem of "not enough milk." *Can Fam Phys* 32:571–4, 1986.

Newman J: Breastfeeding problems associated with the early introduction of bottles and pacifiers. *J Hum Lact* 6:59–63, 1990.

Newton N: Nipple pain and nipple damage: problems in management of breast feeding. *J Pediatr* 41:411–23, 1952.

Newton N, Theotokatos M: Breast-feeding during pregnancy in 503 women: does a psychobiological weaning mechanism exist in humans? In: Carenza L, Zichella L, eds. *Proceedings of the Fifth International Congress on Psychosomatic Obstetrics and Gynecology.* London: Academic, 1979:845–9.

Nicholson WL: Cracked nipples in breast feeding mothers: a randomised trial of three methods of management. *Breastfeeding Rev* 9:25–7, 1986.

Notestine GE: The importance of the identification of ankyloglossia (short lingual frenulum) as a cause of breastfeeding problems. *J Hum Lact* 6:113–5, 1990.

Pascale JA, et al: Breastfeeding, dehydration, and shorter maternity stays. *Neonat Netw* 15:37–41, 1996.

Phillips V: *Successful breastfeeding.* Brisbane, Australia: Nursing Mothers' Association of Australia, 1991:109.

Pittschieler K: Cow's milk protein-induced colitis in the breast-fed infant. *J Pediatr Gastroenterol Nutr* 10:548–9, 1990.

Prosser CG, Saint L, Hartmann PE: Mammary gland function during gradual weaning and early gestation in women. *Aust J Exp Biol Med Sci* 62:215–28, 1984.

Pugh LC, et al: A comparison of topical agents to relieve nipple pain and enhance breastfeeding. *Birth* 23:88–93, 1996.

Quinn A, Kopsell D, Haller S: Breastfeeding incidence after early discharge and factors influencing breastfeeding cessation. *JOGNN* 26:289–94, 1997.

Quinlan PT, et al: The relationship between stool hardness and stool composition in breast- and formula-fed infants. *J Pediatr Gastroenterol Nutr* 20:81–90, 1995.

Rattigan S, Ghisalberti AV, Hartmann PE: Breast milk production in Australian women. *Br J Nutr* 45:243–9, 1981.

Riordan J: The effectiveness of topical agents in reducing nipple soreness of breastfeeding mothers. *J Hum Lact* 1:36–41, 1985.

Riordan J: *A practical guide to breastfeeding.* Boston, MA: Jones and Bartlett, 1990.

Rosanove R: Dangers of the application of lanolin [letter]. *Med J Aust* 146:232, 1987.

Ruvalcaba RHA: Stress-induced cessation of lactation. *West J Med* 146:228–30, 1987.

Said G, Patois E, Lellouch J: Infantile colic and parental smoking. *Br Med J* 289:660, 1984.

Saint L, Maggiore P, Hartmann PE: Yield and nutrient content of milk in eight women breast-feeding twins and one woman breast-feeding triplets. *Br J Nutr* 56:49–58, 1986.

Schneeberg NG, Perloff WH, Israel SL: Incidence of unsuspected "Sheehan's syndrome." *JAMA* 172:70–7, 1960.

Seidman DS, et al: Hospital readmission due to neonatal hyperbilirubinemia. *Pediatrics* 96:727–9, 1995.

Sollid DT, et al: Breastfeeding multiples. *J Perinat Neonat Nurs* 3:46–65, 1989.

Soskolne EI, et al: The effect of early discharge and other factors on readmission rates of newborns. *Arch Pediatr Adolesc Med* 150:373–9, 1996.

Spangler A, Hildebrandt E: The effect of modified lanolin on nipple pain/damage during the first ten days of breastfeeding. *Int J Childbirth Ed* 8:15–20, 1993.

Storr GB: Breastfeeding premature triplets: one woman's experience. *J Hum Lact* 5:74–7, 1989.

Taubman B: Parental counseling compared with elimination of cow's milk or soy milk protein for the treatment of infant colic syndrome: a randomized trial. *Pediatrics* 81:756–61, 1988.

Walker M, Driscoll JW: Sore nipples: the new mother's nemesis. *MCN* 14:260–5, 1989.

Weaver LT, Ewing G, Taylor LC: The bowel habit of milk-fed infants. *J Pediatr Gastroenterol Nutr* 7:568–71, 1988.

Wharton BA, Balmer SE, Scott PH: Faecal flora in the newborn. *Adv Exp Med Biol* 357:91–8, 1994.

Widdice L: The effects of breast reduction and breast augmentation surgery on lactation: an annotated bibliography. *J Hum Lact* 9:161–7, 1993.

Wiessinger D, Miller M: Breastfeeding difficulties as a result of tight lingual and labial frena: a case report. *J Hum Lact* 11:313–9, 1995.

Willis CE, Livingstone, V: Infant insufficient milk syndrome associated with maternal postpartum hemorrhage. *J Hum Lact* 11:123–6, 1995.

Wilton JM: Sore nipples and slow weight gain related to a short frenulum. *J Hum Lact* 6:122–3, 1990.

Woodward DR, et al: Human milk fat content: within-feed variation. *Early Hum Dev* 19:39–46, 1989.

Woolridge MW: Aetiology of sore nipples. *Midwifery* 2:172–6, 1986.

Woolridge MW, Fisher C: Colic, "overfeeding," and symptoms of lactose malabsorption in the breast-fed baby: a possible artifact of feed management? *Lancet* 2:382–4, 1988.

Woolridge MW, Ingram JC, Baum JD: Do changes in pattern of breast usage alter the baby's nutrient intake? *Lancet* 336(8712):395–7, 1990.

Working Group on Cow's Milk Protein Allergy: Cow's milk allergy in the first year of life. *Acta Paediatr Scand Suppl* 348:2–14, 1988.

Ziemer MM, et al: Methods to prevent and manage nipple pain in breastfeeding women. *West J Nurs Res* 12:732–44, 1990.

CHAPTER 111

SLOW WEIGHT GAIN AND FAILURE TO THRIVE

Kathleen G. Auerbach and Jan Riordan

One of the most distressing clinical situations is a breastfeeding baby who is gaining weight poorly or not at all. Because the breastfeeding mother and baby operate as a team, the failure of one partner to do his or her "job" affects the other partner as well. Certain maternal conditions can negatively affect milk production. In some cases, the baby's inability to effectively stimulate the maternal milk supply will result in a gradual reduction of that supply of needed nutrients. In other cases, the baby is unable to suckle appropriately as a result of neurological impairment or other disorders. In rarer situations, the mother's ability to make milk in sufficient quantity to totally nourish her baby at the breast is impaired. Regardless of the cause(s), the outcome remains the same: the baby is growing slowly or gaining poorly or not at all. Both short- and long-term intervention may be needed to resolve the situation satisfactorily while preserving the important breastfeeding relationship and infant access to those elements in human milk that cannot be provided in artificial form.

This chapter discusses clinical situations involving poor weight gain and distinguishes between slow weight gain and failure to thrive. Because there are many reasons for inadequate weight gain, we identify the circumstances that may precede or contribute to this problem, noting whether they are management problems or whether they are infant- or mother-related. In all instances, the nutritional integrity of the baby is the paramount concern.

Normal Growth

Weight norms collected in the last century show that following birth in the hospital, most neonates will lose a small percentage of their birth weight. If the mother has received intravenous fluids during her labor, her infant may appear to lose a greater percentage of his birth weight–often very rapidly– as excess water weight is lost. In such instances, if evaluation of the breastfeeding episodes suggests that mother and baby are doing well, observation may be all that is necessary to verify that such early, rapid weight loss is indeed temporary and is not an indication of a serious problem that requires intervention. Breastfed infants usually regain their birth weight in the second week of life. Generally, babies–regardless of how they are fed–double their birth weight at about five to six months of age and triple their birth weight by one year of age. In some cases, these milestones may be reached earlier without implying infantile obesity.

Weight gain is not the only criterion by which to evaluate normal growth patterns; body length and head circumference are also important parameters of growth. An infant who is 20 inches long at birth can be expected to be approximately 30 inches high at one year of age, or one and a half times his birth length. Brain growth is rapid and, in the first year, an infant's head circumference will increase approximately 7.6 cm (3 inches); it will increase another 7.6 cm in the next 16 years of life. When other growth parameters are met, it is very likely that the child will show age-appropriate behavior as well. This will include reaching such developmental milestones as creeping, crawling, babbling and other verbal activities, and walking within the range of time considered normal for these behaviors.

Breastfed and formula-fed infants do not grow at the same rate at the same time. For example, Butte et al. (1990) found that breastfeeding infants gained about 34.5 gm/day at one month of age, whereas formula-feeding infants gained 34.4 gm/day. By four months of age, breastfeeding babies were taking less milk (18.7 gm/day), whereas the infants receiving artificial baby milk were taking 23 gm/day. Also, by four months of age, the breastfed baby's total daily energy expenditure is less than his formula-feeding counterpart; he takes less milk and he uses it more efficiently (Butte et al., 1985).

Normal growth reflects heredity for the individual infant. Often, mothers (and fathers) of slow-gaining infants, after asking their parents or finding their own infant growth records, learn that they too gained weight slowly as infants. Frequently, the pattern of growth of the first baby will be observed in later children, even if the method of feeding differs. The time at which the baby gains is also governed by heredity. In some families, infants tend to gain weight more rapidly in the second year than in the first, regardless of the timing of supplementary foods or the frequency of breastfeeding. Normal growth in infants may occur in brief—possibly even 24-hour—bursts that punctuate periods during which no measurable growth occurs. Further, growth follows no regular cycle and can occur after "quiet" periods that last as long as several weeks. Although many cultures tend to equate plumpness with well-being, obesity is not a sign of

health. Thus the method of feeding—although an obvious element in the consideration of nutritional intake—is not the only determinant of growth. Assessment of factors that may contribute to the pattern of growth of a young infant or child must include consideration of the contribution of genetic heritage.

Much work has been done in recent years to examine how babies grow and whether their growth differs according to how and what they were fed, thus contributing to our understanding of the differences in growth patterns when fully breastfed infants are compared with babies who are fully bottle-fed using artificial baby milk.

As noted elsewhere, milk production is related more to what the effectively breastfeeding baby takes than to potentially (in)adequate maternal ability to make milk (Dewey & Lönnerdal, 1986; see also Daly et al., 1993) and to the fact that the baby never completely empties the breast (Dewey et al., 1991a). In addition, the total time at the breast in a given 24-hour period appears to be at least as important for milk production as the frequency of breastfeeding episodes in the early weeks of the baby's life (Dewey et al., 1992a).

It is also important to remember that human milk has relatively low levels of protein. However, that low level has not been found to slow the growth of the human infant. In a comparison of babies who were exclusively breastfeeding with those who were also receiving solids, the groups were comparable in length and weight regardless of their protein intake, which is markedly higher in nonhuman milk feeds (Dewey et al., 1996). Finally, infant fatness appears to be unrelated to the lipid level in mother's milk; rather, it is related to the duration of breastfeeding episodes—further evidence that time at the breast is an important parameter to consider when a baby is gaining slowly, poorly, or not at all. Infants of mothers with higher-fat milk took a lower volume of milk (perhaps because of the higher concentration of cream) than did the babies of mothers with lower-fat milk, once more suggesting that it is the baby who determines intake by *how* he breastfeeds (Dewey et al., 1992b).

This intertwining of the threads of need to feed, duration of feeds, and maternal milk production further emphasizes that a baby who is gaining poorly represents a breakdown in the interaction between maternal and infant contributions to the milk-transfer process. Thus, although we may conclude that one or the other partner is not doing her or his "job" adequately, the contribution of each to that interactive modality is affected. The result? Each partner must be assisted to work more effectively with the other.

Growth Charts: How Good Are They?

Breastfed babies grow in a slightly different pattern than do artificially fed babies. Mature human milk changes and more closely reflects the breastfed baby's needs throughout the entire breastfeeding course as well as from the beginning to the end of the feeding, and from the first feeding in the morning to the last feeding at night. None of these changes can be mimicked in commercially made milks.

However, it is from the pattern of growth of primarily artificially fed infants that the growth charts currently in use were standardized. This presents a dilemma when assessing the adequacy of growth of breastfed babies, for they do not exhibit the same pattern of weight gain over time as do their formula-fed age-mates. For example, we know that breastfed babies gain weight rapidly in the first three months of life (Dewey et al., 1991b; Whitehead & Paul, 1984) and then slow their rate of weight gain. Height and head circumference measurements tend to be very similar regardless how babies are fed (Dewey, et al., 1992b). By the end of the first year, the breastfeeding baby is leaner than his formula-fed counterpart (Dewey et al., 1993). Because milk volume intake is substantially higher in the formula-fed infant, particularly after four months of age, Heinig et al. (1993a) suggest that the more rapid growth seen in formula-fed babies represents a less efficient use of the protein that they are receiving and that these higher rates of growth—as reflected in the standardized growth charts, which themselves are based on proprietary milk-fed infants—may be artificially high.

Finally, the amount of milk taken after solid foods are introduced also differs between breastfed and artificially fed babies. Breastfed babies tended to feed less often and to take in less milk if solid foods were given before they reached six months of age. This pattern of feeding suggests that the solid foods

were *replacing,* rather than adding to, the nutrition received through their mother's milk. If solids were introduced after the baby was six months old, breastfeeding frequency was not affected by the addition of those solid food–derived calories. By comparison, although feeding frequency declined, the formula-fed infants continued to take the same amount of formula even after solids were introduced (Heinig et al., 1993b). One must ask whether the constancy of intake by the formula-fed infants is an outcome deriving from the baby's need for the same amount of milk or whether it reflects the greater control of the feeding by the caregiver rather than the baby, who so clearly governs intake when breastfed (Daly & Hartmann, 1995; Daly et al., 1993).

It is appropriate to consider how the standardized growth charts in use today influence our conclusions about the infant's growth when the baby is breastfed. In a comparison of an affluent population (United States) and a poor population (Peru), the breastfeeding babies in Peru were observed to "falter" in their growth after six months. The authors suggested that this was related (potentially) to lower-protein complementary foods that the babies were receiving and to the greater morbidity from infections and diarrhea in the Peruvian sample (Dewey et al., 1992c). Note, however, that the "growth faltering" was identified by using the currently available standardized growth charts representing Western European and North American primarily formula-fed infants.

In yet another study, Dewey et al. (1995) examined seven different data sets, representing studies conducted between 1979 and 1991 in Canada, Denmark, Finland, Sweden, the United Kingdom, and the United States. When a pooled analysis was completed, the investigators found that breastfeeding infants grew more slowly after the first two months of life than was reflected in the current WHO/CDC (Centers for Disease Control) reference data. The authors noted that "Because of this [slowing], their growth often *gives the appearance of faltering* after the first 2 to 3 months, even if they are healthy and thriving" (p. 495, emphasis added by the chapter authors). The investigators concluded that new standardized reference data are needed to adequately evaluate infant growth for fully breastfed infants.

Peerson et al. (1993) also have examined different models designed to describe growth patterns of weight, length, and head circumference in breastfed and artificially fed infants. They found that none of the models closely predicted the weight curve for breastfeeding babies, implying once again that the current growth charts may exact an unfair burden on the breastfeeding baby to "measure up."

Growth charts are often used to record the growth of the individual child; however, they are standards based on percentiles, sometimes called *percentile rank*. In a growth chart based on percentiles, such as the ones shown in Appendix L, all the measurements of a large sample of children are ranked in size, from the smallest to the largest, and are assigned percentiles that correspond to their position in the rank order. For example, the middle measurement, or median, is called the 50th percentile; a percentile of 90 indicates a measurement that is as great or greater than that of 90 percent of the children in the sample. One-half of the children in a normal distribution can be expected to fall between the 25th and 75th percentiles, which are equidistant from the median; 80 percent of the children can be expected to fall between the 10th and 90th percentiles.

Growth can also be expressed in terms of standard deviation (SD), a statistical measure of variability, or the extent to which measurements deviate from the mean (or norm) of all the measurements in the sample. It is expressed as a distance in either direction from the mean, along the baseline of a normal distribution. About 68 percent of growth measurements of children can be expected to fall between +1 and –1 SD from the mean; 95 percent fall between +2 and –2 SD, and 99 percent between +3 and –3 SD.

The most commonly used charts in the United States are from the National Center for Health Statistics (NCHS, 1977), which maintains separate charts for girls and for boys. The charts for children from birth to 36 months of age include measurements of head circumference, body weight by age, recumbent length by age, and weight by length. Unfortunately, none of these charts reflect the normal growth of the breastfed infant. The sample of babies used to create growth charts were predominantly bottle-fed and often included infants who were introduced very early in life to supplementary solid foods (Tanis, 1985). The sample was also limited to white infants from predominantly middle-class families living in Ohio. It is important to keep this in mind when using these charts to evaluate whether a baby is gaining slowly or failing to thrive.

The WHO Working Group on Infant Growth (1994) has since developed growth data that more closely reflect the growth of breastfed children. The international sample of infants in the WHO study received no formula or other milks or any solid foods before four months of age. To illustrate how the absolute weight and length data from the 1994 WHO study compare with the NCHS growth charts, the quartile values for the pooled group of infants breastfed for at least 12 months are shown in Figures 11–1 and 11–2. The shapes of the curves for weight are clearly different, with the breastfed group showing much greater curvature between 3 and 12 months than the NCHS charts seen in Appendix L. The growth data from a subgroup of infants in this study, all of whom were breastfed for at least 12 months, is shown in Figures 11–3 and 11–4.

The Slow-Gaining Infant

The term *slow-gaining infant* has been used to characterize infants whose weight

- shows slow but steady growth and, when charted on a standardized growth chart, remains between the same two percentiles over time;

- exhibits proportional growth for height, length, and weight; and

- reaches developmental milestones within the normal periods.

Although such infants appear to weigh less than many of their age-mates, they are healthy and happy. In short, they are at the low end of the normal range of growth for healthy infants. Often intervention is not necessary, although mismanagement of breastfeeding should be ruled out as a factor contributing to such slow but steady weight gain.

Familial weight and stature are important criteria to consider when evaluating an infant who

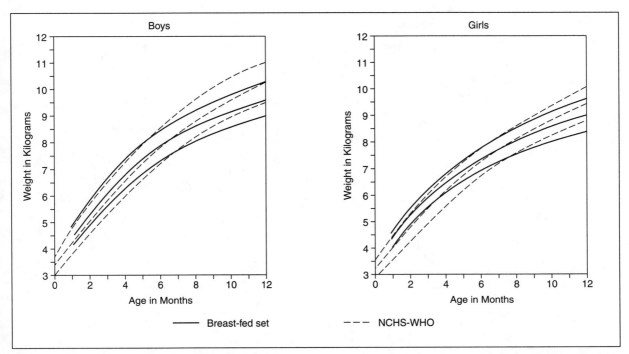

FIGURE 11–1. Weight quartiles on infants breastfed at least 12 months (N = 226) compared with current NCHS-WHO reference data. *(By permission of the Programme of Nutrition, World Health Organization.)*

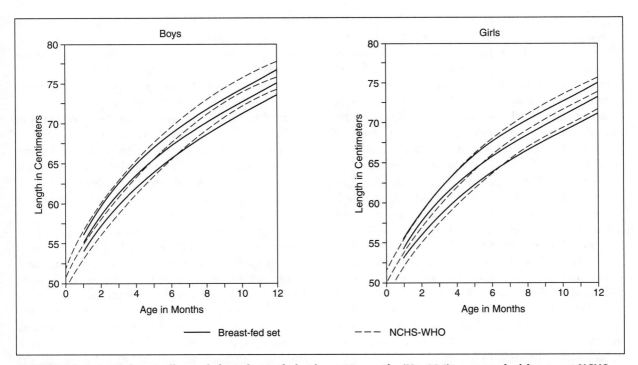

FIGURE 11–2. Length quartiles on infants breastfed at least 12 months (N = 226) compared with current NCHS-WHO reference data. *(By permission of the Programme of Nutrition, World Health Organization.)*

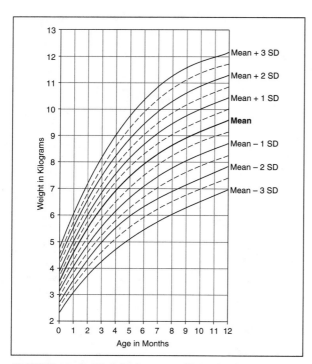

FIGURE 11–3. Weight-for-age of boys in the 12-month breastfed pooled data set. *(By permission of the Programme of Nutrition, World Health Organization.)*

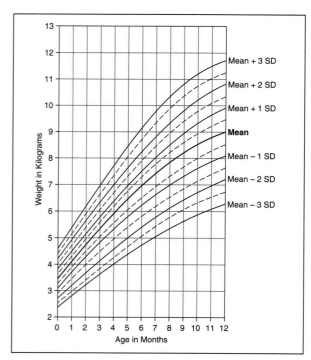

FIGURE 11–4. Weight-for-age of girls in the 12-month breastfed pooled data set. *(By permission of the Programme of Nutrition, World Health Organization.)*

appears to gain weight slowly (Christian et al., 1989). The child of parents who are of small stature should not be expected to be in the ninety-fifth percentile for height, for example. Normal growth parameters of Asian families are not the same as those of northern Europeans, whose adult stature and weight are considerably different from those of the adult Asian. When the average growth rates of American and Chinese children are compared on the standard NCHS growth chart, the mean height and weight for Chinese children fall into the tenth percentile, as compared to the mean growth measurements for white American children, which fall into the 50th percentile (Whaley & Wong, 1989).

Concern has been raised about the effect on growth of breastfed babies who are found to have low levels of vitamin B_6. Heiskanen et al. (1995) reported that those babies with low vitamin B_6 levels experienced a reduced gain in length but not in the rate of gain over the 12 months that these babies were followed.

In addition to genetic heritage, numerous factors–including organic disease–can contribute to

slow weight gain (Box 11–1). Thus any slow-gaining or poorly feeding infant should be evaluated to rule out an underlying illness or some organic problem before feeding method is considered a cause of the problem (Combs & Magino, 1993; Lukefahr, 1990). Certain congenital conditions at birth may contribute to slower-than-expected rates of gain. Babies born with a cleft palate feed more slowly, expend more energy doing so, and thus gain weight more slowly than do babies born without this congenital anomaly, regardless of how they are fed (Avedian & Ruberg, 1980).

In addition, maternal behaviors, illness, or conditions may also have an effect on the infant's rate of gain. For example, Martens, Martin, and Berlin (1990) report a baby failing to continue to gain weight sufficiently after her mother had gastric bypass surgery to correct her morbid obesity. Although the mother had breastfed three previous children with no difficulty, the authors speculate that her substantial weight loss following the surgery (more than 100 lb) may have affected her fat absorption and, secondary to that, the caloric value of her milk. Motil et al. (1994) followed a mother who, at 8 months postpartum, went on a very low-fat diet to resolve an acute episode of cholecystitis. The mother's own body weight decreased by 12 percent as a result of her extreme fat restriction. In addition, her baby dropped from the 25th percentile for length and weight at 6 months to below the fifth percentile for length and weight by 12 months of life. Although the mother was breastfeeding frequently and her milk composition did not change, her milk volume declined markedly, and thus the caloric volume that the baby received was affected. The authors urge careful assessment of maternal dietary adequacy in evaluating a breastfed infant whose rate of gain changes markedly.

Failure to Thrive

Although no universally accepted definition for failure to thrive (FTT) exists, infants are generally considered to be failing to thrive when their weight drops below the third percentile or is 2 SD below the mean on a standardized growth chart. Indications of poor weight gain in the breastfed baby in the first month of life, which may lead to FTT, include either or both of the following: the baby has not regained his birth weight within the first three weeks of life, or the baby is gaining less than four ounces per week.

FTT accounts for 2 to 5 percent of pediatric hospital admissions. FTT is neither a medical nor a nursing diagnosis; instead, it represents a cluster of symptoms occurring concurrently. FTT is classified into three categories:

1. *Organic FTT* is caused by physical factors such as renal disease, congenital defects, and other conditions given in Box 11–1.

2. *Nonorganic FTT* is the absence of physical evidence indicating that organic disease is a cause of weight loss; environmental factors may be inferred, such as insufficient caloric intake or a disturbance in the mother-baby relationship.

3. *Mixed FTT* is a combination of organic and nonorganic factors. For example, if the baby is unable to suckle adequately because of an undiagnosed neuromuscular problem, the mother may feel that her baby's inability to feed well is her fault. This may block the interplay of positive interaction and reciprocal play often associated with feedings.

Most cases of FTT are not caused by a physical problem. However, attempts to rule out the possible role of illness in a downturn in weight-gain rate are appropriate. Of 38 breastfed infants with FTT seen in one pediatric practice, only 7 cases (18 percent) were associated with an underlying physical illness (Lukefahr, 1990). One-half of the babies diagnosed as failing to thrive because of organic illness were taken to the pediatrician at between one and six months of age. About 40 percent of the cases were attributed to maternal misinformation or mismanagement, and 16 percent were thought to be caused by insufficient milk production (primary lactation failure). This study is congruent with an earlier report of organic FTT in 18 percent of the study cases, whether the babies were bottle-fed or breastfed (Sills, 1978).

More recently, numerous lactation consultants in the United States and elsewhere have noted a relationship between babies presenting with markedly slowed weight gain or FTT when their mothers were following a parenting pattern that includes rigid structuring of the timing, duration, and frequency of parent-child interactions, including feedings. Advocated by authors who have linked their work with inferred religious teachings (Ezzo & Ezzo, 1993), this parenting pattern has been expanded into a secular presentation (Ezzo & Bucknam, 1995). The followers of these recommendations are often reluctant to change how they relate to their children. Those proselytizing the program claim to teach "flexibility in feeding," inferring that reported problems are the result of its inappropriate application by some of the parents practicing this method of structured living (Frame, 1998; Giles, 1993; Griffith, *Bradenton Herald,* April 26, 1997; LaMendola, 1997). Reports on use of this approach indicate an increase in the number of infants who have become dehydrated or who have failed to gain weight as expected. Another outcome is early weaning from the breast in favor of bottle-feeding.

Feeding styles of breastfed infants who suffer weight loss also tend to fall into two categories: the fretful, underfed baby and the contented, underfed

---

BOX 11–1

Conditions That May Slow Infant Weight Gain or Contribute to Failure to Gain Weight

Anemia, maternal
Biliary atresia
Central nervous system insult
Cleft palate
Congenital cardiac anomalies
Cystic fibrosis
Food restriction, severe (maternal)
Galactosemia
Glycogen storage disease
Hyperthyroidism (inherited or acquired)
Hypoadrenalism

Hypocalcemia
Hypothyroidism (maternal)
Intestinal malabsorption syndrome
Lupus erythematosus (maternal)
Megacolon
Narcotic addiction (maternal)
Obstruction of gastrointestinal tract
Parasitic infection
Postpartum hemorrhage (maternal)
Renal insufficiency
Urinary tract infection

---

baby (Davies, 1979). The fretful baby is characterized by near-constant crying; irritability associated with frequent, short feedings; and colic. The mother, who is under stress and worried about the baby, may have (or may think she has) a poor let-down reflex, which results in a vicious cycle of ineffective feedings and anxious interactions between mother and infant. The contented baby, on the other hand, is placid and gives the impression of being satiated after feedings. This infant often allows long intervals between feedings. He may begin sleeping through the night in the first week or two. If the mother is waiting for a cue from the baby that he needs to be fed, she may not realize that she needs to initiate more frequent feedings. In general, mothers try to meet the norms of their society or family; thus a mother will heed the common admonition not to pick up her baby so often ("You might spoil him"; "He needs his rest; let him sleep").

It is uncommon to identify maternal deprivation as a factor when the breastfed baby fails to thrive. One likely reason for this is self-selection; the mother who chooses breastfeeding is more likely to be committed to her baby, a commitment that is incompatible with maternal deprivation. Moreover, the holding and skin-to-skin touching

that occur with feeding at the breast in most cases preclude the possibility that the baby will be touch deprived. Because of the intimate interaction that occurs with breastfeeding, these infants usually function within normal developmental limits until their malnutrition becomes extreme, unlike many FTT infants who are not breastfed. Two exceptions to this general rule are:

- the breastfeeding mother who is a victim of sexual abuse–if she links the baby's behavior to abuse that she experienced in the past, feeding behaviors may not be optimal; and

- the mother who is following a highly structured parenting pattern, particularly if espoused by religious teachers or leaders.

Lack of a support system for parents, regardless of their previous experience as parents, is a significant factor in FTT. Breastfeeding mothers of infants for whom inadequate weight gain becomes a severe problem seldom have family or close friends whom they see frequently or who are available to give the mothers the emotional support they need.

When a baby fails to thrive, he must be referred to the direct care of a physician who will conduct a thorough assessment, including a complete physical examination and laboratory studies. The assessment is usually made by a multidisciplinary team, including the nurse, lactation consultants, physician, social worker, dietitian, and psychologist. The first approach is to feed the baby supplementary foods without changing any other aspects of caregiving. If weight gain occurs, the cause is considered to be nonorganic and the result of insufficient caloric intake. The lactation consultant may then be asked for her evaluation of how to assist mother and baby to a more appropriate pattern of feeding that will sustain appropriate growth.

Factors Associated with Inadequate Caloric Intake

Inadequate intake of breastmilk may be caused by a number of factors that may center around the baby, the mother, or breastfeeding management (Table 11–1). In addition, risk factors (red flags) listed in Box 11–2 may help to identify factors that may have contributed to the baby's poor rate of weight gain.

The Maternal-Infant History Form that appears in Appendix 11–1 is a helpful tool for gathering important information about the mother and the baby when the infant has trouble gaining weight. It is important for the clinician to incorporate issues relating to both the baby and the mother and to identify necessary referrals to other health care disciplines as part of a team approach.

Red Flags

Risk factors for poor feeding that pertain to the perinatal period may be an issue only for the first few days after birth. Thereafter, other factors take on more importance. For example, if the baby has been exposed to maternal labor medications that tend to make the baby sleepy, the mother should be taught that the baby may not let her know when he needs to feed, and so she should offer her breast more often. If the baby was dehydrated, care must be taken to avoid overhydrating the baby. Rehydration must be accomplished slowly to avoid this

difficulty (Blackburn & Loper, 1992). If the baby was reported to have difficulty latching on prior to hospital discharge, an assessment should be undertaken to determine whether that problem is still present and, if so, to learn what the mother has already attempted to resolve this difficulty.

Limited Length of Feedings. Inadequate frequency and duration of feedings is a major factor leading to FTT in breastfed babies. Asking how long each feeding usually lasts and who stops it can indicate how advice has influenced the mother's breastfeeding pattern. Howie et al. (1981) found that five- to seven-day-old infants averaged 17 minutes of suckling per feeding period, with a range of 7 to 30 minutes. It is reasonable to assume that newborns will suckle as long as they need to do so and that some feedings will be shorter, whereas others will be longer. If allowed to finish the first breast before being moved to the second breast, the baby may stay on that side for a much longer period than he will remain on the second breast, assuming he takes the second side (Righard et al., 1993). This change in feeding times should not interfere with infant growth, as adequate milk transfer is likely in such a circumstance. Woolridge, Ingram, and Baum (1990) found that volume from one-breast feedings tends to be lower than if the baby takes two breasts; however, the milk obtained was creamier and thus actual caloric intake was only 10 percent less than that found in the higher-volume but less fat-rich feedings obtained when both breasts were used. In both cases, encouraging the mother to look to the baby for cues regarding when to end the feeding is more appropriate than is suggesting an arbitrary time limit.

When a mother restricts breastfeeding time (often because she has been told that her breasts contain a finite amount of milk or that the baby gets all that he needs within a particular time frame) and then supplements her infant, she unwittingly begins the process of weaning. The breasts receive less stimulation, and the milk supply begins to decrease (Frantz, 1980).

McNeilly et al. (1983) have substantiated multiple let-down responses through successive bursts of oxytocin release during the same breastfeeding episode. Although the infant of an experienced breastfeeding woman with a very active let-down

Table 11–1

SUMMARY OF PROBLEMS WITH AND INTERVENTIONS FOR SLOW WEIGHT GAIN WHEN ORGANIC CAUSES HAVE BEEN RULED OUT

	Assessment	Intervention	Rationale
Mismanagement	Mother removes baby before he finishes feeding.	Encourage mother to let infant self-limit feeding by monitoring swallows. Teach her the swallow sounds. Explain to mother who overdresses her infant that the baby may need to be awakened to finish the feeding.	Breastfed newborns need some long feedings. Length of feeding is proportional to quality of suckle. Overheated infants decrease their suckling; swaddled newborns assume a sleep state.
	Long interval between feedings (4 hr or more)	Suggest baby be allowed to feed often.	Breastfed newborns feed every 2 to 3 hr. Some newborns "cluster" feed (i.e., many feedings after a long sleep).
		Discourage pacifier use in the beginning weeks of breastfeeding.	Baby's desire to suckle is a survival mechanism and indicates need to feed. Keeping all suckling at breast helps to establish good maternal milk supply.
	Infant sleeping longer than a 4-hr stretch at night before 8–12 weeks. Mother promotes long sleep at night.	Teach parents not to expect a young infant to "sleep through the night."	Sleeping 6 hr usually occurs after six weeks.
		Suggest additional waking if infant sleeps a long period.	Prolactin levels are highest from 10 PM to 2 AM, and infants feed best at night.
	Mother offering water to reduce jaundice.	Suggest that water be discontinued in favor of more frequent breastmilk feeding.	Milk feedings lower bilirubin levels faster than do water feedings.
Disorganized suck	Infant feeds with eyes closed.	Encourage mother to clothe baby lightly for feedings.	Infants often find mother's arms "womblike" and assume a state of near-sleep.
	Suckles and swallows audibly only during let-downs;	Have mother monitor nutritive suck-swallow	Fast milk flow improves suckle.

	rest of feeding is a non-nutritive suckling pattern.	pattern and have her switch breasts when swallows cease.	
	Infant feeds frequently (q1h) or continuously.	Explain that if infant feeds more effectively, he will not feed as often. However, very infrequent feedings will not improve nursing behavior.	Smaller intake results in more frequent feedings. Small bursts of nutritive suckling may not have completed the feeding, and the baby is still hungry.
	Infant fusses when laid down.	Encourage nutritive suckling throughout entire feeding to avoid long periods between bursts of suckling.	
	Infant sleeps long stretches at night.	Encourage mother to wake infant at least q4h at night.	Establish more efficient daytime feedings.
Immature CNS or neuromuscular disorder	Poor suckling caused by poor coordination or muscle tone (hypotonia or hypertonia).	Teach mother to realign infant for postural control. Baby should have chin near chest and flexion of arms, legs, hips, and feet.	Flexion helps organize oromotor function and normalizes tone.
	Breastfeeds continuously and, when put on a 2-hr schedule, loses weight. Mother states she hears swallows only for the first 5 minutes into the feeding.	Teach "switch" nursing; if not effective, suggest use of feeding-tube device.	Tube device organizes a suckle, changes the pattern at the swallow phase, and initiates a sustained coordination. "Switch" nursing may not produce enough flow to sustain a nutritive suckle.
	Use of feeding-tube device causes infant to gain weight and causes a noticeable increase in mother's milk supply within 48 hr. Need for supplement increases or remains the same.	Assist in developing an optimal feeding plan. Evaluate the feeding tube size. It may be too large. Point out the baby's progress. Explain CNS development in infants.	A fast milk flow may overwhelm the infant. Most infants gradually develop organized CNS and neuromuscular abilities on their own by the third month.
	Baby continues to have diminished muscle tone and skill in suckling.	Refer for comprehensive pediatric evaluation. Pediatrician may refer to neurologist.	Degenerative neuromuscular disease often becomes more evident with time.

CNS: central nervous system.

Source: Derived from K Frantz: Slow weight gain. In: J Riordan, ed.: A practical guide to breastfeeding. *St Louis: Mosby, 1983.*

BOX 11–2

Maternal and Infant Risk Factors for an Infant's Failure to Thrive

MATERNAL RISK FACTORS

- Does the mother report little or no change in her breasts during pregnancy?
- Does the mother report having little or no breast fullness in the first week of breastfeeding?
- Does she have a history of breast surgery, or previous inability to exclusively breastfeed? If so, under what circumstances?
- Does she have more than one child younger than 5 years?
- Is she breastfeeding for the first time?
- Is she feeding the baby fewer than eight times per 24 hours?
- Does the mother describe her baby as "good" or "sleepy"?
- Does the mother report that the baby seems satisfied to "nap" at the breast?
- Does she report feeling minimal or no suckling pressure when the baby is feeding?
- Does the mother have a history of any conditions that could negatively affect her milk-production capability?
- Is she hypothyroid?
- Is the mother taking drugs of any kind?
- Does the mother exhibit signs of inadequate glandular tissue?
- Does the mother exhibit or complain of a poor let-down reflex?
- Has the mother been told to limit the length of feedings in order to prevent or cure nipple tenderness; to ensure that the baby will take the second breast; or to get the baby onto a predetermined feeding schedule?
- Is she interpreting the baby's dozing at breast as an indication that the baby has completed the feeding?

- Is positioning during feedings suboptimal? Has the mother been given advice by others regarding positioning? For example, has she been told that the baby's head must be higher than his body (an appropriate suggestion for the bottle-feeding baby)? If she has breastfed a previous infant, is she holding this new little one much as she held the last one when he was nearly weaned?

INFANT RISK FACTORS

- Did the baby have meconium stools through much of the first week of life and transitional stools into the second week of life?
- Did the baby have up to four wet diapers per day after the first week of life?
- Did the baby have up to two stools per day after the first week of life?
- Is the baby continuing to lose weight after hospital discharge?
- Did the baby lose 7 percent of birth weight within the first two to four days of life in the absence of possible reasons for this weight loss?
- Did the baby lose 10 percent or more of birth weight within the first week of life in the absence of possible reasons for this weight loss?
- Was dehydration previously diagnosed in the baby?
- Does the baby ask for (or is he receiving) six or fewer feedings per day?
- What is the baby's suckling pattern? Is it disorganized? random? infrequent? Is it stimulated only when the mother has a milk-ejection response? Has it been influenced by hospital routines? If so, which one(s)? Is the baby fretful when off the

breast but settles quickly into a sleeplike state at the breast, with eyes closed and minimal jaw excursions? Does the baby swallow minimally early in the feeding and rarely more than three to five times in a given feeding period before only sucks occur thereafter? Does the baby appear to "gum" the breast but not to actively suckle?

- Does the baby use a pacifier? If so, when (how often each day and for how long)?
- Has the baby recently been ill with an acute condition?
- Does the mother report that the baby has a chronic condition that may influence

how well or for how long he feeds in order to sustain sufficient nutriment?

- Has the baby a neurological problem that could be affecting the suck pattern and, subsequently, his growth?
- Does the baby have hypertonia or hypotonia?
- Does the baby have a condition that affects his ability to breastfeed effectively?
- Is the baby tongue-tied? The position of the tethering may require time, or clipping, in order to enable the tongue to effectively milk the breast.

response may consume his total feeding quite rapidly–for example, within 5 to 10 minutes–and still gain weight well, this is the exception rather than the rule. The volume of milk received depends on the length of the feeding and the effectiveness of the infant's suckling.

The baby's desire to feed from only one breast, or from both–even more than once–should dictate the feeding pattern. A baby is most likely to seem satisfied with only one breast if no time limit is arbitrarily set. In many cases, a baby who was originally content with one breast will often nurse from both breasts during periods of increased growth. Mothers need to be informed that the pattern for yesterday may not be the pattern for today or tomorrow.

Insufficient Number of Feedings. When the baby is "content to starve" (Davies, 1979), the mother may conclude that lack of interest on the baby's part or his willingness to wait long periods between feedings is an indication that he is satiated. Usually, the number of feedings declines gradually over several days in the first few weeks postpartum, until the baby is nursing five or fewer times in 24 hours. In some cases, an infrequent number of breastfeeding episodes will be combined with overly long periods of what the mother perceives to be suckling but that may be little more than the baby's wetting of the nipple and areola with his saliva. In other cases, infrequent nursings may dwindle into sleep sessions shortly after the baby has received some milk, particularly if the baby has become progressively weaker as his nutritional intake declines.

In the absence of a neurological problem in the baby, a marked increase in breastfeedings, usually in combination with a feeding-tube device that provides extra calories with little effort on the part of the baby, will change the baby's breastfeeding pattern dramatically. Instead of very long, inefficient feedings separated by more than four hours, the baby becomes more obviously wakeful at the breast, obtains more milk in a shorter period, and begins to spontaneously express a desire to nurse. Often, the baby who has not been waking for night feedings will begin to do so. This should be viewed as a positive sign that the baby is now recognizing and responding to hunger signals. In some cases, after the mother has insisted that the baby breastfeed more frequently, she will report, as a new experience, or one that has not occurred since the first week postpartum, a feeling of fullness in her breasts just prior to a breastfeeding. This feeling is an indication of increased milk production in response to increased stimulation through breastfeeding.

Suboptimal Positioning. As already noted in Chapter 9, positioning is an obvious, often overlooked, element in maternal breastfeeding behavior. However, the baby's position at the breast and the mother's own body position and her comfort when holding her baby are important preliminaries to effective breastfeeding.

There is no single "right" position for breastfeeding. There are, however, some positions that seem to work better for most mothers. The lactation consultant should first observe how the mother is already positioning her baby and herself and should then offer one or more suggestions to help the mother become more comfortable and to assist the baby to maintain contact with the breast without slipping off or causing discomfort for the mother.

Positioning difficulties that most often contribute to poor breastfeeding do not provide the baby with an opportunity to suckle comfortably. Usually, his body is at least partially turned away from the mother's, which results in an attempt to suckle "over his shoulder" or in a manner that forces his head to tilt too deeply into or away from the breast. If the baby is falling into the breast or is pressed too closely against it, he will not be able to breathe without periodically pulling his head back. Outcomes include sore or injured nipples for the mother and eventual refusal of the baby to go back to the breast, which he now associates with smothering. If the baby is too far away from the breast or his body is aligned such that only his head faces his food, the baby will tend to slip on and off the breast as he attempts to make and retain contact. If the baby is pressed too closely to the top of the breast and not close enough to that portion under the areola, his receding chin will not be in contact with the mother's breast. Once again, he will have difficulty breathing, and the mother may complain of nipple tenderness on the lower portion of the nipple and areola. In any of these situations, the baby expends a great deal of energy attempting to get comfortable, failing to do so, and coming on and off the breast.

If the mother has breastfed before, she may assume a body position relative to the baby that replicates the way that her previous child suckled when he was weaning or near the end of the breastfeeding course. Although an older baby can suckle in a wide variety of positions as a result of more well-developed musculature and maturity, the newborn is unable to control his body as easily. Thus, when held too low, he cannot reach the breast, can do so barely, or has to hang on by clamping his jaws onto the nipple, much as a climber who is slipping attempts to maintain his position by clinging to the rock. The result is a mother who reports sore nipples and a baby who gains weight poorly, who fusses at the breast, falling off frequently, and who eventually refuses to continue to struggle in order to eat.

Very often, simply helping the mother to more appropriately position the baby for breastfeeding quickly changes the dynamics between mother and baby so that each is more comfortable: the baby is better able to suckle without causing the mother discomfort and without having to struggle to obtain milk. In a situation in which the mother's milk supply is reduced because of poor feedings by a baby who has been poorly positioned for several weeks, the mother will need careful, written instructions to help her unlearn what she has been practicing for so long. Often, a Polaroid photograph or other "instant picture" of the mother feeding the baby in a position that she has assumed after receiving assistance can serve as a visual reminder of what she learned at the lactation consultant's office or the hospital or outpatient clinic where she sought help. The elimination of pain is a strong incentive for her to correct herself when she inadvertently slips into old routines. By the same token, the baby who is finally positioned comfortably for several feedings is more inclined to protest when placed inappropriately at the breast.

Maternal Diet. FTT can also occur when the mother is severely restricting her own dietary intake. Weight reduction associated with dietary restriction of 20 to 30 percent does not appear to interfere with milk production. However, when her energy and protein intakes decline further, lactation can falter (Motil et al., 1994). See Chapter 16 for additional discussion of the relationship between maternal dietary intake and milk production.

Infant Factors

Infant Illness. Although lactation-related difficulties are probably responsible for the majority of FTT cases in breastfed babies, illness, which accounts for almost one case in five (Lukefahr, 1990), must be ruled out. In addition, certain physical conditions have been linked to slower-than-expected rates of gain. Careful history taking, laboratory studies, and observation will establish whether an organic disease has resulted in the infant taking in insufficient calories.

Even when the baby does have an underlying health problem, breastfeeding may ameliorate, rather than worsen, the condition. For example, poor weight gain has been associated with cystic fibrosis and congenital heart disease. Some infants with these conditions, however, have shown a slow but steady weight gain and may even remain asymptomatic throughout the breastfeeding course. In other cases, they have shown only minimal evidence of the disease while being breastfed. The authors of this chapter have worked with families whose infants were diagnosed with cystic fibrosis early in infancy. The infants continued to breastfeed while receiving oral enzyme therapy in addition to milk through a feeding-tube device. This approach controlled symptoms of the disease, improved weight gain, and provided the babies with the all-important immunological protections available only by receiving human milk. The opportunity to continue to provide human milk to infants with cystic fibrosis has only recently been considered in the standard therapy offered to these children (Holliday et al., 1991; Luder et al., 1990).

Disorganized Suckling. Impairment of an infant's suckling will affect how much and what kind of milk he gets. When the infant's pattern of suckling improves, the mother's milk supply will usually increase. The strength of the suckle, and its organized, rhythmic occurrence will facilitate the letdown reflex and help the baby to obtain adequate volume and fat concentrations. The organization of the infant's suck pattern is as important as the frequency or duration of the feedings (Auerbach & Eggert, 1987). Observation of how the baby suckles may reveal that his feedings must be managed differently from those of a baby who gains weight more appropriately.

If the baby has received a pacifier (dummy) or bottle-feedings, he may be attempting to suckle from the breast as from the rubber or silicone nipple set or pacifier to which he has already been exposed. It is possible that the relationship between pacifier use and shortened breastfeeding duration that has been reported (Barros et al., 1995; Newman, 1990; Victora et al., 1993, 1997; Wright et al., 1996) may actually reflect early nipple confusion or nipple preference, which is not identified as a problem until the baby is no longer breastfeeding.

A careful history of the mother's birth experience and early breastfeeding may reveal mismanagement of early lactation in the hospital, combined with lack of sufficient skilled help to identify that her baby's suck is disorganized and requires modification (Klaus, 1987; Livingstone, 1990; Righard & Alade, 1990; Strembel et al., 1991). However, babies born at home, where no hospital routines can interfere with early breastfeeding, may also exhibit a disorganized suck pattern. Thus, although it is important to rule out mismanagement issues that may contribute to the problem of disorganized suckling, one must not be fooled into thinking that the elimination of such issues alone will resolve the problem.

Disorganization of suckling, a temporary condition, is most often seen in infants younger than one month (Neifert, Lawrence, & Seacat, 1995), particularly if the baby was born to a mother who received obstetrical medications. Time and appropriate assistance are required to help the baby to organize what is primarily a reflex action at this time. In most situations, one or more of the following elements is present:

1. *The baby frequently suckles with his eyes closed throughout the feeding.* The baby is not asleep, although he may appear to be. When removed from the breast, he may fuss and cry, prompting the mother to put him back for another round of extended suckling with minimal swallowing. In some cases, the baby may cease fussing and appear to be "content to starve." Menahem (1994) describes a case in which the baby stopped fussing and seemed happy to fall asleep at the breast. The mother concluded that his behavior indicated adequacy of feeding and denied that he was failing to thrive.

2. *The baby may suck and swallow rhythmically one to three times at the beginning of a feeding,* when the mother's body is responding to the baby's grasp of the breast with an initial spurt of milk; however, when lesser milk volumes provide a less obvious stimulus, the baby appears to flutter his tongue. Often the chin can be observed to move rapidly in very brief excursions, which place only minimal pressure on the lactiferous sinuses.

3. *The mother reports that the baby's suck is difficult to feel* or "doesn't feel very strong" or is "very soft." If the mother has previously breastfed an infant who gained weight appropriately, she may compare the relative strength of her first baby's suck with that of this infant. If this is the first baby the mother has breastfed, she may comment either that "it hurts when he nurses" or that "it is hard to tell if he is doing anything."

4. *The mother is unable to identify a swallow* or reports that the baby swallows for a very brief period and then falls asleep.

Over time, the mother's milk supply, which may have been adequate to copious early in the lactation course, will decline as a result of insufficient stimulation. Often the mother has been told that she does not have enough milk, but she has not also been informed that her baby's lack of consistent or effective stimulation is the primary cause of her inadequate milk production. If the mother has happily breastfed a previous baby, she may ask if this baby is doing something wrong. If she is a mother who is breastfeeding for the first time, she may blame herself for attempting to breastfeed, particularly if other relatives, friends, or health care providers question the quality or quantity of her milk.

As noted in Chapter 4, suckling during milk flow occurs at the rate of about one suckle per second; a swallow usually follows each suckle when the mother's milk is actively ejected into the baby's mouth. Although this is the general rule, toward the end of the feeding, nutritive suckling can slow down to one swallow for every three suckles and still be within the normal range (Bowen-Jones et al., 1982).

Nonnutritive suckles have often been described by mothers as "very soft" and observed by lactation consultants as a "quiver" or "fluttering" action on the chin. Milk is usually available to the infants with this suckling pattern only when it leaks out of the breast, when the milk let-down reflex occurs spontaneously, or when the baby momentarily suckles well at the beginning of the feed. Many slow-gaining breastfed infants engage in a pattern of suckling without swallowing. Frequently, the nipple is not drawn well into the baby's mouth.

Whenever an infant is not gaining weight well, it is important for the lactation consultant to observe breastfeeding to determine how the infant suckles and what the mother is doing, as well as what she reports that she is feeling when the baby is at the breast. First, ask the mother for permission to watch her baby feeding at the breast. The mother often feels that she has done something wrong if her infant is gaining weight poorly. The mother's positioning of her own body and her baby's should be noted, as well as the baby's action during the breastfeeding (Escott, 1989). Infant swallows sound like soft exhales. Their frequency, pattern of occurrence, and cessation should be noted. Weighing the baby on an electronic scale before and after a feeding may also verify how much milk is being transferred from the mother to the baby (Meier et al., 1994).

Changing the conditions surrounding suckling will elicit the baby's maximum potential for appropriate behavior. For example, flexing the baby's body may place his head in a position that brings the infant's tongue forward, which is an added advantage for the breastfeeding baby. Allowing the baby to extend his neck slightly may cause him to relax and to feed more comfortably. Adding a liquid flow will organize suckling action by triggering a swallow.

Although assessment of the suckling reflex is part of the neurological portion of the normal examination of newborns, a digital suckling assessment may also be indicated if a breastfeeding problem is identified.

Neurological Dysfunction. In some cases, the baby's suckle is not disorganized but rather exhibits a pattern suggestive of dysfunction. Unlike a disorganized suck, a temporary condition most apt to occur for a relatively brief period after birth and that usually resolves spontaneously, a dysfunctional suckle may be a sign of a mild to severe neurological problem.

Persistent poor suckling, particularly if it is associated with a delay in reaching developmental milestones, suggests neurological dysfunction. Because the tongue, jaws, and lips are operated by muscles that are innervated by the central nervous system, a neurological dysfunction often manifests itself first in a feeding problem (Glass & Wolf, 1994; McBride & Danner, 1987).

In some cases, the neurological problem is transitory and is caused by central nervous system immaturity. As the infant matures, feeding problems disappear spontaneously. A baby who displays hypertonia as a result of immaturity usually responds to postural control measures, such as flexion and calming, while rapidly maturing.

Those infants with hypotonia build muscle tone more gradually than do babies with hypertonia and usually require a feeding-tube device at the breast for an extended period. Examples of how such specialized therapy has been used to assist the slow-gaining breastfeeding infant can be found in Desmarais and Browne (1990).

Referral to a physical therapist who has had specialized training in assessing and treating feeding problems can improve the efficiency of the infant's suckling. The physical therapist or occupational therapist who proves to be most helpful for infants with suckling problems has additional neurodevelopmental treatment training and certification (NDT), based on the research of Morris and Klein (1987), Bobath (1971), and Mueller (1972). Such a therapist assesses and works with the baby's entire body musculature and movements that affect his oromotor function (Glass & Wolf, 1994).

A feeding-tube device may be used for these infants while the mother's milk supply is increasing, simultaneously enhancing the milk let-down response while the baby is learning to suckle more effectively. A physical therapist can further assist the family in maintaining flexion during bathing and diaper changes, as well as in holding the baby and in other daily activities, so that the infant can more easily control his own actions.

Infants with a disorganized suck rarely need a feeding-tube device for their entire breastfeeding course, unless other problems exist. In most cases, the timing of elimination of the feeding-tube device is dictated by the baby's need for less than a few ounces of milk per day. Often, the mother is the first to recognize that the baby's suckle is consistently stronger, from first grasp to last suck into satiated drowsiness. At that time, it is appropriate for the caregiver to encourage the mother to cease using the "coaxer" because it is clear that neither the baby nor she needs it any longer.

In some cases, a mother whose self-confidence has been severely shaken by the baby's previous failure to gain weight appropriately may be hesitant to eliminate the visible message that her baby is receiving milk. After all, she can see what the baby gets from the feeding tube device. The use of a chart that shows how the volumes obtained from supplementation have declined as the baby continued to gain weight well can be important in demonstrating to the mother that her own milk supply is now adequate to continue to meet the baby's needs.

Ankyloglossia (Tongue-Tie). An infant with a short frenulum may or may not be able to suckle efficiently at the breast (Berg, 1990; Marmet et al., 1990; Nicholson, 1991; Notestine, 1990; Ward, 1990; Wilton, 1990). In situations in which the condition prevents the infant from moving his tongue forward sufficiently to support and cup the elongated nipple and areola in order to form it into a teat, maternal nipple soreness is often the first sign that the infant is suckling inappropriately. This sign is followed by poor weight gain in spite of frequent breastfeeding and obvious interest in suckling (Fig. 11–5). In rare cases, the labial frenulum may also be implicated (Wiessinger & Miller, 1995).

When the lingual frenulum is clipped, relief from nipple pain and a markedly changed "feel" of the infant's suckling pattern is noted by the mother. In nearly all cases, the baby whose previous weight gain was minimal improves. In some cases, a short frenulum will, over time, be stretched by the baby's suckling action and other movements of the tongue, so that clipping is not necessary. The degree of severity of both the mother's and the infant's conditions will determine whether poor weight gain secondary to ankyloglossia is an issue that requires intervention rather than the patient application of "tincture of time."

Maternal Factors

The mother's rigid adherence to a demand-feeding philosophy, coupled with the baby's failure to express a need to be fed or to protest when too much time has elapsed between feedings, can be significant factors in failure to thrive (Pfeifer & Ayoub, 1978). If the mother has no previous experience in mothering or breastfeeding, she may not realize that feedings at the breast should be expected to occur frequently, particularly in the early weeks. The problem is compounded if the baby has a passive temperament or if a pattern of infrequent feeding is established that fails to meet the baby's nutritional needs.

If the mother has chosen to feed her baby according to a schedule not determined by the baby, her child's rate of weight gain may slow or cease. Often the mother describes her slow-gaining baby as a "good" baby who responds with quiet smiles, is often active and alert, and has long sleep periods. Pfeifer and Ayoub (1978) note that these mothers often have dependent personalities and spend a great deal of time meeting the needs of their families at the expense of their own needs; often the father's emotional support is minimal.

Physical problems deriving from the mother are less common than problems on the baby's side of the breastfeeding equation; however, maternal problems can include hypothyroidism, drug use, history of breast surgery, and insufficient glandular tissue, among others.

Hypothyroidism. Thyroid-deficient mothers may not produce enough milk; this lack of adequate milk can be one of the diagnostic signs of maternal hypothyroidism. Correcting the mother's dose of thyroid medication will often result in an adequate weight in the infant as a result of a more copious milk supply (Neville & Berga, 1983). If the mother reports a history of thyroid deficiency, she should be reevaluated. The physician will probably order a thyroxine test to measure her thyroid level.

Drug Use. Drugs taken by a woman, particularly estrogen-containing birth-control pills, may decrease her milk supply. Other drugs that are sometimes suspect include antihistamines and sedatives.

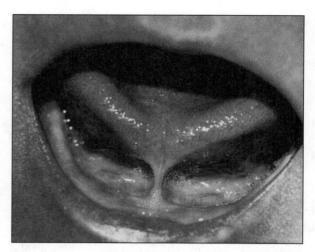

FIGURE 11–5. A severe tongue-tie. *(Courtesy Gregory E. Notestine, DDS.)*

A detailed discussion of the effect of medications on the breastfeeding mother and baby is found in Chapters 6 and 21.

Insufficient Glandular Tissue. Neifert and Seacat (1987) have described women with a congenital lack of glandular breast tissue that led to FTT in their infants. This is a rare phenomenon. Often, but not always, the mother may present with breasts of markedly different shape and size. In addition, she may report never having experienced any breast changes during her pregnancy or minimal or absent "filling" sensations in the days following the baby's birth. Breastfeeding need not be halted because of this problem. A feeding-tube device can be used to make up the difference in milk volume while providing the baby with whatever volume of milk his mother is producing.

Other Factors. Factors reported to interfere with the milk let-down reflex include maternal hormonal problems, fatigue, excessive amounts of caffeine, smoking, postpartum hemorrhage, lupus, maternal anemia, and the effects of certain drugs. In addition, the degree of stimulation (poor or absent) by the baby can play a role. Although many mothers may not be affected by any of these factors, each element is an important consideration when the lactation consultant is attempting to assess factors contributing to poor weight gain in the breastfeeding infant.

Clinical Implications

Whenever a baby is thought to be gaining poorly, a prenatal history, perinatal information, and a feeding history should be obtained. When collecting this information, the lactation consultant must note how the mother talks about her baby as well as the parent-infant emotional relationship. A thorough history may elicit enough information that laboratory testing is not necessary. The health care worker should be empathetic and kind during this interview, avoiding any hint that the parents are to blame for the baby's condition. In the authors' experience, most parents of slow-gaining breastfed babies are already distraught: they feel helpless and guilty and already blame themselves, usually unjustly. After taking the history, the health care worker should ask the mother to breastfeed her baby using both breasts, so that a complete assessment of a feeding can be made. In addition to suckling, the mother's level of comfort, body positions, eye contact, and verbalizations with the infant should be noted. The baby's behavior should also be noted: his willingness to suckle, how he does so, length of time that he remains at the breast, swallowing pattern (if any), and whether and how he indicates that he wishes to continue to feed.

If the baby is severely malnourished or dehydrated, he may have to be hospitalized; in most cases, however, the slow-gaining breastfeeding baby can be treated on an outpatient basis. If the infant is hospitalized, caloric intake should be closely monitored and recorded, and the baby should be weighed at the same time each day, under similar conditions, preferably on an electronic scale, calibration of which reveals consistency and accuracy of output information. An accurate record of intake and output is kept, including weighing the diapers. The nurse records the number, character, color, and consistency of the stools. Serum samples will be drawn from the infant for laboratory testing to rule out organic disease, and the stool may be tested for occult blood as well as for reducing substances. A Denver Developmental Screening Test may be administered to determine the baby's level of developmental maturity and whether a program of structured stimulation is needed to foster his development.

Treatment will depend on the results of assessment and testing. Organic disease, if found, will be treated. In cases in which the mother is simply uninformed about basic breastfeeding, supplementation to preserve the baby's nutritional integrity until the mother's milk supply is adequate, additional stimulation of her breasts through expression, teaching, and close supervision will usually suffice. In other rare cases, the mother (and possibly other family members) will require the assistance of a psychologist or social worker. In almost all circumstances, the mother may continue to breastfeed; feedings may be augmented by expressed breastmilk, formula, or solid foods. Valentine, Hurst, and Schanler (1994) report that pumped hindmilk increased significantly the rate of weight gain of low-birth-weight infants. Optimally, the mother is given a feeding tube or some other device for supplementing the baby's intake at the breast.

Supplementation

Devices

The use of a cup or spoon or a feeding-tube device that cues the baby when to swallow—and requires him to do so when his oral cavity is filled with milk—usually results in a steady and sometimes rapid resolution of the problem. Feeding-tube devices are described in Chapter 13 and are discussed here only in terms of slow weight gain.

Fig. 11–6 shows a commonly used device, the Supplemental Nutrition System (SNS). The use of such a device almost always prompts maternal questions about how much milk the baby must ingest in order to grow and about how she can tell whether her own milk supply will increase when the baby is obviously deriving nutrients from the feeding-tube device. Particularly in the first several days or week of use of a device, the amount of supplemental fluid taken from the feeding tube will climb, sometimes rapidly, because the mother should be told not to limit the amount that the baby receives.

Any mother who is contemplating use of a feeding-tube device should be reminded of the following four points:

1. A general rule is to begin with two to three ounces in the feeding-tube device and to add one-half ounce more than the baby took at the

previous feeding, until he is leaving about one-half ounce in the feeding-tube device for at least three feedings. At this point, the mother need not continue to add fluid to the amount the baby has been taking.

2. After a period that varies from one baby to the next, the amount of milk the baby takes from the feeding-tube device will begin to decline. When this occurs consistently over several feedings, the mother can be instructed to reduce the amount in the feeding-tube device to about one-half ounce more than the baby usually takes. This extra one-half ounce assures that the baby will receive milk rather than air from the tube.

3. Usually the reduced amount of milk taken from the feeding-tube device declines in stages, with plateaus between the stages. In some cases, these plateau periods coincide with the infant's temporary age-appropriate appetite spurts.

4. Remind the mother—usually at each visit and often during phone follow-ups between visits—that the baby is gaining weight during the course of the use of the feeding-tube device, even as the amount being taken from that container declines. The guidelines in Box 11–3 show the approximate amount of milk that the baby should receive in the feeding-tube device to support growth.

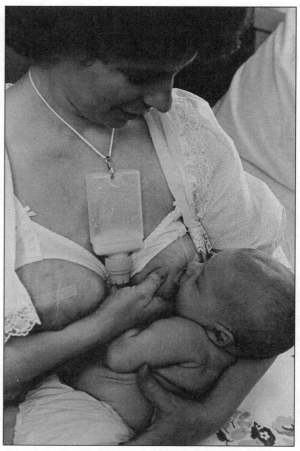

FIGURE 11–6. The Supplemental Nutrition System (SNS) feeding-tube device. *(Courtesy Medela, Inc., McHenry, IL.)*

A baby whose suckling pattern is assisted in becoming more organized simultaneously begins to stimulate the mother's breasts more appropriately while using a feeding-tube device. Such stimulation, in the absence of maternal breast tissue deficits, usually results in an increase in milk production. Often a first sign that the mother reports, usually within days of using the feeding-tube device, is a feeling of breast fullness on waking. Thereafter, she may note spontaneous milk leakage from the contralateral breast when the baby is suckling. If she has never noted this before, it is time for congratulations! At the same time, the mother, who has been instructed about ways to identify swallows, reports that the baby is more consistently and rhythmically swallowing. Usually,

when a rhythmic suck-swallow pattern is established, the baby keeps his eyes open through most of the feeding.

Often, a previously fussy baby is noticeably more relaxed in demeanor and behavior after he is receiving adequate amounts of food. Figure 11–7 shows a two-month-old infant who looked and acted passive. When he went to breast, he immediately closed his eyes and appeared to be asleep; however, he could not be put down, because he continually fussed and cried when not held at breast. Bottle-feedings after breastfeeding brought his weight up temporarily, but because the mother's two previous children had stopped breastfeeding soon after being given bottles because of poor weight gain, the mother was reluctant to continue

BOX 11–3

Guidelines for Using a Feeding-Tube Device

1. The mother should begin using the device when she and the baby are most rested, usually in the morning or at a time when other household or family activities are unlikely to require her attention.

2. Prepare the feeding before the baby becomes hungry or fussy. If the baby is frantic, the mother will become anxious.

3. Fill the device and position the tubing so that it extends slightly past the end of the mother's nipple. Use any kind of hypoallergenic tape to hold the tubing in place. If the baby appears to be sucking only on the end of the tubing, pull it back so that it is flush with the end of the mother's nipple.

4. Most babies will take most of the fluid in the device within the first 30 minutes. If the baby is actively suckling but the device is flowing very slowly or not at all, test it by filling it with water and holding it upside down. If the cap is screwed on too tightly, the tubing flow may be blocked. Check this and then test it again by squeezing the container gently to activate the flow. If the device is working properly, there should be a steady drip from the end of the tubing. In some cases, rapidity of flow can be increased by allowing the unused tubing (that which might be attached to the contralateral breast) to remain "open." Taping the unused tubing end along the side of the container will prevent it from dripping milk but allow air intake into the bottle portion, thereby increasing milk flow from the other tubing.

However, rapidity of flow ideally should be determined by the baby and his suckling pattern. In most cases, increasing the rapidity of flow by opening the other tubing is not necessary.

AMOUNT OF SUPPLEMENT TO USE

If a feeding-tube device is used to assist the baby in gaining weight, both the caregiver and the mother need to know how much supplement the baby must have in order to grow. In the table below, find the weight of the baby and identify in the second or third columns the approximate amount of milk required per day for that weight. Subtract the amount of milk the baby took from the feeding tube per day. The figure remaining is a rough estimate of the amount of breastmilk the baby received.

Infant Weight	Approximate Daily Milk Requirement	
lb	oz	ml
5	13	371
6	16	457
7	19	542
8	21	600
9	24	685
10	27	771
11	29	828
12	32	914

BOX 11–3 *(cont.)*

Example:

(a) Infant weight: 7 lb 2 oz, which means that approximately 19 oz, or 542 ml, of milk is needed per day.

(b) Amount taken from tube device per day = 9 oz of supplemental milk.

(c) 19 oz − 9 oz = approximately 10 oz of breastmilk was taken.

Another method of figuring required intake is to convert into ounces the baby's weight in pounds. Divide that number by six; the result is the total number of ounces of milk the baby needs in 24 hours to secure a 4- to 6-oz gain per week (Petok, personal communication, 1991).

Example:

(a) Infant weight: 7 lb 2 oz = 114 oz.

(b) 114 oz ÷ 6 = 19 oz/day.

(c) 19 oz/day divided into eight feedings (approximately every three hours) suggests that about $2\frac{1}{3}$ oz should be placed in the feeding-tube device for each feeding.

---

artificial feeding. At two months of age, this baby was two ounces below his birth weight; he had gained two pounds on bottle-feedings and then lost that weight again before being seen for breastfeeding evaluation and assistance. Two months later (Fig. 11–8), he was in the 75th percentile for weight and was a happy, smiling baby, who, according to his mother, "almost never cries". In the first week of supplementation using the feeding-tube device at the breast, he gained two pounds; such a pattern of very rapid weight gain early in the supplementation period is nearly always catch-up growth. Thereafter, the rate of gain approaches that which one would expect in a baby who is breastfeeding effectively.

This infant began by receiving 20 oz of supplement in the SNS per day (in addition to milk at the breast). Fig. 11–9 illustrates the usual pattern of intake of supplemental fluid–the mother's own expressed milk, donated human milk, or artificial baby milk–that is placed in the feeding-tube device and thus can be measured. He peaked at 32 oz of supplement in the SNS per day during the week when he gained two pounds. Thereafter, his daily supplementation amount came down steadily, with two- to four-day plateaus between declines that usually lasted approximately one week each. This baby used the SNS for four months.

It may take twice as long as the age of the baby at the time of the first visit to fully correct the presenting problem, but every baby is different. One four-week-old baby (seen by the lactation consultant who assisted the first infant) exhibited an identical suckling pattern but no longer required the SNS after 19 days. One should not attempt to predict how quickly a given baby will no longer need additional milk in order to grow appropriately. As the number of potentially contributing factors that must be corrected or improved goes up, so does the amount of time needed to resolve the difficulty. In the authors' experience, rarely does only one factor contribute to a baby's presentation with FTT.

Other Methods

Sometimes drugs may be given to the mother to increase her milk supply. Chlorpromazine (Thorazine) is known to increase milk production by raising the prolactin level. Metoclopramide (Reglan) has also been found to increase prolactin levels and subsequent milk production in mothers (Ehrenkranz & Ackerman, 1986; Gupta & Gupta, 1985). Expressing milk by hand or breast pump may also be helpful, particularly if low milk supply is secondary to poor infant suckling. However, the degree of emphasis on breast pumping needs to be

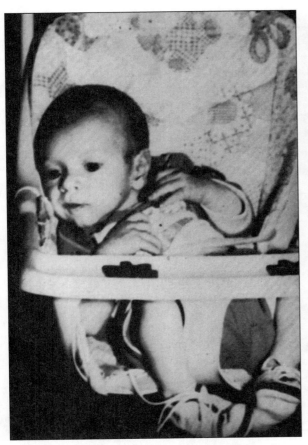

FIGURE 11–7. An infant who was failing to thrive at two months of age due to disorganized suckling.

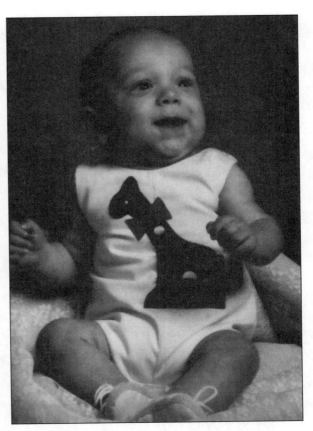

FIGURE 11–8. The same infant as in Figure 11–7 at four months of age, following correction of suckling pattern.

determined within the context of daily living. A mother who has several other children or one very busy toddler and who has no household assistance may decide that having to pump her breasts—in addition to the time she is already spending with each feeding episode—is sufficient to discourage her from continuing with the care plan. Unless a family history of allergies is identified, the judicious use of formula in the feeding-tube device may assist continued breastfeeding, particularly if the mother's milk supply is very low at the time the care plan is begun. The bottom line throughout resolution of FTT is to feed the baby. *How* that is accomplished is less important than that it *is* accomplished. As the baby's weight, strength, and alertness improve, a return to exclusive breastmilk feedings and breastfeedings without supplementation are more likely to be achieved.

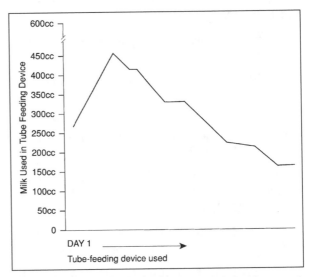

FIGURE 11–9. Characteristic pattern of supplemental milk intake when a baby's disorganized suckling pattern is being improved.

SUMMARY

Breastfeeding is a normal physiological process. However, problems such as poor weight gain occasionally occur. A first step in helping the mother of a baby who is gaining weight poorly is to identify aspects of her experience that differ from the optimal breastfeeding course. Identification and treatment of any underlying illness, feeding the baby, and managing the problem while preserving breastfeeding should be the ultimate goal.

The majority of cases resulting in nutritional FTT derive from nonorganic or environmental barriers that lead to inadequate weight gain. Therefore, when an infant fails to thrive, both mother and baby, as interacting individuals working as a team, must be evaluated together. Assessment and treatment are most effective when they include evaluation of mother and baby during several breastfeeding sessions.

Often the mother's knowledge of breastfeeding is thought to be greater than it is, particularly if she has breastfed more than one baby. Assessing the mother's understanding of the underlying factors contributing to her baby's difficulties with breastfeeding is the first step in helping her to see where her behavior fits into the picture and how her own knowledge of her baby is essential as a care plan is developed to improve the infant's weight gain.

Many mothers have breastfed in the most daunting situations, positions, and surroundings–and their infants thrive. However, when an infant fails to do so, consideration must be given to all the factors that may be contributing to the problem. At the same time, support should be offered for continued breastfeeding by avoiding any treatment option that separates the baby from the mother.

Every mother-infant pair is unique. Close and continuing follow-up care, by telephone and face-to-face visits, not only supports the mother during a stressful, fearful time but also informs the health care provider by enabling her to evaluate the results of her care plan.

REFERENCES

Auerbach KG, Eggert LD: The importance of infant suckling patterns when a breast-fed baby fails to thrive. *J Trop Pediatr* 33:156–7, 1987.

Avedian LV, Ruberg RL: Impaired weight gain in cleft palate infants. *Cleft Palate J* 17:24–6, 1980.

Barros FC, et al: Use of pacifiers is associated with decreased breast-feeding duration. *Pediatrics* 95:497–9, 1995.

Berg KL: Two cases of tongue-tie and breastfeeding. *J Hum Lact* 6:124–6, 1990.

Blackburn ST, Loper DL: *Maternal, fetal, and neonatal physiology: a clinical perspective.* Philadelphia: Saunders, 1992;369.

Bobath B: *Abnormal postural reflex activity caused by brain lesions* (2nd ed). London: Heinemann, 1971.

Bowen-Jones A, Thompson C, Drewett R: Milk flow and sucking rates during breastfeeding. *Dev Med Child Neurol* 24:626–33, 1982.

Butte NF, et al: Feeding patterns of exclusively breast-fed infants during the first four months of life. *Early Hum Dev* 12:291–300, 1985.

Butte NF, Smith EO, Garza C: Energy utilization of breast-fed and formula-fed infants. *Am J Clin Nutr* 51:350–8, 1990.

Christian PS, et al: Relationship between maternal and infant nutritional status. *J Trop Pediatr* 35:71–6, 1989.

Combs VL, Magino BL: A comparison of growth patterns in breast and bottle-fed infants with congenital heart disease. *Pediatr Nurs* 19:175–9, 1993.

Daly SE, Hartmann PE: Infant demand and milk supply: Part 1. Infant demand and milk production in lactating women. *J Hum Lact* 11:21–6, 1995.

Daly SE, Owens RA, Hartmann PE: The short-term synthesis and infant-regulated removal of milk in lactating women. *Exp Phys* 78:209–20, 1993.

Davies DP: Is inadequate breast-feeding an important cause of failure to thrive? *Lancet* 1:541–2, 1979.

Desmarais L, Browne S: *Inadequate weight gain in breastfeeding infants: assessments and resolutions* (Unit 8, Lactation Consultant Series). Garden City, NY: Avery Publishing, 1990.

Dewey KG, Lönnerdal B: Infant self-regulation of breast milk intake. *Acta Paediatr Scand* 75:893–8, 1986.

Dewey KG, et al: Adequacy of energy intake among breast-fed infants in the DARLING study: relationships to growth, velocity, morbidity, and activity levels. *J Pediatr* 119:538–47, 1991a.

Dewey KG, et al: Breast-fed infants are leaner than formula-fed infants at 1 yr of age: the DARLING study. *Am J Clin Nutr* 57:140–5, 1993.

Dewey KG, et al: Do exclusively breast-fed infants require extra protein? *Pediatr Res* 39:303–7, 1996.

Dewey KG, et al: Growth of breast-fed infants [reply]. *J Pediatr* 121:171–2, 1992a.

Dewey KG, et al: Growth of breast-fed and formula-fed infants from 0 to 18 months: the DARLING study. *Pediatrics* 89:1035–41, 1992b.

Dewey KG, et al: Growth of breast-fed infants deviates from current reference data: a pooled analysis of US, Canadian and European data sets. *Pediatrics* 96:495–503, 1995.

Dewey KG, et al: Growth patterns of breast-fed infants in affluent (United States) and poor (Peru) communities: implications for timing of complementary feeding. *Am J Clin Nutr* 56:1012–8, 1992c.

Dewey KG, et al: Maternal versus infant factors related to breast milk intake and residual milk volume: the DARLING study. *Pediatrics* 87:829–37, 1991b.

Ehrenkranz RA, Ackerman BA: Metroclopramide effect on faltering milk production by mothers of premature infants. *Pediatrics* 78:614–20, 1986.

Escott R: Positioning, attachment and milk transfer. *Breastfeed Rev* 14:31–7, 1989.

Ezzo G, Bucknam R: *On becoming babywise.* Sisters, OR: Multnomah Books, 1995.

Ezzo G, Ezzo AM: *Preparation for parenting* (4th ed). Chatsworth, CA: Growing Families International, 1993.

Frame R: Growing criticism. *Christianity Today* (Feb. 9, 1998), 96–97.

Frantz K: Slow weight gain. In: Riordan J: *A practical guide to breastfeeding.* St Louis: Mosby, 1983.

Frantz K: Techniques for successfully managing nipple problems and the reluctant nurser in the early postpartum period. In: Freier S, ed. *Human milk: its biological and social value.* Amsterdam: Exerpta Medica, 1980;314–7.

Giles TS: The brave new baby. *Christianity Today,* (August 16):34–6, 1993.

Glass RP, Wolf LS: Incoordination of sucking/swallowing, and breathing as an etiology for breast-feeding difficulty. *J Hum Lact* 10:185–9, 1994.

Griffith K: Raising babies God's way may not be the right way. *Bradenton Herald* (April 26, 1997), 8–10.

Gupta A, Gupta P: Metaclopramide as a lactagogue. *Clin Pediatr* 24:269–72, 1985.

Heinig MJ, et al: Energy and protein intakes of breast-fed and formula-fed infants during the first year of life and their association with growth velocity: the DARLING study. *Am J Clin Nutr* 58:152–61, 1993a.

Heinig MJ, et al: Intake and growth of breast-fed and formula-fed infants in relation to the timing of introduction of complementary foods: the DARLING study. *Acta Paediatr* 82:999–1006, 1993b.

Heiskanen K, et al: Low vitamin B_6 status associated with slow growth in healthy breast-fed infants. *Pediatr Res* 38:740–6, 1995.

Holliday KE, et al: Growth of human milk-fed and formula-fed infants with cystic fibrosis. *J Pediatr* 118:77–9, 1991.

Howie PW, et al: How long should a breast feed last? *Early Hum Dev* 5:71–7, 1981.

Klaus MH: The frequency of suckling: a neglected but essential ingredient of breast feeding. *Obstet Gynecol Clin North Am* 14:623–33, 1987.

LaMendola B: Time to eat? *Fort Lauderdale Sun-Sentinel,* June 2, 1997, p. 10.

Livingstone VH: Problem-solving formula for failure to thrive in breast-fed infants. *Can Fam Phys* 36:1541–5, 1990.

Luder E, et al: Current recommendations for breast-feeding in cystic fibrosis centers. *Am J Dis Child* 14:1153–6, 1990.

Lukefahr JL: Underlying illness associated with failure to thrive in breastfed infants. *Clin Pediatr* 29:468–70, 1990.

Marmet C, Shell E, Marmet R: Neonatal frenotomy may be necessary to correct breastfeeding problems. *J Hum Lact* 6:117–21, 1990.

Martens WS, Martin LF, Berlin CM: Failure of a nursing infant to thrive after the mother's gastric bypass for morbid obesity. *Pediatrics* 86:777–8, 1990.

McBride MC, Danner SC: Sucking disorders in neurologically impaired infants: assessment and facilitation of breastfeeding. *Clin Perinatol* 14:109–30, 1987.

McNeilly AS, et al: Release of oxytocin and prolactin in response to suckling. *Br Med J* 286:257–59, 1983.

Meier PP, et al: A new scale for in-home test-weighing for mothers of preterm and high risk infants. *J Hum Lact* 10:163–8, 1994.

Menahem S: Conservation-withdrawal reaction in infancy? An underdescribed entity. *Child Care Health Dev* 20:15–26, 1994.

Morris S, Klein M: *Pre-feeding skills.* Tucson, AZ: Therapy Skill Builder, 1987.

Motil KJ, et al: Case report: failure to thrive in a breast-fed infant is associated with maternal dietary protein and energy restriction. *J Am Coll Nutr* 13:203–8, 1994.

Mueller H: Facilitating feeding and pre-speech. In: Pearson PH, Williams CE, eds. *Physical therapy services in the developmental disabilities.* Springfield, IL: Thomas, 1972.

National Center for Health Statistics: *NCHS growth curves for children: birth–18 years.* Public Health Service pub. no. 78-1650. Washington, DC: U.S. Department of Health, Education and Welfare, 1977.

Neifert M, Seacat J: Lactation insufficiency: a rational approach. *Birth* 14:182–8, 1987.

Neifert M, Lawrence R, Seacat J: Nipple confusion: toward a formal definition. *J Pediatr* 126:s125–s9, 1995.

Neville MC, Berga SE: Cellular and molecular aspects of the hormonal control of mammary function. In: Neville MC, Neifert M, eds. *Lactation: physiology, nutrition and breast-feeding.* New York: Plenum, 1983;162–3.

Newman J: Breastfeeding problems associated with the early introduction of bottles and pacifiers. *J Hum Lact* 6:59–63, 1990.

Nicholson WL: Tongue-tie (ankyloglossia) associated with breastfeeding problems. *J Hum Lact* 7:82–4, 1991.

Notestine GE: The importance of the identification of ankyloglossia (short lingual frenulum) as a cause of breastfeeding problems. *J Hum Lact* 6:113–5, 1990.

Peerson JM, et al: Use of growth models to describe patterns of length, weight, and head circumference among breast-fed and formula-fed infants: the DARLING study. *Hum Biol* 65:611–26, 1993.

Pfeifer DR, Ayoub C: Nonorganic failure to thrive in the breastfeeding dyad. *Keep Abreast J* 3:283–6, 1978.

Righard L, Alade MO: Effect of delivery room routines on success of first breast-feed. *Lancet* 336(8723):1105–7, 1990.

Righard L, et al: Breastfeeding patterns: comparing the effects on infant behavior and maternal satisfaction of using one or two breasts. *Birth* 20:182–5, 1993.

Sills R: Failure to thrive. *Am J Dis Child* 132:967–9, 1978.

Strembel S, et al: Breast-feeding policies and routines among Arizona hospitals and nursery staff: results and implications of a descriptive study. *J Am Diet Assoc* 91:923–5, 1991.

Tanis AL: Growth in breastfed babies. *Breastfeed Abstr* 4:13, 1985.

Valentine CJ, Hurst NM, Schanler RJ: Hindmilk improves weight gain in low-birth-weight infants fed human milk. *J Pediatr Gastroenterol Nutr* 18:474–7, 1994.

Victora CG, et al: Pacifier use and short breastfeeding duration: cause, consequence, or coincidence? *Pediatrics* 99:445–53, 1997.

Victora CG, et al: Use of pacifiers and breastfeeding duration. *Lancet* 34(8842):404–6, 1993.

Ward N: Ankyloglossia: a case study in which clipping was not necessary. *J Hum Lact* 6:126–7, 1990.

Whaley LF, Wong DL: *Essentials of pediatric nursing* (3rd ed). St Louis: Mosby, 1989;1094.

Whitehead RG, Paul AA: Growth charts and the assessment of infant feeding practices in the Western world and in developing countries. *Early Hum Dev* 9:187–207, 1984.

Wiessinger D, Miller M: Breastfeeding difficulties as a result of tight lingual and labial frena: a case report. *J Hum Lact* 11:313–6, 1995.

Wilton JM: Sore nipples and slow weight gain related to a short frenulum. *J Hum Lact* 6:122–3, 1990.

Woolridge MW, Ingram JC, Baum JD: Do changes in patterns of breast usage alter the baby's nutritional intake? *Lancet* 336(8712):395–7, 1990.

World Health Organization Working Group on Infant Growth: *An evaluation of infant growth.* Geneva: World Health Organization, Nutrition Unit, 1994.

Wright A, et al: Changing hospital policies to increase the duration of breastfeeding. *Pediatrics* 97:669–75, 1996.

APPENDIX 11-A

MATERNAL-INFANT HISTORY FORM

Infant's Name: _____

Mother's Name: _____

Consultation For: _____

Office Tel.: ( )_____ _____

Or call   -   from

(hours/A.M., P.M.) Weekdays and

(hours A.M., P.M.) Weekends

Date: _____

Phone Number: _____

PART I. PATIENT HISTORY

Please describe in your own words why you have sought this breastfeeding consultation.

_____

_____

_____

_____

_____

_____

Past Maternal Medical History

Yes No   Are you in good health? If not, describe any medical problems.

_____

_____

Are you taking:

Yes No   Birth control pills?

Yes No   Prescription medications?

Yes No   Non-prescription (over-the-counter) medications?

Yes No   Have you had any thyroid problems at any time in your life?

Yes No   Are you taking any thyroid medications *now?* If so, what kind; dosage?

_____

Yes No   Do you have any endocrine ("glandular") problems?

Yes No   Have you had any previous surgery?

Yes No   Have you ever had breast surgery? If so, specify when, what, and for what reason.

_____

Yes No   Do you have any allergies?

Yes No   Did you observe any breast changes during pregnancy? Describe.

_____

Yes No   Did you take any medications during pregnancy? If so, which one(s); what dosage?

_____

_____

Yes No   For this baby and any other breastfed infants, did your milk "come in" on or before the third postpartum day?

Maternal Family History

Has anyone in your family had a history of the following problems? If so, specify below.

Yes No   Breastfeeding problems?

Yes No   Eczema or allergy to food, pollen, or other substances?

Yes No   An infant who had difficulty gaining weight?

Yes No   Metabolic or malabsorption disease?

Yes No   Cardiac or neurologic problems?

_____

_____

_____

Maternal Habits

Yes No Do you smoke? If so, specify brand and number per day.

_____

Yes No Do you drink coffee or tea? If so, specify number of cups per day.

_____

Caffeinated?	Yes _____	No _____
Decaffeinated?	Yes _____	No _____
Herbal?	Yes _____	No _____
Type of herbal tea: _____		

Yes No Do you drink caffeinated sodas? If so, specify number per day; ounces per day.

_____

Yes No Do you drink alcohol? If so, specify what type, and how much per day/week/month.

_____

Yes No Do you use recreational drugs? If so, specify kind and frequency.

_____

Maternal Diet

Yes No Do you eat regular meals?

Yes No How would you rate the food you eat?
     Excellent   Good   Poor

Yes No Do you currently take prenatal vitamins? If so, specify what brand and type.

_____

Yes No Do you take any other vitamins? If so, specify brand(s) and type(s).

_____

Yes No Are you on a restricted diet of any kind (e.g., vegetarian, low sodium)? If so, specify type of restriction and purpose.

_____

Yes No Are you currently on a weight loss diet?

Yes No Are you drinking more fluids now that you are nursing?

Maternal Social History

Are you: single _____ married (how long?) _____
     divorced (how long?)_____

Do you: own _____ rent _____ live with relatives _____

How long have you lived there? _____

Who lives in your household? (list all) _____

_____

Please supply the following information about each of your children?

	Age	Breastfed?	How long?
1st (oldest) child			
2nd child			
3rd child			
4th child			
5th child			
6th child			

How would you describe your relationship with the baby's father?
     Good   Fair   Poor

Yes No Do you have a busy lifestyle? If so, describe. _____

_____

Yes No Do you have any source(s) of anxiety or tension? If so, describe. _____

_____

Yes No Do you have any friends or relatives who have breastfed their babies? If so, describe. _____

_____

Yes No Are any of your relatives or close friends opposed to/nonsupportive of breastfeeding? If so, describe. _____

_____

Breastfeeding Preparation

When did you decide to breastfeed this baby?

_____ before pregnancy

_____ early pregnancy (in the first 4 months)

_____ late pregnancy (in the last 3 months)

_____ after the baby's birth. When was that? Why? Specify reason.

_____

Who most influenced your decision to breastfeed?

_____

How long do you want to breastfeed?

_____ up to 6 weeks

_____ up to 3 months

_____ up to 6 months

_____ up to 1 year

_____ until the baby weans

_____ other (specify) _____

Yes No Have you read anything about breastfeeding? If so, specify.

_____

_____

Yes No Have you attended any classes or support groups for breastfeeding? If so,
when, and by whom?

_____

_____

Yes No During your pregnancy, were your
breasts examined? If so, provide the
names of care provider.

_____

Infant's Birth History

Type of delivery:

　Vaginal: __ augmented __forceps __ suction

　Cesarean: why? _____

Yes No Labor experienced? Length?

_____

Yes No Were medications given during labor or
delivery? If so, what kind?

_____

Yes No Was it a difficult birth? If so, describe.

_____

Yes No Were medications taken after birth? If
so, what kind? For what reason?

_____

Place of birth: home__ birth center__ hospital __
If not at home, where was baby kept?
　　　in nursery__　　rooming in __
If rooming in, what kind of plan? (How many
hours with mother?) _____

Yes No Were you separated from infant for any
length of time? If so, why?

_____

Maternal Feeding Experience

When infant nurses, do you feel:

　　　　　　　　tingling ___ warmth ___

　　　　　　　　burning___ filling _____

leaking on other side ___ nothing ___ other _____

If other, describe. _____

Yes No Do you have a quiet place for nursing?
If not, where do you usually nurse?

_____

Yes No Do you use a rocking chair for nursing?

Have you ever experienced any of the following?

Yes No Sore nipples.

Yes No Plugged duct.

Yes No Breast infection.

Yes No Severe engorgement.

Yes No A feeling of being "softer" after a feeding.

Yes No Discomfort from fullness in the breasts.

Infant Feeding History

First time infant was put to breast was _____
hours after birth.

Yes No Did infant take to nursing easily?

Yes No Has your baby received any bottle-
feedings? If so, when and why?

_____

_____

What was in the bottle(s)? Human milk only_____
Other(?)_____

Yes No Does your baby feed at each breast at
each feeding?
How long on each breast at each feeding?

_____

How many times on each breast at each
feeding?

_____

How long is each feeding, on average?

_____

Yes No Does the infant pause often during a
feeding?

Yes No Do you hear the baby swallowing?

Yes No Does the baby make clicking or popping sounds while nursing?

Yes No Does the baby initiate the end of each feeding?

Yes No Does the baby appear to be satisfied at the end of a feeding?

How would you rate his sucking?

poor___ weak ___ average___ strong___

Yes No Does he burp easily?

When is he burped? _____

What technique is used?

_____

Yes No Does the baby spit up or vomit after a feeding? If so, how often does this occur?

_____

Number of wet diapers per day? _____

Yes No Are paper diapers used?

Number of stools per day?_____

Consistency _____ Color _____

Is infant   placid _____ average _____
            active _____ fussy _____

When during the day/night is the baby awake? _____

What is your baby's longest sleep period?

_____

When? _____

At what time is baby put to bed for the night? _____

Yes No Is this bedtime regular?

Circle the time when feedings begin on a typical day.

Midnight 1 2 3 4 5 6 7 8 9 10 11 AM

Noon 1 2 3 4 5 6 7 8 9 10 11 PM

Yes No Is a pacifier used? If so, what kind?

_____

How often? _____

Yes No Does the baby suck his thumb or fingers?

Yes No Does the baby have "colic"?

Yes No Has the baby begun receiving solid foods? If so, what are they? How often?

_____

Infant Medical History

Infant's Expected Date of Birth: _____

Infant's Actual Date of Birth: _____

Infant's Birth Weight: _____

Infant's Current Weight: _____

Infant's APGAR Scores:

_____ 1 minute   _____ 5 minutes

Yes No Were there any problems with the infant immediately after birth? If so, describe. _____

Yes No Has the infant had any problems since birth? If so, describe. _____

_____

Yes No Was the infant jaundiced? If so, peak bilirubin level? _____ On what day? _____

Yes No Is the infant receiving any medications? If so, what kind? What dosage? Why?

_____

Yes No Is the infant receiving any vitamins? If so, what kind? What dosage? Why?

_____

Yes No Has the infant had any other tests performed (especially for slow weight gain)? If so, what kind? When? Where?

_____

_____

Yes No Does the infant have a milk allergy? If so, to what kind of milk? When did it first appear?

_____

Yes No Does the infant have cystic fibrosis?

PART II: PHYSICAL EXAMINATION

For each structure being examined, assign one of the two following codes: **0** (within normal range), **X** (abnormal). If abnormal, specify problem.

Maternal Examination

Right   Left

Nipple size: _____
Protractility: _____
Other: _____
Notes: _____
_____
_____

Infant Examination

1. Infant behavior at time of exam: _____

_____

2. Measurements:

	Date	Weight	Length	Head Circumference
At birth:				
Discharge date:				
Today:				

Notes: _____
_____

3. Muscle Tone _____
Positions (supine, prone, other) _____
_____

Notes: _____
_____

4. Oral exam:

Notes

Mouth _____

Jaw _____

Tongue: _____

Frenulum: _____

Palate: _____

Digital suck exam: _____

Clinical Data

Enter all data (test, date, results) pertaining to creamatocrit, prolactin, triple prolactin, maternal thyroid, etc. _____

_____

_____

_____

ASSESSMENT SUMMARY

Summarize problems in order of impact upon breastfeeding:

1. _____
2. _____
3. _____
4. _____
5. _____

MANAGEMENT PLAN

Key to above numbers:

1. _____
2. _____
3. _____
4. _____
5. _____

PHYSICIAN FOLLOW-UP

Date _____

Notes: _____

PATIENT FOLLOW-UP

Date _____

Notes: _____

_____

Source: L Desmarais, S Browne: Inadequate weight gain in breastfeeding infants: assessments and resolutions *(Unit 8, Lactation Consultant Series). Garden City, NY: Avery Publishing , 1990. Reprinted with permission.*

Special acknowledgment for the technical assistance of Janet Repucci, BS, MT (ASCP), IBCLC.

CHAPTER

12

JAUNDICE AND THE BREASTFEEDING BABY

Richard A. Guthrie and Kathleen G. Auerbach

Few early experiences of the newborn are as apt to have as deterrent an effect on breastfeeding as does the diagnosis of neonatal jaundice. This diagnosis is a frequent cause of early unnecessary weaning. When this occurs, it represents a failure of health care workers to understand the normal physiology of the neonate and his adaptation to the high-oxygen environment of extrauterine life. Health care personnel have a responsibility to change institutional routines that are related to neonatal bilirubin levels if those routines adversely affect breastfeeding. This chapter reviews the etiology of early-onset jaundice, late-onset jaundice, and the clinical implications of the normal infant's response to extrauterine life.

Early-Onset (Neonatal) Jaundice

After birth, the human neonate must initiate many activities that previously were managed by the placenta. Instead of continuously feeding, as in the womb, the infant feeds intermittently. Waste products are now cleared by the immature liver and kidneys. At the same time, these organs are confronted by a relatively concentrated load of bilirubin caused by the rapid breakdown of red blood cells and the meconium that coats the intestines.

Conjugated, water-soluble bilirubin is excreted by the kidneys in the urine; unconjugated, lipid-soluble bilirubin is excreted by the liver in the bile through the bowel. As the gastrointestinal tract becomes coated and recoated with milk, recirculation of the unconjugated, lipid-carried bilirubin is reduced, and more frequent stooling removes the unconjugated bilirubin.

Jaundice is caused by the accumulation of bilirubin in the tissue, particularly the skin, where it is visible as a yellow pigment. Jaundice in older children and adults is considered a pathological condition, but this is not true for the newborn. As a result of the low level of maternal oxygen in placental blood, the fetus develops a relatively high red-blood-cell count with high hemoglobin of a special kind—*hemoglobin F,* or *fetal hemoglobin.* The high hemoglobin level increases the oxygen-carrying capacity of fetal blood. Fetal hemoglobin takes up oxygen poorly, so more hemoglobin is needed. The normal, full-term baby is born with a relatively high level of red blood cells containing a high level of fetal hemoglobin.

Fetal hemoglobin is well adapted to assisting the fetus in the low-oxygen environment of the uterus. It has a low affinity for oxygen; therefore, it picks up oxygen less well than does adult hemoglobin (which has more need for it). However, it also is better able to release the oxygen to peripheral tissue, thus enabling the fetus to live and grow in a relatively low-oxygen environment.

After birth, the low-affinity fetal hemoglobin is a liability in the high-oxygen environment of lung breathing, so the bone marrow begins producing adult hemoglobin (hemoglobin A). The red blood cells containing fetal hemoglobin can now be broken down and eliminated from the body. Hemoglobin is a complex molecule consisting of heme, globin, and iron. When the hemoglobin molecule is broken down, iron returns to the bone marrow, where it is used in hemoglobin synthesis. Globin, a protein, returns to circulation in the blood. Heme is broken down by the spleen into unconjugated bilirubin.

Unconjugated (indirect) bilirubin is a lipid-soluble compound that is transported from the spleen to the liver by attachment to transporting proteins such as albumin—in a fashion similar to the transport of cholesterol in the blood by apoproteins (lipid-transporting proteins that are synthesized by the liver). In the liver, the indirect bilirubin is detached from the carrier proteins and is conjugated with other compounds, such as glucuronic acid. This results in conjugated (direct) bilirubin, which is water-soluble. Some conjugated bilirubin reenters the circulation and is excreted in the urine. Most, however, is excreted in the bile. Some unconjugated bilirubin is also excreted in the bile. High concentrations of direct bilirubin in serum usually indicate an obstruction of the biliary system; otherwise, this water-soluble bilirubin is not harmful.

It is the unconjugated, or indirect, fat-soluble bilirubin that, in increasing concentrations, causes the baby's skin and sclera to take on a yellowish cast (Table 12–1). The concentration of indirect bilirubin can increase if its production exceeds the protein-carrying capacity of the blood or if excretion is so slow that bilirubin accumulates faster than can be handled by excretion and carrying capacity.

In the fetus, the gastrointestinal tract is sterile. Bilirubin excreted into the gastrointestinal tract throughout fetal life accumulates in the meconium. Much of this bilirubin can be reabsorbed. After the baby's birth, the large load of meconium bilirubin

Table 12–1

RULE OF THUMB OBSERVATION AND ITS RELATIONSHIP TO BILIRUBIN LEVELS

Involvement of the Body	Serum Bilirubin Levels
Sclera	3 mg/dl
Face	5 mg/dl
Upper trunk	5–7 mg/dl
Complete trunk	7–10 mg/dl
Spread to extremities	10–12 mg/dl
Extremities yellow; palms and soles clear	12–15 mg/dl
Palms and soles yellow	> 15 mg/dl

combined with the relatively slow functioning of the liver and the rapid breakdown of fetal hemoglobin may result in an early, temporary exaggeration of serum bilirubin concentration, which manifests itself in yellowing of the sclera and skin during the early neonatal period. This is a natural result of the normal physiological process experienced by every newborn in the early extrauterine period. Moreover, the increase in serum bilirubin may serve a protective function: its antioxidant effects may guard the newborn against the effects of oxygen free radicals (McDonagh, 1990).

Generally, in African and white neonates, a mean serum bilirubin peak of 6 mg/dl occurs on the third or fourth day of life. Thereafter, serum bilirubin levels decline to about 2 to 3 mg/dl by the end of the first week of life and gradually reach the normal adult value (1 mg/dl) by the end of the second week (Gartner et al., 1977; Kivlahan & James, 1984). Higher values of 10 to 15 mg/dl will sometimes occur, and glucose-6-phosphate dehydrogenase deficiency may predispose neonates of

African heritage to higher bilirubin levels within hours after birth (Brown AK, 1992).

Bilirubin levels may remain elevated for weeks with no untoward effects in healthy newborns. Brown et al. (1993) followed 155 normal, full-term white infants. Transcutaneous bilirubinometry was conducted on days 2, 3, 5, 7, 9, 11, and 13 after birth. By day 3, nearly 50 percent of the infants had levels above 10 mg/dl. By day 13, 10 percent of the infants still were classified as jaundiced (bilirubin ≥ 10 mg/dl). The percentage of infants classified as jaundiced was slightly, but not statistically significantly, higher among those with an older sibling who had been diagnosed as jaundiced through day 11. The authors noted that treatment protocols need to take into account the potential for elevated bilirubin levels beyond day 3 in healthy, full-term breastfeeding infants. Protocols should support establishing adequate maternal milk volume and appropriate feeding technique throughout the period when bilirubin levels are likely to be elevated. There is no scientific evidence that bilirubin levels of less than 20 mg/dl in the first week of life and less than 25 mg/dl thereafter have any harmful effect on full-term, healthy infants (Gartner, 1992; Newman & Maisels, 1992).

In 1995, Maisels and Newman reported on 22 babies who had kernicterus and had been breastfed and in whom elevated bilirubin levels were alleged to have been responsible for brain damage. All of these babies had bilirubin levels of 39 mg/dl or higher at 4 to 10 days after birth and most had received more than one exchange transfusion. The authors noted that there was no reliable method for distinguishing these infants from others in the neonatal period and that the feasibility, risks, costs, and benefits of rigorous intervention in order to do so remain to be determined (Maisels & Newman, 1995).

Pathological Jaundice

Pathological jaundice usually falls into three general categories:

1. disease that causes increased red-cell hemolysis (e.g., Rh disease, ABO incompatibility, congenital spherocytosis, and other hemolytic processes);

2. a deficiency of carrier protein or binding sites (such as occurs with prematurity, sepsis, hypoxia, and the use of certain drugs); and

3. liver and metabolic disease (e.g., hepatitis, Crigler-Najjar syndrome, Rotor's syndrome, liver damage from cytomegalovirus, toxoplasmosis, rubella, syphilis, congenital biliary atresia, and metabolic problems such as galactosemia and hypothyroidism).

Usually, diseases causing a deficiency of carrier protein or binding occur after the first week of life and result in late-onset jaundice, which can persist for several weeks.

Factors Associated with Early-Onset Jaundice

The medical and nursing literature is replete with discussions linking the presence or severity of neonatal jaundice to a wide range of variables, including mode of feeding (Rubaltelli, 1993) and hospital practices. Examination of the literature provides no clear picture of how these variables affect jaundice, because feeding groups are rarely defined in the same way and are rarely totally discrete. In addition, other factors (identified by different investigators as important) may have been allowed to vary without considering their potential influence as intervening variables.

Infant Characteristics

Race or Ethnic Group. Different racial groups appear to exhibit neonatal hyperbilirubinemia in varying degrees. Japanese neonates are more than three times as likely as are white newborns to have jaundice, defined as a serum bilirubin level exceeding 10 mg/dl (Fischer et al., 1988; Horiguchi & Bauer, 1975; Maisels et al., 1988). Genetic or environmental factors contributing to an increased rate of heme catabolism may explain the differences between the groups. Similar patterns have occurred when comparing other Asian neonates (e.g., Chinese and Korean) with white infants.

Navajo neonates also have substantially higher serum bilirubin levels than do white infants at two days of age (Johnson, 1992), possibly caused by differences in red-blood-cell metabolism or membrane structure. Saland et al. (1974) controlled for feeding method when they compared Navajo infants with white controls. The Navajo infants exhibited higher serum bilirubin levels in all feeding groups. The highest levels occurred when the Navajo infants were breastfed. Hodgman and Edwards (1992) found that Hispanic infants also had higher bilirubin levels than did white neonates. These investigators caution that guidelines for white babies may substantially overestimate the need for intervention in Hispanic neonates.

Birth Weight. Osborn et al. (1985) noted that lower birth weight was related to the likelihood of hyperbilirubinemia. When Bracci et al. (1989) performed a linear regression analysis of numerous variables, they found that only birth weight and gestational age remained significantly associated with the likelihood of neonatal jaundice . They suggested that "most factors already reported in the literature play a minor role which may not merit attention from a preventive point of view."

Stool Patterns. De Carvalho, Robertson, and Klaus (1985) evaluated 24 exclusively breastfed and 13 exclusively formula-fed infants in the first three days after birth. Stool frequency and volume also varied by feeding group, with the bottle-fed infants stooling more often and in greater volume than the breastfed babies. For them, the amount of stool bilirubin increased as the volume of stools increased through the three-day study period. This was not so for the bottle-fed babies, which may partially explain the greater frequency of jaundice in breastfed babies—so-called breastfeeding jaundice.

Frequent suckling has been found to shorten gut-transit time and to promote stool output in both full-term (Cavell, 1981; Tomamasa et al., 1987; Weaver et al., 1988) and preterm infants (Bernbaum et al., 1981). As breastfed babies increase their stool output, they excrete more stool bilirubin and have lower serum bilirubin concentrations, which suggests that early stimulation of intestinal motility may reduce the likelihood of hyperbilirubinemia (De Carvalho et al., 1982). Thus there is a need for early and frequent breastfeeding in newborn infants. Ince et al. (1995) noted that babies fed fewer than eight times daily in the first three days of life, particularly if three or more

other variables (maternal age 35 years or older, use of oxytocin during labor, male gender, or first feeding occurring 12 hours or more after birth) are present, were significantly more likely to be jaundiced than were babies in whom those variables were not present. That feeding frequency was an issue only when other variables also were present supports the notion that elevated bilirubin levels are related, at least in part, to other factors relating to the mother and baby. Unlike management issues, such as timing of the first feeding and labor medications or aids, several of these factors cannot be controlled by health care providers.

The *expected* higher incidence of neonatal jaundice with earlier dismissal from the hospital was a factor in passing the so-called drive-through delivery legislation by numerous state legislatures and the U.S. federal government (Kotagal & Tsang, 1996). Whether early discharge from the hospital (in the first 24 hours) actually contributes to the likelihood of occurrence of jaundice is unclear. The issue may be not the timing of hospital discharge but rather the absence of sufficient instruction, especially of new mothers, adequate observation by the hospital staff, or correction of poor breastfeeding practices prior to the mother's departure.

Weight Loss. Among hospital-born infants, those who are breastfed have been reported to lose more weight than their artificially fed counterparts (Butler & MacMillan, 1983; De Carvalho et al., 1985; Hall, 1983). De Carvalho et al. (1985) found that throughout the study period, the breastfed group lost significantly more weight than did the bottle-fed babies, but there was no correlation between weight loss and serum bilirubin concentrations. It remains unclear whether weight loss alone contributes to elevated bilirubin levels.

Hospital Routines

Routine care patterns have been implicated as influencing factors both in bilirubin levels and in breastfeeding patterns. For example, Osborn, Reiff, and Bolus (1985) reported that problems during labor and delivery, cesarean delivery, postnatal complications, blood group incompatibility, bruising, and infant feeding method were significantly correlated with jaundice in the neonate.

Type of Feeding. With few exceptions, neonatal jaundice is thought to occur with greater frequency and to rise to higher levels when the baby is breastfed than when he or she is artificially fed. However, Maisels and Gifford (1983) reported that no cause was identified in more than one-half of the cases in which serum bilirubin concentrations exceeded 12 mg/dl in the 264 term infants whom they evaluated.

Dahms et al. (1973) studied 199 full-term infants, dividing them into four groups. Demand breastfeeders and formula-feeders received no supplemental feedings and went to the breast by six hours after birth, nursing six to seven times every 24 hours. Control breastfeeders did not go to breast until 20 hours or more after birth and received four breastfeedings every 24 hours and two formula feedings in the nursery at night. The control bottle-feeders were not fed until 20 hours or more after birth and received six formula feedings every 24 hours. The two control groups also received one or two feedings of 5% dextrose. Bilirubin levels were not statistically different among the four groups.

Frequency of Feeding. De Carvalho et al. (1982) evaluated the relationship between the frequency of breastfeeding and mean bilirubin levels on the third day of life. The infants in their two groups did not differ in length of feedings, weight loss during the first three days of life, or hematocrit readings. However, the 29 infants who composed group 1 had a mean feeding frequency of 6.8 ± 0.8 feedings per 24 hours. The mean serum bilirubin level on day three for this group was 9.3 ± 3.5. By contrast, the 26 infants who composed group 2 had a mean feeding frequency of 10.1 ± 1.6 feedings per 24 hours and a mean serum bilirubin level of 6.5 ± 4.0, a statistically significant difference ($p < .01$). De Carvalho et al. (1982) concluded that "policies that reduce or limit the number of breastfeedings in the first days of life may interfere with normal mechanisms that eliminate bilirubin from newborn infants."

A more recent study (Maisels et al., 1994) compared babies who were breastfed frequently (median, nine feedings per day) with those who were fed on demand (median, six and a half feedings per day). Serum bilirubin levels between 48 and 80 hours were not significantly different between the groups. Unfortunately, at the mother's request, water feedings were given to 11 percent of the frequent feeders and 21 percent of the demand feeders, thus contaminating the results.

Supplemental Feedings. Adams, Hey, and Hall (1985) examined the incidence of hyperbilirubinemia in 223 consecutively born, full-term, healthy infants. In their analysis, breastfeeding was the best predictor of hyperbilirubinemia exceeding 12 mg/dl. However, most babies received fewer than eight feedings in 24 hours. In addition, all of the breastfed infants in the study were complemented with water feedings after breastfeeding, and many received two or three formula feedings as well. These factors raise questions about the degree to which reduced caloric intake (from water feeds), infrequent feedings from the breast, and possible delay in establishing maternal milk supply because of infrequent stimulation may contribute to higher serum bilirubin concentrations.

Water Supplementation. Nicoll et al. (1982) found that most full-term breastfed infants in their sample received supplementary feeds of water, dextrose, or formula during the first days of life. When they compared plasma bilirubin levels in babies grouped by supplemental feeding, those infants having the highest bilirubin levels were those who had received water feedings in addition to breastfeeding. The group receiving dextrose had slightly lower bilirubin levels, whereas those babies who were exclusively breastfed had the lowest bilirubin levels. Although there was no relationship between weight loss and physiological jaundice, the amount of supplemental water or dextrose taken was reported to account for more than one-fourth of the infants' calculated daily fluid requirements; this raises the issue of the degree to which water and dextrose feedings reduce the total daily calories received. Because thirst is the primary drive of infant appetite (Taitz & Byers, 1972), supplementation that depresses the thirst response may reduce neonatal interest in breastfeeding, thereby interfering with lactation.

Glover and Sandilands (1990) found that glucose water supplementation was associated not only with greater weight loss in the first week of life but also with increased length of hospital stay as the total volume of glucose water supplementation increased. One might ask whether bottle-fed babies who develop hyperbilirubinemia may also be receiving more supplemental water feedings than is appropriate. Nicoll et al. (1982) suggest that the practice of supplementing breastfeeding babies should be discouraged. Furthermore, they speculated that not providing prepacked feeds, which have no redeeming benefits for their recipients, would result in a 70 percent savings in hospital costs for breastfeeding infants. Studies by De Carvalho et al. (1981) and Clarkson et al. (1984) confirm these findings.

Laws (1981) reported that whereas supplemented infants lost less weight than did unsupplemented neonates, glucose supplementation appeared not to affect bilirubin levels or the likelihood of subsequent phototherapy for bilirubin concentrations exceeding 12 mg/dl. Instead of being concerned about the temporarily "calorically deprived" breastfed infant (a frequently used rationale for offering supplements), Laws suggested that clinicians should direct their attention to the "'calorically supplemented' (overfed?)" bottle-fed baby, whose rapid bilirubin clearance represents a deviation from the expected norm.

Kuhr and Paneth (1982) studied 135 consecutively born, healthy newborns. Among the breastfed infants, jaundice (defined as a total serum bilirubin level greater than 10 mg/dl in the first four days of life) occurred with greater frequency than among the bottle-fed babies. In a subset of 44 breastfed infants, the investigators examined the effect of complementary glucose water feedings on likelihood and severity of jaundice. As the volume of glucose water intake increased, estimated breastmilk intake declined, prompting the authors to speculate that, because sugar water provides fewer calories for infants, it may contribute to impaired hepatic clearance of bilirubin. Kuhr and Paneth suggest that breastfeeding may not have been the reason that the infants were jaundiced; instead, glucose water supplementation may have been the culprit.

Because prevention of dehydration and thus jaundice is the reason usually given by physicians for ordering supplements or by nurses for giving them, it seems logical from these data to reexamine routine practices, especially glucose water supplements, in hospital and nursery guidelines (Zimmerman & Bernstein, 1996) and in medical and nursing school teaching programs.

Routine Therapy for Early-Onset Jaundice

Current recommendations regarding early-onset jaundice are simple: observe and encourage early, frequent breastfeeding. (Characteristics of early-onset jaundice are summarized in Box 12–1.) Previous therapy for early-onset jaundice has, unfortunately, included interrupting breastfeeding, an action that in most cases is both unnecessary and introduces other negative consequences, including early breastfeeding termination (Elander & Lindberg, 1986; Kemper et al., 1989) and the use of phototherapy. Although exposing the infant's skin to light in the blue range of 460- to 480-nm wavelength appears to break down the bilirubin and render it water-soluble, such therapy is not without risks. Because blue light can damage the cornea and possibly the retina, the baby's eyes must be covered during light therapy (Fig. 12–1). Body-wrap phototherapy may solve this problem, but it may also increase sweat losses. Because the baby tends to sweat under the lights, dehydration can occur, particularly if the baby is left under the lights for long periods. Furthermore, in the absence of phototherapy, serum bilirubin levels drop of their own accord, thereby calling into question the necessity of additional hospitalization to perform phototherapy. In the first week of life, in healthy, full-term infants who are feeding well and voiding regularly, there is no scientific justification for instituting phototherapy for serum bilirubin levels of less than 20 mg/dl (Oski, 1992). Levels between 20 and 25 mg/dl warrant careful assessment of the infant before using phototherapy. Lethargy, poor feeding, and infrequent stooling may contribute to a relatively rapid rise in serum bilirubin concentrations. Under such circumstances, phototherapy may slow the rise; however, improving the baby's feeding pattern is also necessary to increase the frequency of stooling and to break the cycle of continued lethargy.

The preceding discussion relates to continuous phototherapy. Dodd (1993) suggests that intermittent phototherapy, a practice used in the United Kingdom, is as effective as continuous therapy but without the attendant risks of the latter.

Martinez et al. (1993) compared four treatment options in 125 breastfeeding newborns whose serum bilirubin levels exceeded 17 mg/dl by day 3 or 4. The babies were randomized to one of four groups:

group 1: continue breastfeeding and observe
group 2: interrupt breastfeeding and feed formula
group 3: interrupt breastfeeding, feed formula, and administer phototherapy
group 4: continue breastfeeding and administer phototherapy

Serum bilirubin levels dropped most rapidly in group 3, followed by groups 4, 2, and 1, in that order. Most of the infants in each group experienced declines in bilirubin concentrations during the study period. Martinez et al. (1993, p. 472) concluded that "the majority of infants require no intervention and can safely be observed. . . . If a decision is made to intervene, the parents can be given a number of options and can make an informed decision regarding which intervention they prefer."

The American Academy of Pediatrics (AAP, 1994) has reviewed management practices for healthy, full-term newborns with hyperbilirubinemia and suggests observation and careful consideration of the need for nonhuman milk feedings and phototherapy.

Incipient Vulnerable Child Syndrome: One Cost of Overdiagnosis

Rarely has consideration been given to the possible effects of routine treatment for jaundice other than its effect on the bilirubin concentrations. Kemper, Forsyth, and McCarthy (1989, 1990) asked whether the benefits of such treatments might contribute to psychosocial and parenting risks that were previously ignored–risks that they labeled as *incipient vulnerable child syndrome*. In their matched sample of 124 control mothers and 85 mothers whose infants were diagnosed as jaundiced, they found that the mothers of the jaundiced babies were significantly more likely to consider the diagnosis of jaundice as moderately to very serious. This was especially true if the babies had received phototherapy to reduce the bilirubin levels. In addition, as late as one month after discharge, the mothers of the jaundiced babies were not sure that their babies had

| BOX 12–1 |

Characteristics of Early-Onset Jaundice

Affects nearly all newborns

Manifests itself after 24 hours of age

Peaks on the third or fourth day of life

Usually declines steadily through the first month to normal levels

May be more obvious in all infants whose feeding is limited in frequency or duration and with whom nonmilk complements or supplements are used

Is self-limiting in a healthy, full-term infant

Requires no intervention in the majority of infants

recovered. More than twice as many mothers of jaundiced infants had stopped breastfeeding, compared with the breastfeeding termination rate among the control group of mothers whose babies were *not* diagnosed as jaundiced. Obviously, new mothers need better instruction and reassurance. In addition, the decision to use phototherapy must be reassessed.

Interruption of breastfeeding as a treatment for jaundice also played a role in breastfeeding rates at one month. Those infants who experienced an interruption of breastfeeding were only half as likely to be nursing one month after birth if they were diagnosed with jaundice. In those babies with no diagnosis of jaundice, breastfeeding interruption

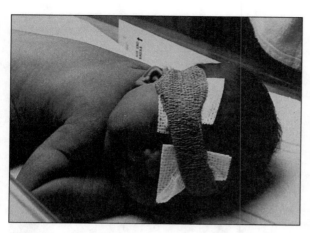

FIGURE 12–1. Phototherapy for jaundice. *The baby's eyes must be covered during light therapy for jaundice.*

resulted in a 40 percent reduction in breastfeeding likelihood at one month.

In addition, the authors found differences between the groups in the frequency with which the mothers sought health care. More than twice as many mothers with jaundiced babies made more than two "well child" visits within the first month and more than one "sick visit" in that same period. Mothers of jaundiced babies were more than five times as likely as control mothers to have used an emergency room for a problem unrelated to jaundice in the baby's first month of life and not to have left their babies in the care of someone else, even another adult family member.

By six months after birth, the mothers of jaundiced babies were still more than twice as likely as control mothers to have used emergency-room care for their baby, but they were also much more likely than the mothers in the control group to have left their babies for 48 hours (Kemper et al., 1990). The authors suggest that separating a mother from her baby or interrupting breastfeeding to treat a self-limiting condition must be considered a risk with potentially significant negative consequences. Does overconcern in the early neonatal period result in an apparent reduction of concern in the postneonatal period—perhaps as a reaction to the stress of the diagnosis and the parental perceptions of vulnerability it engenders? Correction of these perceptions could greatly reduce costs of care for these infants.

James et al. (1993) found that the location of the babies' treatment also influenced the likelihood of discontinuation of breastfeeding. In their study, interruption of breastfeeding occurred nearly five times more frequently when the babies were in the hospital than when they were at home. The authors suggested that phototherapy was safe, far less costly, and harbored fewer side effects at home (Woodall & Karas, 1992) than in the hospital.

In addition to the psychosocial costs of a diagnosis of, and subsequent treatment for, jaundice, other investigators question whether routine evaluations or interventions are appropriate, suggesting that they may be an unnecessary use of increasingly scarce health care funds. Newman et al. (1990) examined the medical records of nearly 2,500 infants born at the University of California, San Francisco. They found that 447 (18 percent) of the babies born between 1980 and 1982 met the standard criteria for "nonphysiologic" hyperbilirubinemia; in 214 (48 percent) of these, no cause of the jaundice was identified. On the basis of their examination, the investigators made five recommendations for determining when blood work for infants is necessary (Box 12–2). The criteria recognize the effect of both feeding method and racial or ethnic heritage; they are aimed at avoiding trauma to the infant and saving the high cost of testing infants who do not actually need these expensive tests, the results of which will yield no useful information.

Late-Onset Jaundice

In an infant with late-onset jaundice, serum bilirubin concentrations characteristically decline in the first week and then rise again, often climbing well above the level at which early-onset jaundice usually peaks. Late-onset jaundice is generally defined as a serum bilirubin concentration exceeding 10 mg/dl in the third week of life (Clarkson et al., 1984; Winfield & MacFaul, 1978). Approximately 2 to 4 percent of all full-term, healthy, breastfeeding non-Asian neonates will exhibit this condition, which is sometimes called *breastmilk jaundice*. Usually, breastfed infants with late-onset jaundice will have had earlier higher serum bilirubin levels than breastfeeding infants of the same age who do not exhibit late-onset jaundice. One study has shown that some normal, healthy, breastfeeding

BOX 12–2

Determining the Need for Laboratory Evaluation of Hyperbilirubinemia

1. If a newborn requires transfusion, search for evidence of hemolysis in the event that the infant shows signs of early-onset jaundice.

2. If a newborn is 24 hours of age or older and has a high bilirubin level, do follow-up tests, taking into account both racial origin and feeding experience. According to 1994 AAP guidelines for treating high bilirubin levels, a full-term, healthy infant is defined according to the following ages and bilirubin levels:

INFANT'S AGE	CONSIDER PHOTOTHERAPY	PHOTOTHERAPY	EXCHANGE TRANSFUSION (IF PHOTOTHERAPY FAILS)
25–48 hr	≥ 12 mg/dl	≥ 15 mg/dl	≥ 20 mg/dl
49–72 hr	≥ 15 mg/dl	≥ 18 mg/dl	≥ 25 mg/dl
> 72 hr	≥ 17 mg/dl	≥ 20 mg/dl	≥ 25 mg/dl

3. If an infant is not anemic and the Coombs test is negative, there is little justification for ordering additional tests.

4. If bilirubin levels continue to rise, it is important to attempt to identify the cause.

5. If an infant is seven days old or older, shows signs of illness, and the jaundice is prolonged, check a direct bilirubin to rule out cholestasis.

6. Avoid direct bilirubin tests otherwise; they are neither helpful nor cost-effective in evaluating jaundice in full-term newborns.

Source: Derived from Newman TB, et al: Laboratory evaluation of jaundice in newborns: frequency, cost & yield. Am J Dis Child 144:364–68, 1990.

infants will have elevated bilirubin levels through the sixteenth day of life. The only difference between these babies and other breastfeeding infants in the study was the levels of bilirubin in the baby's blood and the mother's milk. The authors noted that the babies with high serum bilirubin levels into the third week of life (36 percent of the sample) did not differ from the babies with low serum bilirubin levels with regard to infant age, maternal age, or frequency of breastfeeding per day. The findings from this study imply that elevated bilirubin levels are more likely to be a normal (though as yet incompletely understood) consequence of adjustment to extrauterine life rather than an indication of a potentially serious pathological process that requires intervention (Alonso et al., 1991).

Grunebaum et al. (1991) followed a sample of infants for five years and identified no neurodevelopmental delays or hearing problems in the

BOX 12–3

Characteristics of Late-Onset Jaundice

Affects a very small percentage of breastfed infants

Excludes all pathological causes of jaundice

Infant is thriving, healthy, and gaining weight

Manifests itself in the second week of life

Peaks around the tenth day of life or later

Bilirubin levels remain elevated for some time

Bilirubin levels drop rapidly if other milk is provided along with, or as a temporary substitute for, the mother's milk

Often manifests itself in siblings of the index infant

Requires no intervention in most cases

weight appropriately. Thus the diagnosis of benign late-onset neonatal jaundice is often made after ruling out other explanations for late elevations of serum bilirubin. Characteristics of late-onset jaundice are summarized in Box 12–3.

Investigators have also examined the variability of fat content in human milk. Bevan and Holton (1972) reported that the milk from mothers whose babies had late-onset jaundice inhibited conjugation by the liver and that this inhibition was caused by the free fatty acid concentrations in the milk after refrigeration. However, Odievre and Luzeau (1978, 1982), Odievre et al. (1973), and others (Bevan & Holton, 1972; Hargreaves, 1973) reported that when fresh, unrefrigerated milk from mothers of jaundiced infants was examined, no concentrations of free fatty acids were evident.

The higher fat content in some mothers' milk may be a risk factor for late-onset jaundice, according to Amato et al. (1985). These researchers found that the milk from mothers of babies with hyperbilirubinemia had significantly higher cream content than did the milk from mothers of babies without hyperbilirubinemia. Although elevated serum bilirubin concentrations may continue for several weeks, this finding is not sufficient to warrant the interruption of breastfeeding. In nearly all cases, serum bilirubin concentrations will continue to decline slowly over many weeks, eventually plateauing at the normal adult level of 1 mg/dl. Generally, the likelihood is high that all children of the same mother will exhibit a similar pattern of bilirubin concentration if breastfed.

Clinical Implications

Most infants have elevated serum bilirubin levels in the first week of life. Although a wide variety of variables has been linked to the likelihood of elevated serum bilirubin, including some over which the clinician has no control, many hospital routines also have been implicated, particularly those governing frequency and duration of feeding (Box 12–4).

It is appropriate for the clinician to examine those routines that contribute to hyperbilirubinemia (Auerbach, 1992). Whenever hyperbilirubinemia manifests itself in the first day of life, pathological jaundice should be suspected, and steps should be taken to identify the cause in order to effect

children who had elevated neonatal bilirubin levels. Further, they found no difference in bilirubin levels when comparing those infants for whom breastfeeding was interrupted with those who continued breastfeeding.

Correctly identifying late-onset jaundice first requires that all other causes be ruled out. Obvious causes include organic and functional problems, such as intestinal obstruction, hemolytic disease, hypothyroidism, and transient familial neonatal hyperbilirubinemia (Gartner & Auerbach, 1987). In addition, the infant with late-onset jaundice should be evaluated to determine whether he is thriving, vigorous, and healthy, and is gaining

BOX 12–4

Hospital Routines and Their Effects on the Neonate

HOSPITAL ROUTINES	EFFECT OF ROUTINES ON THE NEONATE
Limited or infrequent feedings	Slowed gastrointestinal tract motility
	Reduced stooling
	Greater frequency, volume of supplementary feedings
	Greater weight loss
	Higher bilirubin levels
Sterile water and glucose feedings	Caloric deprivation, contributory to "starvation-induced" jaundice
	Muting of thirst response
	Reduced neonatal interest in feeding
	Slowed weight gain
	Reduced breastmilk intake
	Slowed bilirubin clearance
	Higher bilirubin levels
Separation of mother and baby	Reduced satisfaction with hospital care
	Increased likelihood of supplementation
	Shorter breastfeeding duration
Phototherapy for jaundice	Increased risk of dehydration
	Separation of mother and baby
	Increased length of hospital stay
	Increased costs of hospitalization
	Shorter breastfeeding duration
	Abnormal caregiving patterns
	Enhanced likelihood of Incipient Vulnerable Child syndrome
	Greater frequency of use of expensive health care facilities after hospitalization.
	Questionable benefit in reducing bilirubin levels
	Shorter breastfeeding duration
Laboratory evaluations	Overall higher cost of hospital care
	More frequent use of additional laboratory test
	Limited benefit for the majority of cases
	Increased parental anxiety

BOX 12–5

Assessing the Relationship of Feeding to Jaundice

1. How often is the infant being put to breast? The total number of such episodes in each 24-hour period, as well as the duration of each episode, should be noted.

2. Is the baby suckling when put to breast? Active suckling should be noted; in particular, the pattern and frequency of swallowing should be recorded.

3. Has the baby begun stooling, and if so, how frequently is this occurring? Early stooling that does not continue may be an early indication of inadequate intake, particularly of a calorically dense fluid such as milk. If stooling is occurring, note the color and explain to the mother how she can verify through changes in stool color that the baby is obtaining milk from the breast.

4. Is the baby receiving complementary or supplementary feedings? Fluids offered after breastfeedings and fluids offered in lieu of breastfeedings may contribute to serious breastfeeding problems; they should be avoided. If additional fluid is deemed medically necessary, the fluid should contain as many calories as does human milk to avoid starvation-induced jaundice from insufficient caloric intake.

5. Is the mother encouraged to nurse her infant at night? To ensure frequent feedings, the lactating mother and her breastfeeding infant should have ample opportunities to breastfeed throughout the 24-hour day.

Source: Derived from KG Auerbach, LM Gartner: Breastfeeding and human milk: their association with jaundice in the neonate. Clin Perinatol 14:89–107, 1987.

---

appropriate treatment while avoiding unnecessary overtreatment. The breastfeeding mother and baby should be observed carefully and helped to begin breastfeeding so that frequent, effective feedings occur. If the baby is feeding poorly or is exhibiting lethargy, supplementation at the breast may be used to break the cycle of lethargy, poor feeding, climbing serum bilirubin concentrations, and more lethargy, which can result in symptoms of jaundice (Auerbach, 1986). The relationship of feeding to jaundice can be assessed using a battery of questions designed to elicit pertinent information (Box 12–5). For most breastfed babies, early-onset jaundice will peak on the fourth or fifth day, to be followed by a gradual decline in serum bilirubin levels as they approach the normal adult level of 1 mg/dl.

To appropriately assess the baby's serum bilirubin levels, the race of the infant and his parents should be noted. In the case of a Native American infant or a baby of Mediterranean extraction, a test for glucose 6-phosphate dehydrogenase should be requested.

Supplemental feedings of sterile water or glucose are not indicated. If the baby is administered phototherapy (which is rarely needed), the mother should be urged to offer feedings frequently, at least every two hours, to reduce the likelihood of dehydration. In situations in which mother and baby are still hospitalized, mobile phototherapy

Table 12–2

CLINICAL CARE PLAN FOR PHYSIOLOGICAL JAUNDICE

NURSING DIAGNOSIS: Deficit of maternal knowledge about physiological jaundice

Case notes: A two-day-old white male neonate has a total bilirubin concentration of 8 mg/dl. At three days, the level is 13 mg/dl. The infant's skin about his head has a yellow cast when pressed above the nose and on the forehead; the rest of his body remains pink. The baby has been vigorous since birth and is breastfeeding effectively. The parents are concerned that "something might be wrong with our baby."

Assessment	Goals	Intervention	Rationale
Bilirubin rising 5 mg/day	Maintain lactation	Increase number of breastfeedings (q3h at night; q2h during day)	Milk intake stimulates bilirubin excretion
Yellowish cast confined to head	Reduce bilirubin levels	Discourage water and glucose feedings	Increase caloric intake
		Place infant near natural light	Natural light breaks down unconjugated bilirubin
Baby alert and vigorous	Prevent neuro complications	Obtain serum bilirubin q24h until levels decline	
		Observe for irritability or lethargy	
Sucking effectively	Maintain adequate hydration	Monitor number of wet diapers and stools (color, consistency)	
Breastfeeding ad lib until satiation 8–12 times/24 hr.		Observe for swallowing during feedings	
Parents express concern, confusion, anxiety about baby's status	Provide emotional support	Explain reason for jaundice and its benign nature	Teaching basic facts about jaundice fosters understanding and relieves unvoiced parental guilt feelings
		Reassure that lactation can and should continue	
		Encourage parents to express their concerns	Verbalization reduces anxiety
		Assure parents that baby's skin color will return to normal	
		Reassure parents that jaundice is not caused by anything they did or did not do; it is a normal occurrence of early neonatal life	

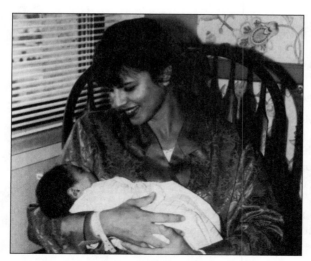

FIGURE 12–2. Neonatal jaundice. *Interruption of breast-feeding is rarely necessary. (Courtesy Debi Leslie Bocar.)*

units placed in the mother's room will enable frequent feeding and more careful monitoring of the baby than occurs in busy nurseries, where crying babies tend to receive the most attention. Body-wrap phototherapy may facilitate mother-baby contact and may enable the baby to receive such treatment at home (Schuman & Karush, 1992).

For the small percentage of infants with late-onset jaundice, organic or functional causes must first be ruled out. If the infant is thriving, frequent monitoring of serum bilirubin levels is recommended to discern whether the levels remain within an acceptable range. Caution dictates that the risk of brain damage be minimized through careful monitoring and intervention in those situations in which serum bilirubin concentrations significantly exceed 20 mg/dl.

With early discharge (within 48 hours of birth), peak bilirubin levels occur while the infant is at home (Brown, 1992). In most cases, the concentra-tion of serum bilirubin will peak and then decline while the baby continues to breastfeed. Discreet observation of the infant and continued support of and reassurance to the mother are all that are necessary. In rare situations in which concentrations of serum bilirubin continue to climb to levels above a 25 or even 30 mg/dl in healthy, full-term infants, a brief period of breastfeeding supplementation may be helpful, but the need for such intervention is rare (Gartner, 1994). Such supplementation can occur at the breast using a feeding-tube device such as the Supplemental Nutrition System (SNS). The addition of such supplemental milk will result in a decline in concentrations of serum bilirubin. When the mother prefers to give her baby only her own milk in the face of significant rises of serum bilirubin concentrations which are suggestive of late-onset jaundice, her expressed milk should be heated to 56°C for 15 minutes and then cooled to body temperature prior to being offered to the baby in a bottle or cup. Such heat treatment appears to alter the milk, so that concentrations of serum bilirubin are reduced.

If the mother prefers to interrupt breastfeeding for 24 to 48 hours and to give the baby some other milk from a bottle, this too will result in a decline in concentrations of serum bilirubin. After such a brief interruption, unsupplemented breastfeeding can continue. An initial small rebound response will occur, followed by gradually declining concentrations of bilirubin. Interrupting breastfeeding even for a few feedings is rarely needed and is discouraged, because other methods of management will usually suffice (Fig. 12–2 and Table 12–2). These measures are not needed in an otherwise healthy, full-term infant unless bilirubin concentrations exceed 20 mg/dl prior to three days of age or 25 mg/dl after three days.

SUMMARY

Jaundice in the newborn, in most cases, is an exaggeration of a normal physiological process that can be managed conservatively and is not a contraindication to breastfeeding. If we understand the normal physiological process and intervene only when absolutely necessary, there is no contraindication to the neonate's consumption of human milk, either by direct suckling at the breast or by tube feeding for those who may be too small or too young to suckle.

Breastfeeding should never be interrupted because of a diagnosis of "physiological" jaundice and should only rarely be interrupted for pathological jaundice. Even in the presence of jaundice that is believed to be brought about by the breast-milk itself, there is no reason to wean the baby. Breastfeeding should be strongly encouraged for all mothers and all babies.

REFERENCES

Adams JA, Hey DJ, Hall RT: Incidence of hyperbilirubinemia in breast- vs. formula-fed infants. *Clin Pediatr* 24:69–73, 1985.

Alonso EM, et al: Enterohepatic circulation of nonconjugated bilirubin in rats fed with human milk. *J Pediatr* 118:425–30, 1991.

Amato M, Howald H, von Muralt G: Fat content of human milk and breast milk jaundice. *Acta Paediatr Scand* 74:805–6, 1985.

American Academy of Pediatrics Provisional Committee for Quality Improvement and Subcommittee on Hyperbilirubinemia. Practice parameter: management of hyperbilirubinemia in the healthy term newborn. *Pediatrics* 94:558–65, 1994.

Auerbach KG: Supportive management of the jaundiced breastfeeding infant. *Rental Roundup* 3:5–6, 1986.

Auerbach KG: When treatment for jaundice undermines breastfeeding. *Contemp Pediatr* 9:105–6, 1992.

Auerbach KG, Gartner LM: Breastfeeding and human milk: their association with jaundice in the neonate. *Clin Perinatol* 14:89–107, 1987.

Bernbaum JC, et al: Enhanced growth and gastrointestinal function in premature infants given non-nutritive sucking. *Pediatr Res* 15:650, 1981.

Bevan BR, Holton JB: Inhibition of bilirubin conjugation in rat liver slices by free fatty acids, with relevance to the problem of breast milk jaundice. *Clin Chim Acta* 41:101–7, 1972.

Bracci R, et al: Epidemiologic study of neonatal jaundice: a survey of contributing factors. *Acta Paediatr Scand* Suppl. 360:87–92, 1989.

Brown AK: Hyperbilirubinemia in black infants: role of glucose-6-phosphate dehydrogenase deficiency. *Clin Pediatr* 31:712–5, 1992.

Brown LP: Breastfeeding and jaundice: cause for concern? *Clin Iss Perin Wom Health Nurs.* 3:615–19, 1992.

Brown LP, et al: Incidence and pattern of jaundice in healthy breast-fed infants during the first month of life. *Nurs Res* 42:108–10, 1993.

Butler DA, MacMillan JP: Relationship of breast feeding and weight loss to jaundice in the newborn period: review of the literature and results of a study. *Cleve Clin Q* 50:263–6, 1983.

Cavell B: Gastric emptying in infants fed human milk or infant formula. *Acta Paediatr Scand* 70:639–41, 1981.

Clarkson JE, Cowan JO, Herbison GP: Jaundice in full term healthy neonates–a population study. *Aust Paediatr J* 20:303–8, 1984.

Dahms BB, et al: Breast feeding and serum bilirubin values during the first 4 days of life. *J Pediatr* 83:1049–54, 1973.

De Carvalho M, Hall M, Harvey D: Effects of water supplementation on physiological jaundice in breastfed babies. *Arch Dis Child* 56:568–9, 1981.

De Carvalho M, Klaus MH, Merkatz RB: Frequency of breast-feeding and serum bilirubin concentration. *Am J Dis Child* 136:737–8, 1982.

De Carvalho M, Robertson S, Klaus M: Fecal bilirubin excretion and serum bilirubin concentrations in breast-fed and bottle-fed infants. *J Pediatr* 107:786–90, 1985.

Dodd KL: Neonatal jaundice: a lighter touch. *Arch Dis Child* 68:529–32, 1993.

Elander G, Lindberg T: Hospital routines in infants with hyperbilirubinemia influence the duration of breast feeding. *Acta Paediatr Scand* 75:708–12, 1986.

Fischer AF, et al: Comparison of bilirubin production in Japanese and Caucasian infants. *J Pediatr Gastroenterol Nutr* 7:27–9, 1988.

Gartner LM: Management of jaundice in the well baby. *Pediatrics* 89:826–7, 1992.

Gartner LM: Neonatal jaundice. *Pediatr Rev* 15:422–32, 1994.

Gartner LM, Auerbach KG: Breast milk and breastfeeding jaundice. *Advances Pediatr* 34:249–74, 1987.

Gartner LM, et al: Development of bilirubin transport and metabolism in the newborn rhesus monkey. *J Pediatr* 90:513–31, 1977.

Glover J, Sandilands M: Supplementation of breastfeeding infants and weight loss in hospital. *J Hum Lact* 6:163–6, 1990.

Grunebaum E, et al: Breast milk jaundice: natural history, familial incidence and late neurodevelopmental outcome of the infant. *Eur J Pediatr* 150:267–70, 1991.

Hall RT, et al: Hyperbilirubinemia in breast-versus formula-fed infants in the first six weeks of life: relationship to weight gain. *Am J Perinatol* 1:47–51, 1983.

Hargreaves T: Effect of fatty acids on bilirubin conjugation. *Arch Dis Child* 48:446–50, 1973.

Hodgman JE, Edwards N: Racial differences in neonatal jaundice: hyperbilirubinemia in Hispanic infants: a survey. *Clin Pediatr* 31:719–22, 1992.

Horiguchi T, Bauer C: Ethnic differences in neonatal jaundice: comparison of Japanese and Caucasian newborn infants. *Am J Obstet Gynecol* 121:71–4, 1975.

Ince Z, et al: Breast milk ß-glucuronidase and prolonged jaundice in the neonate. *Acta Paediatr* 84:237–9, 1995.

James JM, et al: Discontinuation of breast-feeding infrequent among jaundiced neonates treated at home. *Pediatrics* 92:153–5, 1993.

Johnson JD: Jaundice in Navajo neonates. *Clin Pediatr* 31:716–8, 1992.

Kemper K, Forsyth B, McCarthy P: Jaundice, terminating breast-feeding, and the vulnerable child. *Pediatrics* 84:773–8, 1989.

Kemper KJ, Forsyth BW, McCarthy PL: Persistent perceptions of vulnerability following neonatal jaundice. *Am J Dis Child* 144:238–41, 1990.

Kivlahan C, James EJP: The natural history of neonatal jaundice. *Pediatrics* 74:364–70, 1984.

Kotagal UR, Tsang RC: Impact of early discharge on newborns. *J Pediatr Gastroenterol Nutr* 22:402–4, 1996.

Kuhr M, Paneth N: Feeding practices and early neonatal jaundice. *J Pediatr Gastroenterol Nutr* 1:485–8, 1982.

Laws HF: Caloric deprivation questioned in breast milk jaundice [letter]. *Pediatrics* 67:748–9, 1981.

Maisels MJ, Gifford K: Neonatal jaundice in full-term infants: role of breast-feeding and other causes. *Am J Dis Child* 137:561–2, 1983.

Maisels MJ, Newman TB: Kernicterus in otherwise healthy, breast-fed term newborns. *Pediatrics* 96:730–3, 1995.

Maisels MJ, et al: Jaundice in the healthy newborn infant: a new approach to an old problem. *Pediatrics* 81:505–11, 1988.

Maisels MJ, et al: The effect of breast-feeding frequency on serum bilirubin levels. *Am J Obstet Gynecol* 170:880–3, 1994.

Martinez JC, et al: Hyperbilirubinemia in the breastfed newborn: a controlled trial of four interventions. *Pediatrics* 91:470–3, 1993.

McDonagh AF: Is bilirubin good for you? *Clin Perinatol* 17:359–69, 1990.

Newman TB, et al: Laboratory evaluation of jaundice in newborns: frequency, cost, and yield. *Am J Dis Child* 144:364–8, 1990.

Newman TB, Maisels MJ: Evaluation and treatment of jaundice in the term newborn: a kinder, gentler approach. *Pediatrics* 89:809–18, 1992.

Nicoll A, Ginsburg R, Tripp JH: Supplementary feeding and jaundice in newborns. *Acta Paediatr Scand* 71:759–61, 1982.

Odievre M, et al: Effect of fatty acids on bilirubin conjugation. *Arch Dis Child* 48:984, 1973.

Odievre M, Luzeau R: Lipolytic activity in milk from mothers of unjaundiced infants. *Acta Paediatr Scand* 67:49–52, 1978.

Odievre M, Luzeau R: More on breast-milk jaundice [letter]. *J Pediatr* 100:671–2, 1982.

Osborn LM, Reiff MI, Bolus R: Jaundice in the full-term neonate. *Pediatrics* 73:520–5, 1985.

Oski FA: Hyperbilirubinemia in the term infant: an unjaundiced approach. *Contemp Pediatr* 9:148–54, 1992.

Rubaltelli FF: Unconjugated and conjugated bilirubin pigments during perinatal development: IV.

The influence of breast-feeding on neonatal hyperbilirubinemia. *Biol Neonate* 64:104–9, 1993.

Saland J, McNamara H, Cohen MI: Navajo jaundice: a variant of neonatal hyperbilirubinemia associated with breastfeeding. *J Pediatr* 85:271–5, 1974.

Schuman AJ, Karush G: Fiberoptic vs. conventional home photo therapy for neonatal hyperbilirubinemia. *Clin Pediatr* 31:345–52, 1992.

Taitz LS, Byers HD: High calorie osmolar feeding and hypertonic dehydration. *Arch Dis Child* 57:257–60, 1972.

Tomamasa T, et al: Gastroduodenal motility in neonates: response to human milk compared with cow's milk formula. *Pediatrics* 80:434–8, 1987.

Weaver LT, Ewing G, Taylor LC: The bowel habit of milk-fed infants. *J Pediatr Gastroenterol Nutr* 7:568–71, 1988.

Winfield CR, MacFaul R: Clinical study of prolonged jaundice in breast- and bottle-fed babies. *Arch Dis Child* 53:506–7, 1978.

Woodall D, Karas JG: A new light on jaundice: a pilot study. *Clin Pediatr* 31:353–6, 1992.

Zimmerman DR, Bernstein WR: Standing feeding orders in a well-baby nursery: "Water, water everywhere . . ." *J Hum Lact* 12:189–92, 1996.

Breast Pumps and Other Technologies

Marsha Walker and Kathleen G. Auerbach

Special devices have been used for hundreds of years to help breastfeeding mothers to overcome various problems. Examples of someone, or something, other than a baby removing milk from the breasts are cited in medical literature as early as the mid-1500s (Fildes, 1986). Before breast pumps or other instruments were used to withdraw milk from the breasts, children, young puppies, or birth attendants were enlisted to do the job. By the 1500s, the medical literature included discussions of "sucking glasses." These devices allowed women to remove milk themselves and were recommended for relieving engorgement or expressing milk when the nipples were damaged or when mastitis was present. Sucking glasses were also thought to help evert flat and inverted nipples. For the most part, vacuum was generated by mouth, and the devices were made of glass (Fig. 13–1). Women could use a glass, glass vial, or glass bottle heated with very hot water and applied to the breast to draw out milk. French breast pumps in the 1700s resembled smoking pipes but were made of different materials.

As technology advanced, so did breast pump materials and design. Combinations of such materials as brass, wood, glass, and rubber were used to make pumps like the syringe pump (Fig. 13–2), the long-handled lever pump (Fig. 13–3) and the glass and rubber "bicycle horn" pump, all c. 1830. The reasons that women chose to express milk also changed. Today women express their milk for short periods to solve acute problems and for extended periods to continue to provide human milk for their babies while they are employed or following a preterm birth. Although much of this chapter focuses on mechanical means of obtaining milk from the breasts, many of the recommendations for optimal pumping apply as well to hand expression. Thus when we use the term *expression,* we refer to obtaining milk by hand and mechanical techniques. Additional discussion of hand expression can be found in Chapter 10.

Concerns of Mothers

Most mothers want a pump that works efficiently and comfortably and at a reasonable cost. They want pumps that are easily available and easy to use and clean. The amount of milk expressed and the time it takes to obtain it are the two issues most frequently mentioned by mothers when they are choosing or using a breast pump.

Satisfaction with breast pumps, however, is highly individual. In an informal survey of more than 200 mothers, a pump was rated highly if it

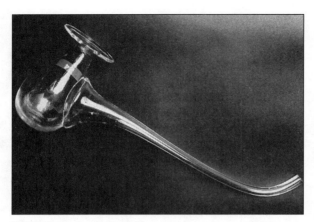

FIGURE 13–1. An American sucking glass, c. 1870.

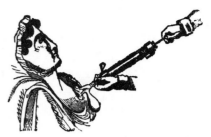

Where the breast is hard, swollen and painful, from inflammation, or the nipple sore from excoriation, the application of this instrument is attended with more ease to the patient than any other means, and she may without difficulty use it herself, by which she can regulate its action agreeably to her own sensations. The flat surface of the glass should be smeared with oil before it is put on, and the bulb preserved in a dependant position to receive the fluid. During the operation the small aperture in the brass socket must be closely covered with the finger, which being removed, admits air into the glass and causes it to be detached from the breast whenever it may be desired.

FIGURE 13–2. Expressing the breasts with a syringe pump, c. 1830.

(1) worked quickly (less than 20 minutes total), (2) obtained two or more ounces of milk from each breast, and (3) did not cause pain. The mothers in this survey suggested pumping techniques to speed the process and to increase the volume of milk per pumping session. Many mothers expressed the most milk before or after the first morning feeding, when their breasts were reported to be fullest (and intra-mammary pressure was the highest); later volumes steadily decreased throughout the day. Many mothers mentioned that if they were not relaxed or if they were uncomfortable or felt rushed, their output dropped by one-third to one-half the usual amount.

The majority of mothers used one or more techniques to increase pumping efficiency. The two most frequently mentioned techniques were eliciting the milk-ejection reflex before starting to pump and massaging the breast while pumping. Both techniques increased pumping speed and milk output. Some mothers were able to double the amount pumped by using both of these techniques at each pumping session.

Stimulating the Milk-Ejection Reflex

Much of the research and literature in the dairy industry supports the importance of eliciting the milk-ejection reflex before starting to express milk. Premilking stimulation of the udder increases serum oxytocin levels (Merrill et al., 1987) and results in shorter "machine-on" time and a higher average rate of milk flow (Dodd & Griffin, 1977; Goodman & Grosvenor, 1983; Gorewit et al., 1983;

Sagi et al., 1980). In the second edition of *Dairy Science,* Petersen (1950) cited five factors that contribute to poor milking: undue excitement at milking time, improper stimulation for the let-down of milk, too long an interval between stimulation of let-down and the beginning of milking, too slow milking, and incomplete withdrawal of milk. His observations regarding proper milking techniques parallel many recommendations of professionals and the expression techniques mothers have discovered on their own. Women are not the same as cows; nevertheless, animal models of lactation provide a frame of reference from which similarities can be drawn and applied. For example, Petersen (1950) recommended certain guidelines that can apply to breastmilk expression:

1. *Avoid undue excitement at milking time.* Many women use specific relaxation techniques and visual imagery before and during pumping. Feher et al. (1989) reported using a guided relaxation audiotape to increase milk output during breast pumping among mothers of preterm infants. Newton and Newton (1948) described the adverse effect of a painful or dis-

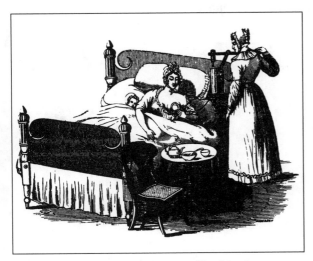

FIGURE 13–3. Expressing breastmilk with a long-handled lever pump, c. 1830.

tracting stimulus during nursing on the milk-ejection reflex.

2. *Elicit the milk-ejection reflex first, one to two minutes before pumping begins; massaging with a hot, wet cloth before milking is the most effective stimulus for let-down.* Mothers have reported using hot compresses, showers, and breast massage before expressing to obtain the best results. Some report that they are most successful if they pump one side while the baby feeds on the other breast (as with pumping in dairy cattle when all teats are milked simultaneously), if the baby elicits the milk-ejection reflex first and they then pump, or if they hand-express first and then pump the breasts.

3. *Massage each quarter of the udder during mechanical milking.* Massaging during breast pumping can markedly increase milk yield. Breast massage may increase fat content and milk yield when a baby is at breast. Bowles et al. (1987) and Stutte et al. (1988) found that infants gained greater amounts of weight and mothers experienced little nipple pain or painful engorgement when the breasts were massaged by quadrant in an alternating pattern with the baby's suckling bursts.

4. *When hand-milking, avoid point compression and digging in with the fingertips, which is likely to cause injury.* The Marmet method of hand expression (Marmet & Shell, 1979) cautioned against this technique when a mother is hand-expressing her milk.

5. *Remove the milking machine as soon as the milk stops flowing.* Stopping the pump when the milk stops flowing reduces tissue injury. Many mothers switch to the other breast when the milk flow slows in the breast being pumped. Some mothers mention that pain is the cue for this switch, indicating a change in the pressure gradient. Auerbach (1990b) found that protracted pumping times did not significantly increase milk yield beyond a certain point. Those who pumped (sequentially or simultaneously) for longer than 16 minutes averaged total milk volumes of 55 ml or less.

The dairy literature includes many recommendations that are applicable to human breast pumping. Even the modern electric breast pumps designed for mothers have similarities to the agricultural milking units. The Whittlestone pump has incorporated the design of the double-chambered teat cups. The suction and rest phases of a milking unit are either 60:40 or 70:30 (percentage of suction to percentage of rest per cycle). There are usually 60 cycles generated per minute (a calf generates about 120 cycles), and negative pressure is around 375 mm Hg (similar to the pressure seen in many breast pumps, including hand pumps).

Breast pumps must also be easy to clean, affordable, and accessible. When recommending a pump, the caregiver should give a specific name and several places to find it. Hospital or medical supply houses may have pumps originally designed as chest aspirators. They are not as suitable for milk expression as those specifically designed for the purpose. Many mothers in the survey complained of the extra expense incurred if their pump broke (common with the battery pumps) and required replacement. Of 97 battery pumps used in the survey, 24 broke or stopped generating suction and had to be replaced (a 25 percent breakage rate). The life of a battery-operated pump is considered to be about 16 weeks (four months) by some companies, a much shorter period than many employed mothers require. Batteries are a major expense for mothers who pump regularly; many purchase an AC adapter to economize. The cost of the accessory kit and daily rental charges for an electric pump can be expensive, even with a long-term rental contract. Some insurance carriers and health maintenance organizations cover the cost of pump rentals only while a baby is hospitalized.

Several mothers in the survey purchased a hand pump solely to cut cost. Some were dissatisfied and purchased a second, more expensive pump that worked better. Pump prices vary considerably, depending on the type of store or organization that sells them (see Fig. 13–4). Some breastfeeding programs provide breast pumps at cost to their clients. Many hospitals give breastfeeding mothers a high-quality hand pump on discharge rather than formula packs. Box 13–1 summarizes recommendations for mothers using a breast pump.

Hormonal Considerations

When milk expression via a pump is necessary, the device must be efficient enough to activate prolactin and oxytocin release and to efficiently remove milk from the breasts.

Prolactin

A steady rise in prolactin during pregnancy prepares the breasts for lactation (Neville, 1983). Prolactin levels will only remain high after the first weeks postpartum if the baby is put to breast or in the absence of breast stimulation by an infant if milk expression mechanically maintains prolactin cycling (de Sanctis et al., 1981; Howie et al., 1980; Noel, Suh, & Frantz, 1974; Weichert, 1980; Whitworth et al., 1984). Basal prolactin levels and the magnitude of the sucking-induced rise in prolactin normally decrease over time as lactation extends beyond three to four months (Whitworth, 1988). This occurs regardless of the frequency of feeding (Battin et al., 1985; Johnston & Amico, 1986) and regardless of whether breast pump stimulation has replaced the sucking infant (Leake et al., 1983).

According to Whitworth (1988, p. 183), "Postpartum, the response threshold [of prolactin] is maintained by frequent suckling, which both releases prolactin and ensures that prolactin-

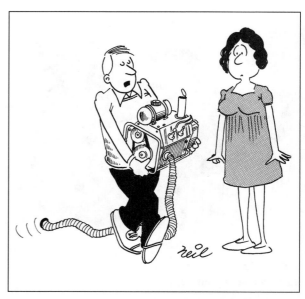

FIGURE 13–4. "They didn't actually have a breast pump . . ." *(Courtesy of Neil Matterson. © 1984, Marion Books, Wooend, Victoria, Australia.)*

release mechanisms remain responsive to future suckling stimuli." Early and frequent breast stimulation causes the mother's serum prolactin levels to rise, which in turn increases milk production. Because of this physiological sequence, the clinician should offer certain specific suggestions if the mother is using a pump during the immediate postpartum period:

- *In the absence of a baby at breast (because of prematurity, maternal or infant illness, or early separation), the breasts should be stimulated eight or more times every 24 hours.* Pumping only once or twice during the day and never at night, when prolactin levels are at their peak, is not helpful. A faltering milk supply in the following weeks may be attributed to the lack of sufficient prolactin receptors and infrequent breast stimulation while lactation is being established.

- *Prevent painful overdistention of the breasts (secondary engorgement).* As alveolar pressure rises, lactation suppression begins. Painful engorgement lasting longer than 48 hours can decrease the milk supply. Therefore, if a baby cannot keep up with a suddenly increased milk supply, the mother should express her milk. When

BOX 13–1

Recommendations for the Mother Who Expresses Her Milk

GENERAL PUMPING RECOMMENDATIONS

1. Read the instructions governing the use and cleaning of a pump before expressing milk with any product.

2. Wash hands before each pumping session.

3. Frequency: For occasional pumping, pump during, after, or between feedings, whichever gives the best results. Most mothers tend to express more milk in the morning. For mothers employed outside the home, pumping should occur on a regular basis for the number of nursings that are missed. For premature or ill babies who are not at breast, the number of pumpings should total eight or more in 24 hours. Initiation of pumping should be delayed no longer than six hours following birth unless medically indicated. This assures appropriate development and sensitivity of prolactin receptors. More frequent pumping will avoid the buildup of excessive backpressure of milk during engorgement. For more information about breast pumping following a premature birth, see Chapter 14.

4. Duration: With single-sided pumping, optimal duration is 10 to 15 minutes with an electric pump and 10 to 20 minutes with a manual pump. If double-pumping with an electric or two battery-operated pumps, 7 to 15 minutes is optimal. Encourage mothers to tailor these times to their situation.

5. Technique:
   - Elicit the milk-ejection reflex before using a pump.

- Use only as much suction as is needed to maintain milk flow.
- Massage the breast in quadrants before or during pumping to increase intra-mammary pressure.
- Allow enough time for pumping to avoid anxiety.
- Use inserts or different flanges if needed to obtain the best fit between pump and breast.
- Avoid long periods of uninterrupted vacuum.
- Stop pumping when the milk flow is minimal or has ceased.

RECOMMENDATIONS FOR SPECIFIC TYPES OF PUMPS

1. Avoid pumps that use rubber bulbs to generate vacuum.

2. Cylinder pumps:
   - When O rings are used, they must be in place for proper suction.
   - Gaskets should be removed after each use for cleaning to avoid harboring bacteria in the pump.
   - The gasket on the inner cylinder may be rolled back and forth to restore it to its original shape.
   - The pump stroke may have to be shortened as the outer cylinder fills with milk.
   - The user may need to empty the outer cylinder once or twice during pumping.
   - Hand position should be palm up with the elbow held close to the body.

3. Battery-operated pumps:
   - Use alkaline batteries.
   - Replace batteries when cycles per minute decrease.

BOX 13–1   *(cont.)*

- Interrupt vacuum frequently to avoid nipple pain and damage.
- Use an AC adapter when possible, especially if the pump generates fewer than six cycles per minute.
- Consider renting an electric pump if pumping will continue longer than one or two months.
- Use two pumps simultaneously if pumping time is limited or to increase the quantity of milk obtained.
- Choose a pump in which the vacuum can be regulated.
- Massage the breast by quadrants during pumping.

4. Semiautomatic pumps:
  - Vacuum may be easier to control if the mother does not lift her finger completely off the hole but rolls it back and forth rhythmically so that the vacuum is efficient but not painful.

5. Automatic electric pumps:
  - Use the lowest pressure setting that is efficient.
  - Use a double setup (simultaneous pumping) when time is limited, to increase milk supply and for prematurity, maternal or infant illness, or other special situations.

milk production begins in the absence of a baby, pumping frequency may need to be temporarily increased to prevent involution of the alveoli caused by the backup pressure of milk and the buildup of suppressor peptides that downregulate milk volume (Akre, 1989). Wilde et al. (1995) have named this peptide the *feedback inhibitor of lactation* (FIL).

- *Early breastfeeding has a critical period during which frequent nipple stimulation and milk removal are necessary for a plentiful milk supply in later weeks.* The clinician should offer management guidelines with this in mind, especially if mother and baby are separated. Always keep in mind Whitworth's (1988) reminder: "Postpartum, the response threshold [of prolactin] is maintained by frequent suckling, which both releases prolactin and ensures that prolactin-release mechanisms remain responsive to future suckling stimuli."

- More recently, Daly et al. (1992, 1993) have shown that *the more thoroughly the breast is drained, the more milk is made.* Daly and Hartmann (1995a, b) noted that breasts with smaller storage capacities may need to be stimulated more frequently than breasts that are

able to store more milk between feedings or expressions, even though most breasts (regardless of size) are capable of synthesizing the same amount of milk in 24 hours.

Oxytocin

Oxytocin is responsible for the milk-ejection reflex. By acting on the myoepithelial processes, oxytocin causes shortening of the ducts without constricting them, thus increasing the milk pressure. Cobo et al. (1967) measured milk ejection by recording intraductal mammary pressure using a catheter placed in a mammary duct. Values were measured at 0.19 plus or minus 0.04 in. per minute and from 0 to 25 mm Hg on recording paper. Ductal contractions last about a minute and occur at about 4 to 10 contractions every 10 minutes. Caldeyro-Barcia (1969) reported that intramammary pressure rose 10 mm Hg after five days postpartum with oxytocin release. Prolactin release occurs in impulses at about one-minute intervals (McNutley et al., 1983). Thus oxytocin release is pulsatile and variable with intermittent bursts. These pressure changes cease when suckling stimulation ends. Oxytocin also responds in the same way to prenursing stimuli and mechanical nipple stimulation by a breast pump. The milk-ejection reflex, initiated by oxytocin release, serves to increase the intraductal mammary pressure and to maintain it at levels sufficient to overcome the resistance of the breast to the outflow of milk (Drewett et al., 1982).

Pumps

Mechanical Milk Removal

A pump does not pump, suck, or pull milk out of the breast. It reduces resistance to milk outflow from the alveoli, allowing the internal pressure of the breast to push out the milk. The milk-ejection reflex produces an initial rise in the intramammary pressure; because of the pulsatile nature of oxytocin release and its short half-life, periodic rises in ductal pressure maintain the pressure gradient over time.

The classic work on breast pumps conducted by Einar Egnell (1956) was based on research in dairy cattle and Egnell's own experiments with a pump that created periodic and limited phases of negative pressure. Egnell assumed that the milk-secreting alveoli of the breast and the cow udder were similar, even though the two organs are anatomically different and do not drain in the same way. The quantity of secreted milk is regulated by the counterpressure it exerts. This counterpressure rises as milk fills the available space; secretion ceases when the pressure reaches 28 mm Hg. Egnell's pump created a maximum negative pressure of 200 mm Hg below atmospheric pressure (760 mm Hg). He based this setting on previous research done with an Abt pump (on human mothers), which produced 30 periods of negative pressure per minute and was reported to rupture the nipple skin in every third breast. Egnell placed his settings well below this level to avoid damaging the human nipple. He calculated the difference between the pressure-filled alveoli and his pump's negative pressure as $760 + 28 - 560 = 228$ mm Hg. He maintained that it was the pressure within the breast that activated milk outflow.

Egnell's original pump operated in four phases per cycle: (1) a phase of increasing suction that is relatively short, (2) a decreasing phase of suction, (3) a resting phase, and (4) a slight amount of positive pressure when the decreased suction phase is finished. Egnell contended that mechanical pumping was safer than manual expression: he feared that the "high" positive pressure generated by "squeezing" the breast could damage the alveoli and ducts. He also speculated that manual expression would leave too much milk in the breast, a common concern in the dairy industry. However, in countries where hand expression is used to obtain mothers' milk when the baby is unavailable, increased breast damage has not been reported.

The Evolution of Pumps

Many pump manufacturers still use Egnell's pressure settings as a guide. However, several hand-operated pumps can generate more suction than that in his calculations. As breastfeeding rates increased and reasons for pumping changed, mothers and professionals demanded products that were safe, efficient, and effective in maintaining a good milk supply. The breast-pump market has exploded in recent years, particularly in the United States; bicycle horn–type pumps and chest aspirators have been replaced by a bewildering array of other devices from which to choose (Frantz, 1993).

In this chapter, three broad classifications of breast pumps are discussed: hand pumps that generate suction manually, battery-operated pumps with small motors that generate suction from power supplied by batteries, and electric pumps in which suction is created by various types of electric motors. Other miscellaneous pumps are also described. (See Appendix 13–1 at the end of this chapter.)

Hand Pumps

Hand pumps are popular, relatively inexpensive, and readily available. Much information on the efficiency of hand pumps is anecdotal; some pumps work quite well, whereas others suffer from poor suction, cylinders that pull apart during pumping, and user fatigue from the repeated motions necessary to work the pumps. A few studies have examined the efficiency of hand pumps and their ability to influence prolactin levels, the volume of milk, and its fat and energy content. These studies are difficult to compare, because study design and methodology vary widely. The results may depend on single or random milk samples, and on measurement of milk components obtained at different postpartum times.

Green et al. (1982) evaluated four methods of milk expression, measuring the milk volume obtained and the fat content with the Evenflo (bulb), the Egnell electric pump, the Loyd-B hand pump, and manual expression. Six mothers with exclusively breastfed, full-term infants who were two weeks of age at the time of the study provided milk samples obtained after 10 minutes of pumping. The percentage of fat content was similar for the four methods, but the Egnell pump obtained the largest volume of milk. Of the two hand pumps evaluated, the Loyd-B obtained the most milk.

Johnson (1983) evaluated eight pumps in eight categories—pressure; pressure control; nipple cup, size and shape; volume; ease of handling; ease of cleaning; visual feedback; and cost—and observed the pumps' use by more than 1,000 mothers. The Egnell electric, the Kaneson, and the Loyd-B pumps scored the highest in overall user satisfaction. The Gomco (continuous-vacuum electric), the Davol, and the Binter (glass bicycle horn) pumps scored lowest, whereas the Evenflo (bulb) and Ora'lac (mouth suction) pumps were frequently ineffective. The Kaneson and the Loyd-B were the highest ranking hand pumps, but the research report gave no description of pumping techniques, days postpartum when pumping occurred, volume of milk pumped, or how long the mothers pumped.

Wennergren, Wiqvist, and Wennergren (1985) studied two manual pumps, the Medela and the Arta Plast (a European cylinder pump similar to the Kaneson). This two-part study involved 13 primiparae and 13 multiparas who evaluated the two pumps during their hospital stay following childbirth. The preferred pump was then used by 30 mothers for a one-month period at home. The Medela manual pump was rated higher by primiparas during their hospital stay and was used for the second part of the study. It was highly rated for relief of engorgement, hypergalactia, and for occasional pumping. Nine of twelve mothers were highly satisfied when the pump was used to increase a low milk supply. The authors concluded that a manual pump can be used to provide efficient milk stimulation. The study is limited in that only two pumps were evaluated during the early period of milk production and only one pump was used for the rest of the study period.

Boutte et al. (1985) compared the Egnell electric pump and the Medela manual pump in nine full-term mothers for one month postpartum. Twenty-four-hour pooled milk samples were evaluated for volume, fat, and energy content. The volume of milk collected by the two pumps was similar, but the energy content of milk obtained by the Egnell electric pump was greater than with the Medela manual pump. Because similar volumes of milk with significantly different energy concentrations were found, the authors suggested that collection method is an important consideration when energy content or other nutrient levels are of interest.

Grams (1988) reported comments from 268 women on 12 pumps (Medela Manualectric, Kaneson, Loyd-B, Faultless, and Evenflo bulb hand pumps; Medela, Egnell, and White River large electric pumps, plus the Gerber small electric model; Gentle Expressions, Mag Mag, and Egnell Lact-B battery-operated pumps). Top rated were the Medela Manualectric, Kaneson, and Loyd-B hand pumps and the Medela and Egnell electric models. The other pumps got mixed reviews. However, all the mothers did not use all 12 pumps and then compare their effectiveness; thus these grouped data are of limited value.

Zinaman et al. (1992) studied differences in the volume of milk obtained and prolactin stimulation by various types of breast pumps and by the mother's baby, in 23 women who were 28 to 42 days postpartum. Their results showed that a double-setup (in which both breasts are pumped simultaneously) electric pump did better in stimulating prolactin levels than did battery or manual pumps or hand expression, when only one breast was stimulated at a time. The White River electric pump was reported to stimulate the highest prolactin levels, cycling at 40 times per minute. Milk volumes were highest with the White River electric pump. Lowest milk volume was with hand expression and the Gentle Expressions battery pump, which produced only 6 to 10 cycles per minute. When mothers rated their satisfaction with the pumps, the White River electric rated as one of the more uncomfortable to use. A singular problem with this study was its comparison of double pumping to breastfeeding a single baby or sequential pumping of one breast at a time. A more complete test of pump desirability would be to control for breast stimulation by using mothers of twins when comparing double pumping–or using other double-pump setups or two pumps simultaneously.

Various types of hand pumps rely on different mechanisms to generate suction:

Rubber-Bulb Models. Barum, Davol, Evenflo, and Goodyear models are rubber-bulb pumps occasionally seen in use. Squeezing and releasing a rubber bulb generates a vacuum in these pumps. In most bicycle-horn pumps, the rubber bulb is attached directly to the collection container. Some manufacturers have separated the bulb from the collection container by modifying the angle at which it is attached to the pump or by adding a length of tubing. These modifications are thought to reduce the high potential for bacterial contamination of the bulb caused by the easy backflow of milk. Backflow risk is reduced when the bulb is separated from the collection container. Vacuum control on these pumps is extremely difficult, thus increasing the likelihood of nipple pain and damage. Even with the use of a blood pressure–type bulb, vacuum control is left to chance. The bicycle-horn pumps are inexpensive but collect only about one-half ounce of milk at a time and must be emptied frequently. The other pumps collect milk in a bottle. Mothers often complain of nipple pain during pumping and of low milk yields, especially if they have used these pumps for more than a few weeks.

Squeeze-Handle Models. Models with squeeze handles include Avent, One Hand (Hollister), and Loyd-B pumps. Squeezing and releasing a handle creates suction in these pumps.

The Loyd-B pump has a small trigger for vacuum release. The milk is collected in a glass baby-food jar or in a standard baby bottle. Two sizes of stoppers accommodate the opening of the collection container used. The earlier version of the Loyd-B used a glass shield; two sizes of plastic shields are now available. A small length of tubing connects the pump handle with the collection container. The Hollister and Avent models have pump handles that attach directly to the bottles. The Loyd-B has been used for more than 20 years by mothers who sometimes find it awkward to oper-

ate, although it efficiently extracts milk and effectively maintains milk supply over time. Some mothers remark that larger hands are required or that their hand tires over time. The One Hand pump is reported to be easy to use and effective. This model is easily cleaned, but its operation may present difficulties for women with hand or arm problems, such as carpal tunnel syndrome. The hand and wrist can tire easily with repeated use.

Cylinder Pumps. Evenflo, Happy Family (also privately labeled as the Ross Deluxe by Ross Labs), Kaneson Comfort Plus, Medela Little Hearts, Medela Manualectric, Gerber, Sears, and White River cylinder pumps are all available on the market. All of these pumps, except the Medela and Evenflo, consist of two cylinders. The outer cylinder generates vacuum as it is pulled away from the body. The inner cylinder with the flange is placed against the breast; a gasket at the other end helps form a seal with the edge of the outer cylinder. Gaskets may have to be replaced occasionally if they dry out, shrink, or lose their ability to form a seal. Gaskets can harbor bacteria and must be removed during cleaning, contrary to some user instructions. When placing the gasket back on the cylinder, roll it back and forth over the cylinder to help restore the shape. Some pumps come with extra gaskets.

Small plastic or silicone inserts can be placed in the inner opening to custom-fit the pump to the breast. Silicone liners are available for some pumps; these are designed to collapse against the breast during the suction phase to provide external positive pressure. These pumps are lightweight, not too expensive, and easily cleaned.

The Hollister One Hand pump interrupts vacuum at maximum squeeze (250 mm Hg). The Medela Manualectric and the Medela Little Hearts pumps have three vacuum settings and automatically interrupt suction at about 240 mm Hg, when the outer cylinder reaches the end of the outward stroke. The Medela Manualectric, the Little Hearts, and the Evenflo Natural Mother pumps use a bottle to collect milk.

Some pumps also provide an extra cylinder for milk storage or have an angled rather than a straight flange. Some mothers report that the angled flange does not work as well as does the straight flange. As the outer cylinder fills with milk, the gasket is repeatedly dunked in the milk. Mothers who express more than three ounces of milk at a time may have to empty these pumps more than once in a single pumping episode.

Efficiency of use varies from brand to brand. The Medela Manualectric and the Hollister can also be adapted for use on the larger electric pumps. Table 13–1 summarizes information on the currently available manually operated pumps. Higher vacuum is generated as the outer cylinder fills with milk. Mothers may need to shorten the outward stroke after collecting more than one ounce.

Battery-Operated Pumps

Evenflo, Gerber, Little Hearts, Mag Mag, Mag Mag Advanced, and Medela battery-operated pumps are available. The Little Hearts uses two D-size batteries. These pumps use a small motor with two AA 1.5-volt batteries to generate suction.

The Evenflo pump uses two size C batteries. The Gerber pump has a dial to raise or lower the vacuum level. It also has a small cup that can be placed in the collection container attached to the motor unit. Called a *trainer cup,* it reduces the amount of air in the system, thereby increasing the vacuum. The Mag Mag pump has no vacuum-adjustment dial. The Mag Mag Advanced pump has a vacuum-control dial and a removable inner collecting bottle for milk storage. Vacuum can take 30 seconds to reach its maximum level and is regulated by how frequently the vacuum is interrupted.

Most of these pumps have a button or bar to press to release the vacuum periodically and to simulate the rhythm of a nursing baby. All take varying periods for the recovery of suction following each release. This limits the number of suction-release cycles per minute to as few as six and may require relatively long periods of vacuum application to the nipple. To compensate for this, some mothers leave the suction on far longer than the pump instructions recommend. Times of 30 to 60 seconds were mentioned by several mothers in one survey. Four women never interrupted the suction during the entire pumping session because they could not get the milk flow restarted following vacuum interruption.

Several pumps have AC adapters to decrease battery use. A major complaint about these pumps is their short battery life. This affects pumping efficiency because fewer cycles are generated as the batteries wear down. Batteries may have to be replaced as frequently as every second or third use. Rechargeable batteries are an option, but they usually require charging each night and may not produce as many cycles per minute as do alkaline batteries. AC adapters usually allow the maximum number of cycles per minute that the motor can produce. Maximum suction after each vacuum release will often continue decreasing in amount throughout the pumping session. The Medela battery pump automatically produces 32 cycles per minute with alkaline batteries, 30 cycles per minute with rechargeable batteries, and 42 cycles per minute with the AC adapter.

Battery pumps require only one hand to operate, are lightweight, and are popular with mothers employed outside the home. Some mothers use two battery-operated pumps simultaneously to decrease pumping time when they are on a tight schedule. Mothers who plan to pump for several months while at work may consider a long-term rental contract for an electric pump, because battery replacement can be very expensive, as can artificial formula if it must be used to substitute for breastmilk. See Table 13–2 for a summary of information about battery-operated breast pumps.

Electric Pumps

Both small semiautomatic pumps, including the Kadan, Mada, Nurture III, and Schuco-Vac models, and large semiautomatic pumps, including Gomco, Schuco-Vac, and White River, are on the market. The large, fully automatic pumps include Egnell Elite, Medela Classic, Medela Lactina, Medela Pump-N-Style, and White River models. The Whittlestone model is not available in the United States.

Various types of electric motors are used in these pumps to generate suction. Semiautomatic pumps require the mother to cycle suction by covering and uncovering a hole in the flange base. By doing so, the mother creates a pumping rhythm designed to simulate the pattern of a suckling baby. These pumps maintain a constant negative pressure. Some lack a dial or mechanism to adjust the amount of suction. The actual amount of vacuum delivered to the nipple is determined by the degree of closure of the hole in the flange base. Many mothers learn to roll their finger three-fourths of the way off the hole rather than to lift the finger completely, to generate vacuum faster for the subsequent cycle by preventing complete interruption of vacuum. However, too much negative pressure or negative pressure applied for too long a period increases the risk of damage to the nipple and underlying vascular structures. The initiation of suction places the greatest pressure on the nipple; thus it is most desirable that a pump generate suction quickly.

Automatic electric pumps are designed to cycle pressure rather than to maintain it. Because Egnell (1956) observed nipple damage when cycles were two seconds long (30 per minute), manufacturers have increased the number of cycles so that they more closely simulate that of a nursing baby. Pressure-setting parameters on these large pumps also attempt to mimic that of an infant. Mean sucking pressures of most full-term infants range from -50 to -155, with a maximum of -220 mm Hg (Caldeyro-Barcia, 1969). In pumps that have a preset pulsed suction (automatic pumps), there is a 60:40 ratio. Negative pressure is applied for 60 percent of the cycle; 40 percent of the cycle is the resting phase. For example, the U.S. model of the Medela electric pump is set so that each cycle lasts 1.15 seconds (suction plus rest); 52 cycles are generated per minute. In Europe, with the same pump, 48 cycles occur each minute because of the difference in the frequency of the electric voltage. The Egnell Elite generates 48 cycles per minute in the United States at 60 Hz and 48 cycles per minute in Europe at 50 Hz. These pumps generally produce a maximum pressure of 220 mm Hg at their normal (high) setting. By comparison, the Nurture III semiautomatic pump produces 220 mm Hg after about 2.5 seconds using a single collecting kit (approximately 24 cycles per minute). With the double collecting kit, this same pump takes about 3.25 seconds to achieve this level, generating about 18 cycles per minute.

Negative pressure is a function of the volume of air in the accessory kit. Negative pressure increases as the bottle fills with milk. The pressure generated varies with different-sized bottles (collecting containers) and from one manufacturer to another. When double-pump setups are used (two collecting containers simultaneously), the potential for very low negative pressure exists if the containers are empty; negative pressure increases as the bottles fill. Some accessory kits attempt to compensate for this to keep the pressure levels constant (Rental Roundup, 1986b). For example, the Medela Manualectric accessory kit has a valve head and membrane that separate the collection containers from the power source, thereby creating a closed system. Thus the amount of air in the system remains constant regardless of the amount of fluid in the collection container. If a mother is using an accessory kit or pump without a similar feature, she can compensate by using a smaller collection bottle (Vol-u-feeders fit on some pumps), turning down the vacuum as the bottle fills, emptying the bottle more frequently, or cycling the suction more frequently on the hand- or battery-operated pumps or on the semiautomatic pumps. Unfortunately, most instructions do not include these cautions.

All of the automatic electric pumps now have collection kits for simultaneous pumping of both breasts. Neifert and Seacat (1985) reported the experiences of 10 mothers who were two to seven months postpartum. The women alternated between sequentially pumping each breast for 20 minutes and then pumping both breasts simultaneously for 10 minutes. Milk yield was about the same with both techniques but was obtained in one-half the time with lower pump suction (320 mm Hg versus 260 mm Hg) when pumping was simultaneous. They also found a significantly higher prolactin rise with double pumping. This is similar to Tyson's (1977) report, which cited a doubling in prolactin rise when two infants were put to breast simultaneously, and echoes the findings of Saint et al. (1986), who reported larger milk volumes in mothers of twins (up to double that of singleton mothers). Auerbach (1990b) studied 25 mothers with babies between 5 and 35 weeks of age. She investigated the amount of milk obtained with single and double pumping, whether it takes longer to pump with a single setup as compared to a double setup, and whether the milk fat varies between the two methods of pumping. Results showed that highest milk yields with single pump-

Table 13–1

MANUALLY OPERATED PUMPS

Type	Brand	Vacuum Source	Flange	Contamination
Bicycle horn	Barum Davol Evenflo	Squeezing and releasing a rubber bulb makes vacuum control very difficult.	One size. No adaptors. Barum is made of glass.	Easy backflow of milk into rubber bulb. Bulb is difficult to clean or sterilize and can harbor bacteria. Potential for contamination is high.

Risks of Use/Caution: No instructions. Less than 1/2 oz. reservoir. Must be emptied frequently. Potential for tissue and vascular damage is very high. Poor efficiency is reported from users.

Squeeze handle	Avent Gerber One Hand (Ameda- Egnell/ Hollister)	Squeezing and releasing a handle generates suction. Loyd-B has a trigger for vacuum release. A short length of tubing connects handle to collection container (baby-food jar or bottle). Others have handles that attach directly to standard bottle. Vacuum control is moderate to somewhat difficult to manage.	Loyd-B has two sizes, glass and plastic. Avent has a thin membrane that fits over the flange. Gerber uses a soft silicone flange.	Contamination risk is lower than with rubber bulb pumps. Pumps are easy to clean. Reduced potential for backflow of milk.

Risks of Use/Caution: Loyd-B can be awkward and tire the hands. Its trigger can be hard to reach but is reported to be effective. Tissue damage potential is lower than for rubber-bulb pumps, and most women find these devices comfortable to use. Mothers with a history of carpal tunnel injury may risk exacerbation of this condition when using a squeeze-handle pump.

Cylinder (piston)	Comfort Plus (Kaneson) Evenflo Gerber	Movement of outer cylinder away from the body. Vacuum is easier to control but can become excessive if not properly instructed. Medela automatically releases suction at end of outward stroke	Hard plastic with two silicone or two plastic adaptors and two sizes of flanges. Gerber has soft plastic flange. Happy Family has two angled	Contamination potential is lower; however, the gasket must be removed during cleaning to prevent bacteria from collecting under it.

Table 13–1

Happy Family Infa Little Hearts (Medela) Mini-Manual (White River, distributed by Ross Laboratories) Ross Deluxe Sears Spring Express (Medela) White River	(220 mm Hg) and has three vacuum settings. Its collection bottle is separate from the handle unit. Evenflo has swivel handle separated from collection bottle. User may need to roll gasket back and forth several times when reattaching it to inner cylinder after cleaning to restore its original shape and efficiency to improve suction. Evenflo has a suction valve to increase vacuum. Users of White River report difficulty in maintaining contact between soft flange and breast when attempting to create suction. flanges. Spring Express uses a spring to push rather than pull outward to generate suction. Pump release is automatic. Sears angled soft flange can be rolled back to adjust for different-sized breasts. White River has silicone flange.

Risks of Use/Caution: Potential for tissue damage is moderate, as high levels of vacuum can be generated unless mothers are fully instructed. The outer cylinder can come off during the outward stroke on some pumps. Some types of gaskets can lose their seal from repeated boiling or cleaning. Some come with extra gaskets, all of which must be oriented properly for optimum suction. O rings must be in place on the pumps that use them for a tight seal. Efficiency varies among these devices. White River Mini-Manual breast pump is distributed by Ross Laboratories in their formula-containing hospital discharge kit. The outer cylinder shows a Ross logo and the names of two commercial milk products. This may make the pump unsuitable for those institutions abiding by the International Code of Marketing of Breast-Milk Substitutes.

Table 13–2

BATTERY OPERATED PUMPS

Brand	Vacuum	Flange or Adaptor	Cleaning	Contamination
Evenflo	2 C batteries; suction level selector; swivel handle	Silicone flange with two silicone adapters		Must avoid tilting to prevent backflow into motor
Gentle Expressions	2 AA batteries, 1.5-volt batteries; dial to adjust vacuum; small cup inserted into bottle to increase suction	Hard plastic flange; two silicone inserts; Lactostim silicone liner	Easily cleaned	Fluid can be drawn into motor, which eliminates vacuum
Mag Mag	2 AA batteries; no vacuum adjustment; takes 30 seconds to reach maximum vacuum	Hard plastic flange with two inserts		
Mag Mag Advanced Little Hearts (Medela)	Vacuum adjustment 2 D batteries; optional AC adapter. Automatically interrupts vacuum; vacuum adjustment	Insert with ridges Hard plastic flange		
Mini-Electric (Medela)	2 AA batteries; AC adapter. Variable vacuum adjustment	Hard plastic flange with insert		

Risks of Use/Caution: Nipple pain or damage can occur with all battery-operated pumps unless instructions are given that stress the importance of frequent interruption of vacuum (if this does not occur automatically), massaging while pumping, and eliciting the milk-ejection reflex before applying suction. Batteries must be fresh to generate near the maximum number of cycles/minute. AC adapter will allow maximum number of cycles per minute. Nipple damage potential is low on Medela pumps because they generate 32 cycles per minute with automatic vacuum interruption. All battery-operated pumps suffer from short battery life and work best with alkaline batteries. Most also have AC adapter capability. These may be a good choice for mothers with an abundant milk supply and a quick milk-ejection reflex. These pumps are not a good choice for mothers with slow or erratic milk ejection, sore nipples, low milk supply or who need to pump more than occasionally. All pumps in this group can be noisy.

ing occurred over 10 to 15 minutes. With double pumping, maximum milk volumes were seen in 7 to 12 minutes. Maximum yield overall occurred with double pumping. Milk fat concentrations were only slightly higher for double pumping sessions with no time limits. However, the mothers preferred double pumping three to one. Mothers' preferences regarding pumping regimens usually predicted how they obtained the highest yields. Groh-Wargo et al. (1995) studied 32 preterm mothers, half of whom pumped each breast in sequence; the other half pumped both breasts simultaneously. Daily frequency of pumping in both groups ranged from three to nearly five times. The single-pumping group averaged 24 minutes for each pumping session; the bilateral pumping group expressed milk for an average of 16 minutes per session. There was no statistically significant difference in milk obtained or in pre- and postexpression prolactin levels.

Most electric pumps have hard plastic shields or flanges, except for the White River, the Whittlestone, and the Gerber battery with an AC adapter. All White River products use a flexible silicone flange to achieve a degree of positive pressure and massage over a larger area of the areola and breast. Hughes et al. (1989) compared three pumps, manual expression, and infant sucking. They showed that the White River double-setup pump generated a 117 percent rise over baseline prolactin levels as compared to a singleton baby at breast and other pumps used sequentially on one breast at a time. This pump is capable of generating very high vacuum levels, but the flange is designed to distribute pressure over a wider area of the breast, thus avoiding nipple damage that might otherwise occur. Mothers have reported that the flange will occasionally pinch the nipple as it collapses.

The Whittlestone Breastmilker is a New Zealand pump with a double-pumping flange design based on milking techniques used by the dairy industry. The early mechanical milking devices used on domestic animals consisted of a single-chambered teat cup attached to a vacuum source that withdrew milk by simple suction (Woolford & Phillips, 1978). This design was inefficient, and the cows objected to the discomfort. A teat cup is now used, consisting of a metal

case lined with soft rubber. The milking apparatus produces a regular collapsing of the rubber liner against the teat to cause stimulation. The Whittlestone breast cups consist of a solid casing attached to a pulsating vacuum source. A foam pad in the cup case is held in place by a liner. When negative pressure occurs in the cup case, the liner moves against the pad, and the nipple and areola are drawn down into the conical portion of the liner (Whittlestone, 1978). Mothers report that this pump is comfortable and efficient.

Johnson (1983) measured several aspects of flanges, including the diameters of the outer opening (flare), the inner opening, the depth of flare, and the length of the shank. She measured negative pressure at the inner opening of the flange and reported that the smaller the nipple cup, the greater the pressure exerted on the tip of the nipple. The larger and deeper flanges may provide greater stimulation of the areolar region of the breast. Zinaman (1988) repeated the same measurements on 11 manual pumps, 4 battery pumps, and 7 electric pumps. Comparing these measurements among pumps highly rated in the other studies showed that diameter of the flange ranged from 60 to 69 mm, depth ranged from 25 to 30 mm, and the inner opening was between 21 and 26 mm for the manual pumps. The Schuco-Vac pump has the smallest inner opening—6 mm (1/4 AE)—and generates relatively high vacuum levels; it was also reported to cause noticeable discomfort in many women. A woman with a large or wide nipple may have difficulty with a flange that has a small opening or a narrow slope.

Because no size flange fits all breasts, many manufacturers either provide two sizes of flanges (soft plastic or silicone flexible flanges) or small inserts that are placed at the level of the inner opening to narrow the diameter. The Hollister/Ameda-Egnell pump has a silicone Flexiflange that lines the entire flange, as does the Gerber pump, which features the Lact-Stim. Inserts and silicone liners placed in the flanges are designed to provide a better fit between pump and breast. In general, a pump is more likely to be effective when it fits the anatomical configuration of the breast. To help with this fitting process, many health professionals who have access to autoclaving or similar sterilizing facilities offer mothers the opportunity to try several different brands of breast pumps to ascertain optimal fit before they purchase or rent a pump. Tables 13–3 and 13–4 summarize some features of electric breast pumps. See also Table 13–5 for technical information.

Product Effectiveness and Safety

Whenever a product is used, its effectiveness must be assessed. For example, if a lactation consultant is assisting a mother using a breast pump that causes pain, or does not work according to the information in the packaging, the consumer has recourse (Box 13–2).

Miscellaneous Pumps

Juice-Jar Breast Pump

The concept of the juice-jar breast pump is reminiscent of the bottles mentioned at the beginning of this chapter. A 1.5-quart jar is filled with hot water and then is emptied. The nipple and areola are inserted into the jar's opening, and a cool wash cloth is rubbed around the outside of the jar. As the hot air in the jar cools, it creates a gentle suction. Leaning over the jar may be uncomfortable for some women, and the water must be reheated for each breast. It is an inexpensive method of obtaining milk and may be helpful for women with sore nipples. However, it is time consuming (Rees, 1977).

Ora'lac

The Ora'lac pump generates suction by the mother's sucking on a plastic, tubelike straw. It is the modern plastic version of the early sucking glasses. A second tube is attached to the flange, and a saliva trap prevents saliva from entering the bottle. It takes only one hand to operate and can be used even when the mother is lying down. The amount of suction varies and may not be efficient enough for regular pumping. It takes practice to use and may work better for women who have a large milk supply and an easily elicited milk-ejection reflex.

Venturi Breast Pump

The Venturi pump (Fig. 13–5) generates a vacuum as a stream of running water passes through the

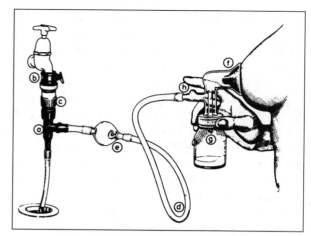

FIGURE 13–5. Venturi water-powered breast pump. *(a) Connected to water tap via universal screw-on adaptor (b), which may be left in place, and click-on connector (c) (Hozelock UK, Ltd.) that allows easy removal of pump between feedings. Tubing (d) transmits suction to milking apparatus, and safety trap (e) prevents backflow of water vapor. Breast cup (f) is applied to areolar skin, and evacuation of milk bottle and breast cup is achieved when valve (h) is occluded by mother's finger. Expressed milk enters bottle via internal channel (g). Pulsatile sucking action is created by repeated light touch and release of finger valve. (From W Sponsel: Simple and effective breast pump for nursing mothers. Br Med J 286:1680, 1983.)*

faucet attachment. The faster and harder the water flows, the more suction is generated. A hole in the flange base is covered and uncovered to generate and release the vacuum. Unless the water is saved and reused, this method of pumping wastes a lot of water. The mother must have access to a sink with running water to use the pump. The parts are inexpensive (Sponsel, 1983).

Medela Pedal Pump

The Medela pedal pump is relatively new on the market and is designed to enable the user to generate pressure by using her feet. The leg muscles tend to be stronger than are hand and arm muscles; thus muscle fatigue is less an issue with this pump. This pump works well in households where hand expression is not practiced, where a hand pump is not preferred, or where electricity is unavailable.

As of late 1997, its effectiveness in comparison to other pumps on the market was unknown.

Clinical Implications Regarding Breast Pumps

The concerns of health professionals vary considerably from those of mothers and typically center around safe collection techniques and the maintenance of low bacteria counts in the expressed milk. Of equal importance are choosing the right pump for each individual situation, providing appropriate pumping instructions, and tempering all this with a consideration of the emotional toll that pumping can sometimes exact.

The professional literature includes reports of bacterial contamination of breastmilk and breast pumps. Factors related to nipple cleansing, hand washing, collection technique, type of pump, feeding method of preterm infants, pump-cleaning routines, and gestational age of the baby have all been identified as contributing to concern over high bacteria counts in expressed milk. Expressed breastmilk is not sterile (El-Mohandes et al., 1993b). There is considerable disagreement over what constitutes an acceptable bacteria count, especially if the recipient of the milk is a preterm infant (El-Mohandes et al., 1993a). Caution must be exercised in reviewing the literature, because certain institutional practices may increase the likelihood of contamination problems with expressed milk.

With the increased use of both hand and electric pumps in the 1970s, many reports described contaminated milk as one source of bacteremia, but the reports lacked conclusive epidemiology. Hand expression of breastmilk showed lower bacteria counts than did breastmilk obtained by manual or electric pumps when pumps first began to be commonly used. Donowitz et al. (1981) reported an outbreak of *Klebsiella*-caused bacteremia in a neonatal intensive care unit (NICU). The electric breast pump was grossly contaminated and lacked proper bacterial surveillance. Once gas sterilization of pump parts was required between each mother's use of the equipment, the problem disappeared. However, all five affected babies in the report were fed milk by the nasoduodenal route, which delivers the milk directly to the small bowel, thus bypassing the protective action of gastric acid in the stomach.

Four of the five infants had received broad-spectrum antibiotic therapy prior to the contaminated feedings and therefore received contaminated milk in a bowel with altered protective gastrointestinal flora. Such a practice predisposes an infant to infection, with even small challenges from bacteria.

Gransden et al. (1986) reported an outbreak of *Serratia marcescens* in an NICU via inadequately disinfected breast pumps (Kaneson manual and Egnell electric models). Kaneson pump parts (after being washed) were soaked in a solution of hypochlorite. Egnell pump parts were washed with the metal parts soaked in a solution of 0.5% chlorhexidine in 70% ethyl alcohol. The pumps were soaked for 1.5 hours in a 1% hypochlorite solution, and the solution was changed every 24 hours. Bacteria were isolated from the soaked pump parts and from the hypochlorite solution itself. When the Egnell pump parts were autoclaved and the Kaneson pumps were washed at 80°C, the problem was resolved. Often, the available chlorine in these chemical solutions is readily inactivated by small amounts of organic matter. The original disinfection technique in this study had several faults, including failure to completely dismantle the hand pump, failure to remove the rubber gasket, and failure to totally immerse the pump components.

Moloney et al. (1987) reported isolation of *Serratia marcescens, Staphylococcus aureus,* and *Streptococcus faecalis* from hand-operated and electric breast pumps. The pumps were disinfected in a hypochlorite solution, as in the previous study. It is well known that there are infection risks from electrically operated breast pumps. With proper surveillance and sterilizing by autoclaving, gas (ethylene oxide), or high-temperature washing (rather than by chemical sterilization), the risk of overgrowth and transmission of pathogenic bacteria can be substantially reduced. If pumps or pump parts are heat-sensitive, consideration should be given to using pumps that do not depend on chemical sterilization.

Asquith, Sharp, and Stevenson (1985) compared Medela hand and electric pumps to manual expression to measure the amount of bacterial contamination. Boiling the personal-use kits for 10 minutes worked well. The disposable kits were washed in hot soapy water and used for only one

Table 13–3

SEMIAUTOMATIC ELECTRIC PUMPS

Type	Brand	Vacuum	Flanges	Contamination and Cleaning
Small semiautomatic	Gerber	Continuous vacuum, cycles by covering and uncovering hole in collection funnel; vacuum not adjustable	Hard and soft flanges; small angled flange can be uncomfortable	Vacuum release hole is positioned in funnel, permitting milk to flow over the user's finger. Increases risk of bacteria into milk.
	Nurture III	Adjustable vacuum; continuous suction	Hard plastic; no adapters; double set of flanges for simultaneous pumping	
Large semiautomatic	Gomco	High continuous vacuum	Small inner opening of flange	
	Schuco-Vac	High continuous vacuum; vacuum adjustable	Narrow opening of glass flange; capable of simultaneous pumping	
	White River	Continuous vacuum; vacuum adjustable	Flexible silicone flange distributes vacuum over larger area of breast	

Risks of Use/Caution: Gerber: Moderate potential for nipple pain; strength of suction regulated by the degree of closure of the mother's finger over the hole in the flange base. Nurture III: Very short electric cord

Risks of Use/Caution: Gomco: Poor vacuum control knob; glass flange and collection chamber; Schuco-Vac: high pressures are best controlled by interrupting vacuum every 1–2 seconds; occasionally, mothers report pinching of the nipple. All pumps in this group have potential for nipple damage if vacuum is not cycled quickly. Vacuum increases as containers fill.

Table 13–4

FULLY AUTOMATIC ELECTRIC PUMPS

Type	Brand	Vacuum	Flanges	Contamination and Cleaning
Large automatic	Ameda-Egnell/Hollister	Rate and amount of vacuum adjustable	Flexi-shield silicone liner can take up room in hard plastic flange; provides areolar stimulation	Hygieni-kit isolates vacuum source from milk and prevents outside air from being drawn into the pumping system; comes completely assembled
	Lactina (Medela)	Has rechargeable battery option; preset suction; adjustable vacuum; the Select model allows user to adjust recycling speed	Uses same accessory kit as Pump-In-Style and Classic pumps; capable of simultaneous pumping	
	Classic (Medela)	Preset pulsed suction; adjustable vacuum	Hard flanges with inserts, can be used with Pump-In-Style and Lactina; filter system prevents backflow of milk into pump; capable of simultaneous pumping	
	Pump-In-Style (Medela)	Preset pulsed suction; adjustable vacuum	Same accessory kit as the Lactina pump; capable of simultaneous pumping	
	White River	Preset pulsed suction; adjustable vacuum	Flexible flange; capable of simultaneous pumping	

Risks of Use/Caution: Pump-In-Style may not be optimal choice for mothers of premature infants or when mother has been ill or hospitalized. White River users report pinching of the nipple as soft flange collapses.

Table 13–5

SELECTED TECHNICAL DATA REGARDING PUMPS

Type/Brand	Maximum Pressure Range: Empty (mm Hg)	Pressure with 1 oz. (mm Hg)	Pressure with 2 oz. (mm Hg)	Cycles per Minute	Double Setup Empty (mm Hg)	Double Setup 1 oz. (mm Hg)	Double Setup 2 oz. (mm Hg)
Manual							
Rubber bulb[a]							
Barum	120			Erratic			
Davol	76–229			Erratic			
Evenflo	81–127			Erratic			
Squeeze-handle[b]							
Avent	200–260	200–260	200–260	Variable			
Ameda-Egnell/ Hollister One Hand	0–250	0–260	0–260	Variable			
Loyd-B	380–650	620	620	Variable			
Cylinder[c]							
Ameda-Egnell/ Hollister	0–420	460–500	Spillage with 2 oz. during testing	Variable			
Evenflo	60–120	40–100	80–140	Erratic (owing to differing number of pulls to reach maximum pressure)			
Happy Family (also private label Ross Labs)	320	250	340	Variable			

Table 13-5

			Spillage with 2 oz. during testing	
Infa	400	380–500	Spillage	Variable
Kaneson	420–440	480–500	460–480 (spillage)	Variable
Little Hearts (Medela)	L 200 M 280 H 280	220 240 280	220 240 280	Variable
Manualectric (Medela)	L 120–140 H 140–180 H 235–250	140–220 180–220 240–270	160–180 200–220 260–280	Variable
Mini-Manual (White River/Ross distributed)	300	400	380	
Spring Express (Medela)	Untested	Untested	Untested	Variable
Sears	360	380	440	Variable
White River	240–320	180–260	200–260	Variable
Battery[d]				
Evenflo	L 40–94 M 90–140 L 160–180	70–90 120–140 160–200	60–95 95–140 160–220	10–28
Gentle Expressions	L 20 M 140 H 180	40 180 180	20 140 180	9–13
Little Hearts (Medela)	Unknown[e]			

Table 13–5 *(cont.)*

Type/Brand	Maximum Pressure Range: Empty (mm Hg)	Pressure with 1 oz. (mm Hg)	Pressure with 2 oz. (mm Hg)	Cycles per Minute	Double Setup Empty (mm Hg)	Double Setup 1 oz. (mm Hg)	Double Setup 2 oz. (mm Hg)
Mag Mag	110	110	120	15			
Mag Mag Advanced	L 60 M 120 H 260	60 120 260	60 140 260	13 (with AC adapter)			
Little Hearts (Medela)	L 200 M 280 H 280	220 240 280	220 240 280	Variable			
Medela	L 60 M 140 H 200	60 160 200	60 160 200	42 (with AC adapter)			
Electric							
Small semiautomatic[f]							
Gerber	20	20	40	18			
Kadan	580	580	580	11			
Nurture III	L 120–180 M 160–200 H 180–220	140–180 160–200 200–220	140–190 180–220 200–240	9–20	L 160–220	160–220	180–220
Schuco-Vac	120	200	180	52	H 200–250	195–250	200–260
Large semiautomatic							
Schuco-Vac	L 260 M 360 H 360	360 350 360	280 360 360	10–12			
White River	L 370–400 M 440–460 H 320–540	300–400 460–470 560–650	390–420 460–480 560–650	12–42	L 300–320 M 380 H 400–440	320 360–390 440–460	300–320 340–360 380–460

Table 13-5

Large automatic							
Ameda-Egnell/ Hollister SMB	70–250	—	—	48	H 180–200	H 200–220	H 220–240
Ameda-Egnell/ Hollister Elite	70–250	—	—	—	—	—	—
Ameda-Egnell/ Hollister Lact-E	—	—	—	—	—	—	—
Medela Classic	L 140 / M 160 / H 160	160 / 160–170 / 160–180	160–210 / 160–210 / 160–210	46	L 210–220 / M 220–270 / H 240–280	220–260 / 240–270 / 240–270	220–260 / 240–270 / 240–280
Medela Lactina	0–250	—	—	—	0–225	—	—
Medela Pump-In-Style	—	—	—	—	—	—	—

aCycles per minute depends on number and speed of squeezes on the rubber bulb.

bCycles per minute depends on number and duration of squeezes.

cCycles per minute varies depending on number and duration of outward strokes.

dCycles per minute depends on how frequently and for how long the vacuum is interrupted and on how quickly the vacuum can regenerate after interruption. Cycles are also influenced by the type of battery, whether the batteries are partially worn down, and whether an AC adapter is used.

eFlange was too small for independent vacuum gauge testing.

fCycles per minute depends on how frequently and for how long vacuum is interrupted and on how quickly vacuum can regenerate after interruption.

Note: All results are approximate. Hand-held vacuum gauge made by MacDaniel Controls, Inc. Long dash (–) indicates that pumps were unavailable for independent vacuum testing.

BOX 13–2

When Products Generate Problems

In the United States, the Food and Drug Administration (FDA) maintains a medical products reporting program that enables health professionals and consumers to report problems with marketed products. These reports have resulted in changing labels to provide accurate information, placing warnings in the package insert to alert potential users to specific risks, and recalling or withdrawing products.

A product problem can relate to any concern regarding the quality, performance, or safety of the item in question, including its suspected contamination (as in a formula can), questionable stability, defective components or parts, poor packaging or labeling, a suspected problem with the potency of a medication (either too potent or not potent enough), or a malfunction of the product (such as infant formula, which falls under the

category of special nutritional products) or device (such as a breast pump, which falls under the category of medical devices).

The report should include identification of the adverse event or product problem, when it occurred, the brand name of the product, what it is, and the manufacturer's name and address. Information about the person using the device (health professional, client or patient, etc.) also should be given. The reporter of such a problem, if different from the person who was injured or otherwise experienced the problem, is also identified; if the FDA chooses to look into the report or complaint, information about the reporting person(s) is kept confidential. Such reports should be made directly to MEDWatch at 5600 Fishers Lane, Rockville, MD 20852-9787 (fax: 1-800-332-0178).

day. In some hospitals, a fresh sterile kit is used for each pumping session.

Other approaches to reducing the bacterial count in expressed breastmilk have included expressing techniques and various breast-nipple cleansing routines. Asquith et al. (1984) noted that the bacterial content of milk was high when expression first began, regardless of collection technique. Asquith and Harod's earlier work (1979) recommended that stripping and discarding the first 10 ml of expressed milk would decrease total bacteria counts. They observed that bacterial contamination was high within the first 24 hours after birth or after initiation of pumping, whether or not the first 10 ml was discarded. Asquith et al. (1984) suggested that delayed expression of breastmilk is associated with high bacterial counts of nonnursing

mothers of NICU infants: "Milk stasis and breast engorgement may provide an opportunity for bacteria, including 'normal flora' or pathogenic species, to incubate in the breast." Their recommendations for mothers of hospitalized newborns include initiation of expression as soon as possible on a frequent and regular basis, thereby avoiding excessive engorgement, and the discarding of the first 10 ml of milk with each pumping. Some mothers may get only 10 ml of colostrum or milk at first, so care should be taken to determine the necessity of discarding this early milk.

Pittard et al. (1991) found no difference in the number of heavily contaminated (>10,000 colony-forming units/ml [cfu/ml]) milk cultures when a clean versus a sterile collection container was used, or when manual versus mechanical collection techniques were employed. They did not observe increased levels of bacteria in the initial milk removed from the breast.

According to Meier and Wilks (1987), acceptable bacteria levels in expressed breastmilk are difficult to define and vary between healthy full-term infants and preterm, high-risk babies. Healthy full-term infants can tolerate some pathogens and relatively high levels of nonpathogenic bacteria (>104 cfu/ml of milk). Preterm or high-risk infants with immature immune systems who are not nursing directly from the breast may be at greater risk from the same level of bacterial growth. The investigators' criteria for acceptable bacteria levels for preterm infants is the absence of any pathogens and a maximum concentration of 104 cfu/ml. Mothers in their study were instructed in hand washing, especially under and around the fingernails. The nipples and areolae were cleaned with pHisoDerm soap before each pumping session. Increased nipple soreness was not noticed in this study but the number of weeks of pumping was not specified. Using these guidelines, 74 of 84 expressed milk specimens had concentrations of less than 104 cfu/ml. It is not known whether this type of cleansing increases the risk for problems, other than topical soreness, such as dry areolar skin, which is susceptible to breakdown and infection, or a change in the pH of the skin, which affects the secretions of the glands of Montgomery.

Costa (1989) reported significantly lower bacterial counts when preterm mothers washed their nipples and areolae with pHisoDerm soap prior to each pumping session. Although Costa noticed no skin breakdown with this routine, it is unknown what adverse affects would be encountered from using this soap six to eight times a day over an extended period.

Wilks and Meier (1988) described guidelines for care of hospital breast-pump equipment that included scrubbing collection kits and tubing with instrument-cleaning solution after each use and autoclaving each item. The exterior of the pump should be cleaned with antiseptic solution each day, and the pump should be cultured monthly. They also described other factors that may influence the amount of nonpathogens that a preterm baby can tolerate. These include the baby's clinical condition, the use of bolus feedings every two hours rather than continuous feedings, the use of refrigerated rather than frozen milk to retain active antiinfective properties, and feeding the baby directly from the breast as much as possible to provide unaltered antiinfective properties, thereby further decreasing the risk of infection.

Nwankwo et al. (1988) showed that colostrum inhibited bacterial growth more than did mature milk—full-term colostrum even more so than preterm colostrum. At room temperature (27–32°C; 74–96°F), mature milk from full-term mothers could be stored without a significant increase in bacterial counts for six hours. Preterm milk could be stored for four hours at room temperature before bacterial counts exceeded 104 cfu/ml or became significantly higher than initial counts at the time of expression. Colostrum was obtained within six days of delivery and mature milk at six weeks or more postpartum. The authors suggested caution in the storage of preterm milk. This should also be kept in mind for situations of continuous versus bolus tube feedings. Milk-storage guidelines for term infants, particularly employed mothers, are more lenient. Hamosh et al. (1996) offered the following suggestions for short-term storage of human milk:

38°C (100°F): safe for less than 4 hours
25°C (77°F): safe for 4 hours
15°C (59°F): safe for 24 hours. (This is the temperature in a cooler with an ice pack.)

In addition, amylase and bile-salt-stimulated lipase, key digestive enzymes, remain stable at 15°C for 24 hours, thus providing the same compensatory digestive activity as when the breastmilk is fed fresh to the infant (Hamosh et al., 1997).

During each year, many pumps are changed or have features added (especially the electric type) that reduce the chance of milk backflow and contamination. Most models use filters in the pump; some use overflow bottles, and others have filters or protection against overflow in the accessory kit. When choosing a pump for milk collection for preterm babies, the professional should know whether the pump or accessory kit guards against contamination. For example, the Hollister/Ameda-Egnell kit is designed to prevent milk from entering the tubing. Outside air cannot be drawn into the pumping system. The Medela Classic uses a filter barrier to protect against cross-contamination. Although air passes through the filter, liquid will not. If the filter comes into contact with any liquid, the filter becomes impermeable. Only after being washed and dried or autoclaved will it work again. The large Schuco-Vac model has no device in the accessory kit to prevent backflow, but has a bacterial filter just outside the air-intake port on the pump. If a pump depends on an overflow bottle, it is mandatory that the bottle be used at each pumping session and that it be properly cleaned after each use.

Concern over obtaining bacterially safe breastmilk is only one aspect of managing milk expression to be considered when mothers and infants are separated. Forte et al. (1987) collected data from 51 mothers of hospitalized neonates, noting that more than 50 percent of the sample identified the need for additional information about breastfeeding on hospital discharge. Some mothers received no written guidelines before or after discharge and lacked information about pumping frequency, how to increase milk production, and pumping and storage techniques. Women in this sample used hand expression (12 percent), a manual pump (17 percent), an electric pump (55 percent), or an electric pump in combination with other methods (16 percent). Of these mothers, 35 percent pumped only two to four times in 24 hours, 41 percent expressed five to six times, and 24 percent pumped seven to eight times in 24 hours. The number-one reason for discontinuing breastmilk collection was obtaining insufficient milk, followed by the complaint that pumping was too time consuming. More than one-half of the women delayed expression until two to five days postpartum. Only 33 percent of the mothers identified hygienic practices as important in the collection of breastmilk. These findings from four different hospitals show the prevalence of practices unlikely to promote an optimal supply of bacterially safe breastmilk. According to Forte, Mayberry, and Ferketich (1987), "A lack of perceived support may reduce the number of mothers who are attempting to maintain lactation."

Morse and Bottorff (1988) observed 61 nursing mothers and their emotional experiences related to expressing milk. Many were surprised that the ability to express their milk was not automatic. They often found that verbal and written instructions were unclear and confusing; many learned by trial and error. Mothers in this study stressed that "instructions for one mother did not necessarily work for all." Some were embarrassed, and others were frustrated when they obtained only small amounts of milk. Although success with expression increased a mother's self-confidence, women who perceived expression to be an important aspect of breastfeeding but who were unable to express milk displayed heightened feelings of inadequacy. The authors suggested modifying how expression is taught to include not only explicit "how-to" instruction but the encouragement of private exploratory practice and (when appropriate) the use of humor by the instructor to reduce embarrassment.

Many mothers receive only the pump insert instructions to use as a guide in learning milk expression and handling. These instructions vary widely in their recommendations on pumping techniques and even on the cleaning of the pump. Further confusion is possible if a mother uses more than one type of pump, especially if she fails to read all of the instructions carefully or if the instructions from one manufacturer conflict with those from another.

The concerns of mothers are rarely addressed in the professional literature on breast pumps and milk expression. Clinicians must remember that the best pump will do little for a mother whose emotional needs are not met and who lacks the guidelines necessary to use the equipment properly for optimal results (see Table 13–6 for a selected comparison of pump instructions). These directions are taken directly from the literature provided with the pumps and can vary considerably.

Sample Guidelines for Pump Recommendations and Pumping Techniques

The health care professional needs to base pumping recommendations on many factors and to take into account each mother's situation. For example, a mother whose premature infant is younger than 30 weeks of gestation and is not taking oral feedings needs instructions very different from those for a mother who is pumping during her hours of employment or one who is only occasionally expressing milk. The mother of the premature infant needs a pump that embodies many basic features:

- Removes milk quickly
- Pumps both breasts simultaneously
- Promotes physiological prolactin cycling
- Obtains milk with a high energy content
- Has an easily controlled vacuum
- Permits the vacuum to be applied for short periods to avoid tissue damage
- Produces high milk yields
- Is easy to use
- Is heat resistant for high-temperature sterilization
- Is durable (will not stop working or break easily)
- Is economical
- Is accessible

A reasonable option for long-term pumping is an electric pump with a double collecting kit that is leased on a long-term basis. The mother should begin pumping as soon after the birth as possible and should do so at least eight times each 24 hours (Hill et al., 1996).

The mother who has a healthy two- to three-month-old infant and is returning to full-time employment outside the home may have different needs. Although battery pumps are popular, using an AC adapter will help to increase efficiency and decrease the cost of replacement batteries. This mother might also consider a long-term lease of an electric pump. If this mother chooses to use a manually operated cylinder pump, instructions should include proper hand positioning to avoid developing lateral epicondylitis (i.e., tennis elbow; Williams et al., 1989). These instructions emphasize shoulder adduction, with the elbow lying against the body, the forearm in supination (turned up), and the wrist slightly flexed. A mother with carpal tunnel syndrome or other hand, wrist, arm, or shoulder problems may need to use an electric pump rather than a manual or battery-operated pump to avoid exacerbation of her symptoms.

A mother who expresses only small amounts of milk or who has a low milk supply should be advised to elicit the milk-ejection reflex by allowing baby suckling, looking at a picture of her baby, listening to guided relaxation tapes, or practicing slow chest breathing before applying the pump and to massage the breast by quadrants throughout the pumping session. She may need to sit in a quiet area that permits relaxation with a minimum of interruptions. Pumping early in the morning or on the opposite breast while the baby is nursing may also prove helpful. In the absence of an abundant milk supply and a reliable milk-ejection reflex, the use of a battery-operated pump may not prove to be the best choice. The mother should also be advised to express milk after each breastfeeding to drain the breasts as much as possible.

Common Pumping Problems

The most common pumping problems seen by clinicians are sore nipples, obtaining only small amounts of milk per pumping session, erratic or delayed milk-ejection reflex, and dwindling milk supply over a long-term course of pumping (Walker, 1987). Sore nipples caused by breast pumps can be minimized by certain techniques: using the lowest amount of vacuum that works to obtain milk, applying vacuum only after the breast has begun to release its milk, interrupting the vacuum frequently to avoid or decrease pain while still maintaining milk flow, switching from side to side frequently as the milk flow slows (when using single-sided pumping), ensuring proper flange fit with an inner opening that is not too small for the nipple entering it or too large to be effective, and pumping for shorter periods.

Obtaining only small amounts of milk per pumping session occurs most often when the milk-ejection reflex has not been elicited. Mothers complain that the milk drips but does not spray out and that it takes more than 45 minutes to accumulate 0.5 to 1.0 oz. As a result of this frustration, pump vacuum levels are often increased and maintained for long, uninterrupted periods. This contributes more to sore nipples than to increased milk yields. To elicit the milk-ejection reflex, some mothers have reported using a hot shower or hot compresses, having their partner massage their breasts, or establishing a pumping routine (activities performed prior to each pumping session that elicit milk flow). Increasing fluid intake does not usually increase milk yield. Some mothers pump

Table 13–6

SELECTED USER INSTRUCTIONS

Cylinder	Elicit Milk Ejection Before Pumping	Massage Breast	Sterilizing	Technique	Cleaning	Sanitizing	Miscellaneous
Hand Pumps							
Evenflo Natural Mother	Yes	Yes	3–5 minutes in boiling water.	Nipple in exact center; move handle in and out in a steady rhythmic motion. Can increase suction by inserting suction valve. Interrupt suction at end of outward stroke.	Warm soapy water, rinse well. Dishwasher-safe in top rack. Leave seal on during cleaning.		Hand position pronated in picture.
Ross Deluxe (Happy Family)	Yes	Yes—before pumping.	No	Slowly push and pull cylinder back and forth; when flow decreases, massage and repeat.	Remove gasket during cleaning; use hot soapy water, rinse well. Safe in upper rack of dishwasher, except for gasket and sealing disk.		Hand position supine; flared end of basket must point up.
Sears Naturally Soft	Yes	Yes—before pumping to decrease pumping time.	No	Move outer cylinder to and from breast; as outer cylinder fills, shorten pump stroke.	Clean with warm water and mild detergent.	Sanitize in boiling water for 10 seconds after cleaning. Before first use boil for 10 seconds.	Rinse nipples with plain water; flared end of gasket faces breast; hand supine.
Medela	No	No	Prior to first use and before first use in the morning. Disassemble and boil for 20 minutes.	Slow rhythmic intervals; pull piston full length of cylinder with every stroke.	After each use wash in lukewarm soapy water and rinse well.		Breast cleaned with damp cloth prior to pumping; hand supine with elbow close to body.

Table 13-6

Ameda/ Egnell	No	No	Can be boiled briefly prior to first use. Sterilize in upper rack of dishwasher.	Pull pump cylinder slowly down.	No–gasket can be left on during cleaning.	No. Hand supine.
Kaneson	Yes–to decrease pumping time.	Yes–for 2 minutes to promote let-down.	Sterilize in boiling water for 5 minutes before first use. Rubber gasket may remain on.	Nipple in center of adapter, outer cylinder moved away from body. As milk fills outer cylinder, shorten length of stroke to avoid gasket coming in contact with milk.	After each use rinse with warm water and clean with mild detergent.	
Infa	Yes	Yes–for a minute or two to stimulate milk flow.	Presterilize all parts in boiling water 3–4 minutes.	Slowly pull the outer cylinder creating suction with a gentle pumping action.	Wash in warm soapy water after each use; dishwasher safe.	Assembly instructions do not include how to attach gasket.
White River						
Squeeze-handle manual						
Loyd-B	No	No	With shield in stopper, boil for 15 minutes.	Center nipple in shield; pump to comfort level; leave under vacuum 30–45 seconds, then release. Hold and release in this cycle for 3 minutes each side twice.	No	
Avent	Yes–by hand expressing.	No	Sterilize by boiling.	Pump gently, occasionally holding handle down for 2–3 seconds to maintain vacuum.	Wash in warm soapy water.	Clean the breast.
Ameda/ Egnell (one hand)	Yes–warm wet compresses.	Yes–light circular massage.	Sterilize before use by boiling for 20 minutes.	Adjust speed and intensity of hand movements to control vacuum.	After use, large parts can go in dishwasher; small parts hand washed.	Attachment for electric pump not packed in all kits.

Table 13-6 (cont.)

SELECTED USER INSTRUCTIONS

Cylinder	Elicit Milk Ejection Before Pumping	Massage Breast	Sterilizing	Technique	Cleaning	Sanitizing	Miscellaneous
Battery-operated							
Evenflo Sof-Touch Ultra	Yes—to promote easier milk flow and prevent soreness.	Yes—for 1-2 minutes.	Before first use, sterilize in boiling water for 3–5 minutes.	Nipple in exact center; allow suction to increase to a comfortable level. Depress and release button to comfort.	Wash in warm soapy water and mild detergent, rinse well.		Has AC adapter.
Ameda/Egnell Lact-B	No	No	Sterilize in boiling water for 20 minutes before first and after each use; or place in upper rack of dishwasher.	4–6 seconds of suction followed by 1–2-second interruption to elicit let-down and for entire pumping session.	Wash in soapy water after each use.		Cautions that continuous suction may hurt the breast.
Mag Mag	No	Massage during pumping for better suction.	Sterilize in top rack of dishwasher or boil for 3–5 minutes.	Allow suction to build for as long as 30 seconds. Release button for 1–2 seconds.			
Mag Mag Advanced	Yes	Yes—for more fluent suction.	Stir boil for 3–5 minutes.	Determine comfortable suction; release button pushed for 2–3 seconds.	Hand wash all parts; or place in top rack of dishwasher.		Four raised areas in hard nipple adapter claimed to stimulate milk glands. Caution about tilting pump because of danger of milk flowing down into motor. Can flush motor with backed-up milk.

Table 13-6

Gentle Expressions	Yes—or can nurse baby on one side while pumping the other.	Yes—to encourage let-down.	Before first use; hot soapy water; rinse; boil 5–15 minutes to sterilize; dishwasher safe.	Center the nipple; use the suction-release button frequently after adjusting the suction regulator for comfort.	Wash and sanitize after each use.	Clean breast with damp cloth prior to pumping. As batteries wear down, vacuum held longer causing possible discomfort. Reduce vacuum level and replace batteries.
Medela (Mini electric)	No	No	No instructions.	Relax and alternate between breasts.	Disassemble and clean all parts separately.	
Small semiautomatic electric						
Precious Care	Yes—to decrease pumping time.	Yes—to push milk down into ducts.	Before first use, wash in hot water and mild detergent; then sanitize in boiling water for 10 seconds.	Center the nipple; cover vacuum-release hole and release the vacuum to suit your comfort. Some mothers leave the vacuum steady while others create a pulsing or sucking action by covering and uncovering the hole.	After use, clean with mild detergent and sanitize for 10 seconds in boiling water.	Rinse nipples with clear water. Allow unit to run for 45 seconds before using.

Table 13-6 (cont.)

Cylinder	Elicit Milk Ejection Before Pumping	Massage Breast	Sterilizing	Technique	Cleaning	Sanitizing	Miscellaneous
Nurture III	No—towel soaked in warm water and applied to breasts helps with let-down.	No		Begin pumping with low setting; tap hole to make and break suction; vary time interval during which finger covers hole. To further control suction, roll finger back and forth over tap hole rather than lifting it off completely.	Wash before use.		Can also pump both sides simultaneously.
Schuco Model #400	No	No	Disinfect once a day in boiling water for 2–3 minutes.	Center the nipple; regulate pressure by partially or fully covering the vent hole of the suction bell with finger; cover and open vent hole for natural suction.	Clean with water and rinse before each use. Clean after each use; add a few drops of soap to water for cleaning.		Drink fluids as much as possible to stimulate production of milk. Use only 4-oz. collection container and empty at 3½ oz.
Large semiautomatic electric							
Mada #174	No	No	Before first use; boil for 20 minutes.	Close and open aperture for repeated suction and relaxation by lifting finger or partially closing and opening hole.	After each use; warm soapy water, rinse in lukewarm water.		If mother does not get milk after several minutes of initial pumping, stop and try again in 20 minutes.
Schuco-Vac Easy Flow Expressor	No	No	No	Center breast shield; press index finger on control to seal. Hold finger over fingertip control for 10–20 seconds and release for 2–5 seconds.	No	No	Should soreness or irritation occur, discontinue use and consult a physician.

Table 13-6

Large automatic electric

White River	Yes—to encourage milk to move down to milk sinuses.	Yes—before and when pumping begins.	To sterilize, boil for 20 minutes.	Moisten flexible flange with water; center nipple in flange; cover and release the valve 7 times per 5 seconds.	Breast and surrounding area should be cleaned with damp cloth.
Medela	No	No	Prior to first use and before first use in the morning; boil for 20 minutes.	Adjust vacuum to personal comfort.	After each use, wash in lukewarm soapy water.
Ameda/Egnell	No	No	Can disinfect by boiling for at least 20 minutes.	Adjust pressure to personal comfort.	After use, wash in warm soapy water.
The Rose				Place on low suction to begin and increase to comfortable level.	

Source: Data in this chart were derived directly from instructional inserts provided with the pumps by the manufacturers.

whenever they experience a spontaneous milk ejection. Timing pumping sessions may also help some women, particularly if they find it difficult to obtain much milk immediately after the baby has fed. Pumping midway between feedings may alleviate this situation. Morning pumping sessions also tend to yield more milk. Mothers who are employed full-time report that pumping sessions early in the week also tend to yield more milk than do those later in the week (Auerbach & Guss, 1984).

Oxytocin (Syntocinon) has been used prior to each pumping session as a temporary boost to milk ejection. Although this agent is no longer available as a nasal spray, compounding pharmacies can purchase oxytocin and mix it into a nasal spray form (Gross, 1995). Oxytocin has been used by mothers during the first week of pumping following a preterm birth with promising results. In one study, primiparous mothers showed a 3.5-fold increase in milk production, and multiparous mothers a 2.5-fold increase compared to mothers who did not use oxytocin nasal spray prior to each pumping session (Ruis et al., 1981).

Medicine and technology are saving infants as young as 23 weeks' gestational age. Mothers of extremely premature infants will likely be expressing their milk for many weeks or months. They can encounter difficulties in maintaining an optimal milk supply through artificial means. A flexible pumping plan should be developed for optimal milk production (Auerbach & Walker, 1994). Faltering milk production is not unusual with extended pumping. In addition to the guidelines in this chapter, additional interventions include the use of metoclopramide (Ehrenkranz & Ackerman, 1986), domperidone (Motilium), acupuncture (Clavey, 1996), and human growth hormone (Gunn et al., 1996).

Factors other than the type of equipment used also affect milk flow. Morse and Bottorff (1988, p. 170) stated, "Understanding the complex feelings towards expressing and the experimental nature of learning to express has important implications for the way that expression is taught." An erratic or delayed milk-ejection reflex is common when a mother must respond to a mechanical device rather than to her baby, particularly when she is first learning to use a pump. If the milk-ejection reflex is not triggered quickly, the nipples and breast tissue are exposed to high levels of vacuum over an inefficient pressure gradient. This can result in low milk yields, sore nipples, and frustration with the pumping process. Although pumps are capable of eliciting milk ejection and their instructions often advise applying the pump for this purpose, some women will have difficulty in releasing their milk. This may be caused by inhibitory messages received by the hypothalamus. Embarrassment, tension, fear of failure, pain, fatigue, and anxiety may block the neurochemical pathways required for milk ejection. If these factors appear to interfere with milk ejection, ask the mother how she feels about pumping. A negative attitude does little to contribute to milk flow. One mother, when offered the option of double pumping, said it made her feel like a cow. Single-sided pumping was more appealing to her. When the clinician elicits the mother's feelings and attitudes about pumping, guidelines can be individually created for each situation.

It is not unusual for the milk-ejection reflex to take longer to trigger as the lactation course increases. What works early in lactation may change over time. Some mothers report improved results later in lactation after they change to a different pump or use a different flange that fits the breast better.

Expressing milk has different meanings for each mother. Some see it as a way to continue providing breastmilk in their absence, especially in families with a history of allergies. Some women prefer to hand-express and can obtain as much or more milk than other mothers who are using a mechanical device (see Chapter 10 for additional information about hand expression). Other mothers view pumping as part of a grieflike reaction that is reinforced every two to three hours when they must use a pump in the absence of a baby at breast. Sound recommendations for expressing milk—however it is accomplished—with instructions based on a clear understanding of the anatomy and physiology of the breast and knowledge of the lactation process will enable many women to give their infant the best possible nutritional and emotional start.

Nipple Shields

Nipple shields appeared in the medical literature as early as the mid-1600s. Scultetus describes shields made of silver and used so that ". . . nurses may suckle the infants without trouble which, when children were breast-fed until long after their front teeth were cut, must have been very necessary" (Bennion, 1979). Shields were first used to evert flat nipples and to protect nipples from the cold and rubbing against clothing between feedings. Shields were made of lead (which caused brain damage in babies), wax, wood, gum elastic, pewter, tin, horn, bone, ivory, silver, and glass. The gum elastic shield in Fig. 13–6 was used for babies to nurse on. Maygrier (1833) stated that "This mode is difficult and generally the child is unwilling."

The design of nipple shields has changed little since the 1500s. By the 1800s, rubber shields began appearing. The Maw's shield (Fig. 13–7) was constructed with a rubber lining, a glass shank, and a rubber teat. In the 1980s, this design was still used with a glass or plastic shank and a rubber teat (Davol). Rubber versions of the silver and wood shields also began appearing. The early shields were composed of thick rubber with a firm nipple cone (The Mexican Hat, Macarthy's Surgical, Ltd.). One U.S. version, the Breast-Eze, was a modified rubber nipple on a rubber base with thick rubber ribs lining the inside to help "stimulate" the breast and has been reported to be very painful to use. The rubber shields gradually became thinner (Evenflo) and were replaced with thin latex (Lewin Woolf, Griptight, Ltd.) and silicone (Cannon Babysafe) seen today (Fig. 13–8).

Shields are currently used during feedings to assist baby and mother in various ways:

- To latch onto flat nipples
- To latch onto nipples that are everted but that the baby does not actively draw into his mouth (Elliott, 1996)
- To latch on when he has experienced difficulty from the previous use of artificial nipples
- To latch onto an engorged breast in which the nipple is surrounded by noncompressible areolar tissue

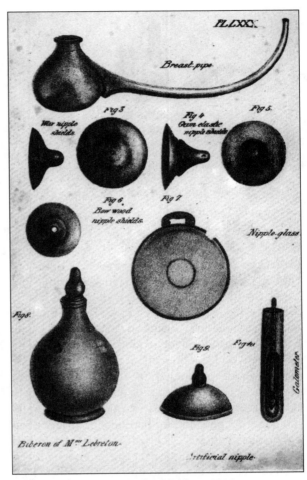

FIGURE 13–6. Early nipple shields, c. 1833.

- To ease feeding when a weak, disorganized, or dysfunctional suck is present (in the case of special babies with neurological problems, following preterm birth, or Down syndrome) (Clum & Primomo, 1996)
- To protect sore or damaged (cracked) nipples during a breastfeeding
- To prevent sore nipples (claimed by manufacturers but not proved)

Although the idea of protecting the nipple may be made in good faith, the ramifications of nipple shield use can be both destructive to the course of lactation and risky to the health of the baby (Desmarais & Browne, 1990).

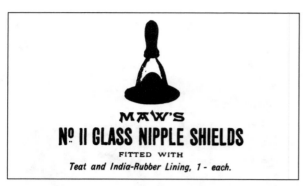

FIGURE 13–7. Nipple shield and breast glass, c. 1864.

Review of the Literature

Woolridge et al. (1980) studied the effect of the all-rubber shield (Macarthy-Mexican Hat) and a thin latex shield on the sucking patterns and milk intake of five- to eight-day-old babies of mothers with problem-free lactation experiences. The Macarthy-Mexican Hat reduced milk transfer by 58 percent and changed infant sucking patterns by increasing the sucking rate and the time spent pausing. This is a pattern typically seen when milk flow decreases. The thin latex shield reduced milk intake by 22 percent and had no significant effect on sucking patterns. The babies observed in this study had no difficulty in latching onto mothers' nipples, and no nipple soreness was reported by the mothers in the study. If these problems existed, milk transfer and sucking patterns could be further compromised with the use of any shield. Using the same thin latex shield, Jackson et al. (1987) showed a 29 percent decrease in milk transfer during their study of nutrient intake in healthy, full-term newborns.

Amatayakul et al. (1987) measured plasma prolactin and cortisol levels in mothers, with and without a thin latex nipple shield in place. They found that prolactin and cortisol levels were unaffected by the shield but that milk transfer was decreased by 42 percent when the shield was in place during feedings. They postulate that this effect on milk volume is attibutable to an interference with oxytocin release.

Auerbach (1990a) studied changes in pumped milk volume with and without the use of a thin silicone shield (Cannon Babysafe). Twenty-five mothers used a breast pump (Medela electric model) to provide milk samples, which prevented any change in infant sucking patterns from affecting milk volume amounts. Milk volume was significantly reduced when a shield was in place. Seventy-one percent of the total milk obtained was recorded when no shield was used. Pumping without a shield resulted in mean volumes five to seven times greater than when a shield was in place.

More recent discussions of nipple-shield use report beneficial outcomes. Key to such use is experienced assessment by a skilled lactation consultant, continuing assistance, and careful follow-up. Thus babies who might not otherwise continue to milk the breast made the transition to breastfeeding without having to continue to use the device. Woodworth & Frank (1996) described a baby who refused to continue to breastfeed following inappropriate assistance in the hospital that included forcing the baby onto the breast. In this case presentation, nipple shield use in conjunction with long-term support of the mother's efforts to bring the baby back to the breast enabled the mother and baby to continue breastfeeding, ultimately without the shield.

Wilson-Clay (1996) reported the experiences of 32 mothers who used nipple shields to resolve breastfeeding problems. The majority of these women continued to breastfeed after using nipple shields. Brigham (1996) reviewed the experiences of 51 mothers. In 86 percent of the cases, these women reported positive experiences with the nipple shields to resolve the problems that they were encountering. In the ten cases reported by Bodley and Powers (1996), infant weight gain was appropriate during and after the period of nipple shield use. These authors concluded, "In some special situations, the use of a nipple shield can permit breastfeeding to continue, provided the lactation consultant carefully follows up, and the baby is weighed regularly" (Bodley & Powers, 1996, p. 303).

Risks

Besides reducing milk-volume transfer, all shield designs have drawbacks that may compromise the breastfeeding course for the mother attempting to use them. For this reason, their use should be carefully monitored to enhance their likelihood of

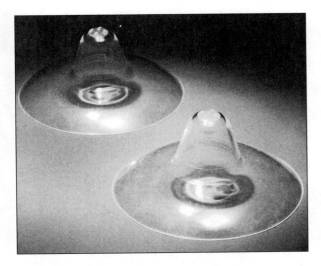

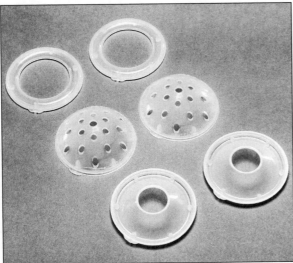

FIGURE 13–8. Modern nipple shields (top) and breast shells (bottom). *(Courtesy Medela, Inc., McHenry, IL)*

in by the infant, thus reducing the likelihood that the baby will learn correct latch-on

- Change the sucking pattern to a nonnutritive mode (typically seen when milk flow decreases at the end of a breastfeeding)

- Reduce stimulation of the nipple-areolar complex, potentially interfering with prolactin and oxytocin release

- Temporarily or permanently reduce the milk-producing capacity of the breasts, and contribute to slow, low, or no weight gain in the baby, which results in acute dehydration, failure to thrive, and weaning

- Prevent proper extension of the nipple back into the baby's mouth (Minchin, 1985)

- Pinch the nipple and areola, thus causing abrasion, pain, skin breakdown, and internal trauma to the breast

- Create nipple-shield addiction (DeNicola, 1986), after which the baby will not feed at breast without the shield in place

- Predispose the nipple to damage when the baby is put to breast without the shield, as he may chew rather than suckle

- Relay the message to the mother that she or her baby may not be good enough to feed her baby unless a barrier is placed between the two

Standard Bottle Nipples or Bottle Nipples Attached to a Glass or Plastic Base. In addition to the problems just listed, these bottle-nipple types of shields place the baby and his mouth one to two inches away from the mother's nipple, significantly altering positioning at breast. This does not permit compression of the milk sinuses or skin-to-skin stimulation of the nipple-areolar complex and may alter prolactin cycling. Milk may pool in the base that holds the artificial nipple and may never reach the baby or may simply leak out the sides.

Latex and Silicone Shields. Latex and silicone shields are extremely thin, flexible shields shaped like the rubber shields. Only the nipple portion is firm, about 2 cm long with four holes in the tip. Because the silicone is so thin, more stimulation reaches the areola, and milk volume is not as

appropriate assistance and to reduce the likelihood of problems additional to those they were meant to alleviate.

All-Rubber Shield. Before recommending the use of all-rubber shields, remember that they can result in detrimental side effects:

- Interfere with positioning baby properly at breast

- Present a firm nipple portion that can be inserted into baby's mouth rather than being drawn

seriously depleted as with the other designs (Auerbach, 1990a). Furthermore, the mother's ability to feel the infant suckling may encourage her to continue to attempt breastfeeding when difficulties have already occurred. In addition, rewarding with his mother's milk the baby who suckles the breast with a nipple shield in place may encourage the baby to continue to breastfeed. Over time, continued use of the shield may enable both mother and baby to move to direct breastfeeding once each is working well with the other.

Because of increasing reports of latex allergy in the general population, the clinician needs to ascertain whether the mother is sensitive to latex before suggesting use of this product.

Responsibilities of Health Care Professionals

The health care professional has certain responsibilities regarding breastfeeding women and nipple shields:

1. *Understand the risks of using such a device.* Hospital-based providers must be aware of the previously mentioned long-term consequences when shields are given to mothers. Research-based hospital protocols should clearly state the rationale behind avoiding the routine use of shields.

2. *Assess the situation before recommending a shield* (Auerbach, 1989). Shields used as a quick fix to ensure infant feedings before early discharge, particularly in the absence of an opportunity for follow-up, may act as a kind of "Band-Aid therapy," appearing to solve the problem without addressing its cause. Identify and take steps to correct the problem rather than issuing a shield as the initial therapy. Box 13–3 shows a chart summarizing alternatives to shield use.

3. *Employ informed consent* (Kutner, 1986) and sensitize providers to the risks of shields if a mother wishes to use them. A consent form should be signed by the mother, the father (if available), and the provider who is recommending the shield. This will assure that everyone knows the risks of using a shield and knows how to use it so that its dangers are minimized.

A consent form used in this manner also serves as a teaching aid to professionals who are unaware of potential long-range problems. A copy should be given to the mother, another copy retained in the medical record, and a third sent to the pediatrician.

The consent form should specify the reason the shield has been recommended. It should clarify that the shield is for temporary use; warn that continuous use at each feeding can cause a decreased milk supply, low weight gain, and acute dehydration; note that the baby's weight needs to be monitored twice a week; and state that the mother may need to express milk to maintain an adequate supply.

4. *Realize that the risks of nipple shield use have legal implications* for the hospital and for the professional who recommends them. A malpractice case was lodged against a nurse and her employing hospital after a nipple shield was dispensed without warning the parents of the potential consequences of its use (Bornmann, 1986).

5. *Provide proper instructions and referrals* if a shield is used as an interim recommendation to assist with breastfeeding. Written instructions should explain that shield use is often temporary and that it should be discontinued as soon as possible. It can be used to assist with latch-on and removed when the baby has established rhythmic nutritive suckling. The baby should be put directly to breast as much as possible and may accept the breast better when in a state of light sleep. If a mother is discharged from the hospital using a shield, a community referral should be made to a lactation consultant or the nurse practitioner at the pediatrician's office for daily follow-up and assistance in breastfeeding without the shield when it is appropriate to do so. Frequent weight checks should be obtained. The pediatrician should be alerted to the problem that required use of the shield in the first place and should be aware of suggestions for discontinuing its use. If the mother continues to use the shield long term, regular weight checks should be included in the care plan to ensure that the infant continues to gain weight and reaches developmental

BOX 13-3

Alternatives to Nipple Shield Use

SITUATION	MANAGEMENT
Sore or cracked nipples	Observe and correct maternal and infant positioning. Document a correct nutritive suckling pattern and tongue placement of baby at breast. Assist baby to latch on with a wide-open mouth if necessary and hand-express colostrum or milk to prevent build-up of negative pressure.
Flat or retracted nipples	Roll and shape the nipple prior to feeding. Pump briefly before each feeding to evert nipples. Consider use of breast shells between feedings.
Engorgement	Hand-express to increase compressibility of areolar tissue, followed by use of an electric pump if necessary prior to feedings for easier latch-on.
Difficulty or failure of baby to latch onto the breast	In addition to the foregoing, or if the baby requires more assistance, incentives at breast to promote latch-on should be attempted (i.e., feeding-tube device, syringe, or dropper to place or dribble fluid into or near the baby's mouth). Finger-feeding can be done by either parent to establish appropriate nutritive suckling patterns.

milestones as expected. Although the preceding cautions may seem less necessary when a thin latex or silicone shield is used, remaining vigilant regarding potential adverse outcomes may reduce the likelihood of their occurrence.

Weaning from a Shield

Weaning a baby from a shield can be a lengthy process (Bodley & Powers, 1996). If a thick rubber shield is being used or a bottle nipple has been placed over the mother's nipple, switch to a thin latex shield as soon as possible. Once the baby has shown that he will appropriately suckle at the breast at each feeding with the shield in place, it may be time to begin attempting to remove it. In some cases, the baby will make clear that the shield is no longer necessary.

When attempting to wean the baby from the shield, allow him to use the shield for a minute or two or until there is a pause in his suckling pattern; remove the shield and ask the mother to quickly bring the baby back to her breast. This technique may help draw flat nipples out far enough for the baby to grasp without the shield (Auerbach, 1987).

A feeding tube can be secured to the outside or inside of the shield with a supplement running to promote latch-on and to deliver expressed breastmilk or formula to a calorie-deprived baby. Sometimes a quick removal of the shield, with the supplement delivered by a tube taped to the areola under the shield, orients the baby to the breast more quickly.

Ongoing assessment and management to eliminate the original cause for use of the shield should continue. Rarely, a situation may arise in which a shield can be used temporarily to eliminate the need to wean the baby from the breast. The authors have used a silicone shield with a mother who presented with weeping eczema on the areola of her right breast. The mother had been advised to wean because the orange discharge would "make the baby sick." Instead of weaning, she began pumping that breast, which exacerbated the damage to the areola and created much pain with each pumping session. After referral, we secured a thin silicone shield on which the baby nursed at each feeding; pumping of the right breast was discontinued. The shield was thoroughly cleaned between uses while cortisone therapy resolved the eczema. The baby went back to the involved nipple and areola with no problems.

Postpartum units that are reluctant to discontinue stocking nipple shields may benefit from a product evaluation form describing the drawbacks of shields, along with copies of documentation from the breastfeeding literature (Shrago, 1988). The occasional use of thin nipple shields may be appropriate but cannot replace thorough assessment of the presenting problem.

Breast Shells

Breast shells are two-piece plastic devices worn over the nipple and areola to evert flat or retracted nipples. Historically, these shells were called *nipple glasses* (see Fig. 13–7) and were used to protect the mother's clothing from leaked milk or were applied if the mother had "too much" milk. Some brands are still marketed as a device for catching leaked milk between feedings. Shells are not recommended for this use, although many mothers find them helpful for collecting dripped milk from one breast while nursing or pumping on the opposite side. Some clinicians also recommend their use for engorgement, as their gentle pressure encourages milk to leak. The milk collected between feedings should be discarded because of potential high bacteria counts. If dripped milk is collected during a feeding or pumping session, it can be stored as usual.

Inverted nipples are identified when the areola is compressed behind the base of the nipple and the nipple retreats into the surrounding skin. Lawrence (1989) calls this a *tied nipple,* which is caused by the presence of the original invagination of the mammary dimple. Prenatally, breast shells were worn for increasingly longer periods throughout the day and were removed at night. The constant gentle pressure around the base of the nipple was thought to release the adhesions anchoring the nipple, thus allowing it to protrude when the baby latched onto the breast. Shells can be worn between feedings after the baby is born if nipple flattening or retraction is identified postpartum or if the nipples still need correction. Current information shows that little correction of the nipple takes place prenatally and that some women do not like using these devices (Alexander et al., 1992).

Several brands of shells are available, all of which have a dome that is placed over a base through which the nipple protrudes when worn under a bra. Depending on the brand, the dome may have one or many ventilation holes. The domes with only one or two holes may not provide adequate air circulation to the nipple and areola. The retained moisture and heat (especially in hot weather) can create a miniature greenhouse effect that promotes soreness and skin breakdown. Extra holes can be drilled in the top of the dome. Some brands have many holes in the dome to help with this problem. Both the Hollister/Ameda-Egnell shells and the Medela shells have absorbent pads that are placed in the bottom of the shell under the areola to absorb leaked milk and moisture. It is not known whether this padding provides a reservoir for bacterial buildup. They also have a pad that is placed between the shell and skin to decrease skin irritation or discomfort. The Medela shell is well ventilated and somewhat narrower than is the Hollister/Ameda-Egnell shell. A breast pad may be worn between the shell and bra with the Medela shell, because there are vent holes in the bottom of the dome as well.

Recommendations on Breast Shells

Prenatal use of breast shells has been suggested for nipples that appear retracted or severely flattened. Although research shows that they are not effective (Alexander et al., 1992), some mothers insist on using them. When the LC is instructing the expectant mother in the prenatal use of breast shells, she should advise her to:

- wear the shells for one or two hours a day, gradually increasing the time until they are worn all day, remove the shells before going to bed, wash them well, rinse, and air dry overnight;

- in hot weather or if moisture buildup occurs, remove the shells for 20 minutes at a time, two or three times a day, and dry the shells well;

- if the nipple does not fit completely through the hole in the base, use a brand with a larger opening or a shallower-sloping base.

When instructing a mother in the use of breast shells postpartum, the LC should advise her to

- wear the shells for 30 minutes prior to each feeding or for the entire time between feedings, whichever gives the best results;

- use only the drip milk that collects during a feeding or pumping session, discarding any milk that is collected between feedings;

- wear shells to relieve excess milk buildup in the lactiferous sinuses by inducing slow leaking;

- wash the shells in hot, soapy water and rinse well before using them to collect drip milk if they have been worn between feedings;

- remove the shells at bedtime or for naps so that areas of the breast do not become obstructed;

- use shells with well-ventilated domes;

- obtain a snug-fitting shell; if painful rings occur on the areola, consider changing to a larger bra or increase the cup size of the bra.

Feeding-Tube Devices

Feeding-tube devices are a recent addition to the options for help in special breastfeeding situations. Judicious use of these devices enables many mothers and babies to breastfeed who otherwise would have lost this unique opportunity.

Description

Feeding-tube devices consist of a container to hold breastmilk or formula and a length of thin tubing that runs from the container to the mother's nipple. The tube is secured in place by nonallergenic tape or sterile dressing material, and as the baby suckles at breast, supplement is simultaneously delivered. Providing milk in this manner may be a novel idea to both the mother and her nurse or physician. Careful explanations should include how the feeding tube device is used and the expected outcomes. Some mothers are put off by the thought of feeding their babies in what they consider "a nonnatural" way that at first appears complicated. Explaining that the device is a temporary aid in establishing the baby at breast while ensuring adequate nutrition helps the mother to accept tube feeding. Several commercial devices are on the market; in addition, noncommercial devices can be constructed from bottles or syringes and tubing.

Lact-Aid (USA). Developed in 1971 for nursing the adopted baby, the Lact-Aid device created a breastfeeding experience for those mothers and babies who previously had no choice in terms of feeding methods. It is a closed system consisting of a presterilized, disposable four-ounce bag to hold milk, with a cap through which a length of fine tubing extends to the nipple. The bag hangs around the mother's neck on a cord. Air is squeezed out of the bag to facilitate milk flow. Powdered or meat-based formulas will not flow readily through the device.

Supply Line (Australia). In Australia, this device uses two 140-ml feeding bottles worn around the neck in a pouch with a double length of tubing. The tubing is threaded through a hole in the bottle lid.

D-I-Y Nursing Supplementer (United Kingdom). A regular bottle and nipple are used with a length of tubing inserted through the nipple into the bottle. The mother must hold the bottle and regulate the flow by changing the height of the bottle.

Axi-Care Nursing Supplementer (United Kingdom). The Axi-Care device uses a plastic bottle, tubing, and a roller clamp (as on an intravenous setup) to control supplement flow. Reports indicate that the bottle will sometimes collapse, because it is not a completely vented system.

Supplemental Nutrition System (United States) Medela, Inc. The Supplemental Nutrition System consists of a five-ounce plastic bottle with a cap through which a length of tubing is secured to each breast. A smaller version also is available. This two-tube unit allows the tubing to be set up on both breasts at the same time and comes with three different sizes of tubing. It is a vented system with a cap that has notches for pinching off both tubes while setting up the unit and securing one tube as the baby is feeding from the other side. Flow rates are influenced by the size of the tubing used (small, medium, large), the height of the bottle, and whether the opposite tube is pinched off during the feeding.

Situations for Use

Feeding-tube systems can be recommended and used in many situations where other measures have failed or to prevent further complications.

Infant Sucking Problems. Babies with weak, disorganized, or dysfunctional sucking are candidates for feeding-tube systems. This group includes

- hyperactive or hypoactive infants
- infants with Down syndrome
- preterm infants
- infants with cardiac problems
- infants with cleft lip or palate
- infants who have experienced perinatal asphyxia
- nipple-confused infants
- neurologically impaired infants
- infants with low, slow, or no weight gain, or experiencing weight loss due to ineffective suckling
- lethargic infants in the hospital who are at risk for inadequate food or fluid intake, bilirubin levels, or supplementation with sugar water using an artificial nipple

Maternal Situations. Several groups of mothers can benefit from the use of feeding-tube devices, including

- adoptive nursing (induced lactation) mothers (Auerbach & Avery, 1981; Sutherland & Auerbach, 1985)

- mothers who are relactating (i.e., inducing a milk supply after a separation or interruption of breastfeeding) (Auerbach & Avery, 1980; Bose et al., 1981)
- mothers who have had breast surgery, especially breast-reduction mammaplasty that included moving the nipple
- mothers who suffer from primary lactation insufficiency (i.e., not enough functional breast tissue to support a full milk supply) (Neifert & Seacat, 1985)
- mothers with severe nipple trauma
- mothers who have recently discontinued short-term medications contraindicated for a nursing infant
- mothers who are suffering from an illness or undergoing surgery or hospitalization
- mothers who have flat or inverted nipples and a baby who cannot latch on

Generally, a feeding-tube device is used to maintain a mother's milk supply, to deliver sufficient or extra nutrients to the baby, and to create a behavior-modification situation that shapes the baby's suckling pattern to one suitable for obtaining milk from the breast (or prevents the suckling pattern from changing). These devices allow feedings to be done at breast when formerly, in certain situations, bottles with nipple sets were used. Because these devices are used only in special situations, it is imperative that the professional who recommends their use follow up closely (daily if necessary) to ensure adequate milk intake by the baby, correct use by the mother, and weaning from the device when it is appropriate to do so.

For a baby to use a feeding tube at breast, he must be able to latch on and execute some form of suckling. For babies who are unable at first to do this because of strong extensor positioning, hypotonia, or lethargy, finger-feeding with the device can be used as an interim measure (Bull & Barger, 1987). The mother can place a tube on the pad of her index finger or whichever finger is closest in size to her nipple. She allows the baby to draw the finger into his mouth. Correct suckling will cause the milk to flow and will reward the desired behavior. This is a teaching technique that rewards only correct suckling; no milk is removed if the baby bites the finger like an artificial nipple. This also allows the father or other caregiver to feed the baby. Finger-feeding in this manner may help to bring the baby back to the breast faster than if artificial nipples were used to feed the baby.

Clinical Implications

In-hospital situations—such as the infant's reluctance to latch on, poor or frustrating feedings, few wet diapers, inefficient feedings at breast with minimal intake, increased bilirubin levels, and inability to establish baby at breast before discharge—may benefit from the assistance of a feeding-tube device. Edgehouse and Radzyminski (1990) described a device made from a 20-cc or 30-cc syringe and 12-inch tubing formed from a butterfly needle. The tubing is taped in place on the areola at each feeding and serves as a "coaxer," delivering colostrum, breastmilk, water, or formula to effect latch-on and suckling. If the baby cannot cause fluid to flow at first, the plunger can be depressed slightly as an incentive. A nurse or lactation consultant should remain with the mother at each feeding until efficient suckling and swallowing is documented independent of the device.

Newman (1990) described another type of tube feeding. He used a feeding bottle filled with expressed breastmilk or formula and a 36-inch length of No. 5 feeding tube. The bottle is set on a table at the level of the baby's head, and the tubing is taped in place on the breast. Gravity at this level is sufficient to move the milk from the bottle though the tubing when the baby suckles. Newman used this to prevent or treat hypoglycemia and to encourage latch-on so that artificial nipples can be avoided during a temporary situation. When a baby will latch onto the breast but is unable to suckle properly or long enough to maintain good intake and weight gain, a feeding-tube device can be used with a written feeding plan provided to the mother. Consistent use is important in establishing the baby at breast and in reducing the mother's confusion in using the device (see the case study in Box 13–4).

Finger-feeding can be used to take the edge off the baby's hunger before putting him to breast. A feeding plan to establish these babies at breast involves finger-feeding for a few minutes to establish correct and rhythmic sequencing of a suck-swallow pattern. This is followed by putting the baby to breast and repeating the process for a period (determined by the mother and baby) at each feeding, until either the mother or baby become frustrated or the baby latches on and feeds. These practice sessions at breast may last no longer than 10 minutes before the feeding at breast ends and the feeding is completed by finger-feeding with a tube device. Box 13–5 lists some principles regarding the use of feeding tubes.

For long-term use with the Supplemental Nutrition System, some mothers may want to have two or three of the plastic bottles with lids so they can be prefilled with breastmilk or formula for the day. If using other devices, a backup set of tubing or bags or bottles should be available. Mothers may appreciate contact with other women who have used such a device for support and understanding of the conflicting feelings they may experience at different times during the use of the device.

BOX 13–4

Case Study: A Feeding-Tube Device for Baby Cara

Three-week-old baby Cara was referred after failing to regain her birth weight and after showing a loss of two ounces at a three-week weight check. She had been readmitted into the hospital after discharge for two days of phototherapy when her bilirubin levels reached 17 mg/dl on day 4. During her two-day stay, Cara was taken off breastmilk and fed formula every three hours by bottle and artificial nipple. Cara's mother pumped her milk after being told it was contributing to the infant's jaundice. She froze it for use at a later date. Cara's mother described feedings at the breast prior to phototherapy as taking at least one hour, followed by Cara's fussiness when removed from the breast. After discharge, Cara would frequently refuse the breast, and her wet-diaper count fell to five in each 24 hours. Fearing that she was not getting enough milk, Cara's mother began giving her one bottle of formula in the early evening, which was quickly increased to two bottles per day. Pediatric advice called for topping off each feeding with a bottle of formula.

This perpetuated a downward cycle of poor feeding at breast and a decreased milk supply. Observation of a breastfeeding session revealed that the baby had a large, resolving cephalohematoma from a vacuum extraction delivery. Digital examination of Cara's mouth revealed that she bunched her tongue in the middle, but a rhythmic suck with a cupped tongue was established with gentle massage of the tongue and hard palate. At breast, Cara displayed 8 to 10 nonnutritive sucks before one nutritive suck and swallow. With the milk-ejection reflex, this changed to a 4 : 1 ratio but soon reverted back to 8 to 10

sucks for each swallow. Alternate massage (massage and compression of the breast during the pauses between sucking bursts) improved this ratio somewhat but not enough to significantly increase milk intake. A Supplemental Nutrition System was recommended because of the baby's weight loss and the mother's distress.

The feeding plan included the following protocols:

- Feed 8 to 10 times each 24 hours.

- Fill the supplementer with 3 to 4 oz. of breastmilk or formula.

- Use middle-sized tubes with the bottle at a level above the breasts.

- Tape the tubes in place so that they extend to the end of the nipple.

- Use the supplementer at each feeding for three days and obtain a weight check.

- If the weight gain is good and the sucking has improved, run the supplementer to the end of each feeding; obtain another weight check in three days. If the sucking has not improved, the supplementer will continue to be used with each feeding.

- Keep a log and record at each feeding how much supplement was offered and how much the baby took. Note the weekly changes in amounts, record the number of wet diapers and bowel movements each 24 hours, and note when the breasts begin to feel fuller and more supplement is being left in the device. Also record the weight of the baby at each check and note when stool reverts to a predominantly breastmilk consistency and color.

BOX 13–4

- When the growth rate is appropriate and the supplement has decreased, change to the smallest-sized tube. Run the supplementer at the end of every other feeding if weight gain continues to be appropriate.
- Pump the breasts if no breast changes have been observed in three days of use

at each feeding and if supplement is still being completely drained after one week.

- Finger-feed with the two large tubes if Cara does not feed well at breast, if more feedings are necessary than the mother can initially cope with, or if she will not be available for a feeding.

BOX 13–5

Guidelines on the Use of Feeding Tubes

When considering using a feeding-tube device, the clinician should note the following guidelines:

- They can be used to temporarily assist the baby at breast but are generally not necessary if the baby is gaining weight adequately.
- In situations of adoptive nursing, breast-reduction surgery, primary lactation insufficiency, and certain genetic, anatomical or neurological problems in an infant, these feeding devices may require long-term use with or without breast pumping.
- Feeding tubes are not always easy to use, either physically or psychologically, for the mother. Not all women will accept their use or use them as instructed.
- Close follow-up is mandatory with short- or long-term use.
- Because the baby controls the flow, he will not aspirate or be overwhelmed by the fluid he receives. When he swallows

or releases the vacuum, the milk flows backward, and the baby must initiate another suck to start the flow. If he cannot initially do this, the bottle or bag of supplement can be squeezed or the plunger of the syringe can be pushed slightly. The milk will not continuously drip or flow, as with a bottle and artificial nipple.

- Risks of use include "addiction" to the device by the clinician, mother, or baby. The mother and baby should be weaned from the device as quickly as is appropriate. Some mothers may have difficulty in believing that they can support a milk supply without the device and may not trust themselves to provide for the baby. The clinician should avoid routine use of tube-feeding devices except where necessary. Some clever babies learn to suck only on the tube, in which case it should be placed so that it does not extend beyond the end of the mother's nipple. If the baby has become accustomed to the

---

BOX 13–5   *(cont.)*

feel of the tubing, it can be moved to the corner of his mouth and gradually removed. One mother finally taped a one-inch length of the tube to her areola and withdrew it after her baby latched on.

- The football (clutch) position may be easier to use at first because the mother has greater control of the infant's head.

- A gavage setup with a No. 5 feeding tube can also be used as a feeding device.

- Tubing from a butterfly needle can also be used as it is smaller and softer than is gavage tubing.

- A baby can also be fed by dropper, spoon, cup, or bowl if tubing is not available.

- If a mother needs a tube-feeding device but cannot afford to buy a commercial one, it can be loaned to her, and the tubing can be replaced with each new user.

- Powdered formulas and special formulas may clog the smaller tubes if the formula is not mixed well.

- If special formulas are used, larger sizes of tubing may be necessary to prevent clogging.

- The device should be rinsed in cold water after each use and then filled with warm, soapy water, which is squeezed through the tubing and rinsed well. Sterilization can be performed once a day, usually by placing it in boiling water for 20 minutes. In the hospital, some of the devices can be steamed or autoclaved (*Rental Roundup,* 1986a).

- Feeding in public may be more difficult or obvious. The mother may prefer to use alternatives to tube feeding when she is away from home.

SUMMARY

Ideally, the health care professional recommends the use of any breastfeeding technology only after careful consideration. Too often, a breastfeeding mother may see a device advertised as an aid to breastfeeding and assume that she needs to use it. If she then attempts to do so without thoroughly understanding the risks and benefits, she could unwittingly interfere with the lactation course or the baby's ability to breastfeed. This is particularly true if she obtains the device from a person or institution not specializing in lactation management.

Nipple shields are most apt to be used when they are not necessary, in part because of their wide availability and in part because of their attractiveness in busy hospitals or practices, where health care workers offer the devices because they appear to "make the baby nurse." As noted in this chapter, however, the design of the nipple shield can, in some cases, cause sore nipples when they did not previously exist. Thus, when a health care provider considers offering any device to a mother, careful instructions and emphasis on the expected temporary nature of its use must be offered.

Breast shells are less easily misused because they must be removed for the baby to feed. However, collecting milk in the cups without careful attention to the cleanliness of the shell and the time period over which the drip milk was obtained can create other problems, not the least of which is offering the baby contaminated milk.

Feeding-tube devices are more complex and may be more intimidating to the mother than are either breast shells or nipple shields. There are women, however, who insist on using the device because they are convinced that their own milk supplies are inadequate to support infant growth; they need careful follow-up. Too often, the mother misinterprets the instructions or reads only enough to know how to put the device together and to clean it. The manner in which the device should be used is rarely completely understood from a single reading of the package instructions. In addition, observation and assessment of the breastfeeding encounter–with and without the device–is necessary if the health-care provider is to make appropriate recommendations for an optimal outcome.

In most cases, a tube-feeding device is necessary when additional nutrition for the baby is critical and the mother is very anxious. The lactation consultant, nurse, or other health care worker can expect that working with such a mother and baby will be time-consuming and will require many more hours of follow-up time than is the case for other situations. (For additional discussion of the use of a feeding-tube device, see Chapter 11.)

Whenever a breastfeeding device is used, the benefits of the device must be weighed against the risks of interfering in the breastfeeding relationship, just as bottle-feeding represents a risk of varying degrees for different mothers and their babies. Anticipating the emotional response of mothers to devices and discussing them in a straightforward manner helps to determine whether and when to suggest a particular device and how to help the mother to stop using it when it is no longer necessary. As with all other care, the use of a breastfeeding device of any kind must first be found to "do no harm"; thereafter, its benefits must outweigh the risks for the breastfeeding relationship to truly be supported.

REFERENCES

Akre J, ed: Infant feeding:the physiological basis. *Bull WHO* 67:(suppl) 22, 1989. (entire issue)

Alexander JM, et al: Randomized controlled trial of breast shells and Hoffman's exercises for inverted and non-protractile nipples. *Br Med J* 304 (6833):1030–2, 1992

Amatayakul K, et al: Serum prolactin and cortisol levels after suckling for varying periods of time and the effect of a nipple shield. *Acta Obstet Gynecol Scand* 66:47–51, 1987.

Asquith M, et al: The bacterial content of breast milk after early initiation of expression using a standard technique. *J Pediatr Gastroenterol Nutr* 3: 104–7, 1984.

Asquith M, Harod J: Reduction of bacterial contamination in banked human milk. *J Pediatr* 95: 993–4, 1979.

Asquith M, Sharp R, Stevenson D: Decreased bacterial contamination of human milk expressed with an electric breast pump. *J Calif Perin Assoc* 4:45–7, 1985.

Auerbach KG: *Breastfeeding techniques and devices*, Unit 17 (Lactation Consultant Series). Garden City Park, NY: Avery Publishing Group, 1987.

Auerbach KG: The effect of nipple shields on maternal milk volume. *JOGNN* 19:419–27, 1990a.

Auerbach KG: Sequential and simultaneous breast pumping: a comparison. *Int J Nurs Stud* 27:257–65, 1990b.

Auerbach KG: Using nipple shields appropriately. *Rental Roundup* 6:4–5, 1989.

Auerbach KG, Avery JL: Induced lactation: a study of adoptive nursing by 240 women. *Am J Dis Child* 135:340–3, 1981.

Auerbach KG, Avery JL: Relactation: a study of 366 cases. *Pediatrics* 65:236–42, 1980.

Auerbach KG, Guss E: Maternal employment and breastfeeding: a study of 567 women's experiences. *Am J Dis Child* 138:958–60, 1984.

Auerbach KG, Walker M: When the mother of a premature infant uses a breast pump: what every NICU nurse needs to know. *Neonat Netw* 13:23–9, 1994.

Battin D, et al: Effect of suckling on serum prolactin, luteinizing hormone, follicle-stimulating hormone, and estradiol during prolonged lactation. *Obstet Gynecol* 65:785–8, 1985.

Bennion E: *Antique medical instruments.* Berkeley, CA: University of California, 1979:271.

Bodley V, Powers D: Long-term nipple shield use–a positive perspective. *J Hum Lact* 12:301–4, 1996.

Bornmann P: *Legal considerations and the lactation consultant–USA,* Unit 3 (Lactation Consultant Series). Garden City Park, NY: Avery Publishing Group, 1986.

Bose C, et al: Relactation by mothers of sick and premature infants. *Pediatrics* 67:565–8, 1981.

Boutte C, et al: Comparison of hand- and electric-operated breast pumps. *Hum Nutr Appl Nutr* 39A:426–30, 1985.

Bowles B, Stutte P, Hensley J: Alternate massage in breastfeeding. *Genesis* 9:5–9, 1987.

Brigham M: Mothers' reports of the outcome of nipple shield use. *J Hum Lact* 12:291–7, 1996.

Bull P, Barger J: Fingerfeeding with the SNS. *Rental Roundup* 4:2–3, 1987.

Caldeyro-Barcia R: Milk ejection in women. In: Reynolds M, Folley S, eds. *Lactogenesis, the initiation of milk secretion at parturition.* Philadelphia: University of Pennsylvania, 1969.

Clavey S: The use of acupuncture for the treatment of insufficient lactation (Que Ru). *Am J Acupunct* 24:35–46, 1996.

Clum D, Primomo J: Use of a silicone nipple shield with premature infants. *J Hum Lact* 12:287–90, 1996.

Cobo E, et al: Neurohypophyseal hormone release in the human: II. Experimental study during lactation. *Am J Obstet Gynecol* 97:519–29, 1967.

Costa K: A comparison of colony counts of breast milk using two methods of breast cleansing. *JOGNN* 18:231–6, 1989.

Daly SEJ, et al: The determination of short-term breast volume changes and the rate of synthesis of human milk using computerized breast measurement. *Exp Phys* 77:79–87, 1992.

Daly SEJ, et al: The short-term synthesis and infant regulated removal of milk in lactating women. *Exp Phys* 78:209–20, 1993.

Daly SEJ, Hartmann PE: Infant demand and milk supply. Part 1: Infant demand and milk production in lactating women. *J Hum Lact* 11:21–6, 1995a.

Daly SEJ, Hartmann PE: Infant demand and milk supply. Part 2: The short-term control of milk synthesis in lactating women. *J Hum Lact* 11:27–37, 1995b.

DeNicola M: One case of nipple shield addiction. *J Hum Lact* 2:28–9, 1986.

de Sanctis V, et al: Comparison of prolactin response to suckling and breast pump aspiration in lactating mothers. *La Ric Clin Lab* 11:81–5, 1981.

Desmarais L, Browne S: *Inadequate weight gain in breastfeeding infants: assessments and resolutions,* Unit 8 (Lactation Consultant Series). Garden City Park, NY: Avery Publishing Group, 1990.

Dodd F, Griffin T: *Milking routines, machine milking.* Reading, England: National Institute of Research on Dairying, Shinfield, 1977;179–200.

Donowitz L, et al: Contaminated breast milk: a source of *Klebsiella* bacteremia in a newborn intensive care unit. *Rev Infect Dis* 3:716–20, 1981.

Drewett R, Bowen-Jones A, Dogterom J: Oxytocin levels during breastfeeding in established lactation. *Horm Behav* 16:245–8, 1982.

Edgehouse L, Radzyminski S: A device for supplementing breast-feeding. *MCN* 15:34–5, 1990.

Egnell E: The mechanics of different methods of emptying the female breast. *J Swed Med Assoc* 40:1–8, 1956.

Ehrenkranz RA, Ackerman BA: Metoclopramide effect on faltering milk production by mothers of premature infants. *Pediatrics* 78:614–20, 1986.

El-Mohandes AE, et al: Aerobes isolated in fecal microflora of infants in the intensive care nursery: relationship to human milk use and systemic sepsis. *Am J Infect Cont* 21:231–4, 1993a.

El-Mohandes AE, et al: Bacterial contaminants of collected and frozen human milk used in an intensive care nursery. *Am J Infect Cont* 21:226–30, 1993b.

Elliott C: Using a silicone nipple shield to assist a baby unable to latch. *J Hum Lact* 12:309–13, 1996.

Feher S, et al: Increased breastmilk production for premature infants with a relaxation/imagery audiotape. *Pediatrics* 83:57–60, 1989.

Fildes V: *Breasts, bottles and babies*. Edinburgh: Edinburgh University, 1986:141–3.

Forte A, Mayberry L, Ferketich S: Breast milk collection and storage practices among mothers of hospitalized neonates. *J Perinatol* 7:35–9, 1987.

Frantz K: *Breastfeeding product guide, 1994*. Sunland, CA: Geddes Productions, 1993.

Goodman G, Grosvenor C: Neuroendocrine control of the milk ejection reflex. *J Dairy Sci* 66:2226–35, 1983.

Gorewit R, et al: Current concepts on the role of oxytocin in milk ejection. *J Dairy Sci* 66:2236–50, 1983.

Grams M: *Breastfeeding source book*. Sheridan, WY: Achievement Press, 1988;100–42.

Gransden W, et al: An outbreak of *Serratia marcescens* transmitted by contaminated breast pumps in a special care baby unit. *J Hosp Infect* 7:149–54, 1986.

Green D, et al: The relative efficacy of four methods of human milk expression. *Early Hum Dev* 6:153–9, 1982.

Groh-Wargo S, et al: The utility of a bilateral breast pumping system for mothers of premature infants. *Neonat Netw* 14:31–6, 1995.

Gross MS: Letter. *ILCA Globe* 3:5, 1995.

Gunn AJ, et al: Growth hormone increases breast milk volumes in mothers of preterm infants. *Pediatrics* 98:279–82, 1996.

Hamosh M, et al: Breastfeeding and the working mother: effect of time and temperature of short-term storage on proteolysis, lipolysis, and bacterial growth in milk. *Pediatrics* 97:492–8, 1996.

Hamosh M, et al: Digestive enzymes in human milk: stability at suboptimal storage temperatures. *J Pediatr Gastroenterol Nutr* 24:38–43, 1997.

Hill PD, Aldag JC, Chatterton RC: The effect of sequential and simultaneous breast-pumping on

volume and prolactin levels: a pilot study. *J Hum Lact* 12:193–9, 1996.

Howie P, et al: The relationship between suckling-induced prolactin response and lactogenesis. *J Clin Endocrinol Metab* 50:670–3, 1980.

Hughes V, et al: *Acute prolactin stimulation in breast-feeding women using three commercial breast pumps, manual expression and natural infant suckling*. Presentation at the Congress for International Federation for Family Life Promotion, Nairobi, Kenya, 1989.

Jackson D, et al: The automatic sampling shield: a device for sampling suckled breast milk. *Early Hum Dev* 15:295–306, 1987.

Johnson C: An evaluation of breast pumps currently available on the American market. *Clin Pediatr* 22:40–5, 1983.

Johnston J, Amico J: A prospective longitudinal study of the release of oxytocin and prolactin in response to infant suckling in long-term lactation. *J Clin Endocrinol Metab* 62:653–7, 1986.

Kutner L: Nipple shield consent form: a teaching aid. *J Hum Lact* 2:25–7, 1986.

Lawrence R: *Breastfeeding: a guide for the medical profession*. St Louis: Mosby, 1989;183–5.

Leake R, et al: Oxytocin and prolactin response in long-term breast-feeding. *Obstet Gynecol* 62:565–8, 1983.

Marmet C, Shell E: *Marmet technique of manual expression of breastmilk*. Encino, CA: The Lactation Institute, 1989.

Maygrier J: *Midwifery Illustrated*. Philadelphia: Carey & Hart, 1833:173.

McNeill AS, et al: Release of oxytocin and prolactin response to suckling. *Br Med J* 286(6361): 257–9, 1983.

Meier P, Wilks S: The bacteria in expressed mothers' milk. *MCN* 12:420–3, 1987.

Merrill W, et al: Effects of premilking stimulation on complete lactation, milk yield and milking performance. *J Dairy Sci* 70:1676–84, 1987.

Minchin M: *Breastfeeding matters*. Victoria, Australia: Alma Publications, 1985;142–5.

Moloney A, et al: A bacteriological examination of breast pumps. *J Hosp Infect* 9:169–74, 1987.

Morse J, Bottorff J: The emotional experience of breast expression. *J Nurse Midwifery* 33:165–70, 1988.

Neifert MR, et al: Lactation failure due to insufficient glandular development of the breast. *Pediatrics* 76:823–8, 1985.

Neifert M, Seacat J: *Milk yield and prolactin rise with simultaneous breast pumping.* Presentation at the Ambulatory Pediatric Association Meeting, Washington, DC, May 7–10, 1985.

Neville M: Regulation of mammary development and lactation. In: Neville M, Neifert M, eds. *Lactation: physiology, nutrition and breast-feeding.* New York: Plenum, 1983:118.

Newman J: Breastfeeding problems associated with the early introduction of bottles and pacifiers. *J Hum Lact* 6:59–63, 1990.

Newton M, Newton N: The let-down reflex in human lactation. *J Pediatr* 33:698–704, 1948.

Noel G, Suh H, Frantz A: Prolactin release during nursing and breast stimulation in postpartum and nonpostpartum subjects. *J Clin Endocrinol Metab* 38:413–23, 1974.

Nwankwo M, et al: Bacterial growth in expressed breast-milk. *Ann Trop Paediatr* 8:92–5, 1988.

Petersen W: *Dairy science: principles and practice.* Philadelphia: Lippincott, 1950;373–87.

Pittard W, et al: Bacterial contamination of human milk: container type and method of expression. *Am J Perinatol* 8:25–7, 1991.

Rees D: Juice-jar breast pump. *Keep Abreast J* 2:225, 1977.

Rental Roundup: New product, SNS. 3:1–3, 1986a.

Rental Roundup: Warning: these devices can hurt a woman. 3:9–12, 1986b.

Ruis H, et al: Oxytocin enhances onset of lactation among mothers delivering prematurely. *Br Med J* 283:340–2, 1981.

Sagi R, Gorewit R, Zinn S: Milk ejection in cows mechanically stimulated during late lactation. *J Dairy Sci* 63:1957–60, 1980.

Saint L, Maggiore P, Hartmann P: Yield and nutrient content of milk in eight women breast-feeding twins and one woman breast-feeding triplets. *Br J Nutr* 56:49–58, 1986.

Shrago L: Product evaluation: nipple shields. *J Hum Lact* 4:169, 1988.

Sponsel W: Simple and effective breast pump for nursing mothers. *Br Med J* 286:1676–84, 1983.

Stutte P, Bowles B, Morman G: The effects of breast massage on volume and fat content of human milk. *Genesis* 10:22–5, 1988.

Sutherland A, Auerbach KG: *Relactation and induced lactation,* Unit 1 (Lactation Consultant Series). Garden City Park, NY: Avery Publishing Group, 1985.

Tyson J: Nursing and prolactin secretion: principle determinants in the mediation of puerperal infertility. In: Crosignani P, Robyn C, eds. *Prolactin and human reproduction.* New York: Academic, 1977:97–108.

Walker M: How to evaluate breast pumps. *MCN* 12:270–6, 1987.

Weichert C: Prolactin cycling and the management of breastfeeding failure. *Adv Pediatr* 27:391–407, 1980.

Wennergren M, Wiqvist N, Wennergren G: Manual breast pumps promote successful breast-feeding. *Acta Obstet Gynecol Scand* 64:673–5, 1985.

Whittlestone W: The physiologic breastmilker. *NZ Fam Phys* 5:1–3, 1978.

Whitworth N, et al: The effect of fetal genotype on the human maternal PRL response to labor, delivery and breast stimulation. *Abstr Proc Int Cong Prolactin* 4:60, 1984.

Whitworth N: Lactation in humans. *Psychoneuroendocrinology* 13:171–88, 1988.

Wilde CJ, et al: Breast-feeding: matching supply with demand in human lactation. *Proc Nutr Soc* 54:401–6, 1995.

Wilks S, Meier P: Helping mothers express milk suitable for preterm and high-risk infant feeding. *MCN* 13:121–3, 1988.

Williams J, Auerbach K, Jacobi A: Lateral epicondylitis (tennis elbow) in breastfeeding mothers. *Clin Pediatr* 28:42–3, 1989.

Wilson-Clay B: Clinical use of silicone nipple shields. *J Hum Lact* 12:279–85, 1996.

Woodworth M., Frank E: Transitioning to the breast at six weeks: use of a nipple shield. *J Hum Lact* 12:305–7, 1996.

Woolford M, Phillips D: Evaluation studies of a milking system using an alternating vacuum level in a single chambered teatcup. In: *Proceedings of the International Symposium on Machine Milking*. National Mastitis Council, 1978:125–49.

Woolridge M, Baum J, Drewett R: Effect of a traditional and of a new nipple shield on sucking patterns and milk flow. *Early Hum Dev* 4:357–64, 1980.

Zinaman M: Breast pumps: ensuring mothers' success. *Contemp Obstet Gynecol* 32:55–62, 1988.

Zinaman M, et al: Acute prolactin, oxytocin response and milk yield to infant suckling and artificial methods of expression in lactating women. *Pediatrics* 89:437–40, 1992.

APPENDIX 13-A

Manufacturers and Distributors of Breastfeeding Devices

Avent America, 5161 Thatcher Road, Downers Grove, IL 60515

Bailey Medical Engineering, 2020 11th Street, Los Osos, CA 93402 (Nurture III small semiautomatic breast pump)

Cannon Babysafe Ltd., Lower Road, Glemsford, Suffolk, England CO10 7QS (Avent squeeze-handle breast pump, silicone nipple shields)

CEA of Greater Philadelphia, 127 Fayette Street, Conshohocken, PA 19428 (Comfi-Dri Milk Cups)

D.A. Kadan, Inc., 10100 Industrial Drive, Pineville, NC 28134 (Kadan small semiautomatic electric pump)

Evenflo Products Co., P.O. Box 1206, 771 North Freedom Street, Ravenna, OH 44266–1206 (cylinder pump, battery pump)

Gerber Products Co., 445 State Street, Fremont, MI 49412 (cylinder pump, small semiautomatic electric pump)

Graham-Field, Inc., 400 Rabro Drive, East Hauppauge, NY 11788 (Gentle Expressions battery pump, The Rose automatic electric pump, breast shells)

Hollister/Ameda-Egnell, 755 Industrial Drive, Cary, IL 60013 (automatic electric breast pump, battery pump, cylinder pump, breast shells, nipple shields)

International Design/Manufacturing, Inc., 305 Avenue G, Redondo Beach, CA 90277 (Happy Family cylinder pump)

Lact-Aid, P.O. Box 1066, Athens, TN 37303 (tube-feeding device)

Lopuco Ltd., 1615 Old Annapolis Road, Woodbine, MD 21797 (Loyd-B squeeze-handle pump)

Mada Medical Products, Inc., 60 Commerce Road, Carlstadt, NJ 07072 (small semiautomatic pump)

Medela, Inc., 4610 Prime Parkway, P.O. Box 660, McHenry, IL 60051 (automatic electric pump, manual pump, battery pump, Lactina pump, breast shells, nipple shield, Supplemental Nutrition System feeding-tube device)

Netsy Company, 34 Sunrise Avenue, Mill Valley, CA 94941 (breast shells)

Omron Marshall Products, Inc., 300 Lakeview Parkway, Vernon Hills, IL 60061 (Kaneson cylinder and Mag Mag battery pumps)

Ora'lac, Inc., 204 East A Street, No. 1, Moscow, ID 83843 (Ora'lac pump)

Pharmics, 1878 South Redwood Road, Salt Lake City, UT 84104 (breast shells)

Ross Laboratories, 625 Cleveland Avenue, Columbus, OH 43216 (cylinder pump)

Sassy, Inc., 1534 College S.E., Grand Rapids, MI 49507 (Infa cylinder pump)

Schuco, Inc., 1419 Expressway Drive, North Toledo, OH 43608 (small and large semiautomatic electric pumps)

Sears, Roebuck and Co., Chicago, IL 60684 (cylinder pump)

Trigon Industries, Ltd., 12 Maidstone Street, CPO Box 3674, Auckland 2, New Zealand (Whittlestone automatic electric pump)

White River Concepts, 924 Calle Negocio, San Clemente, CA 92673 (cylinder pump, semiautomatic and automatic electric pumps)

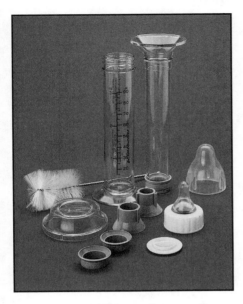

Comfort Plus™ Kaneson (Courtesy Omron Healthcare, Inc., Vernon Hills, IL)

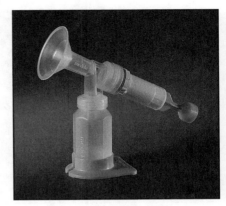

Hand pump (Courtesy Medela, Inc., McHenry, IL)

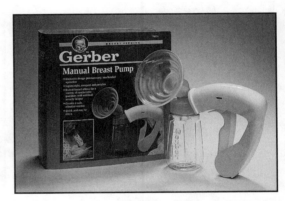

Hand pump (Courtesy Gerber Products Company, Fremont, MI)

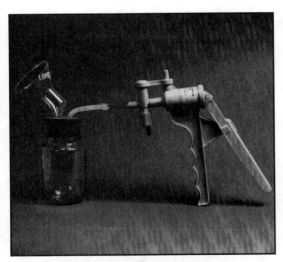

Loyd-B squeeze-handle manual pump (Courtesy Lopuco Ltd., Woodbine, MD)

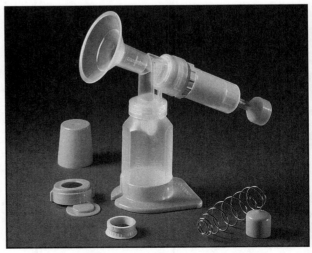

Spring Express™ (Courtesy Medela, Inc., McHenry, IL)

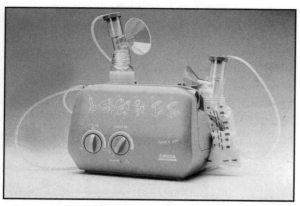

Elite hand pump (Courtesy Hollister/Ameda-Egnell, Cary, IL)

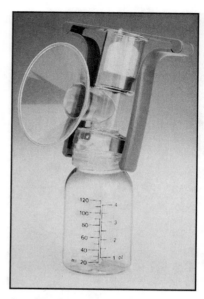

One-hand pump (Courtesy Hollister/Ameda-Egnell, Cary, IL)

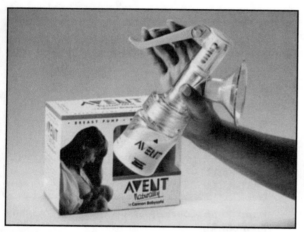

Avent squeeze-handle manual pump (Courtesy Cannon Babysafe Ltd., Suffolk, England)

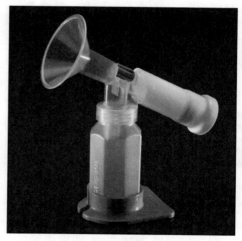

Little Hearts™ hand pump (Courtesy Medela, Inc., McHenry, IL)

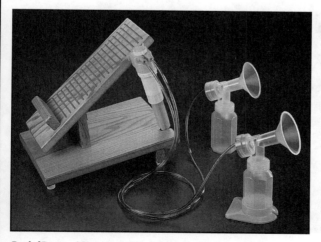

PedalPump (Courtesy Medela, Inc., McHenry, IL)

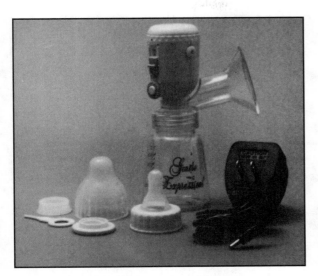

Gentle Expressions battery pump (Courtesy Graham-Field, Hauppague, NY)

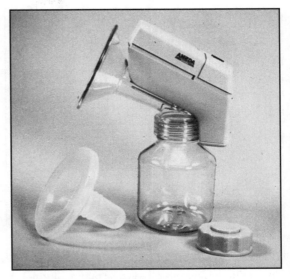

Lact-B battery-operated pump (Courtesy Hollister/Ameda-Egnell, Cary, IL)

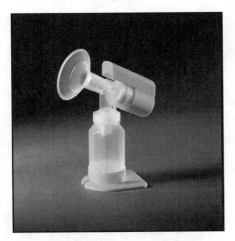

Mini-Electric battery-operated pump (Courtesy Medela, Inc., McHenry, IL)

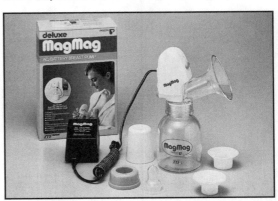

Mag-Mag battery-operated pump (Courtesy Omron Marshall Products, Vernon Hills, IL)

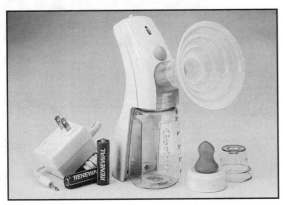

Battery-operated pump (Courtesy Gerber Products Company, Fremont, MI)

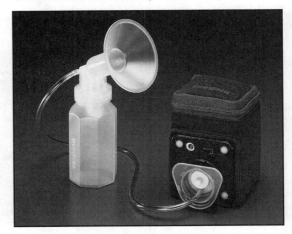

Little Hearts™ electric pump (Courtesy Medela, Inc., McHenry, IL)

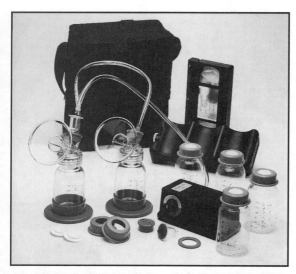

Nurture III semiautomatic electric pump (double) (Courtesy Bailey Medical Engineering, Los Osos, CA)

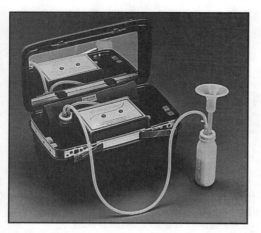

Electric breast pump (single) (Courtesy White River Natural Technologies, Laguna Hills, CA)

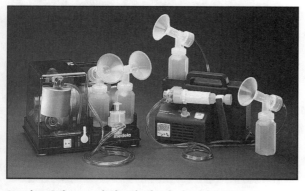

Lactina Select and Classic (both double) (Courtesy Medela, Inc., McHenry, IL)

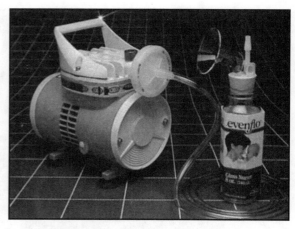

Semiautomatic electric pump (Courtesy Schuco, Inc., Carle Place, NY)

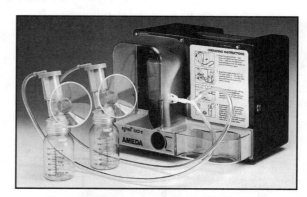

Lact-E (Courtesy Hollister/Ameda-Egnell, Cary, IL)

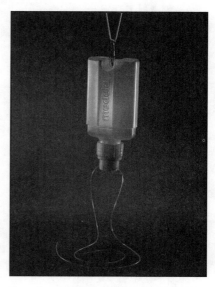

Supplemental Nutrition System (Courtesy Medela, Inc., McHenry, IL)

14

Breastfeeding the Preterm Infant

Paula P. Meier, Linda P. Brown, and Nancy M. Hurst

Mothers of preterm infants encounter numerous well-documented barriers to breastfeeding that are not experienced by mothers of healthy, full-term infants. Recent studies suggest that these barriers exist in both developed and developing countries, as reflected in lower worldwide rates of breastfeeding initiation and duration for preterm and low-birth-weight infants than for full-term, healthy babies (Meier & Brown, 1996). Lower breastfeeding rates for this vulnerable population are of particular concern because preterm infants and their mothers receive unique benefits from breastfeeding that cannot be duplicated in feeding with commercial infant formulas.

To improve these breastfeeding outcomes, clinicians must use research-based strategies that target specific barriers to breastfeeding initiation and duration for mothers and their preterm infants. In the past decade, numerous scientific reports have focused on delineating and studying these barriers (Baker & Rasmussen, 1997; Blaymore-Bier et al., 1993; Brennan-Behm et al., 1994; Charpak et al., 1994; deMonterice et al., 1992; Hurst et al., 1997; Jaeger et al., 1997; Jennings et al., 1997; Kavanaugh et al., 1995, 1997; Lang et al., 1994; Meier, 1995, 1996; Meier & Brown, 1996, 1997a, c; Meier et al., 1993, 1994, 1996; Nyquist et al., 1996; Nyquist &

Sjöden, 1993; Nyquist et al., 1996; Ramasethu et al., 1993; Schanler & Hurst, 1994.

Cumulatively, these studies indicate that preterm infants are not just "small term infants" with respect to breastfeeding management. Instead, they have maturity-dependent physiological and metabolic differences that require integration. Similarly, mothers of preterm infants experience unique physiological and emotional challenges, such as maintaining lactation for several weeks and coping with extreme vulnerability about infant intake during breastfeeding. These barriers adversely affect breastfeeding initiation and duration rates for this population.

Preterm Infants

Compositional differences between the milk produced by mothers who deliver prematurely and that from those that deliver at term have been postulated since the 1950s (Crosse et al., 1954; Stevens, 1969) and are documented in controlled trials (Atkinson et al., 1981; Atkinson et al., 1983; Gross et al., 1981). Compared to term milk, preterm milk is theoretically more suited to the growth and immunological needs of preterm infants and has significantly higher concentrations of several components, including sIgA and other antiinfective properties, protein, fat, sodium, chloride, and iron (Dawodu, 1989; Goldman et al., 1994; Groer & Walker, 1996; Mathur et al., 1990; Schanler, 1995; Schanler & Hurst, 1994; Steichen et al., 1987; Udosen & Ebong, 1992). Additionally, the within-lipid profile differs significantly from full-term milk, with preterm milk having higher concentrations of medium-chain triglycerides and long-chain polyunsaturated fatty acids (Armand et al., 1996; Hamosh, 1994). These prematurity-specific lipid differences may provide substrate for short-term energy needs and for longer-term neurological and visual development.

The clinical significance of these gestationally dependent differences in milk composition is apparent when short- and long-term health outcomes are compared for preterm infants receiving either human milk or formula-feedings. These outcomes, summarized in Table 14–1, suggest that human milk may provide optimal "nutritional programming" for preterm infants and may be protective against several prematurity-related health conditions (Brown et al., 1996; Buescher, 1994; DeCurtis, 1987; Lucas, 1980; Lucas & Cole, 1990; Lucas et al., 1990a, b; Meier & Brown, 1996; Morley, 1996; Neu, 1996; Schanler, 1995; Schanler & Hurst, 1994; Tudehope & Steer, 1996).

For most of these studies, human-milk feedings were supplemented with commercial formulas. In some studies, infants received donor rather than own-mothers' milk (OMM) and, in most reports, commercial human milk fortifiers were used. However, the documented advantages were consistent across these studies, providing strong scientific support for a link between type of feeding and health outcome (Meier & Brown, 1997c). Few data are available in which these outcomes have been studied for preterm infants who received exclusive OMM feedings. Given the recently documented differences in term and preterm milk, these studies are essential for understanding the true relationship between type of feeding and the measures of infant outcome.

Mothers of Preterm Infants

Reports in the historical literature emphasize the psychological significance of milk expression and breastfeeding for mothers of preterm infants (Budin, 1907; Lundeen, 1939). In addition, breastfeeding is described as a contribution to infant care that only the mother can make (Auerbach, 1977; Cohen, 1987; Ehrenkranz & Ackerman, 1986; Gotsch, 1991; Neifert & Seacat, 1988) and as one aspect of "natural" caregiving that is not forfeited because of preterm birth (Meier et al., 1993).

These clinical impressions were confirmed and extended in a recent study of 20 mothers of preterm infants who were interviewed in the home one month after infant discharge from the neonatal intensive care unit (NICU) (Kavanaugh et al., 1997). These women, who received research-based in-hospital breastfeeding services (Meier et al., 1993), reported that "the rewards outweigh the efforts" in describing their breastfeeding experiences during the first month that their infants were at home.

The mothers from this study delineated and exemplified five rewards of breastfeeding their preterm infants. Most frequently reported was "knowing that they had given their infants a good start in life," with references to the health benefits of breastfeeding for premature babies followed by the mothers' enjoyment of the physical closeness and intimacy of breastfeeding, and their perception that their infants "preferred" the breast to bottle-feedings of expressed milk. A fourth reward was "making a unique contribution to infant care," but mothers circumscribed this reward to the NICU stay when other caregiving opportunities were limited. Finally, the mothers felt that even with the extra effort of feeding and continued milk expression in the home, breastfeeding was "convenient" for them.

Thus the literature suggests that breastfeeding affords unique advantages for this vulnerable population that stand in addition to the health benefits of breastfeeding for mothers and full-term, healthy infants. These important findings provide scientific justification for the allocation of resources to improve breastfeeding outcomes for this vulnerable population.

Rates of Breastfeeding Initiation and Duration

Although breastfeeding statistics vary for individual countries, worldwide data suggest that mothers

Table 14–1

HEALTH ADVANTAGES OF HUMAN MILK FEEDING FOR PRETERM INFANTS

Benefit	References
Greater enteral feeding tolerance and more rapid achievement of full enteral feedings.	Armand et al., 1996 Gross, 1983 Simmer et al., 1997 Uraizee & Gross, 1989
Reduced risk and severity of infection (short- and long-term)	El-Mohandes et al., 1993, 1997 Narayanan et al., 1981, 1982, 1984 Uraizee & Gross, 1989
Reduced risk and severity of necrotizing enterocolitis	Albanese & Rowe, 1995 Buescher, 1994 DeCurtis et al., 1987 Gross, 1983 Kleigman et al., 1979 Lucas & Cole, 1990 Neu, 1996
Reduced risk of atopic disease for infants with family risk histories	Chandra, 1997 Lucas et al., 1990a
Enhanced retinal maturation and visual acuity	Carlson et al., 1986 Faldella et al., 1996 deAndreca & Uauy, 1995 Uauy et al., 1990
Enhanced developmental and neurocognitive outcome	Carlson et al., 1986 deAndreca & Uauy, 1995 Lucas et al., 1990a, b, 1990 1992, 1994 Morley, 1996 Morley et al., 1988 Pierrat et al., 1996
Greater physiological stability during breastfeeding than bottle-feeding	Blaymore-Bier et al., 1993 Bosque, et al., 1995 Meier, 1988, 1996 Meier & Anderson, 1987

of preterm infants initiate and sustain breastfeeding at rates lower than those of the general population (Byrne & Hull, 1996; Ehrenkranz et al., 1985; Gamble, 1993; Hill et al., 1994; Hill et al., 1997; Jaeger et al., 1997; Kaufman & Hall, 1989; Lefebvre & Ducharme, 1989; Meberg et al., 1982; Meier & Brown, 1996; Meier et al., 1993; Nyqvist & Ewald, 1997; Richards et al., 1986; Ryan et al., 1991; Simmer et al., 1997; Trause et al., 1986; Verronen, 1985; Yip et al., 1996). Several conclusions and practice priorities can be drawn from this body of worldwide studies:

- Breastfeeding initiation rates appear to be increasing for this population (*Updated Breastfeeding Trends,* 1996), presumably because promotion efforts have made mothers aware of the health benefits of human milk.

- The duration of breastfeeding for mothers and preterm infants is typically shorter than the mothers' initial goals.

- Rates for breastfeeding initiation and duration can be improved if mothers are provided with research-based, comprehensive breastfeeding services.

Thus a prerequisite for research and practice is to address the documented barriers to breastfeeding for mothers and preterm infants through the use of evidence-based strategies. These barriers and strategies are summarized in Table 14–2.

Providing Research-Based Breastfeeding Services

In 1993, Meier et al. published a research-based model for providing breastfeeding services in the NICU. It included specific interventions within a four-phase temporal model:

phase 1: expression and collection of mothers' milk
phase 2: gavage feeding of mothers' milk
phase 3: in-hospital breastfeeding
phase 4: postdischarge breastfeeding management.

Since 1993, this model has been expanded and refined and has served as the basis for several clinical and research programs (Baker & Rasmussen, 1997; Brown et al., 1995; Hurst et al., 1997; Meier & Brown, 1996, 1997c). A central feature of this model is that breastfeeding services are directed or coordinated by a nurse or physician with expertise in both lactation and intensive preterm infant care.

The Decision to Breastfeed

Until recently, health care providers took the position that preterm infant feeding was a matter of parental choice. Professional responsibility was limited to implementing a parent's decision.

However, Meier & Brown (1997c) have challenged this perspective by emphasizing the importance of sharing research-based health benefits of breastfeeding with parents, so that they can make informed decisions about feeding methods. Specifically, this information should include factual verbal and written materials and alternatives to exclusive, long-term breastfeeding for women who do not want to make these commitments.

Facilitating an Informed Decision

All mothers who are hospitalized for preterm labor should be approached by a health care professional who can provide information about breastfeeding. If the mother has already given birth, breastfeeding should be discussed as soon after delivery as the mother is able to converse. The clinician should use specific information about the baby–such as maturity or health condition–and share with the mother the breastfeeding research that is relevant to her baby's situation.

One barrier to providing mothers with this information is concern among some health care providers that mothers will be made to feel guilty if they elect not to breastfeed. However, in other areas of NICU care, professionals do not withhold factual information that may influence a parent's decisions about infant management plans. Withholding such information would be considered unethical if it involved respiratory care or a surgical procedure. Providing parents with research-based options for infant feeding should be handled in a manner consistent with NICU policies for other decisions about infant management.

Alternatives to Exclusive, Long-Term Breastfeeding

Many mothers, especially those who had not intended to breastfeed, remain indecisive or reluctant to begin milk expression if they feel they must make a commitment to exclusive breastfeeding for several months. Additionally, they may have been advised by health care providers or family members that breastfeeding is "too much" for them at a time when they are consumed with discomfort, anxiety, stress, and fatigue. These women should be encouraged to begin milk expression immediately after birth, when the hormonal milieu is

Table 14–2

GUIDELINES FOR COLLECTING, TRANSPORTING, STORING, AND FEEDING OWN MOTHERS' MILK

Mother

Milk Collection

1. Sterilizes all milk collection equipment once daily, either by boiling for 20 minutes or in the dishwasher with a sani-cycle.

   a. Washes equipment thoroughly with soap and hot water after each milk expression.

   b. Allows equipment to air-dry between uses.

2. When preparing to express milk, washes hands thoroughly with soap and water before handling milk collection equipment.

   a. Takes care not to sneeze or cough on equipment.

   b. Washes the breasts once daily during the bath or shower. No other breast cleansing is required unless instructed.

3. Places collection devices on the breasts, taking care not to touch the inside of the flange area. Expresses milk for approximately 15 minutes or until milk droplets have ceased flowing for two consecutive minutes.

4. Transfers milk into sterile specimen containers, taking care not to separate foremilk and hindmilk unless instructed to do so.

5. Uses a separate container for each milk expression, because adding warm milk to cold or frozen milk can alter the milk.

6. Labels containers with infant's name, time and date of expression, and any medications consumed within the past 24 hours.

7. Places a colored sticker on the lid of the container to designate the type of milk collected:

   – Green (fresh, refrigerated milk, never frozen)

   – Blue (frozen milk)

   – White (colostrum: milk collected within the first 3–4 days after birth); also using green or blue dot

Nurse

1. Ensures that mother has written information outlining procedures for milk collection, storage, and transport of milk.

2. When mother expresses milk at the bedside, ensures that she is able to maintain appropriate milk expression technique.

4. Provides the mother with sterile specimen containers, remembering that some mothers need as many as 20–25 per day. Ensures that each mother has at least an extra day's supply of containers in the home.

7. Provides mother with appropriate colored stickers.

Table 14–2 *(cont.)*

Mother	Nurse

Mother

Milk Collection

  – Yellow (hindmilk); also using green or blue dot

  – Red (foremilk); indicating do not use–freeze until infant is discharged

8. Refrigerates or freezes milk until it is transported to the hospital for infant feeding.

Transporting Milk to SCN

1. Transports milk to the SCN in the insulated bags provided by the nurse.

2. Brings all milk to the SCN, except for foremilk, which can be kept at home for use after infant discharge.

Milk-Storage Conditions

1. Whenever possible, OMM should be fed *fresh,* not frozen, to retain maximum nutritional and infection-fighting properties.

2. *Frozen* OMM retains many important antibodies, is nutritionally superior to commercial formula for feeding of preterm infants, and should be fed when fresh milk is not available.

Nurse

Transporting Milk to SCN

1. Provides mothers with transport bags before hospital discharge. If an infant has been transported from another hospital, gives mother the bag at the time of the first SCN visit.

2. When the mother arrives with refrigerated or frozen milk for her infant, takes the milk from her, and

   a. Checks that (1) the milk is labeled with name, date and time, and any medications taken; (if not, do not label the milk–ask the mother to do so), and that (2) a colored sticker has been placed on the lid to designate the type of milk in the container.

   b. Places the milk in the infant's plastic storage bin in either the refrigerator or freezer. (If no bin has been allocated, label one for the infant.)

Milk-Storage Conditions

1. Keeps *fresh,* unrefrigerated milk at room temperature for up to 2 hours or refrigerates it ($\leq 4^{\circ}C$) for up to 48 hours. Discards any milk unused after 48 hours.

2. Stores *frozen* OMM at $\leq -20^{\circ}C$ until thawed for infant feeding. After thawing, stores milk in the refrigerator for up to 24 hours. Discards any milk unused after 24 hours.

3. Does *not* instruct mothers to leave milk at home or to take extra milk home unless the infant is to be discharged within a few days. All expressed milk should be stored in a hospital freezer or refrigerator.

Feeding OMM

1. Provides and labels milk that is prescribed for infant feeding.

2. Assists nurses by ensuring that milk in the plastic storage bins is properly labeled and (if indicated) numbered, so that it can be fed in a particular order.

3. Prepares and administers infant's feeding, seeking assistance from nurses as needed.

1. Refers to the infant's kardex and institutional protocols for differentiating among procedures for colostrum, composite, and hind-milk feedings.

2. When removing OMM from the refrigerator for feeding, verifies that the mother's name is clearly written on the milk label and that milk has not been stored longer than the times outlined in Milk Storage Conditions (above).

   Never feed unlabeled milk to an infant, even if it is in an infant's plastic storage bin.

3. After removing the milk from the refrigerator, handles it according to institutional protocols.

   a. Warms milk to body temperature over $\frac{1}{2}$–1 hour, in a warm-water bath or in the infant's incubator.

   b. Encourages mothers to prepare and administer their infants' feedings after bringing milk from the refrigerator.

OMM: own-mother's milk; SCN: special-care nursery

Source: Courtesy Rush-Presbyterian-St. Luke's Medical Center, Chicago, Illinois.

---

optimal, so their infants can receive colostrum. Mothers should be told that they can cease milk expression at any time they desire and that professional help is available to help them to discontinue pumping.

When women are indecisive and their initial plans include a day-by-day commitment to breastfeeding, several issues can help women to make these important choices. For example, mothers who are unenthusiastic about pumping often ask how long they must provide milk for their infants. The practitioner can use infant milestones to make the recommendations more real for mothers. For example, a mother can be told that the most important time for the preterm infant is the introduction and advancement of early feedings and that her colostrum is ideal for this purpose. This translates

into milk expression for approximately one week. The clinician can add that providing milk until the baby reaches his full-term, corrected age is especially beneficial because of the unique nature of the lipids in preterm milk. Most mothers are willing to consider short-term "contracts" of this nature when they understand the day-by-day importance of their milk for their infant.

Some mothers will express milk with a breast pump but do not want to feed their infants at the breast. The practitioner can introduce this option by stating, "Some women decide that they will use a breast pump to express milk and then feed it to their babies by bottle. Is this something that you would consider?" This approach informs mothers about this option and reassures them that other women have chosen it.

When the mother of a preterm infant selects an alternative to exclusive, long-term breastfeeding, the breastfeeding specialist and NICU staff must not imply that her choice is "second best." Instead, the previously indecisive mother should be praised for her commitment and respected for her choice. The mother should be made aware of resources to help her if she changes her breastfeeding goals in the future.

Milk Expression and Collection

Mothers of preterm infants must initiate and maintain lactation with a breast pump until their infants are able to regulate intake from the breast. This universally frustrating experience may last from several days to a few months, and mothers need research-based advice and support to persevere with their breastfeeding goals during this time.

Principles of Milk Expression

No published reports have focused on the mother's physiological response to exclusive, long-term breast pump use. Thus the principles of lactation that have been studied for the healthy population are commonly applied to the mother who initiates and maintains lactation with a breast pump. Although giving birth prematurely does not appear to limit milk production, several factors surrounding the birth experience–prolonged bed rest, maternal complications, fatigue, stress, and irregular breast emptying–are documented prolactin-inhibitors and can adversely affect milk volume (Brown et al., 1991; Cohen, 1987; Ehrenkranz & Ackerman, 1986; Fehrer et al., 1989; Lawrence, 1994; Schanler & Hurst, 1994).

The available research supports the practice of beginning milk expression with a hospital-grade electric breast pump as early as possible after delivery (Hill, et al., 1996; Meier & Brown, 1996; Neifert & Seacat, 1988). Frequent pumping and milk flow during the first week postbirth stimulate prolactin and optimize milk yield (deCarvalho et al., 1985; Hill et al., 1995). Hopkinson et al., (1988) report that establishing an adequate milk volume was associated with at least five milk expressions and 100 minutes of pump use each day.

Clinically, advising mothers to express milk more frequently (e.g., 8–10 times daily) during the first week to 10 days postbirth may result in a milk volume approximating 750 to 1,000 ml/day. Mothers can be informed that establishing an abundant milk yield provides a "reserve" against diminishing milk volume later in lactation. With a daily milk volume of 1,000 ml, the mother's milk volume can decrease by 50 percent, but she will still have enough milk to feed her preterm infant at discharge.

Selecting a Breast Pump

Mothers who initiate long-term milk expression need a hospital-grade electric breast pump with a double collection kit (Auerbach, 1990b; Auerbach & Walker, 1994; Hill et al., 1996; Neifert & Seacat, 1985; Zinaman et al., 1992; see also Chapter 13). Controlled clinical trials have demonstrated that these pumps are the most effective in maximizing milk volume.

The clinical challenge is ensuring that these breast pumps are available to mothers who need them. These pumps may be rented through pharmacies, lactation consultants, and home health agencies, but low-income mothers may be unable to incur the rental expense. A letter, such as the one in Figure 14–1, should be prepared on a hospital letterhead, signed by a neonatologist or the NICU lactation specialist, and given to mothers for reimbursement purposes. Even with such a letter, the rental expense may be rejected by third-party payors, with an explanation that the mother can use a less expensive battery-operated model or that breastfeeding is "elective" and formula-feeding is cheaper.

Reimbursement

It is helpful to have a packet of research-based materials (such as the following documents) that parents can use to challenge these decisions:

- an official letter on an institutional letterhead that is specific to the infant's condition and the mother's breastfeeding needs

- research reports that demonstrate the superiority of electric breast pumps and double collection kits (Auerbach, 1990b; Hill et al., 1996; Zinaman et al., 1992)

- official statements and data that endorse the importance and short- and long-term health

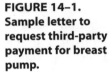

FIGURE 14–1.
Sample letter to request third-party payment for breast pump.

RUSH-PRESBYTERIAN-ST. LUKE'S MEDICAL CENTER   1653 WEST CONGRESS PARKWAY, CHICAGO, ILLINOIS 60612-3833 • 312.942.6640
RUSH UNIVERSITY   RUSH MEDICAL COLLEGE

⟨𝕴⟩ RUSH
SECTION OF NEONATOLOGY
DEPARTMENT OF PEDIATRICS

Date

Insured:

Policy Number:

Re: Electric Breast Pump Rental

To Whom It May Concern:

Dr. _____, a neonatologist in the Special Care Nursery at Rush-Presbyterian-St. Luke's Medical Center has prescribed human milk feedings for _____, who was born on _____,and whose parents are _____. Because this infant is too small and/or ill to feed at the breast, the mother must remove her milk with an electric breast pump, store it, and transport it to the Special Care Nursery so that it can be fed to her infant using a gavage tube.

A hospital grade electric breast pump with a double collection kit is necessary for extracting milk under these circumstances. Randomized controlled trials have shown that manual and/or battery-operated pumps, intended for occasional use by mothers of healthy infants, are inadequate for mothers who must initiate and maintain lactation in the absence of a nursing infant. Although hospital grade electric pumps can be purchased (approximately $900), they are more economical to rent on a short-term basis. We estimate that this mother will require use of the pump for approximately _____.

I trust that this information will expedite insurance coverage of the electric pump rental for this mother and infant. Should there be additional questions, please contact me at the above address/telephone.

Sincerely,

Paula P. Meier, RN, DNSc, FAAN
NICU Lactation Program Director

---

outcomes of human-milk feeding for preterm infants

Milk-Expression Technique

The mother's milk-expression technique can influence the composition and the bacterial count of the milk to be fed to her infant. For this reason, mothers need detailed verbal and written information about the specific components of the procedure and its underlying rationale.

Mothers should be informed of how their expression technique can influence the amount of lipid and calories in their milk. Because lipids provide at least 50 percent of the calories in human milk, and lipid concentration increases over a single milk expression (Brennan-Behm et al., 1994; Harzer et al., 1983; Jensen, 1989), it is essential that mothers be instructed to pump until all milk droplets cease flowing, which usually takes 10 to 15 minutes. The last few drops of milk are very high in lipids and can contribute a substantial proportion of the calories in the entire milk sample.

Similarly, mothers should understand that all milk from a single milk expression should be thoroughly mixed before it is placed into sterile containers for storage. Mothers who produce large volumes of milk may have to empty the collection containers during milk expression to avoid overflow of the bottles. Typically, the first part of the expression will have lower fat and calories than will the latter. If the specimens are not mixed, the infant can receive feedings with markedly different fat and caloric values, affecting metabolic processes and overall weight gain (Brennan-Behm et al., 1994). An exception to this principle is the intentional feeding of hindmilk only, which is discussed later in this chapter.

Even with meticulous technique, no mothers' milk is sterile (Botsford et al., 1993; El-Mohandes et al., 1993; Hamosh et al., 1996; Law et al., 1989; Lemons et al., 1983; Meier & Wilks, 1987). Mothers' attention to hand washing and cleansing of milk-expression equipment is extremely important in reducing colonization by pathogens other than normal skin flora.

Milk-Expression Schedule

Mothers must understand the importance of frequent milk expression during the early days and weeks postbirth, when the lactation hormones support optimal milk production. The actual number of daily milk expressions will depend on each mother's breastfeeding goals. Mothers who need to produce maximal volumes of milk to achieve their goals should plan to express milk 8 to 10 times daily. Included in this group are women who want to breastfeed exclusively at the time of infant discharge and to provide hindmilk for infant feedings or have given birth to multiples. Mothers who plan to provide milk for a limited time (e.g., until an infants' expected birth date) or those who plan to combine formula and breastfeeding can pump less frequently. Instructing "short-term" breastfeeding mothers to express milk more than five or six times daily is unnecessary and may discourage them from pumping at all.

The NICU staff can make it possible for mothers to accomplish frequent milk expression by modifying the nursery environment to meet mothers' needs. Mothers who spend time traveling to and from the NICU often prefer to be with their infants rather than in a separate room where they can express milk. As a result, these mothers may pump only before and after leaving home, and several hours elapse when their breasts are not stimulated.

One NICU enables mothers to remain at their infants' bedside while expressing milk with the electric breast pump. Mothers bring their collection kits to the hospital, and an electric breast pump is brought to the infant's bedside. The mother can see, touch, or hold her infant while expressing milk. Mothers use the pump on arrival in the NICU, every two hours thereafter, and immediately before departure. Bedside pumping incorporates the scientific literature on the use of relaxation and imagery in enhancing milk volume (Brown et al., 1991; Fehrer et al., 1989) and is convenient for the mother and staff. Additionally, the expectation that mothers will provide milk while in the NICU highlights their indispensable role in infant care. Anecdotally, mothers have reported that they express more milk at their babies' bedsides, especially when combined with skin-to-skin (STS) care and nonnutritive sucking at the breast, and that bedside pumping gives them a purpose for frequent and lengthy NICU visits.

Preventing Low Milk Volume

Most mothers of preterm infants experience a decrease in milk volume during the second month of milk expression (Brown et al., 1991; Ehrenkranz & Ackerman, 1986; Fehrer et al., 1989; Hill et al., 1995; Hill et al., 1994; Hopkinson et al., 1988; Hurst, 1997; Neifert & Seacat, 1988). Although no published studies have examined the physiology of this phenomenon, data from studies with term infants may be helpful. Daly & Hartmann (1995a, b) have documented that maternal milk volume is limited primarily by infant demand rather than by a finite capacity of the mother to produce milk. These findings suggest that, over days or weeks, the milk-expression procedure may be ineffective in stimulating an optimal milk supply for mothers of preterm infants. In particular, a breast pump does not mimic the infant's physical closeness and responsiveness, which may be essential for optimal hormonal regulation of milk volume. Thus encouraging infant contact during and after milk expression in the NICU may represent a promising intervention in preventing and improving low milk volume.

Skin-to-Skin Care

A series of worldwide studies have documented the safety of skin-to-skin (STS; kangaroo) care and its effectiveness in promoting physiological stability in preterm infants (Anderson, 1989, 1991; Bergman & Jurisoo, 1994; Charpak et al., 1994; Gale et al., 1993; Legault & Goulet, 1995; Ludington-Hoe & Swinth, 1996; Ludington-Hoe et al., 1994; Ludington-Hoe et al., 1991; Mondlane et al., 1989; Sloan et al., 1994; Wahlberg et al., 1992; Whitelaw, 1990; Whitelaw & Liestol, 1994). Although the relationship between STS care and lactation has been studied less systematically, the duration of breastfeeding appears to be higher for STS infants than for incubator controls (Anderson, 1991; Charpak et al., 1994; Ludington-Hoe & Swinth, 1996; Wahlberg et al., 1990; Whitelaw, 1990).

Furthermore, STS holding may trigger the production of maternal milk antibodies to specific pathogens in the infant's environment through mechanisms in the enteromammary pathway (Hurst et al., 1997). In this study, mothers' milk volume at one, two, three, and four weeks after delivery was compared for two groups of women: 8 mothers who participated in STS holding and 15 mothers who did not. Even with just 30 minutes daily of STS holding mothers in the STS group had a significantly greater increase in milk volume between two and four weeks than did mothers in the control group. At four weeks after delivery, mothers in the STS group produced significantly more milk each day than did control mothers (647 ml versus 530 ml, respectively).

Mothers whose infants are in STS care have reported the infants' making rooting and mouthing movements and moving toward the nipple during STS sessions (Hurst et al., 1997). Mothers frequently note feelings of milk ejection and leaking, and many report that they express the largest milk volumes immediately following STS care.

Although a complete review of procedures for STS holding is beyond the scope of this chapter, several principles can be summarized:

- Infants can be safely placed in STS care while very small and mechanically ventilated (Gale et al., 1993).

- There is no scientific reason to restrict the duration of STS care, unless an infant becomes physiologically unstable while on the mother's chest. Typically, an STS care session is ended based on the mother's availability rather than on infant criteria.

- The position of the infant in STS care is important in maintaining physiological stability, and recliners are ideal for achieving this position. The infant should be placed upright between the mothers' breasts, with the side of the face against the internal surface of one breast. The recliner is angled back to allow the infant's body to remain at a 45- to 60-degree angle from the floor. STS sessions of two or more hours are ideal, and it is not uncommon for infants to display behaviors that suggest autonomic instability when returned to the incubator following STS care (Bosque et al., 1995; Ludington-Hoe et al., 1991; Ludington-Hoe & Swinth, 1996).

Nonnutritive Suckling

Controlled clinical trials have demonstrated many benefits of nonnutritive suckling (NNS) with a pacifier for preterm infants (Anderson et al., 1983; Bernbaum et al., 1983; McCain, 1992; Schwartz et al., 1987). Theoretically, these same benefits should extend to the preterm infant's suckling at the mother's recently pumped breast, an experience that may also maximize the mother's milk production (Narayanan, 1990). Initiating NNS at the emptied breast provides a maternal stimulus that is different from routine breast pump use and, as such, may increase milk yield. In addition, mothers receive instant reinforcement from infants' behaviors that reflect enjoyment and physiological stability while at the breast.

For small infants (<1,000 gm), the mother completely expresses milk from the breast just prior to the infant's being placed in STS care at the breast. The infant should be supported in the football hold or across the chest, so that his entire ventral surface is in direct contact with the lateral aspect of the mother's breast. The infant's temperature can be monitored noninvasively if this is a concern. Although the infant should be held in proximity with the breast, no attempt should be made to "position" the infant's mouth and gums over the nipple and areola. Instead, licking and suckling on the nipple tip is all that is expected of very small preterm infants. In one NICU, NNS may begin as soon as small infants are extubated. Infants on Neonatal Continuous Positive Airway Pressure (NCPAP) can participate in NNS; positioning across the lap with tubings delivering oxygen directed upward and over the breast is most effective (Fig. 14–2). For larger infants, the mother can combine NNS at the emptied breast with administering her freshly expressed milk by gavage (Fig. 14–3).

Management of Low Milk Volume

No previous research has examined the physiology of long-term milk expression for mothers of preterm infants. Therefore, strategies to manage low milk volume for such mothers have focused on pharmacological and nonpharmacological enhancement of prolactin secretion (Ehrenkranz & Ackerman, 1986; Gunn et al., 1996; Neifert & Seacat, 1985, 1988).

The use of oral contraceptives may diminish milk volume in mothers of preterm infants who are expressing milk with a breast pump. Although these women are usually advised by the obstetrician that "low-dose" contraceptives will not interfere with lactation, the mothers' experiences indicate that that this may not be true for a less-established "vulnerable" milk supply. Mothers report that milk volume diminishes markedly within days of starting oral contraceptives and returns to baseline shortly after they are discontinued. This phenomenon has to be explored in controlled studies. In the interim, clinicians should ask about oral contraceptive use if mothers report a rapid decline in a previously adequate volume.

Gavage Feeding of Mothers' Milk

In most countries, preterm infants receive their mothers' milk by gavage until they are able to consume feedings directly from the breast. At this

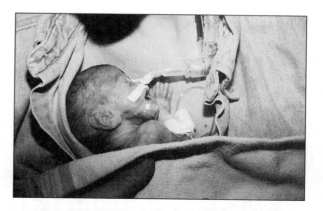

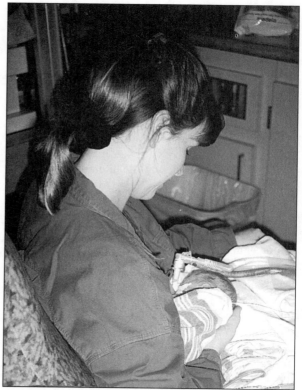

FIGURE 14–2. Infants with NCPAP tubes positioned across mothers' lap.

time, infants are small and vulnerable to problems that can occur when mothers' milk is administered artificially. Four bodies of research are relevant when mothers' milk is administered mechanically:

1. minimizing bacterial growth and nutritional changes in the milk during storage and feeding
2. fortifying or modifying the milk to prevent nutritional deficiencies or promote weight gain

3. transfer of maternal medications into milk that is fed to small preterm infants

4. standards for storing and feeding milk in the NICU

Expressed mothers' milk (EMM) contains a variety of bacteria that can grow rapidly during handling and slow-infusion feeding. Proper techniques for milk expression, storage, and handling may be as effective as bacterial surveillance programs (Botsford et al., 1986; El Mohandes et al., 1993; Law et al., 1989; Lemons et al., 1983; Meier & Wilks, 1987). Guidelines for refrigerating, freezing, and thawing mothers' milk are summarized in Table 14–3. Techniques for limiting the ingestion of bacteria during human milk feeding are seen in Table 14–4.

The scientific literature supports feeding with fresh (unfrozen) milk when possible, because the antiinfective properties are maximally preserved (American Academy of Pediatrics, 1985; Hamosh et al., 1996; Williamson & Murti 1996). Ideally, preterm infants should receive at least one daily feeding of milk that has been pumped at the bedside and fed without refrigeration. This milk retains all of its antiinfective properties and has been subjected to minimal handling and temperature changes.

Many mothers will ensure that their infants have fresh milk available for feedings if they understand the rationale behind this practice. The staff can support this plan by developing a sequence of using the milk so it can be received within 48 hours of expression or alternated with frozen milk when necessary. Additionally, it is important to emphasize to the mother that frozen milk still retains most of its antiinfective properties and is nutritionally superior to formula.

A series of studies provides strong scientific support for the administration of EMM by intermittent rather than slow-infusion continuous gavage (Brennan-Behm et al., 1994; Brooke & Barley, 1978; Narayanan et al., 1984). In particular, milk lipids that comprise 50 to 60 percent of the calories in EMM adhere to the lumen of infusion tubings, and their loss results in a relatively dilute, low-calorie feeding (Brennan-Behm et al., 1994). The greatest lipid loss occurs during the slowest infusion (Greer et al., 1984; Stocks et al., 1985). Clinically,

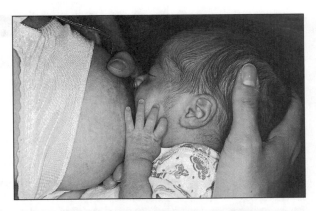

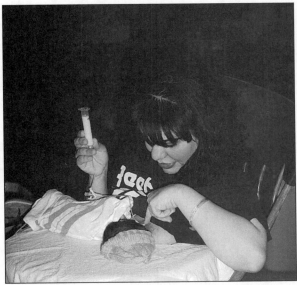

FIGURE 14–3. Nonnutritive suckling with administration by gavage.

this means that the smallest babies, for whom caloric requirements are the highest, will receive EMM at the slowest infusion rates, resulting in low-calorie milk. For this reason, EMM should be administered by slow, intermittent bolus rather than by continuous gavage infusion.

Rapid heating, especially microwaving, has been demonstrated to adversely affect both the immunological and the nutritional properties of EMM (Asquith et al., 1987; Hamosh et al., 1996; Jensen, 1989; Quan et al., 1992; Williamson & Murti, 1996). Refrigerated or frozen EMM should be gradually warmed (over 30 minutes to 1 hour) to approximately body temperature before being fed to small preterm infants. For the smallest infants, the feeding volume can be withdrawn into

Table 14–3

GUIDELINES FOR STORING EXPRESSED MOTHER'S MILK FOR PRETERM INFANT FEEDING

Milk Type	Feeding Parameters	Warming or Thawing	Special Considerations
Fresh, unrefrigerated	1 hour	Not necessary	Extra milk can be refrigerated or frozen after 1 hour at room temperature.
Fresh, refrigerated	24–48 hours	1. Warm slowly (over ½ hour) to approximately body temperature (≤36°C). Do *not* overheat. 2. Do not microwave.	1. Literature indicates milk is suitable for 48 hours with refrigeration at ≤4°C. However, in a large NICU, 24 hours may be a better criterion, so it is consistent with the 24 hours for *thawed frozen* milk. 2. "Cream" layer separates with refrigeration, so milk should be shaken vigorously before use. 3. Milk remaining after the 24- to 48-hour criterion should be discarded, not frozen.
Frozen	24 hours after thawing	1. Thaw gradually (over 1 hour), warming to approximately body temperature (≤36°C). Do *not* overheat. 2. Do not microwave. 3. Take care not to contaminate milk with water if warm-water bath is used.	1. Do not refreeze milk. 2. Do not add any fresh milk to bottles of frozen milk. Use separate containers. 3. Discard unused milk after 24 hours of refrigeration.

Source: Courtesy Ross Products Division.

a syringe that is placed in the infant's incubator for gradual warming.

Fortifying and Modifying EMM
Commercial Additives

EMM is deficient in protein and selected minerals needed to support optimal growth and bone min-eralization for small preterm infants (Schanler, 1995; Schanler & Hurst, 1994; Simmer et al., 1997; Steichen et al., 1987). Thus, for most preterm infants, these additional nutrients are provided in the form of commercial milk fortifiers. However, recent studies have raised concern that these commercial liquids and powders may affect the bioavailability and function of human milk components (Lucas et al., 1996; Quan et al., 1994;

Table 14–4

MINIMIZING BACTERIAL COLONIZATION AND GROWTH IN HUMAN MILK

- Give mothers institution-specific written instructions for expressing and storing milk. Include the following principles:

    Wash your hands thoroughly with soap and water before handling your breasts or the milk-expression equipment.

    Cleanse or sterilize pumping equipment according to institutional guidelines.*

    Hand-express and discard the first few drops of milk (about ½ teaspoonful) before using the breast pump.

    Place milk from each pumping into separate sterile containers. Do not mix milk from separate pumpings unless instructed to do so.

    Refrigerate or freeze the milk, and transport it to the nursery in a cooler with ice.

- Ensure that temperatures for milk storage in the NICU are monitored and recorded on a regular basis. Recommended temperatures are as follows:

    ≤4°C for refrigerated milk
    ≤−15°C for frozen milk

- Take care not to contaminate milk as it is prepared for gavage infusion, especially if it is thawed in a warm-water bath.

- Feed fresh (unfrozen) milk when it is available.

- Feed milk by intermittent, rather than continuous, gavage if possible.

- If continuous gavage feedings are used:

    Administer milk by the most rapid rate that is considered safe.

    Change the entire infusion system (tubings and syringe but not the nasogastric tube) at least every 4 hours.

Although most standards include soap-and-water cleansing and air-drying for pumping equipment, these practices reflect feasibility and practicality rather than conclusive research. In certain instances, the NICU may want mothers to sterilize pumping equipment.

Source: Courtesy Ross Products Division.

Schanler, 1996; Schanler & Hurst, 1994; Schanler et al., 1997).

In particular, a study by Lucas et al. (1996) confirmed a clinical observation of NICU nurses: that commercial fortifiers were associated with "hard stools" and other symptoms of reduced gastrointestinal tolerance of human milk feedings. In a related study, investigators quantified the relationship between stool hardness and type of feeding for full-term and preterm infants (Quinlan et al., 1995). Hard stools are extremely rare among exclusively breastfed infants but occur commonly in formula-fed babies. The investigators concluded that the differences in stool consistency for the two feeding methods may be a function of the calcium and fatty-acid patterns for breast- and formula-fed infants. These findings may be relevant to changes in stool consistency when commercial fortifiers are added to EMM for preterm infant feeding.

Hindmilk Feeding

The feeding of the hindmilk-only fraction of EMM has received increasing interest among clinicians (Valentine et al., 1994). The lipid and caloric content of hindmilk is greater than that of foremilk or composite milk (e.g., a full pumping that includes foremilk and hindmilk). By fractionating the hindmilk portion of a milk expression, mothers can provide a high-lipid, high-calorie milk that promotes accelerated infant growth (Valentine et al., 1994). Although hindmilk feeding holds remarkable potential for preterm infant nutrition, the technique has not yet been subjected to randomized controlled trials.

There is tremendous within- and between-mother variation in lipid content. Thus a standard procedure for collecting hindmilk does not ensure a standard outcome. Clinically, the lipid and caloric content of milk can be estimated with the creamatocrit, a technique that involves centrifuging a milk specimen that has been drawn into a capillary tube (Jensen, 1989; Lucas et al., 1978; Lemons et al., 1980; Polberger & Lönnerdal, 1993). The creamatocrit, or the percentage of total volume in the capillary tube that is equivalent to lipid, can be converted to an estimate of lipid and caloric content using one of the published regression graphs (Jensen, 1989; Lemons et al., 1980; Lucas et al., 1978). However, creamatocrits performed in this manner represent only a relative estimate of lipid and calories. A more accurate quantification of lipid and calorie content requires that the creamatocrit be standardized with one of the direct measures of total milk lipid, such as the Folch technique (Jensen, 1989).

Hindmilk and commercial fortifiers and additives are not interchangeable, a point that is often misunderstood. Although commercial fortifiers provide small amounts of calories in the form of carbohydrates, their primary purpose is to supplement essential nutrients that are thought to be deficient in human milk. In contrast, hindmilk does not "concentrate" these nutrients (Valentine et al., 1994) but does provide an extremely efficient energy source by concentrating the endogenous milk lipids. Thus the use of hindmilk does not replace the need for mineral supplementation, and commercial fortifiers are a relatively inefficient means of supplying extra calories.

Finally, the needs of the mother must be considered whenever her composite milk is not used exclusively. It is easy for mothers to infer that their milk is not "adequate" for their infants when it must be fortified or fractionated for hindmilk feedings. Mothers should be informed that their milk is ideal with respect to immunological and nutritional properties but that the rapid growth of their very small infants requires temporary supplementation with commercial fortifiers or hindmilk.

Lactoengineering of own mothers' milk (OMM) through a combination of hindmilk and creamatocrit measures can be empowering for mothers of preterm infants (Jennings et al., 1997).

Specifically, mothers are assisted in expressing milk with a creamatocrit value that meets their individual infant's growth needs. When their infants demonstrate the desired weight-gain pattern, mothers recognize that their milk modifications supported the desired growth. This program, which includes empowering mothers of preterm infants through breastfeeding, includes a study in progress that examines the accuracy with which mothers can perform creamatocrits on their expressed milk.

Maternal Medications and Small Preterm Infants

When small preterm infants receive OMM by gavage, extra care must be taken to ascertain that maternal medications in the milk can be tolerated safely. Preterm infants, especially those who are at extremely low birth weight, have immature metabolic and excretory pathways. As a result, drugs that may be safely given to mothers of term, healthy infants may have adverse consequences for more vulnerable infants. Although a detailed description of these issues is beyond the scope of this chapter, several principles should be considered when a mother of a preterm infant must take medications:

- The medication should be considered "safe" for healthy term infants (American Academy of Pediatrics Committee on Drugs, 1994); if this is not the case, the medication should not be considered safe for the small preterm infant.

- If the medication or its metabolites has been shown to accumulate in newborn body tissues, its accumulation may be even more exaggerated for the preterm infant.

- Many mothers of preterm infants will have had complicated births or health conditions that necessitate a combination of medications.

- The infant may be receiving medications or other therapies that could interact with the maternal medications. The safety of these combinations—rather than the individual medications—must be considered.

- Extra caution is needed when lipid-rich hind-milk is being fed: medications that are lipophilic may cross readily into the milk.

Advice concerning the safety of medications for small, preterm infants should be provided only by health care professionals who have expertise in lactation, pharmacology, and neonatal care. When doubt arises about a specific medication or combination of medications, a national expert should be consulted. In all instances, any information about maternal medications should be reviewed with the neonatologist who is responsible for the infant's care, and mothers should record on the individual milk container any medications they have consumed.

Standards for Storing and Handling Milk in the NICU

Few published standards exist for the handling of OMM in the NICU. In general, these standards are limited to temperature, duration of storage, and type of storage container and are inadequate for ensuring that OMM is handled according to the research literature. Several principles should be considered when OMM is stored and handled in the NICU:

1. *Human milk is a living fluid, not unlike blood, and should be handled as such.* This means that each milk container should be carefully labeled by the mother and checked by the nurse prior to preparing the feeding. Anecdotally, it is well recognized that errors occur in which infants receive another mother's milk. Considering the host-defense nature of human milk and the extent to which viruses can be transferred via milk, administering the wrong milk to an infant is a serious error. The NICU nurse should never administer a container of unlabeled milk to an infant under any circumstances.

2. *All milk that is to be used for infant feeding should be stored in the hospital under controlled conditions.* All too often, mothers are told to store their expressed milk at home because of insufficient storage space in the NICU freezer. However,

this approach would not be recommended for medications or blood, and expressed milk should be handled no differently. When milk is out of sight of the NICU staff, there is no assurance that it has remained completely frozen and unopened before it is subsequently fed to small, preterm infants.

3. *Ensure that OMM in the NICU is not subject to tampering.* There are no clear guidelines as to whether refrigerators and freezers should be locked or have restricted access, but this is a very important issue. Anecdotally, NICU staff have expressed concerns that suggest that OMM should be kept in an environment that eliminates the potential for tampering.

Feeding at the Breast in the NICU

Feeding at breast in the NICU incorporates two principal topics: the science and practice of initiating and advancing direct breastfeedings, and the measurement and facilitation of milk transfer.

The Science of Early Breastfeeding

Early breastfeeding is less physiologically stressful than is early bottle-feeding for preterm infants (Blaymore-Bier et al., 1993; Bosque et al., 1995; Meier, 1996; Meier & Anderson, 1987). In 1988, Meier demonstrated that preterm infants who served as their own controls for breastfeeding and bottle-feeding had more stable measures of transcutaneous oxygen pressure and body temperature during breastfeedings than during bottle-feedings. Blaymore-Bier et al. (1993) and Bosque et al. (1995), using measures of oxygen saturation, noted similar findings. These data suggest that the more stable patterns of oxygenation for breastfeeding than for bottle-feeding are a result of less interruption of breathing during breastfeeding.

To test this theory, Meier (1996) studied a cohort of clinically stable preterm infants who served as their own controls for serial breastfeeding and bottle-feedings from the time of oral feeding initiation until NICU discharge. The following variables were monitored and recorded continuously on an eight-channel polygraph: sucking event, respiratory event, body temperature, and oxygen saturation during each feeding session. Volume of intake was measured by test weighing. Previous research validated the instruments that were used for the measurement of sucking (deMonterice et al., 1992) and milk intake (Kavanaugh et al., 1990; Kavanaugh et al., 1989; Meier et al., 1990) in this research.

Analysis of the results of this study revealed that during bottle-feedings, preterm infants frequently did not breathe during sucking bursts; instead, they alternated short bursts of sucking with pauses during which they breathed rapidly. Oxygen saturation measures in response to this suck/breathe patterning varied. For most, but not all, infants who maintained short sucking bursts (e.g., minimal durations of not breathing), oxygen saturation remained relatively stable. For infants who attempted longer sucking bursts or for those who demonstrated long durations of breath holding following short sucking bursts, oxygen saturation declined significantly. Examples of these patterns of suck/breathe coordination are depicted in Figure 14–4.

During breastfeedings, these same infants integrated breathing with sucking bursts (Fig. 14–5). A maturational trend was seen, in which less mature infants demonstrated brief episodes of breath holding within long sucking bursts. As the infants approached 34 to 35 weeks' adjusted gestational age, the suck/breathe patterning approximated a ratio of 1:1.

These findings are consistent with those of previous researchers who described more stable patterns of oxygenation during breastfeedings than during bottle-feedings for preterm infants. However, these findings explain the mechanism for this stability: less interruption in breathing during breastfeeding. Meier (1988) concluded that differences in suck/breathe patterning for bottle-feeding and breastfeeding may be due to the infant's ability to control the flow of milk during breastfeeding by subtle alterations in the suck mechanism. These alterations, consisting of the infant's manipulation of intrasuck and intersuck intervals to accommodate breathing, may not be clinically apparent but were detected during this research (see Fig. 14–5). Infants did not demonstrate similar suck/breathe patterning during bottle-feedings until they were several weeks older.

The ability to remain physiologically stable during feedings occurs earlier for breastfeeding preterms than for bottle-feeding preterms. Thus waiting to initiate breastfeedings until the infant demonstrates the ability to consume entire bottle-feedings is not a research-based criterion of readiness to breastfeed. For clinical purposes, all infants should be monitored for physiological stability during early oral feedings, regardless of method.

Initiating Early Breastfeeding

There are no universally agreed-upon criteria for when breastfeeding should be initiated for preterm infants. Instead, several commonly used criteria–minimal body weight or ability to consume entire feedings by bottle–are not research based.

When infants are placed at the breast for daily nonnutritive sucking opportunities, the transition to nutritive feedings can be gradual. When it is determined that the infant should consume some low-flow milk, the mother can express some (but not all) of the milk from the breast. In this way, the preterm infant is introduced to small droplets of milk, which do not necessitate prolonged closure of the airway for swallowing. As the infant matures, the mother can regulate the milk flow by pumping the amount of milk necessary to reduce the post-milk-ejection flow. When the infant demonstrates the ability to coordinate sucking and breathing, the mother no longer needs to express milk prior to the feeding. This progressive increase in the rate of flow during breastfeeding is consistent with recommendations from a recent study in which suction and expression pressures were measured during low-flow bottle-feedings for low-birth-weight infants (Lau et al., 1997). These data suggest that less mature preterm infants could initiate feedings safely, provided that milk flow was restricted.

Positions for Early Breastfeeding

The preterm infant should be breastfed in a position that affords support to the head and neck, such as the football or the across-the-lap hold. The head of the preterm infant is heavy in relation to the weak musculature of the neck, and undirected head movements can easily collapse the airway, with resultant apnea and bradycardia. Use of these positions will help the preterm infant to obtain milk

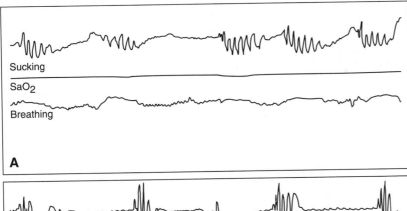

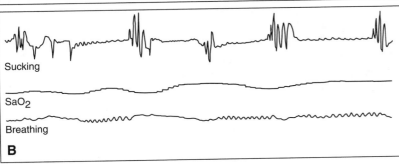

FIGURE 14–4. *A. Polygraphic recording demonstrating suck/ breathe patterning and oxygenation during bottle-feeding for preterm infants. In this recording, the infant alternates short sucking bursts with breathing but does not breathe within sucking burst. Oxygen saturation remains stable. B. Polygraphic recording demonstrating suck/breathe patterning and oxygenation during bottle-feeding for a preterm infant. Oxygen saturation fluctuates, with values as low as 78 percent during short sucking bursts. (Reproduced by permission of Royal Society of Medicine Press, London.)*

from the breast. Specifically, the data from nonnutritive sucking and bottle-feeding studies reveal that suction pressures are maturationally dependent (Anderson et al., 1983; Anderson & Vidyasagar, 1979; Lau et al., 1997; Weaver & Anderson, 1988). With this limitation, the small preterm infant needs to be "placed" and "kept" on the nipple, because the limited suction pressures do not permit the infant's bringing the nipple into the correct position for milk extraction (Figs. 14–6, 14–7).

Milk Transfer for Preterm Infants

After preterm infants have been introduced to unrestricted milk flow during breastfeeding, it is important to evaluate milk transfer. Milk transfer is a function of the interaction of maternal milk volume, milk ejection, and infant suckling (Kavanaugh et al., 1995; Meier & Brown, 1997a, b, c). Mothers and their preterm infants may experience problems with any or all of these components. Conversely, because these components are interactive, a problem with one (e.g., ineffective suckling) can be compensated for by adequacy in the other components. Application of this framework to intake-related

questions and problems is essential in determining the appropriate clinical intervention.

For example, most but not all preterm infants experience ineffective or marginally effective suckling during early breastfeeding experiences. Typically, these infants suckle in short bursts and fall asleep quickly at the breast (Kavanaugh et al., 1995; Nyqvist et al., 1996; Nyqvist et al., 1996). However, some infants can still consume an adequate quantity of milk during breastfeeding, because the mothers have a copious milk volume, and it flows readily. Thus milk volume and ejection can compensate for marginally effective suckling.

Mothers and health care professionals are unable to use clinical indices to accurately estimate milk intake for preterm infants (Kavanaugh et al., 1995; Meier et al., 1993, 1994, 1996). However, clinicians are concerned that more accurate measures of milk intake are either too stressful for mothers or unnecessary for preterm infants (Driscoll & Sheehan, 1985; Meier, 1995; Walker, 1995). Similarly, many care providers are unaware that accurate measurement of milk intake for preterm infants is possible.

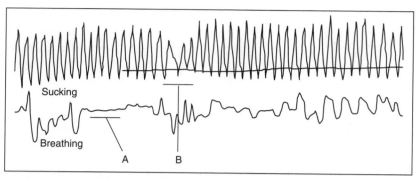

FIGURE 14–5. Polygraphic recording demonstrating suck-breathe patterning and oxygenation during breastfeeding for an infant of 33 weeks' gestational age. *The infant breathes within this long (104 sucks) suckling burst until phase A, when breathing is interrupted for several sucks. In phase B, the infant alters the duration and amplitude of individual sucks, apparently to reinstitute a more regular breathing pattern, which continues through the remainder of the burst. (Reproduced by permission of Royal Society of Medicine Press, London.)*

Test Weighing

The most accurate clinical technique for estimation of milk intake is test weighing, a procedure in which the clothed infant is weighed before and after breastfeeding under identical conditions (Woolridge et al., 1985). The weight gain (in grams) after the feeding is equivalent to the volume (in milliliters) of milk consumed. Several research reports have demonstrated the accuracy of test weighing for term and preterm infants when electronic (but not mechanical) scales are used (Meier et al., 1990, 1994).

Test weighing should be introduced in the NICU when it appears that milk transfer has occurred or discharge is imminent. For smaller preterm infants, the test-weight estimate permits individualized complementation of breastfeedings, so that 24-hour fluid and caloric requirements can be met. For larger infants awaiting NICU discharge, test weights can be used to diagnose milk-transfer problems. For example, the infant may suckle marginally, but the mother's milk volume is adequate. It is impossible to know whether the mother's milk flow can compensate for the infant's suck unless volume of intake is measured.

Unlike full-term, healthy infants, preterm infants do not demonstrate predictable demand feeding behaviors until close to term-corrected age (Meier, 1997b, d; Nyqvist et al., 1996). Thus infants may consume minimal volumes at a breastfeeding and still sleep for several hours, if undisturbed. The use of test weights permits the emergence of demand feeding behaviors while retaining a safeguard against slow weight gain or dehydration in the days before NICU discharge.

When the infant has demonstrated the ability to consume all feedings orally, the neonatologist or neonatal nurse practitioner can prescribe a 24-hour minimal milk intake for the infant. The 24-hour volume can then be subdivided into six- or eight-hour volumes to permit a modified demand feeding schedule. For example, if a 1,700-gm infant needs a minimum of 300 ml/day, the mother and nurse can plan to feed 100 ml every eight hours. Then the infant is allowed to feed on demand but must receive the prescribed 100-ml volume within an eight-hour period. Test weights are measured with each breastfeeding, and the volume of complements and supplements is recorded. Thus if the 1,700-gram infant consumes 15 ml, 12 ml, and 18 ml, respectively, within a period of two hours, he has been given the opportunity to self-regulate sleep and feeding. However, the infant still must consume the remaining 55 ml over the next six hours. NICU nurses can help mothers to implement this plan in the days before infant discharge, so that mothers develop an understanding of how the infant coordinates sleep and feeding.

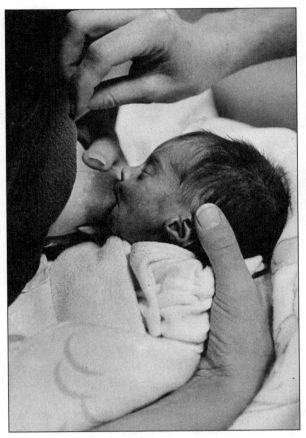

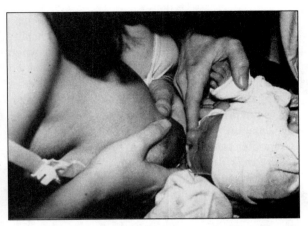

FIGURE 14–7. Use of both hands to support the large breast with flattened nipple for breastfeeding a preterm infant.

FIGURE 14–6. Head support and latching on for a small, preterm infant.

Facilitating Milk Transfer

Seldom does significant milk transfer occur during the first few breastfeedings for preterm infants. However, as NICU discharge approaches, consistently small volumes of intake become a concern that must be evaluated. Selected problems of milk transfer are particularly common among preterm infants.

The single most important factor for mothers who will be breastfeeding a preterm infant at home is maintaining a milk supply that exceeds the baby's requirements at hospital discharge (Meier, 1997; Neifert & Seacat, 1988). With an adequate milk supply, the infant's immature suckling may be less problematic. Mothers can plan for this by expressing their milk an extra time or two in the week before their baby's discharge. For mothers who have a borderline milk supply as NICU dis-

charge approaches, the clinician should consider a regimen of metoclopramide (Ehrenkranz & Ackerman, 1986; Lawrence, 1994) to augment the milk yield. Theoretically, the prolactin stimulus from the medication will be maintained by the infant's direct breastfeeding in the home.

Mothers should be reminded to express milk with the electric breast pump after each breastfeeding in the hospital. NICU staff and mothers seldom appreciate that a preterm infant cannot substitute for the breast stimulation provided by the electric breast pump, especially if the infant consumes only small milk volumes. Mothers frequently question how to coordinate milk expression with demand feedings, because they are concerned that their breasts will be empty when their infants awake to feed. An appropriate strategy in this situation is to emphasize the priority of maintaining the milk yield. If the mothers have emptied their breasts with a breast pump, the infant can still be breastfed with a supplemental nurser, using freshly expressed milk. Unlike a term infant, the preterm infant's suck is unlikely to extract milk that remains after breast pump usage.

Milk Ejection

Many mothers of preterm infants deny feeling the sensations of milk ejection both when using the electric pump and when feeding their infants at breast.

Thus it is often difficult to evaluate the synchronization of milk ejection and infant suckling. Typically, mothers experience a delay in milk ejection when infants are placed at the breast, because the women are conditioned to the sensations of the breast pump. It is not uncommon for milk flow to begin just as the preterm infant falls asleep at the breast. If this situation persists for more than a few feedings, the mother can use the electric breast pump to initiate the milk flow. This can be done by placing the infant at one breast and the pump at the other or by first initiating the milk flow with the double collecting kit and then placing the infant at breast.

Infant Suckling

The majority of milk-transfer problems for preterm infants can be related to immaturity and inconsistency in suckling (Kavanaugh et al., 1995; Meier & Brown, 1997a, c; Meier et al., 1996). The relatively low suction pressures and the infants' inconsistent, irregular sucking bursts do not sustain the milk flow needed for effective milk transfer. These phenomena appear to be maturationally dependent. Until the infant achieves full-term, corrected age, strategies to increase the effectiveness of sucking are often necessary:

1. The infant should be fed in the previously described positions that provide support for the head, neck, and torso. The infant's head should be guided onto the breast and kept in this position with gentle pressure. Although care must be taken that the nares are not occluded, the tip of the infant's nose may touch the breast surface to maximize the amount of nipple and areolar tissue in the infant's mouth. Mothers of small preterm infants have repeatedly expressed their initial discomfort with this position, because they are invariably concerned that the breast tissue will suffocate their babies. Anecdotal evidence suggests that correcting this position for a preterm infant can increase milk intake considerably.

2. Although nipple shields are seldom recommended in the clinical literature (Newman, 1990), they may increase milk transfer and duration of breastfeeding for a subpopulation of preterm, low-birth-weight infants (Clum & Primomo, 1996). Clinical indications for nipple shield use among this group are numerous: flat, ill-defined maternal nipple that may also have a large, puffy areola; ability of the infant to place the mouth appropriately over the areola, but not able to sustain regular sucking; and a "difficult" nipple in conjunction with short, ineffective sucking bursts. In these instances, the infant will not transfer adequate volumes of milk without the assistance of a nipple shield.

It has been hypothesized that the nipple shield functions to increase the effectiveness of the infant suck by remaining in correct position within the infant's mouth in the absence of strong suction pressures. This principle is illustrated in Figure 14–8. Then the infant can use expression pressures in combination with relatively weak suction to extract larger quantities of milk. Although an ideal nipple shield for preterm infants has yet to be designed, the smallest, thinnest shield available is indicated for these babies.

The nipple shield is extremely well accepted by mothers because it often represents the first breastfeeding experience in which the infant remains awake, sucks eagerly, and consumes measurable volumes of milk. However, mothers are concerned about providing the gentle pressure necessary to keep the infants correctly positioned over the areola, because of the plastic nature of the shield. Thus mothers need to be shown how to support the breast with the shield in place so that the infant can achieve an effective sucking position while keeping the shield away from the nares.

Clinicians often assume that preterm infants do not take as much milk with the shield in place as they would without its use. This concern seems to be based on data (Auerbach, 1990a) that demonstrated reduced milk transfer when mothers of term infants expressed milk with a breast pump with a nipple shield in place. Although this study addressed an important concept, the findings cannot be applied directly to infants, because milk transfer was measured for milk expression, not for infant feeding. Preterm infants who have no milk transfer prior to nipple shield use actually increase milk intake when the shield is used. Similarly, concern that use of the shield will reduce the milk yield over time is not applicable in this situation. Preterm infants who feed longer and more eagerly with the shield in place provide considerably more breast stimulation than that in breastfeeding without the shield.

3. Clinicians suggest that other feeding techniques, such as cup- or finger-feeding, be used as an alternative to the nipple shield. This approach appears to reflect an unscientific bias against the nipple shield and is especially problematic, because use of the shield means that the infant can feed at the breast. Mothers of preterm infants who have spent weeks or months expressing milk prefer to feed their babies at the breast, even if it entails temporary nipple-shield use. Use of the shield saves time for mothers, because they do not need to offer a complement after breastfeeding, as is the case with cup- or finger-feeding.

4. If the nipple shield is effective in correcting milk-transfer problems in the hospital, its use should be continued after NICU discharge. Additionally, there is no scientific reason for recommending that infants be weaned from the shield as soon as possible. Typically, the infant will require the shield for adequate milk transfer until approximately full-term, corrected age. For most mothers, this coincides with two to three weeks of nipple-shield use, over which time the infant's intake and weight gain can be monitored regularly. Mothers have described their individual approaches to discontinuing the shield, but in no case should they be advised to "cut back" or tamper with the integrity of the shield. Serial test weights are helpful to most mothers as they transfer from the shield to feeding at the breast without the shield.

Breastfeeding Devices

In addition to the nipple shield, other breastfeeding devices are frequently recommended to measure and facilitate milk transfer. A supplemental nurser, as described in Chapter 13, can be helpful for the mother who has a limited milk supply or for the infant who achieves an appropriate position and sucking mechanism at the breast without extracting milk. This device is especially helpful for borderline preterm infants (e.g., those older than 34 weeks of gestation who are not admitted to the NICU). These infants, who are still premature with respect to the ability to extract adequate volumes of milk, can receive the extra milk they need with a supplemental nurser while feeding at the breast.

Many mothers of preterm infants—both borderline babies and those who have been admitted

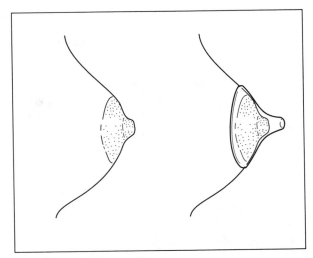

FIGURE 14–8. Nipple shield.

to the NICU—find it reassuring to measure milk intake and serial weight gain in the first days after infant discharge. A portable, battery-operated scale that mothers can rent and use to perform daily weighings in the home is ideal for this purpose. The scale, which weighs to the nearest 2 gm and automatically calculates milk intake from the prefeeding and postfeeding weights, has been demonstrated to measure milk intake accurately for full-term and preterm infants (Meier et al., 1994). This scale can be a useful adjunct to breastfeeding management for mothers and preterm infants during the first week or two after discharge. However, mothers should be introduced to the proper use of the scale prior to NICU discharge.

Alternative feeding devices are frequently recommended by clinicians to avoid "nipple confusion" (Lang et al., 1994; Newman, 1990; Stine, 1990). Although the phenomenon of "nipple confusion" has received little systematic study, it is likely that selected risk factors make it difficult for some infants to alternate breast- and bottle-feedings (Cronenwett et al., 1992; Neifert et al., 1995). Reports from clinicians suggested that these alternative feeding methods are safe when performed by experts (Lang et al., 1994), but no controlled clinical trials have established either safety or effect on breastfeeding outcome for these devices. A significant volume of milk may be spilled during cup-feedings (Narayanan, 1997).

Postdischarge Breastfeeding Management

The United States is different from most developed countries in that preterm infants are typically discharged from the NICU before their expected birth dates, whether or not breastfeeding has been well established. In contrast, in most European countries, preterm infants are discharged only when weight gain on complete breastfeedings has been documented, which may be several weeks later than in the United States. In developing countries, preterm infants are frequently discharged at lower weights, but many of these infants are small for gestational age (Narayanan, 1985; Ramasethu et a., 1993) or are maintained in STS care in the home (Bergman & Jurisoo, 1994; Charpak et al., 1994; Colonna, 1990; Mondlane et al., 1989; Whitelaw & Liestol, 1994).

When these data are considered in combination, it appears that preterm infants remain at risk for underconsumption of milk by exclusive breastfeeding until approximately full-term corrected age (Meier & Brown, 1996; Meier et al., 1996). This is suggested by the low incidence of exclusive breastfeeding in the early weeks after NICU discharge in the United States, the longer hospitalization in European countries so that exclusive breastfeeding is established, and the slow weight gain on exclusive breastfeedings in the first two to four weeks after hospital discharge in developing countries. This commonality probably reflects a problem with the maturationally dependent "infant suckling" component of milk transfer, often expressed by mothers as "getting enough."

Getting Enough: Milk-Transfer Problems

Studies from the United States have examined the phenomenon of getting enough for mothers and preterm infants (Hill et al., 1994; Hill et al., 1997; Kavanaugh et al., 1995). However, clinicians who work primarily with full-term, healthy infants do not always comprehend the difference between getting enough and insufficient milk supply. As a result, mothers of preterm infants are frequently told to breastfeed their babies and to pump more frequently, interventions that are focused on the milk-volume component of milk transfer. These recommendations are inappropriate for most mothers of preterm infants who describe problems with getting enough. These women report that they can express adequate volumes of milk with the breast pump but perceive that their infants do not take all of the milk available to them. Thus effective interventions must focus on the infant suckling component of milk transfer. This distinction has important research and practice implications.

The most fundamental research issue is that accepted nomenclature for describing and classifying the amount of breastfeeding does not fit the breastfeeding patterns for this population (Meier & Brown, 1997a). For example, most mothers of preterm infants complement breastfeedings with their own expressed milk during the early weeks at home, but the Labbok and Krasovec (1990) schema does not accurately capture this pattern. If this pattern is categorized as "exclusive breastfeeding," it overestimates mothers' successes and misrepresents data on duration of breastfeeding. Thus research-based criteria to categorize the amount of breastfeeding for these mothers must be developed and standardized (Brown et al., 1995).

Research addressing the early postdischarge period must also include methods that accurately and reliably distinguish between insufficient milk supply and getting enough (Hill et al., 1997; Kavanaugh et al., 1995; Meier & Brown, 1997a). These studies must incorporate available technology to measure milk volume and infant intake during breastfeeding rather than relying on checklists or clinical indices that have been demonstrated to be inaccurate or unreliable (Hill et al., 1997; Meier et al., 1994, 1996). Similarly, other studies in which milk intake during breastfeeding was not measured have related slow weight gain or the need for continued milk fortification postdischarge to deficiencies in the mothers' milk (Chan et al., 1994; Hall et al., 1993). Thus future postdischarge studies for preterm infants must include accurate instrumentation to differentiate among milk supply, "milk quality," and infant intake.

Practice Implications

Preterm infants are vulnerable to underconsumption of milk during the first weeks after discharge.

This must be acknowledged by clinicians who are accustomed to helping mothers of full-term, healthy infants. Several key principles must be understood and incorporated into postdischarge breastfeeding plans for preterm infants:

- The practitioner must recognize that the clinical indices of intake used for healthy, full-term infants, such as breastfeeding behaviors, wet diapers, frequency of stools, and sleep patterns, are not accurate or reliable for preterm infants. For example, a preterm infant may remain "hydrated" but still not consume enough milk to grow.

- Preterm infants may not consistently "demand," so mothers should not be told, "You'll know when your baby is hungry."

- These infants should not be awakened more frequently than every three hours to breastfeed, because sleep interruption interferes with growth hormone release, retarding weight gain.

- Mothers of preterm infants are not reassured with nonspecific comments, such as "Trust your body." It is important to accept that mothers' concerns about intake are real and not just a reflection of their NICU experience.

In summary, mothers of preterm infants need a "safety net" during the first weeks at home, until their infants have demonstrated the ability to gain weight on exclusive breastfeedings. Milk transfer should be monitored regularly (e.g., every 48–72 hours) and accurately at this time, either through frequent visits to the primary care provider for serial growth measures or by in-home test weighing.

Care should be taken to listen to these women and their feelings of vulnerability with respect to infant intake. They must not be hurried through these processes or told that they are not breastfeeding correctly. For example, if a mother feels that she needs to give bottle supplements of her expressed milk in the first few days, she should not be warned about nipple confusion or told that alternative feedings should be used. Instead, her ability to determine and advocate what she feels is best for her infant should be interpreted as a sign of strength. It is important to remember that breastfeeding is only one activity that these women must deal with; their babies are vulnerable to many conditions, and mothers need time to sort out care priorities.

Similarly, mothers should be encouraged to continue the breastfeeding strategies that worked in the hospital until their infants have demonstrated an acceptable pattern of growth for at least a week or two. For many women, these devices will include a nipple shield or in-home weighing, and there are no data to support withdrawing these aids before the mother is ready. Finally, the mother needs access to both consumer support groups and a professional who is experienced with breastfeeding for preterm infants when discharge approaches.

SUMMARY

In summary, breastfeeding for preterm infants and mothers is different from breastfeeding for healthy populations in many important ways. The vast body of research in this area suggests that these differences are physiological, biological, metabolic, and emotional and that they are common across a variety of national boundaries and cultures. The challenge to researchers and clinicians who work with mothers and preterm infants is to continue to generate new studies and practices that incorporate findings from these scientific publications. Only research-based practices can address the many barriers to breastfeeding initiation and duration for this at-risk population.

REFERENCES

Albanese CT, Rowe MI: Necrotizing enterocolitis. *Sem Pediatr Surg* 4:200–6, 1995.

American Academy of Pediatrics: Nutritional needs of low-birth-weight infants. *Pediatrics* 75:976–86, 1985.

American Academy of Pediatrics Committee on Drugs: Transfer of drugs and other chemicals into human milk. *Pediatrics* 93:137–50, 1994.

Anderson GC: Current knowledge about skin-to-skin (kangaroo) care for preterm infants. *J Perinatol* 11:216–26, 1991.

Anderson GC: Skin-to-skin: kangaroo care in Western Europe. *Am J Nurs* 89:662–6, 1989.

Anderson GC, Vidyasagar D: Development of sucking in premature infants from 0–7 days postbirth as measured with a suck scoring system. In: Anderson GC, Raff B, eds. *Newborn behavioral organization: nursing research and implications.* (National Foundation March of Dimes Birth Defects Original Article Series 15). New York: Liss, 1979:145–71.

Anderson GC, Burroughs AK, Measel CP: Nonnutritive sucking opportunities: a safe and effective treatment for preterm neonates. In: Field TM, Sostek AK, eds. *Infants born at risk: physiological, perceptual, and cognitive processes.* New York: Grune & Stratton, 1983:129–46.

Armand M, et al: Effect of human milk or formula on gastric function and fat digestion in the premature infant. *Pediatr Res* 40:429–37, 1996.

Asquith MT, et al: Clinical uses, collection, and banking of human milk. *Clin Perinatol* 14:173–85, 1987.

Atkinson SA, Bryan MH, Anderson GH: Human milk feeding in premature infants: protein, fat and carbohydrate balances in the first 2 weeks of life. *J Pediatr* 99:617–24, 1981.

Atkinson SA, Raddle IC, Anderson GH: Macromineral balances in premature infants fed their own mothers' milk or formula. *J Pediatr* 102:99–106, 1983.

Auerbach KG: Breastfeeding the premature infant: a symposium. *Keep Abreast J* 2:98–121, 1977.

Auerbach KG: The effect of nipple shields on maternal milk volume. *JOGNN* 19:419–27, 1990a.

Auerbach KG: Sequential and simultaneous breast pumping: a comparison. *Int J Nurs Stud* 27:257–65, 1990b

Auerbach KG, Walker M: When the mother of a premature infant uses a breast pump: what every NICU nurse needs to know. *Neon Netw* 13:23–29, 1994.

Baker BJ, Rasmussen TW: A system for organizing and documenting lactation support of NICU families. *JOGNN* 26:515–21, 1997.

Bergman NJ, Jurisoo LA: The 'kangaroo-method' for treating low birth weight babies in a developing country. *Trop Doc* 24:57–60, 1994.

Bernbaum JC, et al: Nonnutritive sucking during gavage feeding enhances growth and maturation in premature infants. *Pediatrics* 71:41–5, 1983.

Blaymore-Bier J, et al: Breastfeeding of very low birth weight infants. *J Pediatr* 123:773–8, 1993.

Bosque EM, et al: Physiologic measures of kangaroo versus incubator care in a tertiary-level nursery. *JOGNN* 24:210–26, 1995.

Botsford K, et al: Gram-negative bacilli in human milk feedings: quantitation and clinical consequences for premature infants. *J Pediatr* 109:707–10, 1986.

Brennan-Behm M, et al: Caloric loss from expressed mothers milk during continuous gavage continuous infusions of breastmilk. *Neon Netw* 1994;13:27–32.

Brooke OG, Barley J: Loss of energy during continuous infusions of breast milk. *Arch Dis Child* 53:334–45, 1978.

Brown LP, et al: Use of human milk for low birthweight infants. *On-Line J Know Synth Nurs* 3(27), 1996.

Brown LP, et al: Breastfeeding services for low birthweight infants: outcomes and cost. NINR Grant R0111NR03881, September, 1995–June, 2000.

Brown L, Hollingsworth A, Armstrong C: Factors affecting milk volume in mothers of VLBW infants. In: *Abstracts of 1991 Scientific Sessions of the 31st Biennial Convention,* Sigma Theta Tau International, 1991:46.

Budin PC: *The nursling.* London: Claxton Press, 1907.

Buescher ES: Host defense mechanisms of human milk and their relations to enteric infections and necrotizing enterocolitis. *Clin Perinatol* 21:247–62, 1994.

Byrne B, Hull D: Breast milk for preterm infants. *Prof Care Mother Child* 6:39–45, 1996.

Carlson SE, Rhodes PG, Ferguson MG: Docosahexaenoic acid status of preterm infants at birth and following feeding with human milk or formula. *Am J Clin Nutr* 44:798–804, 1986.

Chan GM, Borschel MW, Jacobs JR: Effects of human milk or formula feeding on the growth, behavior and protein status of preterm infants discharged from the newborn intensive care unit. *Am J Clin Nutr* 60:710–16, 1994.

Chandra RK: Five-year follow-up of high-risk infants with family history of allergy who were exclusively breast-fed or fed partial whey hydrolysate, soy, and conventional cow's milk formulas. *J Pediatr Gastroenterol Nutr* 24:380–8, 1997.

Charpak N, Ruiz-Pelaez JC, Charpak Y: Rey-Martinez Kangaroo Mother Program: an alternative way of caring for low birth weight infants? One year mortality in a two cohort study. *Pediatrics* 94:804–10, 1994.

Clum D, Primomo J: Use of a silicone nipple shield with premature infants. *J Hum Lact* 12:287–90, 1996.

Cohen S: High tech-soft touch: breastfeeding issues. *Clin Perinatol* 14:187–96, 1987.

Colonna F: The "Kangaroo-mother" method: evaluation of an alternative model for the care of low birth weight newborns in developing countries. *Int J Gynecol Obstet* 31:335–9, 1990.

Cronenwett L, et al: Single daily bottle use in the early weeks postpartum and breastfeeding outcomes. *Pediatrics* 90:760–6, 1992.

Crosse VM, et al: The value of human milk compared with other feeds for premature infants. *Arch Dis Child* 29:178–95, 1954.

Daly SEJ, Hartman PE: Infant demand and milk supply: Part 1. Infant demand and milk production in lactating women. *J Hum Lact* 11:21–6, 1995a.

Daly SEJ, Hartman PE: Infant demand and milk supply: Part 2. The short-term control of milk synthesis in lactating women. *J Hum Lact* 11:27–37, 1995b.

Dawodu AH: Nutritional composition and volume of milk produced by mothers of preterm infants in developing countries. *J Trop Pediatr* 35:95–6, 1989.

deAndreca I, Uauy R: Breastfeeding for optimal mental development: the alpha and the omega in human milk. *World Rev Nutr Diet* 78:1–27, 1995.

deCarvalho M, et al: Frequency of milk expression and milk production by mothers of non-nursing premature neonates. *Am J Dis Child* 139:483–5, 1985.

DeCurtis M, et al: A case control study of necrotizing enterocolitis occurring over 8 years in a neonatal intensive care unit. *Eur J Pediatr* 146:398–400, 1987.

deMonterice D, et al: Concurrent validity of a new instrument to measure sucking for preterm infants. *Nurs Res* 41:342–6, 1992.

Driscoll JW, Sheehan CS: Breast-feeding and premature babies: guidelines for nurses. *Neon Netw* 4:18–24, 1985.

Ehrenkranz R, Ackerman B: Metoclopramide effect on faltering milk production by mothers of premature infants. *Pediatrics* 78:614–20, 1986.

Ehrenkranz R, et al: Breastfeeding and premature infants: incidence and success [abstract]. *Pediatr Res* 19:199A, 1985.

El-Mohandes AE, et al: Aerobes isolated in fecal microflora of infants in the intensive care nursery: relationship to human milk use and systemic sepsis. *Am J Infect Cont* 21:231–4, 1993.

El-Mohandes AE, et al: Use of human milk in the intensive care nursery decreases the incidence of nosocomial sepsis. *J Perinatol* 17:130–4, 1997.

Faldella G, et al: Visual evoked potentials and dietary long chain polyunsaturated fatty acids in preterm infants. *Arch Dis Child* 75:F108–F112, 1996.

Fehrer S, et al: Increasing breast milk production for premature infants with a relaxation/imagery audiotape. *Pediatrics* 83:57–60, 1989.

Gale G, Franck L, Lund C: Skin-to-skin (Kangaroo) holding of the intubated premature infant. *Neon Netw* 12:49–57, 1993.

Gamble S: Report on breastfeeding in Dunedin Hospital's neonatal intensive care unit. *ACMI J* 6:18–20, 1993.

Goldman AS, et al: Immunologic protection of the premature newborn by human milk. *Sem Perinatol* 18:495–501, 1994.

Gotsch C: One innovation helping breastfeeding mothers of preterm infants. *J Hum Lact* 7:189, 1991.

Greer F, McCormick A, Loker J: Changes in fat concentration of human milk during delivery by intermittent bolus and continuous mechanical pump infusion. *J Pediatr* 105:745–9, 1984.

Groer M, Walker WA: What is the role of preterm breast milk supplementation in the host defenses of preterm infants? Science vs. fiction. *Adv Pediatr* 43:335–58, 1996.

Gross SJ: Growth and biochemical response of preterm infants fed human milk or modified infant formula. *N Engl J Med* 308:237–41, 1983.

Gunn AJ, et al: Growth hormone increases breast milk volumes in mothers of preterm infants. *Pediatrics* 98:279–82, 1996.

Hall RT, Wheeler RE, Rippetoe LE: Calcium and phosphorus supplementation after initial hospital discharge in breast-fed infants of less than 1800 grams birth weight. *J Perinatol* 13:272–8, 1993.

Hamosh M: Digestion in the premature infant: the effects of human milk. *Sem Perinatol* 18:485–94, 1994.

Hamosh M, et al: Breastfeeding and the working mother: effect of time and temperature of short-term storage on proteolysis, lipolysis, and bacterial growth in milk. *Pediatrics* 97:492–8, 1996.

Harzer G, et al: Changing patterns of human milk lipids in the course of lactation and during the day. *Am J Clin Nutr* 37:612–21, 1983.

Hill PD, Aldag JC, Chatterton RT: The effect of sequential and simultaneous breast pumping on milk volume and prolactin levels: a pilot study. *J Hum Lact* 12:193–9, 1996.

Hill PD, Brown LP, Harker TL: Initiation and frequency of breast expression in breastfeeding mothers of LBW and VLBW infants. *Nurs Res* 44:352–5, 1995.

Hill PD, Hanson KS, Mefford AL: Mothers of low birthweight infants: breastfeeding patterns and problems. *J Hum Lact* 10:169–76, 1994.

Hill PD, Ledbetter RJ, Kavanaugh KL: Breast-feeding patterns of low birthweight infants after hospital discharge. *JOGNN* 26:189–97, 1997.

Hopkinson J, Schanler R, Garza C: Milk production by mothers of premature infants. *Pediatrics* 81:315–20, 1988.

Hurst NM, et al: Skin-to-skin holding in the neonatal intensive care unit influences maternal milk volume. *J Perinatol* 17:213–7, 1997.

Jaeger MC, Lawson M, Filteau, S: The impact of prematurity and neonatal illness on the decision to breast-feed. *J Adv Nurs* 25:729–37, 1997.

Jennings T, Meier W, Meier P: High lipid and caloric content in milk from mothers of preterm infants [abstract]. *Pediatr Res* 41:233A, 1997.

Jensen RG: *The lipids of human milk.* Boca Raton, FL: CRC Press, 1989.

Kaufman K, Hall L: Influences of the social network on choice and duration of breast-feeding in mothers of preterm infants. *Res Nurs Health* 12:149–59, 1989.

Kavanaugh K, Engstrom JL, Meier PP: The reliability of weighing procedures for preterm infants. *Nurs Res* 38:178–9, 1989.

Kavanaugh K, et al: Getting enough: mothers' concern about breastfeeding a preterm infant postdischarge. *JOGNN* 24:23–32, 1995.

Kavanaugh K, et al: How reliable are scales for weighing preterm infants? *Neon Netw* 9:29–32, 1990.

Kavanaugh KL, et al: The rewards outweigh the efforts: breastfeeding outcomes for mothers of preterm infants. *J Hum Lact* 13:15–21, 1997.

Kleigman R, Pittard W, Fanaroff A: Necrotizing enterocolitis in neonates fed human milk. *J Pediatr* 95:450–3, 1979.

Labbok M, Krasovec K: Toward consistency in breastfeeding definitions. *Stud Fam Plann* 21:226–30, 1990.

Lang S, Lawrence CJ, Orme RLE: Cup-feeding: an alternative method of infant feeding. *Arch Dis Child* 71:365–9, 1994.

Lau C, et al: Oral feeding in low birth weight infants. *J Pediatr* 130:561–9, 1997.

Law BJ, et al: Is ingestion of milk-associated bacteria by preterm infants fed raw human milk controlled by routine bacteriologic screening? *J Clin Microbiol* 27:1560–6, 1989.

Lawrence R: *Breastfeeding: a guide for the medical profession* (4th ed). St Louis: Mosby, 1994.

Lefebvre F, Ducharme M: Incidence and duration of lactation and lactational performance among mothers of low-birth-weight and term infants. *Can Med Assoc J* 140:1159–64, 1989.

Legault M, Goulet C: Comparison of kangaroo and traditional methods of removing preterm infants from incubators. *JOGNN* 24:501–6, 1995.

Lemons J, et al: Bacterial growth in human milk during continuous feeding. *Am J Perinatol* 1:76–80, 1983.

Lemons J, Schreiner R, Gresham E: Simple method for determining the caloric and fat content of human milk. *Pediatrics* 66:626–8, 1980.

Lucas A: Does early diet program future outcome? *Acta Paediatr Scand* Suppl 365:58–67, 1980.

Lucas A, Cole T: Breast milk and neonatal necrotizing enterocolitis. *Lancet* 336:1519–23, 1990.

Lucas A, et al: Breastmilk and subsequent intelligence quotient in children born preterm. *Lancet* 339:261–4, 1992.

Lucas A, et al: Crematocrit: simple clinical technique for estimating fat concentration and energy value of human milk. *Br Med J* 1:1018–20, 1978.

Lucas A, et al: Early diet of preterm infants and development of allergic or atopic disease: randomized prospective study. *Br Med J* 300:837–40, 1990a.

Lucas A, et al: Early diet in preterm infants and development status at 18 months. *Lancet* 335:1477–81, 1990b.

Lucas A, et al: A randomised multicentre study of human milk versus formula and later development in preterm infants. *Arch Dis Child* 70:F140–6, 1994.

Lucas A, et al: Randomized outcome trial of human milk fortification and developmental outcome in preterm infants. *Am J Clin Nutr* 64:142–51, 1996.

Ludington-Hoe SM, Swinth, JY: Developmental aspects of kangaroo care. *JOGNN* 25:691–703, 1996.

Ludington-Hoe SM, Hadeed AJ, Anderson GC: Physiologic responses to skin-to-skin contact in hospitalized premature infants. *J Perinatol* 11:19–24, 1991.

Ludington-Hoe SM, et al: Kangaroo care: research results, and practice implications and guidelines. *Neon Netw* 13:19–27, 1994.

Lundeen EC: Feeding the premature baby. *Am J Nurs* 39:3–11, 1939.

Mathur NB, et al: Anti-infective factors in preterm human colostrum. *Acta Pediatr Scand* 79:1039–44, 1990.

McCain GC: Facilitating inactive awake states in preterm infants: a study of three interventions. *Nurs Res* 41:157–60, 1992.

Meberg A, Willgraff S, Sande HA: High potential for breastfeeding among mothers giving birth to pre-term infants. *Acta Pediatr Scand* 71:661–2, 1982.

Meier PP: Bottle and breastfeeding: effects on transcutaneous oxygen pressure and temperature in preterm infants. *Nurs Res* 37:36–41, 1988.

Meier PP: Caution needed in extrapolating from term to preterm infants: author's reply [letter]. *J Hum Lact* 11:91, 1995.

Meier PP: *Professional guide to breastfeeding premature infants*. Columbus, OH: Ross Laboratories, 1997.

Meier PP: Suck-breathe patterning during bottle and breastfeeding for preterm infants. David TJ, ed. *Major controversies in infant nutrition* (Inter-

national Congress and Symposium Series 215). London: Royal Society of Medicine Press, 1996: 9–20.

Meier PP, Anderson GC: Responses of small preterm infants to bottle and breastfeeding. *MCN* 12:97–105, 1987.

Meier PP, Brown LP: Limitations of the Labbok and Krassovec breastfeeding classification for preterm infants [letter] *J Nurse Midwif* 42:1259–60, 1997a.

Meier PP, Brown LP: Persevering with breastfeeding after NICU discharge: reflections on Ryan's story. *Breastfeed Abstr* 17:3–4, 1997b.

Meier PP, Brown LP: State of the science: breastfeeding for mothers and low birth weight infants. *Nurs Clin North Am* 31:351–65, 1996.

Meier PP, Brown LP: Strategies to assist breastfeeding in preterm infants. In: David TJ, ed. *Recent advances in pediatrics*. London: Churchill-Livingstone, 1997c:137–50.

Meier PP, Wilks S: The bacteria in expressed mothers' milk. *MCN* 12:20–3, 1987.

Meier PP, et al: The accuracy of test weighing for preterm infants. *J Pediatr Gastroenterol Nutr* 10:62–5, 1990.

Meier PP, et al: Breastfeeding support services in the neonatal intensive care unit. *JOGNN* 22:338–44, 1993.

Meier PP, et al: Estimating milk intake of hospitalized preterm infants who breastfeed. *J Hum Lact* 12:21–6, 1996.

Meier PP, et al: A new scale for in-home test-weighing for mothers of preterm and high risk infants. *J Hum Lact* 10:163–8, 1994.

Mondlane RP, deGraca AMP, Ebrahim GC: Skin-to-skin contact as a method of body warmth for infants of low birth weight. *J Trop Pediatr* 35:321–6, 1989.

Morley R: The influence of early diet on later development. *J Biosoc Sci* 28:481–7, 1996.

Morley R, et al: Mother's choice to provide breast milk and developmental outcome. *Arch Dis Child* 63:1382–5, 1988.

Narayanan I: *Breastfeeding the preterm infant: international perspectives.* Conference sponsored by Rush-Presbyterian St. Luke's Medical Center, Chicago, October 1997.

Narayanan I: Nutrition for preterm and growth retarded infants: developing countries concerns. *Hum Nutr Appl Nutr* 39A:242–54, 1985.

Narayanan I: Sucking on the 'emptied' breast–a better method of non-nutritive sucking than use of a pacifier. *Ind Pediatr* 27:1122–3, 1990.

Narayanan I, Prakash K, Gujral V: The value of human milk in the prevention of infection in the high-risk low-birth-weight infant. *J Pediatr* 99:496–8, 1981.

Narayanan I, Singh B, Harvey D: Fat loss during feeding of human milk. *Arch Dis Child* 59:475–7, 1984.

Narayanan I, et al: A planned prospective evaluation of the anti-infective property of varying quantities of expressed milk. *Acta Pediatr Scand* 71:441–5, 1982.

Narayanan I, et al: Randomized controlled trial of effect of raw and holder pasteurized human milk and of formula supplements on incidence of neonatal infection. *Lancet* 2:1111–3, 1984.

Neifert M, Seacat J: Milk yield and prolactin rise with simultaneous breast pump. In: *Proceedings of the Ambulatory Pediatric Association Annual Meeting,* Washington, DC Ambulatory Pediatric Assoc., May 7–10, 1985.

Neifert M, Seacat J: Practical aspects of breastfeeding the premature infant. *Perin Neonatol* 12:24–30, 1988.

Neifert M, Lawrence R, Seacat J: Nipple confusion: toward a formal definition. *J Pediatr* 126:S125–9, 1995.

Neu J: Necrotizing enterocolitis: the search for a unifying pathogenic theory leading to prevention. *Pediatr Clin North Am* 43:409–32, 1996.

Newman J: Breastfeeding problems associated with the early introduction of bottles and pacifiers. *J Hum Lact* 6:59–63, 1990.

Nyqvist KH, Ewald U: Successful breastfeeding in spite of early mother-baby separation for neonatal care. *Midwifery* 13:24–31, 1997.

Nyqvist KH, Sjöden PO: Advice concerning breastfeeding from mothers of infants admitted to a neonatal intensive care unit: the Roy adaptation model as a conceptual structure. *J Adv Nurs* 18:54–63, 1993.

Nyqvist KH, Ewald U, Sjöden PO: Supporting a preterm infant's behavior during breastfeeding: a case report. *J Hum Lact* 12:221–8, 1996.

Nyqvist KH, et al: Development of the preterm breastfeeding behavior scale (PIBBS): a study of nurse-mother agreement. *J Hum Lact* 12:207–19, 1996.

Pierrat V, et al: Somatosensory evoked potentials in preterm infants with intrauterine growth retardation. *Early Hum Dev* 44:17–25, 1996.

Polberger S, Lönnerdal B: Simple and rapid macronutrient analysis in human milk for individualized fortification: basis for improved nutritional management of very-low-birthweight infants? *J Pediatr Gastroenterol Nutr* 17:283–90, 1993.

Quan R, et al: The effect of nutritional additives on anti-infective factors in human milk. *Clin Pediatr* 325–8, 1994.

Quan R, et al: Effects of microwave radiation on anti-infective factors in human milk. *Pediatrics* 89:667–9, 1992.

Quinlan PT, Lockton S, Irwin J: The relationship between stool hardness and stool composition in breast and formula-fed infants. *J Pediatr Gastro-enterol Nutr* 20:81–90, 1995.

Ramasethu J, Jeyaseelan L, Kirubakaran C: Weight gain in exclusively breastfed preterm infants. *J Trop Pediatr* 39:152–9, 1993.

Richards M, Lang M, MacIntosh C: Breastfeeding the VLBW infant: successful outcome and maternal expectations [abstract]. *Pediatr Res* 20:383A, 1986.

Ryan A, et al: A comparision of breast-feeding data from the national surveys of family growth and the Ross laboratories' mother survey. *Am J Public Health* 81:1049–52, 1991.

Schanler RJ: Human milk fortification for premature infants [editorial]. *Am J Clin Nutr* 64:249–50, 1996.

Schanler RJ: Suitability of human milk for the low-birthweight infant. *Clin Perinatol* 22:207–22, 1995.

Schanler RJ, Hurst NM: Human milk for the hospitalized preterm infant. *Sem Perinatol* 18:476–84, 1994.

Schanler RJ, Schulman RJ, Lau C: Growth of premature infants fed fortified human milk [abstract]. *Pediatr Res* 41:240A, 1997.

Schwartz R, et al: A meta-analysis of critical outcome variables in nonnutritive sucking in preterm infants. *Nurs Res* 36:292–5, 1987.

Simmer K, Metcalf R, Daniels L: The use of breast-milk in a neonatal unit and its relationship to protein and energy intake and growth. *J Pediatr Child Health* 33:55–60, 1997.

Sloan NL, et al: Kangaroo mother method: randomised controlled trial of an alternative method of care for stabilised low birthweight infants. *Lancet* 344:782–5, 1994.

Steichen JJ, Krug-Wispe SK, Tsang RC: Breastfeeding the low birth weight preterm infant. *Clin Perinatol* 14:131–71, 1987.

Stevens LH: The first kilogram: the protein content of breast milk of mothers of babies of low birth weight. *Med J Aust* 2:555–7, 1969.

Stine MJ: Breastfeeding the premature newborn: a protocol without bottles. *J Hum Lact* 6:167–70, 1990.

Stocks R, et al: Loss of breastmilk nutrients during tube feeding. *Arch Dis Child* 60:164–6, 1985.

Trause MA, et al: Successful lactation in mothers of preterms. *J Perinatol* 5:22–9, 1986.

Tudehope D, Steer PA: Annotation: which milk for the preterm infant? *J Paediatr Child Health* 32:275–7, 1996.

Uauy R, et al: Effect of dietary omega-3 fatty acids on retinal function of very-low-birth-weight neonates. *Pediatr Res* 28:485–92, 1990.

Udosen EO, Ebong PE: Milk macronutrient levels during the first month of term and preterm Nigerian mothers. *Trop Geogr Med* 44:256–9, 1992.

Updated breastfeeding trend, 1987–1995. Columbus, OH: Ross Products Division, Abbott Laboratories, 1996.

Uraizee F, Gross S: Improved feeding tolerance and reduced incidence of sepsis in sick very low birthweight infants fed maternal milk [abstract]. *Pediatr Res* 25:298A, 1989.

Valentine CJ, Hurst NM, Schanler RJ: Hindmilk improves weight gain in low-birth-weight infants fed human milk. *J Pediatr Gastroenterol Nutr* 18:474–7, 1994.

Verronen P: Breastfeeding of low birth weight infants. *Acta Pediatr Scand* 74:495–9, 1985.

Wahlberg V, Affonso DD, Persson, B: A retrospective, comparative study using the kangaroo method as a complement to the standard incubator care. *Eur J Public Health* 2:34–7, 1992.

Walker M: Test weighing and other estimates of breastmilk intake [letter]. *J Hum Lact* 11:91–2, 1995.

Weaver KA, Anderson GC: Relationship between integrated sucking pressures and first bottle-feeding scores in premature infants. *JOGNN* 17:113–20, 1988.

Whitelaw A: Kangaroo baby care: just a nice experience or an important advance for preterm infants? *Pediatrics* 85:604–5, 1990.

Whitelaw A, Liestol K: Mortality and growth of low birth weight infants on the Kangaroo Mother Program in Bogota, Colombia. *Pediatrics* 94:931–2, 1994.

Williamson MT, Murti PK: Effects of storage, time, temperature, and composition of containers on biologic components of human milk. *J Hum Lact* 12:31–5, 1996.

Woolridge MW, et al: Methods for the measurement of milk volume intake of the breast-fed infant. In: Jensen RC, Neville MC, eds. *Human lactation: milk components and methodologies*. New York: Plenum, 5–20, 1985.

Yip E, Lee J, Sheehy Y: Breast-feeding in neonatal intensive care. *J Pediatr Child Health* 32:296–8, 1996.

Zinaman MJ, et al: Acute prolactin and oxytocin response and milk yield to infant suckling and artificial methods of expression in lactating women. *Pediatrics* 89:437–40, 1992.

15

BREAST-RELATED PROBLEMS

Jan Riordan and Kathleen G. Auerbach

In nursing or lactation consultant practice, as elsewhere, an ounce of prevention is worth a pound of intervention. Many difficulties women encounter while breastfeeding can be prevented by the self-care measures and breastfeeding education discussed in preceding chapters. When a woman fully understands how her body works, she is at less risk for frustration and failure when she encounters a barrier to breastfeeding. This chapter deals with specific breast problems and identifies how health professionals can help.

Clinicians who work with breastfeeding women agree that breast and nipple problems can be common barriers to breastfeeding. During prenatal visits, women should be screened for unusual-looking breasts, areolas, or nipples, and lack of breast enlargement. Any of these, coupled with previous breastfeeding difficulties, are high-risk indicators for breastfeeding problems (Livingstone, 1990).

Before discussing the more clinical aspects of breast-related problems, including surgery, it is important to address the emotional significance of the female breasts. Breasts are part of a woman's internalized body image that she develops around adolescence and carries with her for the rest of her life. They represent a woman's deepest sense of womanhood. Any change in her breasts (e.g., breast surgery) threatens this feminine internal view of self and creates a disequilibrium. When a woman's breasts are altered by illness or infection,

it can be a "double whammy": both her femininity and her ability to breastfeed can be threatened.

Nipple Variations

Inverted or Flat Nipples

As pointed out in Chapter 4, the frequency of nipple inversion is unknown, although clinicians have reported that this condition sometimes resolved itself from the beginning to the end of pregnancy. In many cases, the degree of inversion is such that it does not affect the ability of the baby to grasp the areolar tissue and draw the nipple into the mouth, although this action might take longer. Lactation consultants have observed that women who have markedly inverted nipples early in their first pregnancy and who breastfeed have much less inversion with subsequent pregnancies. In some cases, these women have reported that their nipples, which initially inverted between feedings with the first baby, no longer do so with second and later infants.

The degree to which inverted nipples are an impediment to breastfeeding is partially caused by the belief that they prevent breastfeeding. How the nipple looks when it is not in the baby's mouth, however, does not always predict how well it functions. In most cases, as long as the mother positions the baby well back on the areola so that the entire nipple is placed well back in the baby's mouth, there is no reason why a mother with inverted nipples should forgo breastfeeding. During suckling, the nipple elongates to double its "resting" length (Smith et al., 1988). Such reactivity to infant suckling helps to explain by inference why the degree of inversion appears to lessen after weeks or months of repeated suckling by the infant.

When the clinician examines the mother's breasts and nipples in the third trimester of pregnancy, discussion about breastfeeding can continue. If the mother has flat or inverted nipples at that time, she can be taught that following birth, exercising the nipple just before latching on by a newborn appears to loosen the nipple tissue and helps to separate adhesions that cause retraction or inversion. The infant also stretches the nipples during feedings.

Hoffman's exercises (exercises of the nipples during pregnancy) and breast shells, two traditional methods for treating inverted nipples, appear to be ineffective and are no longer recommended. Alexander et al., (1992) found that a sustained improvement in nipple inversion was more common in the group of women who did not use breast shells, although the differences were not statistically significant. The authors of this study wisely pointed out that too much stress on preparation of the breasts may discourage mothers from breastfeeding.

The most effective intervention for treating an inverted or flat nipple is to stimulate and shape the nipple just before the feeding. For a flat nipple (not inverted), massage the nipple or apply a cold cloth to help the nipple to evert outward. For an inverted nipple, instruct the mother to shape her nipple by placing her thumb about one and a half to two inches behind the nipple (with her fingers beneath) and pushing back into her chest. This works best in a side-lying position (Huggins, 1986). Any pump can be used to help pull out the nipple immediately before the infant feeds. Color Plates 19 and 20 are "before and after" photographs showing eversion of an inverted nipple through gentle suction.

Large or Elongated Nipples

Nipples come in assorted sizes and shapes and, like all anatomical structures, are genetically influenced. Clinicians report that Asian women are more likely to have unusually long nipples. Generally, nipples that are larger or longer than normal are less likely to cause problems in breastfeeding than are inverted or flat nipples. In fact, they are often viewed as an anatomical gift that will make breastfeeding easier. Although this is true in many cases, exceptionally long or large nipples may detract from breastfeeding, especially if the infant is small. Infants of mothers with extra-long nipples have been observed to gag after latch-on and to slide back toward the nipple tip, which in some cases causes the mother to develop sore nipples.

Plugged Ducts

No one knows the specific cause of plugged ducts, but they are usually found in mothers who have an abundant milk supply and who do not adequately drain each breast (Livingstone, 1990). Pathological changes within the breast causing the plug are vaguely referred to in the literature as a *stasis, clogging of milk,* or local accumulations of milk or dead cells that have been shed. A plugged duct is indicated by either of these two sets of symptoms: complaints of tenderness, heat, and possible redness in one area of the breast or (if the plug is located in a duct close to the skin) a palpable lump of well-defined margins without a generalized fever. Sometimes, a tiny white milk plug can be seen at the opening of the duct on the nipple. One mother described it as "little bits of a hard white substance" just beneath the surface of milk duct outlets. Color Plate 7 shows a milk plug.

Clinicians are aware of a higher frequency of plugged ducts during the winter season. Although the reason for this is not clear, it may be related to the restricting effects of winter clothing or simply to the cold weather. There is also some evidence that, whereas some women are predisposed to developing plugged ducts, others never encounter it through multiple breastfeeding experiences. Plugged ducts also can lead to mastitis, especially if ignored or untreated. Self-care measures to recommend to a mother with a plugged duct are given in Box 15–1.

In acute situations, stripping the breast effectively dislodges the blocked milk. If a mother has chronically recurring plugged ducts, some physicians elect to open the duct with a sterile needlelike instrument. After this is done, the milk may forcibly shoot out from the duct, and the mother

BOX 15–1

Self-Care for Treating a Plugged Duct

- Continue to breastfeed often. Begin feeding on the affected breast to promote drainage.
- Apply moist heat to the area several times a day, generally before breastfeeding.
- Massage the affected breast before and during feeding to stimulate flow of milk. Support the breast with a cupped hand and use firm massage, starting at the periphery of the breast, using the thumb to encourage milk flow while baby suckles. (Another option is to massage in a hot shower or bath.) Outside of the shower,

- try using an electric vibrator (on low setting).
- Soak the affected breast(s) by leaning over a basin of warm water and gently massaging them.
- Change position of the infant during feedings to ensure drainage of all the sinuses and ductules in the breast. At least one position should result in the baby's nose being pointed toward the site of the plugged duct.
- Avoid any constricting clothing, such as an underwire bra or straps on a baby carrier.

feels relief. However, this procedure can be followed by recurring pain in the affected area and should be done only in extreme cases.

Incomplete drainage caused by a skipped feeding or a constricting bra, poor nutrition, and stress have all been implicated in the development of plugged ducts, but a cause-and-effect relationship has never been substantiated. Assessment should include a review of these possibilities with the mother and a review of events leading up to the plugged duct, especially if the mother has a repeated problem. There is no need for an antibiotic to treat a plugged duct unless a fever and mastitis develop.

Mastitis

Mastitis usually develops after the mother leaves the hospital. Nurses and lactation consultants who practice in the community may be the first to speak with the mother whose symptoms suggest early indication of mastitis. The advice dispensed during this initial call can prevent the condition from advancing to an abscess, especially if the mother

mistakenly thinks she should stop breastfeeding or has already done so.

Mastitis is usually a benign, self-limiting infection, with few consequences for the suckling infant (Ogle & Davis, 1988). The initial symptoms of puerperal mastitis may be fatigue, localized breast tenderness, and a flulike, muscular aching. If a breastfeeding mother calls the clinic or office complaining that she has the "flu," the first consideration is to rule out infectious mastitis. Typically, fatigue, headache, and muscular aching are followed by fever, a rapid pulse, and the appearance of a hot, reddened, and tender area on the breast (see Color Plate 15). The infection is usually unilateral and located in one area (often in the upper outer breast quadrant), although it can occur in any area of the breast. It can occasionally occur in both breasts simultaneously and may involve a large portion of the breast. The infection is also associated with an elevation of sodium and chloride in the milk from an infected breast caused by the temporary opening of the normally tight junctions between secretory cells in the paracellular pathway (Prentice et al., 1985; Thullen, 1988).

After the resolution of mastitis, the affected breast undergoes a temporary "resting" phase and usually produces less milk than it did before the infection occurred.

Among women who breastfeed long term, mastitis is most likely to occur in the first several weeks after delivery, most frequently during the sixth week, among mothers aged 30 to 34, and when the mother works full-time outside the home (Foxman, 1994). About one-third of the cases, however, occur after the infant is six months old. Another one-fourth of the cases occur after 12 months of breastfeeding (Riordan & Nichols, 1990). Symptoms may last from two to four days, followed by resolution. Early reports showed the incidence to be 6 percent or less (Leary, 1948; Marshall et al., 1975; Waller, 1938); these studies, however, counted only those women who returned to a clinic or the physician for treatment. The actual incidence is much higher. Foxman (1994) found that about one-third of mothers with prior breastfeeding experience had a history of mastitis.

A number of factors are thought to predispose a woman to mastitis. These are stress, fatigue, cracked or fissured nipples, plugged ducts, constriction by a tight bra or incorrect sleeping position, engorgement or milk stasis, and abrupt change in frequency of feedings. Foxman (1994) found that women were more likely to report nipple pain, a crack or fissures during the week before mastitis developed. They were also more likely to report they could not take a daytime nap and slept less than did mothers who did not develop mastitis prior to the onset of mastitis. When mothers who had mastitis were asked to list factors present before the breast infection, they rated fatigue, stress, and plugged ducts as most prevalent (Riordan & Nichols, 1990).

The best treatments for hastening recovery are continued breastfeeding, application of moist heat, increased fluids, bed rest, and the judicious use of antibiotics (Table 15–1). It is well established in the medical literature that mastitis is associated with the presence of *Staphylococcus aureus*. Only rarely is a streptococcus involved; when it is, the mastitis may be bilateral (Schreiner et al., 1977). Although untreated cases heal almost as quickly as treated ones, the standard antibiotic for lactation mastitis is a penicillinase-resistant penicillin or a cephalospo-rin that covers *S. aureus* for 6 to 10 days (Matheson, 1988; Ogle & Davis, 1988; Thomsen, 1985).

For chronic mastitis, erythromycin at low doses (regular doses 250–500 mg every six hours) or trimethoprim-sulfamethoxazole (Bactrim, Septra) over a longer period of time has been recommended (Cantlie, 1988). However, staphylococci rapidly develop resistance against erythromycin. Trimethoprim-sulfamethoxazole and erythromycin are also options when the mother is allergic to penicillin. In a case report, trimethoprim-sulfamethoxazole (two tablets per day for ten days) was effective in preventing recurrence of mastitis in a patient with multiple incidences of mastitis who was allergic to penicillin (Hoffman & Auerbach, 1986). These medications can be taken during breastfeeding without known untoward reactions in the infant.

A small percentage of breast infections develop into an abscess. An abscess, like a boil, is basically a collection of pus that must be drained (Color Plates 9, 12, & 13). If the abscess is small, the pus may be aspirated with a fine needle under ultrasound guidance. For a larger abscess, the physician makes an incision and drains the area. According to Love (1990, pp. 99–100)

The surgeon will never sew up a drained abscess; that would lock the bacteria into the abscess, and almost insure the infection's return. I tell my patients to go home and rest; then, after 24 hours, begin taking daily showers; let the water run over the breast and wash away the bacteria, and then put a dressing over it to absorb oozing fluids from the incision.

A drain is placed in the incision to promote drainage; in addition, manual expression helps to eliminate pus and milk. The incision heals from the inside out within a week or two. Treatment of abscesses varies across cultures. Efrem (1995) reported on 285 cases of breast abscess in lactating Nigerian women. Most (85 percent) grew *S. aureus*, 5 percent grew coliforms, and 10 percent grew no organism. All of the cases responded well to treatment by incision and drainage followed by packing daily with ribbon gauze soaked in magnesium sulphate solution (135 cases), Euseol (100 cases), and honey (50 cases).

Table 15-1

SELECTED ANTIBIOTICS FOR MASTITIS

Generic Name	Trade Name	Adult Dosage Ranges
Penicillinase-resistant penicillins		
Cloxacillin	Cloxapen, Tegopen	250–500 mg PO q6h
Dicloxacillin	Dynapen	125–250 mg PO or IM q6h
Oxacillin	Prostaphlin	500 mg–1 gm PO or IM q4–6h
Cephalosporins		
Cephalexin	Keflex	250–500 mg PO q6h
Cepharadine	Anspor, Velosef	250–500 mg PO q6h
Cefaclor	Ceclor	250–500 mg PO q8h

The major share of research on lactation mastitis has focused on pathology, biomedical analysis, and attempts to classify types of mastitis. Gibberd (1953), for instance, described two types of mastitis: cellulitis and adenitis. Cellulitis is thought to involve the interlobular connective tissue that has been infected by the introduction of bacteria through cracked nipples; it is treated with antibiotics. In adenitis, presumably, the breast ducts are blocked, and the clinical symptoms are less severe. Treatment is to get the milk flowing with heat, expression, and pumping. Antibiotics are used only if the infection is not resolving (Livingstone, 1990).

Thomsen et al. (1985) proposed another classification based on leukocyte counts in milk from the infected breast:

- *Milk stasis:* leukocyte count less than 10^6/ml of milk; symptoms lasting for an average of 2.1 days
- *Noninfectious inflammation:* leukocyte count more than 10^6/ml of milk; symptoms lasting about 5.3 days
- *Infectious mastitis:* leukocyte count more than 10^6/ml and bacteria count more than 10^3/ml

Thomsen et al. (1985) recommended that antibiotic treatment be used only for infectious mastitis, the third classification. Although this taxonomy is helpful in theory, laboratory studies on mastitic milk are seldom done in practice. By the time the mother reports the problem to a health care provider, she usually has been ill for several hours, if not a day or two; the peak of the infectious process may already have passed, and she is getting well by the time she seeks medical treatment. Other drawbacks are that the milk sample must be collected before any antibiotics are started, laboratory studies may take several days, and the testing expense may not be covered by health insurance.

Skin Rashes, Lesions, and Eczema

Breast rashes and lesions on the nipple or areolar area are unusual and often difficult to diagnose. They are particularly distressing if they are painful. In one case (Brackett, 1988), a mother described a periodic burning sensation in the breast not related to actual breastfeeding. Most of the mother's areola was itchy, flaky, and red. The family lived without air conditioning during hot, humid weather. In addition, the mother swam in a chlorinated pool each day, often wearing her bathing suit for some time after returning home. Thrush was ruled out. The mother stopped swimming, and her rash resolved within two weeks.

Eczema is a type of dermatitis with redness and crusting and oozing papules. Amir (1993) described a case in which a breastfeeding mother with celiac disease developed red, scaly, and cracked nipples. The mother appeared to have eczema, possibly infected, involving most of both breasts. A topical steroid ointment (betamethasone dipropionate 0.05% [Diprosone]) was applied four times daily, and a topical antibiotic was used twice daily. Two weeks later, the eczema had resolved, and the mother was able to continue breastfeeding without pain. See Box 15–2 for precautions for such disorders.

A more severe breast skin problem is redness and itching accompanied by tiny ulcers on the nipple and areola that resemble chicken pox. Breastfeeding is extremely painful. As the ulcers heal, they form scabs. The baby may or may not have similar perioral skin lesions. This condition requires referral to a physician, who should evaluate the mother for a possible staphylococcal or viral infection. Culture of the lesion should be taken during its early stages before the lesion begins to dry and heal over. Color Plate 4 depicts a cracked nipple with a possible bacterial infection.

Treatment will depend on laboratory results of a culture of the lesion and maternal serum antibody titers. If the lesions are herpes simplex and the baby is younger than three weeks (Whitley, 1980), it is advisable for the mother to wean the infant or to pump her milk until the lesions are healed. The mother will be treated with an antiviral ointment.

The breast lesions from herpes (Color Plate 10) were described by the lactation consultant who saw her (L. Zielinski, personal communication, 1987) as looking like chickenpox: the healing lesions were scabbing, the active lesions were oozing ulcerations, and the new lesions were tiny, bright-red flat areas. The mother complained of extreme "razor blade-like" pain during feedings. She was evaluated by two physicians, who offered differing diagnoses. Her pediatrician suggested that it might be herpes virus, whereas her dermatologist thought the mother had a staphylococcal infection. Neither physician obtained a culture or serum antibody titers.

The woman was first treated for a staphylococcal infection, which worsened the problem and then with an antiviral agent (Zovirax). The lesions began to resolve shortly after the mother applied Zovirax to her nipples and areola. The mother interrupted breastfeeding her 10-month-old baby

for two weeks while the lesions healed. During this time, she expressed her milk and later resumed full breastfeeding. The child had "fever blisters" every three or four months for some time after this episode, and the mother developed more breast lesions a few months after the first infection, which she again treated successfully with Zovirax. For more discussion on herpesvirus, see Chapter 7.

Candidiasis (Thrush)

When a mother has persistent sore nipples, candidiasis is likely. It is caused by a yeast, *Candida albicans* (also called *Monilia* or thrush) when it occurs orally. *Candida* thrive in the warm moist areas of the infant's mouth and on the mother's nipples. The infant's mouth can become infected during vaginal birth and can then infect the mother's breast and nipple during breastfeeding (Hancock & Spangler, 1993). Candidiasis should be suspected if the mother has been breastfeeding without discomfort and then rapidly develops extremely sore nipples, burning or itching, and, possibly, shooting pain deep in the breast.

Although *Candida* is a naturally occurring yeast that lives in the mucous membranes of the gastrointestinal and genitourinary tract and on the skin, the use of antibiotics promotes overgrowth (candidiasis); consequently, infants and women who have received antibiotic therapy are more susceptible to candidiasis (Amir, 1991). Mothers with vaginal candidiasis and nipple trauma are also predisposed to candidiasis of the breast (Tanguay, McBean, & Jain, 1994). In checking for candidiasis, inspect the woman's breasts for inflammation of the nipples and areola. The inflammation is usually a striking deep pink, sometimes with tiny blisters (see Color Plate 8). The mother will complain of severe tenderness and discomfort, especially during and immediately after feedings.

The baby may have a diaper rash, with raised, red, sore-looking pustules or red, scalded-looking buttocks. Also examine the child's mouth carefully for white patches surrounded by diffuse redness. The absence of symptoms in the child's mouth, however, does not rule out thrush, because the infant may be asymptomatic. On the other hand, thrush symptoms in the baby (temperament

BOX 15–2

Interventions for Breast Skin Rashes and Infections

- Discontinue irritant.
- Take frequent showers.
- Wear all-cotton bras.
- Expose breasts to sunlight (15 minutes) and to air.
- Apply hydrocortisone cream (available over the counter) on the affected area

twice a day. Remove cream with clean cotton swab if used on nipple-areola.
- Rinse nipple-areola area with warm water after each feeding. Pat dry, then air dry with blow-dryer on the low setting.

---

change, frequent suckling) can go unnoticed or can be attributed to something else. Moreover, treatment may be needed even in the absence of positive cultures in the mother and the infant (Jennison, 1977). Whenever any woman has recurrent yeast infections, her sexual partner should be considered a potential reservoir of infection. Pacifiers and bottle nipples are another source of recurrent thrush infection; they may harbor persistent oral *Candida* colonization (Manning et al., 1985) and should be replaced or boiled after each exposure in the infant's mouth.

Candidiasis is a "family" disease; it spreads quickly among family members, especially with intimate contact involving warm, moist areas of the body, as is the case with breastfeeding and with sexual contact. Candidiasis that develops during breastfeeding can persist and recur unless all areas of possible infection in the baby, mother, and her sex partner are treated promptly and aggressively. The infant's mouth and anal area and the mother's breasts (nipples and areola) and vagina are prime sites for *Candida* infection; all should be treated simultaneously. Treatment for the infant includes placing an antifungal medication in the infant's mouth with a medicine dropper after feedings and swabbing it over the mucosa, gums, and tongue. This treatment should be continued for two weeks.

The mother must apply an antifungal topical cream or lotion to her nipples and breast before

and after each feeding and to the infant's entire diaper area if there is any redness. The mother may also have vaginal yeast infection and should simultaneously use an antifungal intravaginal preparation. Clotrimazole (Gyne-Lotrimin) is an over-the-counter drug in the United States and is available as a vaginal suppository or as a cream. Other recommendations for the mother to use on a case-by-case basis include:

- Expose the nipples directly to the sun for a few minutes twice a day.

- Dry the external genitalia with a blow-dryer on a warm setting.

- Wear 100 percent cotton underpants and bras that can be boiled in plain water for 5 to 10 minutes to kill spores.

- Avoid baths with other members of the family.

- Use condoms during coitus (because cross-infection with a sexual partner is possible).

Nystatin is the most commonly used medication for candidiasis. Nystatin oral suspension should be painted on the baby's oral mucosa and tongue with a large cotton swab after every breastfeeding (see Color Plate 25). In the case of persistent candidiasis, treatment calls for painting ketoconazole suspension on the breast twice a day for five days, followed by prolonged nystatin application.

If the mother has allergies, the health care provider must be aware that Seldane (terfenadine) should *not* be taken in conjunction with antifungal drugs ketoconazole or itraconazole or the antibiotic erythromycin (see Chapter 6). Mixing these drugs can be life-threatening.

For a listing of recommended dosages for commonly used antifungal medications, see Table 15–2. After taking an antifungal medication, mothers need encouragement and follow-up; they may not get immediate relief from pain, because nystatin may not bring instant relief. In fact, after starting treatment the pain may become worse before it begins to fade.

In the case of chronic candidiasis, a restricted diet and prolonged oral nystatin use is an option. A midwife (Clay et al., 1990) suggested a regimen for the mother that combines a strict yeast-free diet with oral nystatin:

- Nystatin (oral), 2 million units three times daily for four weeks, then 1 million units three times daily for the next four weeks, followed by 500,000 units three times daily for four weeks

- Restriction of all alcohol, cheese, bread, wheat products, sugar, honey, and condiments

- Acidophilus (40 million–1 billion viable units, approximately one tablet) daily

If nystatin does not clear the fungal infection, other antifungal medications, such as miconazole (Monistat), clotrimazole (Gyne-Lotrimin), naftifine (Naftin), or oxiconazole (Oxistat), should be tried. Johnstone and Marcinak (1990) reported a case in which nystatin oral suspension was applied to the infant's mouth lesions with a clean cotton swab four times daily for two weeks, and to the mother's nipples immediately after feedings. This treatment was ineffective. The mother then applied clotrimazole gel to her nipples and to the baby's oral lesions every three hours. After five applications, both mother and baby were symptom free. For vaginal candidiasis, a single 150-mg dose of fluconazole is recommended. For early cases, suggest that the mother try warm vinegar soaks (one part vinegar, four parts water) followed by air-drying and an antifungal preparation.

Gentian violet is an old-fashioned antifungal drug that is enjoying a comeback because it works well, is inexpensive, and does not require a prescription. One drawback is that gentian violet stains anything with which it comes into contact, although rubbing with alcohol helps to remove the dye. In advising a mother who is using it, suggest that she keep her sense of humor and wear clothing she can throw away. She should apply the gentian violet (0.25% or 0.5% solution), using clean cotton swabs, in the baby's mouth and diaper area and on her nipples after feedings. When the purple disappears (after about two days in a baby's mouth and daily on his diaper area), it should be reapplied only once or twice. Gentian violet treatment is controversial, because prolonged use of gentian violet can cause irritation and ulceration of the infant's oral mucous membrane (Utter, 1990). One to two days after the gentian violet is applied, the epidermis on both the baby's diaper area and the mother's breasts may peel and become red. A & D ointment may then be applied to any red areas covered by the diaper that are not thrush-related.

Anything that comes into contact with the baby's mouth (pacifiers, rubber nipples, teethers, or toys) or the mother's breasts (breast-pump parts, bras, reusable breast pads) should be washed and boiled daily, because the spores are heat-resistant. Disposable breast pads should be thrown away after each feeding (Danforth, 1990). The expressed milk of a mother with candidiasis should not be saved and frozen, because freezing deactivates yeast but does not kill it.

In one case of candidal infection of the breast (see Color Plate 8), the infant remained symptom-free for the entire four-month period, whereas the mother had repeated episodes of candidiasis. Because her baby's pediatrician would not prescribe treatment for the baby in the absence of a positive culture in his mouth, the mother limited treatment to her nipples. Within four days after resolving the painful blistering and redness, she experienced a new flare-up. After four such episodes in four months, she sought a second opinion and obtained medication for both her infant and herself; after five days of treatments after *every* suckling episode, she was symptom-free and remained so.

When candidiasis infection is severe, it can involve the lower ducts and sinuses of the breast in addition to the outer skin of the nipples and breast.

Table 15–2

Selected Antifungal Preparations

Drug Name	Preparations	Usual Dosage
Clotrimazole (Lotrimin, Mycelex)	Creams, solutions, vaginal cream, and vaginal tablets	Skin cream: apply twice daily vaginal cream or tablet: 100 mg/day for 7 days or 200 mg/day for 3 days
Gentian violet	Adults and children: 0.5%, 1% solution	Topical: infant: two to three times over several days. Use dilute 0.5% solution. Do not repeat.
Fluconazole (Diflucan)		Safe. Cleared for pediatric use.
Itraconazole (Sproranox)		Cleared for adult use only.
Ketoconazole (Nizoral)	Oral tablets	Oral: for adults: 200–400 mg/day, given in single dose; for children weighing less than 20 kg, 50 mg/day; for children weighing 20–40 kg, 100 mg/day
Miconazole (Monistat)	Creams, lotions, vaginal cream, and vaginal suppositories	Skin cream or lotion: apply three to four times per day Vaginal cream or suppository: 100 mg/day for 7 days
Nystatin (Mycostatin)	Suspensions, cream, powders, ointment, and vaginal suppositories	Oral: for adults: 1,500,000–2,400,000 units/day divided into three to four doses; for infants: 400,000–800,000 units/day, divided into three to four doses Topical: 1 million units applied two times per day Duration of therapy: at least two days after symptoms disappear Vaginal: 1–2 million units/day

When the ducts are infected, the mother is very likely to feel a burning sensation deep in the breast, which is distinct from the burning sensation of the breast skin itself. Often the inner burning persists several minutes after the baby has come off the breast. When the mother is treated with oral antifungal medication, the pain subsides (Johnstone & Marcinak, 1990). The more severe the candidiasis infection, the longer it takes for the treatment to work and for the pain to disappear.

Breast Pain

Breast pain that may derive from any number of sources can be both disconcerting and discouraging. In some cases, pressure on the brachial plexus can result in shooting pain in the breast. Identifying the cause of this pressure (e.g., a badly fitting bra or baby-carrier straps that are pulled too tightly across the mother's back) is a key to alleviating such pain (Simkin, 1988).

Women have reported feeling shooting pain that coincided with powerful ejection of milk. Such episodes are most likely to occur in the first month of the breastfeeding course. When the milk-ejection reflex subsides, the pain often subsides as well. This temporary pain tends to occur more often in primiparous women; often the same mothers who have experienced it with a first breastfeeding baby do not experience a recurrence with later infants. This pain may reflect distention of the milk ducts, which is more obvious in the early first breastfeeding course than at later periods.

In cases in which the mother reports very intense pain coincidental with a vigorous milk-ejection response, the caregiver should encourage the mother to gently massage her breasts before putting the baby to breast to enhance the likelihood of some initial leaking of milk before the baby's active suckling stimulates milk ejection. When the milk begins to drip freely, sprays, and then subsides, subsequent suckling is less likely to result in such intense discomfort. By the end of the first month, such pain is usually no longer present when the milk-ejection reflex is activated.

Two recent studies examined psychosocial variables surrounding breastfeeding nipple pain. Amir et al. (1996) studied the distress and depression levels of mothers when they were experiencing nipple pain. They found that these women were highly anxious and distressed. However, once the pain resolved, their distress also resolved. Heads & Higgins (1995) looked at nipple trauma in relation to nipple pain between three and five days postpartum. Visible evidence of nipple damage and nipple trauma was observed in 38 (55 percent) of the 69 women in the study. Damage occurred most commonly in the form of minor grazes (61 percent) or blisters (23 percent). Although the authors found a positive relationship between nipple damage and the level of reported pain, women who had a greater desire to breastfeed had less continuing pain that was unrelated to the amount of nipple trauma. It appears that women who have a strong personal commitment to breastfeed their baby report less nipple pain than do those who are not so strongly committed.

Vasospasm

In breast vasospasm, the nipple appears blanched after the feeding, sometimes turning blue or red before returning to its normal color. The mother feels extreme pain during the "spasm." This cluster of symptoms is often referred to as *Raynaud's of the nipple*. Raynaud's phenomenon (an intermittent ischemia usually affecting fingers or toes) is more prevalent in women.

In a report of five women with this problem, Lawlor-Smith and Lawlor-Smith (1997) described blanching of the nipple not only during and immediately after feedings but also between feedings. Exposure to cold precipitated nipple blanching and pain in all of the women. Two mothers showed the classic triphasic color change of Raynaud's phenomenon (white, blue, and red) in their nipples, and three showed biphasic color change (white and blue). Two of the women gave a history of Raynaud's phenomenon before their first pregnancy, affecting not only their fingers and toes but also their nipples. Two gave a family history of Raynaud's phenomenon affecting a parent. Four of the five reported nipple trauma. None of the women smoked.

Some maternal medications, such as fluconazole and oral contraceptives, may be associated with vasospasm (Escott, 1994). Ibuprofen and warmth applied to the breasts, either by a warm shower or by covering the breasts with a heating pad, help to alleviate discomfort. Topical nitroglycerine and low doses of nifedipine (5 mg three times per day for one week) have been reported as effective for treating vasospasm (Gross Shirley._Vasospasm_{Online from LACTNET}, 4 October 1995). Nifedipine is a calcium channel blocker used to treat hypertension; its transfer through breastmilk to the baby is not significant (Penny & Lewis, 1989). Dietary supplementation of calcium (2,000 mg/day) and magnesium (1,000 mg/day) for mothers experiencing nipple vasospasm while breastfeeding an older baby has also been advised.

Milk Blister

Infrequently, a milk blister, a whitish, tender area, develops on the upper areola. This blister is thought to be caused by nipple-pore milk that has been sealed over by the epidermis and has triggered an inflammatory response. This obstruction then prevents the duct system from draining, so milk buildup behind the occlusion causes symptoms of a blocked duct (Noble, 1991). The spot may be white or yellow, depending on how long it has been present. The skin on and around the area may be reddened. See Color Plate 7.

Persistent and very painful during feeding, it can remain for several days or weeks and then spontaneously heal by a peeling away of the epithelium over the affected area. An effective treatment is to break the epithelial tissue using a sterile needle, sometimes along with a sterile tweezers and small sharp scissors to entirely remove the excess skin. Aspiration may be necessary to draw out the fluid. According to Noble (1991), in some cases complete removal of this overgrowth is needed to prevent recurrence. A less invasive treatment is rubbing the area with a damp cloth after softening the skin by immersion in warm water. With ice packs, an analgesic to relieve discomfort, and a topical antibiotic, breastfeeding can continue, and healing is rapid.

In addition to the larger blister, tiny blisters that appear to have a whitish fluid, possibly milk, within may appear on nipples. These blisters are sore and painful. Vitamin E ointment (applied sparingly and wiped off before feedings) and weaning breast shells (to relieve the pressure from clothing on the nipples) relieve discomfort and possibly aid healing.

Mammoplasty

Breast augmentation and reduction are increasingly common surgical procedures. Since 1960, 2 million women have received breast implants; during 1988 alone, 70,000 breast augmentations were performed in the United States. Although augmentation is performed for cosmetic effect, reduction of very large breasts is often performed to reduce discomfort from neck and back pain.

Sooner or later, the clinician will see a client who has had breast augmentation or reduction and who wants to know whether she will be able to breastfeed her baby. The ability to breastfeed after these surgeries depends on the type of surgery, the specific technique used, whether neural pathways were severed, and the amount of breast tissue removed. Generally speaking, full breastfeeding is possible with augmentation surgery but usually not after reduction surgery, unless feedings are supplemented; however, exceptions occur in both instances with any breast surgery. An explanation of the differences in the operative procedures is crucial to understanding the subsequent effect on lactation.

Breast Reduction

The ability to breastfeed after breast reduction depends on whether the surgeon deliberately tries to leave nerve pathways and blood supply intact or whether tissue is removed without regard for these structures (Soderstrom, 1993). Women with the least amount of glandular tissue removed have a greater opportunity to lactate (Marshall, Callan, & Nicholson, 1994), particularly if the fourth intercostal nerve that branches to the breast and areola is left intact (see Chapter 4).

The two techniques used for breast reduction are the *pedicle* technique and the *free-nipple* technique. With the pedicle technique, the nipple and areola remain attached to the breast gland on a pedicle, and the tissue is "reduced." A wedge is removed from the sides of the underside of the breast (Fig. 15–1). Because the breast, its ducts, its blood supply, and some nerves remain intact, breastfeeding has been possible after this operation.

The free-nipple technique (autotransplantation of the nipple) involves removing the nipple-areola entirely from the breast and preserving it in saline (much like a graft) while the additional breast tissue (usually fatty tissue) is removed. Then the nipple-areola is stitched back in place. This technique is used for women with extremely large breasts and is designed to reduce risks and complications and to position the nipple approximately on the substantially resculpted breast. Full breastfeeding may be possible with the pedicle technique, but it is rarely possible with the free-nipple technique, because the blood supply of the nipple-areola is completely severed (Barnett, 1990), and damage to the nerves occurs. Breast scars after a reduction are depicted in Color Plate 22. Several cases of spontaneous galactorrhea after reduction mammaplasty are reported in the literature; all of these women had not breastfed for several months before the surgery (Menendez-Graino et al., 1990; Song & Hunter, 1989).

Mastopexy

Mastopexy is a "breastlift" in which sagging breasts are lifted and made firmer (Fig. 15–2). The operation involves removing excess skin and breast tissue and elevating the nipple. It may be done either in the hospital or in the physician's office. Although there may be a very slight loss of sensation in the nipple or areola, the operation should not affect the ability to breastfeed (Love, 1990).

Augmentation

Because augmentation surgery is most often performed on women during their childbearing years, lactation consultants are likely to be asked about it by their clients (Fig. 15–3). Four techniques are used to enlarge the breasts:

- The *infrasubmammary* procedure calls for an incision to be made under the breast and for the implant to be placed under the breast tissue. One disadvantage is that the scar is very visible and is easily irritated by a bra.
- In the *periareolar* technique, an incision is made around the areola-nipple. Although the scar is less visible than in the inframammary procedure, there is often a loss of sensation.

- The *transareolar* technique involves an incision made across the areola-nipple area. This technique is preferred by Asian women, because they are less likely to have severe scarring. Barnett (1990) describes this technique as "unphysiological" and advises against its use. Full lactation is almost always impossible after this procedure, because the glandular tissue, nerve, and blood supply are extensively disrupted. This should be made clear to any woman who contemplates having this procedure.
- An *axillary* enlargement is effected by making an incision underneath the arm and placing the implant below the gland. Although there are few scars and no interference with breast tissue and lactation, this type of implantation makes breast cancer harder to detect, and there is a possibility of contractures. If the implant is placed below the muscle, it interferes less with mammograms (Fig. 15–4).

Hughes and Owen (1993) interviewed 51 women who had reduction or augmentation. Of the 23 women who underwent reduction, only 30 percent were "successful" in that they breastfed for as long as they wished. Most had difficulty establishing breastfeeding, especially those who had the nipple and areola removed and replaced, thereby severing all ducts. Of the 26 women with augmentation surgery, 62 percent were successful. Augmentation had little impact on initial success with breastfeeding. Women who received implants feared that the silicone would leach into the breastmilk and that they themselves might be at increased risk for breast cancer.

The concern that silicone may "bleed" into body tissues or into breastmilk, affect the immune system, and cause toxic reactions in the mother and infant has generated heated debate. In 1994, Levine and Ilowite published a study on a small sample of children with chronic gastrointestinal disorders who were born to women with silicone breast implants. Eight of the children had been breastfed. Six of these children were found to have reduced esophageal motility thought to be due to silicone leakage. Despite the lack of clinical evidence, the authors initially suggested that the motility disorder might be due to scleroderma. The study set off a blitz of media and public discussion

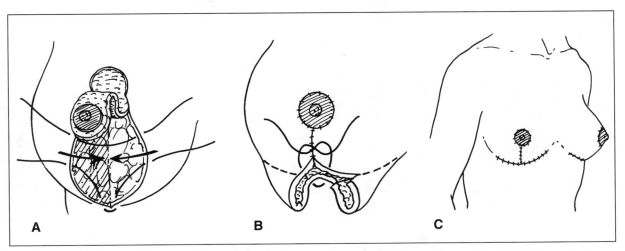

FIGURE 15–1. Breast reduction. *A. Wedge of breast tissue removed, areola pulled up, gap closed. B. Excess tissue removed, skin closed with stitches. C. Postoperative appearance.*

about the safety of silicone implants. Later work resulted in the opposite conclusion (Levine et al., 1996). Case studies describing connective tissue disorders in women with silicone implants continue to be published, some of which found no relationship between the implants and the likelihood of subsequent scleroderma in the women or their offspring (Englert & Brooks, 1994). Most breast implants now are filled with saline water. Silicone implants are available only through enrollment in controlled clinical studies.

A major problem in discerning the effect of silicone is that virtually all people have some silicone in their bodies (Berlin, 1994). Silicone is a major ingredient in such drugs as Di-Gel and is added to processed foods, hand lotion, hair spray, over-the-counter drug preparations, including those given to babies and young children, and other common products—even beer! Measurement of silicone in breastmilk is difficult and may be misleading because of its ubiquitous presence in the environment. Dow Corning assayed silicone in breastmilk, a laborious test that took 10 days to complete, and found that the amount of silicone in the milk of women with implants was not statistically different from that in control samples (Bejarnot & Simmer, 1991). Moreover, the testing requires 10 days and can lead to unnecessary weaning. One breastfeeding mother in Wichita had her milk "tested" for silicone and insisted on weaning her baby when she was told it

was above normal levels. Based on the weaknesses of the Levine and Ilowite study (1994) and other evidence, La Leche League International (Mohrbacher & Stock, 1997) and others (Epstein, 1994) suggested that the benefits of breastfeeding even with silicone breast implants outweigh the risks.

Both Neifert et al. (1990) and Hurst (1996) found that women who had periareolar and transareolar incision experienced greater incidence of lactation insufficiency. Neifert et al. (1990) studied 319 primiparous women who were breastfeeding healthy, full-term infants. Women who had previous breast surgery had a greater than three-fold risk of lactation insufficiency as compared with women who had not had surgery. The mothers with periareolar incisions were more than four times as likely to have insufficient milk than were those with no breast surgery. Women with breast incisions in other locations had no statistically significant increase in risk compared with those who never had breast surgery. Hurst's findings were similar. Of those women among the 42 she followed who had augmentation surgery, 64 percent had insufficient lactation. Of the women who had periaureolar surgery, none lactated sufficiently, compared with 50 percent who made sufficient milk if they had submaxillary or axillary augmentation (Hurst, 1996).

Why do some women with the "right" type of incision for augmentation still have difficulty lac-

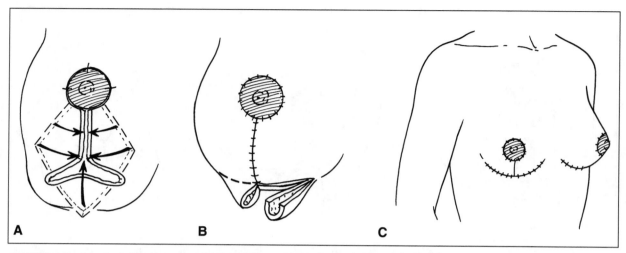

FIGURE 15–2. Breast "lift" or mastopexy *A. Skin edges pulled together. B. Excess tissue removed. C. Postoperative appearance*

tating? In addition to the type of incision, the pressure of the implant must also be considered. Although postpartum breast engorgement occurs despite ductal damage, milk transfer and milk production continue only in part of the breast. Lobes that cannot empty because of severed ducts quickly undergo cellular-wall involution caused by intramammary pressure atrophy, suggesting that increased pressure, when prolonged and unrelieved, can cause an atropy of the alveolar cellular wall and diminished milk production (Hurst, 1996; Neifert, 1992).

Breast Lumps and Surgery

What happens if a breastfeeding mother develops a lump or nodule in her breast? Warnings by the American Cancer Society have made American women keenly aware of breast lumps, and the woman discovering one is usually anxious and perhaps frightened. However, a breast lump in a lactating woman is most often a galactocele, a milk-filled lacteal cyst caused by plugged milk in the ducts (Stevens et al., 1997). A galactocele is usually tender and will atrophy rather rapidly and disappear in a matter of days.

If the lump does not resolve or reduce in size, the lactation consultant should refer the mother to a physician or surgeon for an examination. If the lump appears to be a cystic mass, a needle aspira-tion will determine whether it is fluid-filled. To aspirate a cyst, the physician first cleans and anesthetizes the skin, immobilizes the mass with his or her hand, and inserts a 20- to 22-gauge needle to draw out fluid. This procedure collapses the cyst and solves the problem. Cysts are almost never malignant. If a biopsy is necessary, one of four methods may be used (Love, 1990):

- A fine-needle biopsy, which draws out a few cells;
- A larger-needle ("tru-cut") biopsy, which cuts out a small piece of tissue without an incision;
- An incisional biopsy, which takes a much larger piece of tissue; or
- An excisional biopsy, in which an entire lump is removed.

A breast mass discovered by palpation can be evaluated further, usually by biopsy or ultrasonography, to determine whether it is fluid-filled (cystic or benign) or solid (possibly malignant). Because of the tissue density of the lactating breast, mammography is often inconclusive and not the preferred procedure. Most diagnostic procedures are performed on an outpatient basis either in a freestanding ambulatory clinic or in a minor operating room. Magnetic resonance imagery (MRI) and needle-core biopsy are newer techniques for evaluating breast lesions. Using the lowest dosage possible of local anesthetic minimizes the amount of anesthetic the infant might ingest with the next breastfeeding. When the mother resumes breastfeedings depends on her comfort level and the type of procedure used, but she certainly should be able to resume within 12 hours. Although the area will be tender, resuming feedings needs to be weighed against the discomfort of engorgement and listening to the cries of an unhappy child. If breastfeeding is not resumed within 12 hours, the mother should pump her breasts to relieve the intermammary pressure. Too much milk pressure and stasis could lead to undue stress on the surgical site and infection.

Day (1986) described a case in which a woman underwent biopsy of her right breast after suspicious calcifications were found by xeromammography. Biopsy was accomplished with a wedge-shaped resection at the nine o'clock position through a circumareolar skin incision with excellent cosmetic result. The pathology report indicated a benign "fibrocystic" condition. After the delivery of her next baby, the woman's breasts became engorged symmetrically. By the fourth postpartum day, she noted that her right breast remained engorged after breastfeeding, although her left breast seemed relieved of its milk supply. The client subsequently used warm packs and oxytocin nasal spray, starting feedings on the right side only, and using an electric breast pump in efforts to build up her milk supply in the treated breast. At no time was more than 2 ml of milk obtained from the right breast using the electric pump, although the mother had previously breastfed her first child on both breasts. Day (1986) suggested that the surgeon must weigh the cosmetic considerations of breast surgery against the need for an adequate biopsy and the threat to future milk ejection.

Galactoceles

Galactoceles—milk-filled cysts in the lactating breast—are uncommon. The etiology of galactoceles is not known, but they cause multiple breastfeeding problems. Bevin (1993) described a case in which a mother had a palpable chronic galactocele behind the left areola for 10 years, during which time she breastfed several children. The left breast was the site of many plugged ducts, breast infections (some requiring antibiotics), and a breast

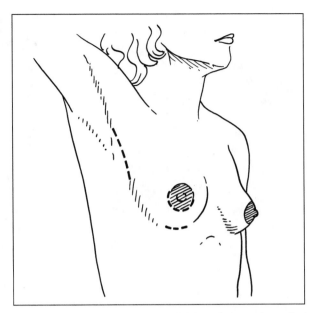

FIGURE 15–3. Breast augmentation. *Incision is made through the armpit, underneath the breast, or under the areola.*

abscess. At various stages, 10 to 20 ml of milky fluid was aspirated, but the lump refilled quickly. No single treatment was helpful. However, on one occasion, antibiotic treatment caused the galactocele to disappear temporarily. Optimal management of a galactocele has yet to be determined.

Fibrocystic Disease

Fibrocystic breast disease (benign breast disorder) is a general term that describes a number of benign breast conditions. It should not be assumed that fibrocystic disease actually refers only to a disorder in those breasts with cysts or nodules; the term is also used to include evidence of hyperplasia, metaplasia, and atypia, among other conditions (Brucker, 1991). The American Cancer Society recommends that clinicians use the term *fibrocystic changes;* nevertheless, the diagnosis of fibrocystic disease is commonly used because it guarantees reimbursement by health care insurers.

About half of all women of childbearing age will develop one of these conditions at some point. Years of menstrual cycling will eventually produce dense or fibrous breast tissue. Women usually develop cysts in their thirties. Because of its

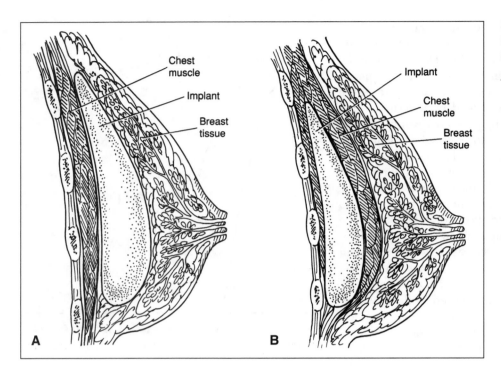

**FIGURE 15–4.
Location of breast
implant.** *A. Implant
placed between
breast and muscles.
B. Implant placed
under muscles.*

occurrence rate, the condition is sometimes referred to as a *nondisease*.

From 50 to 75 percent of all breast biopsies are done because of clinical diagnoses of fibrocystic disease (Norwood, 1989). About one-fourth of women with fibrocystic disease develop gross evidence of a cyst or a fibroadenoma, a smooth, round lump that moves around easily when palpated. Fibroadenomas can vary from the size of a pea to the size of a lemon. A needle aspiration helps to confirm the diagnosis. If no fluid can be aspirated, a fibroadenoma is likely. Tissue is sent to the laboratory to confirm the diagnosis. Fibroadenomas are harmless in themselves and, if the woman is lactating, most surgeons choose to delay surgery at least until lactation ceases and the child is completely weaned. In middle-aged or older women, fibroadenomas are usually removed at the time they are diagnosed. A mother with persistent benign breast disease is commonly advised to reduce or eliminate caffeine (coffee, tea, cola, chocolate) and to take vitamin E supplements.

Bleeding from the Breast

Red-tinged, pink, or rusty breastmilk is relatively rare, but it does occur and causes concern, because it signals the presence of blood. There are several possible antecedent factors that lead to bleeding in the milk ducts. For example, one mother with severely retracted nipples had painless bleeding from her breasts after wearing breast shells late in pregnancy. After she reduced the wearing time of the shells, the bleeding ceased.

In other cases, the etiology of the bleeding is not so clear. Marmet (1990) has worked with several mothers whose milk appears brown or rusty-looking, like rusty water emitted from pipes that haven't been used for a long while. Hence, she calls it the *rusty-pipe syndrome*. This syndrome appears to occur more often in primiparous mothers during the early stages of lactogenesis and is not associated with any discomfort. O'Callaghan (1981) reported 37 cases of this syndrome in the Australian women they followed. Most of these women reported that their breast discharge was either red or brown. Its earliest appearance was during the fourth month of pregnancy and was associated with antenatal breast expression in a little over half of the mothers. Dairy farmers report similar rusty milk from cows calving for the first time and suggest that the reason is slight internal bleeding from edema during the cow's first engorgement.

Bright-red bleeding from the breast in the absence of nipple soreness or cracking indicates that the mother should be assessed for the possibility of an intraductal papilloma. This is a small, benign, wartlike growth on the lining of the duct that bleeds as it erodes. Usually no mass or tumor is palpable, and there may or may not be moderate pain and discomfort. Often the bleeding stops spontaneously without any treatment, but if bleeding continues, the woman should be medically evaluated. The physician will probably remove it surgically to confirm that it is an intraductal papilloma and not something more serious. In any case, the lactation consultant can reassure the mother that the infant is not harmed by the intake of small amounts of serosanguinous discharge.

Breast Cancer

Breast cancer is the most common malignancy among women, affecting more than 175,000 individuals annually. About 25 percent of all women receiving diagnoses of breast cancer are premenopausal and potentially fertile. With the increasing incidence of breast cancer, greater use of breast-conserving therapy, and the trend toward pregnancy later in life, we can expect an increase in the number of women who become pregnant and lactate.

Only 2 to 3 percent of breast cancer overall is diagnosed during pregnancy or lactation (Hoover, 1990). However remote, a tumor or nodule may be malignant during this time. Breastfeeding does *not* prevent breast cancer, although many studies conclude that it provides a protective function (Enger et al., 1997). For a woman who is at risk for breast cancer, prolonged breastfeeding may at least delay its occurrence before menopause. Studies on lactation and breast cancer may be divided into three categories: general protection, protection based on duration, and no protection.

Breastfeeding as Protection Against Breast Cancer. Ing et al. (1977) reported that women in fishing villages near Hong Kong customarily breastfeed only with the right breast. Among these women, they reported a fourfold, "highly significantly increased risk of cancer in the unsuckled breast" after menopause. Byers et al. (1985), in a study of premenopausal women in New York State,

identified a negative association between breastfeeding duration and risk of breast cancer. The protective effect of lactation held after Byers et al. controlled for such factors as age, parity, age at first pregnancy, age at menarche, and education. These authors concluded that a woman's risk of developing premenopausal breast cancer decreases steadily for every 12 months she breastfeeds (Byers, 1985).

McTiernan and Thomas (1986) conducted a case-control study of women in Washington State. Premenopausal women who had lactated had less than one-half the risk of developing breast cancer as compared with the control group. A dose response was noted, with the risk of breast cancer declining as the duration of breastfeeding increased; this was particularly strong among premenopausal women. The protective effect of breastfeeding persisted even after controlling for maternal age, parity, and age at first full-term pregnancy.

Both the length of time that the mother breastfeeds and her age when she first breastfeeds play a role in breast cancer. For premenopausal women, the longer the continuance of lactation, the lower the risk. This may be because ovulation is interrupted or pituitary and ovarian hormone secretions are favorably influenced, particularly if lactation occurs in early reproductive life. Katsouyanni et al. (1996) found a reduction of breast cancer among premenopausal women who had breastfed between 12 and 23 months. Layde et al. (1989) also found that the risk of breast cancer declined in inverse proportion to the duration of breastfeeding. In their analysis of the experiences of 4,599 women, the mother's age at first full-term pregnancy exerted the strongest influence on reducing the risk of breast cancer. Thereafter, the number of births (parity) and the duration of breastfeeding became important elements. Women whose breastfeeding career exceeded 25 months had the lowest risk for breast carcinoma. Likewise, Kvåle and Heuch (1987), Newcomb et al. (1994), Brinton (1995), and Yoo et al. (1992) found that among premenopausal women, lactation at early ages and for long periods was associated with a reduction in risk. A British study estimated that breastfeeding each baby for three months or longer gives the greatest protection (United Kingdom National Case-Control Study Group, 1993).

Romieu et al. (1996) found an inverse dose response not only for premenopausal but also postmenopausal women, possibly because they included in their study so many postmenopausal women who breastfed longer than twelve months.

Inability of Breastfeeding to Protect Against Breast Cancer.

Other studies show that breastfeeding and lactation neither prevent nor delay breast cancer. Siskind (1989) found that Australian women who had breastfed were only slightly less likely to develop breast cancer than were women who had not breastfed. The greatest protective effect occurred if the first child was breastfed. There were no differences in the risk ratio after breastfeeding between premenopausal women and postmenopausal women. Likewise, London et al. (1990) found no independent association between lactation and risk of cancer; however, only 6 percent of the women in the study had breastfed for at least 24 months. Ramon et al. (1996) carried out a case-control study in Spain. Although breast cancer was not significantly associated with lactation duration, the risk of breast cancer decreased with increasing number of births. Yang et al. (1997) found no relationship between breast cancer and duration of breastfeeding in women living in Taiwan. Finally, the authors of several recent case-control studies found no important overall association between breastfeeding and the occurrence of breast cancer (Michels et al., 1996; Negri et al., 1996; Stuver et al., 1997).

Patients with diagnosed breast cancer during pregnancy and lactation are largely in their thirties and forties and often have more advanced disease than do nonpregnant or lactating women (Lethaby et al., 1996; Tretli et al., 1988). They have had multiple pregnancies and relatively few deliveries, and usually there has been a long interval since a previous pregnancy or childbirth (Deemarsky & Semiglazov, 1987). Unlike women who are past menopause (Dunne, 1988), premenopausal women are more likely to have breast cancer that is not hormone dependent.

Most studies in the past 30 years have shown convincingly that poor prognosis of breast cancer found during pregnancy is attributable more to delay in diagnosis and reluctance to treat patients aggressively rather than to any detrimental effect of pregnancy or lactation itself (Donegan & Spratt, 1988; Hoover, 1990; Lethaby et al., 1996; Ribeiro & Palmer, 1977). The delay is due to denial by both the physician and the mother that it occurs in pregnant or lactating women; to breast tenderness; and to lobular hyperplasia, which hides a tumor and hinders its detection, giving it time to grow and spread. Lactating breasts are very dense (see Chapter 4), rendering mammography or sonography of little value in diagnosis.

An experienced lactation consultant, Petok (1995) described several cases of breast carcinoma seen in her consulting practice: lobular carcinoma, ductal carcinoma, and inflammatory breast cancer. Most of these women came for treatment of what they called a *plugged duct* and described a large lump in the breast that had persisted for one to two weeks. The lumps were 4 to 6 cm in diameter and were irregularly shaped. One mass felt like two firm lumps clustered together. The lumps did not change after feedings or after the usual treatments for a plugged duct (hot compresses, frequent feedings, breast massage, pumping, etc.). Only one woman reported feeling pain at the site of the lump. In one woman, slight redness showed on the side of the breast opposite the lump. The redness lasted only a few days and then disappeared, although the lump did not change. This woman later developed peau d'orange (dimples on the breast similar to those on an orange peel). All of the infants were breastfeeding and gaining weight. None of the infants rejected the cancerous breast, although one did show a preference for the noncancerous breast. After diagnosis of breast cancer, two of the three women weaned their infants before beginning chemotherapy. The third woman continued to breastfeed for four months, despite the objections of her physician, before initiating chemotherapy.

Petok (1995) recommends referring the mother to a physician for evaluation for

- any mass that shows no decrease in size after 72 hours of treatment,

- afebrile mastitislike symptoms that are unresolved after a course of antibiotics, or

- recurrent mastitis that appears at the same location.

The initial referral is usually to a primary physician, who then refers to a general surgeon. Hesitation to refer out of fear of causing unnecessary concern by mentioning referral to rule out a tumor in a breastfeeding mother is unwise. One of the authors included consideration of lactation-related experiences in a discussion of breast cancer. A participant in the audience then returned to her physician and insisted he look further for a cause of her unresolving recurrent plugged ducts. An intraductal carcinoma was diagnosed and chemotherapy was initiated, actions that may have saved the woman's life.

Approximately 7 percent of fertile women treated for mammary carcinoma subsequently become pregnant, usually within the first five years. Their survival rate is the same as for women who were never pregnant (Deemarsky & Semiglazov, 1987; Donegan & Spratt, 1988). Previously, it was widely taught that subsequent pregnancy and lactation aggravated the course of mammary cancer; however, outcome and survival rates are similar for both pregnant and nonpregnant women who are of similar age and disease stage at time of diagnosis (Cooper & Butterfield, 1970; Peters & Meaken, 1965). Inflammatory breast cancer can be mistaken for mastitis, because the symptoms of an inflamed, edematous breast are similar. Breast cancer is different from mastitis, because inflammatory carcinoma rarely produces fever, there is no palpable mass, and the symptoms do not respond to antibiotic treatment (Petok, 1995).

As long as the woman remains clinically free of cancer, there is no therapeutic benefit in interrupting the pregnancy. If advanced cancer is diagnosed in the first or second trimester, however, treatment often requires that the pregnancy be terminated, because chemotherapy or radiation or hormone therapy place the fetus at risk (Deemarsky & Semiglazov, 1987). Some women who have had a unilateral mastectomy breastfeed after a subsequent pregnancy. The mother should be encouraged to alter her baby's position frequently to provide optimal stimulation to all portions of the breast.

One of the myths about breastfeeding and cancer is that a baby can receive cancer-causing viral particles in human milk. This is not true; there is no increased incidence of breast cancer in breastfed daughters of women who have had breast cancer (Miller & Fraumenti, 1972; Morgan et al., 1974). In some cases (Goldsmith, 1974; Hadary et al., 1995; Saber, 1996), the infant may reject the breast without apparent reason. Although it is true that most of the time an infant rejects the breast for another reason, close surveillance and perhaps also a search for an occult breast carcinoma in the involved breast may enable earlier diagnosis and improved prognosis.

Pregnant women diagnosed with early breast cancer are treated medically, as are nonpregnant women. Hornstein, Skornick, and Rozin (1982) have outlined a protocol for breastfeeding after a diagnosis of breast cancer.

- If breast cancer is diagnosed toward the end of pregnancy, the woman will undergo immediate surgery. If chemotherapy follows, the mother should not breastfeed.

- If the diagnosis is made during lactation, breastfeeding should be immediately suppressed by medications other than estrogen. Other standard treatments for carcinoma are then begun.

- Following the diagnosis of breast cancer, subsequent pregnancies should be delayed until the period of greatest risk is over (three to five years). After this time, the mother may breastfeed.

Lactation following Breast Cancer. Women who have undergone treatment (surgery, radiation, chemotherapy) for breast cancer and have then become pregnant and delivered report common experiences (David, 1985; Green, 1989; Higgins & Haffty, 1994):

- Little or no enlargement of the treated breast during pregnancy

- Ability to lactate and breastfeed from the untreated breast but less likelihood of having a full milk supply from the treated breast and possible absence of lactation

- Possible difficulty with latch-on, because the nipple on the breast may not extend as completely as might be expected

- Less likelihood of an absence of lactation with a circumareolar incision; lactation from the treated breast is less likely to occur in centrally located lesions (Higgins & Haffty, 1994). The interval from the time of treatment to the time of delivery does not appear to affect adversely lactation from the treated breast.

There are a few anecdotal case reports in literature of women who lactated after breast-conservation surgery and postoperative radiation therapy. Green (1989) reported that a woman who received breast-radiation treatment for an infiltrating ductal carcinoma became pregnant 19 months after the irradiation treatment. After giving birth to a healthy infant, she began breastfeeding. The radiation-treated breast neither enlarged nor produced colostrum. Two days after the untreated breast began leaking milk, the treated breast also leaked milk; however, it never produced the same volume of milk as did the untreated breast, even though the baby suckled from both breasts. Approximately four weeks after lactation began, it ceased in the treated breast; however, lactation continued on the untreated side. Vaison and Yahalom (1991) reported a similar finding.

David (1985) also reported the lactation experience of a woman with a history of fibrocystic disease who was treated with radiation therapy for a small mass in the right breast. One year after completion of the radiation therapy, she gave birth to a healthy infant who suckled well from both breasts. The right breast enlarged during pregnancy but not as much as did the left breast. Following the baby's birth, this mother experienced near-normal lactation from the treated breast.

How does radiation therapy affect lactation? A 30-year-old woman received a dose of between 42 and 45 Gy in 20 fractions, followed by a single iridium implant of an additional 20 Gy. Three years later, the mother successfully lactated from both breasts (Rodger, Corbett, & Chetty, 1989). In a survey of radiologists who treated pregnant women with breast cancer, of 53 patients who became pregnant and delivered after radiation, 18 (34 percent) were able to lactate. Although all 18 patients were able to exhibit some level of lactation, only 13 women chose to breastfeed. Of the five who did not breastfeed, three reported insufficient milk as a reason. Of the 18, 5 described their treated breast as smaller (Tralins, 1995).

Women receiving chemotherapy for breast cancer or for any other cancer should not breastfeed. All chemotherapeutic drugs cross into the milk. Although the levels are low in milk, these compounds are potent antimetabolites, and they are potentially toxic to the infant.

Clinical Implications
Mastitis

A mother with mastitis feels ill, and often she is discouraged. She asks, "Why does this have to happen to me?" and she may contemplate weaning. In addition, her supply of milk in the affected breast may be diminished for several weeks following the infection. She needs mothering herself, a role that the lactation consultant can assume as she reassures the mother that the infection will resolve and that to stop breastfeeding will only increase the risk of infection or recurrence. Tender loving care goes a long way in helping her through this difficult time. She also needs specific advice and a plan for care (Table 15–3) as well as a long-term plan for self-care. A considerable number of mothers develop mastitis more than once during the course of lactation (Riordan & Nichols, 1990). Therefore, certain women may be prone to the condition, and prevention is important. Review with the mother all the possible factors that preceded and may have contributed to her bout(s) of mastitis. Then encourage the mother to seek medical help early if symptoms recur. Some mothers, especially if they are experienced long-term breastfeeders, do not consult their physicians, even though their mastitis warrants medical attention.

Fatigue and Stress. Mothers rate stress and fatigue as major factors leading to mastitis. The effect of stress on the individual's immune defense system has been substantiated. Recounting events leading up to mastitis, a mother explained, "My husband took a new job which meant moving out of state. I also was planning a christening party in order to fit it in before moving away. Everything happened very rapidly, and my baby was only two weeks old."

Typically, mothers who develop mastitis are stressed from overwork or lack of sleep; they

Table 15–3

Mastitis Teaching Plan

Content-Goal	Teaching
Prevention	
To reduce stress and fatigue related to childbearing responsibilities	
Management of work	Prioritize tasks from most important to least important. Encourage other family members to assist in routine household tasks. Delay return to job as long as possible.
Management of socializing	Hold one informal open house for all friends and relatives to see new baby. Use voice machine to filter calls. Turn down social invitations.
Adequate rest and sleep	Take day naps when infant sleeps.
Avoid plugged ducts	Breastfeed often (at least 8–12 times per day). Massage any reddened area of breast, especially while breastfeeding.
Avoid change in number of feedings	Pump or express milk if a feeding is skipped.
Engorgement/stasis	Pump or express milk if breasts become overfull or distended. Wear bras without support underwires.
Care If Mastitis Occurs	
To prevent breast abscess and hasten recovery	
Self-care and relief of discomfort	Recognize early signs and symptoms: redness, fatigue, fever, chills. Rest with infant and fluids at bedside. Continue frequent breastfeedings.
Medical care	Monitor oral temperature. Place moist, warm packs at place of infection and over nipple. Expect slightly reduced milk supply in affected breast postinfection Take antibiotics if needed (may not be necessary if fever is already subsiding). Take antipyretic to reduce fever.

describe themselves as exhausted as a result of circumstances above and beyond the normal stresses of taking care of the infant. A mother wrote, "I was doing too much—just starting to get out with my first baby and trying to get ready for our first Christmas."

Plugged Duct. As discussed, some women repeatedly develop plugged ducts, some of which lead to a full-blown infection. It is not uncommon to be able to see this plug as a white "head" and to feel pressure and tenderness around the plug. Gentle massage above the area of tenderness may help while the baby is breastfeeding from that breast, particularly if the plug is newly formed.

Decrease in Number of Feedings. A sudden reduction in the number of feedings may lead to breast distention. If the number of feedings is reduced for any reason, milk collects in the ducts, and stasis may occur. One mother reported, "We were on vacation 1,000 miles from home. After driving for two days and exclusively breastfeeding, we arrived at our destination, and the feedings were cut back quite a bit. The infection started a few days after this."

Engorgement and Stasis. A decrease in the frequency of feedings presents the potential for engorgement or milk stasis. In one case, a mother whose infant was sleeping 10 hours at night was plagued with repeated mastitis. When she awakened in the morning, her breasts were always hard and sore. As soon as she began waking up her baby for a night feeding, she had no more such problems.

Sore and Cracked Nipple. A breakdown in the epidermis provides an avenue of entry into the breast tissue, although breakdown is not a prerequisite for a breast infection. Mastitis from sore, cracked nipples usually occurs in the first few weeks postpartum.

Other Factors. Other conditions, such as breast trauma, poor maternal nutrition, and vigorous exercise (particularly of the upper arms and chest) have been mentioned anecdotally as factors leading up to mastitis. These also should be noted in the assessment and history in the event that they predispose the mother to mastitis.

Breast Surgery and Abscess

With abscess drainage, lump removal, or biopsy, there is usually no reason the mother should stop breastfeeding. Even when a breast abscess is surgically drained, the mother can breastfeed on the unaffected side and possibly on the affected side, if the incision is far enough from the nipple so that the baby's mouth does not touch it when he breastfeeds (Mohrbacher & Stock, 1997). After a biopsy, protocol at the Lactation Institute in Los Angeles calls for continued feeding on the affected breast as long as the incision and stitches are dorsal to the nipple and areola and the mother does not find this objectionable (Marmet, personal communication, 1991). Sometimes, the baby feeds only from the unaffected breast while waiting for the affected breast to heal, and the mother hand-expresses or pumps milk from the affected side.

If the wound is left open to drain, breastfeeding can be "messy," because milk and other body fluids may leak from the ducts for as long as four weeks or more. The mother should be prepared to replace soiled dressings with clean pads. A consultation with a wound-care specialist (a clinical nurse specialist) might be helpful. Milk leaking from the wound may slow healing. As a result, the mother is at risk for a breast infection or a milk cyst; a low-dose prophylactic antibiotic is sometimes used to avoid infection. A rubber nipple shield with the teat cut off (leaving a doughnut ring of rubber over her nipple) will hold down the bandage and keep the baby's mouth off it. Wounds closer to the nipple-areola and in the lower part of the breast usually take longer to heal. If the problem persists, gradual weaning from the affected side might be necessary while the baby feeds from the unaffected side.

Usually the mother resumes breastfeeding on the affected breast when the drain or stitches are removed and when she can tolerate it. A child's reaction to being prevented from feeding from the affected breast (sometimes his "favorite" breast) varies. Some cooperate without a fuss; others are distraught and actively fight to breastfeed there.

If breast cancer is diagnosed during lactation, subsequent surgery and possible radiation and chemotherapy make continued lactation impossible. Whether a woman should become pregnant again and breastfeed after she has had breast cancer is a medical decision. No studies demonstrate that a subsequent pregnancy accelerates cancer. However, many physicians are reluctant to advise breastfeeding because of limited data regarding the outcomes.

Many mothers have shared their breastfeeding experiences after breast surgery in La Leche League's *New Beginnings,* a rich source of clinical information. One mother (Hart, 1980) had a lump removed as an outpatient. The following day, her breast started swelling with stored milk because her baby had not nursed from that breast. After expressing by hand for 12 days, she began feeding her infant again on the affected breast. Her milk supply in the affected breast returned, though for two to three days nursing was uncomfortable.

Another woman (Paster, 1986) underwent a breast biopsy under general anesthesia for a lump that was deep within her breast. By 12 hours after the procedure, she was able to nurse on the affected side. Although painful at first, by the second or third day, breastfeeding was quite tolerable. The mother found that putting pressure (splinting) on the dressing helped to allay the feeling that the baby would pull the incision apart. At first, there was some lessening of milk production, because about 25 percent of the ducts had been disturbed. Subsequently, the mother nursed another baby without noticing any difference in milk production in the affected breast.

In a third case (Resico, 1990), the nipple was cut during surgery from top to bottom and lifted to remove a golfball-sized lump. The surgeon suggested that the mother not attempt to breastfeed when she became pregnant, because he thought he had severed milk ducts during surgery. Surprisingly, the mother was able to breastfeed from that breast. This suggests one of two possibilities: either some of the ducts were not actually severed, or it is possible for milk ducts to re-canalize after having been severed.

Any woman contemplating breast surgery needs to be fully informed about the procedure and the different techniques that are available. A chart that shows the anatomy and lactational functions of the breast is indispensable for explaining the possible effects of surgery. If the patient is highly motivated to breastfeed, it is the clinician's responsibility to counsel her and suggest techniques that are less disruptive to breastfeeding than are others. If the surgery is very likely to disrupt breastfeeding, that likelihood should be made clear to the woman before the operation. At the same time, it is almost impossible to predict whether breastfeeding will be successful.

Few studies regarding breastfeeding outcomes following breast surgery are available to guide us. Hatton and Keleher (1983) presented two cases of women who breastfed after reduction mammaplasty in which the surgical procedure used was nipple transposition. In the first case, the mother prenatally prepared her breasts for breastfeeding and expressed colostrum, which was very reassuring to her. During her postpartum stay, she breastfed frequently and for long periods. Her follow-up care consisted of frequent phone calls by the nurse-midwives and several office and home visits. At two and one-half weeks of age, the baby weighed two ounces less than at birth, even though he was being breastfed every two hours during the day and every six hours at night. At seven weeks of age, the infant was at the 20th percentile for weight, and the mother started formula supplements. She continued to breastfeed with supplements for several months. Prolactin levels were obtained from this mother before and after breastfeeding her six-week-old infant. Her prebreastfeeding prolactin level was 80 ng/ml; after breastfeeding, it was 245 ng/ml, indicating a normal prolactin response to suckling and an intact neuroendocrine pathway.

The second case report concerned a mother who likewise massaged and prepared her breasts during pregnancy. She was able to express a small amount of colostrum, which greatly encouraged her. Her breasts became fully engorged on the second day after delivery. During the first month, the baby gained weight slowly but continued to nurse frequently. At one month, the baby was just above the 10th percentile for weight and was increasingly fussy. By eight weeks, he had dropped to the fifth percentile, and he was breastfeeding very frequently. The baby was started on formula supplements when he was three months of age. In retrospect, the client remembered feeling guilty for delaying formula supplements, even though she thought that supplements would further decrease her milk production. For these mothers, the necessity of supplements for their babies should be discussed antepartally. If supplements become necessary, a feeding tube could be used, so that the milk production is stimulated by allowing the infant to suckle at the breast while receiving a supplement.

Following the publication of these cases in the *Journal of Nurse-Midwifery,* Schoch (1985) responded with a report of a similar outcome in another woman. This mother also started off well, with both breasts becoming full of milk after delivery. As the breastfeeding course progressed, however, the untreated breast was noticeably larger and produced more milk than did the treated breast. An occasional bottle of formula was started in the third week. During the fourth week, mastitis occurred in the untreated breast, and the mother decided to slowly stop breastfeeding because of the low milk supply of the treated breast and her reluctance to breastfeed with only one breast. This mother did not regret her actions and believed that the baby benefited from the breastfeeding in the first critical weeks; if she has another baby, she intends to breastfeed again. A similar outcome–apparent copious arrival of milk, with early satiation and appropriate growth of the baby, followed by gradual awareness that the baby needs more than the mother's body is providing–has been observed by the authors. The LC who works with mothers who have had breast surgery needs to inform mothers of the possibility that supplementation may be necessary to assure continued infant growth.

If a woman has already had breast surgery and wants to know whether she can breastfeed, it is vital that the caregiver ask about the specific details of the surgery and assess the scarring to try to determine the surgical technique that was used. Following breast surgery, the ability to breastfeed depends on the location of the incision, the techniques employed, and the extent of damage to the tissue, especially to blood and neural pathways. Before any biopsy or breast surgery is performed on any woman of childbearing age, *informed consent dictates that she know the probable effect of the surgery on her ability to breastfeed.*

If the client is able to express colostrum during pregnancy, she may feel optimistic about being able to breastfeed. At the same time, her inability to express colostrum does not necessarily mean that she cannot breastfeed (Hatton & Keleher, 1983). However, not every woman who has milk

after birth will be able to fully lactate. Breastfeeding may go along well for days or weeks with the infant gaining weight until the rapidly growing baby's demand for milk exceeds the mother's ability to produce (E. S. Petok, personal communication, 1990).

Breast-reduction surgery and transareolar-augmentation surgery are particularly damaging to breastfeeding. The mother who has had one of these procedures needs to consult a health professional experienced with such cases. The health professional should provide a forthright discussion about the likelihood of successful lactation and about options for supplemental feedings, especially in the later months. Very few individuals have the expertise to do this. Plastic surgeons, though they may be sympathetic to breastfeeding, are more interested in the surgical technique and the cosmetic results; they are generally uninformed about breastfeeding. The risks of such surgery are high. One of the consequences is reduction or loss of sensation. Courtiss and Goldwyn (1976) found that two years after augmentation mammaplasty, 15 percent of the patients still had decreased sensation in the nipple and areola. In other cases, lactation consultants have been told by their clients that their nipples are "hypersensitive"; none, however, described an improved sensation (C. Marmet & E. Shell, personal communication, 1991).

An experienced lactation consultant (Petok, personal communication, 1990) has worked with many mothers who have had mammaplasty surgery. If the mother has had a reduction surgery, Petok reported, the mother often gratefully accepts whatever extent she can breastfeed without regretting that she had the surgery. If breastfeeding is not at all possible and she had it to do all over again, she would still choose to have the reduction. Marmet and Shell (personal communication, 1991) believe that this percentage is much lower, about 25 percent and that "most women go into reduction surgery uninformed about the consequences of surgery on breastfeeding and their sex lives and later they are angry about this."

Likewise, some women who have had augmentation surgery become angry that their surgeons did not discuss with them the surgery's negative impact on breastfeeding. These women are also angry with themselves for proceeding with the surgery without having been completely informed. Because childbearing and lactation were not a priority at the time of breast surgery, many did not ask the surgeon about their future ability to breastfeed (Hughes & Owen, 1993). Some of these women report that if they had to do it over again, they would not have had the surgery. Some made the decision at a time in their life when they were not feeling good about themselves. They feel guilty about having the implant and are reluctant to tell the pediatrician about their surgery, especially if their baby fails to adequately gain weight because their breasts are not producing enough milk.

Widdice (1993) has written a comprehensive annotated review of published sources on breast reduction and augmentation.

Most of what lactation consultants do for their clients is to give of themselves—the therapeutic self. Therefore, when a mother faces surgery or other procedures on her breasts that are painful and that might also potentially alter or scar her breasts, it is the LC's responsibility to encourage her to openly express her feelings and to answer her questions—and perhaps anticipate her unspoken fears—as completely as possible (Luker et al., 1995).

SUMMARY

Breast-related problems constitute a substantial proportion of clinical breastfeeding counseling. The overuse of antibiotics that leads to candidiasis and the surge in the popularity of cosmetic breast surgery are human-made barriers to breastfeeding and are peculiar to affluent countries. Breast cancer is thus quite likely another disease of the developed world.

Women have the right to be fully informed about any medical procedure, especially a surgical one, because the outcome is apt to be irreversible. Part of the health professional's responsibility is to act as client advocate. The client should know all options available to her (including the right to refuse surgery) and all probable outcomes before consenting to a medical procedure.

Careful consideration of the effects of breast surgery (especially breast augmentation, which is popular among the childbearing age group) is a research priority. Such a study could be done nationwide by collectively pooling data regarding these cases. Education on the effect of lactation in protection against breast cancer is also needed. If women who do not breastfeed or who breastfeed for less than three months were to do so for 4 to 12 months, breast cancer among parous premenopausal women could be reduced by 11 percent, judging from current rates (Newcomb et al., 1994).

REFERENCES

Alexander JM, Grant AM, Campbell MJ: Randomised controlled trial of breast shells and Hoffmans's exercises for inverted and non-protractile nipples. *Br Med J* 304:1030–2, 1992.

Amir LH: *Candida* and the lactating breast: predisposing factors. *J Hum Lact* 7:177–81, 1991.

Amir LH: Eczema of the nipple and breast: a case report. *J Hum Lact* 9:173–5, 1993.

Amir LH, et al: Psychological aspects of nipple pain in lactating women. *J Psychosom Obstet Gynecol* 17:53–8, 1996.

Barnett A: *Breast surgery and breast feeding.* Presentation at the International Lactation Consultant Association Conference, Scottsdale, AZ, July 13–15, 1990.

Bejarnot MA, Simmer MA: *Determination of low levels of silicones in human breast milk by the aqueous silanol functionality test* (rep. no. 1991-10000-36332). Midland, MI: Dow Corning Corporation, 1991.

Berlin CM: Silicone breast implants and breastfeeding. *Pediatrics* 94:546–9, 1994.

Bevin TH, Persok CK: Breastfeeding difficulties and a breast abscess associated with a galactocele: a case report. *J Hum Lact* 9:177–8, 1993.

Brackett VH: Eczema of the nipple/areola area. *J Hum Lact* 4:167–8, 1988.

Brinton LA, et al: Breastfeeding and cancer risk. 6:199–208, 1995.

Brucker MC, Scharbo-DeHaan M: Breast disease: the role of the nurse-midwife. *J Nurse Midwif* 36:63–73, 1991.

Byers T, et al: Lactation and breast cancer: evidence for a negative association in premenopausal women. *Am J Epidemiol* 121:664–74, 1985.

Cantlie HB: Treatment of acute puerperal mastitis and breast abscess. *Can Fam Physic* 34:2221–6, 1988.

Clay LS et al: Chronic moniliasis. *J Nurse Midwif* 35:377–84, 1990.

Cooper DR, Butterfield J: Pregnancy subsequent to mastectomy for cancer of the breast. *Ann Surg* 171:429–33, 1970.

Courtiss EH, Goldwyn RM: Breast sensation before and after plastic surgery. *Plast Reconstr Surg* 58(1):1–12, 1976.

Danforth D: Could it be thrush? *Leaven* 26:56, 1990.

David FC: Lactation following primary radiation therapy for carcinoma of the breast [letter]. *Int J Radiat Oncol Biol Phys* 11:1425, 1985.

Day TW: Unilateral failure of lactation after breast biopsy. *J Fam Pract* 23:161–2, 1986.

Deemarsky LJ, Semiglazov, VF: Cancer of the breast and pregnancy. In: Ariel IM, Cleary JB: *Breast cancer: diagnosis and treatment.* New York: McGraw-Hill, 1987:475–88.

Donegan WL, Spratt JS: *Cancer of the breast.* Philadelphia: Saunders, 1988:685–7.

Dunne CR: Hormonal therapy for breast cancer. *Cancer Nurs* 11:288–94, 1988.

Efrem SEE: Breast abscesses in Nigeria: lactational versus non-lactational. *J R Coll Surg Edinb* 40: 25–7, 1995.

Enger SM, et al: Breastfeeding history, pregnancy experience and risk of breast cancer. *Br J Cancer* 76:118–23, 1997.

Englert HJ, Brooks P: Scleroderma and augmentation mammoplasty: a causal relationship? *Aust NZ J Med* 24:74–80, 1994.

Epstein WA: Silicone breast implants and breast feeding. *J Rheumatol* 24:913–14, 1997.

Escott R: Vasospasm of the nipple: another case [letter]. *J Hum Lact* 10:6, 1994.

Foxman B, Schwartz K, Looman SJ: Breastfeeding practices and lactation mastitis. *Soc Sci Med* 38:755–61, 1994.

Gibberd GF: Sporadic and epidemic puerperal breast infections. *Am J Obstet Gynecol* 65:1038–41, 1953.

Goldsmith HS: Milk rejection sign of breast cancer. *Am J Surg* 127:280–1, 1974.

Green JP: Post-irradiation lactation [letter]. *Int J Radiat Oncol Biol Phys* 17:244, 1989.

Hadary A, Zidan J, Oren M: The milk-rejection sign and earlier detection of breast cancer. *Harefuah* 128:680–1, 1995.

Hancock KF, Spangler AK: There's a fungus among us! *J Hum Lact* 9:179–80, 1993.

Hart J: Nursing after breast surgery. *La Leche League News* 22:10, 1980.

Hatton M, Keleher KC: Breastfeeding after breast reduction mammaplasty. *J Nurse Midwif* 28:19–22, 1983.

Heads J, Higgins LC: Perceptions and correlates of nipple pain. *Breastfeed Rev* 3:59–64, 1995.

Higgins S, Haffty BG: Pregnancy and lactation after breast-conserving therapy for early stage breast cancer. *Cancer* 73:2175–80, 1994.

Hoffman KL, Auerbach KG: Long-term antibiotic prophylaxis for recurrent mastitis. *J Hum Lact* 1:72–5, 1986.

Hoover HC: Breast cancer during pregnancy and lactation. *Surg Clin North Am* 70:1151–63, 1990.

Hornstein E, Skornick Y, Rozin R: The management of breast carcinoma in pregnancy and lactation. *J Surg Oncol* 21:179–82, 1982.

Huggins K: *The nursing mother's companion*. Boston: Harvard Common Press, 1986:46–7.

Hughes V, Owen J: Is breast-feeding possible after breast surgery? *MCN* 18:213–17, 1993.

Hurst N: Lactation after augmentation mammoplasty. *Obstet Gynecol* 87:30–4, 1996.

Ing R, Ho JHC, Petrakis, NL: Unilateral breast-feeding and breast cancer. *Lancet* 2:124–7, 1977.

Jennison RF: Thrush in infancy. *Arch Dis Child* 52:747–9, 1977.

Johnstone HA, Marcinak, JF: Candidiasis in the breastfeeding mother and infant. *JOGNN* 19:171–3, 1990.

Katsouyanni K, et al: A case-control study of lactation and cancer of the breast. *Br J Cancer* 73:814–18, 1996.

Kvåle G, Heuch, I: Lactation and cancer risk: is there a relation specific to breast cancer? *J Epi Commun Health* 42:30–7, 1987.

Lawlor-Smith L, Lawlor-Smith C: Vasospasm of the nipple–a manifestation of Raynauds' phenomenon: case reports. *Br Med J* 314:644–5, 1997.

Layde PM, et al: The independent associations of parity, age at first full term pregnancy, and duration of breastfeeding with the risk of breast cancer. *J Clin Epidemiol* 42:963–73, 1989.

Leary WG: Acute puerperal mastitis: a review. *Calif Med Soc* 68:147–9, 1948.

Lethaby AE et al: Overall survival from breast cancer in women pregnant or lactating at or after diagnosis. Auckland Breast Cancer Study Group. *Int J Cancer* 67:751–5, 1966.

Levine JJ, Ilowite NT: Sclerodermalike esophageal disease in children breast-fed by mothers with silicone breast implants. *JAMA* 271:213–6, 1994.

Levine JJ, et al: Lack of autoantibody expression in children born to mothers with silicone breast implants. *Pediatrics* 97:243–45, 1996.

Livingstone V: Problem-solving formula for failure to thrive in breast-fed infants. *Can Fam Phys* 36:1541–5, 1990.

London SJ, et al: Lactation and risk of breast cancer in a cohort of US women. *Am J Epidemiol* 132:17–26, 1990.

Love SM: *Dr. Susan Love's breast book*. Reading, MA: Addison-Wesley, 1990:32–121.

Luker KA, et al: The information needs of women newly diagnosed with breast cancer. *J Adv Nurs* 22:134–41, 1995.

Manning DJ, Coughlin RP, Poskitt EME: Candida in mouth or on dummy? *Arch Dis Child* 60:381–2, 1985.

Marmet C: *Breast assessment: a model for evaluating breast structure and function*. Presentation at the La Leche League International Annual Seminar for Physicians, Boston, MA, July 11–13, 1990.

Marshall DR, Callan PP, Nicholson W: Breast-feeding after reduction mammaplasty. *Br J Plast Surg* 47:167–9, 1994.

Marshall BR, Hepper JK, Zirbel CC: Sporadic puerperal mastitis: an infection that need not interrupt lactation. *JAMA* 233:1377–9, 1975.

Matheson I, et al: Bacteriological finding and clinical symptoms in relation to clinical outcome in puerperal mastitis. *Acta Obstet Gynecol Scand* 67:723–6, 1988.

McTiernan A, Thomas DB: Evidence for a protective effect of lactation on risk of breast cancer in young women. *Am J Epidemiol* 124:353–8, 1986.

Menendez-Graino F, et al: Galactorrhea after reduction mammaplasty. *Plast Reconstr Surg* 85:645–6, 1990.

Michels KB, et al: Prospective assessment of breastfeeding and breast cancer incidence among 89,887 women. *Lancet* 347(8999):431–6, 1996.

Miller R, Fraumenti J: Does breastfeeding increase the child's risk of breast cancer? *Pediatrics* 49:645–6, 1972.

Mohrbacher N, Stock J: *The breastfeeding answer book* (rev ed). Schaumburg, IL: La Leche League International, 1997.

Morgan RW, Vakil DV, Chipman ML: Breast-feeding family history and breast disease. *Am J Epidemiol* 99:117–22, 1974.

Negri E, et al: Lactation and the risk of breast cancer in an Italian population. *Int J Cancer* 67:161–4, 1996.

Neifert M: Breastfeeding after breast surgical procedure or breast cancer. *Clinical issues in perinatal and women's health nursing* 3:673–82.

Neifert M, et al: The influence of breast surgery, breast appearance, and pregnancy-induced breast changes on lactation sufficiency as measured by infant weight gain. *Birth* 17:31–8, 1990.

Newcomb PA, et al: Lactation and a reduced risk of premenopausal breast cancer. *N Engl J Med* 330:81–7, 1994.

Noble R: Milk under the skin (milk blister)–a simple problem causing other breast conditions. *Breastfeed Rev* 2:118–9, 1991.

Norwood SL: Fibrocystic breast disease. *JOGNN* 19:116–19, 1989.

O'Callaghan MA: Atypical discharge from the breast during pregnancy and/or lactation. *Aust NZ J Obstet Gynaecol* 21:214–6, 1981.

Ogle KS, Davis S: Mastitis in lactating women. *J Fam Pract* 26:139–44, 1988.

Paster BA: Surgery on the nursing breast. *New Beginnings* 2:92, 1986.

Penny WJ, Lewis MJ: Nifedipine is excreted in human milk. *Eur J Clin Pharmacol* 36:427–8, 1989.

Peters MV, Meaken JW: The influence of pregnancy on carcinoma of the breast. *Prog Clin Cancer* 1:471, 1965.

Petok ES: Breast cancer and breastfeeding: five cases. *J Hum Lact* 11:205–9, 1995.

Prentice A, Prentice AM, Lamb WH: Mastitis in rural Gambian mothers and the protection of the breast by milk antimicrobial factors. *Trans Roy Soc Trop Med Hyg* 79:90–5, 1985.

Ramon JM, et al: Age at first full-term pregnancy, lactation and parity and risk of breast cancer: a case-control study in Spain. *Eur J Epidemiol* 12:449–53, 1996.

Resico S: Nursing after breast surgery. *New Beginnings* 6:118, 1990.

Ribeiro GG, Palmer, MK: Breast carcinoma associated with pregnancy: a clinician's dilemma. *Br Med J* 2:1524–7, 1977.

Riordan J, Nichols F: A descriptive study of lactation mastitis in long-term breastfeeding women. *J Hum Lact* 6:53–8, 1990.

Rodger A, Corbett PJ, Chetty U: Lactation after breast conserving therapy, including radiation therapy, for early breast cancer. *Radiother Oncol* 15:243–4, 1989.

Romieu I, et al: Breast cancer and lactation history in Mexican women. *Am J Epidemiol* 143:54–52, 1996.

Saber A: The milk rejection sign: a natural tumor marker. *Am Surg* 62:998–9, 1996.

Schoch RN: Letters to the editor. *J Nurse Midwif* 30:240, 1985.

Schreiner RL, et al: Possible breast milk transmission group B streptococcal infection. *J Pediatr* 91:159, 1977.

Simkin P: Intermittent brachial plexus neuropathy secondary to breast engorgement. *Birth* 15:102–4, 1988.

Siskind V, et al: Breast cancer and breastfeeding: results from an Australian case-control study. *Am J Epidemiol* 130:229–36, 1989.

Smith WL, Erenberg A, Nowak A: Imaging evaluation of the human nipple during breast-feeding. *Am J Dis Child* 142:76–8, 1988.

Soderstrom B: Helping the woman who has had breast surgery: a literature review. *J Hum Lact* 9:169–71, 1993.

Song IC, Hunter JG: Galactorrhea after reduction mammaplasty. *Plast Reconstr Surg* 84:857, 1989.

Stevens K, et al: The ultrasound appearances of galactoceles. *Br J Radiol* 70:239–41, 1997.

Stuver SO, et al: The association between lactation and breast cancer in an international case-control study: a re-analysis by menopausal status. *Int J Cancer* 71:166–9, 1997.

Tanguay KE, McBean MR, Jain E: Nipple candidiasis among breastfeeding mothers. *Can Fam Phys* 40:1407–13, 1994.

Thomsen AD, et al: Course and treatment of milk stasis, noninfectious inflammation of the breast, and infectious mastitis in nursing women. *Am J Obstet Gynecol* 149:492–5, 1985.

Thullen JD: Management of hypernatremic dehydration due to insufficient lactation. *Clin Pediatr* 27:370–2, 1988.

Tralins AH: Lactation after conservative breast surgery combined with radiation therapy. *Am J Clin Oncol* 18:40–3, 1995.

Tretli A, et al: Survival of breast cancer patients diagnosed during pregnancy or lactation. *Br J Cancer* 58:382–4, 1988.

United Kingdom National Case-Control Study Group: Breast feeding and risk of breast cancer in young women. *Br Med J* 307:17–20, 1993.

Utter AR: Gentian violet treatment for thrush: can its use cause breastfeeding problems? *J Hum Lact* 6:178–80, 1990.

Vaison G, Yahalom J: Lactation following conservation surgery and radiotherapy for breast cancer. *J Surg Oncol* 46:141–44, 1991.

Waller HK: *Clinical studies in lactation.* London: Heinemann, 1938:115–35.

Whitley RJ, et al: The natural history of herpes simples virus infection of mother and newborn. *Pediatrics* 66:489–94, 1980.

Widdice L: The effects of breast reduction and breast augmentation surgery on lactation: an annotated bibliography. *J Hum Lact* 9:161–7, 1993.

Yang PS, et al: A case-control study of breast cancer in Taiwan—a low-incidence area. *Br J Cancer* 75:752–6, 1997.

Yoo K-Y, et al: Independent protective effect of lactation against breast cancer: a case-control study in Japan. *Am J Epidemiol* 135:726–33, 1992.

Beyond Postpartum

Although most women are generally healthy during their childbearing years, a mother's nutritional status can affect her health and the lactation course. With adequate social support and prenatal care, pregnancy, birth, and breastfeeding usually go well. Nonetheless, some mothers encounter difficulties, many of which are preventable and nearly all of which can be resolved in a manner that preserves breastfeeding. Major lifestyle concerns for the breast-feeding woman include her child's health, her employment outside the home, and concerns relating to her fertility and her resumption of sexual activity after the birth of her infant.

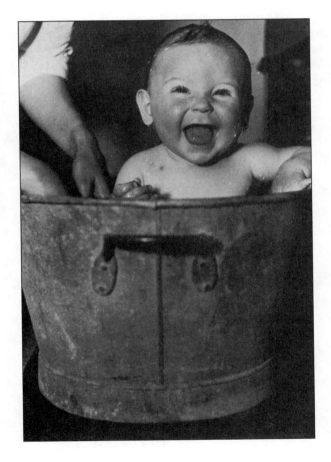

MATERNAL NUTRITION DURING LACTATION

Yvonne L. Bronner and Kathleen G. Auerbach

Breastfeeding is the norm for infant nutrition, and the American Dietetic Association strongly supports breastfeeding. This chapter discusses common concerns that lactating women bring to dietitians–concerns such as weight, exercise, and vegetarian diets. In addition, we examine the effect of supplements (used to maintain or add to nutrient intake in the childbearing woman), caffeine, and food flavorings on both mother and breastfeeding baby, and we explore the development of allergic reactions during lactation. Finally, we offer suggestions related to the questions most frequently asked by mothers who are expecting to breastfeed or who already are breastfeeding their babies.

Pregnant women are usually motivated to eat a more healthful and more varied diet than they ate before they were pregnant. This motivation can be encouraged during lactation as well, although the emphasis on maintaining a "good" diet should be tempered by an understanding that the breastfeeding woman can still breastfeed even if her diet is not ideal. This happens because the body efficiently uses nutrients that are available in the mother even when the mother's diet is limited. Under conditions of chronic malnutrition, nutrients to synthesize breastmilk can be mobilized from maternal stores at the mother's expense.

Worldwide studies, considered together, support the idea that maternal nutrition has only a modest effect on milk production and milk composition. For example, during the "hunger winter" in Holland in 1944–45, women were undernourished as a result of wartime conditions. Dutch infants who were born during this period were found not to be affected by their mothers' inadequate nutritional intake. Slightly less maternal milk was produced than in previous years when the food supply was more ample, but neither duration of breastfeeding nor infant growth patterns were affected (Smith, 1947). Malnourished Brazilian women actually produce milk with a slightly higher fat content than do well-nourished women (Spring et al., 1985), and Nepalese women with protein-calorie malnutrition breastfed babies who were in the low-normal range of weight and length for age yet who appeared healthy; Bangladeshi women who are considered "marginally nourished" maintain an average daily milk production of 750 gm (Brown et al., 1986).

Maternal Caloric Needs

The amount of energy intake needed by lactating mothers continues to be debated. The lactating mother need not maintain a caloric intake that is markedly higher than that maintained prior to pregnancy: in most cases, 200 to 500 calories in excess of that which is needed to maintain the mother's body weight is sufficient. Even though Recommended Dietary Allowance (RDA) levels are thought by many to exceed the levels that women actually need, the RDA is based on the average energy expenditure of moderately active women with an additional 500 calories allowed for lactation. For several reasons, a woman might ingest fewer calories during lactation than are stipulated in the RDA for lactating women:

- She is attempting to return to her prepregnancy weight while breastfeeding her infant.

- She does not have access to sufficient food in a given day.

- She does not wish to gain weight.

- She did not consume this number of calories before pregnancy.

- She is less active than the level used to estimate daily caloric intake.

Basal metabolic rates are higher during lactation but are lower than those during the latter months of pregnancy (Piers et al., 1995). Metabolic efficiency increases during pregnancy, enabling women to use fewer calories more efficiently to sustain themselves during this time. This energy efficiency has not been as well demonstrated during lactation as it has during pregnancy, although women with a wide variety of energy intakes adequately breastfeed their infants. Three recent studies make a case for recommending fewer calories as a base against which to evaluate maternal energy intake during the childbearing years. Other studies using new techniques for measuring energy expenditure are now being conducted on lactating women; thus more, and perhaps better, data will be used for future energy-intake recommendations.

In their prospective study of 458 pregnant women whom they followed for one year, Murphy and Abrams (1993) found that women with lower incomes and African-American women–as compared to women with higher incomes and whites–take in fewer calories, whether they are prepregnant, pregnant, or lactating. Only if they were not breastfeeding did poorer or African-American mothers have higher energy intake than the other women with whom they were compared (Table 16-1). For lactating women in this study, the mean energy intake was considerably lower than recommended levels. Among white and higher-income mothers lactating beyond three months postpartum, energy levels were lower than in the earlier postpartum period. This pattern was reversed among African-American and lower-income women, who increased their energy intake as the infant aged.

Most striking in this study is the substantial difference between RDAs and actual reported energy intake, averaging 700 to 900 kcal lower than levels routinely recommended. Murphy and Abrams (1993) offer two related explanations for this disparity: pregnant and postpartum women (whether lactating or not) have lower energy requirements than were previously computed as a result of their lower average energy expenditures. We agree with the authors that additional studies are needed to track the energy intake of pregnant and lactating women and to note the health outcomes of their infants over time. Only with such studies can we be assured that women can adequately sustain lactation with lower energy levels at no risk to themselves or the babies for whom they are producing milk.

Todd and Parnell (1994) followed 73 women who provided nutrient intake information through 24-hour recalls for three months. Most of the women in this study reported dietary intakes approximately two-thirds the level of the Australian Recommended Nutrient Intake (RNI) for zinc, calcium, folate, and vitamin A. The authors concluded that lactation can be maintained on lower levels of energy intake than are currently recommended, and they suggest reassessment of RNI levels.

The efficiency of conversion of food energy into breastmilk appears to be higher than the 80 percent assumed by the FAO/WHO/UNU joint expert consultation (1985), according to Piers et al. (1995). Frigerio et al. (1991) have proposed that the figure of 95 percent is more appropriate to calculate the energy cost of lactation. These authors argue that use of the value of 95 percent would reduce the energy requirement for milk synthesis in lactation by 96 kcal/day. However, the consen-

Table 16–1

MEAN ENERGY INTAKE (IN KILOCALORIES) OF WOMEN BY RACE AND INCOME LEVEL

| | Race | | Income Level | | Recommended Dietary Allowances |
	White	Black	Above Poverty Line	Below Poverty Line	
Prepregnant	1,569	1,433	1,603	1,440	
Pregnant					2,500
1st trimester	1,616	1,408	1,523	1,683	
2nd trimester	1,854	1,734	1,829	1,851	
3rd trimester	1,830	1,718	1,850	1,779	
Postpartum					
Nonlactating, early*	1,534	1,586	1,535	1,579	2,200
Nonlactating, later	1,600	1,747	1,594	1,690	
Lactating, early*	1,940	1,562	2,023	1,693	2,700
Lactating, later	1,750	1,875	1,807	1,750	

*Infant younger than 90 days.

Source: Derived from SP Murphy, BF Abrams: Changes in energy intakes during pregnancy and lactation in a national sample of U.S. women. Am J Public Health 83:1161–3, 1993.

sus of opinion still suggests that 80 percent is the efficiency value of conversion. The possibility of a systematic underestimation of energy intake in studies reporting a low increment in energy during lactation cannot be ruled out.

Maternal Fluid Needs

Increased fluids also aid the lactating mother's milk production but should not be overemphasized, because excess fluid intake also may result in reduced milk production (Dusdieker et al., 1985, 1990). What the mother drinks will not markedly affect the fluid content of breastmilk. If the mother drinks to meet her own thirst needs, she will drink enough to sustain lactation. The easiest way to ensure adequate fluid intake is to suggest that the mother have something to drink each time she sits down to breastfeed the baby. If a busy mother for-

gets to drink enough fluids as she rushes through her day, she may notice more constipation, one of the first signs of dehydration. Additionally, she can check the color of her urine as she voids through-out the day. With the exception of the first-morning urination, if the mother is drinking enough liquid, her urine will be clear to light yellow.

A woman should be encouraged to follow a diet appropriate to her culture or subculture, eating foods of different colors, flavors, and textures, and in as natural a state as possible. She should avoid processed foods as much as possible, particularly those that contain refined sugars. If the mother does not overeat and maintains a low intake of animal fat, she is unlikely to gain weight while she is breastfeeding, particularly in the early weeks when she is using more energy to make milk for her infant who is breastfeeding exclusively and nursing frequently.

Weight Loss During Lactation

Because thinness is often equated with feminine attractiveness, new mothers may be concerned about their weight. They also may want information about dietary regimens that are compatible with breastfeeding and advice about when they can begin an exercise program postpartum and how strenuously they can exercise.

Generally speaking, breastfeeding women lose more weight postpartum than do their non-breastfeeding counterparts. Kramer et al. (1993) compared the weight-loss patterns of fully breast-feeding, partially breastfeeding, and formula-feed-ing mothers. Both of the breastfeeding groups lost more weight in the first month postpartum than did the formula-feeding women. By six months post-partum, the fully breastfeeding women had attained their prepregnancy weights, but neither the partially breastfeeding nor the formula-feeding mothers had done so.

During the recuperative postpartum period, mothers tend to eat less and to be less active than they were prior to delivery. This pattern of less-ened activity is more pronounced among breast-feeding than among bottle-feeding mothers; in spite of these differences, breastfeeding women lose more weight than bottle-feeding women throughout the first six months postpartum (Bradshaw & Pfeiffer, 1988). Dugdale and Eaton-Evans (1989) contended that postpartum weight loss in the first six months was more likely attribut-able to duration of breastfeeding than to the women's previous body mass. In their study, women who were heavier before pregnancy tend-ed to lose less weight postpartum than women who weighed less at the start of their pregnancy. Dewey et al. (1993) reported that maternal weight loss was greater in the first 12 months postpartum if the mothers breastfed; this weight-loss pattern was most marked in the second six months postpartum and was related to both breastfeeding frequency and duration. Even moderate dieting during breast-feeding can achieve a 4- to 5-lb weight loss per month (Dewey & McCrory, 1994). Fornes and Dorea (1995) reported that breastfeeding mothers begin losing fat from the fifteenth day postpartum. The relationship between maternal weight loss and lactation is summarized in Box 16–1.

A portion of the energy stored during pregnan-cy will be mobilized to accommodate milk produc-tion. For example, if a woman gains 24 to 26 lb (11 to 12 kg) during pregnancy, she can expect that a reserve of about 4 to 7 lb (2 to 3 kg) is used at the rate of 100 to 150 kcal/day to support lactation (Institute of Medicine, 1989). If all goes well, this mobilized fat will be associated with a gradual but steady weight loss until the client reaches her prepregnant weight or "healthy weight" (the weight achieved when the client is eating wholesome foods and engaging in at least 30 minutes of physical activity on most days of the week) (Meisler & St. Jeor, 1996).

Gradual weight reduction has no deleterious effect on lactation and is attainable with lower ener-gy intakes than usually are recommended (Butte et al., 1984; van Raaij et al., 1991). Women who have a caloric intake of 2,600 kcal/day experience no weight loss, whereas those taking in fewer than 2,200 kcal/day gradually lose weight. Mothers with less than 20 percent body fat do not produce less milk than do heavier mothers; however, they do consume more energy. In addition to weight loss from using stored energy reserves, weight loss during lactation is best achieved by lowering the fat content of the diet and exercising. Weight loss is more likely to occur when the fat content is reduced to 20 to 25 percent of calories. Modest weight loss (approximately 1 lb/week) appears to have no adverse effect on the quantity or quality of the breastmilk (Dusdieker et al., 1994). Strode et al. (1986) reported that a modest intake of 1,500 kcal/day in the first six months post-partum did not adversely affect milk production. With this nutritional intake, prolactin levels remained unaffected, and the nursing mothers lost approximately 1 lb/week.

The mother who chooses to diet while lactating should be encouraged to avoid crash or fad diets that promise marked, rapid weight loss, because fat-soluble environmental contaminants and toxins stored in body fat are released into the milk when caloric intake is severely restricted. Additionally, a marked reduction of caloric intake can result in fussiness in some babies. Modest food intake (1,500 kcal/day) does not adversely affect milk produc-tion; however, a rapid, severe weight loss will neg-atively affect infant weight gain. Motil et al. (1994) reported a case in which a breastfed infant failed to thrive at 8 months postpartum as a result of the mother's seriously fat-restricted dietary regimen. Thereafter, the volume of milk declined markedly, although milk composition was unaffected. A safe maternal weight-loss regimen includes careful analysis of the mother's prepregnancy caloric needs accompanied by a plan that enables her to maintain her own nutritional needs while total calories are gradually reduced. In most cases, a weight loss of no more than 1 to 1.5 lb/week can be sustained during lactation without compromising the baby's milk supply or cream content.

Exercise

Regular exercise is healthful at any time during life, including during lactation. Even 45 minutes of aerobic exercise five times weekly has no adverse effect on maternal lactation or on the baby's feeding pattern (Dewey et al., 1994). Lovelady et al. (1990) followed eight exercising and eight sedentary women who were exclusively breastfeeding their 9- to 24-week-old infants. No difference in plasma hormones or milk energy, lipid, protein, or lactose content of the milk was noted between the groups. However, the subjects who were exercising gained less weight during their pregnancy, made more milk, expended more energy, and ate more than the nonexercising women. In no way was lactation adversely affected by these women's moderate exercise regimen.

Alternatively, exercising to exhaustion may increase lactic acid levels to the point at which the baby refuses to breastfeed (Wallace et al., 1992). Removing milk from the breasts prior to exercise and giving this milk to the baby might be one way to reduce the likelihood of infant refusal or even difficulty accepting milk with elevated lactic acid. The authors speculated that, when the breasts are not emptied in advance of vigorous exercise, lactic acid increases rapidly and then decreases steadily throughout the postexercise recovery period. Dewey and Lovelady (1993) noted that such elevated lactic acid levels are not seen when moderate exercise is practiced.

Calcium Needs and Bone Loss

In addition to concerns about weight loss after the birth of a baby, some women fear that breastfeeding

> **BOX 16–1**
>
> ## Relationship Between Maternal Weight Loss and Lactation
>
> - Breastfeeding mothers tend to be less active and to eat less in the early postpartum period than do their non-breastfeeding counterparts.
> - Breastfeeding mothers lose more weight in the second six months postpartum than in the first six months.
> - Mothers who breastfeed more frequently will lose more weight than those mothers who breastfeed infrequently.
> - Mothers who breastfeed for a longer period will lose more weight than those mothers whose lactation course is shorter.
> - Moderate exercise should not affect the mother's milk or her baby's reaction to it.

will cause sufficient bone loss to place them at risk for developing osteoporosis later in life. These fears are unfounded. In fact, the opposite is true: bone density is restored after weaning, although the mother suffers slight bone loss while she is lactating. Before we describe the research literature on this topic, it is helpful to look at calcium needs in general.

Prentice (1994) reviewed the RDAs for calcium in different countries and found that they vary widely. Similarly, calcium intake varies widely, Finland having the highest levels, whereas black women in South Africa were reported to have the lowest calcium intakes. Clearly, these findings reflect dietary differences that occur in these countries. However, Prentice points out that for postmenopausal osteoporosis to occur, the woman must not have achieved maximum bone mass during her young adult life. Furthermore, calcium intake by the mother is not closely related to her breastmilk calcium secretion. In fact, no relationship has been found between breastmilk calcium concentrations and maternal calcium intake through food or calcium supplements (Kirksey et al., 1979; Vaughn et al., 1979). Furthermore, increasing calcium intake may result in increased risk of kidney stones and urinary-tract infections and may result in reduced absorption of other minerals, including iron, zinc, and magnesium (Prentice et al., 1994).

Outcomes of bone-loss studies during lactation are relatively consistent and favor breastfeeding. Specker et al. (1991) compared 26 lactating women with 32 nonlactating postpartum controls over the first year postpartum. Lactating women were more likely to mobilize bone during lactation and to recover bone mass during and after weaning, whether that occurred before or after six months postpartum. Cumming and Klineberg (1993) asked whether there was a relationship between parity, breastfeeding, age at menarche and menopause, and the risk of hip fracture among Australian women aged 65 years and older. As duration of breastfeeding increased, the risk of hip fracture decreased in a dose-response relationship ($p < .01$). Additionally, parous women who breastfed all their children were at lower risk for hip fracture than were parous women who had never breastfed their children.

Sowers et al. (1993) followed 101 women through the first 12 months after the birth of their children. They examined bone mineral density (BMD) of the proximal femur at 2 weeks, 2 months, 4 months, 6 months, and 12 months, and BMD of the lumbar spine at 2 weeks, 6 months, and 12 months. Women who breastfed longer than 6 months had mean BMD losses of 5.1 percent of the lumbar spine and 4.8 percent of the femoral neck. Women who breastfed one month or less lost no BMD at either site. The bone loss noted was not explained by differences in maternal age, diet, body size, or physical activity. In addition, among

the women who breastfed six months or longer, there was a return to baseline BMD levels at 12 months postpartum. The authors stated that health care providers should be aware that transient bone loss can occur with several months of lactation. They also noted, however, that there was little evidence to justify therapeutic intervention.

Sowers et al. (1995) also reported 5 percent short-term bone loss among breastfeeding women, followed by recovery of lost bone within the first 18 months after parturition. Predictive factors were lactation status and the number of months to resumption of menses. These authors concluded that menstrual activity, rather than diet, dietary calcium intake, or physical activity, is the primary factor in bone mass recovery after initial bone loss during lactation.

Kalkwarf and Specker (1995) followed 65 lactating women and 48 nonlactating women for five to six months postpartum. The breastfeeding women lost significantly more bone in the total body (2.8 percent versus 1.7 percent) and lumbar spine (3.9 percent versus 1.5 percent) than did the nonbreastfeeding women. However, after weaning, the breastfeeding women gained significantly more bone in the lumbar spine (5.5 percent versus 1.8 percent) than did the nonbreastfeeding women. These investigators also found that earlier resumption of menses was associated with small amounts of bone loss during lactation and with greater increase of bone after weaning. They concluded that lactation may result in a transient loss of bone for which compensation occurs that may exceed the loss.

Although dietary calcium intake does not explain calcium recovery after lactation, Kalkwarf et al. (1996) suggest that calcium and phosphorus levels are higher in breastfeeding women and that this becomes apparent after weaning and resumption of menses. These researchers suggest that serum calcium concentrations are maintained or elevated by calcium that is metabolized from bone owing to low blood estrogen concentrations. Prentice et al. (1995) found that providing supplements for women whose calcium levels were initially low did not increase these women's calcium intake during lactation or their bone mineral content. Specker et al. (1994) suggest that calcium intake increases during lactation and is greater in women with low-calcium diets. They contend that calcium needs for milk production are met by decreased urinary excretion of calcium and increased bone resorption.

Vegetarian Diets

People choose vegetarianism for religious, economical, cultural, and ecological reasons. Lacto-ovo vegetarians eat milk, eggs, and plant food. Lactovegetarians eat milk and plant food. Usual vegetarian diets supply a balance of nutrients but may be low in energy owing to their low fat and high fiber content. The vegan diet generates the greatest concern because it is very restricted. Some practitioners of this diet are called *fruitarians* and eat only dried fruits, nuts, and honey. Women practicing this diet should be encouraged to take in adequate calories and complementary protein combinations and to consume foods rich in iron, calcium, and vitamins D, B_{12}, and riboflavin to ensure adequate intake. Special attention should be given to vitamin B_{12} intake, because it is available only from animal sources, fortified soy and meat analogues, or B_{12} supplements (Institute of Medicine, 1989).

The milk of breastfeeding vegetarians is generally nutritionally adequate. However, women on a macrobiotic diet who avoid meat, poultry, dairy products, and sometimes fish may produce milk with decreased levels of calcium, magnesium, and vitamin B_{12}. Although taurine is a bit lower in the milk of vegans than in that of omnivores, the level is still 30 times higher than that found in cow's milk–based formulas (Rana & Sanders, 1986; Rassin et al., 1977).

Dietary Supplements

Nutrient needs during lactation vary by the volume of breastmilk produced and the mother's postpartum nutritional status. Generally, if the mother is consuming the recommended calories from a variety of foods, her nutrient needs will be met from food alone. The Institute of Medicine (1989) report includes recommendations that nutrient needs be met from food and that nutrition counselors suggest ways to help women consume adequate food to meet their nutritional needs. If insufficient resources to purchase food of adequate quantity or quality is a problem, WIC and other similar programs should be recommended and referrals made. For women whose income level qualifies them, WIC provides food supplements for lactating mothers. This program supports breastfeeding by providing additional food to the breastfeeding mother for up to the first year of the baby's life, should the mother breastfeed that long. In addition to food, nutrition education and suggestions about how to select and prepare foods for optimal food value are offered. If the mother is restricting her caloric intake to fewer than 1,800 kcal/day in order to lose weight while nursing, she should be encouraged to eat nutrient-dense foods–that is, foods that supply a large proportion of nutrients relative to their calorie content. Vegetables and legumes are good examples of nutrient-dense foods.

If a nutrient deficiency is identified, a balanced multivitamin supplement that supplies iron to 100 percent of RDAs may be recommended on an individual basis. Women who avoid dairy products and other calcium-rich food sources may need a calcium supplement of 600 mg/day of elemental calcium taken with meals. Likewise, the mother's avoidance of vitamin D–enriched foods and the baby's limited exposure to sunlight may lead to inadequate levels of vitamin D in the baby (Specker et al., 1985, 1987). For example, dark-skinned infants given minimum exposure to sunlight (30 minutes per week in a diaper only or two hours per week fully clothed) should receive a supplement of 5 to 7.5 μg/day of vitamin D (Mahan & Escott-Stump, 1996).

Foods That Pass Through Milk
Caffeine

Caffeine-containing foods or fluids have been questioned as an appropriate item for breastfeeding mothers. Mothers often report that their very young babies seem to react when caffeinated beverages or foods are part of the maternal diet. Berlin et al. (1984) evaluated caffeine levels in the milk of 15 mothers. In 11 women, measurable amounts of caffeine were noted in their milk. However, the amount of caffeine available to the infant was 0.06 to 1.5 percent of the maternal dose. No caffeine was detected in the infants' urine, which was collected for five hours after the first nursing period. These investigators concluded that maternally ingested caffeine in moderate amounts presents no significant dose to the normal full-term infant.

Ryu's findings (1985a, b) are also reassuring for parents who regularly consume caffeinated beverages. For young neonates, even five daily cups of coffee ingested by the mother over a five-day period altered neither infant heart rate nor sleep time. Concentrations of caffeine in the term infants' serum were slightly elevated, but by day 9, caffeine levels in the mothers' milk and their babies' serum were below the limits of detectability. LeGuennec and Billon (1987), however, cautioned that babies born prematurely exhibit a delay in eliminating caffeine. This suggests that maternal intake of caffeine may have variable effects on preterm or sick infants as compared to healthy, full-term neonates.

Food Flavorings

Mennella and Beauchamp (1991) carefully examined the effects of maternally ingested garlic and learned that breastfeeding babies suckled longer and obtained more milk when it was garlic-flavored. They speculated that formula-feeding may represent a deficient sensory experience in that the milk always tastes the same. Sullivan and Birch (1994; see also Mennella & Beauchamp, 1997) reported that breastfed babies were more accepting of solids at their introduction than were formula-fed infants. These investigators suggested that the varied flavor cues to which the breastfeeding babies are exposed may facilitate acceptance of new foods. Furthermore, "learning" the taste of foods acceptable to the mother may also facilitate later independent appropriate food selection by the young child (Mennella, 1995).

Vanilla, a potent food flavoring, also alters infant feeding behavior (Mennella & Beauchamp, 1996). Breastfeeding babies suckled longer when first exposed to vanilla-flavored milk. Bottle-feeding babies similarly exposed fed longer when

the milk was flavored but did not continue to do so over time, suggesting that the change in flavor, but not the flavor itself when repeated, may trigger altered feeding behavior. For the breastfeeding baby, continued flavor changes enable the child to become familiar with the flavors represented in his family's foodways.

Goal of the Maternal Diet During Lactation

Food intake during lactation should ensure nutritional adequacy for the maternal postpartum period and support breastmilk production to promote optimal growth and development of the infant. Certain demographic, lifestyle, and environmental factors may place a client at increased nutritional risk during lactation. The most important of these factors are listed in the Box 16–2.

Nutrition During Pregnancy and Lactation: An Implementation Guide was developed to help deliver high-quality nutritional care during lactation (Institute of Medicine, 1992). Single copies of this guide are available from the National Maternal and Child Health Clearinghouse, 8201 Greensboro Drive, Suite 600, McLean, VA 22102. This guide contains:

A sample nutrition questionnaire to help identify women at nutritional risk (Box 16–3)

Answers to questions in the nutrition questionnaire

General strategies for providing effective nutritional care

Dietary assessment and nutritional guidance

Guidance for assessing weight change using the body-mass index chart (which help in evaluating whether the lactating woman is underweight, overweight, or in the average weight range)

A chart of indications for vitamin and mineral supplementation

Supplementary information for nutrition referrals and resources to help you meet the comprehensive nutritional needs of clients

The nutrition questionnaire will help to evaluate the client's (1) eating behavior (meal patterns, food

BOX 16–2

Steps to Successful Dietary Counseling

1. Acknowledge that the client is doing something right.
2. Use the Food Guide Pyramid (Fig. 16–1) to help the client identify areas of the diet that need to be improved.
3. Review the food intake goals for each section of the pyramid and let the client help develop a plan to improve her food intake.
4. Problem solve with the client to determine exactly how the plan will be implemented.
5. Identify facilitators to more appropriate food intake and barriers to same.
6. Determine a time for follow-up, so that progress toward meeting the dietary goals can be evaluated.

BOX 16–3

Assessing Maternal Nutritional Risk: Screening Questions

1. Do you have trouble getting adequate food on a regular or periodic basis? For example, do you run out of food before the end of the month? Do you have problems getting to the store to purchase food? Do you use money allocated for food for other purposes?
2. Does your diet contain calcium-rich foods such as dairy products, fish with edible bones, greens (collards, turnip, etc.), tofu, and broccoli?
3. To lose weight, are you restricting your food intake?
4. If you practice vegetarianism, which of these foods do you exclude from the diet: all meat, fish, poultry, eggs, and dairy products?
5. Are you on some type of special diet that causes you to limit your food intake?
6. Within a week, do you regularly eat five fruits and vegetables?
7. Are you exposed to sunlight on a regular basis? If not, do you regularly consume vitamin D–fortified milk or cereal products?
8. How would you describe your weight status–underweight, overweight, average weight?

Source: Derived from Institute of Medicine, Committee on Nutritional Status During Pregnancy and Lactation, Food and Nutrition Board: Nutrition during pregnancy and lactation: an implementation guide. *Washington, DC: National Academy Press, 1992.*

intake patterns); (2) food security (the ability to get enough food); (3) actual food intake; and (4) lifestyle issues related to nutritional status (smoking, alcohol and other drug use). Answers provided on the questionnaire will help to focus nutrition counseling. After reviewing the steps to successful dietary counseling in Box 16–2, the lactation consultant can begin the counseling session. She should bear in mind that certain factors place mothers and babies at nutritional risk during lactation (Box 16–4).

Nutrition Basics

Nutrition consists of several different elements, including energy; macronutrients, such as carbohydrates, protein, and fat; and micronutrients. We examine each in turn.

Energy

Energy is the capacity to do work. The sun provides the source of energy through plant photosynthesis. Humans gain energy by eating plants or animals that have eaten plants. Several factors influence the total daily amount of energy needed by the body: (1) the basal metabolic rate (BMR), which represents the amount of energy needed for mechanical activities of the body, such as breathing, heart muscle activity, and maintaining body temperature; (2) physical activity; and (3) the thermal effects of food, such as digestion and metabolism. Energy needs are individualized, and studies suggest that there may be some adaptive conservation adjustments in energy expenditure during lactation (Illingsworth et al., 1986; Paul et al., 1979; Schutz et al., 1980). The RDA for energy during lactation is specified by age and represents the average energy expended for light to moderate activity (Institute of Medicine, 1989).

The following quick method may be used to calculate energy need:

1. **Convert "desirable" body weight in pounds to kilograms (kg) by dividing weight in pounds by 2.2.**

Example: desired body weight = 130 pounds/ 2.2 = 59 kg

2. **Use Table 16–2 to select the factor that represents the client's activity level or energy expenditure factor. For this example, let us assume a moderate activity level: moderate energy expenditure factor (MEEF) = 37. Add 500 kcal/day during lactation. Using this figure and the client's "desirable" body weight in kilograms, calculate caloric estimate for the day.**

Example: 59 kg × 37(MEEF) = 2,183 kcal/day + 500 kcal (lactation) = 2,683 kcal/day

The 500 additional calories recommended during lactation can be obtained in the form of a sandwich (~300 to 350 kcal), fruit (60 to 80 kcal), and a glass of skim milk (90 kcal).

This calculation assumes 10 hours of rest and 14 hours of moderate activity.

The preceding calculation would appear to require more calories than most women need while avoiding weight gain. This formula may assume an activity level higher than is applicable to most women in the early postpartum weeks. The health care worker must keep this variability in mind when recommending caloric intake. The recommendation of an additional 500 kcal during lactation, to account for energy needs in making milk, is now considered the upper level of a range of additional calories.

Macronutrients

Carbohydrates. Food intake during lactation is designed to provide the nutritional needs of the mother while enabling her to produce adequate milk for the baby. Most nutritional needs increase during lactation. Carbohydrates are the main energy source for all body functions and are classified as monosaccharides (glucose, fructose, galactose), disaccharides (sucrose, lactose, maltose), and polysaccharides (starch, glycogen, dietary fiber, dextrin). Low carbohydrate intake is associated with fatigue, dehydration, and energy loss. Carbohydrates provide 4 kcal/gm. When carbohydrate is in short supply, protein is broken down to replace it as a source of energy (Mahan, 1996).

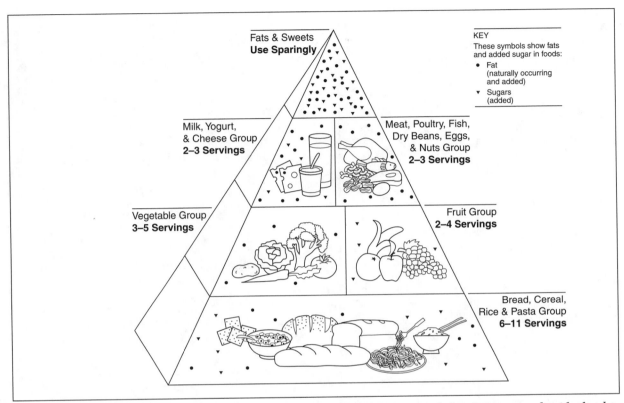

FIGURE 16-1. Food Guide Pyramid. *The pyramid is an outline of what to eat each day. It is a general guide that lets you choose a healthful diet that is right for you. The pyramid calls for eating a variety of foods to get the nutrients you need and, at the same time, the right amount of calories to maintain a healthy weight. The food guide pyramid emphasizes foods from the five food groups, shown in the three lower sections of the pyramid. Each of these food groups provides some, but not all, of the nutrients you need. Foods in one group cannot replace those in another; no one food group is more important than another: for good health, you need them all. (Source: U.S. Department of Agriculture and the U.S. Department of Health and Human Services.)*

Carbohydrates should make up 55 percent of total calories, with a minimum intake of 100 gm/day for lactating women. Lactating women should obtain their carbohydrates from whole-grain breads and cereals, fresh fruits, and vegetables. Simple sugars found in soft drinks, tea, and products labeled *drinks* should form a minimal portion of the daily diet.

The diet should also contain 25 gm/day of dietary fiber. The carbohydrates just recommended, in the form of soluble or insoluble fiber, will help lactating women to reach this goal. Soluble fiber such as pectins and gums (found in fruits–apples, citrus fruits, strawberries, etc.) helps to reduce serum cholesterol levels and cardiovas-

cular disease. Insoluble fiber, such as cellulose and hemicellulose (found in fruit and vegetable pulp and skins) helps to prevent constipation and to reduce the incidence of colon cancer.

Protein. Proteins, which build muscle tissue, enzymes, hormones, and antibodies, are made up of 22 amino acids, 8 of which are essential for adults because the body cannot produce adequate quantities to meet physiological needs; therefore, they must be supplied from the diet. Food proteins are considered complete and of high quality when they contain all 8 of the essential amino acids. Protein from animal sources contain all of the essential amino acids; protein from vegetable

BOX 16–4

Nutritional Risk Factors During Lactation

1. *Maternal age younger than 17 years.* Teens may often have less-than-adequate dietary habits. Therefore, a careful assessment of their food intake is important, using a simple tool such as the Food Guide Pyramid (see Fig. 16–1). Often such assessment will reveal low intake of calcium-rich food and fruits and vegetables rich in vitamins and fiber.

2. *Economic deprivation.* WIC, the Commodity Supplemental Food Program, food stamps, and the Expanded Food and Nutrition Education Program (EFNEP) are examples of U.S. federally funded food and nutrition programs that may meet the needs of economically deprived mothers.

3. *Past restrictive dietary practices or unsound current dietary practices.* Some breastfeeding women severely restrict caloric intake in order to lose weight shortly after pregnancy. Use the Food Guide Pyramid (see Fig. 16–1) to screen for less-than-adequate food intake, especially the omission of an entire group of foods.

4. *Multiple gestation.* The mother of multiples should be encouraged to eat to appetite and drink to thirst while getting as much rest as possible.

5. *Maternal weight less than 85 percent of suggested height and weight* (Institute of Medicine, 1989).

6. *Suboptimal weight gain during pregnancy,* resulting in a low postpartum body mass index (< 19.8)

7. *Rapid weight loss while breastfeeding.*

8. *Pregnant while breastfeeding.* Breastfeeding one infant while pregnant with another necessitates that the mother eat to appetite and drink to thirst while getting as much rest as possible.

Note: Items 5 through 7 in this list relating to weight should receive careful assessment by the health care team. A preliminary step should include a rapid dietary intake assessment using the Food Guide Pyramid and recommendations based on the findings.

Source: Derived from the American Dietetic Association: Manual of clinical dietetics. *Chicago: Chicago Dietetic Association and the South Suburban Dietetic Association, 1996.*

---

sources may be low in one or more of the essential amino acids. Eating at one meal combinations of cereals and legumes–which are low in lysine and methionine, respectively–results in a mixture of amino acids that are adequate for protein synthesis. When caloric intake is adequate, vegetarian diets containing a variety of nutrient-dense foods provide enough essential amino acids for protein metabolism.

Rice contains all of the essential amino acids but in less-than-optimal quantities. When rice is mixed with small quantities of meat or fish, amino acids become adequate for protein synthesis. Complete proteins can be mixed with incomplete proteins or with each other to provide adequate amounts of the essential amino acids. Adding milk to cereal is an example (Mahan, 1996).

The average daily dietary protein requirement is influenced by many factors such as age, digestibility, rate of protein synthesis, and carbohydrate and fat levels (DeSantiago, 1995). The current recommendation is 65 gm/day of protein intake for the mother during lactation during the first six months and 62 gm/day during the second six months (Food and Nutrition Board, 1984). Protein, like carbohydrates, provides 4 kcal/gm.

Fat. Of all the nutrients in human milk, lipids are most affected by the mother's food intake (Butte et al., 1984; Nommsen, 1991). Fats carry the fat-soluble vitamins A, D, E, and K, as well as the essential fatty acid linoleic. Fats provide elements for tissue structure, cell metabolism, and nerve-impulse transmission. They are a concentrated source of energy–9 kcal/gm, as compared to 4 kcal/gm from carbohydrates and protein. Fat should supply no more than 30 percent of the total calories consumed daily. No more than 7 to 10 percent of calories should be from saturated fat (available primarily from animal sources [milk, meat] and coconut and palm oils), more than 10 percent should be monounsaturated, and 10 percent should be polyunsaturated fats (from vegetable sources, nuts, and seeds) (Mahan, 1996).

The overall recommended distribution of calories from the macronutrients for lactating women is as follows:

> **Carbohydrates:** 50 to 55 percent of calories
> **Protein:** 12 to 15 percent of calories
> **Fat:** < 30 percent of calories

Macronutrients are required in large amounts, and they compose most of the body's weight, whereas micronutrients are required in smaller quantities and make up a small percentage of body weight.

Micronutrients

Vitamins. Traditionally, vitamins have been best known by diseases that are caused by their deficiencies (e.g., vitamin A deficiency causes blindness; vitamin C deficiency causes scurvy, etc.). More recent recommendations for vitamin intake are based on principles of health promotion and disease prevention. An example is increasing folate during the periconceptional period to protect against neural-tube defect.

Vitamins are organic, noncalorigenic food substances that are required by the body in small quantities and contribute to the regulation of metabolic processes. Fat-soluble vitamins (A, D, E, and K) are stored by the body in fatty tissue, whereas

Table 16–2

WOMEN'S* TOTAL ENERGY NEEDS AT VARIOUS LEVELS OF PHYSICAL ACTIVITY

Level of General Activity	Energy Expenditure (kcal/kg body wt/day)
Very light	30
Light	35
Moderate	37
Heavy	44
Exceptional	51

*Women aged 19–50 years.

Source: Derived from Institute of Medicine, Food and Nutrition Board, National Research Council: Recommended dietary allowances *(10th ed)*. Washington, DC: National Academy Press, 1989:29.

water-soluble vitamins (B complex and C) are not stored for long periods and need to be supplied in the diet more frequently.

As a mother's intake of water-soluble vitamins increases, the vitamin level in her milk will also increase, but it will reach a plateau that is not raised by giving additional vitamin supplements. Water-soluble vitamin levels in human milk are more likely to be associated with maternal diet or supplement intake than are fat-soluble vitamins or minerals. For example, vitamin B_6 is essential to normal neurological development. The concentrations in breastmilk vary with the vitamin B_6 nutritional status of the mother. Therefore, mothers whose dietary intake of vitamin B_6 is low may be at risk of secreting milk in less-than-adequate quantities (Borschel et al., 1986; West & Kirksey, 1976) (Table 16–3).

Even though vitamin K is fat-soluble and passes more slowly into human milk, oral supplements of vitamin K in exclusively breastfed infants does elevate plasma levels and may be an alternative method of supplementation in situations in which parents refuse intramuscular newborn vitamin K prophylaxis at the time of birth. In addition, maternal oral supplements at the time of birth should be considered, given the decreased intake of breastmilk during the first few days of life and the risk of hemorrhagic disease of the newborn (Greer et al., 1997; see also Victora and van Haecke, 1998).

Minerals. Minerals are inorganic substances that build body tissues and activate, regulate, and control metabolic processes. They also transmit neurological messages.

There is no consensus regarding the exact amount of calcium required during lactation (Prentice et al., 1995). The recommendation for calcium is 1,200 mg/day, an amount that can generally be achieved with generous quantities of dairy products and green, leafy vegetables. Even in countries in which calcium intake is chronically low, Fairweather-Tait et al. (1995) report no effect on the efficiency of calcium absorption by type or amount of calcium supplementation or stage of lactation. This finding suggests that body calcium is mobilized to meet additional needs during lactation.

Clinical Implications

Optimal food patterns to maintain health emphasize intake of grains, fruits, and vegetables and small amounts of low-fat meat and legumes and low-fat dairy products. When making recommendations related to eating, the lactation consultant must consider such factors as the client's or family's culture, environment, socioeconomic status, and energy and nutrient needs. Food labels and the Food Guide Pyramid help mothers to apply the principles from the *U.S. Dietary Guidelines for Americans* when purchasing food and planning meals (see Fig. 16–1, the Food Guide Pyramid). The *U.S. Dietary Guidelines* emphasize seven general recommendations, each of which applies to all members of the family.

1. *Eat a variety of foods.* Different foods are rich in varying nutrients. Therefore, it is important to eat foods from each of the five food groups in the Pyramid and to explore new foods to increase their variety. Vegetarians can obtain adequate nutrients if they eat a variety of foods and take in adequate calories. Vegans, who eat only foods from plant origin, need to ensure that they take a vitamin B_{12} supplement or eat foods fortified with the vitamin.

2. *Balance the food eaten with physical activity.* Physical activity will help to maintain appropriate weight. Although it is important to select foods wisely, it is also necessary to watch portion sizes. The Food Guide Pyramid identifies the number of daily servings appropriate in the daily diet. For example, a hamburger roll is two servings of bread; 1 cup raw or cooked vegetables equals one serving. Three ounces of meat (about the size of the palm of the adult hand) equals one serving. People who restrict their total calorie intake need to eat nutrient-dense foods (high portion of nutrients per calories). Lactating women need to eat a diet rich in calcium (low-fat dairy products, dark-green, leafy vegetables, tofu, canned fish with soft bones) and iron (low-fat meat, fish, and poultry, leafy greens, legumes, and iron-enriched grain products). To maintain a healthy weight, food intake should be balanced with exercise.

3. *Choose a diet with plenty of grain products, vegetables, and fruits.* Most calories should come from grain products, fruits, and vegetables. These foods are high in nutrients and fiber and low in fat.

4. *Choose a diet low in fat, saturated fat, and cholesterol.* Total and saturated fat is highly correlated with serum cholesterol. Therefore, eating low-fat dairy products and meat and increasing the number of meatless meals by using legumes as the main dish is recommended. Monounsaturated and polyunsaturated fats found in olive and canola oils are recommended over butter and fats that are hard at room temperature (such as lard). Limit the number of meals containing egg yolks, organ meats, and other meats to decrease cholesterol intake. Total cholesterol intake should be kept below 300 mg/day.

5. *Choose a diet moderate in sugar.* Sugars alone are not associated with diabetes or becoming overweight, but people who eat large quantities of sweet foods (which are often high in fat) will consume too many calories, which can lead to overweight and obesity.

Table 16-3

RECOMMENDED VITAMIN AND MINERAL INTAKE DURING LACTATION

Nutrient	1–6 mo	7–12 mo	Source	Comments	Lactation Effects
Fat-soluble vitamins					
Vitamin A (μg RE)	1,300	1,200	Liver, kidney, milk fat, fortified margarine, egg yolk, yellow and dark-green leafy vegetables, apricots, cantaloupe, peaches	Essential for normal growth, development, and maintenance of epithelial tissue. Essential to the integrity of night vision. Helps provide for normal bone development and influences normal tooth formation. Toxic in large quantities.	While the efficiency with which a well-nourished mother transfers vitamin A is unknown, in chronically malnourished women, dietary supplements increase milk concentrations.
Vitamin D (μg)	10	10	Vitamin D milk, irradiated foods, some in milk fat, liver, egg yolk, salmon, tuna fish, sardines. Sunlight converts 7-dihydrocholesterol to cholecalciferol.	Really a prohormone. Essential for normal growth and development: important for formation of normal bones and teeth. Influences absorption and metabolism of phosphorus and calcium. Toxic in large quantities.	The increase during lactation is recommended for women beyond age 24 years to maintain calcium balance.
Vitamin E (mg alpha-tocopherol equivalents)	12	11	Wheat germ, vegetable oils, green leafy vegetables, milk fat, egg yolk, nuts	A strong antioxidant. May help prevent oxidation of unsaturated fatty acids and vitamin A in the intestinal tract and body tissues. Protects red blood cells from hemolysis. Role in reproduction (in animals). Role in epithelial tissue maintenance and prostaglandin synthesis.	This allowance accounts for incomplete absorption and individual variability in need. No documented deficiency when fat intake is adequate.
Vitamin K (μg)	65	65	Liver, soybean oil, other vegetable oils, green leafy vegetables, wheat bran. Synthesized in the intestinal tract.	Aids in production of prothrombin, a compound required for normal clotting of blood. Toxic in large amounts.	Lactation poses little additional need beyond pregnancy and is usually not a problem since consumption usually exceeds the RDA.

Table 16-3 (cont.)

Water-soluble vitamins

Nutrient	1-6 mo	7-12 mo	Source	Comments	Lactation Effects
Vitamin C (mg)	95	90	Acerola (West Indian cherry-like fruit), citrus fruit, tomato, melon, peppers, greens, raw cabbage, guava, strawberries, pineapple, potato	Maintains intracellular cement substance with preservation of capillary integrity. Cosubstrate in hydroxylations requiring molecular oxygen. Important in immune responses, wound healing, and allergic reactions. Increases absorption of nonheme iron.	Concentration in human milk varies widely depending on the dietary intake.
Thiamin (mg)	1.6	1.6	Pork, liver, organ meats, legumes, whole-grain and enriched cereals and breads, wheat germ, potatoes. Synthesized in the intestinal tract.	As part of cocarboxylase, aids in removal of CO_2 from alpha-keto acids during oxidation of carbohydrates. Essential for growth, normal appetite, digestion, and healthy nerves.	The allowance is set to account for thiamin loss in milk and increased energy consumption during lactation.
Riboflavin (mg)	1.8	1.7	Milk and dairy foods, organ meats, green leafy vegetables, enriched cereals and breads, eggs	Essential for growth. Plays enzymatic role in tissue respiration and acts as a transporter of hydrogen ions. Coenzyme forms FMN and FAD[a].	The allowance is set to account for the amount secreted in human milk.
Niacin (mg NE)	20	20	Fish, liver, meat, poultry, many grains, eggs, peanuts, milk, legumes, enriched grains. Synthesized by intestinal bacteria.	As part of enzyme system, aids in transfer of hydrogen and acts in metabolism of carbohydrates and amino acids. Involved in glycolysis, fat synthesis, and tissue respiration.	The allowance accounts for increased energy expenditure to support lactation.
Vitamin B_6 (mg)	2.1	2.1	Pork, cereal bran and germ, milk, egg yolk, oatmeal, and legumes. Synthesized by intestinal bacteria.	As a coenzyme, aids in the synthesis and breakdown of amino acids and in the synthesis of unsaturated fatty acids. Essential for conversion of tryptophan to niacin. Essential for normal growth.	Concentration in milk reflects the nutritional status of the mother.

Nutrient			Functions	Food Sources	Comments
Folate (µg)	280	260	Appears essential for biosynthesis of nucleic acids. Essential for normal maturation of red blood cells. Functions as a coenyzme: tetrahydrofolic acid.	Green leafy vegetables, organ meats (liver), lean beef, wheat, eggs, fish, dry beans, lentils, cowpeas, asparagus, broccoli, collards, yeast. Synthesized in the intestinal tract.	If intake is chronically low, maternal reserves may be depleted to maintain levels in human milk.
Vitamin B_{12} (µg)	2.6	2.6	Involved in the metabolism of single carbon fragments. Essential for biosynthesis of nucleic acids and nucleoproteins. Role in metabolism of nervous tissue. Involved with folate metabolism. Related to growth.	Liver, kidney, milk and dairy foods, meat, eggs. Vegans require supplement.	Human milk and serum concentrations are similar. Deficiency has been noted in infants of women on a strict vegetarian (no animal food source) diet in the absence of supplements.

Minerals

Nutrient			Functions	Food Sources	Comments
Calcium (mg)	1,200	1,200	Dietary surveys indicate that many diets do not meet recommended dietary allowances for calcium. Because bone serves as a homeostatic mechanism to maintain calcium level in blood, many essential functions are maintained, regardless of diet. Long-term dietary deficiency may be a factor responsible for development of osteoporosis in later life.	Milk and milk products, sardines, clams, oysters, kale, turnip greens, mustard greens, tofu	Absorption rate may increase during lactation but may not adjust for chronically low intake. There is no correlation between bone health and number of pregnancies and lactation history. However, the allowance should be taken for optimal health maintenance.
Phosphorus (mg)	1,200	1,200	Dietary inadequacy not likely to occur if protein and calcium intake are adequate.	Cheese, egg yolk, milk, meat, fish, poultry, whole-grain cereals, legumes, nuts	Precise requirement is not known but is usually set equal to calcium.
Magnesium (mg)	355	340	Dietary inadequacy considered unlikely, but conditioned deficiency often seen in clinical medicine, associated with surgery, alcoholism, malabsorption, loss of body fluids, and certain hormonal and renal diseases.	Whole-grain cereals, tofu, nuts, meat, milk, green vegetables, legumes, chocolate	The allowance is set to cover individual variability in needs.

Table 16-3 (cont.)

Nutrient	1-6 mo	7-12 mo	Source	Comments	Lactation Effects
Iron (mg)	15	15	Liver, meat, egg yolk, legumes, whole or enriched grains, dark green vegetables, dark molasses, shrimp, oysters	Iron-deficiency anemia occurs in women in reproductive years and in infants and preschool children. May be associated in some cases with unusual blood loss, parasites, and malabsorption. Anemia is last effect of a deficient state.	The loss for lactation is less than normal menstrual loss, which may be absent during lactation. Allowance is similar as that for nonpregnant women.
Zinc (mg)	19	16	Oysters, shellfish, herring, liver, legumes, milk, wheat bran	Extent of dietary inadequacy in this country not known. Conditioned deficiency may be seen in systemic childhood illnesses and in patients who are nutritionally depleted or who have been subjected to severe stress, such as surgery.	Zinc is important to maintain immune status; thus the allowance is inflated to account for poor absorption.
Iodine (µg)	200	200	Iodized table salt, seafoods, water and vegetables in nongoitrous regions	Iodization of table salt is recommended, especially in areas where food is low in iodine.	The addition for lactation is based on the needs of the infant rather than loss in milk.
Selenium (µg)	75	75	Grains, onions, meats, milk. Vegetables variable, depending on the selenium content of soil.	Keshan disease is a selenium-deficient state. Deficiency has occurred in patients receiving long-term TPN without selenium.	The allowance is set to prevent depletion in the mother, given individual variability in absorption.

[a] FMN, flavin adenine mononucleotide; FAD, flavin adenine dinucleotide; TPN, total parenteral nutrition.

Source: Adapted from Institute of Medicine, Food and Nutrition Board, National Research Council: Recommended dietary allowances (10th ed). Washington, DC: National Academy Press, 1989:29; Institute of Medicine, Committee on Nutritional Status During Pregnancy and Lactation, Food and Nutrition Board: Nutrition during pregnancy and lactation: an implementation guide. Washington, DC: National Academy Press, 1992; and LK Mahan, S Escott-Stump: Krause's food, nutrition, and diet therapy (9th ed). Philadelphia: Saunders, 1996:1194.

6. *Choose a diet moderate in salt and sodium.* Processed and prepared foods often contain high amounts of salt and sodium. In addition, some people add salt at the table and during food preparation. Enjoy the natural taste of food by eating fresh fruits and vegetables rather than versions that have added salt or sugar. If you are salt-sensitive, you must limit your intake. The daily value for sodium is 2,400 mg/day. Reading food labels can help you to determine when a food is high in sodium.

7. *If alcoholic beverages are used, do so in moderation.* Any alcohol taken during lactation can cross into the milk; the effect on the infant is dose-related. Alcohol is not recommended during lactation, but if it is taken, it should be ingested in small amounts, with meals, and at a time when breastfeeding is less likely to be compromised.

The dietitian or clinician who is assisting the breastfeeding family to eat in an optimal fashion may wish to refer to one or more of many nutrition information resources now available, in addition to information included in the Food Guide Pyramid shown in Figure 16–1. In the United States, these resources include the following:

Institute of Medicine, *Nutrition During Lactation: Report and Summary.* Washington, DC: National Academy Press, 1991

Institute of Medicine, *Nutrition During Pregnancy and Lactation: An Implementation Guide.* Washington, DC: National Academy Press, 1992

USDA/DHHS, *U.S. Dietary Guidelines for Americans,* 1995

Some questions that mothers commonly ask about nutrition and lactation are reviewed in Box 16–5.

BOX 16–5

Questions Mothers Often Ask About Nutrition and Lactation

1. *Am I at risk for bone loss when I breastfeed my baby?* No. Breastfeeding for six months or longer is the best protection against bone loss. Although calcium is mobilized during breastfeeding, hormones increase calcium absorption and limit the amount of calcium that is excreted. A diet that includes low-fat dairy products and green, leafy vegetables will provide adequate calcium; taking in plenty of sunshine will ensure an adequate supply of vitamin D, which also is important in bone health.

2. *Can I provide sufficient vitamin D to protect my breastfeeding baby against rickets?* Yes. Even in the northern hemisphere where sunlight may be severely limited for several months of the year, there is no need to be concerned (Specker et al., 1994). Human milk contains small amounts of vitamin D, and some sunshine exposure is usually sufficient to maintain appropriate levels of vitamin D in the breastfeeding baby.

3. *I am a teen mother, and I am still growing. Can I still make milk that will help my baby grow?* Yes. Only minimal differences exist between milk samples from teenage mothers and older mothers (Lipsman et al., 1985). If you are capable of sustaining a pregnancy, you can also make sufficient milk to nourish your baby.

BOX 16–5   *(cont.)*

4. *What about folic acid? I have been told this is important for the growing infant.* Folate deficiency and subsequent anemia is highly unlikely in the breastfeeding baby. Breastfeeding babies nearly always have higher folate levels than their formula-feeding age-mates (Salmepera et al., 1986).

5. *If I eat high-fat foods, will I also produce high-fat milk?* To some degree. The specific dietary fatty acids that you consume will be reflected in the milk your baby receives. However, foods low in fat will not prevent you from making milk with sufficient creamy portions.

6. *If I have low levels of vitamin B_6, will this affect my milk supply?* Vitamin B_6 deficiency in a mother may contribute to lethargy in her infant. In one study, a baby with this deficiency also was difficult to console when distressed (McCullough et al., 1990).

7. *What if I am anemic? Will this mean that my baby will have low iron levels, too?* Breastfed babies use the iron in their mother's milk more efficiently than do babies who are fed iron-fortified commercial formulas; thus your baby is at lower risk for anemia when breastfed (Duncan et al., 1985).

8. *Is it true that caffeine makes breastfed babies jittery?* Most studies do not support this expectation. The amounts of caffeine found in infants are usually very small; in other cases, they are undetectable (Berlin et al., 1984).

9. *Will I make enough milk if I don't eat "right"?* Your diet does not have to be perfect in order for you to breastfeed. Caloric intake is what enables a mother to make milk. Even if you eat foods that are higher in sugar or fats than would be considered appropriate, you will still make milk that can nourish your baby. However, it is to your advantage to select foods wisely not only because you are breastfeeding, but because you are feeding yourself, your body, and your future, and because you are responsible for modeling healthful eating for your baby. Selecting foods based on the Food Guide Pyramid (see Fig. 16–1) is good insurance for now and the future.

10. *How will I know my milk is "rich" enough or "not too rich" for my baby?* Nature has made the nutritional composition of your breastmilk just right for your baby. In particular, your milk has an abundant supply of the fatty acids that will lead to optimal nerve and brain development in your child. The milk you make will vary from one feeding to the next, throughout the day, and throughout the baby's entire breastfeeding period. Some feedings will be richer than others, but all will meet the baby's needs.

11. *I am a vegetarian. Can I still breastfeed?* People who practice vegetarianism eat a variety of foods, and most of them are healthful. Nutritionists and other health professionals recommend five or more fruit and vegetable servings per day for everyone. As long as you consume enough calories to maintain an appropriate weight and you use a variety of foods, including legumes and other forms of protein, you will do well. If you are a vegan–consuming only plant foods–you may need to take a vitamin B_{12} supplement. If you express milk after eating a large amount of dark green vegetables, your milk may have a slight green tinge, but the baby will not care!

12. *I hate to drink milk. Does this mean I cannot breastfeed?* Drinking milk and mak-

ing breastmilk are not related. Think about the nutrients available from milk and get them from other foods. You can get calcium, for example, from other low-fat dairy products, green, leafy vegetables, and canned fish with soft bones.

13. *What do you mean by "drink to thirst"? How much should I drink?* This depends in part on where you live. A hot, dry climate may cause you to drink more than another climate would. Your body needs water to make optimal use of the foods you eat. If you drink sufficiently, your urine will be pale in color. If you are thirsty, drink water; it is a thirst-quencher. Sugar-added fluids tend to make you feel more, not less, thirsty.

14. *How soon can I resume my previous exercise plan now that I am breastfeeding? Is it true that exercise will make my milk sour?* You can begin a previous exercise plan as soon as you feel ready to do so. However, it is wise to breastfeed shortly before doing any exercise that causes the breasts to bounce. Wear a support bra. Your milk will not be affected by exercise unless you are exercising to exhaustion; most women report no such effects (Dewey & McCrory, 1994).

15. *I was told I could not begin a weight-reduction program while breastfeeding, but I need to lose weight–and more than a few pounds, too!* Some of the weight you gained during pregnancy is designed to be mobilized and used during lactation. Most of the reputable weight-reduction programs have a plan geared to pregnant and breastfeeding women. They are safe. Increasing fiber and the number of fruit and vegetable servings, using low-fat cooking methods, and decreasing the number of meals that are high in fat, sodium, and calories but low in fiber also will help you lose weight. In addition, daily exercise helps with weight reduction. Frequent breastfeeding has been shown to help women lose weight, particularly in the early weeks and months when the baby is most likely to be fully breastfeeding (Dewey et al., 1993).

16. *I have never been one to take pills, even vitamins. How important are extra vitamins if I breastfeed?* If you eat a healthful diet based on the Food Guide Pyramid and you and your baby get plenty of sunshine (30 minutes per week), there should be no need for extra vitamins.

17. *What special foods should I eat in order to breastfeed?* You do not need to eat any special foods in order to breastfeed. Eating a variety of nutrient-dense foods should be your goal–before, during, and after you are pregnant or lactating.

18. *What foods should I avoid in order to breastfeed?* Most babies and mothers do well with most foods. Sometimes babies will react to certain foods in the mother's diet. Experiment if this happens to you: eliminate the suspected food to determine whether the difficulty disappears. If so, eliminate this food for a while. In most cases, a baby who seems to react to a food when he is very young may not have a problem with that same food when he is older, even if still breastfeeding. Remember too that babies have been found to like highly flavored milk, such as occurs when the mother uses garlic (Mennella & Beauchamp, 1991). Do not be afraid to enjoy highly flavored foods when you eat. Variety seems to be the spice of life for breastfed babies, too!

SUMMARY

During pregnancy, what a woman eats will influence not only her physical well-being but that of her fetus. During lactation, how well she eats has less effect on her ability to make milk than on her well-being. Nevertheless, it is appropriate for clinicians who are offering suggestions pertaining to food intake to encourage the breastfeeding mother to eat in a manner that will support her optimal health. Dietitians have extensive education in infant and maternal nutrition and so are well equipped to educate lactating women; yet, they remain a rarely tapped resource in breastfeeding management (Helm et al., 1997).

Stressing that the mother must eat properly in order to breastfeed places an unnecessary burden on the mother and will likely result in reluctance by some to feed their babies naturally, out of fear that their own established eating habits are not appropriate during breastfeeding. Food choices that the client is already making that support and sustain energy should be praised, and suggestions should be offered within the context of established food patterns. Because food intake–including food selection, meal planning and preparation, and serving–reflects a social behavior that has significance far beyond its nutritional and life-sustaining roles, remaining sensitive to this understanding will enable the clinician to make suggestions that are more likely to be accepted and acted on. Providing examples of nutrient-dense foods that are low in fats and cholesterol will assist the mother in learning to make additional or new food choices. Enabling her to breastfeed by encouraging her to view her milk production as the optimal food for her growing baby and child may help her to make changes in her own dietary choices that will sustain her health as well as that of her children.

REFERENCES

American Dietetic Association: *Manual of clinical dietetics*. Chicago: Chicago Dietetic Association and the South Suburban Dietetic Association, 1996.

Berlin CM, et al: Disposition of dietary caffeine in milk, saliva, and plasma of lactating women. *Pediatrics* 73:59–63, 1984.

Borschel MW, Kirksey A, Hannemann RE:. Effects of vitamin B_6 intake on nurture and growth of young infants. *Am J Clin Nutr* 43:7–15, 1986.

Bradshaw MK, Pfeiffer S: Feeding mode and anthropometric changes in primiparas. *Hum Biol* 60:251–61, 1988.

Brown KH, et al: Lactation capacity of marginally nourished mothers: infants' milk nutrient consumption and patterns of growth. *Pediatrics* 78:920–7, 1986.

Butte NF, et al: Effect of maternal diet and body composition on lactational performance. *Am J Clin Nutr* 39:296–306, 1984.

Cumming RG, Klineberg RJ: Breastfeeding and other reproductive factors and the risk of hip fractures in elderly women. *Int J Epidemiol* 22:684–91, 1993.

DeSantiago S, et al: Protein requirements of marginally nourished lactating women. Unidad de Investigacion en Nutricion, Hospital de Pediatria, Centro Medico Nacional. *Am J Clin Nutr* 62:364–70, 1995.

Dewey KG, Lovelady C: Exercise and breastfeeding: a different experience [letter]. *Pediatrics* 91:514–5, 1993.

Dewey KG, McCrory MA: Effects of dieting and physical activity on pregnancy and lactation. *Am J Clin Nutr* 49(suppl):446s–8s, 1994.

Dewey KG, et al: Maternal weight-loss patterns during prolonged lactation. *Am J Clin Nutr* 58:162–6, 1993.

Dewey KG, et al: A randomized study of the effects of aerobic exercise by lactating women on breastmilk volume and composition. *N Engl J Med* 330: 449–53, 1994.

Dugdale AE, Eaton-Evans J: The effect of lactation and other factors on post-partum changes in body-weight and triceps skinfold thickness. *Br J Nutr* 61:149–53, 1989.

Duncan B, et al: Iron and the exclusively breast-fed infant from birth to six months. *J Pediatr Gastroenterol Nutr* 4:421–5, 1985.

Dusdieker LB, et al: Effect of supplemental fluids on milk production. *J Pediatr* 106:207–11, 1985.

Dusdieker LB, et al: Is milk production impaired by dieting during lactation? *Am J Clin Nutr* 59: 833–40, 1994.

Dusdieker LB, et al: Prolonged maternal fluid supplementation in breast-feeding. *Pediatrics* 86: 737–40, 1990.

Fairweather-Tait S, et al: Effect of calcium supplements and stage of lactation on the calcium absorption efficiency of lactating women accustomed to low calcium intakes. *Am J Clin Nutr* 62:1188–92, 1995.

FAO/WHO/UNU: *Report of a joint expert consultation: energy and protein requirements* (Tech. Rep. series 724). Geneva: WHO, 1985.

Food and Nutrition Board, National Research Council: *Recommended dietary allowances* (9th ed). Washington, DC: National Academy of Sciences, 1984.

Fornes NS, Dorea JG: Subcutaneous fat changes in low-income lactating mothers and growth of breast-fed infants. *J Am Coll Nutr* 14:61–5, 1995.

Frigerio C, et al: Is human lactation a particularly efficient process? *Eur J Clin Nutr* 45:459–62, 1991.

Greer F, et al: Improving the vitamin K status of breastfeeding infants with maternal vitamin K supplements. *Pediatrics* 99:88–92, 1997.

Helm A, Windham CT, Wyse B: Dietitians in breastfeeding management: an untapped resource in the hospital. *J Hum Lact* 13:221–5, 1997.

Illingsworth PJ, et al: Diminution in energy expenditure during lactation. *Br Med J* 292:437–41, 1986.

Institute of Medicine, Committee on Nutritional Status During Pregnancy and Lactation, Food and Nutrition Board: *Nutrition during pregnancy and lactation: an implementation guide.* Washington, DC: National Academy Press, 1992.

Institute of Medicine, Food and Nutrition Board, National Research Council, National Academy of Sciences. *Recommended dietary allowances* (10th ed). Washington, DC: National Academy Press, 1989.

Kalkwarf HJ, Specker BL: Bone mineral loss during lactation and recovery after weaning. *Obstet Gynecol* 86:26–32, 1995.

Kalkwarf HJ, et al: Intestinal calcium absorption of women during lactation and after weaning. *Am J Clin Nutr* 63:526–31, 1996.

Kirksey A, et al: Influence of mineral intake and use of oral contraceptives before pregnancy on the mineral content of human colostrum and of more mature milk. *Am J Clin Nutr* 32:30–9, 1979.

Kramer FM, et al: Breast-feeding reduces maternal lower-body fat. *J Am Diet Assoc* 93:429–33, 1993.

LeGuennec J-C, Billon B: Delay in caffeine elimination in breast-fed infants. *Pediatrics* 79:264–8, 1987.

Lipsman S, Dewey KG, Lönnerdal B: Breast-feeding among teenage mothers: milk composition, infant growth, and maternal dietary intakes. *J Pediatr Gastroenterol Nutr* 4:426–34, 1985.

Lovelady CA, et al: Lactation performance of exercising women. *Am J Clin Nutr* 52:103–9, 1990.

Mahan LK, Escott-Stump S: *Krause's food, nutrition, and diet therapy* (9th ed). Philadelphia: Saunders, 1996:1194.

McCullough AL, et al: Vitamin B_6 status of Egyptian mothers: relation to infant behavior and maternal-infant interaction. *Am J Clin Nutr* 51:1067–74, 1990.

Meisler JG, St. Jeor S: Summary and recommendations from the American Health Foundation's Expert Panel on Healthy Weight. *Am J Clin Nutr* 63(suppl):474s–7s, 1996.

Mennella JA: Mother's milk: a medium for early flavor experiences. *J Hum Lact* 11:39–45, 1995.

Mennella JA, Beauchamp GK: The human infants' response to vanilla flavors in mother's milk and formula. *Infant Behav Dev* 19:13–9, 1996.

Mennella JA, Beauchamp GK: Maternal diet alters the sensory qualities of human milk and the nursling's behavior. *Pediatrics* 88:737–44, 1991.

Mennella JA, Beauchamp GK: Mothers' milk enhances the acceptance of cereal during weaning. *Pediatr Res* 41:188–92, 1997.

Motil KJ, et al: Case report: failure to thrive in a breast-fed infant is associated with maternal dietary protein and energy restriction. *J Am Coll Nutr* 13:203–8, 1994.

Murphy SP, Abrams BF: Changes in energy intakes during pregnancy and lactation in a national sample of US women. *Am J Public Health* 83:1161–3, 1993.

Nommsen LA, et al: Determinants of energy, protein, lipid, and lactose concentrations in human milk during the first 12 months. *Am J Clin Nutr* 53:457–65, 1991.

Paul AA, Muller EM, Whitehead RG: The quantitative effects of maternal dietary energy intake on pregnancy and lactation in rural Gambian women. *Trans R Soc Trop Med Hyg* 73:686–92, 1979.

Piers LS, et al: Changes in energy expenditure, anthropometry, and energy intake during the course of pregnancy and lactation in well-nourished Indian women. *Am J Clin Nutr* 61:501–13, 1995.

Prentice A: Maternal calcium requirements during pregnancy and lactation. *Am J Clin Nutr* 59(suppl):477s–83s, 1994.

Prentice A, et al: Calcium requirements of lactating Gambian mothers: effects of a calcium supplement on breast-milk calcium concentration, maternal bone mineral content, and urinary calcium excretion. *Am J Clin Nutr* 62:58–67, 1995.

Prentice AM, Goldberg GR, Prentice A: Body mass index and lactational performance. *Eur J Clin Nutr* 48(suppl 113): S78–S89, 1994.

Rana SK, Sanders TAB: Taurine concentrations in the diet, plasma, urine and breast milk of vegans compared with omnivores. *Br J Nutr* 56:17–27, 1986.

Rassin DK, Sturman JA, Gaull GE: Taurine in developing rat brain, subcellular distribution and association with synaptic vesicles of (35s) taurine in maternal, fetal and neonatal rat brain. *J Neurochem* 28:41–50, 1977.

Ryu JE: Caffeine in human milk and in serum of breast-fed infants. *Dev Pharmacol Ther* 8:329–37, 1985a.

Ryu JE: Effect of maternal caffeine consumption on heart rate and sleep time of breast-fed infants. *Dev Pharmacol Ther* 8:355–63, 1985b.

Schutz Y, Lechtig A, Bradfield RB: Energy expenditures and food intakes of lactating women in Guatemala. *Am J Clin Nutr* 33:892–902, 1980.

Salmepera L, Perkeentupa J, Siimes MA: Folate nutrition is optimal in exclusively breast-fed infants but inadequate in some of their mothers and in formula-fed infants. *J Pediatr Gastroenterol Nutr* 5:283–89, 1986.

Smith CA: Effects of maternal undernutrition upon the newborn infant in Holland (1944–45). *J Pediatr* 30:229–43, 1947.

Sowers MF, et al: Biochemical markers of bone turnover in lactating and nonlactating postpartum women. *J Clin Endocrinol Metab* 80:2210–6, 1995.

Sowers MF, et al: Changes in bone density with lactation. *JAMA* 269:3130–5, 1993.

Specker BL, Tsang RC, Ho ML: Changes in calcium homeostasis over the first year postpartum: effect of lactation and weaning. *Obstet Gynecol* 78:56–62, 1991.

Specker BL, et al: Calcium kinetics in lactating women with low and high calcium intakes. *Am J Clin Nutr* 59:593–9, 1994.

Specker BL, et al: Effect of race and diet on human-milk vitamin D and 25-hydroxyvitamin D. *Am J Dis Child* 139:1134–7, 1985.

Specker BL, et al: Effect of vegetarian diet on serum 1,25-dihydroxyvitamin D concentrations during lactation. *Obstet Gynecol* 70:870–4, 1987.

Spring PCM, et al: Fat and energy content of breast milk of malnourished and well nourished women, Brazil 1982. *Ann Trop Paediatr* 5:83–7, 1985.

Strode MA, et al: Effects of short-term caloric restriction on lactational performance of well-nourished women. *Acta Paediatr Scand* 75:222–9, 1986.

Sullivan SA, Birch LL: Infant dietary experience and acceptance of solid foods. *Pediatrics* 93:271–7, 1994.

Todd JM, Parnell WR: Nutrient intakes of women who are breastfeeding. *Eur J Clin Nutr* 48:567–74, 1994.

United States Dept. of Agriculture/Dept. of Health & Human Services. U.S. Dietary Guidelines for Americans. USDA: Washington, DC, 1995.

van Raaij J M, et al: Energy cost of lactation, and energy balances of well-nourished Dutch lactating women: reappraisal of the extra energy requirements of lactation. *Am J Clin Nutr* 53:612–9, 1991.

Vaughn LA, Weber CW, Kemberling SR: Longitudinal changes in the mineral content of human milk. *Am J Clin Nutr* 32:2301–6, 1979.

Victora CG, van Haecke P: Vitamin K prophylaxis in less developed countries: policy issues and relevance to breastfeeding promotion. *Am J Public Health* 88:203–9, 1988.

Wallace JP, et al: Infant acceptance of postexercise breast milk. *Pediatrics* 89:1245–7, 1992.

West KD, Kirksey A: Influence of vitamin B_6 intake on the content of the vitamin in human milk. *Am J Clin Nutr* 29:961–9, 1976.

Women's Health and Breastfeeding

Jan Riordan and Kathleen G. Auerbach

This chapter discusses acute and chronic maternal health problems that are considered to have an effect on lactation. The health of a mother has a direct impact on her ability (both emotional and physical) to care for her infant. During their childbearing years, most women tend to be healthy and fit. Illness is usually episodic: a head cold or a case of influenza. Breastfeeding empowers women to stay healthy by providing a variety of such health benefits as a reduction in the likelihood of carcinoma-in-situ of the uterine cervix (Brock et al., 1989), endometrial cancer (Rosenblatt et al., 1995), rheumatoid arthritis (Brun et al., 1995), and obesity (Hammer et al., 1996). The health care provider usually does not see the more serious health conditions described here. When she does, she needs a working knowledge of these conditions and the ability to develop a plan of care based on the wishes and needs of the breastfeeding mother who has a health problem.

Alterations in Endocrine and Metabolic Functioning

Anything that affects control of the endocrine system can also affect the production of breastmilk.

The following discussion of diabetes mellitus, thyroid problems, and pituitary dysfunction explains uncommmon conditions that may affect the breastfeeding mother's milk supply. Any woman with symptoms that suggest she might have an altered metabolic functioning should be referred to a physician for further evaluation and treatment.

Type 1 Diabetes

Diabetes is a chronic disease of impaired carbohydrate metabolism caused by insufficient insulin or the inefficient use of insulin. Diabetes mellitus is classified into two main categories: type 1 diabetes, or insulin-dependent diabetes mellitus (IDDM), and type 2 diabetes (of late onset and usually not insulin dependent). Gestational diabetes, a glucose intolerance that occurs in 10 to 12 percent of pregnancies, manifests itself only during pregnancy. Most women with gestational diabetes will revert to normal status and be reclassified as impaired glucose tolerant following the birth of the baby. Women with gestational diabetes are twice as likely (9.4 percent versus 4.2 percent) to develop type 1 diabetes if they do not lactate following the birth of the baby whose pregnancy provoked gestational diabetes, according to Kjos et al. (1993). Lactation–

even for a short duration—improves glucose metabolism, and is a low-cost intervention that may reduce or delay IDDM in these women.

With improvement in the monitoring and control of maternal blood sugar, women with IDDM who are in good diabetic control can usually look forward to a safe and relatively healthy pregnancy and birthing experience. At the same time, an insulin-dependent pregnant woman is considered a high-risk obstetric patient. During pregnancy, her blood glucose levels should be maintained below 130 mg/dl as much as possible. During labor, delivery, and for some time after delivery, blood-glucose levels must be closely monitored. The glycated-hemoglobin laboratory test reflects blood-glucose levels from the preceding three months (American Diabetes Association, 1997). The mother receives insulin in intravenous dextrose and Ringer's solution, carefully regulated by an infusion pump or secondary intravenous site. Cesarean deliveries continue to be much more likely for the mother with diabetes (about 70 percent; Ferris et al., 1993).

The woman with type 1 diabetes not only can but should be encouraged to breastfeed her infant, despite the necessary technology required to bring the diabetic mother and her infant safely through childbirth (Engelking & Page-Lieberman, 1986). Colostrum helps to stabilize the infant's blood sugar and, although breastfeeding should begin as soon after birth as possible, this is usually not the case. Babies of diabetic mothers are considered high-risk infants and are routinely placed in the special or intensive care unit immediately after delivery. The effect of anesthesia with a cesarean birth and the mother's additional discomfort cannot be discounted in delaying breastfeeding. Even if breastfeeding is delayed, the mother should be encouraged to begin expressing her milk as soon as she feels able.

Lactogenesis II, or "coming in," of the milk for mothers with IDDM occurs about one day later than for mothers without type 1 diabetes (Arthur et al., 1994; Bitman et al., 1989; Hutt, 1989; Miyake, 1989). They also have lower milk prolactin concentrations than do women without diabetes (Ostrom & Ferris, 1993). Therefore, these mothers and their neonates need additional attention and care if they are to establish lactation. Early, frequent breastfeeding and keeping the mother and baby together increase the prevalence of mothers still breastfeeding at three months (Whichelow & Doddridge, 1983). Pumping to stimulate the milk supply is advised as well. It may be necessary to supplement the neonate during the first two to three days. Formula is often given in the interim until the mother's milk comes in, which brings up the issue of a potentially destructive autoimmune response in an infant who already has an increased risk of developing diabetes (American Academy of Pediatrics, 1994). Rather than give artificial milk supplements, one pregnant mother with IDDM stored donor breastmilk that she later used to supplement her baby during the first few days postpartum.

During the immediate postnatal period, sudden but normal hormonal changes cause marked fluctuation in maternal blood-glucose levels. Maternal hypoglycemia can be expected to occur immediately postbirth, lasting five to seven hours after delivery; thereafter, insulin requirements usually decrease abruptly. In addition, lactose excretion in the urine drops to a low level two to five days after birth and then rises rapidly. These sudden metabolic shifts require close monitoring. Some women report erratic blood-glucose levels and an increase in insulin reaction. Juggling the feeding schedule of the infant and the amount of milk taken at each feeding are factors to be considered in maintaining good diabetic balance (Gagne et al., 1992).

Lactose is reabsorbed from the breast and is normally excreted in the urine; therefore, nurses and mothers should be aware that in testing the urine after delivery, the presence of lactose may result in a false-positive test if copper-reducing urine testing (Clinitest) is used. For this reason, testing with Testape or Diastix, which measures only glucose, is the preferred method. Once she is physiologically stable, the patient can return to subcutaneous injection insulin or to injection via a portable infusion pump.

Blood-glucose meters are reliable for testing blood glucose by the mother at home. By keeping a daily record of blood-glucose levels, the mother can self-monitor day-to-day changes. Once the blood-glucose level stabilizes, it is generally lower during lactation. Ferris et al. (1988) compared 30 mothers with IDDM with 30 controls and found that fasting plasma-glucose levels during the exclusive breastfeeding period were significantly lower than were the glucose levels of the women with IDDM who had stopped breastfeeding or who had never breastfed, even in the face of markedly higher caloric intake by the breastfeeding mothers. Given the continuous conversion of glucose to galactose and lactose during milk synthesis, less insulin is required when the mother breastfeeds. Davies et al. (1989) showed that women with diabetes may need to reduce their prepregnancy insulin dose by about 27 percent to avoid hypoglycemic reactions.

Breastmilk nutrients vary slightly during the first several days postpartum. In the mother with IDDM, lactose levels in breastmilk are reduced, as compared with the nondiabetic mother on days 1, 2, and 3 after birth, implying that lactose synthesis is not proceeding normally. Between day 3 and day 4, the levels of glucose abruptly increase to levels similar to or higher than those in milk from nondiabetic mothers (Arthur et al., 1994). Nitrogen content in the milk of women with IDDM, higher at two to three days postpartum, reflects delayed lactation and returns to levels of the nondiabetic by day seven (Neubauer et al., 1993). Breastmilk fat content, especially the medium-chain fatty acids, appears to be slightly lower in women with diabetes than that in nondiabetic women (Bitman et al., 1989). Concentrations of total nitrogen, lactose, vitamin E, fat, and energy are indistinguishable from concentrations in the milk of nondiabetic women; however, glucose concentrations and sodium in the milk of the women with diabetes are higher and more variable (Butte et al., 1987; Lammi-Keefe et al., 1995).

In addition to providing the known physiological advantages of breastfeeding for the infant, breastfeeding helps to fulfill the mother's need to feel normal in spite of her diabetic condition. An advantage of working with these women is their keen awareness of their body functions and the importance of diet. They are more knowledgeable than the average woman about physiology and are quick to notice changes that may forewarn of problems.

Women with IDDM have difficulty establishing lactation and tend to discontinue breastfeeding more often in the first week postpartum than do women without IDDM. Any sudden drop in blood glucose appears to affect milk production because of the secretion of epinephrine that accompanies hypoglycemia. For example, one mother's blood-glucose level suddenly dropped to 19 mg/dl eight days after a cesarean birth. For the next 24 hours, she was unable to express any milk using an electric pump, but after her return home, she began to rebuild her milk supply. Alternatively, in a study of 33 women with IDDM and 33 controls, once lactation was established, there was no difference in the frequency of breastfeeding at three months postpartum (Ferris et al., 1993). Women with IDDM are able to establish lactation despite postpartum separation from their infants, delays in the start of breastfeeding, reduced frequency of feeding, increased use of supplemental feedings, and their high rate of cesarean section.

Mothers with diabetes may be more susceptible to mastitis, especially if they are not well controlled (Ferris et al., 1988; Gagne, Leff, & Jefferis, 1992). Any infection will quickly raise the level of blood glucose. Self-care teaching should emphasize recognizing early symptoms of mastitis and seeking prompt treatment while continuing to breastfeed. Mothers with diabetes are also at risk for candidiasis if blood-glucose levels are elevated. Preventing this problem involves careful control of blood glucose, drying the nipple after breastfeeding, and being aware of the early symptoms (see Chapter 15).

Once lactation is established, most women who have IDDM report that their breastfeeding experiences are no different from those of mothers without diabetes (Gagne et al., 1992). The mother with diabetes needs additional calories while breastfeeding. As her child begins to wean, the mother will again need to make alterations in her diet and insulin intake to compensate for a decrease in milk production. If weaning is gradual, fewer problems and adjustments arise.

Thyroid Disease

The thyroid gland controls the body's metabolism and promotes normal growth of central nervous system development. It produces three hormones: thyrosine (T_4), triiodothyronine (T_3), and calcitonin. T_3 and T_4, which are chemically similar, are known as *thyroid hormones*. Postpartum thyroid dysfunction is a quite common event, occurring in some 17 percent of women. The disease is usually transient, lasting one to four months, and is most likely to occur in the first eight months postpartum. Disorders of the thyroid gland have prompted some clinicians to recommend against breastfeeding for mothers with hypothyroidism or hyperthyroidism. Although maternal hypothyroidism can be reflected in poor weight gain in the baby (see Chapter 11), hyperthyroidism has no such effect.

Many thyroid tests are available for screening lactating women who are suspected of having thyroid disease. The most cost-effective, safe, and sensitive test is the FT_4I test. If the results of the FT_4I test are high, an FT_3I test is ordered to confirm a diagnosis of hyperthyroidism. No special patient preparation is required for these laboratory tests; a peripheral venous blood sample is drawn. The radioactive iodine uptake test is not recommended during lactation because radioactive iodine transfers into and concentrates in the breastmilk; breastfeeding must be interrupted for at least 48 hours.

Hypothyroidism. Maintaining full-term pregnancy is rare in untreated women who suffer from hypothyroidism; therefore, most breastfeeding women with a history of hypothyroidism are already receiving medical care.

For the untreated breastfeeding woman, hypothyroidism can result in a reduced milk supply. Other symptoms in the mother are thyroid swelling or nodules (goiter), cold intolerance, dry skin, thinning hair, poor appetite, extreme fatigue, and depression. When the thyroid deficiency is not known, these problems are often attributed to postpartum hormonal changes and changes in lifestyle (notably, constant care of the baby) and remain undiagnosed—at least for a time. When the infant of one mother suddenly and completely weaned, the mother, subsequently receiving a diagnosis of hypothyroidism, reported that she "never experienced any fullness in the breast—it was as though I'd dried up overnight."

These complaints, sometimes coupled with the infant's failure to gain weight satisfactorily on breastmilk alone, should alert the nurse or lactation consultant to the possibility of thyroid deficiency and to the reality that the mother needs further medical diagnostic evaluation. If replacement therapy of thyroid extract with synthetic T_4 (thyroxine, sodium levothyroxine, or Synthroid) or other thyroid preparation is adequate, the relief of the symptoms

and an increase in the milk supply can be quite dramatic. The daily replacement dose of thyroid is 0.25 to 1.12 mg of sodium levothyroxine or equivalent doses of other thyroid preparation. Women whose replacement therapy was determined before pregnancy should be reevaluated after the baby's birth to determine whether adjustment is necessary.

Hyperthyroidism. An excess of thyroid hormone is characterized by loss of weight (despite an increased appetite), nervousness, heart palpitations, and a rapid pulse at rest. A well-developed case of hyperthyroidism with exophthalmos (bulging eyes) is called *Graves' disease.* Hyperthyroidism, a common disorder thought to affect 2 percent of women typically in their mid-twenties or -thirties, can develop for the first time postpartum. The ability to lactate does not appear to be affected, although the mother's nervousness may complicate her ability to cope with the daily caregiving of her infant.

Generally, laboratory diagnosis of hyperthyroidism can be established by values from just two laboratory tests: serum TSH and serum free T_4 index (Franklyn, 1994). According to Romney, Nicoloff, and Esser (1989), hyperthyroidism and thyroiditis can be reliably diagnosed with pertechnetate imaging in combination with clinical symptoms and plasma hormone levels. However, these authors claim that radioiodine studies should not be performed in women who want to continue breastfeeding. Although radioiodine uptake may be considered necessary to establish the treatment dose for hyperthyroidism, the uptake dose and agent then become irrelevant, because breastfeeding must be discontinued when the woman is treated. When evaluation of the thyroid using a radioactive substance is deemed essential, technetium-99m pertechnetate is the preferred agent (Table 17–1).

Treatment usually involves giving an antithyroid drug to lower the maternal thyroid level. If needed, propylthiouracil (PTU) given orally (50–300 mg daily) is the treatment of choice for the lactating woman with hyperthyroidism. Although the infant may be monitored for thyroid function, PTU appears to have little effect on the thyroid functioning of the infant (Kampmann, 1980; McDougall & Bayer, 1986; Momotani et al., 1989).

Table 17–1

ISOTOPE USE IN BREASTFEEDING MOTHERS

Radio Pharmaceutical	Original (No. of Cases) or Review*	Recommendation	Comment	Reference
$^{99m}Tc04$ (pertechnetate)	Review	Interrupt nursing and measure milk activity. Resume when activity < 1 mSv	Time to reduce to EDE < 1 mSv is 36 hr	3
	Original (1)	Discard milk during first 12 hr after tracer administration	EDE to infant < 1 mSv	8
	Original (1)	Discard milk during first 12 hr after tracer administration	Mean effective $t\,^{1}/_{2} = 3.2$ hr; total fraction of injected activity excreted into breast milk = 10.8×10^{-2}	1, 2
	Original (2)	Discard milk during first 24 hr after tracer administration	Recommendation made for doses up to 1.5 mCi*	9
	Original (1)	Discard milk during first 48 hr after tracer administration		10
	Original (2)	Wait until breast milk activity is < 6×10^{-3} µCi/ml	$^{1}/_{10}$ ICRP drinking water standard for ^{99m}Tc; level reached 20–32 hr after tracer administration	6
	Original (1)	Discard milk during first 72 hr after tracer administration levels	Waited until breast milk activity reached background	7
^{99m}Tc-MAA (macroaggregated albumin)	Review	Discard milk during first 6 hr after tracer administration	EDE to infant < 1 mSv	3
	Original (6)	Discard milk during first 12 hr after tracer administration	Mean effective $t\,^{1}/_{2} = 37$ hr; total fraction of injected activity excreted into breast milk = 3.2×10^{-2}	1, 2
	Original (4)	Discard milk during first 24 hr after tracer administration	Cumulative dose to infant = 0.2 mrad if nursing is resumed after 24 hr	11
	Original (1)	Discard milk during first 24 hr after tracer administration	Whole-body dose to infant = < 0.05 mrem	12

* Indicates whether recommendation is based on original data or on a review of previously published/gathered data.

mSv: milliSievart; µCi: microCurie; mCi: milliCurie; mrad: millirad; mrem: millirem; EDE: Effective Dose Equivalent; ICRP: International Commission on Radiological Protection.

Source: Originally appeared in B Fulton, L Moore: Radiopharmaceuticals and lactation. J Hum Lact *6:181–4, 1990. Reprinted with permission.*

Table 17–1 (cont.)

Radio Pharma-ceutical	Original (No. of Cases) or Review	Recommendation	Comment	Reference
	Original (1)	Discard milk during first 24 hr after tracer administration	Also gave 99mTc-DTPA aerosol	13
	Original (1)	Discard milk during first 24 hr after tracer administration	Estimated 24-hr infant exposure if nursed = 0.3 mrad	14
	Original (1)	Interruption not essential		15
	Original (1)	Discard milk during first 24 hr after tracer administration	Estimated dose to infant thyroid if nursed after 24 hr < 1 mrad	16
99mTc-RBC (erythrocytes)	Review	Interrupt nursing and measure milk activity	Time to reduce to EDE < 1 mSv is approximately 13 hr Resume when activity < 1 mSv	3
	Original (1)	Discard milk during first 24 hr after tracer administration	Mean effective $t^{1/2} = 7.7$ hr; fraction of injected activity excreted into breast milk = 6.1×10^{-5}	1, 2
99mTc-DTPA (diethylene-thiamine pentacetic acid)	Review	Interruption not essential	EDE to infant, 1 mSv	3
	Original (1)	Discard milk during first 4 hr after tracer administration	Mean effective $t^{1/2} = 3.7$ hr; total fraction of injected activity excreted into breast milk = 1.5×10^{-4}	1, 2
	Original (1)	Discard milk during first 4 hr and tracer administration	Total activity ingested was approximately 0.1% of ICRP annual limit for 6.6 kg infant nursing not interrupted	17
99mTc-DMSA	Review	Interruption not essential	EDE to infant < 1 mSv	3
99mTc glucoheptonate	Original (1)	Discard milk during first 4 hr after tracer administration (although not essential)	EDE to infant < 1 mSv	3, 8
99mTc-MDP (methylenedi-phosphonate)	Review	Interruption not essential	EDE to infant < 1 mSv	3
	Original (2)	Discard milk during first 4 hr after tracer administration	Mean effective $t^{1/2} = 4.2$ hr; total fraction of injected activity excreted into breast milk = 1.9×10^{-4}	1, 2
99mTc-HDP	Review	Interruption not essential	EDE to infant < 1 mSv	3

Table 17–1 (cont.)

Radio Pharmaceutical	Original (No. of Cases) or Review	Recommendation	Comment	Reference
[123]I-iodide	Review	Interrupt nursing and measure milk activity. Resume when activity < 1 mSv	Time to reduce to EDE < 1 mSv approximately 5 hr	3
	Review	Avoid breastfeeding	Permissible milk concentration = 1.9×10^{-6} µCi	18
	Review	Avoid breastfeeding	112-day delay following 100-µCi dose	19
	Original (1)	Discard milk during first 36–72 hr after tracer administration	Biological $t^{1/2}$ = 10.4 hr	20
	Review	Discard milk during first 48–72 hr after tracer administration	Based on extrapolated ^{131}I data	4
^{123}I-IOH	Review	Interrupt nursing and measure milk activity. Resume when activity < 1 mSv	Time to reduce EDE to < 1 mSv approximately 8 hr	3
^{125}I-IOH	Review	Interrupt nursing and measure milk activity. Resume when activity < 1 mSv	Time to reduce EDE to < 1 mSv approximately 18 hr	3
	Original (1)	Discard milk during first 12 hr after tracer administration	Mean effective $t^{1/2}$ = 4.3 hr; total fraction of injected activity excreted into breast milk = 2.4×10^{-2}	1, 2
^{125}I-HSA	Review	Avoid breastfeeding	Time to reduce EDE to < 1 mSv approximately 206 hr	3
	Original (2)	Discard milk during first 10 days after tracer administration		21
[125]I-fibrinogen	Review	Avoid breastfeeding	Time to reduce EDE to < 1 mSv is 540 hr	3
	Original (1)	Avoid breastfeeding	$t^{1/2}$ in milk = 80 hr	22
[131]I-iodide	Review	Avoid breastfeeding	Time to reduce EDE to < 1 mSv approximately 1,727 hr	3
	Review	Avoid breastfeeding	Biological $t^{1/2}$ = 21.9 days	19
	Review	Discard milk during first 8 weeks after tracer administration	Standard = $^{1}/_{10}$ yearly permissible dose of ICRP Dose = 5 µCi	4
	Original (2)	Discard milk during first 12 days after tracer administration	ICRP drinking water standard	6
	Original (1)	Discard milk during first 24 hr after tracer administration		23

Table 17–1 (cont.)

Radio Pharmaceutical	Original (No. of Cases) or Review	Recommendation	Comment	Reference
	Original (2)	Avoid breastfeeding	Biological $t\,{}^{1\!/_2}$ of radioiodine = 7 days in thyroid gland	24
^{131}I-IOH	Review	Interrupt nursing and measure milk activity. Resume when activity < 1 mSv	Time to reduce EDE to < 1 mSv approximately 30 hr	3
	Review	Discard milk during first 45 days after tracer administration		4
	Original (6)	Discard milk during first 12 hr after tracer administration	Mean effective $t\,{}^{1\!/_2} = 4.5$ hr total fraction of injected activity excreted into breast milk $= 2.8 \times 10^{-2}$	1, 2
[75]Semethionine	Review	Avoid breastfeeding	Time to reduce to < 1 mSv approximately 467 hr	3
	Original (1)	Avoid breastfeeding		25
[67]Ga-citrate	Review	Avoid breastfeeding	Time to reduce to < 1 mSv approximately 427 hr	3
	Review	Interrupt nursing for 4 weeks	Standard $= {}^{1\!/_{10}}$ of yearly permissible dose by ICRP	4
	Original (1)	Avoid breastfeeding	Biological $t\,{}^{1\!/_2}$ in milk = 9 days	26
[111]In-leukocytes	Original (1)	Interruption not essential	Maximum EDE to infant = 1 mSv	27
[51]Cr-EDTA	Review	Interruption not essential	Maximum EDE to infant = 0.001 mSv	3
	Original (2)	Discard milk after first 4 hr after tracer administration	Mean effective $t\,{}^{1\!/_2} = 6$ hr; total fraction of injected activity excreted into breast milk $= 4.0 \times 10^{-4}$	1, 2

References

1. Ahlgren L, et al: Excretion of radionuclides in human breast milk after the administration of radiopharmaceuticals. *J Nucl Med* 26:1085–90, 1985.

2. Ahlgren L: Error in table [letter]. *J Nucl Med* 27:151, 1986.

3. Mountford PJ, Coakley AJ: A review of the secretion of radioactivity in human breast milk: data, quantitative analysis and recommendations. *Nucl Med Commun* 10:15–27, 1989.

4. Romney BM, et al: Radionuclide administration to nursing mothers: mathematically derived guidelines. *Radiology* 160:549–54, 1986.

5. Karjalainen P, Penttila IM, Pystynen P: The amount and form of radioactivity in human milk after lung scanning, renography, and placental localization by ^{131}I labelled tracer. *Acta Obstet Gynecol Scand* 50:357–61, 1971.

6. Wyburn JR: Human breast milk excretion of radionuclides following administration of radiopharmaceuticals. *J Nucl Med* 14:115–7, 1973.

7. Vagenakis AG, Abreau CM, Braverman LE: Duration of radioactivity in the milk of a nursing mother following Tc-99 administration. *J Nucl Med* 12:188, 1971.

8. Mountford PJ, Coakley AJ: Breast milk radioactivity of ^{99m}Tc-pertechnetate and ^{99m}Tc-glucoheptonate. *Nucl Med Commun* 8:839–45, 1987.

Table 17-1 (cont.)

9. Ogunleye O: Assessment of radiation dose to infants from breast milk following the administration of Tc[99m]-pertechnetate to nusring mothers. *Health Phys* 45:149–51, 1983.

10. Pittard WB III, Bill K, Fletcher BD: Excretion of technetium in human milk. *J Pediatr* 94:605–7, 1979.

11. Cranage R, Palmer M: Breast milk radioactivity after [99m]TC-MAA lung studies. *Eur J Nucl Med* 11:257–9, 1985.

12. Heaton B: The buildup of technetium in breast milk following the administration of [99m]Tcm04 labelled macroaggregated albumin. *Br J Radiol* 52:149–50, 1979.

13. Mountford PJ, et al: Breast milk radioactivity after a Tc-[99m] DTPA aerosal/Tc-[99m] MAA lung study. *J Nucl Med* 25:1108–10, 1984.

14. Pittard WB III, Merkatz R, Fletcher BD: Radioactivity excretion in human milk following administration of technetium Tc[99m] macroaggregated albumin. *Pediatrics* 70:231–4, 1982.

15. Tribukati B, Swedjemark GA: Secretion of [99m]Tcm in breast milk after intravenous injection of marked macroaggregated albumin. *Acta Radiol Oncol* 17:379–82, 1978.

16. Berke RA, et al: Radiation dose to breast-feeding child after mother has [99]Tcm MAA lung scan. *J Nucl Med* 14:51–2, 1973.

17. Mountford PJ, Coakley AJ, Hall FM: Excretion of radioactivity in breast milk following injection of [99]Tcm DTPA. *Nucl Med Commun* 6:341–5, 1985.

18. Romney B, Nickoloff EL, Esser PD: Excretion of radioiodine in breast milk. *J Nucl Med* 30:124–6, 1989.

19. Dydek GJ, Blue PW: Human breast milk excretion of iodine-131 following diagnostic and therapeutic administration to a lactating patient with Graves' disease. *J Nucl Med* 29:407–10, 1988.

20. Hedrick WR, DiSimone RN, Keen RL: Radiation dosimetry from breast milk excretion of radioiodine and pertechnetate. *J Nucl Med* 27:1569–71, 1986.

21. Bland EP, et al: Radioactive iodine uptake by thyroid of breast-fed infants after maternal blood volume measurements. *Lancet* 1:1039–40, 1969.

22. Palmer KE: Excretion of ^{125}I in breast milk following administration of labelled fibrinogen. *Br J Radiol* 52:672–3, 1979.

23. Weaver JC, Kamm ML, Dobson RL: The excretion of radioiodine in human milk. *JAMA* 173:872–5, 1960.

24. Nurnberger CE, Lipscomb A: Transmission of radioiodine (I[131]) to infants through human maternal milk. *JAMA* 150:1398–1400, 1952.

25. Taylor DM, McCready VR, Cosgrove DO: The transfer of L-seleno-methionine-75SE to human milk and the potential radiation dose to a breast-fed infant. *Nucl Med Commun* 2:8083, 1981.

26. Tobin RE, Schneider PB: Uptake of ^{67}Ga in the lactating breast and its persistence in milk. *J Nucl Med* 17:1055–6, 1976.

27. Mountford PJ, Coakley AJ: Excretion of radioactivity in breast milk after an Indium-111 leukocyte scan. *J Nucl Med* 26:1096–97, 1985.

Another antithyroid drug, carbimazole, which is widely used in Great Britain, is converted by body metabolism to methimazole (Tapazole). In a case report of a mother being treated with carbimazole for hyperthyroidism, (Rylance et al., 1987) neither of her breastfeeding twins showed any effects of the medication being taken by the mother; she continued breastfeeding.

Pituitary Dysfunction

Severe postpartum hemorrhage and hypotension may result in the pituitary gland's failure to produce gonadotropins, which leads to a condition known as *panhypopituitarism* or *Sheehan's syndrome*. Initial weight gain postpartum, followed by weight loss, loss of pubic and axillary hair, intolerance to cold, breast-tissue atrophy, low blood pressure, and vaginal-tissue atrophy are symptoms of Sheehan's syndrome. Milder cases of pituitary disruption may occur, with less severe symptoms and delay in milk synthesis. DeCoopman's discussion (1993) of lactation following pituitary resection suggests that the role of the pituitary gland may be temporary in the early establishment of lactation rather than an essential requirement throughout its course.

Prolactinomas (prolactin-secreting adenomas) are pituitary tumors that stimulate the secretion of prolactin and produce secondary amenorrhea and galactorrhea. Women with prolactinomas may breastfeed. In a study of 46 women with prolactinomas, Ikegami et al., (1987) reported the results of 51 pregnancies experienced by these women and their subsequent postpartum course. The women were in one of three treatment groups: surgery, surgery plus bromocriptine, and bromocriptine only. Although prolactin levels declined in all three groups after delivery in 87 percent of the patients, more women were breastfeeding from the group whose prolactinoma had been treated with bromo-criptine. Moreover, no woman showed a sharp increase in prolactin levels during the postpartum period, and there were no symptoms of tumor enlargement. The authors suggested that breast-feeding should not be restricted in patients with prolactinomas. Holmgren et al. (1986) also studied women with prolactinoma. In the group of 35 women whom they followed, lactation did not appear to affect the secretory activity of the tumor, and breastfeeding proceeded uneventfully.

Cystic Fibrosis

Cystic fibrosis (CF) is a generalized hereditary dis-order of infants, children, and young adults. It is associated with the widespread dysfunction of the exocrine glands and is marked by signs of chronic pulmonary disease, obstruction of the pancreatic ducts, and pancreatic enzyme deficiency. In the past, children with the disease rarely lived to adult-hood. Early treatment has enabled young women with CF to marry, to give birth, and to breastfeed without evidence of the disease. The median life expectancy is 28 years for women with CF, and more than 1,000 women with this disease have become pregnant and given birth to healthy infants (Shiffman et al., 1989).

Generally, mothers with CF should be encour-aged to breastfeed as much as any other mother, although Luder et al. (1990) report that centers for CF treatment are less likely to report recommend-ing breastfeeding when the mother has CF than when her infant has the condition. Concern about breastfeeding involves the possible risk to the mother's own health status while breastfeeding and caring for a young infant, rather than the quality of the breastmilk. Although there are some differ-ences in lipid composition, the breastmilk of moth-ers with CF contains nutrients sufficient to supply the energy needs of the nursing infant (Bitman et al., 1987).

Shiffman et al. (1989) reported two cases in which the mothers breastfed for one month and two months, respectively, during which time the babies grew at appropriate rates. In both cases, the concentrations of milk sugar, electrolytes, sodium, potassium, and chloride were within normal limits. At the same time, concentrations of milk proteins, fat, and IgA appeared to decrease during periods of pulmonary exacerbations. Michel and Mueller (1994) documented five women with cystic fibrosis who breastfed; four of their five infants maintained adequate growth. The fifth infant's mother, who exclusively breastfed him for six months, added supplemental foods when it became apparent that his growth slowed.

Although these women may breastfeed, they need close nutritional monitoring. Because the nutritional status of the person with CF is already compromised, the extra calories needed for breast-milk production may cause excessive weight loss. One early case presentation (Welch et al., 1981) dis-cussed the breastfeeding course of a 20-year-old woman with CF. Her early breastfeeding course was normal, and the baby grew appropriately through the first 10 weeks postpartum. Thereafter, the mother continued to lose weight, and her respiratory status began to worsen. She began antibiotic therapy and stopped breastfeeding. A later case report (Golembeski & Emergy, 1989) documented the normal growth of an infant through six weeks of exclusive breastfeeding by a 24-year-old mother with CF. These authors concluded that breastfeeding was an "acceptable option" for women with the disease as long as the maternal diet was closely monitored and vitamin and caloric sup-plementation was offered when necessary.

Breastfeeding has another advantage for the mother with CF. Because individuals with CF are chronic carriers of bacterial pathogens (such as *staphylococcus aureus, Pseudomonas*), breastmilk lym-phocytes sensitized to the bacterial pathogens car-ried by the mother protect the infant against these infections.

Acute Illness and Infections

Common illnesses, such as colds and upper-respiratory-tract infections or gastroenteritis, are not contraindications for breastfeeding. For most infections, the key word is *self-limiting*. Usually, such infections are not life-threatening; further-more, the infected mother provides antibody protection to her infant through continued breast-feeding, thereby decreasing her baby's exposure or modifying the illness. Interruption of breastfeeding renders the infant more susceptible to the maternal illness, exposes him unnecessarily to the hazards of artificial baby milks, and removes an important source of comfort for him (Coates & Riordan, 1992).

Postpartum infections expose the breastfeeding dyad to potential delayed breastfeeding, prolonged hospital stay, and possible separation. Urinary-tract infection (UTI) is the most common problem in women seen by primary care providers. Many women, especially if they are sexually active, suffer from multiple recurrence of UTI. *Escherichia coli* is the most common pathogen associated with UTI. Breastfeeding women with a UTI are treated with antibiotics; thus concern relates to the safety of taking a medication while they are breastfeeding.

Timethroprim, 100 mg every 12 hours for three days, is an effective and commonly prescribed treatment for UTIs. Quinolones (norfloxacin, ciprofloxacin), used to treat a broad spectrum of gram-positive and gram-negative infections, are also used to treat UTIs. Both drugs are considered safe during breastfeeding (Hale, 1997). Women should ask their physician for a "standing" prescription at home that will allow them to begin medication as soon as they experience symptoms. Uro-sticks, which detect white cells in the urine, can be purchased for women to use in self-diagnosis. Self-treatment also includes drinking at least six to eight glasses of water a day, drinking cranberry juice, avoiding caffeine, and urinating immediately after having sex.

Antibiotics are commonly used to treat postpartum infections. When given to the mother, they pose no danger to the infant and thus should not be used to justify an unnecessary interruption or cessation of breastfeeding. In addition to UTIs, other postpartum infections that are treated with antibiotics are mastitis (see Chapter 15 for a detailed discussion), puerperal infections (puerperal fever, metritis), wound infections from cesarean incisions, and episiotomies (Clark, 1995).

Approximately one-third of tuberculosis cases in the United States occur in people younger than 35 years of age. The rising incidence of tuberculosis in women in their childbearing years reflects other coexisting influences, such as drug abuse associated with conditions of urban poverty and the influx of immigrants from areas of the world where there is a high prevalence of tuberculosis

(Simpkins et al., 1996). According to the American Academy of Pediatrics, Report of the Committee on Infectious Diseases (1997), women with tuberculosis who have been treated appropriately for two or more weeks (and who are otherwise considered to be noncontagious) may breastfeed. Women with tuberculosis should be encouraged to breastfeed; separation of the mother from her infant is rarely justified. Drug therapy for women with active cases may be initiated in the second trimester of pregnancy; the risk of drug toxicity to an infant breastfed by a mother taking antituberculosis medication is minimal. Snider and Powell (1994) found that such a newborn might receive 6 to 20 percent of the therapeutic dose of isoniazid and 1 to 11 percent of other drugs, such as rifampin, ethambutol, and streptomycin. Moreover, infants exposed to tuberculosis are themselves treated with a therapeutic dose of isoniazid.

If a breastfeeding mother becomes acutely ill, breastfeeding may have to be interrupted. The mother's breasts should not be allowed to become engorged; a staff member should arrange for the mother to express her milk so that the woman's breasts remain comfortable. Supporting the mother in a side-lying position if she cannot sit upright will help the milk to flow more easily during expression. The baby can be fed with a cup or feeding bottle using the expressed breastmilk until the mother can return to breastfeeding (Coates & Riordan, 1992).

Dysfunctional Uterine Bleeding

Normal uterine bleeding (lochia) following birth ceases in about three to five weeks. The median duration of lochial flow for breastfeeding women is 27 days (Visness, Kennedy, & Ramos, 1997). Nearly half of women who fully breastfeed experience some vaginal bleeding or spotting between six and eight weeks postpartum (Visness et al., 1997). Abnormal bleeding can inhibit breastmilk synthesis. Willis and Livingstone (1995) described 10 cases of insufficient milk following severe postpartum hemorrhage. In the early weeks, excessive bleeding may be due to placental fragments retained in the uterus (Neifert et al., 1981).

Bleeding caused by a relaxed uterus occurs less often in the breastfeeding woman, because the oxytocin released by the suckling infant causes the uterus to contract during each suckling episode. Later bleeding may result from miscarriage or the irregular onset of hormonal function. Treatment includes hormonal therapy or nonsteroidal anti-inflammatory drugs (NSAIDs). If bleeding is excessive, prolonged, or unexplained, curettage of the uterine lining may be necessary.

For excessive postpartum bleeding, the physician usually orders several doses of methylergonovine maleate (Methergine), a derivative of an ergot alkaloid. Methergine can be given orally, intramuscularly, or intravenously. Unlike crude ergot preparations, no adverse effects have been reported following the use of methylergonovine by nursing mothers. Methylergonovine does not suppress lactation. If the therapy is prolonged (beyond five days), the infant's pulse and blood pressure should be monitored.

Anxiety always accompanies excessive bleeding. Nursing intervention should focus on relieving the mother's anxiety and assisting in determining the cause of the bleeding while maintaining breastfeeding. The mother should be referred to a physician for an immediate appointment or, if the bleeding is especially severe and a physician is not available, she should be taken to the hospital emergency room. Because leaving her alone only increases her fear, someone should stay with her until she can be medically evaluated. A dilation and curettage (D&C), if required, can usually be performed in an outpatient setting, which reduces the likelihood and duration of mother-infant separation.

Occasionally hormone therapy, either estrogens or progesterone or a combination of both, may be necessary to control bleeding. If hormone therapy is advised, its risks and benefits must be considered in relation to continued breastfeeding. In such cases, the mother may want to seek a second medical opinion for other options. The nurse or lactation consultant can act as a sounding board in assisting her to make this decision.

Surgery

Surgery of any kind is a stressful experience; surgery that is scheduled when the mother is breastfeeding and caring for a small child or infant raises the possibility of separation from the baby and the inability to care for him. The mother who enters the hospital in advance of a surgical procedure may have sufficient time to make plans. If she knows on which floor she will be housed, she can learn the visitation policy for that floor in that hospital (whether her baby and other minor children will be allowed to visit her), how long she will be in the hospital, the availability of a fully automatic breast pump, and the staff's knowledge and experience with breastfeeding mothers.

Getting in touch with a lactation consultant in the hospital may be the first step in ensuring that someone knowledgeable is aware of her concerns about preserving lactation and the breastfeeding relationship. This person may be able to arrange for a breast pump to use in advance of the surgery (and immediately thereafter if needed). Guidelines for helping the breastfeeding mother who undergoes surgery are summarized in Box 17–1.

Generally, surgery is likely to result in a temporary reduction in a woman's milk supply as measured by expressing. However, once the mother is fully awake, she may feel uncomfortably full. If the surgery involved the breast, pumping should begin as soon as possible to avoid putting further pressure on the operative site from engorgement and to relieve the mother's discomfort. Usually, a hand-operated pump or hand-expression will be sufficient, unless she cannot use her hands. If the staff has limited experience in assisting breastfeeding women, a referral should be made to the in-hospital lactation consultant so that she can provide care for the mother. Most hospitals allow a breastfeeding infant to stay with the mother after the surgery, if another adult is present to take care of the infant. If this is not possible, the baby can be brought to the hospital to be breastfed.

During her hospitalization, the mother may be receiving one or more medications. If she must be separated from her baby, she needs to determine whether she will express and discard her milk or send it home with a family member to be given to the baby. In some cases, mothers are reluctant to use milk that they consider to be tainted by even small amounts of medications. This is the mother's choice. If she has decided not to provide her milk during the period of medication use, she may

BOX 17–1

Surgery and the Breastfeeding Mother: Guidelines for Care

- Encourage the mother to plan for help at home after surgery to allow time to recuperate.
- Use an outpatient surgical facility rather than an inpatient facility.
- Arrange for breastfeeding of the baby immediately before the surgery.
- Assist the mother in breastfeeding as soon as she awakes from anesthesia.
- Make rooming-in arrangements for the breastfeeding child, if an inpatient facility is required. (Most hospitals require that another adult be present to care for the baby.)

- Express and freeze a supply of breastmilk before the surgery (if needed).
- Aid the mother in conditioning the baby to cup-feedings before surgery if it is determined that temporary supplementary feedings will be necessary.
- Encourage mother to take postoperative analgesia to alleviate pain. (The infant will receive only a small dose through breastmilk.)
- Show the mother how to "splint" the surgical area with pillows if abdominal surgery is performed. Cover the incision area with dressings.

choose to stockpile milk in advance of her surgery to avoid having the baby fed with artificial baby milk in her absence.

Once the mother is at home, how her baby will react to her depends on several factors, including the length of time the mother was absent, how the baby was fed in her absence, and the baby's age at the time of the separation. One of the authors assisted a mother who had gallbladder surgery and later complications that required three hospitalizations. The baby managed the first two separations easily. The third hospitalization lasted for six weeks, and when the mother returned home, the baby–who was now three months old–acted as though she had never breastfed. This reaction was most distressing to the mother, who had been looking forward to returning to breastfeeding. In this case, special assistance was required to bring the baby back to the breast, a task that was accomplished over the course of an additional month.

Relactation

Relactation is the process of restimulating lactation. It can occur days, weeks, or months after lactation has ended (Waletzky & Hermann, 1976). Brown (1977) notes that in the developing world, when war and other civil disorganization have destroyed families, the key elements to relactation are a mother who is adequately nourished, a baby with a good sucking reflex, and a support system. At South African medical centers, relactation is routinely initiated as part of the rehydration therapy that is offered to ill and seriously malnourished infants and young children whose nutritional difficulties start after weaning from the breast, when the baby develops diarrhea (Olango & Aboud, 1990) after bottle-feedings are introduced. In these centers, the mothers receive additional foods, the babies are put to breast frequently and for long periods, and they are fed other foods only after suckling. The mothers live at the center with other mothers receiving the same assistance, and they become a mutual support system along with the staff, who strongly support the importance of reestablishing breastfeeding. In nearly all cases, the mothers relactate fully, and the babies' health status is improved.

In the developed world, the purpose of relactation and induced lactation is to enable breastfeeding after an untimely weaning or to initiate breastfeeding that has been delayed by neonatal or maternal illness or prematurity (Auerbach, 1981; Auerbach & Avery, 1980; Seema & Satyanarayana, 1997; Thompson, 1996). Relactation is also an option for a mother who bottle-feeds at first but has a change of mind or discovers that her infant cannot tolerate infant formula.

Generally, relactation is easier for the mother to accomplish if the interval between the end of the pregnancy or the last day of previous breastfeeding (or pumping) is short. A milk supply can be reestablished with sufficient, regular stimulation. Although metoclopramide has been used to assist mothers following a premature birth (Ehrenkranz & Ackerman, 1986) and to assist mothers of hospitalized infants (Seema & Satyanarayana, 1997), hormonal preparations are neither necessary nor appropriate in all cases. Furthermore, an important but often neglected consideration is the baby's willingness to accept the breast. In situations in which the baby has never been put to breast, the age of the infant at the time this is attempted makes a difference. The younger the baby, the greater the likelihood that he will be willing to suckle, particularly within the first three months of life. If the baby has breastfed previously, the chances are greater, but in all cases, promptly rewarding the baby when he first attempts to breastfeed will increase the likelihood that the baby will continue to suckle.

The reason for relactation is important. If the baby is intolerant of all or most of the available human milk substitutes, the mother may be more committed to resuming breastfeeding or to increasing her milk supply. However, placing emphasis *only* on her milk as evidence of success can result in increasing her anxiety and thereby inhibiting her milk production and ejection reflex. Thus the clinician needs to weigh carefully—with plenty of discussion with the mother—both the benefits and the more problematic elements of relactation (Box 17-2). The clinician should encourage the mother both at the beginning and throughout her relactation experience but should also caution that reality may not follow her expectations.

Many health workers assume that if the mother has recently been lactating, all she needs to do is to allow the baby to suckle and her breasts will promptly respond to renewed stimulation by producing ample amounts of milk. This assumption must be tempered by knowledge of the reason for the termination of breastfeeding in the first place. If the mother was ill or injured, her own health status may influence how quickly her body responds to suckling stimulation. If the baby was ill or injured, his health status will determine how often and how vigorously he is able to suckle. Additionally, his age at the time he stopped breastfeeding and his age when it is resumed will determine how willing he is to do so. Generally, a baby younger than three months old can usually be coaxed back to the breast. Between three and six months of age, individual infants may be more or less willing to do so; after six months, most babies cannot be convinced that the breast will provide either nutrition or nurturing. This fact points out poignantly that breastfeeding is a two-person activity; failure to keep this point continuously in mind in assisting the mother to relactate is likely to result in disappointment and a sense of failure that is avoidable. Realistic expectations are especially important with relactation, because many unknowns characterize the situation. Although Phillips (1993) reported six cases in which babies returned to breastfeeding after they had been weaned for an extended period of time, these babies initiated the return—again pointing out the importance of the baby in the process.

An infant seen by one of the authors screamed inconsolably when he was put to breast after six weeks of being bottle-fed. The relactation process started with finger-feeding the baby with the feeding-tube device secured to the mother's largest finger under a silicone nipple shield, which felt like a bottle nipple. After a few days, the mother was able to eliminate the nipple shield. Several days later, she moved the feeding tube to her breast and provided the infant with additional milk while her

Questions for the Mother Prior to Relactation or Induced Lactation

1. What is the *primary* reason for relactation or induced lactation?

2. What is the baby's age at the time of relactation or induced lactation?

3. How much time has elapsed since the baby's birth (if never put to breast) or since the last breastfeeding or pumping?

4. How does the mother expect to judge whether she is "successful"?

5. If the mother obtains less than a full milk supply, how does she think she will feel? How will this influence her self-esteem and acceptance of herself as a good mother?

6. Are any immediate family members strongly opposed to her attempt to relactate? If so, how does she plan to confront such opposition?

7. How does she feel about using a device or artificial formula to preserve the baby's nutritional integrity while establishing her own milk supply?

8. Are any immediate family members insisting that she relactate or induce lactation? If so, how does she feel about this?

9. How important to the mother is any increase in her milk supply?

10. If she is planning to induce lactation, does she feel that lack of a previous (successful) pregnancy or birth means she *must* breastfeed to think that she is a "normal" mother? (This is a danger signal.)

11. If she is planning to induce lactation, how does she respond when it is suggested that she consider any milk she obtains as a bonus rather than the primary reason for attempting to induce lactation?

---

milk supply began to build. Three weeks after that, she was able to eliminate the feeding-tube device completely and to breastfeed exclusively.

Induced Lactation

Sutherland and Auerbach (1985) described what they call *pseudo-induced lactation* to distinguish the mother who is still breastfeeding a birth baby while attempting to breastfeed an adopted baby. They note that some of the features of relactation apply in such a situation but that some of the same cautions applicable to adoptive mothers are also rele-

vant. A milk supply initially established by a birth baby is not a guarantee either of the establishment of a complete milk supply or of a more rapid increase in any milk supply (Auerbach & Avery, 1981). This assumption is often misunderstood, particularly by those who have experienced unrestricted biological breastfeeding and who very much want to duplicate this experience with the adopted baby. Expecting that it will be easy to breastfeed another baby in addition to a birth baby can result in frustration and an end to the induced lactation experience. Preliterate peoples have long known that it is possible to induce lactation (Jelliffe & Jelliffe, 1972).

More recently, Nemba (1994) described induced lactation by 37 women in Papua New Guinea, 34 of whom developed a milk supply. Most of these women had birthed a baby but had chosen not to breastfeed it. Others had breastfed a previous child but had not lactated for at least four months (up to several years). Perhaps because most of the women had had a previous pregnancy, which hormonally "primes" the breast for breast-feeding, their induced lactation efforts were successful. The women who had never previously lactated were given a single priming dose of intra-muscular med-roxyprogesterone (Depo-Provera), 100 mg, one week prior to being given chlorpro-mazine, 25 mg four times daily, and metoclo-pramide (Emery, 1996), 10 mg, four times daily, "until adequate lactation" was established. It is unclear how effective the medications were in assist-ing in initiating or continuing milk production. All of the women in this study were urged to put their babies to breast frequently. Support for their efforts was offered by family members and by the health workers who were assisting them. Nemba conclud-ed that high motivation, family and medical support, and encouragement were central to their success.

Defining success as the presence of milk (Hormann, 1977) continues to influence caregivers and their clients as they prepare to breastfeed the adopted infant. Except in cases in which the adopt-ed infant is found to be completely intolerant of all artificial formulas, such an emphasis is usually misplaced. It can contribute more to a sense of failure than to the enhancement of the attach-ment process, which should be the primary con-sideration for breastfeeding an adopted infant.

In some cases, the adopted baby will switch from bottle to breast fairly easily. In preparation for adopting a baby, one mother pumped her breasts for eight weeks, working up to four times a day when the baby arrived (Anderson, 1988).

When we picked up Elissa I tried nursing her right away, but she wanted nothing to do with it. We had hoped she had been with a nursing foster mother but that had obviously not been the case, and she was very definite about preferring the bottle over the breast. The next night we persuaded Elissa to take the breast by using a rubber nipple shield with a nursing supplementer tube inside the shield. Since *this seemed similar to her bottle nipple, she was willing to try it. The following day she decided the shield was too much trouble and willingly took my breast. We became a nursing couple with a mini-mum of problems. I had been expecting it to take about a month to switch from bottle to breast, and we did it in three days. I started to notice milk in my breasts after we had been nursing about four months, but the amount is minimal. I know, the most important thing is the closeness of the nursing relationship. Breastmilk is an added luxury.*

Other mothers, however, have found that adopted babies will not go to breast. One mother who obtained a baby from an overseas agency was told that her new daughter had been suckled by her birth-mother. Although the baby was then housed for five months in an orphanage and bottle-fed before being placed with her adoptive family, her new mother offered the breast. She reported that her baby reacted "in horror, as if she remem-bered having been nursed, but not by me!" It became clear that breastfeeding would not work. This mother continued to offer as much body con-tact and touching as the baby would tolerate with bottle-feedings.

With a newborn or a baby younger than one month, the usual experience is that the baby will, with little encouragement, root at and accept the breast, especially if rewarded for such behavior. Most mothers find that avoiding bottles and using a feeding-tube device that enables her to feed the baby at (if not from) the breast is all that is neces-sary to teach the baby to breastfeed. In many cases, a portion of the baby's total fluid nutritional needs will be obtained, particularly if the mother enhances opportunities for suckling stimulation with frequent breastfeedings and does not become so concerned about milk production as an indica-tor of "success" that her own anxiety inhibits her milk-ejection reflex. Many such mothers often report mild to moderate changes in menstrual cycling, some breast changes (including a feeling of fullness, a change in breast shape, and occasional leaking of milk), and other indicators of increasing milk production in the early adoptive nursing peri-od when breastfeeding occurs very frequently. These changes are an indication of rises in prolactin and oxytocin hormone levels in response to infant suckling (Amico & Finley, 1986).

Another obvious indication of an increasing supply of breastmilk is the change in infant stooling: less stool odor, a softening of the stool so that it more closely resembles the nearly liquid breastmilk stool, and a resultant lightening of the color from dark brown to mustard yellow. Because these stool changes usually occur gradually, the health care worker assisting the adoptive mother needs to remind her that they are an indication of an increase in the proportion of human milk versus artificial formula that the baby is receiving.

In a few instances, mothers have reported a cessation of menstrual bleeding, although such a response is rare; it probably reflects a highly responsive mother and a baby whose suckling pattern is both vigorous and frequent. One mother laughingly reported, "If *your* baby sucked like a vacuum cleaner, you'd get milk in a week, too!" Often the adoptive mother will find that as solid feedings increase in frequency and volume, the amount of necessary supplemental fluid declines, thereby enabling her to be like many other breastfeeding mothers whose babies suckle with varying frequency and who also enjoy solid foods and sips from a cup as they approach their first birthdays.

Even the highly motivated adoptive mother cannot be assured that she will produce milk. To do so without the benefit of a pregnancy that prepares her breasts for milk production, she more obviously depends on the suckling style of her baby: the frequency with which he is put to breast, the strength of his suckling, and the duration of each suckling episode.

The adoptive mother needs to be reminded that a recent birth and breastfeeding experience prior to the arrival of the adoptive baby is no guarantee that she will make sufficient milk to sustain the adoptive baby exclusively at the breast. The age of the birth baby, the frequency of suckling, the use of solid food use for either baby, and the age and frequency of suckling of the new baby—separately or in combination—are insufficient to explain why most women who attempt to tandem-breastfeed a birth baby and an adopted baby are unable to develop a milk supply large enough to sustain the (usually younger) adopted baby (Auerbach & Avery, 1979). One explanation may rest with the age of the birth baby for whom the milk was originally produced. The mother's milk supply and its pattern of volume increase, plateau, and gradual decline over time is a reflection of the older baby's physiological needs. In a situation in which an adopted baby is introduced and offered an opportunity to suckle, the milk-production pattern continues to "age" in concert with the older birth baby's maturation. Thus, if the mother is already at a stage where her milk volume has plateaued (which occurs at around the fourth month postpartum; Butte et al., 1984) or is declining, it may be increasingly difficult to markedly change that decrease in volume, even with the additional stimulation of a younger baby.

Keeping one's priorities clear from the outset can provide the mother and baby with a unique relationship built on the special closeness that characterizes the breastfeeding experience. The clinician who assists a family with relactation or induced lactation is in a position to observe how mother and baby must truly work together to enjoy that which cannot be duplicated with any other method of feeding. The intimacy that mother and baby derive directly from induced lactation cannot be underestimated; often, all family members benefit from the experience as they make this baby "theirs" in a way that cannot be ignored.

Autoimmune Diseases

Systemic Lupus Erythematosus

Systemic lupus erythematosus (SLE), an autoimmune disease of the connective tissues, primarily affects women of childbearing age; therefore, lactation consultants not infrequently are called upon to care for women with this problem. Because pregnancy worsens the symptoms of lupus, the diagnosis is often made at that time. The clinical presentations of lupus are remarkably diverse and include arthritic symptoms of joint redness and swelling and a butterfly rash on the cheeks and nose. Women with lupus have higher rates of miscarriage and infant prematurity. Raynaud's phenomenon is present in about 30 percent of cases. Fatigue is a major symptom, and the diagnosis of chronic fatigue syndrome and fibromyalgia may also be made concomitantly.

These women often report having an insufficient milk supply. One mother who has lupus stated that she "had never had enough milk" with all of her four children and always found it necessary to supplement feedings. Moreover, well-intentioned advice that she would have enough breastmilk if only she would breastfeed more often was frustrating to her, because she was already breastfeeding frequently. Another mother with lupus had an adequate supply of breastmilk for her first two children. She was diagnosed with lupus after the birth of her third child. This infant, unlike her other children, failed to gain adequate weight despite the fact that she was able to suckle effectively at the breast. With supplementation using a tube-feeding device, the infant started gaining weight. The mother continued supplementing her baby's breastfeedings until he was about five months old, when he began taking solid foods.

There is no single medication appropriate for lupus patients; their health problems are managed in a problem-oriented fashion. NSAIDs and corticosteroids are a widely prescribed mainstay of therapy. Breastfeeding is especially encouraged for mothers with lupus who usually suffer from fatigue; it conserves their strength and is one way to space pregnancies (Gelman, 1993).

Multiple Sclerosis

Multiple sclerosis (MS) is a progressive degenerative neurological disorder that includes such symptoms as weakness, fatigue, incoordination, paralysis, and speech and visual disturbances. It affects twice as many women as men, and the diagnosis usually is made during the reproductive years (ages 20–40). The condition is known for its unpredictability and the variability of its prognosis and symptoms; the cause is unknown. Breastfeeding for these mothers is especially important, because some element of breastmilk, perhaps the essential fatty acids, appears to protect their children from subsequently developing multiple sclerosis (Pisacane, 1994).

Pregnancy and the number of births a woman has experienced have no effect on long-term disability from MS (Poser & Poser, 1983). Studies consistently report remission of symptoms during pregnancy, followed by substantially increased exacerbation (deterioration) in the postpartum period, especially in the first three months (Worthington et al., 1994). The presence of an immunosuppressive factor in the maternal serum during the pregnancy may be protective; the subsequent drop in serum hormonal levels after birth may provoke exacerbations.

Women with MS who breastfeed are no more likely than women who do not breastfeed to alter the risk or timing of the exacerbation in the postpartum period (Nelson et al., 1988). Fatigue and exhaustion from care of the infant is a particular problem in all cases, regardless of feeding method. According to one mother (Kirshbaum, 1990, p. 864),

I was nursing every two and one-half hours around the clock; I was totally exhausted. Also I had insomnia and sometimes couldn't get back to sleep after nursing. . . . I had a bad exacerbation and my doctor prescribed a nurse who took care of both of us for two months. After that I used a babysitter, and now day care. I've recovered, but I'm still more fatigued than before my pregnancy.

Disrupted sleep, compromised nutrition, excess weight, and lack of supportive household help—all risks during the postpartum period—are more likely to result in a worsening of the disease, regardless of how the mother is feeding her baby. These mothers, especially, need household support. Acute exacerbations are often treated with adrenocorticotropic hormone and methylprednisolone. Both drugs appear in breastmilk in low concentrations.

Rheumatoid Arthritis

Rheumatoid arthritis (RA) is a chronic inflammatory disease thought to be caused by a genetically influenced autoimmune response. Symptoms include pain and swelling of the joints, pain on movement, and fatigue. RA symptoms usually go into remission during pregnancy and then relapse postpartum. The problem is greater for breastfeeding women, probably owing to their hyperprolactinemic state; prolactin has been shown to act as an immunostimulator (Brennan & Silman, 1994).

NSAIDs are used as first-line therapy to decrease pain and inflammation. Due to their erosive effect on the gastrointestinal tract, the mother also may be anemic from blood loss. Methotrexate therapy, used for severe cases, is contraindicated with breastfeeding, according to the American Academy of Pediatrics (see Chapter 6). However, only very small amounts of this drug are secreted into breastmilk (Hale, 1997). Women with RA often feel overwhelmed with fatigue both during pregnancy and postpartum (Carty et al., 1986). If the mother's hands and fingers are stiff, breastfeeding is simpler than is artificial feeding, which requires more complex movements. Although this mother needs additional rest, she still needs to continue range-of-motion exercises. Periodic rest periods and the wearing of removable braces or splints to support joints will help to reduce fatigue (Carty, Conine, & Hall, 1990).

Disabilities and Impairments

Increasing numbers of women who are physically impaired are choosing to become pregnant and to breastfeed. For physically impaired women, breastfeeding is more than the giving of good nutrition; it helps to normalize this aspect of their life experience. According to one, "You feel a fierce determination, particularly if you have a permanent disability, to show the world that you can manage on your own and prove to everyone that you are a 'competent' mother" (Nursing Mothers' Association of Australia, 1982, p. 15). Breastfeeding builds the mother's confidence and self-esteem by proving that her body is capable of nourishing her baby even though she may be able to do little else quite as easily (Minami, 1990).

In some disorders involving impaired mobility, especially those that are immunologically mediated (e.g., RA, MS, and myasthenia gravis), pregnancy may bring a period of remission followed by postpartum relapse. Often, women suffering from such a disease feel so good during their pregnancy that they take it for granted that their condition has improved. When the condition worsens after birth, it is doubly difficult because additional energy now is required to care for a new baby.

For mothers who are blind and cannot rely on visual cues, breastfeeding is a way to communicate with their infant nonvisually through touch, smell, sound, and even intuitive sensitivity (Martin, 1992). *The Womanly Art of Breastfeeding* and other materials published by La Leche League International* are available on audiotape for mothers who are visually impaired.

Clinical Implications

Disabled parents are adaptive and even ingenious in devising ways to carry out basic baby care activities. A case study (Thomson, 1995) of a mother with a congenital below-elbow limb absence describes how the mother positioned her baby at the breast. "Using her right hand, she held her breast between her thumb and fingers in the same plane as the baby's mouth, when closed. She then placed her breast in the baby's mouth by leaning forward. This mother had her older daughter help her to attach for about four months. After this, the baby was able to 'hop on' by herself." The September 1995 issue of the *Journal of Human Lactation* (vol. 7, issue 3) contains several helpful articles that describe how breastfeeding women have coped with different disabilities.

The lesson for the nurse and lactation consultant assisting mothers with disabilities is simple: creativity counts. Often the mother with a disability knows better than anyone else how important flexible thinking is in solving a problem or overcoming what may seem to be an insoluble problem. Ask for the mother's help in thinking through the situation. Together, a solution may be found. For example, three years before her baby's birth, one mother suffered a debilitating stroke, one outcome of which was substantial loss of arm and hand control and strength. She and her lactation consultant experimented with a variety of slings that the mother could put on with one hand and wear to keep her baby close to her. This was especially important when the mother had to move the baby from one room to another or out of the house, for she was fearful when she could not hang onto a handrail when going downstairs, for example. After practicing with several different positions, the lactation consultant and the mother identified alternate ways to present the breast to the baby that enabled both to be comfortable and

---

*La Leche League International, P.O. Box 4079, Schaumburg, IL 60168-4079, USA.

required a minimum of movement by the mother. By the time the baby was three months old, he had learned to help his mother by scooting up to the breast himself when placed on the bed next to her.

Good parenting occurs even when the parent is severely disabled, as long as psychosocial functioning is not a problem. Generally, these parents find that breastfeeding is more convenient than is bottle-feeding. Breastfeeding also renders caring for the infant simpler, because there is nothing to measure, prepare, pour, or sterilize. Yet friends and relatives may react negatively, concerned that the mother should not breastfeed due to her limited energy or abilities. These mothers need compassionate support and guidance more than those with normal mobility. Suggestions for the physically disabled mother and her family on breastfeeding and baby care are listed in Box 17–3.

The hospital birthing experience can be traumatic. Kopala (1989) interviewed seven mothers with mobility impairments including spina bifida, spinal-cord injury, postpolio syndrome and MS, about their birth experience in the hospital. One mother, a paraplegic, felt that her knowledge about her body and its limitation was not respected by the staff. Less than 24 hours after undergoing a cesarean section, she was told to get out of bed. She knew that without the use of both her arms—she had an intravenous line in one—she was "dead weight" and was therefore afraid of being dropped or hurt.

Because the disabled mother usually is under continuing medical care and has so many needs, the health professional working with the disabled breastfeeding mother may find her role expanding to that of a case manager; she coordinates medical, family, and community support and services (Bowles, 1991). If the mother has someone to help her with the physical tasks, diplomatically arrange for that person to take over the household jobs and care of older children and let the mother take care of her baby. Everyone loves to take care of the new baby (rather than mopping the floor), but when others take over such care, the mother's role and her self-confidence diminish.

Because many of these mothers are already on medications, the physician should be consulted about the safety of taking specific medications while breastfeeding. Most medications are compatible with breastfeeding (see Chapter 6), especially with short-term use. If the physician recommends weaning, the health care provider should research the drug using up-to-date references and, if necessary, act as an advocate for the mother in her desire to continue to breastfeed.

For peer support, set up group sessions that include any woman who has a disability and has given birth in the last five years. The purpose of these sessions is to provide information about coping with the demands placed on them by pregnancy, birthing, and early infant care and about allowing the more experienced women to serve as mother-to-mother role models for those women having a first child.

When first encountering a disabled mother who needs help with breastfeeding, it is easy for the caregiver to feel overwhelmed and inadequate. Having had the disability for a long time, the mother usually is more knowledgeable than anyone else about her problem (both her abilities and limitations); the health care provider may not be. The reality of these feelings should be shared with the mother. The majority of disabled women do not require frequent hospitalizations; thus nurses typically lack experience with these clients (Kopala, 1989). If they have experience in working with disabled individuals, it usually is in an institutional setting. Nurses and health professionals can learn a great deal from the mother who has developed extraordinary survival skills to work around inconveniences. For example, a mother known to the authors has no left hand and lower arm, yet she tends to breastfeed her baby on her left side, propping her baby against her upper left arm so that her right hand is free. This mother also needs a battery or electric pump, not a hand-operated device, to express her milk.

Reinforcing the disabled mother's abilities while supporting her against possible negative attitudes can make a positive difference. When the nurse assists the aforementioned mother in the home, she, rather than the mother, is the guest. This requires a role change that may take some adjustment. Self-care presumes an optimal level of functioning as its goal. Functioning at an optimal level can occur for the physically disabled mother who desires to breastfeed her infant as much as for any mother.

BOX 17–3

Baby Care Guidelines for Physically Disabled, Breastfeeding Mothers

- Mothers with some upper-body strength who are confined to a wheelchair can use a harness or a wide belt with long strip of Velcro to lift and retrieve a crawling baby from the floor.
- Set up one or two special "feeding nests" for breastfeeding that are easily accessible and comfortable for the mother. Group together a crib or other sleeping place for the infant, diaper-changing supplies, and a comfortable place to breastfeed.
- If the baby is small, he can be laid diagonally across the mother's knees on a pillow to breastfeed. Put other pillows under the mother's arms for support. Elevate the mother's feet on a footrest to keep the infant secure during the feeding.
- A mother who cannot elevate her feet can rest her forearm holding the infant on a pillow placed across her knees. This arrangement ensures that if the infant rolls, he will roll toward the mother.
- Changing tables and cribs can be adapted so that they are accessible to a wheelchair, and the room can be arranged so that moving about is minimized. A low-sided pram or baby stroller makes it easier to slide the baby out onto the mother's lap without requiring much lifting.
- A baby sling allows the mother's arms to be free while ensuring that the baby is safe and supported during breastfeeding. This is also helpful when the mother has unilateral weakness or paralysis (e.g., as from a stroke).
- A bell tied to the baby's shoes keeps track of where the mobile child is.
- A toddler will quickly learn to climb on his mother's knee for a ride and to sit still while the chair is moving.
- The baby can be given extra cuddling, such as touching at night in bed, if there are barriers to physical contact during the day.
- A baby clothed in overalls with crossed straps can be picked up fairly easily.
- The mother's use of a nursing bra that opens in the front instead of the back, one with an easy-to-fasten clip or Velcro that can be handled with one hand, will facilitate breastfeeding. The usual clip for opening and closing the bra flap can be replaced with Velcro. Some all-elastic bras are easily pulled down to allow the baby to breastfeed.
- Maternity clothes can be altered to incorporate Velcro openings or large ring zippers. Antique buttonhooks are helpful to manipulate the small buttons found on many garments.
- The mother should plan rest periods during the day and should sit to work whenever possible.
- The mother can sleep with the infant or have the father or someone else bring the baby to her to nurse during the night.
- Use of an intercom system that picks up the sound of the baby crying is helpful. If the mother is deaf, the sound can be transformed into flashing light signals.
- If the mother cannot lift both the baby and herself, she might spend the day on

the floor (preferably carpeted) feeding, changing, and playing with him. This enables her to roll the baby to her, instead of lifting him, when he needs attention. A beanbag will provide support for breastfeeding.

Source: Derived from: TA Conine, E Carty, PH Safarik: Aids and adaptations for parents with physical or sensory disabilities. *Vancouver, BC: School of Rehabilitative Medicine, University of British*

Columbia, 1988:67–71; Nursing Mothers' Association of Australia: Where there's a will, there's usually a way—breastfeeding when the mother has a disability. *Hawthorn, Victoria, Australia: The Association, 1982; M Kirshbaum: The parent with a physical disability. In: JM Auvenshine, MG Enriques:* Comprehensive maternity nursing: perinatal and women's health. *Boston: Jones & Bartlett, 1990; J Minami: Helping mothers with chronic illness,* Leaven *26:52–3, 1990; MM Coates, J Riordan: Breastfeeding during maternal or infant illness.* Clin Iss Perin Wom Health Nursing; *3:683–94, 1992.*

Until recently, limited information was available regarding breastfeeding (and all other aspects of childbearing) among women with disabilities. Unfortunately, society's general view remains that women with a physical disability are not capable of having or caring for a child. Even now, only a few resources for these families exist. Two are La Leche League International and Nursing Mothers' Association of Australia. Both organizations have educational materials, including audiocassette tapes and braille material, for the physically disabled mother who is breastfeeding. These organizations will also refer the mother to another woman who has had a similar experience.

Seizure Disorders

Seizure disorders are now classified into two major classes: partial and generalized. Partial or focal seizures begin in a specific area of the brain and produce symptoms ranging from simple repetitive movements to more complex abnormal movement and bizarre behavior. Generalized seizures have no specific point of origin in the brain. The most common type is a major motor seizure, formerly called *grand mal epilepsy.* Anticonvulsants appear in human milk in much reduced concentrations, as compared with maternal serum. Breastfeeding should be encouraged, keeping in mind that neonatal sedation can occur if the mother is receiving high doses of phenobarbitone, primidone, or one of the benzodiazepines. Brodie (1990) recommended that anticonvulsant therapy be tapered off prior to conception to avoid the higher risk of teratogenicity that such drugs pose.

Seizure disorders can be so well controlled by medications that seizures are rarely a problem for the lactating mother. However, nurses need to know about the effect of the medication on the breastfed infant. The physician will prescribe antiseizure medications on the basis of diagnosis of the seizure and its pattern of occurrence and on the tolerance and response of the mother to the prescribed drug.

Most antiepileptic drugs are generally considered compatible with breastfeeding. Common medications are phenytoin (Dilantin), carbamazepine (Tegretol), primidone (Mysoline), and phenobarbital. Phenobarbital taken in higher-than-average amounts (50–100 mg two or three times daily), however, may cause drowsiness in infants or mothers; primidone may also cause sedation in the infant. For example, an estimated maximal dose of carbamazepine that the breastfed baby would consume in breastmilk is 3 to 5 percent of the weight-adjusted maternal dose, an amount similar to other drugs, such as phenytoin and valproic acid. Consensus guidelines among neurologists state that taking antiepileptic drugs (except for such sedatives as phenobarbital, primidone, or benzodiazepine) does not constitute a contraindication for breast-feeding (Delgado-Escueta & Janz, 1992). Although monitoring the infant is important for detecting idiosyncratic reactions, the risk of these reactions appears to be outweighed by the benefits of breast-feeding (Ito et al., 1995).

In the unusual case in which the mother has seizures, breastfeeding is in no way contraindicated. Dropping or harming the infant during a seizure is no more probable during breastfeeding than it is during bottle-feeding. Usually, a prodromal warning (aura) alerts the mother of an impending seizure, and she is able to take safety precautions to protect her infant (Box 17–4). Despite the view in favor of breastfeeding for women with seizure disorder, women receiving antiepileptics tend to choose formula feeding. Even when they begin breastfeeding, its duration is shorter than usual (Ito et al., 1995). In this same study, the mother was more likely to choose breast-feeding if she was encouraged by her physician to do so.

Headaches

Migraine headaches, hormonally sensitive headaches of an episodic nature, tend to worsen during the first trimester of pregnancy, improving through the course of pregnancy (Silberstein, 1993). Postpartum headaches can be caused by oral contraceptives or by having epidural or spinal anesthesia during childbirth, or they can occur for no apparent reason. Some women, for example, have a brief but intense headache when they have an orgasm. It is thought that rise in blood pressure and heart rate during intercourse are similar to the physiological process that produces migraine.

Several case reports associate breastfeeding with postpartum headaches. No specific pattern of causation emerges from these reports. Thorley (1997) reported a case in which the mother had chronic migraine headaches that appeared to be related first to overfulness of the breast and later to her menstrual cycle. This mother had a history of whiplash injury some years before. Trigger factors for migraine headaches in breastfeeding women have been described as oxytocin surge at let-down (Askmark & Lundberg, 1989; Lawrence, 1989), baby sleeping through the night (Thorley, 1997),

> **BOX 17–4**
>
> ## Guidelines for a Breastfeeding Mother with a Seizure Disorder
>
> 1. Have available on each level of the house a playpen in which to quickly place the baby when a seizure seems imminent.
> 2. Pad with extra pillows and cushions for protection the arms of the rocker or chair where the mother usually breastfeeds.
> 3. Place guardrails padded with pillows around the mother's bed if she customarily takes her infant to bed to breastfeed.
> 4. Attach to the baby and to the stroller or baby carrier tags stating that the mother has a seizure disorder, along with other pertinent information, whenever she is away from home.

and breastfeeding twins (Wall, 1992). Rest and ice packs should be tried before resorting to medications. Propranolol (Inderal) and NSAIDs are standard drugs used for migraine headaches. Scharff et al. (1996) studied the effects of nonpharmacological treatment (biofeedback, relaxation training, and physical therapy) on pregnant women who suffered from headaches. Both the breastfeeding and nonbreastfeeding women in the study who were treated experienced fewer headaches postpartum.

Postpartum Depression

Postpartum depression is a generic term that describes three types of disorders (the word *depression* is probably a misnomer, because anxiety and agitation are just as common with postpartum mood disorder as are typical signs of depression, such as withdrawal and lethargy):

- *The postpartum "blues":* About 70 to 80 percent of women experience a transient depression following birth, usually starting on the third postpartum day and lasting for a few days. The "blues" is temporary, accompanied by lability of mood, tearfulness, and negative feelings and is more common in women having their first child.

- *Postpartum depression:* As many as 20 percent of postpartum women have mild to moderate depression. Symptoms are tearfulness, despondency, feelings of inadequacy, suicidal ideation, sadness, reduced appetite, insomnia, feelings of helplessness and hopelessness, anxiety, and despair. Because every new mother experiences at least some of these symptoms that may be wrongly interpreted as clinical depression, this percentage may be inflated. This type of depression lasts at least two weeks but usually longer.

- *Postpartum psychosis:* The most severe of the postpartum disorders, psychosis typically begins within two to four weeks postpartum. The mother with postpartum psychotic depression may have insomnia, irrational ideas, feelings of failure, self-accusatory thoughts, depression, fatigue, and hallucinations; sometimes, she may threaten to commit suicide.

New mothers with high levels of life stress and few supportive relationships (especially with husband or partner) suffer more from postpartum depression. There is no consistent evidence that the mother's age, the number of children she has, or complications during the pregnancy and delivery are associated with the appearance of depression. Although mothers of preterm infants are more anxious and depressed than are mothers of term infants in the first week following birth, this difference does not last beyond the first week (Gennaro, 1988).

Postpartum hormonal shifts, although dramatic, appear to play no clear role in postpartum depression (Beck, 1993). To ascribe depression to biological variables is to miss the point: we need to look at society's failure to give adequate social support to mothers. Maternal hormonal levels during lactation represent the *normal postpartum state;* thus breastfeeding women should be at no greater risk for postpartum depression because their hormone levels are different from those in nonlactating women (Auerbach & Jacobi, 1990), particularly if this pattern of mothering is supported. Prolonged maternal depression has an adverse effect on children's general behavior and developmental functioning (Cogill et al., 1986).

One Australian study (Astbury et al., 1994) found that having a first child when the mother was older than 34, having an assisted delivery (cesarean, forceps, or vacuum extraction), bottle-feeding, dissatisfaction with some aspect of her care during pregnancy, having unwanted people present at the birth (such as medical students), lacking confidence in her ability to care for the baby on hospital discharge, and not having an active say in decision making (losing control) were all significantly associated with depression in the postpartum period. Tamminen (1989) noted that breastfeeding per se did not appear to be a problem for the mothers in the sample who had symptoms of depression. Rather, these mothers reported having more difficulty with breastfeeding than did the nondepressed mothers. Having twins—particularly if one dies—may contribute to postpartum depression, according to Thorpe et al. (1991). In their study, a significantly higher proportion of mothers of twins were depressed than was the case of mothers who had singletons, even if the singletons were closely spaced, presumably because of additional stress. Increased obstetric risk, congenital abnormalities, perinatal mortality of one of the babies, and the like may have long-term effects on the mother's emotional health.

Beck (1992) conducted a phenomenological study of the lived experience of women with postpartum depression. Eleven themes emerged from interviews with mothers:

loneliness
obsessive thinking
insecurities

anxiety attacks
loss of control
guilt
diminished concentration
fear that life would never be normal again
loss of interest in hobbies or goals
lack of all positive emotion
contemplation of death

Through further study, Beck (1993) found that loss of control was the basic social psychological problem in postpartum depression. One mother said, "I had absolutely no control and that was the scariest thing because I always had control." Another woman said, "I just couldn't get out of the pain. It's like you hurt so bad and you don't want to be that way and yet you lost all control of everything."

Women who experienced postpartum depression attempted to cope with the problem of loss of control through a four-stage process: encountering terror, dying of self, struggling to survive, and regaining control. When depression started, these mothers felt trapped with no foreseeable escape. "One night I had my first severe panic attack. I felt like everything was closing in on me. Something just snapped in me, and there was no going back." Mothers described this period as "going to the gates of hell and back," and "your worst possible nightmare." As the mothers regained control, gradually the number of good days experienced increased; yet they mourned the lost time they would not be able to recapture with their infants. When the mothers recovered, they talked about how their symptoms just eventually faded away. "When I was sick, I didn't want my baby. I didn't love my husband. I didn't want to work. I hated everything. When I got better, it all melted away" (Beck, 1993).

Psychotic depression or psychosis is rare, occurring in about one or two of every 1,000 women who have a child (Lindstrom et al., 1984). The onset of the psychosis occurs within a few days to two weeks after delivery, and symptoms peak at about six weeks postpartum.

Hardly any problem is more distressing to all concerned than a mother suffering from postpartum depression psychosis. The family is in a state of severe crisis and disequilibrium and suffers from lack of sleep. If the mother is breastfeeding, the consulting therapist often insists that the mother wean her baby because of undue concern about a prescribed medication passing through the breastmilk. If the mother needs constant observation, there is the additional threat of hospitalization and separation, because most psychiatric facilities do not allow the infant to remain with the mother.

The decision whether to hospitalize this mother or to wean the baby is agonizing. Care of the infant and possibly other children is an immediate concern. A severe maternal depression also can have a dramatic effect on the infant. Following a suicide attempt by his mother, a 12-month-old toddler suddenly refused any nourishment other than what he received from breastfeeding. All attempts to entice him into eating foods that he had formerly enjoyed were firmly refused for several months. He may have sensed that his becoming totally dependent on his mother for food would ensure her continued presence.

Clinical Implications

Postpartum depression tends to occur when the maternal-infant bond is being formed. Every effort should be made to foster this crucial bond and breastfeeding as well. The mother with depression suffers a loss of maternal identity and self-esteem. When the infant stays with the mother, the mother recovers more quickly and has a lower relapse rate (Waletzky, 1981).

Mothers at risk for postpartum depression usually display emotional problems very soon after the birthing experience. In fact, experienced maternity nurses can usually identify the mothers who are likely to become depressed. Typically, this mother has difficulty bonding with her baby and will make self-accusatory remarks, such as, "I am a terrible person" or "I have a lovely baby, a lovely house, and a lovely husband, and I know I should be happy, yet I feel awful." Kitzinger (1989) reminds us that

Few women are prepared for the resentment, the sense of inadequacy, the guilt, anger and murderous feelings we have as mothers. There is delight, discovery and joy, and sometimes sheer ecstasy, too, and that makes it all worth while. But the trouble is that the image of motherhood is romanticized.

With early postpartum discharge, however, the hospital staff is only able to assess the problem;

their most helpful intervention is to refer the family for follow-up care. Several screening tools are available. Affonso et al. (1990) developed a standardized interview that differentiates postpartum symptoms and pregnancy from postpartum clinical depression. Their interview is especially helpful, because it separates normal and abnormal changes and stresses of childbearing. Certain factors appear to increase the risk of a mother's developing postpartum depression: the greater the number of these factors present, the greater the risk. Beck (1996) also developed a screening tool to identify women who are at risk for depression. Kendall-Tackett and Kantor (1993) offered a model of multiple possible causes of postpartum depression:

- Stressful life events during pregnancy and postpartum
- Postpartum pain and negative birth events
- Constant fatigue and lack of sleep
- A history of maladjustment or inability to cope with stress
- Lack of caring support from a partner or husband
- Lack of a network of social support from relatives or close friends
- A colicky, "difficult" infant (infant temperament)

Health professionals vary in their knowledge about postpartum depression. Nurses tend to be more aware of postpartum depression than are physicians in that they better understand the disorder's impact on the mother and her family. For a clinical care plan for depression, see Table 17–2. Younger, female physicians tend to be more aware of the psychosocial antecedents to postpartum depression than are older, male physicians (Lepper et al., 1994). If the mother has severe symptoms, she should be referred to a psychiatrist, psychologist, or advanced-practice nurse who will probably initiate drug therapy. The risks and benefits of any particular agent must be carefully evaluated. Most of these medications do not pass into the breastmilk in quantities sufficient to harm the infant.

Medications commonly used to control symptoms of postpartum depression are fluoxetine (Prozac), sertraline (Zoloft), and paroxetine (Paxil). These drugs are serotonin-selective reuptake inhibitors (SSRIs) that inhibit neuronal reuptake of serotonin. Their advantages include wide therapeutic range, a greater margin of safety, and fewer side effects than other drugs used to treat depression. Unlike tricyclics, which have an ascending dose curve, the SSRIs have a flat dose curve; thus the starting dose is often the same as the therapeutic dose. Sertraline has the least drug-interaction potential among the SSRIs. Venlafaxine (Effexor), another drug often used in postpartum depression, combines the SSRI action with that of norepinephrine reuptake inhibitors, such as desipramine. A list of medications used in postpartum depression is found in Table 17–3.

Such phenothiazines as perphenazine (Trilafon), such antianxiety drugs as alprazolam (Xanax), and such tricyclic antidepressants as imipramine (Tofranil) or nortriptyline (Pamelor) are also used for postpartum depression. With the exception of monoamine oxidase (MAO) inhibitors, these medications appear to be relatively safe for short-term therapy. The dosage of tricyclics is slowly increased over several days to minimize side effects. Sedation and other side effects may begin at once, but the antidepressant response occurs only after 10 to 21 days at full therapeutic dosage. MAO inhibitors may produce a mild stimulation effect almost at once, but again, full therapeutic benefit may take two to six weeks. Antidepressants need not be continued indefinitely, and the drug will be discontinued after the mother has been asymptomatic for several weeks. Both tricyclics and MAO inhibitors are highly toxic in overdose. As a general rule, the health care provider will limit the prescription to a 7- to 10-day supply.

Chlorpromazine (Thorazine), a tranquilizer, has been prescribed for manic disorders in breastfeeding mothers. Chlorpromazine passes into the milk in minute quantities and may actually increase milk production by blocking the prolactin-inhibitory factor. Lithium, sometimes prescribed for manic-depressive states, may be used with caution if the mother's and infant's serum levels are closely monitored (Schou, 1990).

Social support is a critical intervening variable in the relationship between postpartum depression

Table 17–2

CLINICAL CARE PLAN

Assessment	Intervention	Rationale
History of postpartum depression	Listen to mother describe her feelings	Postpartum depression is likely to recur with subsequent births.
Beyond first week postpartum: tearfulness, mood swings, feelings of failure, insomnia, fatigue, anxiety, suicidal thoughts	Maintain a supportive and non-judgmental attitude	Clinical depression occurs in about 20 percent of mothers.
	Maintain mother's privacy and let her cry	Role changes and increased responsibilities cause stress.
	Assist in providing social support and physical help for mother and infant	
Possible disinterest in baby	Monitor baby's weight gain and general well-being	Infant may not be receiving adequate nurturing and care due to mother's depression.
Depression worsens	Refer to therapist for counseling and evaluation for medication therapy	Antidepressant or antianxiety drugs are effective in treating depression.
Mother taking medication for depression and wants to continue breastfeeding	Research the effect of the medication on the breastfeeding infant; recommend optional medications, if necessary	Most medications are safe to take while breastfeeding.

Note: Nursing diagnosis: Coping, ineffective individual, related to stress or potential complications of perinatal period and to life changes.

and breastfeeding (Wolman et al., 1993). A support group of women with postpartum depression introduces the mother to women who have recovered from postpartum depression and helps to counter the isolation and loneliness these mothers feel. This support is especially crucial for mothers who are relatively housebound and likely to be drained by the demands of child care. A friend of the mother, a neighbor, a La Leche League chapter, or a church group are all possible supports.

Many countries already have supportive systems for these mothers built into their health care. Handford (1985) describes an effective Canadian system of self-help support programs for mothers suffering from postpartum depression. In Australia, hospital-based postnatal groups are offered (Stamp et al., 1995). Support people not only provide individual help, but also play a key role in facilitating the mother's peer relationship with other mothers. Reducing the social isolation of the depressed mother reinforces her identity and ability to cope. The quality of the marital relationship is of primary importance in the mother's postpartum adaptation, especially for first-time mothers. Because the father plays a key role, he should also be counseled and supported. If the mother or father are sleep deprived, every effort should be made to devise a plan by which they may sleep for at least six hours and thus benefit from the restoration of sleep.

Table 17–3

DRUGS USED FOR POSTPARTUM DEPRESSION

Drug Name	Usual Daily Oral Dosage (mg)	Use in Breastfeeding Mother and Safety Level
Serotonin-selective reuptake inhibitors		
Fluoxetine (Prozac)	10–40	Infants receive 5–9% of maternal dose; one case report of infant colic and fussiness
Paroxetine (Paxil)	20–50	Effect not known as yet
Sertaline (Zoloft)	50–150	No apparent adverse effects reported
Serotonin-norepinephrine reuptake inhibitor		
Venlafaxine (Effexor)	75–300	Effect not known as yet
Antianxiety drugs (benzodiazepines)		
Aprazolam (Xanax)	0.75–0.4	Use with caution; may accumulate in infant; do not use in first week.
Diazepam (Valium)	0.5–40	Same as for aprazolam
Tricyclics		
Amitriptyline (Elavil)	50–300	Safe; no effects on infants reported; no apparent accumulation in nursing infant.
Desipramine (Norpramin)	50–300	Relatively safe
Imipramine (Tofranil)	50–300	Relatively safe; infant would receive approximately 0.04 mg/kg/day; recommended initial therapeutic dosage for children, 1 mg/kg/day
Nortriptyline (Pamelor)	25–100	Safe; not detected in serum of infant
Monoamine oxidase inhibitors		
Phenelzine (Nardil)	15–90	Contraindicated; inhibits lactation
Tranylcypromine (Parnate)	10–30	Use with caution
Phenothiazines		
Chlorpromazine (Thorazine)	30–1000	Relatively safe if average dosage; one report of infant drowsiness with high dosage; may increase mother's milk supply
Mesoridazine (Serentil)	100–400	Relatively safe
Perphenazine (Trilafon)	4–6	Safe; dose passed to child through milk is only 0.1% that given the mother
Thioridazine (Mellaril)	150–800	Relatively safe

Source: Data from J Riordan: Drugs excreted in breastmilk. In: L Pagliaro, AM Pagliaro: Problems in pediatric drug therapy *(2nd ed). Drug Intelligence, 1987; T Hale:* Medications and mothers' milk *(6th ed). Pharmasoft Medical Publishing, 1997; GB Lipkin: Drug therapy in maternal care. In: RT Spencer, et al:* Clinical pharmacology and nursing management *(3rd ed). Philadelphia: Lippincott, 1989:1132–70.*

Asthma

About 1 percent of pregnant women have active asthma that may improve, worsen, or remain unchanged during pregnancy (D'Alonzo, 1990). The course of asthma appears to be influenced by the gestational time; it is likely to worsen during the late second trimester, improve during the last four weeks of pregnancy, and revert back to the prepregnancy course within the first three months postpartum.

Lactation appears to influence the course of asthma. The main concern is the effect of medications taken by the mother to control her asthma. Asthma therapy should be continued during lactation and generally does not have to be altered (D'Alonzo, 1990). The two central classes of anti-asthmatic medications are corticosteroids and bronchodilators, including beta-agonists and theophyllines. Beta-agonists (terbutaline, metaproterenol, isoproterenol) are used to treat acute exacerbations and to prevent exercise-induced asthma. Most antiasthma medications are administered by metered-dose inhalers that avoid systemic side effects by delivering the drug directly to the lungs. Metered aerosol inhalers deliver a given amount of a drug, and the likelihood of overdose is small. Halogenated corticosteroids given by inhalation provide selective topical effects that lessen the amount of corticosteroids transferred into breastmilk. Although theophylline is secreted in breastmilk, the infant receives only a small percentage (<10 percent) of the maternal dose (Ellsworth, 1994). Theophylline (Tho-Dur, Slo-BID, Slo-phyllin) taken by the breastfeeding mother may occasionally result in infant irritability and insomnia, necessitating a decrease in the maternal dosage or temporary withdrawal (Yurchak, 1976).

Smoking

Smoking is an addiction; it affects the mother's general health and reduces the amount of milk she makes (Horta et al., 1997; Said et al., 1984; Vio et al., 1991; Widström et al., 1991). Furthermore, women who have a preterm baby and who smoke not only produce less milk over time but often find that their production declines rather than increases. When Hopkinson et al. (1992) measured the fat content of the milk of smoking and nonsmoking mothers of preterms, they found that the creamy portion of the milk was lower in the milk of the smoking mothers. They speculated that both production problems and lower fat content in the milk of mothers who smoke may contribute to earlier weaning. Another potential consequence is slower infant rate of weight gain as the number of cigarettes smoked by the mother increases (Nafstad et al., 1997).

Although nursing mothers tend to take fewer drugs of any kind than do nonbreastfeeding women, weaning occurs earlier when the mother is a smoker, usually exhibiting an inverse dose relationship (Matheson et al., 1990; Woodward & Hand, 1988). Even the milk of nonsmokers has been found to include nicotine through passive exposure to the smoke of others (Trundle & Skellern, 1983). Nicotine concentrations—and those of its metabolite, cotinine—increase markedly in breastmilk immediately after smoking (Dahlström et al., 1990). The half-life of nicotine in milk is 97 ± 20 minutes (Luck & Nau, 1984). Steldinger and Luck (1988) reported that levels of nicotine are higher in the mother's milk than in her serum; although both levels decline over time, the investigators recommend that breastfeeding mothers prolong the period between cigarette smoking and breastfeeding to reduce the amount of nicotine to which the baby is exposed.

The mother who smokes also exposes her infant to second-hand smoke that raises inhaled carbon monoxide to unsafe levels, aggravates allergies, and increases the risk of respiratory illnesses (Bonham & Wilson, 1981; Horta et al., 1997; Luck & Nau, 1985). Maternal cigarette smoking is associated with a 20 to 35 percent increase in respiratory illnesses and may have a deleterious effect on children's growth (Rona et al., 1981). She is also at greater risk for breast abscess (Bundred, 1992).

In many cases, women who have been moderate or heavy smokers will use their pregnancy as a motivation to reduce or stop smoking. Black women are more likely to quit when they become pregnant. In a study of pregnant women who smoked, 35 percent of the less-educated black women stopped smoking during their pregnancy, whereas only 13 percent of less-educated white women quit (O'Campo & Faden, 1992). The negative influence of smoking on breastfeeding needs to

BOX 17–5

Reducing an Infant's Radiation Exposure from the Breast-feeding Mother

1. Ensure that the investigation is essential; avoid unnecessary tests.

2. Request that the physician reduce the dose to the minimum required to obtain a diagnostic result.

3. Change the radiopharmaceutical to one with less concentration in the milk or other more favorable dosimetric properties, including a shorter half-life.

4. Balance the inconvenience and disadvantage of interrupting breastfeeding against the potential risk of exposure to the infant.

5. Consider interruption of breast-feeding rather than weaning baby from the breast.

Source: AJ Coakley, PJ Mountford: Nuclear medicine and the nursing mother. Br Med J *291(6489): 160, 1985.*

frequency of their smoking. This may be important to consider when attempting to rule out factors that may contribute to inadequate milk production or compromised infant growth.

Diagnostic Studies Using Radioisotopes

The degree of interference with lactation from radioactive drugs depends in part on the proposed dose and on the radioactive element to be used. Such elements as iodide are selectively concentrated in human milk; thus their use may interrupt breastfeeding for a longer period (Romney et al., 1989). Studies using radioactive isotopes usually require that breastfeeding be interrupted until nearly all radioactivity is excreted, to avoid its passage to the infant. Most studies use an isotope such as technetium 99, which has a short half-life (four hours) (Evans et al., 1993). Iodine isotopes (^{123}I and ^{131}I) have much longer half-lives, and breastfeeding has to be interrupted for a longer period (Robinson et al., 1994).

Gallium-67 requires two weeks before nursing is safe to resume. In one study, pumping the breasts did not appreciably reduce the radioactivity of the milk during the period when the mother had to interrupt breastfeeding for her baby's protection against the radioisotopes to which the mother was exposed (Weiner & Spencer, 1994). In some cases, transmission can occur directly from the mother even when she cuddles the baby (Coakley & Mountford, 1985). Ways to reduce the effects of radiation therapy are seen in Box 17–5. A list of radiopharmaceuticals and the approximate length of time they are present in human milk is given in Table 17–1.

The Impact of Maternal Illness and Hospitalization

Hospitalization of a mother is a traumatic experience for all members of the family. A mother faced with separation from her infant, whether brief or prolonged, is a mother in crisis. For the breastfeeding woman and her infant, it is essential that ongoing, intimate, and regular contact be maintained. A mother with an acute illness is now more likely to be treated as an outpatient rather than to be hospitalized. As a result, separation because of hospital-

be shared with the mother; such knowledge may serve to strengthen her resolve to continue to reduce her use of nicotine or to stop altogether. Self-reports of nicotine use tend to correlate poorly with laboratory tests (Little et al., 1986), suggesting that these women are not always truthful about the

ization is not as frequent a barrier to breastfeeding as it was a few years ago.

During a postpartum illness, the baby should be allowed to room-in with the mother or at least be brought to her for breastfeeding at frequent intervals during her hospitalization. Nurses and lactation consultants can be advocates for changing policies and for relaxing hospital restrictions that place an unnecessary additional hardship on families. For example, when the mother has a postpartum depression, denying the disturbed woman access to her infant can trigger a justifiable paranoia in addition to whatever thought disorder is already present.

A mother who is chronically or acutely ill may find that the decisions about her health care and advice regarding breastfeeding are divided among her obstetrician, the baby's pediatrician, and the medical specialist. Sometimes, such other health care professionals as the dietitian, the nurse practitioner, or the physician's assistant are involved. Even when all agree that breastfeeding is desirable, childbirth may be riskier for the mother and infant, and they are more likely to be separated postpartum. Although it is possible to establish breastfeeding after an initial separation, it can be more difficult, especially if the separation lasts more than a few days (Coates & Riordan, 1992). Moreover, when an illness such as lupus or hypothyroidism is associated with a reduced milk supply, the mother is further traumatized when she is lectured about breastfeeding more often and about "supply and demand" when the care provider does not first assess the total picture and the possibility that she is already breastfeeding frequently.

Chronic illnesses present a somewhat different potential dilemma for the breastfeeding mother and the clinician assisting her. In some cases, the nature of the chronic illness and its effect on the mother's functioning may interfere to a greater or lesser extent with her ability to breastfeed. In other cases, creative alternatives to "usual" solutions are all that is needed to give the mother the opportunity to experience the same infant feeding as do other mothers who do not have a chronic illness. Additionally, drug therapy, particularly because it is likely to be long-term, may pose risks to the breastfeeding infant that are not an issue if the mother has an acute, self-limiting illness. Thus the clinician needs to look beyond the illness itself and examine how the condition is being managed and what the mother wants to do, given complete information relating to the risks and benefits of breastfeeding to herself and her baby in light of her chronic illness. In many cases, the therapy of choice need not be changed, because it poses no dangers for the suckling infant.

Care must be taken to accurately interpret the mother's desire to begin or to continue breastfeeding when faced with uncommon difficulties or situations. Occasionally, when an illness or a breastfeeding problem occurs, health professionals may be asked to give permission to wean to a woman who no longer wants to continue breastfeeding. Even if there is no reason to wean, a relatively minor difficulty can occasionally present a mother with a socially acceptable "out" from a situation that she finds emotionally uncomfortable or finds inconvenient for her lifestyle. For the health care worker who is enthusiastic about breastfeeding, personal feelings and the knowledge of the benefits of breastfeeding may conflict with the subtle response from the client that suggests she would rather wean. Typically, the comment–that the physician, lactation consultant, or nurse "told me to wean" because of a problem–may partially reflect the mother's own desires. Avoiding judgmental responses and encouraging her to air conflicting feelings may enable the mother to place her breastfeeding experience in context, so that she can focus on the positive aspects of her experience rather than on its more problematic elements.

SUMMARY

This chapter reviewed health conditions that relate to the lactating mother and suggested interventions that facilitate the lactation process. Admittedly, this discussion does not include the full range of acute or chronic disease that the health professional will find in practice. To find information on other health problems that the mother may develop while she is lactating, we recommend several excellent gynecological and medical-surgical texts for physicians and nurses that more thoroughly discuss the conditions described here and others not addressed.

REFERENCES

Affonso D, et al: A standardized interview that differentiates pregnancy and postpartum symptoms from perinatal clinical depression. *Birth* 17:121–30, 1990.

AAP 1997 Red book: Report of the Committee on Infectious Diseases, 24th ed. Elk Grove Village, IL: AAP, 1997.

American Academy of Pediatrics: Work Group on Cow's Milk Protein and Diabetes Mellitus: Infant feeding practices and their possible relationship to the etiology of diabetes mellitus. *Pediatrics* 94:752–4, 1994.

American Diabetes Association: Clinical practice recommendations. *Diabetes Care* 20(suppl)S5–41, 1997.

Amico JA, Finley BE: Breast stimulation in cycling women, pregnant women and a woman with induced lactation: pattern of release of oxytocin, prolactin and luteinizing hormone. *Clin Endocrinol* 25:97–106, 1986.

Anderson K: Nursing my adopted daughter. *New Beginnings* 4:108, 1988.

Arthur PG, Kent JC, Hartman PE: Metabolites of lactose synthesis in milk from diabetic and non-diabetic women during lactogenesis II. *J Pediatr Gastroenterol Nutr* 19:100–8, 1994.

Askmark H, Lundberg PO: Lactation headache–a new form of headache? *Cephalalgia* 9:119–22, 1989.

Astbury J, et al: Birth events, birth experiences and social differences in postnatal depression. *Aust J Public Health* 18:176–84, 1994.

Auerbach KG: Extraordinary breast feeding: relactation/induced lactation. *J Trop Pediatr* 27:52–5, 1981.

Auerbach KG, Avery JL: Induced lactation: a study of adoptive nursing by 24 women. *Am J Dis Child* 135:340–3, 1981.

Auerbach KG, Avery JL: Nursing the adopted infant: report from a survey. *RHNI Monograph 5,* 1979.

Auerbach KG, Avery JL: Relactation: a study of 366 cases. *Pediatrics* 65: 236–42, 1980.

Auerbach KG, Jacobi A: Postpartum depression in the breastfeeding mother. *Clin Iss in Perin Wom Health Nurs* 1:375–84, 1990.

Beck CT: Screening methods for postpartum depression. *JOGNN* 24:308–12, 1996.

Beck CT: Teetering on the edge: a substantive theory of postpartum depression. *Nurs Res* 42:42–48, 1993.

Beck CT: The lived experience of postpartum depression: a phenomenological study. *Nurs Res* 41:166–70, 1992.

Bitman J, et al: Lipid composition of milk from mothers with cystic fibrosis. *Pediatrics* 80:927–32, 1987.

Bitman J, et al: Milk composition and volume during the onset of lactation in a diabetic mother. *Am J Clin Nutr* 50:1364–9, 1989.

Bonham GS, Wilson RW: Children's health in families with cigarette smokers. *Am J Public Health* 71:290–3, 1981.

Bowles BC: Breastfeeding consultation in sign language. *J Hum Lact* 7:21, 1991.

Brennan P, Silman A: Breast-feeding and the onset of rheumatoid arthritis. *Arthr Rheum* 37:808–13, 1994.

Brock KE, et al: Sexual, reproductive and contraceptive risk factors for carcinoma-in-situ of the uterine cervix in Sydney. *Med J Aust* 150:125–30, 1989.

Brodie MJ: Management of epilepsy during pregnancy and lactation. *Lancet* 336:426–7, 1990.

Brown RE: Relactation: an overview. *Pediatrics* 60:116–20, 1977.

Brun JF et al: Breast feeding, other reproductive factors and rheumatoid arthritis. A prospective study. *Br J Rheumatol* 34:542–46, 1995.

Bundred NJ, et al: Breast abscesses and cigarette smoking. *Br J Surg* 79:548–59, 1992.

Butte NF, et al: Human milk intake and growth in exclusively breast-fed infants. *J Pediatr* 104:187–95, 1984.

Butte NF, et al: Milk composition of insulin-dependent diabetic women. *J Pediatr Gastroenterol Nutr* 6:936–41, 1987.

Carty E, Conine TA , Hall L: Comprehensive health promotion for the pregnant woman who is disabled. *J Nurse Midwif* 35:133–42, 1990.

Carty E, Conine TA, Wood-Johnson F: Rheumatoid arthritis and pregnancy: helping women to meet their needs. *Midw Chron* 99:254–7, 1986.

Clark RA: Infections during the postpartum period. *JOGNN* 24:542–8, 1996.

Coakley AJ, Mountford PJ: Nuclear medicine and the nursing mother. *Br Med J* 291(6489):159–60, 1985.

Coates MM, Riordan J: Breastfeeding during maternal or infant illness. *Clin Iss Perin Wom Health Nurs* 3:683–94, 1992.

Cogill S, et al: Impact of maternal postnatal depression on cognitive development of young children. *Br Med J* 292:1165–7, 1986.

Dahlström A, et al: Nicotine and cotinine concentrations in the nursing mother and her infant. *Acta Paediatr Scand* 79:142–7, 1990.

D'Alonzo GE: The pregnant asthmatic patient. *Sem Perinatol* 14:119–29, 1990.

Davies HA, et al: Insulin requirements of diabetic women who breast feed. *Br Med J* 298:1357–8, 1989.

DeCoopman J: Breastfeeding after pituitary resection: support for a theory of autocrine control of milk supply? *J Hum Lact* 9:35–40, 1993.

Delgado-Escueta AV, Janz D: Consensus guidelines: preconception counseling, management, and care of the pregnant woman with epilepsy. *Neurology* 42(suppl 5):149–60, 1992.

Ehrenkranz RA, Ackerman BA: Metoclopramide effect on faltering milk production by mothers of premature infants. *Pediatrics* 78:614–20, 1986.

Ellsworth A: Pharmacotherapy of asthma while breastfeeding. *J Hum Lact* 10:39–41, 1994.

Emery MM: Galactogogues: drugs to induce lactation. *J Hum Lact* 12:55–7, 1996.

Engelking C, Page-Lieberman J: *Maternal diabetes and diabetes in young children: their relationship to breastfeeding,* Unit 5 (Lactation Consultant Series). Garden City Park, NY: Avery Publishing Group, 1986.

Evans JL, et al: Secretion of radioactivity in breast milk following administration of 99Tc^{m}-MAG3. *Nucl Med Commun* 14:108–11, 1993.

Ferris AM, et al: Lactation outcome in insulin-dependent diabetic women. *J Am Diet Assoc* 88: 317–22, 1988.

Ferris AM, et al: Perinatal lactation protocol and outcome in mothers with and without insulin-dependent diabetes mellitus. *Am J Clin Nutr* 58:43–8, 1993.

Franklyn JA: The management of hyperthyroidism. *N Engl J Med* 330:1731–8, 1994.

Fulton B, Moore L: Radiopharmaceuticals and lactation. *J Hum Lact* 6:181–4, 1990.

Gagne MG, Leff EW, Jefferis SC: The breast-feeding experience of women with type I diabetes. *Health Care Wom Int* 13:249–60, 1992.

Gelman JR: Breastfeeding mothers who have lupus. *New Beginnings* Nov–Dec 1993:175–6.

Gennaro S: Postpartal anxiety and depression in mothers of term or preterm infants. *Nurs Res* 37:82–5, 1988.

Golembeski DJ, Emergy MG: Lipid composition of milk from mothers with cystic fibrosis [letter]. *Pediatrics* 31(suppl):631–2, 1989.

Hale T: *Medications and mothers' milk* (6th ed). Amarillo, TX, Pharmasoft Medical Publishing, 1997.

Hammer R, et al: Low-fat diet and exercise in obese lactating women. *Breastfeed Rev* 4:29–34, 1996.

Handford P: Postpartum depression: what is it, what helps? *Can Nurs* 81:30–3, 1985.

Holmgren U, et al: Women with prolactinoma—effect of pregnancy and lactation on serum prolactin and on tumor growth. *Acta Endocrinol* 111:452–9, 1986.

Hopkinson JM, et al: Milk production by mothers of premature infants: influence of cigarette smoking. *Pediatrics* 90:934–8, 1992.

Hormann E: Breast feeding the adopted baby. *Birth Fam J* 4:165–72, 1977.

Horta BL, et al: Environmental tobacco smoke and breastfeeding duration. *Am J Epidemiol* 146:128–33, 1997.

Hutt P: The effects of diabetes on lactation. *Breastfeed Rev* 14:21–5, 1989.

Ikegami H, et al: Relationship between the methods of treatment of prolactinomas and the puerperal lactation. *Fertil Steril* 47:867–9, 1987.

Ito S, et al: Initiation and duration of breast-feeding in women receiving antiepileptics. *Am J Obstet Gynecol* 173:881–6, 1995.

Jelliffe DB, Jelliffe EFP: Non-puerperal induced lactation [letter]. *Pediatrics* 50:170–1, 1972.

Kampmann JP: Proplythiouracil in human milk: revision of a dogma. *Lancet* 1 8171:736, 1980.

Kendall-Tackett K, Kantor GK: Postpartum depression. Newbury Park, CA: Sage Publications, 1993.

Kirshbaum M: The parent with a physical disability. In: Auvenshine JM, Enriques MG, eds. *Comprehensive maternity nursing: perinatal and women's health*. Boston: Jones & Bartlett, 1990.

Kitzinger S: *The crying baby*. New York: Penguin Books, 1989.

Kjos SL, et al: The effect of lactation on glucose and lipid metabolism in women with recent gestational diabetes. *Obstet Gynecol* 82:451–5, 1993.

Kopala B: Mothers with impaired mobility speak out. *MCN* 14:115–9, 1989.

Lammi-Keefe CJ, et al: Vitamin E in plasma and milk of lactating women with insulin-dependent diabetes mellitus. *J Pediatr Gastroenterol Nutr* 20:305–9, 1995.

Lawrence RA: Breastfeeding and medical disease. *Med Clin North Am* 73:583–603, 1989.

Lepper HS, DiMatteo R, Tinsley, BJ: Postpartum depression: how much do obstetric nurses and obstetricians know? *Birth* 21:149–54, 1994.

Lindstrom LH: CSF and plasma beta-Casomorphin-like opioid peptides in postpartum psychosis. *Am J Psychiatry* 141:1059–66, 1984.

Little RE, et al: Agreement between laboratory tests and self-reports of alcohol, tobacco, caffeine, marijuana and other drug use in post-partum women. *Soc Sci Med* 22:91–8, 1986.

Luck W, Nau H: Nicotine and cotinine concentrations in serum and milk of nursing smokers. *Br J Clin Pharmacol* 18:9–15, 1984.

Luck W, Nau, H: Nicotine and cotinine concentrations in serum and urine of infants exposed via passive smoking or milk from smoking mothers. *J Pediatr* 107:816–20, 1985.

Luder E, et al: Current recommendations for breastfeeding in cystic fibrosis centers. *Am J Dis Child* 144:1153–6, 1990.

Martin DC: LLL and the mother who is blind. *Leaven,* Sept–Oct 1992:67–8.

Matheson I, Kristensen K, Lunde PKM: Drug utilization in breast-feeding women. A survey in Oslo. *Eur J Clin Pharmacol* 38:453–9, 1990.

McDougall IR, Bayer MF: Should a woman taking propylthiouracil breast-feed? *Clin Nucl Med* 11:249–50, 1986.

Michel SH, Mueller DH: Impact of lactation on women with cystic fibrosis and their infants: a review of five cases. *J Am Diet Assoc* 94:159–65, 1994.

Minami J: Helping mothers with chronic illness. *Leaven* 26:52–3, 1990.

Momotani N, et. al: Recovery from fetal hypothyroidism: evidence for the safety of breast-feeding while taking propylthiouracil. *Clin Endocrinol* 31:591–5, 1989.

Miyake A, et al: Decrease in neonatal suckled milk volume in diabetic women. *Eur J Obstet Gynecol Reprod Biol* 33:49–53, 1989.

Nafstad P, et al: Weight gain during the first year of life in relation to maternal smoking and breast feeding in Norway. *J Epidemiol Commun Health* 51:261–5, 1997.

Neifert M, McDonough S, Neville M: Failure of lactogenesis associated with placental retention. *Am J Obstet Gynecol* 140:477–8, 1981.

Nelson LM, et al: Risk of multiple sclerosis exacerbation during pregnancy and breast-feeding. *J Am Med Assoc* 259:3441–3, 1988.

Nemba K: Induced lactation: a study of 37 non-puerperal mothers. *J Trop Pediatr* 40:240–2, 1994.

Neubauer SH, et al: Delayed lactogenesis in women with insulin-dependent diabetes mellitus. *Am J Clin Nutr* 58:54–60, 1993.

Nursing Mothers' Association of Australia: *Where there's a will, there's usually a way–breastfeeding when the mother has a disability.* Hawthorn, Victoria, Australia: The Association, 1982.

O'Campo P, Faden RR: The impact of pregnancy on women's prenatal and postpartum smoking behavior. *Am J Prev Med* 8:8–13, 1992.

Olango P, Aboud F: Determinants of mothers' treatment of diarrhea in rural Ethiopia. *Soc Sci Med* 31:1245–9, 1990.

Ostrom KM, Ferris AM: Prolactin concentrations in serum and milk of mothers with and without insulin-dependent diabetes mellitus. *Am J Clin Nutr* 58:49–53, 1993.

Phillips V: Relactation in mothers of children over 12 months. *J Trop Pediatr* 39:45–8, 1993.

Pisacane A, et al: Breast feeding and multiple sclerosis. *BMJ* 308:1411–2, 1994.

Poser S, Poser, W: Multiple sclerosis and gestation. *Neurology* 33:1423–7, 1983.

Robinson PS, et al: Iodine-131 in breast milk following therapy for thyroid carcinoma. *J Nucl Med* 35:1797–1801, 1994.

Romney BM, Nickoloff EL, Esser PD: Excretion of radioiodine in breast milk. *J Nucl Med* 30:124–6, 1989.

Rona RJ, et al: Parental smoking at home and the height of children. *Br Med J* 283:1361, 1981.

Rosenblatt KA, Thomas DB: Prolonged lactation and endometrial cancer. *Int J Epidemiol* 24:499–503, 1995.

Rylance GW, et. al: Carbimazole and breastfeeding [letter]. *Lancet* 1(8538):928, 1987.

Said G, Patois E, Lellouch J: Infantile colic and parental smoking. *Br Med J* 289:660, 1984.

Scharff et al: Maintenance of effects in the nonmedical treatment of headaches during pregnancy. *Headache* 36:285–90, 1996.

Schou M: Lithium treatment during pregnancy, delivery, and lactation: an update. *J Clin Psychiatry* 51:410–13, 1990.

Seema PAK, Satyanarayana L: Relactation: an effective intervention to promote exclusive breast-feeding. *J Trop Pediatr* 43:213–16, 1997.

Shiffman ML, et al: Breast-milk composition in women with cystic fibrosis: report of two cases and a review of the literature *Am J Clin Nutr* 49:612–7, 1989.

Silberstein SD: Headaches and women: treatment of the pregnant and lactating migraneur. *Headache* 33:533–40, 1993.

Simpkins S, Hench CP, Bhatia G: Management of the obstetric patient with tuberculosis. *JOGNN* 25:305–2, 1996.

Snider DF, Powell KE: Should women taking anti-tuberculosis drugs breast feed? *Arch Intern Med* 144:589–90, 1984.

Stamp GE, et al: Evaluation of antenatal and postnatal support to overcome postnatal depression: a randomized controlled trial. *Birth* 22:138–43, 1995.

Steldinger R, Luck W: Half lives of nicotine in milk of smoking mothers: implications for nursing [letter]. *J Perinat Med* 16:261–2, 1988.

Sutherland A, Auerbach KG: *Relactation and induced lactation,* Unit 1 (Lactation Consultant Series) Garden City Park, NY: Avery Publishing, 1985.

Tamminen T: The impact of mother's depression on her breastfeeding attitudes and experiences. *J Psychosom Obstet Gynaecol* 10:69–78, 1989.

Thompson NM: Relactation in a newborn intensive care setting. *J Hum Lact* 12:233–5, 1996.

Thomson, VM: Breastfeeding and mothering one-handed. *J Hum Lact* 11:211–15, 1995.

Thorley V: Lactational headaches. *Breastfeed Rev* 5:23–5, 1997.

Thorpe K, et al: Comparison of prevalence of depression in mothers of twins and mothers of singletons. *Br Med J* 302:875–7, 1991.

Trundle JI, Skellern GG: Gas chromatographic determination of nicotine in human breast milk. *J Clin Hosp Pharmacol* 8:289–93, 1983.

Vio F, Salazar G, Infante C: Smoking during pregnancy and lactation: its effects on breast-milk volume. *Am J Clin Nutr* 54:1011–6, 1991.

Visness CM, et al: Fertility of fully breast-feeding women in the early postpartum period. *Obstet Gynecol* 89:164–7, 1997.

Visness CM, Kennedy KI, Ramos R: The duration and character of postpartum bleeding among breast-feeding women. *Obstet Gynecol* 89:159–63, 1997.

Waletzky L: Emotional illness in the postpartum period. In: Ahmed P, ed. *Pregnancy, childbirth and parenthood.* New York: Elsevier, 1981.

Waletzky LR, Herman EC: Relactation. *Am Fam Phys* 14:69–74, 1976.

Wall VR: Breastfeeding and migraine headaches. *J Hum Lact* 8:209–12, 1992.

Weiner RE, Spencer RP: Quantification of gallium-67 citrate in breast milk. *Clin Nucl Med* 19:7653–65, 1994.

Welch MJ, Phelps DL, Osher, AB: Breast-feeding by a mother with cystic fibrosis. *Pediatrics* 67:664–6, 1981.

Whichelow MJ, Doddridge, MC: Lactation in diabetic women. *Br Med J* 287:649-50, 1983.

Widstrom AM, et al: Somatostatin levels in plasma of non-smoking and smoking breast-feeding women. *Acta Paediatr Scand* 80:13–21, 1991.

Willis CE, Livingstone V: Infant insufficient milk syndrome associated with maternal postpartum hemorrhage. *J Hum Lact* 11:123–6, 1995.

Wolman WL, et al: Postpartum depression and companionship in the clinical birth environment: a randomized, controlled study. *Am J Obstet Gynecol* 168:1388–94, 1993.

Woodward A, Hand K: Smoking and reduced duration of breast-feeding [letter]. *Med J Aust* 148:477–8, 1988.

Worthington J, et al: Pregnancy and multiple sclerosis–a 3-year prospective study. *J Neurol* 241:228–33, 1994.

Yurchak AM, Jusko WSJ: Theophylline secretion into breast milk. *Pediatrics* 57:518–20, 1976.

MATERNAL EMPLOYMENT AND BREASTFEEDING

Kathleen G. Auerbach

The decision to continue breastfeeding following return to part-time or full-time employment may represent a significant departure from the decisions of a woman's mother and grandmother. She may be the first woman in her family to return to work before her child is in school; she may also be the first mother in the family to have chosen to breast-feed, and she is very likely to be the first to have chosen to combine both roles. As such, she is a pioneer; like those who preceded her across the plains, she may feel that she is facing innumerable unknowns for which she is woefully unprepared.

Why Women Work

Most women work for financial and social rewards. In 1995, nearly 6 of 10 women age 16 or older were in the labor force (U.S. Department of Labor, 1996). Many more women today than in previous years are the sole supporter of their families: some are married to men who are underemployed; others are putting their partners through school. When the paycheck arrives, these women receive tangible evidence that what they do counts for something. More importantly, the paycheck enables them to keep a roof overhead and food on the table, even though 1995 median weekly earnings of women were only 75.5 percent those of men. This disparity is only partly related to the work done by men and women (U.S. Department of Labor, 1996). For example, in 1972, women accounted for only 17 percent of physicians and 4 percent of attorneys in the United States. By 1990, 35 percent of physicians and 21 percent of attorneys were women (U.S. Department of Labor, 1991).

Many women also work because they gain self-esteem by being valued for their marketable skills. In addition, the social rewards of the time spent with other adults on the job helps these women to feel good about themselves–to feel as if they are improving the skills for which they sought higher education (of whatever level) and that they (and their skills) are not going to stagnate or become outdated from lack of use.

Number of Women Who Work

How many women work outside the home? This question is difficult to answer, because what one chooses to count influences the answer. More than half of all women with children under the age of three are in the labor force, and most of these woman work full-time (U.S. Department of Labor, 1991). Working wives and mothers are the rule rather than the exception, and many of these women will return to work during the period when they are most likely to be breastfeeding. In spite of this reality, women continue to complain that the workplace culture neither supports nor respects families. Many women report that neither their employers nor public policy adequately recognizes or supports women's family responsibilities (U.S. Department of Labor, 1994).

Four factors influence whether breastfeeding can be combined with maternal employment:

- the nature of the mother's work (whether it is physically demanding or potentially hazardous);
- whether she can arrange breaks for feeding or expressing her milk);
- the baby's age; and
- the amount and type of support the mother has from family, child-care people, and others whose opinions she considers important (Shepherd & Yarrow, 1982).

Being employed, particularly for more than 20 hours per week, has a significant negative influence on breastfeeding duration (Auerbach & Guss, 1984; Gielen et al., 1991). Hence many women who must consider both working and breastfeeding choose not to breastfeed at all (Livingstone & Grams, 1985) or to wean the baby in advance of returning to paid employment outside the home. Although breastfeeding is possible after the mother returns to work, survey results continue to conclude that the employed mother is less likely to breastfeed as long as does the woman who chooses to stay at home during her baby's early infancy (Bourgoin et al., 1997). Ryan and Martinez (1989) found that initiation of breastfeeding was as likely among women planning to return to work as among those who were planning to stay home; however, only 10 percent of the employed mothers were breastfeeding six months later, as compared with 24 percent of unemployed women who were breastfeeding their six-month-old infants. Visness and Kennedy (1997) reported that the decision to breastfeed was not associated with maternal employment but that duration of breastfeeding was shorter if the mother returned to work within one year of her baby's delivery. The longer the dura-

tion of exclusive breastfeeding, the longer the duration of any breastfeeding (Hills-Bonczyk et al., 1994; Piper & Parks, 1996). In addition, when mothers viewed breastfeeding as a special time with the baby that she did not want to give up, she was more likely to breastfeed longer.

Lindberg (1996) used a role-incompatibility model to explain why some employed women breastfeed and others do not. She noted that women working part time were more likely than full-time workers to breastfeed and that more women quit breastfeeding in the same month that they returned to work, supporting her contention that these two behaviors–breastfeeding and working–are viewed by many as being incompatible. The longer women delayed their return to work, the lower the negative effect of employment on their breastfeeding experience.

Most worldwide studies, particularly those conducted in developing countries, report that working negatively affects breastfeeding (Al-Sekait, 1988; Marshall, 1988; Thimmayamma et al., 1980). On the other hand, an Israeli study found that women who worked outside the home during their pregnancy were more likely to breastfeed than were nonworking pregnant women (Birenbaum et al., 1989). This chapter examines these and other issues related to breastfeeding and employment and offers specific guidelines for the health care worker who is asked to counsel or to inform women who are anticipating a return to work outside the home while their babies are breastfeeding.

This chapter is divided into two parts. The reader interested in the "how-to's" of assisting an employed breastfeeding mother may wish to read only the first part, which focuses on how the health care provider can assist the employed breastfeeding mother from pregnancy onward, highlighting those elements that have proved successful for others. The second part discusses some of the contextual issues surrounding breastfeeding and employment, including legal issues, the pull between home and work, and the experiences of health care workers.

Prenatal Planning and Preparation

Just as pregnancy is a time of planning that focuses on caring for and feeding the baby, pregnancy is the best time to plan for one's return to the employment scene. Most women have already decided how they will feed the baby, often before they become pregnant. Many myths exist about breastfeeding, and some view combining breastfeeding (a "home activity") with employment as inappropriate. Thus the health care worker who has contact with the employed pregnant woman does her a great service simply by asking how she plans to combine the two tasks after the baby's arrival. In many cases, the mother's reply to such a question will identify fallacies that need to be debunked and areas of information that need to be shared.

First, the health care worker should encourage the pregnant woman to learn as much as she can about breastfeeding. Discussing breast changes that most mothers observe during pregnancy is a good way to help a mother realize that such physical changes require consideration of other kinds of changes that are going to occur. Primary among them is the baby's need for the mother and how this need can be met, even if they must be separated for many hours on a regular basis.

Next, the health care provider can help the mother to begin planning for her baby and for breastfeeding when she returns to work. The employed breastfeeding mother will want to determine whether she can use her work breaks to nurse her baby and whether lunchtime breastfeeding will be permitted in the center or at the day-care worker's home. If she is entitled to two small "coffee" breaks daily, can they be combined into a single longer period that will enable her to see her baby and either breastfeed or take a more leisurely period for expressing her milk? In some settings, "baby breaks" at the job site are a possibility. In situations in which the father works nearby, a family lunch break may be enjoyed: both parents and baby can meet for some quiet midday contact.

Another question that the health care provider might ask is whether the day-care worker is familiar with human milk and how to warm it, whether it can be refrigerated or frozen at the day-care center and, if facilities for these processes are provided, whether the milk will be used. In addition, the mother needs to ask how babies are fed at the day-care center–specifically, are they given a bottle to hold while lying alone in a crib or on a pad on the floor, or are they held? Women who have bottle-fed other infants may be unaware that most breastfeeding babies younger than three months of age have no idea how to hold a bottle. The mother should insist that her baby be held in arms when fed, if this is important to her.

The Puerperium

The timing of women's return to work is influenced by a number of factors. In most cases, the duration of paid or unpaid maternity leave plays a major role. In the case of the birth of a premature baby, the additional and unexpected costs of extended hospital care may also contribute to the decision. Youngblut et al. (1990) found that women who had already planned to return to work were very apt to do so after the birth of a premature infant. The employed women were less satisfied with their situation than the unemployed women, suggesting that the decision to return to work in the face of increased financial need did not entirely redirect their concerns away from the baby during this period.

If she expects to express milk after her return to work, the new mother may bring a breast pump to the hospital. Assisting her in its use at this time can reduce future difficulties. If she wishes to learn how to express milk, the hospital stay is a good time to introduce hand-expression techniques. However, neither breast pumping nor expression should be viewed as a necessary daily activity. Simply knowing that she can do it and that the time for more active involvement in perfecting these skills will come a bit later is all that is necessary for the mother during the hospital stay. Placing too much emphasis on practicing these skills before the mother's milk supply is well established is self-defeating, unless her baby is ill or born prematurely and she must use these techniques as a substitute for regular breastfeeding. With a healthy, full-term infant, the mother's best preparation for an ample milk supply when she returns to work is frequent, unlimited breastfeeding and getting to know her baby before they must be separated.

Returning to Work

The day on which a mother returns to work, even when she has prepared for it throughout her time at home after the baby's birth, is often characterized by the emotional and physical tugs she feels, the tears that slide unbidden down her cheeks, and the many times she pulls out pictures of the baby to share with her coworkers. Rarely is this day one in which she is as productive as she was prior to the baby's birth.

Informing the mother that her first day back is one for showing off the baby photos and straightening her desk so that her infant's picture is prominently displayed is one way to let her know that things will not be the same and that, however prepared she thinks she is, it may be one of the most difficult days she will experience. The depth of her attachment to the baby means that regardless of the baby's age, this day simply will be one to "get through." Reported one employed mother, "It was no easier with my second than it was with my first. The only reason I was not a basket-case with my third was that I brought her with me. Believe it or not, I got just as much work done as before–precious little!"

The timing of return to work, particularly if it is full time, will influence the breastfeeding-specific problems that the mother encounters and the length of time that she may have to deal with them (Auerbach & Guss, 1984; Kearney & Cronenwett, 1991). In one study, breastfeeding difficulties tended to cluster in the first four months of the baby's life (Auerbach, 1984). The sooner the mother returned to work, the longer she had to deal with one or more of these problems, which included

- concern about an inadequate or fluctuating milk supply

- engorgement

- leaking

- emotional lability

- the need to express or pump milk (its frequency, duration, and likelihood over time)

- the baby's need for frequent feedings, particularly if he was very young when she returned to work

- the baby's frequently changing feeding patterns, including appetite spurts and nighttime nursings

Added to these difficulties is her low reserve of energy, a problem endemic to all new mothers. The helping professional should inform the mother that each of these difficulties will resolve over time and that the longer she is home with the baby, the less likely is it that any of these issues will prove insurmountable. None of these issues are major obstacles after the baby is older than four months; pointing this out may encourage her to see that these difficulties need not reduce breastfeeding duration when the mother returns to work very soon after her baby's birth. This information may also assist her in making decisions about the length of her leave from work, if she has an opportunity to extend it beyond the usual four to six weeks (Frederick & Auerbach, 1985).

Helping the mother to maintain realistic expectations about her first days on the job will enable her to see that most of the problems she encounters will not be specific to breastfeeding (Thompson & Bell, 1997); rather, they are specific to the overworked woman with a family. However, how she plans to breastfeed can make a difference. For example, Morse et al. (1989) interviewed 61 mothers who intended to continue breastfeeding after they returned to work. The strategies the mothers selected for breastfeeding influenced how long they did so. Those women who practiced demand breastfeeding were more likely to breastfeed longer, even though they tended to return to work sooner. Strategies least likely to result in longer duration of breastfeeding included using formula routinely or switching from demand feedings to minimal breastfeeding (one or two per day). In addition, proximity of the baby to the work site significantly influenced the duration of breastfeeding. Those mothers whose babies were nearby had a mean breastfeeding duration of 21.6 weeks, as compared with those whose babies were not nearby; breastfeeding duration averaged only 17 weeks in the latter group.

There are many ways in which breastfeeding can be continued after the mother returns to work: hand expressing one's milk, breast pumping, having the baby brought to the mother during meal breaks, or substituting formula for those feedings that occur during the mother's workday (Broome, 1981). Each of these alternatives represents an option that deserves discussion. In cases in which a family history of allergies has been identified, formula use should be avoided for as long as possible. Setting up the right care situation for the baby may solve many of the problems that the mother feels certain will negatively affect her baby's growth and development. For example, several women in one international study reported resenting deeply the time that the day-care provider had with the baby (Auerbach, 1984). The opportunity to see the baby during the day resolved this difficulty for some of these women (Fig. 18–1).

Hand-Expressing and Breast Pumping?

Prior to the mother's return to work, the lactation consultant or other health worker who is counseling the mother will want to discuss the need to express milk when she is away from her baby. An older baby who nurses infrequently will not require that the mother express her milk as frequently as she would if she had a younger baby who was still feeding very frequently. A mother whose work shift coincides with her baby's usual sleep time may not need to express milk at all while she is at work.

Based on reports of their respondents, Auerbach and Guss (1984) suggest that a week to 10 days before the mother returns to work is a good time for her to begin practicing expression and pumping and to begin stockpiling milk in order to

- learn how to relieve physical discomfort from overfull breasts
- obtain milk for the baby's other feedings
- maintain her milk supply at an optimal level

As a general rule, the earlier in the postpartum period the mother returns to full-time work, the more frequently she will need to express or pump her breasts. Expressing milk at work to give the baby human milk feedings in the mother's absence is only one reason for doing so. The mother is also protecting her baby from infections and allergies, as discussed in Chapters 5 and 19. In addition, the mother who is comfortable on the job is a more efficient worker. If she feels, as one mother put it, "that [she is] going to explode and gallons would flood the room," she cannot concentrate on her

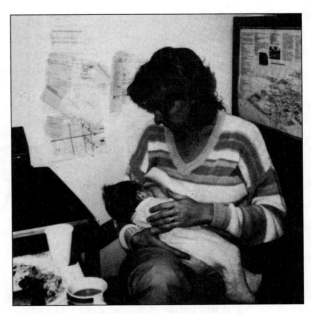

FIGURE 18-1. Breastfeeding in the workplace.

work. Furthermore, painful engorgement contributes to embarrassing leaking, an increased risk of mastitis from milk stasis, and reduction of her milk supply from overfullness.

For a baby who is younger than two months old, 1 to 2 oz. for each feeding will usually be sufficient. When she begins expressing milk, the mother may be dismayed that she obtains so little (sometimes barely enough to cover the bottom of a small 4-oz. bottle). However, each time she expresses, she will probably obtain more milk. Just as she had to learn to breastfeed, her body needs to learn to respond to the stimulation of hand expression or breast pumping in order to trigger milk ejection. (See Chapter 10 for techniques for maximizing milk ejection.) The author usually tells each mother who is planning to return to work to expect no more than 0.5 oz. with the first several pumping or expression sessions. Because most mothers will obtain more than this, especially after several sessions, such a comment results in a feeling of accomplishment for the mother, who may view how much milk she obtains as an indicator of the adequacy of her supply. If she exceeds what "the expert" has told her to expect, surely she will succeed!

During practice sessions, the mother should express or pump in the morning, when she is more likely to feel rested, rather than later in the afternoon or evening. Usually two practice sessions, timed about one hour after each of two consecutive morning breastfeedings, are sufficient to develop her milk-expression skills. Mothers who feel particularly full late in the evening have also found that expressing at this time helps to build up a sizable stockpile of milk. Remind a mother that the milk she obtains in this way is "excess," not an indication of the amount of milk the baby obtains. Furthermore, milk is still present in the breasts after all breastfeedings, regardless of the rate at which the baby is growing (Daly & Hartmann, 1995).

When planning pumping sessions, ask the employed mother to practice the *5-15-5 rule*. The first and last fives refer to two very short, pump-for-comfort sessions in the midmorning and midafternoon. Rarely do such periods last longer than five minutes. Some mothers will choose simply to excuse themselves to the women's room, where they express briefly into the sink until the breast fullness that they are feeling has subsided; they then return to their work station. Other women will save this milk and combine it with the outcome of a later, longer pumping session. At a meal break, the mother then expresses or pumps her breasts for 10 to 20 minutes and saves this milk for later use. As the mother becomes adept at expressing or pumping and as her baby gets older, she may find that she can reduce the duration of each expression period or the number of pumpings to two and then to one per day. Some women have combined the midmorning and midafternoon coffee breaks into a single longer period that is more conducive to breast expression.

When babies are cared for near the workplace, mothers often use this time, as well as lunchtime, to go to the baby for a relaxed midday nursing; sometimes they have the baby brought to them. In either case, breastfeeding stimulates the breasts more effectively than do the best electric pumps or the accomplished mother who hand expresses her milk. Furthermore, both parties enjoy their time together; more than one mother has commented on how much easier it was to return to work after having "touched base" with the baby while grabbing a quick sandwich at the babysitter's house or the day-care center.

If the mother is more comfortable using a breast pump than hand expressing, she will need to rent or purchase this equipment. The breast-pump market has expanded rapidly in recent years (see Chapter 13 for more information about breast pumps). To guide the mother who is planning to pump her breasts, the questions in Box 18-1 are useful.

The first important consideration in selecting a breast pump is that it must be easy to clean. If the user cannot be assured that cleaning is possible at home, with or without a dishwasher, the pump should not be purchased. Generally, any pump with a bulb-syringe attachment is difficult to clean and should be avoided.

The pump should be easy and comfortable to use. No single pump works optimally for every mother. This may relate to the closeness of fit of the pump flange on the mother's breast, to the angle of "pull" of cylinder-style pumps, and other factors as yet undiscovered. The angle of the flange varies from one pump to another, as do the shape, size, and degree of fullness of each mother's breasts. Optimally, the mother should experiment with several pumps before purchasing one. The next best alternative is for her to talk with other mothers who are successfully pumping and compare the efficiency and reported comfort of different pumps. However, it is important to keep in mind that what works for one mother may not work for another.

The length of pumping experience may be more important to obtaining breastmilk than duration of a given pumping session. One mother who used the hospital "Lactation Station" obtained 15 oz. in 20 minutes, during which time she had to empty the collection bottles at least once to avoid their overfilling! Another mother, who used the same equipment, obtained only 6 oz. in 20 minutes. Other mothers averaged 7 to 9 oz. after 15 minutes of pumping. Still another mother sometimes obtained as much as 10 oz. and other times as little as 5. All mothers obtained less milk at the end of the work week than they did at the beginning.

The lesson learned from these mothers is that efficiency needs to be gauged by whether the mother is comfortable with the pump during its use, whether her breasts feel softer after using the pump, and whether, over time, the amount of milk she obtains tends to increase. When she begins offering solid foods, breastfeedings become less frequent or shorter. At that time, the amount obtained

BOX 18–1

Questions to Ask a Mother Who Is Planning to Use a Breast Pump

- Is the pump easy to clean?
- Is the pump easy to use?
- Is the pump physically comfortable to use?
- Is the pump effective in obtaining milk quickly?
- Are the instructions accompanying the pump understandable, accurate, and easy to follow?
- What is the cost (initial investment and daily, weekly, or monthly rental fee) of using the pump?
- Are extra or replacement parts available without having to purchase a new kit?
- What options for expressing her milk are available in the mother's community or workplace?
- Are both single and double pumping options available if desired?

- What is the experience of other women who have used breast pumps in the mother's community or workplace?
- What have other mothers reported about using specific equipment?
- Does the mother feel emotionally and psychologically comfortable pumping her milk? If she does not, has she considered expressing her milk by hand or breastfeeding without expressing her milk for the periods when she is separated from her baby?

Source: Derived in part from KG Auerbach: Assisting the employed breastfeeding mother. J Nurse Midwif *35:26–34, 1990.*

by pumping usually declines. If the foregoing criteria are met, the pump can be considered efficient.

The health care worker who assists the mother should be familiar with instructions for all pumps so that she can clarify instructions that are incomplete, unclear, or written in an unfamiliar language. Additionally, pump instructions should be reviewed to determine whether pictures demonstrating use of the equipment are accurate. In one study, the instructions of several hand-operated pumps included illustrations and recommendations that resulted in tennis elbow (Williams et al., 1989).

If the mother cannot obtain replacement parts or extra pieces without purchasing an entirely new kit, the cost of using the pump may become prohibitive. The same is true if she plans to use a battery-operated pump with cost-effective batteries or a rechargeable battery pack. The least expensive

breast pumps tend not to have replacement parts. Because double pumping is more effective in obtaining milk quickly than is pumping each breast separately, electric pumps that do not offer this option should be carefully considered (Auerbach, 1990).

Storage

Human milk is a dynamic substance that kills bacteria. This ability is highest in the first several hours after expression, even when it is unrefrigerated (Barger & Bull, 1987; Hamosh et al., 1996, 1997; Nwankwo et al., 1988; Pittard et al., 1985), and some investigators have reported that colony counts remain low in such milk for at least 48 hours (Hamosh et al., 1996; Larson et al., 1984; Sosa & Barness, 1987). For this reason, when women use clean containers in which their own fresh milk is stored for less than six to eight hours prior to

---

BOX 18–2

General Guidelines for Storing Human Milk

- Always use a clean container.
- Label each container with date and time of the earliest contribution to the container, particularly if "layering" different expressions into the same container.
- Store milk in the approximate quantities that the baby is likely to need for one feeding.
- If refrigerated within six to eight hours, store in a clean, tightly capped container for the unrefrigerated interim period.
- If refrigerated, use within eight days.*
- If frozen in a refrigerator freezer section, use within one month.*
- If frozen in a deep-freezer, use within six months.*

- Discard any remaining milk that was not used at the feeding for which it was thawed and warmed.
- Match the "age" of the milk as closely as possible to the baby's age in order to optimize the degree of fit between the baby's needs and the properties of the milk.

These general guidelines require cleaning the milk containers and caps well after each use, paying particular attention to removing any milk or soap residue and ensuring that the milk is not mixed with other milk during storage.

Shake while thawing to remix the creamy portion that separates during storage.

---

refrigeration, they are not endangering their healthy babies. (See the list of guidelines in Box 18–2.) Other mothers who prefer to refrigerate their milk should do so in a clean, capped container and use the milk within a few days after it has been refrigerated.

Mothers who express milk on a Friday to use the following Monday often freeze their milk. Milk stored in the freezer compartment of a refrigerator (top, bottom, or side models) should be placed as far away from the door as possible; most mothers use frozen milk within one month of the date when it was expressed. If a deep-freezer is used to store it, the milk can be used up to six months after the date of expression. The mother should be reminded that human milk is a substance that is matched to the baby's age: milk obtained when the baby was three months old will not as completely meet that same baby's needs when he is six months old.

If she finds that her milk changes in odor or consistency after storage, or if the baby begins to refuse it, the mother may need to reduce the stor-age time and freeze rather than refrigerate in order to retard any changes occurring in the milk that might contribute to her baby's adverse reaction.

Once the milk has been refrigerated or frozen, it should be thawed and warmed to body temperature by placing it under the faucet in a sink and running gradually warmer water over the container. It is inappropriate to thaw milk overnight; this practice enables bacteria to multiply in the milk. Neither should it be heated very quickly on a stove or in a microwave oven. Vitamin C and other properties, including IgA (Sigman et al., 1989), are easily destroyed when milk is heated too hot; the protein is altered as well. Additionally, microwave heating nearly always results in uneven distribution of the heat, which usually goes unnoticed because the container rarely feels as warm as the center portion of the fluid (Hibbard & Blevins, 1988; Nemethy & Clore, 1990); thus the milk can be too hot in some spots and substantially cooler in others. Even water-warmed milk should be mixed well and tested on the inside of the caregiver's wrist before offering it to the baby. Mixing should be done not only for heat distribution but also to ensure that the creamy portion of the milk is resuspended. The fat content of milk is altered with refrigeration as well as when the milk is frozen and then thawed for reuse (Silprasert et al., 1986). Loss can be minimized when the container is shaken well before offering its contents to the baby.

Feeding Options

Bottle-Feeding. Most people think that a baby must be bottle-fed when he or she is not breastfed. Many a working mother worries that her baby will reject a bottle in her absence. To avoid this, some women have been told to begin bottle-feeding once a day immediately after the baby's birth. The clinical experiences of many lactation consultants who have worked with breastfeeding mothers suggest that this works only rarely. First, early introduction of a bottle is more likely to result in nipple confusion or preference for the more obvious cue of a bottle teat; even when this problem does not arise, the baby may still reject the bottle, particularly when he reaches two and one-half to three months of age. If the baby is older than four weeks when the bottle is introduced, the risk of nipple preference is reduced and the likelihood of rejection is low, provided that someone other than the mother introduces the bottle and patiently helps the baby to learn how to use it.

A week or 10 days before the mother returns to work allows plenty of time to reassure her that her baby will not starve in her absence and that her baby will learn how to use a bottle without difficulty. If the baby's father is the designated teacher of bottle-feeding, it is important that he select a time when the mother is not around. Ask the father to prepare the bottle about half an hour before the baby may want to feed, because a bottle is apt to be rejected if the baby is famished. The father should then place the baby in his arms, sitting in a place other than where the mother usually breastfeeds the baby. The father should keep the baby's head somewhat higher than the rest of his body and present the bottle so that the teat is well into his mouth–centered on the tongue but not so steeply held as to cause choking. The father should talk or sing to the baby as he patiently waits for him to

accept this new feeding method. Very often, the baby will, after a few tentative sucks, begin to empty the bottle.

Because bottle-feeding is more likely to cause the baby to swallow air, frequent burping (often after each ounce ingested) will be necessary. By stopping and starting the baby on the bottle, feedings last somewhat longer and are more likely to include the socializing behavior that is such a natural part of breastfeeding.

Caution the bottle-feeding caregiver to use a towel or other absorbent cloth under the baby to catch spills. Remind the mother or caregiver that nonhuman milk will stain and smell to a greater degree than will human milk. Finally, reassure the bottle-feeding caregiver that it is acceptable if the baby takes only a small amount of milk; there is no need to empty the bottle. On the other hand, if the baby drains the bottle in very short order, this is not necessarily an indication that the baby needs more. Rather the hole in the rubber teat may be too large, or the steepness of the bottle may be such that the baby has no choice but to drain the container to avoid choking.

Some babies will express clear preferences for particular rubber nipples or teats. If one nipple is rejected, try others. Teats that have been warmed under hot tap water are more likely to be accepted.

Cup-Feeding. If the baby is nearing three months when the mother returns to work, she may wish to forgo using a bottle entirely and have the baby's father teach the baby how to use a cup. Because adults use cups and babies happily imitate the actions of their parents, most babies will eagerly use a cup.

The age of the baby when cup-feeding is begun will affect how the baby accomplishes it. Very young infants, including preterms who are cup-fed, have been observed to extend the tongue and lap the milk (Lang et al., 1994). Older infants adopt a sipping action much like that used by a child or an adult. Often first exposure to cup-feeding triggers a lapping response as the baby is first attracted to the odor of the milk and then tastes it. Sipping responses often follow in short order.

The father or caregiver should sit the baby up in his or her arms, supporting the baby's head and neck. He or she should lean the baby forward slightly and tip the cup into the baby's mouth so that a small amount of fluid is presented. Because sipping is different from suckling, nipple confusion is unlikely to occur. After the first sip, the baby who has sufficient coordination and hand control usually reaches forward and grasps the cup on either side, an indication that he is interested in continuing the activity. Any cup will serve the purpose. Parents who prefer spouted ones often do so because of less spillage. Dropperlike containers that contain liquid baby medicines are a good beginning "cup." A wide variety of small cups, including plastic specimen cups and shot glasses, have been reported to work well. Premature babies have been taught to cup-feed prior to beginning to breastfeed (Armstrong, 1987); parents should be reassured that their baby can learn to cup-feed early, even before he is able to sit (Davis et al., 1949). More than one parent has proudly viewed early cup-feeding as evidence of how bright his or her child is.

Spoon-Feeding. Spoon-feeding proceeds much like cup-feeding, except that the fluid is poured into the spoon, or the spoon is dipped into the liquid, and is offered to the baby. It involves a sipping action and thus eliminates nipple confusion. Very small infants have been taught to spoon-feed. It takes a bit longer than cup- or bottle-feeding but is well accepted by infants.

Loss of Sleep

Fatigue is an issue for all parents. Other frequently mentioned concerns are no free time (for the mother), feelings of unhappiness or guilt about leaving the baby to go to work, and loss of nighttime sleep (Auerbach, 1984).

Sleep deprivation is a fact of life for nearly all parents of very young infants. Many an employed breastfeeding mother who works during the day finds that her baby's sleep pattern changes after her return to work. Instead of taking short naps during the day and sleeping longer at night, the baby begins to sleep for very long periods during the day and to remain awake later into the evening. This may be a coping behavior that enables the baby to tolerate many hours away from his mother, and it leads to "reverse-cycle breastfeeding." Often, the baby's waking time with his mother may alternate between short breastfeeding episodes and simply nestling in her arms. Such behavior need not mean that the mother loses still more sleep. In fact, what better built-in "excuse" than breastfeeding does a mother have for lying down on the couch when she gets home? Sleep-saving techniques that families have found work well include any one of a variety of co-sleeping arrangements, such as keeping the baby's cradle or crib in the parents' room; creating an extension on the parents' bed; graduating from a double to a queen- or even king-size mattress; and placing a spare mattress on the floor of the baby's room for late-night cuddling and nursing away from other family members (McKenna et al., 1997). This last option works best for those near-toddlers and larger babies who tend to "sing" when they eat, sometimes loudly enough to awaken nearby sleepers.

The Triple Breeder-Feeder-Producer

Women's productivity is rarely considered until they leave the home (Boulding, 1976). Only recently have women's contributions as homemakers been a topic of discussion that takes into consideration its economic and other values. The result, however, is rarely a decision to pay housewives to stay at home to continue their role full time. Instead, women have been sold the notion that they can "have it all, all at the same time" (Gilbert et al., 1981). That most women have discovered the inherent falsity of such a premise only adds emphasis to Boulding's (1976) conclusion:

When women have too heavy a work burden with the triple breeder-feeder-producer role, the whole society suffers. Women suffer role strain, men suffer role deprivation, and children suffer from inadequate experiences of relating to the human community.

Given acceptance of the notion that we expect too much of women when we ask them to be full-time mothers and full-time workers simultaneously, part-time employment may be the answer during children's early years. In more than one study, part-time workers, male or female, blue-collar or white-collar, expressed greater satisfaction with their situation and more interest in their jobs than did full-time employees (Ferree, 1976). Increasingly, women are choosing to return to paid work on a part-time basis before resuming full-time employment. Factory workers have reported being able to arrange additional break time to rest when they could not delay their return to work. Sometimes this break was used to express milk; in other cases, women took catnaps.

Working at home is an option for some mothers, particularly where electronic linking to the job via computer modems and fax machines is possible. Telecommuting offers an opportunity for parents who previously worked elsewhere to continue employment while remaining at home with an infant or young child. It also enables the new mother to practice resuming an organized way of life while she learns that a freer form to the day, the norm when a baby's needs come into play, has its own rewards. Television advertisements (such as the catchy phrase, "I e-mail over oatmeal") that tout the joys of telecommuting suggest that it is increasingly accepted as just another way of working, and one that the new mother may wish to explore if it has not yet been incorporated into her employment setting. One mid-1997 television news program examining the frequency of telecommuting found that many companies now make this option available to male and female employees already noted for their self-discipline and their ability to work well in isolation. However, even these workers come into the office at least part of the week to participate in meetings and to share their work with others in face-to-face encounters. When preparing to engage in telecommuting, mothers are often asked to retain established child-care arrangements in order to maintain some degree of separation between home and work activities, even if the site is the same.

Still another option is job-sharing. Advantages to the employer include greater productivity, greater worker satisfaction, and lower turnover. Job-sharing is an alternative to full-time work that seems especially viable for nurses (Lindeke & Iverson, 1986). More than one pair of lactation consultants has made such an arrangement with their hospital employer.

Job-sharing works best if each partner informs the other about work issues before the first partner leaves for home. In most cases, each is more rested than a full-time worker and is thus more efficient during her four-hour workday than either would be for half of a full workday. The flexibility of job-sharing may be appropriate for an employee who wishes to maintain work skills while avoiding stress and burnout, which may occur with having young children.

The Continuing "War" Between Work and Home

Although the discomfort with what today's woman has chosen is less visible today than in previous years, the lack of understanding and empathy that exists between employed women and at-home women remains. On the one hand, the mother at home often feels ignored and devalued. Her feelings are justifiable, because our society rarely values that which is not paid for. Precisely because she is not paid, the at-home mother remains economically invisible. In fact, social scientists often place them in a separate category and ignore them in most analyses, especially those relating to economic contributions.

The employed mother who is struggling to maintain her equilibrium while she simultaneously attempts to be all things to all people may also feel ignored and devalued. She, too, is justified in feeling this way. Although she brings home a paycheck for the work she does at the office or factory, her at-home work does not go away. Rarely is it fully shared by her spouse or partner (Hochschild & Machung, 1989). In spite of the fact that most married households in the country include two workers, it is the wife who still schedules a plumber to fix a broken pipe or an electrician to check a faulty wire; one quickly gains a sense of the degree to which working women feel continually pulled in different directions.

The mother at home may both envy and resent her employed counterpart. The mother at work may both envy and resent the mother at home. Each woman wants to think that she is managing her life the "right" way, even though she may feel that the other alternative has many benefits. The mother at home is attempting to live the myth of the intact American family that never really existed for the majority of women. Today's working woman is attempting to live out yet another myth that suggests that women can and should be able to "have it all": marriage, career, and children.

Neither woman is entirely right or wrong; each is doing the best for her family and each struggles with what often seem to be insoluble problems and unresolvable situations. Each needs the support of the other; each shares far more similarities than differences with the other. Most important among those shared similarities is that both groups of women are caring for children and trying to do the best for them in an environment that values women at far less than their real worth–and that values children even less. The at-home mother deserves to be valued for her truly priceless (not valueless) activity: rearing and caring for children. The working mother needs to be valued sufficiently so that her special procreative and nurturing capabilities are not ignored simply because she goes out of the house to earn a living (Fig. 18–2).

What has this to do with breastfeeding? The relative invisibility of the economic value of breastfeeding (Meershoek, 1993) in today's world is symptomatic of the relative invisibility of most women's accomplishments. Women must value one another and recognize how each affirms female existence and women's contribution to life. Only through such valuation will the barriers they encounter be burned on the bonfire of enlightened self-interest (Table 18–1).

The Importance of Social Support

The employed breastfeeding mother is a pioneer insofar as there is no precedent for what she is trying to do, so it is unlikely that any of her older female relatives have experienced it. Thus she and her partner are setting out on an adventure that places their family at the cutting edge of social change.

Such a position is likely to be unsettling, precisely because there are few established rules governing action. Until they find peers who have done the same thing–and lived to laugh about the inevitable potholes of life that will surely trip them up–the employed breastfeeding mother and her spouse will need the support of other family members, friends, and colleagues whose opinions matter to them. Who will fill these key support roles

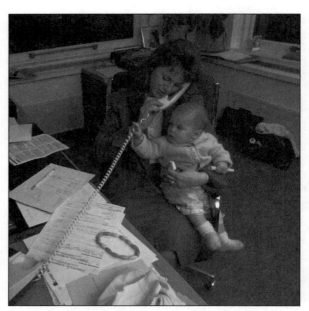

FIGURE 18-2. Baby goes to work with mom.
(© Frank Siteman/Stock Boston/PNI.)

varies by ethnic group. Littman et al. (1994) report that the male partner is the most important person for the white mother. However, among black women, a close friend was most influential, whereas Mexican-American mothers sought the support of their own mothers (Baranowski et al., 1983).

When combining breastfeeding and employment, the mother needs several types of social support, specifically

- a person who cares about her and what she wants for her baby
- a role model
- a knowledgeable advisor
- a person who obviously values breastfeeding
- a person on whose shoulder she can lean or cry

A person who cares about her and what she wants for her baby is most often the baby's father, but not all fathers are supportive of breastfeeding. Most white mothers, however, will look first to the baby's father for support.

A role model is a person who has breastfed her own baby while employed, has enjoyed her experience, and focuses more on the positive aspects of breastfeeding while helping the mother to work

Table 18–1

BARRIERS TO BREASTFEEDING WHILE EMPLOYED, AND SUGGESTED STRATEGIES

Barriers	Short-Term Strategies	Long-Term Strategies
Lack of child care at or near workplace	Ensure that information about child care is located near worksite Establish child-care information and referral system	Establish government policies enabling most employers to subsidize child care
Conditions of work environment	Provide breastfeeding breaks for mothers Provide a place for mothers to express or pump their milk and store for later use	Provide options for flex-time, job-sharing, part-time work at the worksite Provide options to work from home, either part-time or full-time Provide options to bring a non-mobile infant to the worksite with mother
Employer policies: inadequate maternity insurance program	Encourage legislation for disability insurance in states in which it does not yet exist	Establish a national maternity policy with job-protected maternity leave featuring full or partial wage replacement plus health coverage
Societywide attitudes about breastfeeding	Develop public education programs for school-age children	Develop educational attitudes and programs about breastfeeding
Mother's lack of information about breastfeeding	Establish worksite prenatal programs about working, maternity leave, and breastfeeding	Integrate material knowledge with information about employer policies and options
Lack of understanding and knowledge of health professionals about breastfeeding and employment	Develop professional education programs for health care workers at all levels	Integrate material on lactation into curricula in professional training programs at undergraduate and graduate levels

Source: Derived in part from Barber-Madden R, Petschek MA, Pakter J: Breastfeeding and the working mother: barriers and intervention strategies. J Public Health Pol *8:531–41, 1987.*

through the difficult situations that inevitably arise from time to time. The friend who has breastfed can be a particularly powerful ally for Hispanic women or women from low-income groups (Barron et al., 1988).

A knowledgeable advisor might be a lactation consultant, a natural in this role, as is any other health care provider who has counseled other successful breastfeeding and working mothers (Corbett-Dick & Bezek, 1997). Least likely to be an appropriate choice here is a health care worker whose personal experience of combining breastfeeding and working was more negative than positive (Auerbach & Guss, 1985).

A person who values breastfeeding might be a La Leche League leader or Nursing Mothers counselor. Such a person will be enthusiastic and knowledgeable about breastfeeding. Her support and information can be critical to the working mother, who chooses to nurture her baby in a manner that is not supported by all family members or friends.

A person on whose shoulder the mother can lean or cry should probably *not* be the partner. Too often, when the mother complains that things are not going well, her partner–in a sincere desire to give her permission to make her life easier–may suggest that she stop breastfeeding if it is causing so much hassle. He may not want her to do so, but he may feel that this is the only suggestion he can provide that gives them some control. The role model or knowledgeable advisor may better provide that shoulder on which the mother can lean. So also may the person who values breastfeeding. In some cases, this person may be a sister or a dear friend whose familiar voice over the long-distance phone lines may be just the tonic to rejuvenate the new mother as she struggles with one more new experience and feels so alone. Regardless of who this person is, simply knowing that the shoulder is available may give the mother sufficient strength of purpose to persevere. Most often, it is this person who can help her distinguish between baby-related and sitter-related problems.

The more people who support the mother's actions, the more likely she is to feel that she can maintain her equilibrium during the rough spots in her journey through motherhood (Lancaster, 1975; Saunders & Carroll, 1988). Although commitment is clearly necessary whenever a person takes on a

new role (Coreil & Murphy, 1988), the support of others cannot be underestimated, particularly when there is little shared past experience.

Lactation Programs at Work

Among the frequently mentioned features of a company that is considered to be family friendly are work at home, job sharing, flextime, and phase-back options, Family Leave Act–related options, nursing mothers' rooms, and the availability of a breast pump at the work site. In this author's review of the "100 Best Companies" named in the most recent five years of *Working Mother* magazine (October issue), it was clear that breastfeeding-specific items were least likely to be included, even when limiting the survey to the top 10 companies mentioned. Nevertheless, other options also help the breastfeeding mother, particularly those that govern when she must return to work and whether she can return on a part-time basis or use a tele-commuting site in lieu of returning to her previous office-based employment site.

It is costly for a company when an employee–already trained and knowing how to get the job done–opts not to return to work because she feels she must choose between the welfare of her child and her job. If a mother values her baby's needs more than her job, her former employer must recruit and train a replacement. Those costs average more than $2,000 if she is not in management and more than $25,000 if she holds a managerial position. A mother's missing a day of work because her baby is ill is also costly for the employer. The Los Angeles Department of Water and Power estimated that for a $15/hour employee, one day of lost work costs $360, which includes cost for loss of the worker's time as well as for the day and a half of additional work required by someone else to do that employee's job. Clearly, it is in the employer's best financial interest to retain trained workers and to enable them to continue to breastfeed.

People at the work site itself can serve multiple roles in supporting the newly returned employee. Cohen and Mrtek (1994) found that of women working in settings where lactation programs were in place, 75 percent who returned to work still breastfeeding continued to do so for six months or longer. In addition, when formula-feeding and

Table 18-2

EXPERIENCES OF BREASTFEEDING PHYSICIANS AND NURSES

Were more likely to ...	Physicians	Nurses
Return to work	Full time	Part time
Express their milk	Rarely	Often
Substitute for missed breastfeedings	Formula	Human milk
Introduce solid foods	Early	Later
Have contact with support groups	Negative	Positive
Wean the baby	Before 6 months	After 12 months
Consider as the effect of their work on breastfeeding	Impeded	Did not impede

breastfeeding infants of employees were compared, 75 percent of illnesses occurred among the formula-feeding group. Of the 28 percent of infants who had no illnesses in their first year of life, 86 percent were breastfed (Cohen et al., 1995). These findings translated into far fewer employee absences related to infant illness and thus less lost time to the company that employed them.

Health Care Workers: A Special Case?

Health care workers, particularly physicians, midwives, and nurses, are often asked for their assistance when a breastfeeding mother is planning to return to work. Therefore, it is important to examine their experiences, which often form the basis of professional recommendations (Freed et al., 1995; Miller et al., 1996).

Auerbach and Guss (1985) found differences among three health care worker groups: physicians, technicians, and nurses. These findings have been substantiated in later surveys (Miller et al., 1996). A summary of these groups' experiences reveals why physicians tended to encounter more difficulty when attempting to combine breastfeeding with working (Table 18-2).

The degree to which physicians may be frustrated by the feeling that breastfeeding is easier for

others to schedule is reflected in Freed et al.'s (1992) review of pediatric house staff attitudes relating to breastfeeding, attitudes that reflected what they had (or had not) learned about breastfeeding during their professional training. An examination (Balk et al., 1990) of the perceived effect of residency workload on pregnancy–on the mother and her baby as well as on breastfeeding–makes clear that many physicians do not believe that breastfeeding can be combined with employment without serious negative effects on both the mother and the baby. A more recent study (Miller et al., 1996) examined some of the specifics of residency training that interfere with continued breastfeeding, such as nights away from the baby and long hours on call.

Yet the difficulties identified by health care workers can be resolved. Katcher and Lanese (1985; see also Rogers & Banchy, 1994) reported that the availability of an electric breast pump in an accessible location in a hospital, along with supportive professional advice, resulted in longer breastfeeding duration and a slightly earlier return to work.

Said one nurse, "It makes a difference where you work when pumping your breasts. As a nurse, no one makes a big deal of it when I pump and put my milk in the refrigerator. But my friends in business jobs tell me that they wouldn't do that–pumping milk on the job makes them less a businesswoman." At least one group of attorneys would disagree. In their office supply closet next to a stack of legal pads is a pile of breast pads! Such an image suggests that breastfeeding has become just one more experience that working mothers can share.

The Day-Care Dilemma

Whether to use a day-care facility, where such care will be provided, when the baby will be enrolled and for how many hours and days, and the effects of such care on both the child and her or his parents are issues that figure in decision making of the early postpartum period (U.S. Department of Labor, 1994). In some cases, the father may take on such care, particularly when the parents' work hours differ or when the father's work is flexible and he can rearrange his schedule to accommodate his partner's job situation. In other families, however, the mother may not have a partner who is available, or she may be a single parent. Other relatives may not be potential caregivers, because of geographical distance, disinclination to provide such assistance, physical or psychological incapacity, and many other reasons. When a relative is not available or is not considered appropriate, the parents must decide what kind of care the child will receive and where he or she will receive it.

Brazelton and Als (1979) have speculated that four months of close mother-baby interaction is essential for the maternal-infant bond to be cemented and for optimal infant development to be achieved. It is difficult to see how such development can be attained when mothers and babies are separated for long hours many days a week, beginning soon after the baby's birth.

In addition to attachment issues, the likelihood of childhood illness as a result of out-of-home care during the early years must be addressed by parents. Fleming et al. (1987) found that among those children attending day care full time, 31 percent of upper-respiratory-tract infections and 66 percent of ear infections were attributable to day-care attendance. Reves et al. (1993) reported similar findings and noted as well that risk of diarrhea was highest in the first month of day-care enroll-

ment. Another factor, independent of day-care attendance, that also contributes to risk of diarrheal disease is failure to breastfeed.

Bell et al. (1989) reported that children in day-care were four and a half times more likely to be hospitalized than were children who received care in other settings. Many of these hospitalizations were for placement of tympanostomy tubes for recurrent ear infections. These authors also noted that childhood illness accounted for 40 percent of parental absenteeism from work. Parents whose children went to day-care settings outside the home required more than one-half day per month at home because of illness, compared with one-third day at home because of illness for children who received care in other settings. In the study by Bell et al. (1989), most of the children younger than 12 months who were being breastfed were also being cared for in their own homes when the mothers were employed. Hospitalization occurred for 1.7 percent of the children cared for in their own homes but for more than three times as many (5.7 percent) who were cared for at a day-care center.

The frequency with which the young child will become ill has implications for where he can receive care. Generally, when an infant or young child becomes ill, the usual day-care arrangement is no longer available to him (Jones & Matheny, 1993; see also Furman, 1991), thus forcing the family to use an alternative arrangement. Often that arrangement is the mother's loss of one or more days at work because she must stay home to care for the baby.

Alternatives to infant day-care need to be developed and supported by government. One such alternative is a system that enables–perhaps even encourages–parents to remain with their infants during the first few months of life. This could be accomplished with paid infant-care leaves, not to be confused with maternity leaves, which are often viewed as a form of disability. The People's Republic of China, which has a long history of group child rearing, does not allow infants to be placed in such group care during the first four months of life. In Sweden, a mother may receive up to one year of paid leave–and take another six months of unpaid leave–without fear of losing her job. In Denmark, women receive paid maternity leave for the first six months after birth. Most babies enter day care in their seventh month of life, when their mothers return to full-time employment. The mean age at which breastfeeding was stopped for the Danish babies who were placed in day care was six months (Weile et al., 1990).

Clinical Implications

When providing information about breastfeeding and employment, the lactation consultant is wise to sprinkle such information throughout several discussions of breastfeeding, maintaining a matter-of-fact attitude and establishing a positive expectation that this combination of roles is possible. The LC should discuss breastfeeding with the mother well in advance of her return to work (Greenberg & Smith, 1991). She may also suggest that options exist about which her client may be unaware. Is she the first person with her job to continue breastfeeding? Is there a place at work where she can express milk and store it for later use at home or at the sitter's home? Who will be a support system for her? Have some of her breastfeeding coworkers returned to work later than she may have thought was required? Have some of them chosen not to return to work or found ways to rearrange their work so that they could continue it at home, perhaps by telecommuting? One reason for this exodus from the traditional work setting is the increasing recognition by parents of the importance of being with their children when they are young.

The role overload ("superwoman") of the full-time employed mother necessitates that she learn how to organize her time for maximum efficiency (Vaughn & Wittig, 1980). In breastfeeding, she has found an ideal combination for meeting the physical and psychological needs of her young child. In returning to work, she need not feel that she must shorten the period of lactation that she had planned.

A frank discussion of the different ways in which women have chosen to structure their breastfeeding is necessary. There is no "right" way to do things. For example, some women will choose to give their babies only human milk during their absence. Such a decision requires that the mother begin to obtain additional milk before her return to work; in addition, she may need to arrange to express her milk more than once daily in order to maintain a supply that meets her baby's needs as completely as possible. (See the review of decisions in Box 18–3).

Other mothers may choose not to express their milk at all. These women will need to know that expressing for comfort, at least during the first week or two, may be necessary if they are to avoid unpredictable, potentially embarrassing leak spots while their body is adjusting to no breast stimulation during the workday. Additionally, these mothers should be encouraged to have someone introduce a bottle or cup of artificial formula to the baby well in advance of the mother's first day at work in order to make other plans if the baby develops an allergic reaction.

Some mothers will choose to return to work as soon as possible, often because they are financially unable to do otherwise; other women will make every effort to delay returning to work. The type of job that the woman has, the degree of involvement of coworkers and bosses, and her relationship with them, her seniority, and a wide array of other factors will influence these decisions. The health care worker can provide information about maternal employment and breastfeeding, but only the mother can implement them.

The lactation consultant can share with the mother how other women have coped with similar situations and should answer her questions based on study findings, whenever possible (Table 18–3). Decisions relating to day-care are those most likely to be fraught with high emotion. Babies do know when a mother is not available and adapt to her absence by altering sleep patterns. Changes in wakeful and sleepy periods are typical in families in which the mother works at times when the baby has previously been awake a great deal. Increased breastfeeding frequency when the mother is home (reverse-cycle nursing) is a common reaction, particularly in very young babies who breastfeed often. Such a pattern needs to be pointed out to the sitter; the mother should ask that the sitter not wake the baby for feedings. Instead, the sitter should let the baby tell her when he should be fed during the day. These reverse-cycle nursing episodes do not always increase during the mother's nighttime sleeping hours; rather, they tend to be more frequent during the early daytime hours when she is preparing to leave for work and during the evening hours after she has returned home.

BOX 18–3

Decisions the Employed Breastfeeding Mother Must Make

WHEN TO RETURN TO WORK

1. *Never (or at least not for a long while).* This situation occurs more often as the number of children a mother has increases. Often the mother feels that she lost or missed something by returning to work after the birth of her first baby, so she makes different decisions with later-born offspring. Thus a woman who remains in the workforce, or who returns very soon after her first child's birth, will often reduce the time she spends working outside the home after the birth of her second or third child. This is particularly true if the woman is married and her husband earns a salary sufficient to fully sustain the family.

2. *Later than six months.* This situation occurs very rarely, usually in situations in which the woman is a private practitioner or entrepreneur and chooses to be a full-time mother rather than a paid worker for this period.

3. *Between four and six months.* Some female workers are looking on the early months of mothering as "earned" time off, during which they can concentrate on enjoying their new, exciting role without having to worry about planning for an immediate return to work. In the United States, most such leaves are unpaid; thus their likelihood of occurrence is low, unless the woman exercises a great deal of control at work, is highly placed in the company, or runs her own business.

4. *Between six weeks and three months.* Often such a planned return can be arranged, particularly if the mother is a highly valued employee and the cost of training a replacement would be more than the cost of simply waiting for the original employee to return. Many mothers who have negotiated a return at three months or later have done so by offering to begin to work at home ahead of that time.

5. *As soon as maternity leave is over, or when the employer asks or insists.* In some cases, the employer will ask the mother to return as early as three weeks postpartum. In other cases, often out of fear of loss of employment, the woman will return even earlier. This is inappropriate. As a countertactic, a mother might learn when employees (female and male) who have had abdominal surgery are expected to return to full-time employment.

HOW LONG TO BREASTFEED

1. *Until the baby shows no more interest in breastfeeding.* Cues to lack of interest need to be identified so that the mother does not assume weaning is occurring when the baby is cutting teeth or engaging in a nursing strike.

2. *Until the baby gets teeth or reaches a certain age.* The significance of developmental milestones varies by ethnic and social group as well as by the expectations of immediate family members. Many mothers who had decided to breastfeed for a very short period may select later milestones after their baby has "captured" them in the early breastfeeding period.

3. *Until she returns to work.* Many uninformed women begin at this point, and

change their minds after they learn something about how to combine breastfeeding with employment.

WHEN TO EXPRESS OR PUMP MILK

1. *Regularly,* often more than once per day, for as long as the mother chooses to supply this milk to her baby. These mothers are most likely to find that their employment has minimal effect on the duration of their breastfeeding experience.

2. *Once per day.* Many of these mothers often find that the first week or so following their return to work is the most difficult to manage, because one expression session per day is not sufficient to prevent painful overfilling of the ducts and spontaneous leaking, which draws attention to them as breastfeeding mothers. Thereafter, fullness usually does not continue, but they may also find that their milk supply declines more rapidly than they had anticipated. Often, they regret their decision not to express milk more often; however, by the time they realize what has happened, the baby is no longer interested in breastfeeding, and an untimely weaning–one that occurs before the mother wished–has occurred.

3. *For only a brief period after returning to work,* until the body adjusts and breast fullness no longer occurs. Many mothers often assume that they will not be permitted an opportunity at the job site to express milk or to pump their breasts, without having determined whether this is true. It is rare that employees are not allowed to go to the rest room throughout the workday. Explaining that expressing milk need not be time consuming may help them to see that such activity can be incorporated into their workday with minimal disruption.

4. *Never!* Many mothers are initially uncomfortable with handling their breasts and may convey this in their reluctance to learn how to express milk (Morse & Bottorff, 1988).

WHEN TO USE ARTIFICIAL BABY MILK FOR MISSED FEEDINGS

1. *Never!* Those mothers who are aware of the risks of artificial feeding and the unique benefits of breastfeeding subscribe to this principle. In many cases in which the mother expresses milk more than once throughout her working day, the period of exclusively human milk feedings–even in the mother's absence–can extend past the period when the baby is introduced to solid foods. As the baby's needs begin to outstrip the mother's ability to meet them, other nonhuman milk feedings may have to be introduced.

2. *For those feedings for which the mother's expressed milk is not available or has been used up earlier.* Many women with babies older than four months are in this category. Often the mother's milk supply begins to decline at about the time the baby has another appetite spurt and a rapid growth period. Although previously obtained milk can be substituted for most missed breastfeedings, the caregiver may be required to use formula for other feedings if the supply of human milk is depleted. One option that these mothers often use is the substitution of some solid foods for milk feedings, to extend the period when the baby receives only human milk as fluid nourishment.

3. *For all feedings as soon as the mother returns to work.* Women who follow this principle are also the least likely to express their milk. Often, they view human milk as a

BOX 18–3   *(cont.)*

more convenient way of feeding when they are home but see no real benefit in providing their milk if the baby cannot breastfeed directly. In addition, they often perceive that their work environment is not conducive to expressing and storing their milk for later use. Many physicians fall into this group.

WHERE THE BABY WILL BE CARED FOR

1. *In the mother's own home.* This is the most expensive form of care and the least likely to occur unless the substitute caregiver is a relative. The mother who contemplates such care needs to be aware of IRS regulations governing employment of a person on the employer's premises, which also dramatically increase the cost of such care.

2. *In the home of a neighbor or friend.* Such care is often arranged informally. It can work well if the arrangement is maintained in a businesslike manner. Problems tend to arise when differences of opinion regarding discipline and other aspects of child care occur. However, such care may be beneficial to the child, who is not removed from his own neighborhood and who has access to playmates with whom he will share many experiences.

3. *In the home of a stranger who provides day-care services.* Many such homes are unlicensed; others are licensed by the city or state in which they operate. Parents need to find a home that provides what the mother wants for her child, including a minimum number of children of the same age. However, when the child being cared for is less than one year of age, expecting one person to also care for more than two older babies is less than optimal. Older children can be a blessing or a curse, depending on their behavior toward the youngest one.

4. *In a day-care center.* This is the most visible portion of day-care in the United States. Although most media coverage of such centers has focused on the nightmares of alleged (and actual) abuse and neglect, parents must carefully evaluate a center before placing a child, particularly an infant, there. They should assess the staff-to-child ratio, the cleanliness and safety features of the facility, and opportunities for structured and unstructured learning and seek the opinions of previous users of the center. If a center operator cannot (or will not) provide the names of several previous clients, the parents considering such a center should run rapidly out the door!

Many mothers find that setting the alarm an hour earlier than they plan to be up reminds them to offer the baby the breast while they snooze before heading for the shower or the kitchen to start the day. If she is encouraged to see this as the baby's touching and social time, the mother is more likely to view such behavior as a sign of the baby's attachment to her.

No "magic bullet" will resolve day-care issues. Unlike other countries, in which government sub-

sidies enable many mothers to stay home for a substantial period following the birth of their babies, the United States has no federal policy supporting paid maternity leave. At the same time, increasing numbers of families make economic choices that mandate a two-worker household. In addition, day-care workers, often because they are so poorly paid, represent a workforce that has a high turnover, inadequate training, and lack of job commitment.

Table 18–3

STUDY FINDINGS AND RECOMMENDATIONS FOR THE EMPLOYED BREASTFEEDING MOTHER

Study Findings	Recommendations to Share
Successful, employed breastfeeding mothers	
. . . were most anxious about the baby and breast-feeding in the first week of employment.	Arrange to return to work late in the week in order to look forward to a weekend that is only a day or two away.
. . . waited until the baby was four months old or older before returning to work.	Stay home as long as possible.
. . . used part-time or flex-time options when they first returned to work.	Return on less than a full-time schedule in the beginning.
. . . expressed milk during their absences: (a) especially in the first month (b) to remain physically comfortable (c) to reduce the likelihood of leaking (d) to collect milk for later use	Learn how to express or pump milk.
. . . obtained less milk at the end of the work week than at the beginning.	Increase fluids near the end of the work week; to avoid overfullness on Mondays, restrict fluids slightly.
. . . complained most often about exhaustion.	Use breastfeeding as a "break" from home chores.
. . . viewed breastfeeding as the key to continued "connection" with the baby in spite of separations.	Enjoy the closeness that breastfeeding represents–especially after a day-long separation.

Source: Derived from KG Auerbach: Assisting the employed breastfeeding mother. J Nurse Midwif *35:28, 1990.*

SUMMARY

The role of the health care worker is to inform the mother that she is not alone and that what she is likely to encounter has, in most cases, been faced by other women. In some cases, the mothers found partial solutions; in other cases, their solutions enabled them, and will enable others, to proceed with breastfeeding with minimal interruption. Whatever the mother's individual situation, the person providing information needs to do so from a perspective of what has worked for others, recog- nizing that each mother's situation has unique strengths and pitfalls.

In settings in which institutionalized day-care is well organized and carefully supervised, many families' concerns can be set aside. In other day-care situations, the increased illness rates and other issues related to meeting the infant's and child's many needs warrant considerable concern. At-home care is both more expensive and more diffi- cult to obtain; in addition, it provides no guarantee that some of the problems that have surfaced in group settings, including child neglect or abuse, will not also occur.

The length of time that a child breastfeeds (even if it is two years) represents a very small amount of the total time that the child will live in the parents' home. The length of the mother's employment is likely to last far longer than her child's infancy. The longer the mother is home during the baby's early weeks and months, the shorter the time that breastfeeding is most likely to be negatively affected by that employment.

REFERENCES

Al-Sekait MA: A study of the factors influencing breastfeeding patterns in Saudi Arabia. *Saudi Med J* 9:596–601, 1988.

Armstrong H: Breastfeeding low birthweight babies: advances in Kenya. *J Hum Lact* 3:34–7, 1987.

Auerbach KG: Assisting the employed breastfeeding mother. *J Nurse Midwif* 35:26–34, 1990.

Auerbach KG: Employed breastfeeding mothers: problems they encounter. *Birth* 11:17–20, 1984.

Auerbach KG: Sequential and simultaneous breast pumping: a comparison. *Int J Nurs Stud* 27:257–65, 1990.

Auerbach KG, Guss E: Health care workers who breastfeed: implications for patient management. *J Am Med Women's Assoc* 40:111–5, 1985.

Auerbach KG, Guss E: Maternal employment and breastfeeding: a study of 567 women's experiences. *Am J Dis Child* 138:958–60, 1984.

Balk SJ, Christoffel KK, Bijur, PE: Pediatricians' attitudes concerning motherhood during residency. *Am J Dis Child* 144:770–7, 1990.

Baranowski T, et al: Social support, social influence, ethnicity and the breastfeeding decision. *Soc Sci Med* 17:1599–1611, 1983.

Barber-Madden R, Petschek MA, Pakter J: Breastfeeding and the working mother: barriers and intervention strategies. *J Public Health Pol* 8:531–41, 1987.

Barger J, Bull P: A comparison of bacterial composition of breast milk stored at room temperature and stored in the refrigerator. *Int J Child Educ* 2:29–30, 1987.

Barron SP, et al: Factors influencing duration of breast feeding among low-income women. *J Am Diet Assoc* 88:1557–61, 1988.

Bell DM, et al: Illness associated with child day care: a study of incidence and cost. *Am J Public Health* 79:479–84, 1989.

Birenbaum E, Fuchs C, Reichman B: Demographic factors influencing the initiation of breast-feeding in an Israeli urban population. *Pediatrics* 83:519–23, 1989.

Boulding E: Familial constraints on women's work roles. *Signs* 1:95–117, 1976.

Bourgoin GL, et al: Factors influencing the duration of breastfeeding in the Sudbury region. *Can J Public Health* 88:234–41, 1997.

Brazelton TB, Als H: Four early stages in the development of mother-infant interaction. *Psychoanal Study Child* 34:349–69, 1979.

Broome M: Breastfeeding and the working mother. *JOGN Nursing* 10:201–2, 1981.

Cohen R, Mrtek MB: The impact of two corporate lactation programs on the incidence and duration of breast-feeding by employed mothers. *Am J Health Prom* 8:436–41, 1994.

Cohen R, Mrtek MB, Mrtek RG: Comparison of maternal absenteeism and infant illness rates among breast-feeding and formula-feeding women in two corporations. *Am J Health Prom* 10:148–53, 1995.

Corbett-Dick P, Bezek SK: Breastfeeding promotion for the employed mother. *J Pediatr Health Care* 11:12–19, 1997.

Coreil J, Murphy JE: Maternal commitment, lactation practices and breastfeeding duration. *JOGNN* 17:273–8, 1988.

Daly SEJ, Hartmann PE: Infant demand and milk supply: The short-term control of milk synthesis in lactating women. *J Hum Lact* 11:27–37, 1995.

Davis HV, et al: Effects of cup, bottle and breast feeding on oral activities of newborn infants. *Pediatrics* 23:549–58, 1949.

Ferree MM: Working-class jobs: housework and paid work as sources of satisfaction. *Soc Prob* 23:431–44, 1976.

Fleming DW, et al: Childhood upper respiratory tract infections: to what degree is incidence affected by day care attendance? *Pediatrics* 79:55–60, 1987.

Frederick IB, Auerbach KG: Maternal-infant separation and breast-feeding: the return to work or school. *J Reprod Med* 30:523–6, 1985.

Freed GL, et al: Attitudes and education of pediatric house staff concerning breast-feeding. *South Med J* 85:483–5, 1992.

Freed GL, et al: National assessment of physicians' breast-feeding knowledge, attitudes, training, and experience. *JAMA* 273:472–6, 1995.

Furman L: Infirmary-style sick-child day care: do we need more information? *Pediatrics* 88:290–3, 1991.

Gielen AC, et al: Maternal employment during the early postpartum period: effects on initiation and continuation of breast-feeding. *Pediatrics* 87:298–305, 1991.

Gilbert LA, Holahan CK, Manning L: Coping with conflict between professional and maternal roles. *Fam Rel* 30:419–26, 1981.

Greenberg CS, Smith K: Anticipatory guidance for the employed breast-feeding mother. *J Pediatr Health Care* 5:204–9, 1991.

Hamosh M, et al: Breastfeeding and the working mother: effect of time and temperature of short-term storage on proteolysis, lipolysis, and bacterial growth in milk. *Pediatrics* 97:492–8, 1996.

Hamosh M, et al: Digestive enzymes in human milk: stability at suboptimal storage temperatures. *J Pediatr Gasteoenterol Nutr* 24:38–43, 1997.

Hibbard R, Blevins R: Palatal burn due to bottle warming in a microwave oven. *Pediatrics* 82:382–4, 1988.

Hills-Bonzcyk SG, et al: Women's experiences with breastfeeding longer than 12 months. *Birth* 21:206–12, 1994.

Hochschild A, Machung A: *The second shift: working parents and the revolution at home*. New York: Viking Penguin, 1989.

Jones EG, Matheny RJ: Relationship between infant feeding and exclusion rate from child care because of illness. *J Am Diet Assoc* 93:809–11, 1993.

Katcher A, Lanese MG: Breastfeeding by employed mothers: a reasonable accommodation in the workplace. *Pediatrics* 25:644–7, 1985.

Kearney MH, Cronenwett L: Breastfeeding and employment. *JOGNN* 20:471–80, 1991.

Lancaster J: Coping mechanisms for the working mother. *Am J Nurs* 75:1322–3, 1975.

Lang S, Lawrence CJ, Orme RLE: Cup feeding: an alternative method of infant feeding. *Arch Dis Child* 71:365–9, 1994.

Larson E, et al: Storage of human breast milk. *Infect Control* 5:127–30, 1984.

Lindberg LD: Women's decisions about breast-feeding and maternal employment. *J Marr Fam* 58:239–51, 1996.

Lindeke LL, Iverson SL: Job sharing: an employment alternative for nurse practitioners. *Pediatr Nurs* 12:101–4, 1986.

Littman H, et al: The decision to breastfeed: the importance of fathers' approval. *Clin Pediatr* 33:214–9, 1994.

Livingstone VH, Grams GD: Breast-feeding and the working mother. *Can Fam Phys* 31:1685–93, 1985.

Marshall L: Breastfeeding and its alternatives among Papua New Guinea career women–an issue in economic development. *Ecol Food Nutr* 20:311–22, 1988.

McKenna J, Mosho S, Richard C: Bedsharing promotes breastfeeding. *Pediatrics* 100:214–19, 1997.

Meershoek S: The economic value of breastfeeding. *Breastfeed Rev* 2:354–7, 1993.

Miller NH, et al: Breastfeeding practices among resident physicians. *Pediatrics* 98:434–7, 1996.

Morse JM, Bottorff JL: The emotional experience of breast expression. *J Nurse Midwif* 33:165–70, 1988.

Morse JM, Bottorff JL, Boman, J: Patterns of breastfeeding and work: the Canadian experience. *Can J Public Health* 80:182–8, 1989.

Nemethy M, Clore ER: Microwave heating of infant formula and breast milk. *J Pediatr Health Care* 4:131–5, 1990.

Nwankwo MU, et al: Bacterial growth in expressed breast-milk. *Ann Trop Paediatr* 8:92–5, 1988.

Piper S, Parks PL: Predicting the duration of lactation: evidence from a national survey. *Birth* 23: 7–12, 1996.

Pittard WB, et al: Bacteriostatic qualities of human milk. *J Pediatr* 107:240–3, 1985.

Reves RR, et al: Child day care increases the risk of clinic visits for acute diarrhea and diarrhea due to rotavirus. *Am J Epidemiol* 137:97–107, 1993.

Rogers B, Banchy P: Establishing an employee breast pumping facility. *J Hum Lact* 10:119–20, 1994.

Ryan AS, Martinez GA: Breast-feeding and the working mother: a profile. *Pediatrics* 83:524–31, 1989.

Saunders SE, Carroll J: Post-partum breast feeding support: impact on duration. *J Am Diet Assoc* 88:213–5, 1988.

Shepherd SC, Yarrow RE: Breastfeeding and the working mother. *J Nurse Midwif* 27:16–20, 1982.

Sigman M, et al: Effects of microwaving human milk: changes in IgA content and bacterial count. *J Am Diet Assoc* 89:690–2, 1989.

Silprasert A, et al: Effect of storage on the creamatocrit and total energy content of human milk. *Hum Nutr Clin Nutr* 40C:31–6, 1986.

Sosa R, Barness L: Bacterial growth in refrigerated human milk. *Am J Dis Child* 141:111–2, 1987.

Thimmayamma B, Vidyavati M, Bhavani B: Infant feeding practices in working mothers in an urban area. *Ind J Med Res* 72:834–9, 1980.

Thompson PE, Bell P: Breast-feeding in the workplace: how to succeed. *Iss Comp Pediatr Nurs* 20: 1–9, 1997.

U.S. Department of Labor: *Working women: a chartbook* (bull. no. 2385). Washington, DC: Bureau of Labor Statistics, August 1991.

U.S. Department of Labor: *Working women count! A report for the nation.* Washington, DC: U.S. Department of Labor, Women's Bureau, 1994.

U.S. Department of Labor: *Facts on working women* (no. 96–2). Washington, DC: U.S. Department of Labor, Women's Bureau, September 1996.

Vaughn LS, Wittig MA: Occupation, competence, and role overload as evaluation determinants of successful women. *J Appl Soc Psychol* 10:398–415, 1980.

Visness CM, Kennedy KI: Maternal employment and breast-feeding: findings from the 1988 National Maternal and Infant Health Survey. *Am J Public Health* 87:945–50, 1997.

Weile B, et al: Infant feeding patterns during the first year of life in Denmark: factors associated with the discontinuation of breast-feeding. *J Clin Epidemiol* 43:1305–11, 1990.

Williams JM, Auerbach KG, Jacobi A: Lateral epicondylitis (tennis elbow) in breastfeeding mothers. *Clin Pediatr* 28:42–3, 1989.

Youngblut JM, Loveland-Cherry CJ, Horan M: Factors related to maternal employment status following the premature birth of an infant. *Nurs Res* 39:237–40, 1990.

CHAPTER

19

CHILD HEALTH

Jan Riordan

Breastfeeding has long been considered health promoting, and the positive effect of breastfeeding on the health of the baby has been the subject of extensive study and review. Even the cost of not breastfeeding has been calculated: one estimate is more than $1 billion for four medical diagnoses alone (Riordan, 1997). Another recent study found that breastfed infants enrolled in WIC saved $478 in WIC costs and Medicaid expenditures in the first six months, compared with formula-fed infants. Even after considering savings to WIC from formula manufacturers' rebates, breastfeeding babies still represented a savings of $161 (Montgomery & Splett, 1997). Multiplying these figures by the millions of infants enrolled in WIC makes clear how much money breastfeeding represents. Attention has focused on breastfeeding as a means of reducing infections; the effects of breastfeeding in preventing chronic disease and on child development are not as yet recognized.

This chapter reviews child health issues. Discussion begins with the fundamentals of normal growth and development of infants and children and then reviews prominent theories of child development. The rich textures of mother-infant social interaction, woven from the sophisticated sensory abilities of the newborn, creates a lifelong bond. Next, such children's health issues as immunization and dental health answer questions that care providers are frequently called on to provide.

The chapter concludes with the practical considerations of introducing solids and a discussion of weaning.

Developmental Outcomes and Infant Feeding

Before addressing specific elements of growth and development, it is useful to consider studies that compare developmental outcomes between breastfed and bottle-fed babies. A few studies now decades old (Broad, 1972; Hoefer & Hardy, 1929; Rogerson & Rogerson, 1939) found that the cognitive and developmental status of children who were breastfed was higher than that of those who were fed with other milks. However, the authors failed to control for socioeconomic and educational factors (e.g., the education of the mother), thus calling these findings into question. Later studies whose authors did control for these factors confirmed that breastfeeding appears to have a significant positive effect on standardized intelligence tests, a small but significantly positive effect on development, but no effect on motor skills.

Rodgers (1978) analyzed U.K. National Survey of Health and Development data and discovered a small but significant advantage for the children who were breastfed. Fergusson et al. (1982) examined the relationship between breastfeeding and childhood intelligence and development in New Zealand children. Even when the mother's intelligence and education, the family's socioeconomic status, and the baby's birth weight and gestational age were taken into account, breastfed children had slightly higher intelligence test scores than did bottle-fed infants. Two years later, Taylor and Wadsworth (1984) found a positive correlation between duration of breastfeeding and children's performance in vocabulary and visual-motor coordination tests.

Finally, Morrow-Tlucak et al. (1988) compared the cognitive development in breastfed and bottle-fed children living in Ohio. The investigators used rigorous covariate analysis, including controlling for the home environment (HOME scale), to determine whether the previously discerned advantage to breastfed children was evident early in development. In their sample, breastfed infants scored significantly higher on the Mental Development Index of the Bayley Scales at one and two years of age. At six months of age, the breastfed babies scored higher than did the bottle-fed infants, although the difference did not reach significance.

These results raise questions: What elements of breastfeeding play a role in promoting development and intelligence? Is it the nutritional or immunological aspects of breastmilk, or is it the interactions between the mother and infant during breastfeeding? Lucas et al. (1992) controlled for maternal interaction by studying preterm infants who received their mothers' milk via tube feedings and compared them with children who got formula or children whose mothers intended to provide them with breastmilk but did not. Because all the infants were fed only by tube, the effects of breastmilk per se were separate from the normally intertwined effect of intimate maternal contact. The IQ scores of the children fed human milk were 8.5 points higher than those of the groups not fed human milk.

Gale & Martyn (1996) challenged the validity of the beneficial effect of breastfeeding on adult intelligence. Study participants who had been exclusively breastfed had slightly higher IQ scores than did those who had been exclusively bottle-fed or received mixed feedings. IQ was lower in participants who had used a pacifier (dummy) in infancy, in those whose fathers were in manual occupations at the time of their birth, and in those whose mothers were young at the time they were born. After adjusting for the effect of all other variables, no association was found between adult intelligence and method of feeding. Pacifier use, number of older siblings, maternal age at birth of participant, and the father's occupational class remained independent predictors of adult intelligence, suggesting that later intelligence has more to do with social influence than with the nutritional qualities of human milk. This same study was later criticized for selection bias. Presumably, less than 50 percent of the original sample took the IQ test; moreover, the use of pacifiers is detrimental to breastfeeding, thus masking the true effect of breastfeeding (Cockburn et al., 1996). Recent research outcomes on breastfeeding and child intelligence are described in Table 19–1.

If human milk and breastfeeding are linked with higher intelligence, the mechanism of this effect on brain development is unknown at this time. It has been suggested that the presence of longer-chain polyunsaturated fatty acids, particularly arachidonic and docosahexanoic acid in human milk but not in most artificial baby milks, is responsible. These fatty acids are essential nutrients for infants, because they are present in structural lipids in brain and nervous tissue (Farquharson et al., 1992). As discussed in Chapter 5, differences in visual performance between breastfed and formula-fed full-term infants, for example, are thought to result from the provision of arachidonic and docosahexanoic acid in breastmilk (Birch et al., 1993; Makrides et al., 1994).

Growth and Development
Physical Growth

Infant and child growth is affected by genetic makeup, general health, and nutrition. Infants and children vary in their tempo of growth and development, which tends to be marked by spurts of growth separated by plateaus. Still, there are universal patterns of growth for all children. These universal patterns include cephalocaudal growth (growth that proceeds from head to foot), proximodistal growth (growth that occurs from the center outward), and general-to-specific movements.

Table 19–1

STUDIES OF BREASTFEEDING AND CHILDREN'S INTELLIGENCE

Studies	Subjects and Methods	Major Findings
Johnson et al., 1996 (United States)	204 children measured at 3 years of age; Stanford-Binet, Hollingshead Index of Social Status; controlled for socioeconomic status, mother's intelligence, smoking behavior, gender, and birth order of child	Initiation of breastfeeding predicted scores on intelligence tests at age 3. Breastfeeding was associated with 4.6-point higher mean in intelligence.
Florey et al., 1995 (United Kingdom)	592 first-born infants; Bayley Scales of Infant Mental and Motor Development	Higher mental development (3.7–5.7 points) was significantly related to breastfeeding at 2 weeks after discharge after controlling for social and demographic factors. No differences were seen for psychomotor development or behavior.
Temboury et al., 1994 (Spain)	364 healthy infants measured between 18 and 29 months of age; Bayley Scales of Infant Development; controlled for maternal age, number of children, educational level, social class, job, psychosocial risk, and infant variables	Lower results on the Index of Mental Development were associated with bottle-fed infants, lower-middle and lower social class, elementary education of the mother, temper tantrums, and having siblings. Lower results on the Index of Motor Development were associated only with lower and lower-middle social class.
Rogan & Gladen, 1993 (United States)	855 newborns; Bayley Scales of Infant Development; McCarthy Scale; prospective case control	Statistically significant but small increases were noted in scores among breastfed children on cognitive skills, not motor skills. Slightly higher English grades on report cards were noted after adjusting for confounding variables.
Lucas et al., 1992 (United Kingdom)	926 low-birth-weight infants tube-fed with human milk or formula; measured at 8.5 years of age; Weschler Intelligence Scale for Children; randomized controlled trial of feeding mode; controlled for maternal contact, social class, and education	A dose-response relationship was noted between proportion of mother's milk and IQ. Children receiving human milk scored 8.3 points higher.
Morley, et al., 1988 (United Kingdom)	771 low-birth-weight infants; Bayley Mental Scale; Developmental Profile 11; measured at 18 months postterm; randomized controlled trial of feeding mode	The children who received their mothers' milk had a significant 8-point advantage on the Bayley mental developmental index over the children of mothers who received only formula. After adjustment for social and demographic influences, the advantage was 4.3 point ($p < .005$).

The infant's head accounts for about one-fourth of the infant's length at birth and illustrates cephalo-caudal direction of growth. Maturation of motor skills also follows the cephalocaudal pattern: an infant masters control of his head before he masters arm and trunk control, which is followed by leg control (Fig. 19–1).

Proximodistal and general-to-specific development is illustrated by the sequence of muscle control: infants control large muscles before they control small muscles. For example, the child is able to wave "bye-bye" before he is able to grasp with his whole hand and before he is able to hold a small object with his thumb and forefinger (pincer grasp). There is some evidence that breastfeeding has a beneficial effect on neurological development in children. Lanting et al. (1994) found a small advantageous effect of breastfeeding on the neurological status of children nine years of age.

Weight and Length

Change, rather than stability, is the hallmark of infancy; weight increases faster in infancy than at any other time of life. The average neonate weighs about 3,000 to 4,000 gm (6.5–8.5 lb). Because full-term infants are born with excess fluid, they lose 5 to 10 percent of their birth weight following birth and then stabilize within a few days. Generally speaking, infants double their birth weight by about five months of age, triple it by one year of age, and quadruple it by two years of age.

As discussed in Chapters 10 and 11 in this book, weight patterns of formula-fed infants differ from those of infants who are fed exclusively at the breast. Their weights are similar for the first few months, but at three to four months, formula-fed infants begin to weigh more than do their breastfed counterparts. This appears to hold cross culturally: formula-fed Japanese babies six to eight months old weigh significantly more (135 gm) than do those breastfed (Yoneyama et al., 1994). As discussed in Chapter 5, Butte et al. (1990) reported that North American breastfed babies gain an average of 35 gm (approximately 1 oz.) per day at one month and 19 gm (0.6 oz.) per day at four months, whereas formula-fed infants gain an average of 34.4 gm/day at one month and 23 gm/day at four months. Despite their slightly slower weight gain,

breastfed infants at four months have more body fat (Butte et al., 1995).

Length at birth is about 50 to 53 cm (20–21 in.) and, on the average, male infants tend to be 5 oz. heavier and 0.5 in. longer than females. A baby grows about 1 in. each month for the first six months and about 0.5 in. per month for the next six months. By the infant's first birthday, his length has increased by 50 percent. Length and head-circumference growth are similar for both breastfed and formula-fed infants (Butte et al., 1990). The weight of the baby's brain increases most rapidly during infancy as nerve cells enlarge, become longer and branched, and gain myelin sheathing. By 18 months of age, the infant's brain is 75 percent of its adult weight. If the infant becomes malnourished, the first growth factor to be affected is weight. Only when malnourishment is severe and long standing are the infant's length or head circumference compromised.

Senses

Neonates and young infants have remarkably well-developed sensory capabilities. At birth, the infant's auditory nerve tracts have sufficient myelin sheathing to allow them to hear well; they can differentiate various tastes and smells. This ability to selectively respond through their senses enhances the infant's early attempts to locate and attach to the nipple and to distinguish between his own mother and other individuals.

Within several days after birth, breastfeeding infants respond preferentially to breast or axillary odors from their mother. In striking contrast, bottle-feeders display no evidence of recognizing axillary odors from their mothers. While feeding at the breast, the neonate's nostrils are in close proximity with the mother's bare skin, which provides the opportunity to become familiar with her characteristic odor (Makin & Porter, 1989).

As early as two months before birth, hearing develops in the womb. The fetus is already responding to both internal sounds from the mother and to noises outside the mother. Some young infants, for instance, appear to recognize their mother's favorite soap opera when it comes on television. Neonates discriminate between differences in pitch and can detect the direction of the source of sound (Levanthal & Lipsitt, 1964; Weir, 1976).

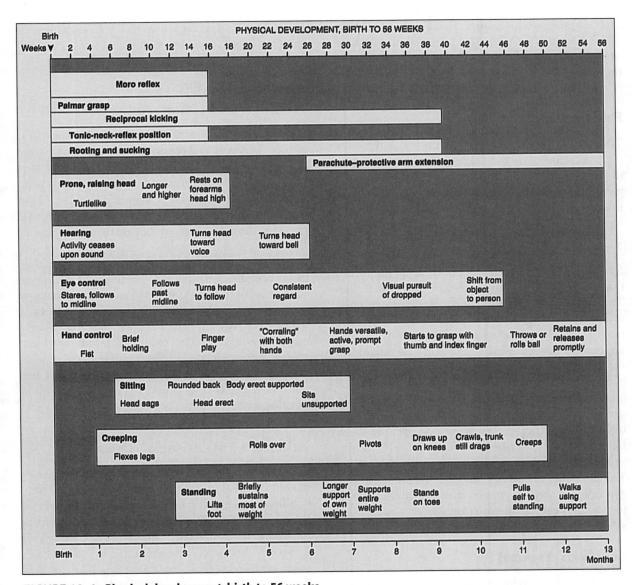

FIGURE 19–1. Physical development, birth to 56 weeks.

Loud, low sounds are likely to disturb and alarm the infant, whereas soft, high-pitched sounds have a calming effect; therefore, the higher-range tones of the female voice tend to quiet and focus the baby's attention. In a nursery when one baby starts crying, others will do the same. Newborns respond to sound by differentiating the caregiver's voice from that of strangers. They also sense heat, cold, pressure, and pain.

The neonate's vision is less developed because retinal structures and the optic nerve are not yet complete. A neonate focuses mainly on large objects close to his face and sees best at a range of 8 to 12 in., with 9 in. as the optimum–just about the distance between the baby's face and the mother's face while the baby is being held at the breast level. Neonates are able to follow and track a moving object with their eyes and prefer moving objects to stationary ones (Kessen et al., 1970).

Babies seem to have an innate visual preference. They prefer more complex stimuli, such as the human face, to a plain surface and will look at a face longer than at other visual patterns (Fantz, 1965; Kagan, 1966; Lewis, 1969). All infants have dark, smoky eyes at birth. Their lids are puffy, and the tear ducts do not function. Eye muscles may occasionally drift to a crossed position.

Reflexes

The fragile appearance of neonates belies the sophistication of their reflexes, which are designed to enhance survival. Reflexes protect the infant and give the central nervous system and brain time to mature and to begin to govern coordinated behaviors (Table 19–2).

Rooting, suckling, swallowing, and gag reflexes are directly applicable to breastfeeding. The rooting reflex initiates the act of suckling milk from the mother's breast and is considered vital to life. The suck swallow reflex is presumably developed at 34 weeks of gestation. Synchronized coordination of suckling and swallowing with breathing appears to be achieved consistently by infants of more than 37 weeks postconception age (Bu'Lock et al., 1990), but in Chapter 14, Meier reported that some infants of 32 weeks' gestation can briefly suckle at the breast. By three to four months after birth, the rooting reflex begins to diminish. In Chapter 4, we described the infant's oral/suckling capabilities as the cockpit of the nervous system. The presence of rooting, sucking, swallowing, and gag reflexes are barometers that indicate an intact, functioning central nervous system.

Levels of Arousal

Young infant behavior can be described by several levels of arousal states (Gill et al., 1988; Prechtl & Beintema, 1975). The Anderson Behavioral State Scale (Gill et al., 1988) lists 12 categories, with states ranging from very quiet sleep to hard crying (Box 19–1). The infant's most complex interaction with his environment is made in the quiet awake state; at this time, the neonate fixates on and follows objects and turns his head toward any sound. The neonate becomes more alert when he senses a new stimulus; if it is repeated, the infant responds less or habituates to the stimulus (Als & Brazelton, 1981). This decrement in response allows the neonate to control his behavioral state. Overactive

infants are said to lack this ability to habituate or respond less to repeated stimuli.

Theories of Development

Nature Versus Nurture

Which is more important in a child's development, nature (genes, heredity) or nurture (environment)? At one end of the spectrum, how a child develops is thought to be determined at conception; at the other end, development is seen as a product of the environment. Although we can demonstrate that breastfeeding appears to optimize development, the issue is still complex. For example, are the overall parenting patterns of a woman who chooses to breastfeed different from those of a woman who chooses to bottle-feed? We cannot say that any one aspect of child development is determined exclusively by either nature or nurture; clearly each plays a role. The extent of influences from nature versus nurture differ among developmental theorists. How these two issues interact are addressed in two popular theories about child development.

Erikson's Psychosocial Theory

Eric Erikson (1963, 1968) identified eight stages of development that center around conflicts. These conflicts are central issues of crucial importance to the personality at each stage of life. Characteristics of the first two stages (infant and toddler) of Erikson's theory are shown in Table 19–3. Each stage requires resolution of its particular conflict, and each stage widens the social radius of the infant's influence. The first conflict is trust versus mistrust. According to Erikson, the first year is when confidence in having one's needs met and feeling physically safe results in the infant's either trusting or mistrusting his environment.

Once trust, as opposed to mistrust, is established, the toddler moves into the next stage, in which autonomy must be mastered over shame and doubt. By then (one and a half to three years of age), he walks, runs, and expresses himself verbally, eagerly exploring his exciting new world but still needing reassurance and returning to his mother for "emotional refueling." If an infant is lovingly fed and

Table 19–2

REFLEXES OF THE NEONATE

Reflex	Stimulus/Description	Appears/Disappears
Rooting	Stroke infant's cheek/head will turn toward stimulus	Birth/disappears by 3–4 mo when awake and by 7–8 mo when asleep
Sucking	Stroke infant's lips; place clean finger in infant's mouth/elicits strong sucking movement	Birth/12 mo
Swallowing	Place liquid on posterior tongue/swallow follows	Persists throughout life
Gag	Stimulate posterior pharynx with object	Persists throughout life
Extrusion	Touch infant's tongue/tongue thrusts outward	Birth/2–4 mo
Moro (startle)	Loud noise; jarring/lowering infant's head	Birth/1–4 mo
Tonic neck	Rotate infant's head to one side while infant lies on back/arm and leg extend on the side that the infant faces; opposite arm and leg are flexed	Birth to 2 mo/4–6 mo
Babinski	Gentle stroking on the sole of the foot/produces fanning and extension of toes	Birth/about 18 mo

his biological needs are cared for, he develops a sense of trust in the world. Being left hungry or crying for long periods results in a sense of mistrust of the world. Breastfeeding for nourishment becomes breastfeeding for reassurance and comfort in this stage. The process of individuation, a realization that he is a separate individual, unfolds gradually as the child begins to assert control over his life.

Piaget's Cognitive Theory

Piaget (1952) stressed the major periods through which humans pass in the course of intellectual maturation. The first is the sensorimotor stage, in which an infant's knowledge of the world comes primarily through his sensory experiences and motor activities. This period begins with the reflex stage and lasts until the child is two years old; its main features are seen in Table 19-3.

As infants experience sensory and motor activities, they construct schemas (concepts or models) for dealing with information and experiences. These schemas are put into play through complementary processes of assimilation and accommo-

dation. Assimilation refers to the process of absorbing new information from the environment and using current structures to deal with the information. Accommodation refers to the process by which the infant alters his behavior and adjusts existing schemas to the requirements of objects or events to integrate new learning with old (and thus adapt to his ever-expanding environments). Hayes (1987) offered the following example:

If a child is breastfed, and a pacifier is given to him for the first time, the pacifier nipple may be sufficiently different so that the old sucking patterns do not work well. When this happens, disequilibrium occurs, and the child must restructure the existing view of suckling so that it fits with the new information or experience. This process is accommodation. Through these processes, schemas are developed and refined.

The concept of object permanence is a feature of the sensorimotor period. Piaget (1952) suggested

BOX 19–1

Anderson Behavioral State Scale: Behavioral States

Sleep
Very quiet sleep
Quiet sleep
Restless sleep
Very restless sleep
Awake
Drowsy
Alert inactivity
Quiet awake
Restless
Restless awake
Very restless awake
Fussing
Crying
Hard crying

Source: Derived from NE Gill, et al: Effect of nonnutritive sucking on behavioral state in preterm infants before feeding. Nurs Res *37:347–50, 1988.*

separation from different caretakers. The ability roughly coincides with diminishing separation anxiety and with Erikson's establishment of trust progressing to the beginnings of autonomy.

Piaget's preoperational period characterizes toddlers and children from about two to seven years of age. During this period, children develop new abilities to think about situations rather than to just behave in them. The acquisition of expressive language marks the beginning of the preoperational stage of intellectual development. Children in this age group view everything in relation to themselves and are unable to take the role of another; this is called *egocentrism*. This egocentricity leads them to believe that their thoughts and actions are shared by others.

Social Development

As infants grow, their periods of waking and socializing lengthen. By six to eight weeks of age, a baby smiles spontaneously to pleasurable stimuli, particularly at human faces. Babies coo and babble to their parents and other fascinated adults who coo and babble back. By three months, the infant is interested in his environment and playfully reaches out to grasp objects, including breasts, nipples, noses, and hair. By six months of age, the infant reaches out to be picked up, squeals with pleasure at recognition of his mother, and enjoys games such as peek-a-boo (Table 19–4).

Language and Communication

Because infants hear well from birth, they are able to discriminate between different intonations and between vowels and consonants. This ability to understand the spoken word is called *passive,* or *receptive, language.* The ability to produce meaningful utterances is called *expressive language.* The speech center in the brain borders on the areas of the motor cortex that control both mouth-tongue movement and hand movement. This proximity explains why we tend to express ourselves with both our hands and our mouths. Infants as well use many gestures in association with sounds and expressive language. Children consistently acquire language communication in a definable sequence:

that the infant younger than six to nine months of age lacks the ability for mental representation of the unseen. For instance, when an object such as a toy is out of sight, it ceases to exist, and the infant does not search for it. With the ability for mental representation, the infant realizes that an object or person continues to exist when out of sight, and he searches for a hidden object. It is now quite certain that person permanency precedes object permanency; an infant does recognize his mother, father, or caretaker long before eight months and thus experiences loss or anxiety when an all-important person is not present. Later, as the child broadens the ability to recognize a separate existence from his mother, he begins to tolerate brief periods of

Table 19–3

THEORIES OF DEVELOPMENT

Theorist	Infant	Toddler
Erikson (psychosexual)	Trust versus mistrust (birth–1 yr)	Autonomy versus shame and doubt (1–3 yr)
	Requires basic needs (food, comfort, warmth) to be met	Increasing independence in eating, dressing, toileting, and bathing
	Learns to trust self (and environment)	Father becomes important
	Mutual giving and getting between self and caregivers	Limits (firm and consistent) lead to security
	Mistrust results if needs not met consistently or inadequately	Acquires "will"; feeling of self-control, bias for self-esteem
Piaget (cognitive)		Excessive criticism and expectation of perfection leads to shame and doubt about ability to control self and world
	Sensorimotor (birth–2 yr); uses senses, motor skills, reflexes to explore	Proconceptual (2–7 yr)
		Self-centered; other centeredness begins
	Object performance	Perception from own point of view
	Trial and error	Use of symbols, especially language
	"Insight" problem solving	Literal interpretation of works and action
	Able to think before acting (18–24 mo)	Judges thing for outcome, consequence to self
		Transductive reasoning

Source: Derived from E Erikson: Childhood and society. *New York: W.W. Norton, 1963; and J Piaget, B Inhelder:* Psychology of the child. *New York: Basic Books, 1969.*

1. Crying: from birth; different rhythms signifying emotions and needs (hunger, anger, pain)

2. Cooing and gooing: after two weeks; a wide variety of meaningless speech sounds (Fig. 19–2)

3. Babbling: 3 to 12 months ("mama-mama," "dada-dada")

4. Holophrasing: 12 months; one-word sentences

5. Telegraphic speech: 18 months; subject-verb-object

6. Complete sentences: two years

The duration of a baby's crying during the early months of life typically increases until about six weeks of age, followed by a gradual decrease until four months of age (Bernal, 1972; Brazelton, 1962; Rebelsky & Black, 1972; Wessel et al., 1954). Infants cry more and are more wakeful during the late afternoon and evening (Emde et al., 1976; Rebelsky & Black, 1972). If the infant is carried during fussy periods, crying and fussing decrease, but the number of feedings and the duration of his sleep do not change (Hunziker & Barr, 1986; McKenna et al., 1997).

Although infants differ in the number of hours of sleep, each baby gets as much sleep as he needs.

Table 19–4

CHARACTERISTICS OF INFANTS' THINKING: SENSORIMOTOR STATE

Major Task

Conquest of object
Throughout this stage, infants are unable to think. Intelligence proceeds from directly acting, as a whole, on the environment to more goal-directed attending to and action on particular objects to make specific events occur. All the senses and motor skills are actively used to define and interpret objects and events.

Perception

Birth–3 months: View of world and self undifferentiated; unconscious of self.
4–6 months: View of world centered around body: self-centered.
After 6 months: View of world as centered around objects.
6–12 months: Self seen as separated from objects.
12–18 months: Objects seen to have constancy and permanence.
18–24 months: Represents spatial relationships between objects and between objects and self (e.g., knows smaller things fit inside larger things).

Thought

Birth–3 months: Not present. Uses inborn reflexes and senses.
4–6 months: Questions presence of thought. Uses combination of reflexes and senses purposively. Develops habits.
6–12 months: Knows objects by how he or she uses them. Knows objects have constant size before knows objects have same form; serially acts out two previously separate behaviors in goal-directed sequences.
12–24 months: Object permanence stimulates purposive, intentional use of behaviors to find hidden objects and to cause event via trial and error–problem solve via "insight": can now see effect when given the cause (e.g., knows where train will come out when goes into tunnel). Symbolism and memory begin–uses deferred imitation to discover new ways of acting (e.g., when "pretends" sleep means "know" symbolic sleeping).

Reasoning

Birth–6 months: Not present.
6–24 months: Syncretism (1) perceives "whole"–impression without analysis of parts or synthesis of relations, (2) lacks systematic exploratory behavior until end of stage, (3) begins to connect series of ideas into a confused whole.

Language

Birth–3 months: Undifferentiated cry. Use of different intensities, patterns, and pitches of cry for different feelings (e.g., pain, hunger, fatigue).
6–8 weeks: Cooing: contented and happy sounds.
3–6 months: Babbling: repeated various sounds for sensation of pleasure. Laughing: when happy or excited.
6–12 months: Spontaneous vocalization: imperfect imitation. Echolalia: conscious imitation of sounds.
12–18 months: Expressive jargon: use for information, rhythms, and pauses to imitate sentence sounds. Holophrases: use of one word to convey meaning. Gestures: substitute for or add meaning to speech.
18–24 months: Telegraphic speech: use of noun and verb to convey many meanings.

Play

Birth–6 months: Exercise play: repetition of actions and sounds for pleasure (e.g., rolling over, babbling).
6–12 months: Exploratory play: pleasure from causing effect and reconfirming skill (e.g., "peek-a-boo," "drop and retrieve," "pat-a-cake").
12–24 months: Deferred imitation: imitates previously observed actions (not reasons for or purposes of actions) from memory (e.g., pretends to be "Daddy" and goes through getting dressed, shaving, then walks outside, and gets in the "car").

Source: From J Servonsky, SR Opas: Nursing management of children. *Boston: Jones and Bartlett, 1987:22.*

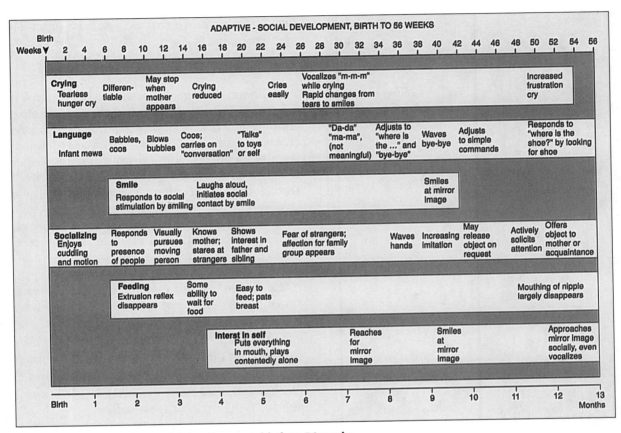

FIGURE 19–2. Adaptive-social development, birth to 56 weeks.

Newborns sleep an average of 16.5 hours per day; some sleep a total of about 10 hours, others sleep up to 23 hours. Generally, infants fuss and cry before falling asleep. The sleeping pattern of breastfed infants differs from that of formula-fed infants. Breastfed infants wake more often during the night and have shortened sleep patterns (Carey, 1974; Elias et al., 1986; Mosko et al., 1996, 1997). The expression "He sleeps just like a baby" simply is not true during the first few months of life for any infant. The typical pattern is one of frequent, short periods of sleep interrupted by crying and fussing. This occurs night and day. The so-called infant sleep disorders being diagnosed today are not disorders at all but normal sleep patterns.

Mothers and babies interact with one another using a variety of communications that are visual, vocal, tactile, and postural. Babies coo, goo, and babble whenever they are alert and content. These sounds change from week to week and are elicited by the smiling faces of adults, by voices, or by touch. Any mother who has breastfed knows that feeding at the breast is a prime time for her baby to communicate actively with coos, babbling, and speech sounds as he looks into the eyes of his mother (Fig. 19–3). These exquisite sensory interchanges further bond the mother and baby. Epstein (1993) videotaped breastfeeding mothers and their babies during feedings to investigate maternal-infant interactions. These videos were later observed and analyzed (p. 100):

The interactions between the mother and infant were elaborate and complex, with each breastfeeding dyad interacting with its own individual style. All of the mothers and babies looked at their partners' bodies, not just at their faces, during the breastfeeding session. All of the mothers had happy and affectionate expressions on their faces as they watched their babies, yet the amount of time they maintained the positive expression differed between mothers.

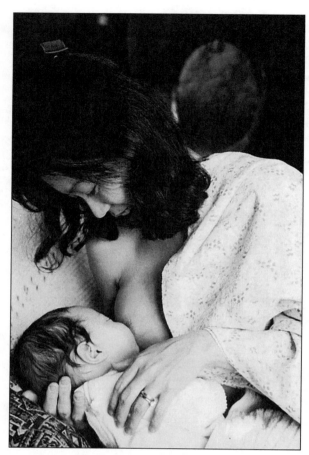

FIGURE 19–3. Mutual caregiving promotes the maternal role-taking process.

Certain babies in the study even smiled and laughed with their mother's nipples in their mouths. Babies and mothers were observed vocalizing to one another. In some dyads, intricate vocal interactions occurred. Babies made sounds that their mothers initiated and this resulted in the babies continuing to make sounds and the mothers continuing to imitate them. In all of these cases, the sounds that the babies made seemed to be expressions of pleasure.

Mothers speak to their infants in a universal dialogue that Sears (1987) calls "motherese." According to Sears (p. 31),

They instinctively use exaggerated upbeat tones and facial gestures to talk to babies. Mothers use slowly rising crescendo and decrescendo allowing the baby time to process each short vocal package before the next communication arrives. How a mother talks to her baby is more important than what she says.

This sing-song quality of the mother's speech is tailored to the baby's listening abilities. Smiling, grasping, and talking all play important roles in the attachment process (i.e., the reciprocal development of an affectional tie between the mother or caregiver and the baby) (Pridham & Chang, 1992). During these interactions, the mother not only gives care to her infant but the newborn gives care back to his mother. For this reason, Anderson (1977) called the mother and infant "mutual caregivers" (p. 53):

As the mother holds her infant to her breast, assumes the en face position, and talks to her newborn, her eyes are the optimal distance away and her head, mouth and eyes move slowly and within a closely circumscribed range. Her newborn will also be sending stimuli, such as changes in facial expression, vocalizations, and eye-to-eye contact. The mother's response to such stimuli is immediate.

In a review of the theoretical framework for studying factors that affect the maternal role, Mercer (1981) emphasized the role of the infant in his mother's maternal role-taking process. The newborn's ability to see, hear, and track the human face shows socialization capabilities at birth that allow the infant to be an active partner with the mother in the attachment process. Pridham and Chang (1992) demonstrated that each new infant presents a challenge to maternal adaptation and that previous experience with infants makes little difference to becoming the parent of a new child. Moreover, the transition process of being mother to a new infant is different in the second and third months from the process in the first month.

The infant uses play as a part of the communication process. During the earliest (sensorimotor) stage of life, infants begin with exercise play, such as repeating newly learned actions for pleasure. Stick out your tongue at a young infant, and he will stick out his tongue at you. Next, they play using exploration of their skills: crawling backward down the stairs, for example, or pushing their finger into mother's mouth while breastfeeding and then squealing with glee when she pretends to bite the finger (Fig. 19–4). Table 19–5 shows infant psychosocial and breastfeeding behaviors at certain points of development. The older baby's playful activities as he breastfeeds are a part of communication and attachment with his mother. Deferred imitation play begins at around 18 months of age, when toddlers begin to imitate the behavior and language they see and hear. For example, little girls, who are already adopting the gender role of their mothers, will very seriously and readily "nurse" their dolls at their breasts (Fig. 19–5).

Attachment and Bonding

This exquisite dance of reciprocal reinforcement in the mother-infant dyad leads to the mother's "taking-in" her maternal role, cementing the mother-infant bond. Early theorists paved the way for understanding the processes of bonding and attachment. Konrad Lorenz (1935) noted the behavior and imitation of the mother animal by the young, which is necessary for survival, and labeled it *imprinting*. It is believed that attachment and bonding are the human equivalent of imprinting.

In the early 1950s, Bowlby (1951) emphasized the importance of an infant's developing a primary attachment to a caring, responsible adult. A decade later, Harlow and Harlow (1965) demonstrated the importance of contact comfort for the attachment and emotional well-being of the newborn rhesus monkey. When presented with "surrogate" mothers—one formed out of unpadded chicken wire and equipped with milk-filled bottles, the other made out of padded terry cloth but without bottles—the baby monkeys spent much more time with the warm, cloth-covered mothers, going only briefly to the bottles for food.

Mothers who room-in with their infants after birth touch their infants' face and head more often than do mothers who have minimal contact with their newborn (Prodromidis et al., 1995). Rubin (1967) showed a progressive attachment that results from touching: a mother first explores her newborn's extremities with her fingertips, rapidly moves to the baby's arms and legs, and finally caresses the trunk with the palm of her hand. Rubin (1977) preferred the term *binding-in* to *bonding* because it more accurately describes the forma-

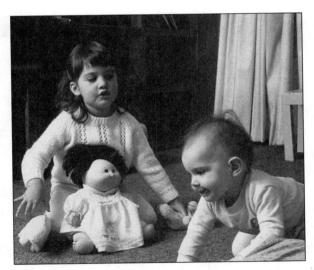

FIGURE 19–4. Developing motor skills by exploring the environment.

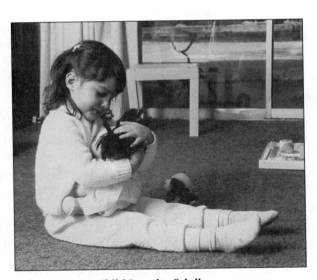

FIGURE 19–5. Child "nursing" doll.

tive stages of the maternal-child relationship as a process, not a state (p. 67):

A conceptual model for the binding-in processes might well be like the weaving of a tapestry. Not a cord, nor a bond, nor a welding job, rather a large creative work, framed between the child and the mother's own significant social world, systematically and progressively developed for durability against time and stress to form the substance of her own

Table 19–5

INFANT PSYCHOSOCIAL AND BREASTFEEDING BEHAVIORS BY AGE

Age	Psychosocial Behavior	Breastfeeding Behavior
First day postpartum	Quiet alert state after birth, followed by long sleep.	May or may not feed following delivery. Sleepy, learning how to suckle.
1 mo	Follows objects with eyes; reacts to noise by stopping behavior or crying.	Becoming efficient at suckling; feedings last approximately 17 minutes. Feedings now 8–16 times per day.
2 mo	Smiles; vocalizes in response to interactions.	Easily pacified by frequent breastfeedings.
3 mo	Shows increased interest in surroundings. Voluntarily grasps objects. Vocalizes when spoken to. Turns head as well as eyes in response to moving object.	Will interrupt feeding to turn to look at father or other familiar person coming into room and to smile at mother.
4–5 mo	Shows interest in strange settings. Smiles at mirror image.	Continues to enjoy frequent feedings at the breast.
6 mo	Laughs aloud. Shows increased awareness of caregivers vs. strangers. May become distressed if mother or caregiver leaves.	Solids offered. Fewer feedings. Feeds longer before sleep for the night. May begin waking to nurse more often at night.
7–8 mo	Imitates actions and noises. Responds to name. Responds to "no." Enjoys peek-a-boo games. Reaches for toys that are out of reach.	Will breastfeed anytime, anywhere. Actively attempts to get to breast (i.e., will try to unbutton mother's blouse).
9–10 mo	Distressed by new situations or people. Waves bye-bye. Reaches for toys that are out of reach.	Easily distracted by surroundings and interrupts feedings frequently. May hold breast with one or both hands while feeding.
11–12 mo	Drops objects deliberately to be picked up by other people. Rolls ball to another person. Speaks a few words. Appears interested in picture books. Shakes head for "no."	Tries "acrobatic" breastfeeding (i.e., assumes different positions while keeping nipple in mouth).

12–15 mo	Fears unfamiliar situations but will leave mother's side to explore familiar surroundings. Shows emotions (e.g., love, anger, fear). Speaks several words. Understands meaning of many words.	Uses top hand to play while feeding: forces finger into mother's mouth, plays with her hair, and pinches her other nipple. Pats mother's chest when wants to breastfeed. Hums or vocalizes while feeding. Verbalizes need to breastfeed–may use "code" word.
16–20 mo	Has frequent temper tantrums. Increasingly imitates parents. Enjoys solitary play or observing others. Speaks 6–10 words.	Verbalizes delight with breastfeeding. Takes mother by the hand and leads her to favorite nursing chair.
20–24 mo	Helps with simple tasks. Has fewer temper tantrums. Engages in parallel play. Combines 2 or 3 words. Speaks 15–20 words.	Stands up while nursing at times. Nursing mostly for comfort. Feeding before bedtime is usually last feeding before weaning. When asked to do so by mother, willing to wait for feeding until later.

personal identity and the fabric of her relationship with this particular child.

Ainsworth et al. (1978) studied brief infant separation from mothers in a laboratory situation to measure the degree of attachment. Mothers defined by the researchers as "securely attached" to their infants were most sensitive to their baby's needs, whereas mothers identified as "insecurely attached" to their infants were less emotionally expressive, felt more aversion to close body contact with the babies, and were more frequently irritated, resentful, and angry.

A multitude of circumstances affect the mother-child relationship, which begins before the child is born; even though the baby is unseen, the mother imagines or fantasizes about her child. According to Clark (1976, p. 96):

Her perceptions of the "dream child" and, subsequently, her relationship with that child will not only be influenced by her self-concept but also by her total life experience. Her culture, social relationship, economic status, and state of health can all add to or detract from her relationship with her unborn child. If she experiences social isolation and economic deprivation during her pregnancy, her emotional reserves will be lowered. If she experiences physical discomfort and ill health, her physical stamina may be depleted. Thus, the support she receives during pregnancy and from her total environment will affect her acceptance and readiness for mothering.

The infant's birth forces the mother to compare her real-life baby with her dreams, fantasies, and expectations. If reality and expectations are congruent, attachment begins soon after birth; if they are divergent, the mother must first work through the loss of the "dream child" and strive to fall in love with this stranger who bears little resemblance to the child of her fantasies.

Klaus and Kennell (1975) moved the concept of attachment one step further by popularizing the existence of a sensitive period for attachment shortly after birth. Barring excessive medication of the mother during delivery, a newborn will normally be in an alert state for at least one hour following birth. During this period, the mother will spend a significant amount of time gazing en face (face to face) into her infant's eyes, touching, and stroking. The neonate is born in a state of readiness for this human interaction. The infant's remarkable perceptual and sensory abilities (hearing, seeing, smelling, and tasting) at birth facilitate the attachment process. As attachment becomes established, the newborn is observed to move his arms and legs in rhythm to the cadences of the mother's voice, in a synchronous pattern that may be the foundation for later speech (Condon & Sander, 1974). Such interaction is known as *entrainment,* and its effects carry over into later life (Fig. 19–6).

An active partner in the attachment process, the infant initiates about one-half of parent-infant interaction. Through predictable and clear-cut transmission of cues or nonverbal signals, neonates are capable of producing the desired behavior in the parent and selectively reinforcing parent behavior. In many ways, the infant is as competent as the parents, "perhaps even more so than young, inexperienced parents" (Anderson, 1981; Bell, 1974).

The baby's cry (impossible to ignore) is his cue for attention, and his mother responds by picking up, feeding, or carrying him. The perceptive mother is attuned to her baby's cues and reacts to them appropriately. If he coos and smiles, she reacts happily to his pleasure. The infant's contentment or irritability signal the mother to increase or decrease stimulation. If parents are aware of these cues as a method of communication for their infant, they respond by viewing their infants as individuals. Informing mothers about the behavioral characteristics of their babies is an effective means of enhancing the interaction between mothers and their infants (Anderson, 1981; Clark, 1976). Breastfeeding, with its frequent touching, holding, and eye-to-eye contact, offers enhanced opportunities for attachment and responding to infant cues. Certainly, the frequency of subjective verbal responses by mothers who state that they "feel closer" to the breastfed child merits serious consideration. Through breastfeeding, the infant may exert more control: for example, the decision to end the feeding is a shared decision between the mother

and baby when the mother "reads" and responds to her baby's behaviors. In bottle-feeding, on the other hand, the mother is chiefly responsible for ending the feeding.

The 1970s social movement to incorporate rooming-in and mother-baby care into hospital maternity care spawned many studies of maternal-infant attachment and bonding. Most of these studies demonstrated that increased mother-baby contact was associated with stronger attachment (Anisfeld et al., 1990; Anisfeld & Lipper, 1983; Klaus et al., 1970; Kontos, 1978; Thomson et al., 1979). It was also shown that children who have minimal separation from their mother after birth have higher levels of parental interaction and personal health in later years (deChateau & Wiberg, 1977; O'Connor et al., 1979). This proliferation of research about attachment and the benefits of rooming-in ceased in the 1980s, because rooming-in and mother-baby care was incorporated by most hospitals and because of criticisms that other maternal factors (e.g., age, education, and socioeconomic status) explained more of the variance in maternal attachment than did early contact (Campbell & Taylor, 1979; Lamb, 1983; Siegel et al., 1980; Svejda & Campos, 1980). Hedberg-Nyqvist and Ewald (1997) found that Swedish infants who were separated from their mothers on the first day because they were ill or because of a complicated delivery breastfed for as many months as did those who had immediate contact with their mother.

Currently, though immediate postpartum mother-child contact is desirable, it is no longer considered critical. Almost all parents are attached to their babies, even if they experience marked disruption of the early parent-child contact, which most healthy mothers and babies now take for granted (see Chapter 9). Parents should be assured that not having the opportunity to interact and bond with their baby soon after birth will not cause irreparable damage to their child (Klaus & Kennell, 1982; Wolff, 1970).

Temperament

During the past two decades, researchers have studied the temperament of the infant and how it influences parenting. The longitudinal work of Thomas and Chess (1977) and Thomas et al. (1963)

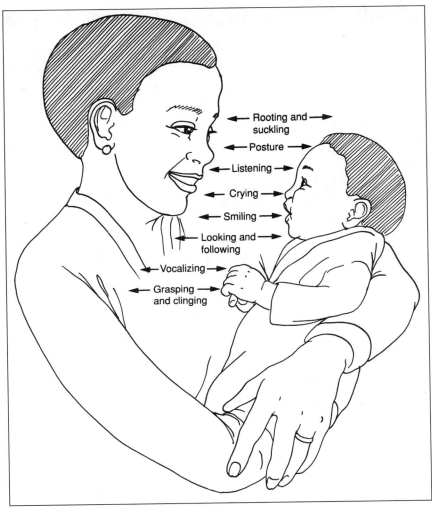

FIGURE 19–6. Components of attachment and their interaction in specific areas. *(From S Mott, NF Fazekas, SR James: Nursing care of children and families. Menlo Park, CA: Addison-Wesley, 1985:206.)*

Labels in figure:
Rooting and suckling
Posture
Listening
Crying
Smiling
Looking and following
Vocalizing
Grasping and clinging

suggested that every child exhibits a particular temperament from birth and that (1) infants have individual characteristics even as newborns, (2) these characteristics differentiate infants one from another, and (3) they remain constant over time. Categories of response that influence a child's temperament include activity level, regularity of body functions, adaptability, response to new situations, sensory threshold, intensity of reaction, quality of mood, distractibility, and attention span and persistence. These characteristics were rated for three temperaments: the easy child, the difficult child, and the slow-to-warm-up child (Thomas & Chess, 1977). Characteristic temperament styles of each are seen in Table 19–6.

Sears (1987) reduced these three temperament characteristics into two categories in which he identified *high-need* and *low-need* babies and popularized the concept for parents to understand and use. High-need babies are fussy, seem to breastfeed "all the time," and cry if put down; low-need babies are content and cuddly and do not need constant carrying or attention. Two questionnaires or tools for assessing the temperament of an infant or child are the Infant Temperament Questionnaire (ITQ) for infants 4 to 12 months of age (Carey & McDevitt, 1978) and the Toddler Temperament Scale for children one to three years of age (Hegvik et al., 1982). The ITQ scores identify a child's temperamental style; the results may be used as an opportunity for

Table 19–6

CHARACTERISTICS OF TEMPERAMENT STYLES IN CHILDREN

Factor	Easy Child	Slow-to-Warm-Up Child	Difficult Child
Activity level–amount of physical activity during sleep, feeding, play, dressing	High	Medium	Low
Regularity–of body functions in sleep, hunger, bowel movements	Fairly regular	Variable	Fairly irregular
Adaptability to change in routine–ease or difficulty with which initial response can be modified in socially desirable way	Generally adaptable	Variable	Generally slow to adapt
Response to new situations–initial reaction to new stimuli, foods, people, places, toys, or procedures	Approach	Variable	Withdrawal
Level of sensory threshold–amount of external stimulation, such as sounds or changes in food or people, necessary to produce a response	High threshold (much stimulation needed)	Medium threshold	Low threshold (little stimulation needed)
Intensity of response–energy content of responses regardless of their quality	Generally intense	Variable	Generally mild
Positive or negative mood–energy content of responses regardless of their quality	Generally positive	Variable	Generally negative
Distractibility–effectiveness of external stimuli (sounds, toys, people) in interfering with ongoing behavior	Easily distractible	Variable	Nondistractible
Persistence and attention span–duration of maintaining specific activities with or without external obstacles	Persistent	Variable	Nonpersistent
Percentage of all children	40%	15%	10%

Source: WB Carey, SC McDevitt: Revision of the infant temperament questionnaire. Pediatrics 61:735–9, 1978.
From J Servonsky, SR Opas: Nursing management for children. Boston: Jones and Bartlett, 1987:180.

making parents aware of their child's temperament and for suggesting appropriate parenting skills.

Stranger Distress

As the infant grows older, the significance of his major caregiver is recognized, and, during the second half of the first year of life, another develop-

mental phenomenon appears: stranger distress. The infant who up to that time has been curious about everything in his environment, including strangers, suddenly frowns and cries and may even attempt physical escape when a stranger approaches. Stranger distress appears quite suddenly as early as six months but more commonly at eight months. It is more pronounced when the mother or primary caretaker is not present. As a consequence, exposure to a variety of strangers is disruptive to an infant at this age. Although stranger distress occurs at about the same period of development as that of separation anxiety, it is a separate phenomenon.

Separation Anxiety

As mother or father leaves the room, anxious eyes follow. Almost instantly, the child's face is contorted by rage; he cries loudly and may throw himself wildly about, kicking and screaming. No action brings solace at this point. This behavior is the first phase of separation anxiety, a phenomenon that emerges toward the middle of the first year of life, peaks from 13 to 20 months, and decreases after the second birthday. Separation anxiety, according to psychoanalytic theory, is the painful effect of anxiety engendered by the threat of actual separation from a loved one. Bowlby (1973) and Robertson (1958) delineated three phases of separation anxiety in young children: protest, despair, and denial.

Protest. In an angry and yearning attempt to recover his mother or primary caregiver, the child violently cries and throws himself about, kicking and screaming. He is angry with the world and with his mother for leaving him. He feels that she must be angry with him also, because she left him. The protest phase can last from a few hours to several days, depending on the energy of the child, his age, his relationship with his mother, and the quality of the new environment.

Despair. Gradually, the child moves into quiet grieving and mourning as he begins to accept his fate. He shows little interest in his environment but suffers intensely; his expression is one of great sadness. Regressive behavior, such as thumb-sucking, occurs as the child turns inward for solace.

Detachment or Denial. The child develops a defense mechanism to deal with his loss by detaching himself from the importance of his mother's love. He gradually begins to interact with others, approaching anyone and even appearing cheerful. This stage is often misinterpreted as adapting or "settling in."

Actually, he is coping with his loss by indiscriminately attaching to caretakers. When he is reunited with his mother at this point, he may appear uninterested and may not seem to recognize her.

Clinical Implications

Deviations from normal patterns of attachment signal that a problem may be present; hence assessing the infant's or child's growth and developmental level–and being able to apply a working knowledge of developmental patterns–is as important as knowing the specifics of a child's health problem. If a baby is being examined, for example, the close proximity of his mother helps to reduce stranger distress. Although "friendly-" (nonwhite-) appearing clothing helps to ameliorate the baby's distress, by no means does it prevent his crying and avoidance behavior as the examiner approaches him, especially for the first time.

How can health care workers who are strangers to the child minimize this fear? First, take advantage of his attachment to his mother by relating to the mother first in the presence of the child. During this interaction with his mother, the child is carefully observing her response to and acceptance of the "stranger" and will take cues from her. Even body position is important; turning slightly sideways away from the child to avoid en face contact while talking with the mother is less threatening to the child. Spitz (1946) demonstrated in one of his films that when a stranger approaches with his back to the child, the child becomes curious and will even reach out after a bit and tug at the stranger. Using a soft, low voice rather than loud or high-pitched tone is more pleasing to the child and facilitates his acceptance of this new person in his life.

Nursing and medicine have made great progress in recognizing and applying development theories in practice. Because a comprehensive listing and discussion of developmental assessment and screening tools is not within the scope of this book, we refer the reader to the many excellent references that discuss child development in detail. In addition, we remind the reader of the use of assessment tools, such as the Bayley Scale of Infant Development, the Denver Development Screening Test, and the Brazelton Neonatal Behavior Assessment Scale.

Immunizations

Immunizations have greatly reduced the incidence of childhood diseases worldwide. Many infections that contributed to high infant mortality in the past can now be prevented through a series of immunizations. Smallpox, for example, has been eliminated and poliomyelitis, rubella, and rubeola have decreased markedly since the rigorous enforcement of a series of immunizations.

In the United States, the recommended age for beginning primary immunizations of infants is at birth. The usual schedule is for three immunizations for DTaP/Hib or DTP/Hib vaccine (diphtheria, tetanus, pertussis, and *Haemophilus influenzae* type b). DTaP is the preferred vaccine because it produces fewer side effects. A combination product containing measles, mumps, and rubella vaccine (MMR) is administered at 12 to 15 months of age, with a second dose recommended for school-age children. The *H. influenzae* type b vaccine has been approved by the Food and Drug Administration for use at 2, 4, and 6 months of age, with a booster at 15 to 18 months of age. Children aged 6 to 12 months are at highest risk of *H. influenzae* type b infection. The exact timing of the immunizations is not nearly as important as the fact that the child eventually receives all of the immunization doses (Table 19-7).

Hepatitis B is a major public health problem in the western Pacific and in central and southern Africa. Of the estimated 300 million chronic carriers of hepatitis B virus (HBV) in the world, about 80 percent live in Asia and Oceania. Many countries and areas in the western Pacific region, including China, have started routine HBV immunization of newborns. In 1992, the American Academy of Pediatrics recommended universal immunization of newborns in the United States against the HBV. Although the schedule calls for the initial vaccine to be given to all newborns soon after birth, again at 1 to 2 months of age, and at 6 to 18 months of age, not everyone agrees with this recommendation, claiming that this decision marks the first time that a vaccine is recommended for children to prevent a disease that primarily occurs in adults. The incidence of HBV in children not exposed to the virus in utero is very low; except for those infants so exposed, the effect of the vaccine will probably not be needed until adolescence (Clay LS, 1993).

Generally, vaccines that contain attenuated "live" organisms are more effective than are inactivated or "killed" vaccines. Live vaccines induce long-lasting immunity, but they are also likely to cause adverse reactions. Although killed vaccines are noninfectious and can be prepared in a purified form, they usually induce a shorter period of protection; therefore, booster injections may be needed. Most vaccines are given parenterally; an exception is the live oral polio vaccine (OPV).

When a measles-mumps-rubella vaccine is given during the immediate postpartum period in the rubella seronegative woman, the live attenuated virus will be found in her breastmilk. This poses no harm to the infant (Wolfe, 1990). Krogh et al. (1989) compared breastfed and formula-fed infants of a group of mothers who had been immunized with the rubella vaccine postpartum with a second group of naturally immune women who were seropositive for rubella and did not receive immunization after childbirth. Subsequent immunization with rubella vaccine of breastfed infants whose mothers had received postpartum immunization resulted in a serum antibody response that was similar to the response observed in formula-fed infants or the infants of naturally immune mothers who had not received immunization. Thus early neonatal exposure to the rubella virus in breastmilk neither enhances nor suppresses subsequent responses to rubella vaccination in early childhood.

Breastfed infants are also successfully immunized with the OPV while receiving breastmilk, and it is not necessary to withhold breastfeeding after administration of the OPV. The same is true for the oral rotavirus vaccine (Deforest et al., 1973; John et al., 1976; Rennels, 1996; WHO, Collaborative Study, 1995) (Fig. 19-7).

In fact, breastfeeding may enhance immunity in some cases. Pabst et al. (1989) found that infants who were breastfeeding had enhanced cell-mediated immune response to bacillus Calmette-Guérin vaccine given at birth. In another study by the same group of investigators, breastfed infants immunized with *H. influenza* type b vaccine had higher antibody levels at 7 months and at 12 months of age–strong evidence that breastfeeding enhances the active immune response in the first year of life. One Swedish study found that breastfed children were less likely to experience H. influenza virus. This protection was dose-related to duration of exclusive breastfeeding and persisted beyond the period of breastfeeding (Silfverdal et al., 1997).

Dental Health

The first primary (deciduous) teeth to erupt are the lower central incisors, which appear at about six to eight months of age. By two and a half years of age, children have a full set of primary teeth that will be replaced by permanent teeth. Although breastfeeding helps to protect the teeth, healthy dental practices should in no way be neglected because the child is breastfeeding.

Nursing-bottle caries is a term applied to progressive dental caries aggravated by sucking on a bottle while sleeping and is associated with a high count of lactobacilli in dental plaque (Matee et al., 1992). In developed countries, the prevalence is reported to vary between 1 and 12 percent (Milnes, 1996). Decay usually starts with the maxillary (upper) incisors and often spares the mandibular (lower) incisors. Overall, breastfed children have less dental decay than do those who are fed otherwise (Al-Dashti et al., 1994; Tank & Storvick, 1965). The probable reasons for this include the mechanical differences between breastfeeding and bottle-feeding. Drawn deep into the child's mouth, the human nipple rests at the junction of the hard and soft palate during breastfeeding, posterior to the child's teeth. A suckle is automatically followed by a swallow, thus preventing the teeth from being bathed in pooled milk. By contrast, the milk from a bottle flows out spontaneously with only the slightest pressure into the anterior part of the mouth, permitting stagnation of the milk on and around the teeth (Abbey, 1979).

Brams and Maloney (1983), Gardner et al. (1977), and Kotlow (1977) have reported a condition similar to nursing-bottle caries that occurred in breastfed children, especially those who breastfed for two to three years and spent long, uninterrupted periods at the breast. Although these cases represent a small percentage of young children who breastfeed, nursing caries is associated with the practice of breastfeeding at night "at will" after six months of age (Al-Dashti et al., 1994; Matee et al., 1994).

As the numbers of breastfeeding toddlers increase, however, it is reasonable to expect that

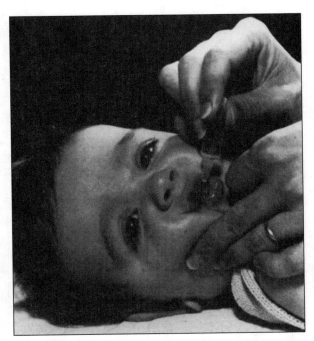

FIGURE 19–7. Receiving polio protection. *(Courtesy WHO/PAHO/C.)*

some of them will develop dental disease, especially after the introduction of solids that often contain sugar. Dental caries is also thought to be an inherited trait; therefore, these children probably represent a group who are more susceptible, and prolonged nocturnal exposure to human milk becomes a risk factor. It could be argued that some breastfed children develop caries not because they were breastfed but in spite of it. The susceptibility of the child's teeth to decay cannot be clinically predicted, and caries may be extensive before they become evident.

Orofacial development is a health issue in which breastfeeding has a measurable impact. The orofacial development of a child is affected by feeding methods, swallowing patterns, and finger sucking (Sanger & Bystrom, 1982). The mechanisms by which bottle-feeding might contribute to the development of malocclusion include a forward thrusting of the tongue, which in turn leads to underdevelopment of the masseter and buccinator muscles (Stanley & Lundeen, 1980; Straub, 1960), abnormal swallowing patterns, and increased prevalence of nonnutritive sucking. Two studies suggested that breastfeeding prevents malocclusion.

Table 19-7

RECOMMENDED CHILDHOOD IMMUNIZATION SCHEDULE, UNITED STATES, JANUARY–DECEMBER 1997

Vaccines[1] are listed under the routinely recommended ages. Bars indicate range of acceptable ages for vaccination. Shaded bars indicate *catch-up vaccination*: at 11–12 years of age, hepatitis B vaccine should be administered to children not previously vaccinated, and varicella virus vaccine should be administered to unvaccinated children who lack a reliable history of chickenpox.

Age ▶ / Vaccine ▼	Birth	1 mo	2 mo	4 mo	6 mo	12 mo	15 mo	18 mo	4–6 yr	11–12 yr	14–16 yr
Hepatitis B[2,3]	Hep B-1	Hep B-2			Hep B-3					Hep B[3]	
Diphtheria, tetanus, pertussis[4]			DTaP or DTP	DTaP or DTP	DTaP or DTP	DTaP or DTP[4]			DTaP or DTP	Td	
H. influenzae type b[5]			Hib	Hib	Hib[5]	Hib[5]					
Polio[6]			Polio[6]	Polio		Polio[6]			Polio		
Measles, mumps, rubella[7]						MMR			MMR[7]	or MMR[7]	
Varicella[8]						Var				Var[8]	

Approved by the Advisory Committee on Immunization Practices (ACIP), the American Academy of Pediatrics (AAP), and the American Academy of Family Physicians (AAFP). Copyright © 1997 by the American Academy of Pediatrics.

[1]This schedule indicates the recommended age for routine administration of currently licensed childhood vaccines. Some combination vaccines are available and may be used whenever administration of all components of the vaccine is indicated. Providers should consult the manufacturer's package inserts for detailed recommendations.

[2]**Infants born to HBsAg-negative mothers** should receive 2.5 μg of Merck vaccine (Recombivax HB) or 10 μg SmithKline Beecham (SB) vaccine (Engerix-B). The second dose should be administered ≥1 mo after the first dose.
Infants born to HBsAg-positive mothers should receive 0.5 ml hepatitis B immune globulin (HBIG) within 12 hr of birth, and either 5 μg of Merck vaccine (Recombivax HB) or 10 μg of SB vaccine (Engerix-B) at a separate site. The second dose is recommended at 1–2 mo of age and the third dose at 6 mo of age.
Infants born to mothers whose HBsAg status is unknown should receive either 5 μg of Merck vaccine (Recombivax HB) or 10 μg of SB vaccine (Engerix-B) within 12 hr of birth. The second dose of vaccine is recommended at 1 mo of age and the third dose at 6 mo of age. Blood should be drawn at the time of delivery to determine the mother's HBsAg status; if it is positive, the infant should receive HBIG as soon as possible (no later than 1 wk of age). The dosage and timing of subsequent vaccine doses should be based on the mother's HBsAg status.

[3]Children and adolescents who have not been vaccinated against hepatitis B in infancy may begin the series during any childhood visit. Those who have not previously received three doses of hepatitis B vaccine should initiate or complete the series during the 11- to 12-year-old visit. The second dose should be administered at least 1 mo after the first dose, and the third dose should be administered at least 4 mo after the first dose and at least 2 mo after the second dose.

[4]DTaP (diphtheria and tetanus toxoids and acellular pertussis vaccine) is the preferred vaccine for all doses in the vaccination series, including completion of the series in children who have received at least one dose of whole-cell DTP vaccine. Whole-cell DTP is an acceptable alternative to DTaP. The fourth dose of DTaP may be administered as early as 12 mo of age, provided 6 mo have elapsed since the third dose, and if the child is considered unlikely to return at 15–18 mo of age. Td (tetanus and diphtheria toxoids, adsorbed, for adult use) is recommended at 11–12 yr of age if at least 5 yr have elapsed since the last dose of DTP, DTaP, or DT. Subsequent routine Td boosters are recommended every 10 yr.

[5]Three H. influenzae type b (Hib) conjugate vaccines are licensed for infant use. If PRP-OMP (PedvaxHIB [Merck]) is administered at 2 and 4 mo of age, a dose at 6 mo is not required. After completing the primary series, any Hib conjugate vaccine may be used as a booster.

[6]Two poliovirus vaccines are currently licensed in the United States: inactivated poliovirus vaccine (IPV) and oral poliovirus vaccine (OPV). The following schedules are all acceptable by the ACIP, the AAP, and the AAFP, and parents and providers may choose among them:
1. IPV at 2 and 4 mo; OPV at 12–18 mo and 4–6 yr
2. IPV at 2, 4, 12–18 mo, and 4–6 yr
3. OPV at 2, 4, 6–18 mo, and 4–6 yr
The ACIP routinely recommends schedule 1. IPV is the only poliovirus vaccine recommended for immunocompromised persons and their household contacts.

[7]The second dose of MMR is routinely recommended at 4–6 yr of age or at 11–12 yr of age but may be administered during any visit, provided at least 1 mo has elapsed since receipt of the first dose and that both doses are administered at or after 12 mo of age.

[8]Susceptible children may receive varicella vaccine (Var) during any visit after the first birthday, and unvaccinated persons who lack a reliable history of chickenpox should be vaccinated during the 11- to 12-year-old visit. Susceptible persons 13 yr or older should receive two doses at least 1 mo apart.

Although some researchers have shown minimal differences (Myers & Hertzberg, 1988) or no difference (Humphreys & Leighton, 1950) in the frequency of malocclusion based on the method of feeding, Adamiak (1981) in Czechoslovakia found that the longer the duration of breastfeeding, the lower the incidence of malocclusion anomalies. Among those breastfed fewer than three months or not at all, 36 percent had anomalies, whereas 24 percent of those breastfed for longer than six months had anomalies. Labbok and Hendershot (1987) analyzed data from the Child Health Supplement of the 1981 National Health Interview Survey and also found that increased duration of breastfeeding was associated with a decline in the proportion of children with malocclusion. This trend was constant for all variables tested and remained even when adjusted for age and maternal educational level as a proxy of socioeconomic status.

Solid Foods

For every breastfed infant, a point is reached when breastmilk alone no longer fulfills his nutritional needs. If breastfeeding is continued exclusively, the baby will eventually become malnourished. How long exclusive breastfeeding can satisfy the nutrient needs of babies is a crucial public health issue, especially in areas with an unsafe water supply and poor sanitation, where early supplements are likely to be associated with infections (Naing & Co, 1991).

Introducing Solid Foods

Solid foods are not necessary, nor are they recommended, before the baby is four to six months of age (AAP, 1980, 1981, 1997). Developmental cues for introducing solid foods to the infant are the fading of his tongue-extrusion reflex, eruption of teeth, the ability to sit, and purposeful movement of the baby's hands and fingers, all of which normally occur during the middle months of the first year of life. Also, in the full-term baby, the prenatal storage of iron acquired during the last trimester of pregnancy gradually begins to diminish by four to five months of age, and external sources of iron are needed. In a study of exclusively breastfed infants at nine months, storage iron was found to absent in 27.8 percent of the breastfed infants versus none in the

formula-fed infants (Calvo et al., 1992). Of 30 infants who had been breastfed until their first birthday without receiving solids or supplements, 30 percent were anemic (Pisacane et al., 1995).

Most infants will at first actively resist the advances of even the most enterprising mother in her attempts to spoon-feed them during the early months of life. Before six months of age, a baby has a tongue-extrusion reflex and is unable to push food to the back of his mouth. Developmentally speaking, the ability to tolerate solids offers no evidence that their early introduction is advantageous. In fact, the practice may initiate a chain of disadvantages that include allergies and obesity.

Early introduction of solids is still a common practice in the United States, even though the American Academy of Pediatrics' Committee on Nutrition (1981) has consistently held that no nutritional advantage results from the introduction of supplemental foods prior to four to six months of age. In fact, mothers sometimes competitively seek to outdo one another in initiating solid food, as if how soon an infant eats adult food is a measure of his maturity (Parrago et al., 1988). Skinner et al. (1997) found that mothers who introduced cereal earliest (<4 mo.) were more likely to have weaned the baby to formula feeds by that time, to feed cereal in a bottle, to be first-time mothers, and to be working outside the home.

Despite official recommendations and a concerted effort to teach parents to delay solids, many infants still receive solid foods during their first few months of life. The first solid food is usually cereal, which is given in the evening because some parents wrongly believe or have been told that feeding solids to the baby will help him sleep through the night. However, feeding infants solids prior to bedtime is not related to evening sleep patterns; according to well-controlled studies, babies who receive solids before bedtime have the same sleep patterns as do babies who are not given solids (Keane et al., 1988; Macknin et al., 1989).

Energy-intake patterns between breastfed and formula-fed infants discussed earlier in this text indicate that breastfed infants maintain energy-intake levels below those of formula-fed infants. These patterns persist even after solid foods are introduced. If breastfeeding infants are given solids at from three to six months, their milk intakes decline significantly; the energy from solids generally replaces that from breastmilk. Although the infant breastfeeds fewer times during the day, the frequency of night feedings remains the same (Heinig et al., 1993). This is not true for formula-fed infants, who continue to take about the same amount of formula when early solids are given. In industrialized countries, infants fed solids early appear to have about the same incidence of illness as do infants who are fed solids later. In developing countries, however, the risk of diarrhea is such that the risks of introducing solids before six months outweighs any potential benefits (Cohen et al., 1994).

Choosing the Diet

If solids are started after six months of age, the sequence of foods is not critical. If solids are introduced earlier, the following order is suggested: fruits, meats and cereals, yellow vegetables, and (last) legumes. For cereal that requires mixing with a liquid, breastmilk (rather than cow's milk) avoids any potential allergic reaction. Egg yolk, if carefully separated from the white (which is highly allergenic), is high in protein and iron, is hypoallergenic, and is therefore safe.

Infants need additional water when solids are started because of their added osmolar load. Juices, which are good sources of vitamin C, can be introduced when the child can drink from a cup. Using one with a tight-fitting lid or a straw at first prevents excessive spilling.

A basic rule is to feed the infant foods in as close to a natural state as possible: pieces of raw, peeled apples, slices of banana, toasted whole-wheat bread, orange sections, and a chicken leg with the skin removed are all good choices. They can be picked up and held and are tasty, nutritious, and satisfying to chew. Small amounts at first, followed by gradually increased amounts (along with continued breastfeeding), avoids constipation. Mothers should be prepared for changes in consistency, odor, and frequency of stool when solids are begun. Generally, all foods eaten by the family can be given to the infant in a consistency that he can handle. The beginning eater enjoys foods of all kinds and relishes the tactile pleasures of squeezing, smearing, and crushing his food–an activity he should be allowed with impunity, because it is also a learning experience. General guidelines for initiating solid foods are found in Table 19–8.

Breastfed babies are exposed to a variety of flavors of a diet that are transmitted in their mothers' breastmilk (Mennella, 1995). As a result, it seems likely that they would be more accepting of novel flavors in solid foods than are formula-fed infants who are not so exposed. To test this assumption, Sullivan and Birch (1994) compared acceptance of vegetables by four- to six-month-old infants. These infants were randomly assigned to be fed 1 vegetable on 10 occasions for 10 days. They found that breastfeeding infants ate more vegetables than did formula-fed infants. Thus breastmilk may facilitate the acceptance of solid foods during the important transition from suckling to feeding solids. Mennella and Beauchamp (1997) found that babies who were given cereal were more accepting of it if it was mixed with mother's milk rather than water. And, in situations in which families are unable to provide high-quality solids, continued breastfeeding beyond one year of age is recommended to enhance linear growth in toddlers (Marquis et al., 1997).

If additional baby food needs to be mashed or blended, foods prepared at home are not only more wholesome and nutritious but cost less than do commercially prepared baby foods. Carrots and applesauce, for example, cost about one-half the store price when prepared at home. Beef and chicken blended in the kitchen provide more nutrients by weight than do their commercial counterparts, chiefly because they contain less water. With the aid of an electric blender, food mill, or grinder, preparing baby food is easily accomplished. The foods should be selected from high-quality fresh or frozen fruits, vegetables, or meats, with special attention to hygienic preparation and storage. For convenience, small individualized portions can be stored safely in the refrigerator or freezer for reasonable periods. A list of foods that can be quickly and easily prepared appears in Box 19–2.

Some parents prefer to buy commercial baby food rather than to make their own. Commercial baby food is generally produced by pulverizing fruit, grain, vegetable, and meat ingredients with water and adding filler ingredients. In the typical selection of strained foods purchased by the average mother, about 80 percent of the calories are carbohydrates in the form of modified starch and

Table 19-8

INTRODUCING SOLID FOODS INTO A BREASTFED INFANT'S DIET

When to Introduce	Approximate Total Daily Intake of Solids*	Description of Food and Hints About Giving Them
6–7 mo if infant is breastfed	Dry cereal. Start with ½ tsp (dry measurement), gradually increase to 2–3 Tbsp. Vegetables: Start with 1 tsp; gradually increase to 2 Tbsp. Fruit: Start with 1 tsp; gradually increase to 2 Tbsp. Divide food among four feedings per day (if possible).	Cereal: Offer iron-enriched baby cereal. Begin with single grains. Mix cereal with an equal amount of breastmilk. Vegetables: Try a mild-tasting vegetable first (carrots, squash, peas, green beans). Stronger-flavored vegetables (spinach, sweet potatoes) may be tried after the infant accepts some mild-tasting ones. Fruits: Mashed ripe banana and unsweetened, cooked, bland fruits (apples, peaches, pears) are usually well liked. Apple juice and grape juice (unsweetened) may be introduced. Initially, dilute juice with an equal amount of water. Introduce one new food at a time and offer it several times before trying another new food. Give a new food once daily for a day or two; increase to twice daily as the infant begins to enjoy the food. Watch for signs of intolerance. Include some foods that are good sources of vitamin C (other than orange juice).
6–7 mo if infant is breastfed	Dry cereal. Gradually increase up to 4 Tbsp. Fruits and vegetables: Gradually increase up to 3 Tbsp of each. Meat: Start with 1 tsp and gradually increase to 2 Tbsp. Divide food among four feedings per day (if possible).	Meat: Offer pureed or milled poultry (chicken or turkey) followed by lean meat (veal, beef); lamb has a stronger flavor and may not be as well liked initially. Liver is a good source of iron; it may be accepted at the beginning of a meal with a familiar vegetable. Continue introducing new cereals, fruits, and vegetables as the infant indicates he is ready to accept them, but always one at a time; introduce legumes last.

███████████████████████████

7–9 mo if infant is breastfed	Dry cereal: Up to ½ c. Fruits and vegetables: Up to ¼ to ½ c. of each. Meats: Up to 3 Tbsp. Divide food among four feedings per day (if possible).	Soft table foods may be introduced; for example, mashed potatoes and squash and small pieces of soft, peeled fruits. Toasted whole grain or enriched bread may be added when the infant begins chewing. If introduction of solids is delayed until now, it is not necessary to use strained fruits and vegetables. Continue using *iron-fortified* baby cereals.
8–12 mo	Dry cereal: Up to ½ c. Bread: About 1 slice. Fruits and vegetables: Up to ½ c. of each. Divide food among four feedings per day (if possible).	Table foods may be added gradually. Cut table foods into small pieces. Start with foods that do not require too much chewing (cooked, cut green beans and carrots, noodles, ground meats, tuna fish, soft cheese, plain yogurt). If fish is offered, check closely to be sure there are no bones in the serving. Mashed, cooked egg yolk and orange juice may be added at about 9 months of age. Sometimes offer peanut butter or thoroughly cooked dried peas and beans in place of meat.

*Some infants do not need or want these amounts of food; some may need a little more food.

Source: Modified from CW Suitor, MF Hunter: Nutrition principles and applications in health promotion. *Philadelphia: Lippincott, 1980.*

sucrose. The Center for Science in the Public Interest, an advocacy group in Washington, DC, challenges the claims of commercial baby-food producers that parents "cannot buy a better baby food" than their product. They charge that Gerber adds sugar, modified food starch, and salt and that Heinz adds sugar and modified food starch. Earth's Best, a producer of organic baby food, and Growing Healthy do not add these ingredients. Salt and sugar are ingredients that babies do not need; if given to them, they develop a taste for such foods early on and tend to want them all their lives.

Choosing Feeding Location

The best place to feed a baby is at the family table at mealtime, in a high chair or on someone's knee. Young children love to be considered one of the family and to sit at the same height as the rest of the family. Even before the infant is ready to take solids, he enjoys being nearby during meals and

BOX 19–2

Quick, Easy-to-Prepare Infant Foods

- Yogurt (low-fat)
- Fresh fruit: cut-up apples, pears, oranges, bananas, grapes, or any fruit in season
- Cheese, cut into chewable pieces
- Toast of whole grain bread, cut into strips
- Chicken: leg, wing, or cut-up pieces
- Egg: soft-boiled; hard-boiled as finger food
- Vegetables: mashed; whole (e.g., peas); in strips or pieces as finger food
- Crackers: whole grain; with peanut butter or cheese spread
- Custard
- Cottage cheese
- Dried fruit: apples, dates, figs, prunes (pitted)
- Liver, sauteed and cut into strips
- Tuna: drained; with grated cheese

started on solid food early (before five to six months) and who have a family history of allergy are more likely to develop atopic disease (allergic asthma, allergic rhinitis, atopic dermatitis, food allergy). Total solid food elimination for the first six months of life, in addition to exclusive breastmilk feeding, appears to reduce atopic disease in children who are at hereditary risk. The protective effect against eczema afforded by solid-food postponement lasts up to one year of age.

IgE, which is associated with allergy, rises in direct time sequence to the introduction of solid foods. IgE is also associated with allergy verified by a positive skin test later in life. Before the age of six months, the infant's intestine lacks the necessary digestive enzymes to completely digest complex proteins and starches down to amino acids and simple sugars. At the same time, the infant's intestinal mucosa is permeable to some intact proteins and starches. These incompletely digested peptides and starches can be absorbed and serve as sensitizing agents to the infant's immune system. IgE is then produced, and allergy results in some (perhaps many) infants. Withholding solids, especially wheat, egg whites, pork, and legumes, from the potentially allergic child until the immature immunity period has passed, minimizes or even prevents the symptoms (Glaser, 1973). At age six months, the infant produces sufficient IgA antibody to prevent absorption of food antigens through the intestinal wall, thus reducing food allergy.

Because there is a tendency for mothers to force food on the baby by encouraging him to finish the jar of baby food without taking cues of satiation from him, it was thought that the potential for obesity increases with the giving of early solids. However, research has not shown a relationship between obesity during infancy and the time at which solid foods were introduced (Davies et al., 1977; Kramer, 1981; Read & Boling, 1982; Yeung et al., 1981). Nevertheless, teaching the young child to eat beyond satiation may contribute to later food problems and should be avoided.

Obesity

Obesity affects between 11 and 19 percent of American children (Wishon & Kinnick, 1986). Is an obese infant likely to become an obese adult? It

can "join in" by chewing on such food as a bread crust or a carrot.

Delaying Solid Foods

According to Finnish studies (Kajosaari & Saarinen, 1983; Saarinen et al., 1979), babies who are

depends on who is asked. Several investigators claim that fat babies have an increased risk of obesity during adulthood (Brook et al., 1975; Fisch et al., 1975; Kramer, 1981; Shulka et al., 1972), whereas others deny that infant obesity usually leads to adult obesity (Roche, 1981; Zack et al., 1979). There is some evidence of a genetic component: that is, children of obese parents are more likely to be overweight themselves (Copeland & Baucon-Copeland, 1981; Dietz, 1983; Taitz, 1977). On the other hand, it is possible that overweight mothers are likely to be more anxious about food and push their children into eating more, creating a persistent food reward system that can lead to overeating for the rest of the individual's life.

Baranowski et al. (1990a, b, 1992) found no relationship between breastfeeding and the subsequent height, obesity, or cardiovascular function in children. Cholesterol levels in breastfeeding children are higher (4 mg/dl) at one year of age than those of children who were never breastfed. This is expected, because human milk has more cholesterol than does artificial baby milk. By four years of age, however, children who had been breastfed had a mean cholesterol level that was 3 mg/dl lower than that of other children (Freedman et al., 1992).

A major obstacle in these studies has been confounding factors (e.g., the mother's nutritional awareness) and methodological problems (e.g., operational definitions of obesity, the distinction between a "breastfed" infant versus a "bottle-fed" infant, and the timing of feedings). Kramer (1981) conducted a case-control study of 639 young patients 12 to 18 years of age living in Montreal. He sought to control bias by

- classifying each subject as either obese, overweight, or nonobese on the basis of both relative weight and skinfold criteria;

- obtaining feeding and family history and demographic data "blindly" by telephone;

- operationalizing the definition of *breastfed* to mean having received no more than one bottle-feeding per day; and

- statistically controlling for confounding effects of family history.

His results suggested that breastfeeding provides a twofold to fourfold protective effect against subsequent obesity that persists at least through adolescence. The protection appears to rise slightly with increased duration of breastfeeding. Delayed introduction of solid food, on the other hand, had little if any additional benefit. Breastfeeding had a far weaker effect on obesity, however, than did genetic, racial, socioeconomic, and behavioral factors.

Weaning

In the United States, weaning usually takes place during the first year of life. Women who breastfeed longer than this have difficulty with acceptance by relatives, peers, and health professionals (Morse & Harrison, 1987). If "baby-led weaning" is practiced, weaning usually takes place between the child's second and fourth birthdays (Sugarman & Kendall-Tackett, 1995). To counteract social pressures for early weaning, women with breastfeeding toddlers find peer support for each other, sometimes changing their circle of friends. In a study by Wrigley and Hutchinson (1990) of 12 mothers who practiced long-term breastfeeding, one mother reported that "her obstetrician told her anyone who breastfed an infant past six months of age was 'perverted.' Another said that her father thought she was 'strange.' Many health care workers, who wholeheartedly support breastfeeding and would never advocate taking a security blanket away from a baby reel in horror when a mother breastfeeds a walking child.

Ideally, the time for weaning is a joint decision (Greiner, 1996), in which both the mother and baby reach a state of readiness to begin weaning around the same time; however, this is not always the case. The child may be ready before his mother; more often, the mother is ready before her child. Sometimes, the decision is made to wean quickly. Although the literature offers considerable advice about gradual weaning, there is little information for the anxious mother in a situation in which weaning must be rapid and will necessarily be traumatic. Rago (1991) reported that the following nondrug therapies may make deliberate weaning easier and at the same time avert plugged ducts or mastitis:

- Shower and allow the warm water to run over the breasts, or soak the breasts by lying down in the tub.
- Use a breast pump or manual expression to relieve breast fullness.
- Wear a supportive, comfortable bra.
- Observe for signs of plugged ducts or a breast infection.
- Expect to feel very emotional during this time, and seek support from people who will listen sympathetically.
- Give the baby extra cuddling and holding.
- It may take several days before the mother finds it is no longer necessary to express breastmilk for comfort. As described earlier in this book, an Australian method for reducing engorged breasts is to wear cool raw cabbage leaves in the bra. Doing so has been reported to quickly relieve engorgement, thereby increasing the mother's comfort.

Clinical Implications

Care providers assume responsibility for educating families in optimal infant-feeding practices and for providing rationale and support when they are needed. Chapter 2 pointed out that the introduction of foods other than breastmilk is culturally influenced and common worldwide. Some mothers encourage their babies to eat as much as possible, believing that a plump baby represents the picture of health. Competition among mothers can also lead to the early introduction of baby foods. Mothers who feel pressure to give their babies solids may misinterpret the baby's cries as hunger, when the baby merely needs stimulation by holding and interacting.

Several important points should be shared with new parents:

- Continue frequent breastfeedings with lots of cuddling and holding.

- Crying is not always a sign of hunger–it can mean that the infant has nonfood needs–e.g., to be held, rocked, and soothed.
- Delay the introduction of solid foods until around the middle of the first year of life when the baby indicates that he is ready for them.
- Prepare foods for the infant in a setting as close as possible to a natural state.
- Have easy-to-prepare foods available for quick meals for the infant (see Box 19–2).
- Bring the baby to the family meal table whenever possible.

It is not unusual for children, usually from about two years of age, to become very fussy about food and refuse to eat certain items; they may especially dislike vegetables. Children will go through periods of eating very little for a period from as short as a week to as long as a few months; then they gradually start eating more again. The mother should be reassured that "this too shall pass" and that her child will start eating again. Meanwhile, she should make the food he does like easily available and neither force the child to eat nor mask his natural appetite by offering sugary foods.

Choices about weaning should be based on the mother's own wishes rather than on the expectations of others and should call for active listening to her feelings. If the mother enjoys breastfeeding but feels pressure to wean, pointing out the advantages of continued breastfeeding and the cultural differences in weaning practices may be all the reinforcement she needs. On the other hand, if she expresses resentment each time her baby breastfeeds and is impatient for each feeding to end, she is entitled to know options for safe and comfortable weaning techniques. Some women report that after weaning their baby, they experienced improvement in mood and sexuality and felt less fatigue (Forster et al., 1994).

SUMMARY

Imperative to assisting a breastfeeding family is recognition and knowledge of a wide array of areas of child health. Taking the holistic view, breastfeeding is but one aspect of the child's overall health and welfare. This chapter has offered readers basic information derived from research findings and clinical experiences. Teaching parents and incorporating research findings into the daily lives of families are the linchpins of effective practice.

REFERENCES

Abbey LM: Is breastfeeding a likely cause of dental caries in young children? *J Am Dent Assoc* 98:21–23, 1979.

Adamiak E: Occlusion anomalies in preschool children in rural areas in relation to certain individual features. *Czas Stomat* 34:551–5, 1981.

Ainsworth MDS, et al: *Patterns of attachment.* Hillsdale, NJ: Lawrence Erlbaum, 1978.

Al-Dashti AA, Williams SA, Curzon MEJ: Breast feeding, bottle feeding and dental caries in Kuwait, a country with low-fluoride levels in the water supply. *Commun Dental Health* 12:42–7, 1994.

Als H, Brazelton, TB: A new model of assessing the behavioral organization in preterm and full-term infants. *J Am Acad Child Psychol* 20:239, 1981.

American Academy of Pediatrics, Committee on Nutrition: Nutritional aspects of obesity in infancy and childhood. *Pediatrics* 68:880–3, 1981.

American Academy of Pediatrics, Committee on Nutrition: On the feeding of supplemental foods to infants. *Pediatrics* 65:1178, 1980.

American Academy of Pediatrics Work Group on Breastfeeding: Breastfeeding and the use of human milk. *Pediatrics* 100:1035–39, 1997.

Anderson CJ: Enhancing reciprocity between mother and neonate. *Nurs Res* 30:89–93, 1981.

Anderson GC: The mother and her newborn: mutual caregivers. *JOGN Nursing* 6:50–55, 1977.

Anisfeld E, et al: Does infant carrying promote attachment? An experimental study of the effects of increased physical contact on the development of attachment. *Child Dev* 61:1617–27, 1990.

Anisfeld E, Lipper E: Early contact, social support, and mother-infant bonding. *Pediatrics* 72:79–83, 1983.

Baranowski T, et al: Ethnicity, infant feeding practices and childhood adiposity. *J Dev Behav Pediatr* 11:234–9, 1990a.

Baranowski T, et al: Height, infant-feeding practices and cardiovascular functioning among 3 or 4 year old children in three ethnic groups. *J Clin Epidemiol* 45:513–18, 1992.

Baranowski T, et al: Infant feeding practices and childhood stature. *Am J Hum Biol* 2:283–90, 1990b.

Bell RQ: Contributions of human infants to caregiving and social interaction. In: Lewis M, Rosenblum LA, eds. *The effect of the infant on its caregiver.* New York: Wiley, 1974:1–19.

Bernal J: Crying during the first ten days of life. *Dev Med Child Neurol* 14:362–72, 1972.

Birch E, et al: Breastfeeding and optimal visual development. *J Pediatr Ophthalmol Strabismus* 30:33–8, 1993.

Bowlby J: *Attachment and loss:* Separation, vol 2. New York: Basic Books, Inc, 1973.

Bowlby J: *Maternal care and mental health.* Geneva: World Health Organization, 1951.

Brams M, Maloney J: "Nursing bottle caries" in breast-fed children. *J Pediatr* 103:415–16, 1983.

Brazelton TB: Crying in infancy. *Pediatrics* 29:579–88, 1962.

Broad B: The effects of infant feeding on speech quality. *NZ Med J* 76:28–31, 1972.

Brook CG, et al: Influence of heredity and environment in determination of skinfold thickness in children. *Br Med J* 2:719–21, 1975.

Bu'Lock F, Woolridge MW, Baum JD: Development of co-ordination of sucking, swallowing and breathing: ultrasound study of term and preterm infants. *Dev Med Child Neurol* 32:669–78, 1990.

Butte NF, et al: Energy utilization of breast-fed and formula-fed infants. *Am J Clin Nutr* 51:350–8, 1990.

Butte N, et al: Influence of early feeding mode on body composition of infants. *Biol Neonate* 67:414–24, 1995.

Calvo EB, Galindo AC, Aspres NB: Iron status in exclusively breast-fed infants. *Pediatrics* 90:375–9, 1992.

Campbell SBG, Taylor PM: Bonding and attachment: theoretical issues. *Sem Perinatol* 3:3–13, 1979.

Carey WB: Night waking and temperament in infancy. *J Pediatr* 84:756–8, 1974.

Carey WB, McDevitt SC: Revision of the Infant Temperament Questionnaire. *Pediatrics* 61:735–9, 1978.

Clark AL: Mother-child relationships. *MCN* 2:94–9, 1976.

Clay LS: Universal hepatitis B immunization. *J Nurse Midwif* 38:129–31, 1993.

Cockburn F, Tappin D, Stone D: Breastfeeding, dummy use, and adult intelligence [Letter]. *Lancet* 3476 (9017):1764–6, 1996.

Cohen RJ, et al: Effects of age of introduction of complementary foods on infant breast milk intake, total energy intake, and growth: a randomised intervention study in Honduras. *Lancet* 343:288–93, 1994.

Condon WS, Sander LW: Neonate movement is synchronized with adult speech: interaction participation and language acquisition. *Science* 183:99, 1974.

Copeland ET, Baucon-Copeland S: Child obesity: a family systems view. *Am Fam Phys* 24:153–7, 1981.

Davies DP, et al: Effects of solid foods on growth of bottle-fed infants in the first three months of life. *Br Med J* 2:7–8, 1977.

deChateau P, Wiberg B: Long term effect on mother-infant behavior of extra contact during the first hour postpartum. *Acta Paediatr Scand* 66:137, 1977.

Deforest A, et al: The effect of breast-feeding on the antibody response in infants to trivalent oral poliovirus vaccine. *J Pediatr* 83:94–5, 1973.

Dietz WH: Childhood obesity: susceptibility, cause, and management. *J Pediatr* 103:676–86, 1983.

Elias F, et al: Sleep/wake patterns of breast-fed infants in the first 2 years of life. *Pediatrics* 77:322–9, 1986.

Emde RN, Gaensbauer TJ, Harmon RJ: Emotional expression in infancy: a biobehavioral study. *Psychol Issues* 10:xxx, 1976.

Epstein K: The interactions between breastfeeding mothers and their babies during the breastfeeding session. *Early Child Dev Care* 87:93–104, 1993.

Erikson EH: *Childhood and society* (2nd ed). New York: Norton, 1963.

Erikson EH: *Identity, youth and crisis*. New York: Norton, 1968.

Fantz RL: Visual perception from birth, as shown by pattern sensitivity. *Ann NY Acad Sci* 118:739–814, 1965.

Farquharson J, et al: Infant cerebral cortex phospholipid fatty-acid composition and diet. *Lancet* 340:810–13, 1992.

Fergusson DM, Beautrais AL, Silva, PA: Breast-feeding and cognitive development in the first seven years of life. *Soc Sci Med* 16:1705–8, 1982.

Fisch RO, et al: Obesity and leanness at birth and their relationship to body habits in later childhood. *Pediatrics* 56:521–8, 1975.

Florey C du V, Leech AM, Blackhall A: Infant feeding and mental and motor development at 18 months of age in first born singletons. *Int J Epidemiol* 24(suppl 1):S21–6, 1995.

Forster C, et al: Psychological and sexual changes after the cessation of breast-feeding. *Obstet Gynecol* 84:872–6,1994.

Freedman DS, et al: Serum cholesterol levels in a multiracial sample of 7,439 preschool children from Arizona. *Prev Med* 21:162–76, 1992.

Gale CR, Martyn CN: Breastfeeding, dummy use, and adult intelligence. *Lancet* 347(9008):1072–5, 1996.

Gardner DE, Norwood JR, Eisensen JE: At-will breastfeeding and dental caries: four case reports. *J Dent Child* 44:186–91, 1977.

Gill NE, et al: Effect of nonnutritive sucking on behavioral state in preterm infants before feeding. *Nurs Res* 37:347–50, 1988.

Glaser J: *Prophylaxis and allergic disease in infancy and childhood: allergy and immunology in children.* Springfield, IL: Thomas, 1973.

Greiner T: The concept of weaning: definitions and their implications. *J Hum Lact* 12:123–28, 1996.

Harlow HF, Harlow M: The affectional systems. In: Schrier A, Harlow H, Stollnitz F, eds. *Behavior of nonhuman primates,* vol 2, New York: Academic, 1965.

Hayes JS: Theories of child development. In: Servonsky J, Opas SR, eds. *Nursing management of children.* Boston: Jones and Bartlett, 1987:230–61.

Hedberg-Nyqvist K, Ewald U: Successful breast feeding in spite of early mother-baby separation for neonatal care. *Midwifery* 13:24–31, 1997.

Hegvik R, McDevitt SC, Carey W: The Middle Childhood Temperament Questionnaire. *J Dev Behav Pediatr* 3:197–200, 1982.

Heinig MJ, et al: Intake and growth of breast-fed and formula-fed infants in relation to the timing of introduction of complementary foods: the DAR-LING study. *Acta Paediatr* 82:999–1006, 1993.

Hoefer C, Hardy MC: Later development of breast-fed and artificially fed infants. *JAMA* 92:615–19, 1929.

Humphreys HG, Leighton BC: A survey of antero-posterior abnormalities of the jaws in children between the age of two and five and a half years of age. *Br Dent J* 88:3–15, 1950.

Hunziker UA, Barr RG: Increased carrying reduces infant crying: a randomized controlled trial. *Pediatrics* 77:641–8, 1986.

John TJ, et al: Effect of breast-feeding on serore-sponse of infants to oral poliovirus vaccination. *Pediatrics* 57:47, 1976.

Johnson DL, et al: Breast feeding and children's intelligence. *Psychol Rep* 79:1179–85, 1996.

Kagan J: Infant's differential reactions to familiar and distorted faces. *Child Dev* 36:519–32, 1966.

Kajosaari M, Saarinen UM: Prophylaxis of atopic disease by six months' total solid food elimination. *Acta Paediatr Scand* 72:411–14, 1983.

Keane V, et al: Do solids help baby sleep through the night? *Am J Dis Child* 142:404–5, 1988.

Kessen W, Haith MM, Salapatek PH: Human infancy: a bibliography and guide. In: Mussen PH, ed. *Carmichael's manual to child psychology.* New York: Wiley, 1970.

Klaus M, et al: Human maternal behavior at first contact with her young. *Pediatrics* 46:187–92, 1970.

Klaus MH, Kennell JH: *Maternal-infant bonding: the impact of early separation and loss on family development.* St Louis: Mosby, 1975.

Klaus MH, Kennell JH: *Parent-infant bonding* (2nd ed). St Louis: Mosby, 1982.

Kontos D: A study of the effects of extended mother-infant contact on maternal behavior at one and three months. *Birth Fam J* 5:133–40, 1978.

Kotlow LA: Breast-feeding: a cause of dental caries in children. *J Dent Child* 44:192–3, 1977.

Kramer MS: Do breast-feeding and delayed introduction of solid foods protect against subsequent obesity? *J Pediatr* 98:883–7, 1981.

Krogh V, et al: Postpartum immunization with rubella virus vaccine and antibody response in breast-feeding infants. *J Lab Clin Med* 113:695–9, 1989.

Labbok MH, Hendershot GE: Does breast-feeding protect against malocclusion? An analysis of the 1981 Child Health Supplement to the National Health Interview Survey. *Am J Prev Med* 3:227–32, 1987.

Lamb M: The bonding phenomenon: misinterpretations and their implications. *J Pediatr* 102:249–50, 1983.

Lanting CI, et al: Neurological differences between 9-year-old children fed breast-milk or formula-milk as babies. *Lancet* 344:1319–22, 1994.

Levanthal AS, Lipsitt LP: Adaptation, pitch discrimination and sound localization in the neonate. *Child Dev* 35:759–67, 1964.

Lewis M: Infant's responses to facial stimuli during the first year of life. *Dev Psychol* 1:75–86, 1969.

Lorenz KZ: The companion in the environment of the bird. *J Ornithol* 83:137–215, 289–413, 1935.

Lucas A, et al: Breast milk and subsequent intelligence quotient in children born preterm. *Lancet* 339:261–4, 1992.

Macknin ML, Medendorp SV, Maier MC: Infant sleep and bedtime cereal. *Am J Dis Child* 143:1066–8, 1989.

Makin JW, Porter RH: Attractiveness of lactating females' breast odors to neonates. *Child Devel* 60:803–10, 1989.

Makrides M, et al: Fatty acid composition of brain, retina, and erythrocytes in breast-fed and formula-fed infants. *Am J Clin Nutr* 60:189–94. 1994.

Marquis GS, et al: Breast milk or animal-products foods improve linear growth of Peruvian toddlers consuming marginal diets. *Am J Clin Nutr* 66:1102–9, 1997.

Matee MIN, et al: Mutans streptococci and lactobacilli in breast-fed children with rampant caries. *Caries Res* 26:183–7, 1992.

Matee MIN, et al: Nursing caries, linear hypoplasia, and nursing and weaning habits in Tanzanian infants. *Commun Dent Oral Epidemiol* 22:289–93, 1994.

McKenna J, Mosko S, Richard C: Bedsharing promotes breastfeeding. *Pediatrics* 100:214–19, 1997.

Mennella JA, Beauchamp GK: Mothers' milk enhances the acceptance of cereal during weaning. *Pediatr Res* 41:188–92, 1997.

Mennella JA: Mothers' milk: a medium for early flavor experiences. *J Hum Lact* 11:39–45, 1995.

Mercer R: A theoretical framework for studying factors that impact on the maternal role. *Nurs Res* 30:73–7, 1981.

Milnes AR: Description and epidemiology of nursing caries. *J Public Dent* 56:38–50, 1996.

Montgomery DL, Splett PL: Economic benefit of breast-feeding infants enrolled in WIC. *J Am Diet Assoc* 97:379–85, 1997.

Morley R, et al: Mother's choice to provide breast milk and developmental outcome. *Arch Dis Child* 63:1382–5, 1988.

Morrow-Tlucak M, Haude RH, Ernhart CB: Breastfeeding and cognitive development in the first 2 years of life. *Soc Sci Med* 26:635–9, 1988.

Morse JM, Harrison M: Social coercion for weaning. *J Nurse Midwif* 32:205–10, 1987.

Mosko S, et al: Infant arousals in the bedsharing environment: implications for infant sleep development and SIDS. *Pediatrics* 100:841–49, 1997.

Mosko S, et al: Infant sleep architecture during bedsharing and possible implications for SIDS. *Sleep* 19:677–84, 1996.

Mott S. Fazekas NF, James SR: *Nursing care of children and families.* Menlo Park, CA: Addison-Wesley, 1985.

Myers A, Hertzberg J: Bottle-feeding and malocclusion: is there an association? *Am J Orthod Dentofacial Ortho* 93:149–52, 1988.

Naing K-M, Co T-T: Growth and milk intake of exclusively breast-fed Myanmar infants. *Eur J Clin Nutr* 45:203–7, 1991.

O'Connor S, et al: How does rooming-in enhance the mother-infant bond? *Soc Pediatr Res* 13:336, 1979.

Pabst HF, et al: Effect of breast-feeding on immune response to BCG vaccination. *Lancet* 1:295–6, 1989.

Parrago IM, et al: Feeding patterns of urban black infants. *J Am Diet Assoc* 88:796–800, 1988.

Piaget J: *The origins of intelligence in children* (M Cook, trans). New York: International Universities Press, 1952.

Pisacane A, et al: Iron status in breast-fed infants. *J Pediatr* 127:429–31, 1995.

Prechtl J, Beintema D: *The neurological examination of the full term infant* (Child Development Medical Series, 12). Philadelphia: Lippincott, 1975.

Pridham KF, Chang AS: Transition to being the mother of a new infant in the first 3 months: maternal problem solving and self-appraisals. *J Adv Nurs* 17:204–16, 1992.

Prodromidis M, et al: Mothers touching newborns: a comparison of rooming-in versus minimal contact. *Birth* 22:196–200, 1995.

Rago JL: Helping a mother wean with the electric breast pump. *Rental Roundup* 8:8–9, 1991.

Read MH, Boling MA: Effect of feeding practices on the incidence of iron deficiency anemia and obesity in a native American population. *Nutr Rep Int* 26:689–702, 1982.

Rebelsky F, Black R: Crying in infancy. *J Gen Psychol* 121:49–57, 1972.

Rennels MB: Influence of breast-feeding and oral poliovirus vaccine on the immunogenicity and efficacy of rotaviru vaccine. *J Infect Dis* 174(suppl 1):S107–11, 1996.

Riordan J: The cost of not breastfeeding: a commentary. *J Hum Lact* 13:93–7, 1997.

Robertson J: *Young children in hospital*. New York: Basic Books, 1958.

Roche AF: The adipocyte-number hypothesis. *Child Dev* 52:31–43, 1981.

Rodgers B: Feeding in infancy and later ability and attainment: a longitudinal study. *Dev Med Child Neurol* 20:421–6, 1978.

Rogan WJ, Gladen BC: Breast-feeding and cognitive development. *Early Hum Dev* 31:181–93, 1993.

Rogerson BFC, Rogerson CH: Feeding in infancy and subsequent psychological difficulties. *J Ment Sci* 85:1163–82, 1939.

Rubin R: Attainment of the maternal role. *Nurs Res* 16:237–42, 1967.

Rubin R: Binding-in in the postpartum period. *MCN* 6:67–75, 1977.

Saarinen UM, et al: Prolonged breast-feeding: a prophylaxis for atopic disease. *Lancet* (8135):163–6, 1979.

Sanger R, Bystrom E: Breastfeeding: does it affect oral facial growth? *Dent Hygiene* 56:44–7, 1982.

Sears W: *Growing together*. Franklin Park, IL: La Leche League International, 1987:30, 71.

Servonsky J, Opas SR: *Nursing management for children*. Boston: Jones and Bartlett, 1987.

Shulka A, et al: Infantile overnutrition in the first year of life. *Br Med J* 4:507, 1972.

Siegel E, et al: Hospital and home support during infancy: impact on maternal attachment, child abuse and neglect and health care utilization. *Pediatrics* 66:183–90, 1980.

Silfverdal SA, et al: Protective effect of breastfeeding on invasive *Haemophilus influenzae* infection: a case-control study in Swedish preschool children. *Int J Epidemiol* 26:443–50, 1997.

Skinner JD, et al: Transitions in infant feeding during the first year of life. *J Am Coll Nutr* 16:209–15, 1997.

Spitz R: Anaclitic depression. *Psychoanal Study Child* 2:313–42, 1946.

Stanley E, Lundeen D: Tongue thrust in breast-fed and bottle-fed school children: a cross-cultural investigation. *Int J Oral Myol* 6:6–16, 1980.

Straub W: Malfunction of the tongue. *Am J Orthodont* 46:404–24, 1960.

Sugarman J, Kendall-Tackett KA: Weaning ages in a sample of American women who practice extended breastfeeding. *Clin Pediatr* 34:642–47, 1995.

Suitor CW, Hunter MF: *Nutrition principles and applications in health promotion.* Philadelphia: Lippincott, 1980.

Sullivan SA, Birch LL: Infant dietary experience and acceptance of solid foods. *Pediatrics* 93:271–7, 1994.

Svejda MJ, Campos J: Mother-infant "bonding": failure to generalize. *Child Dev* 51:779, 1980.

Taitz LS: Obesity in pediatric practice: symposium on nutrition in pediatrics. *Pediatr Clin North Am* 24:107, 1977.

Tank G, Storvick CA: Caries experience of children of one to six years old in two Oregon communities. *J Am Dent Assoc* 70:101, 1965.

Taylor B, Wadsworth J: Breastfeeding and child development at 5 years. *Dev Med Child Neurol* 26:73–80, 1984.

Temboury MC, et al: Influence of breast-feeding on the infant's intellectual development. *J Pediatr Gastroenterol Nutr* 18:32–36, 1994.

Thomas A, Chess S: *Temperament and development.* New York: Brunner/Mazel, Inc, 1977.

Thomas A, et al: *Behavioral individuality in early childhood.* New York: New York University, 1963.

Thomson M, Hartsock T, Larson C: The importance of immediate postnatal contact: its effect on breastfeeding. *Can Fam Phys* 25:1374–8, 1979.

Weir L: Auditory frequency sensitivity in the neonate: a signal detection analysis. *J Exp Child Psychol* 21:219–25, 1976.

Wessel MA, et al: Paroxysmal fussing in infancy. *Pediatrics* 14:421–34. 1954.

Wishon PM, Kinnick VG: Helping infants overcome the problem of obesity. *MCN* 11:118–21, 1986.

Wolfe MS: Vaccine for foreign travel. *Pediatr Clin North Am* 37:757–69, 1990.

Wolff PH: "Critical periods" in human cognitive development. *Hosp Pract* 11:77–87, 1970.

World Health Organization Collaborative Study Group on Oral Poliovirus Vaccine: Factors affecting the immunogenicity of oral poliovirus vaccine: a prospective evaluation in Brazil and the Gambia. *J Infect Dis* 171:1097–1106, 1995.

Wrigley EA, Hutchinson SA: Long-term breastfeeding: the secret bond. *J Nurse Midwif* 35:35–41, 1990.

Yeung DL, et al: Infant fatness and feeding practices: a longitudinal assessment. *J Am Diet Assoc* 79:531–5, 1981.

Yoneyama K, Nagata H, Asano H: Growth of Japanese breast-fed and bottle-fed infants from birth to 20 months. *Ann Hum Biol* 21:597–608, 1994.

Zack PM, et al: A longitudinal study of body fatness in childhood and adolescence. *J Pediatr* 95:126–30, 1979.

The Ill Breastfeeding Child

Jan Riordan

The care of a breastfeeding infant differs from that of an infant artificially fed, and these differences require special consideration when the breastfeeding baby or young child is ill. Also, the crucial role of nursing in direct primary care of a child with a health problem often makes the difference between unnecessary weaning and continued breastfeeding. Despite the many advantages of breastfeeding, many health care professionals assume that it must be terminated when a serious illness strikes. Even when breastfeeding continues, a disruption of the established patterns is inevitable. Nurses and health care workers must know when and how to intervene effectively to improve a child's health status without unnecessarily disrupting the breastfeeding course.

This chapter discusses selected health problems that affect breastfeeding. There are obviously far more pediatric health problems than those presented here. Pumps and other lactation technologies described in Chapter 13 will often be an integral part of nursing interventions.

Infections

The infant is exposed to a variety of pathogens in his environment. Breastfeeding enhances the infant's immune system and thus helps to protect him from infections. During the past two decades, numerous research studies have documented the protection that breastfeeding affords against many infections during infancy and childhood. This protective effect appears to be more striking and easier to demonstrate in settings in which poverty, malnutrition, and poor hygiene are prevalent (Kramer, 1988).

Two studies (Chen, 1994; Chen et al., 1988) have reported the effect of artificial feeding on hospitalization rates in China, the world's most populous country. After controlling for potentially confounding factors (infant gender, infant weight, parent education, smoking), these authors established that artificially fed infants were twice as likely as were breastfed infants to be hospitalized for respiratory infections and about one-third more likely to be hospitalized for gastroenteritis or other infections during the first 18 months of life.

Two years later, Howie et al. (1990) examined breastfeeding and infant illness in Dundee, U.K.; like Chen et al., they also controlled for confounding variables. In their study, however, the data were collected prospectively by the health visitors as they made home visits. Their results were similar to those of Chen et al.: babies who were breastfed for 13 weeks or more had about one-half the incidence of gastrointestinal illness of those who were bottle-fed from birth for the first 13 weeks of life. Dewey et al. (1995) found similar outcomes in children living in the United States. Although breastfeeding is protective, this protection is not complete, and health care professionals are sometimes called on to care for a breastfeeding child with an infection.

Gastrointestinal Infections

The infant may have diarrhea with the flu; however, because the breastfed infant's stools are normally loose, what is thought to be "diarrhea" by an uninformed individual may be a normal stool pattern. Vomiting and diarrhea are common in children but far less common in breastfed children, particularly during the period of exclusive breastfeeding (Clemens et al., 1993; Haffejee, 1990; Huffman & Combest, 1990; Popkin et al., 1990). Although the primary cause is viral or bacterial invasion of the gastrointestinal (GI) tract, vomiting and diarrhea also occur as a result of infections and disorders of other body systems. The stools of babies are also looser when their mothers are taking antibiotics (Taddio et al., 1995). All infants "spit up" occasionally; this does not necessarily mean that the infant is ill. An infant with persistent vomiting, however, should be examined for other problems if an infection is ruled out.

Water is lost from the body through urine, feces, and evaporation from the skin and lungs. Because the infant has a relatively greater body surface area compared with body mass, larger amounts of fluid are lost through the skin. If the baby is nauseated, he will take less fluid, and vomiting will cause direct fluid loss. If he also has diarrhea, fluid loss may be profound, and dehydration is a real threat. Excessive GI losses, particularly diarrhea, involve losses of sodium and potassium along with water. The risk of dehydration and acidosis increases if losses are extensive; prompt fluid replacement with oral rehydration solution is necessary to prevent the need for intravenous replacement therapy and hospitalization.

Following birth, newborns have an excess amount of body fluids that gradually disappear in two or three days. After that time, infants are vulnerable to rapid and extreme disturbances in hydration, because they have such a small extracellular fluid reserve. Until the infant is about two years of age, he has a relatively larger percentage of extracellular fluid and a greater fluid intake and output than does the adult. The daily exchange of fluid volume for an infant is about 40 percent. For example, an infant who weighs seven kilograms has an extracellular fluid volume of 1,750 ml. This baby will drink about 700 ml and excrete about 700 ml daily. An adult, on the other hand, will exchange only about 14 percent of extracellular fluid daily. Thus after the newborn period (when the baby has excess fluid), fluid loss in an infant who does not eat or drink for a day is more critical than in an adult who does not eat or drink in the same period.

Hydration can be assessed by observing the infant's general responsiveness and skin turgor. Dehydrated babies are listless and look and act sick. The degree of dehydration is best determined by the extent of rapid body weight loss. If a baby weighed 10 kg and now weighs 9 kg, he has had a 10 percent loss, which is considered moderate dehydration. Weight loss up to 15 percent is considered severe dehydration. Other evidence of dehydration includes

- depressed or sunken anterior fontanel
- dry mucous membranes
- small urinary output, few wet diapers (oliguria); urine specific gravity greater than 1.030
- cool, clammy extremities, especially the fingers and toes
- rapid pulse, lowered blood pressure, and capillary filling time of greater than two to three seconds
- absence of tears in infant older than three months of age

Normally, six to eight cloth diapers wet with urine in a 24-hour period is an indication of adequate hydration; however, frequent stools confuse estimates of urine output. With dehydration, the specific gravity of the urine (normal, 1.010–1.020) will be high, indicating a diminished water intake. Children younger than two years of age are less able to concentrate urine; a specific gravity of 1.020 reflects a more serious situation than if the child were older.

Treatment for dehydration requires replacement of lost fluids and electrolytes. At home, extra fluids can be given with a spoon or dropper if the infant has not yet begun to drink from a cup. The parents should also place the infant on his side to prevent aspiration if he is regurgitating. If the baby is willing to take anything by mouth, it should be breastmilk (Ruuska, 1992). Even partial breastfeeding reduces the severity and duration of diarrhea episodes—and the likelihood of mortality from diarrhea (Sachdev et al., 1991; Scariati et al., 1997). In the past, many health professionals advised that even breastfed infants should be taken off milk products in the event of vomiting and diarrhea; however, this is no longer thought to be true, nor is human milk part of, or identical to, cow's milk and other dairy products. Because infants digest breastmilk rapidly, even one who is vomiting regularly will absorb some of the nutrient and fluids of the milk before it is regurgitated. The most appropriate management includes continued breastfeeding with or without solids, as determined by the child's willingness to eat. Only a fully formula-fed infant requires a reduction or elimination of milk feedings if the diarrhea persists or worsens (Brown, 1991).

If breastmilk is not available, oral rehydration solution with 75 to 90 mEq/liter of sodium should be used. Solutions of Rehydrate and WHO Oral Rehydration Salts are excellent for rehydration, Pedialyte or Infalyte for maintenance (Straughn & English, 1996). Sodas or Jell-O water offer little in the way of nourishment and none of the immunities of breastmilk. After being told to interrupt breastfeeding because her infant was vomiting and had a mild fever, a mother who is also a nurse reported:

He needed to breastfeed and refusing him for 24 hours would have been devastating. I walked him around to quiet him, waiting as long as I could between feedings. The breastmilk stayed down about 20 minutes before he vomited it up, but at least I felt like he was getting something.

Acute diarrhea continues to be a cause of hospitalization in young children, and deaths from it still occur. Ruuska and Vesikari (1991) followed 336 Finnish children from birth to two and a half years of age to determine the incidence of acute diarrhea. More than 50 percent of the children had no diarrhea, 26 percent had one episode, and 19 percent had two or more episodes of diarrhea. One

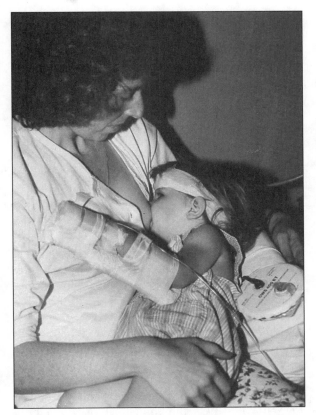

FIGURE 20–1. Comfort at breast while receiving an intravenous infusion. *(Courtesy Debi Leslie Bocar.)*

case-control study in Nigeria found that persistent diarrhea and underweight status was significantly lower in breastfeeding infants than in nonbreastfed children (Clemens et al., 1993; Meremikwu et al., 1997). Rotavirus was by far the most common pathogen. About two-thirds of the infants were breastfed over six months; breastfeeding for less than six months was associated with a higher incidence of rotavirus diarrhea between 7 and 12 months of age but not thereafter.

If severe gastroenteritis develops during weaning, the baby can be brought into a clinic or hospital for intravenous replacement of fluids. Usually, a 5% dextrose-containing solution with added sodium and potassium is given for 24 to 48 hours (Fig. 20–1). Before potassium is added, however, it must be determined that the infant's renal system is functioning, because accumulation of potassium in the system is life-threatening.

Respiratory Infections

Infection of the respiratory tract, the most common cause of illness in infancy and childhood, is usually caused by a virus. Infants with few outside contacts develop fewer respiratory infections than do children in day-care settings. Breastfeeding has a protective effect against respiratory illness, even when important confounding variables (birth weight, number of siblings, maternal age, smoking) are controlled (Beaudry et al., 1995). If a breastfeeding infant develops a respiratory infection, it is usually upper respiratory and less likely to be serious, and he is less likely to be hospitalized (Beaudry et al., 1995; Cunningham et al., 1991; Lopez-Alarcon et al., 1997). The protective effect of breastfeeding against lower-respiratory-tract infections is greatest for children exposed to environmental tobacco smoke (Nafstad et al., 1996, 1997; Horta et al., 1997).

Although newborns may have an infection without a fever, children from six months to three years of age will readily develop a fever, sometimes before any other sign of a respiratory problem is apparent. If the temperature rises rapidly to more than 104°F (40°C), the child is at risk for febrile convulsion with tonic-clonic characteristics. Other symptoms of a respiratory infection include tachypnea, wheezing, hoarseness, cough, nasal flaring; the presence of abnormal respiratory chest sounds, such as rhonchi, rales, and hyperresonance; and the absence of normal lung sounds. Care can be given at home, unless the child's symptoms worsen. Those helping the family of a breastfed child with a respiratory infection should inform them that the baby's previous feeding patterns will be altered during the illness.

Rather than the usual response of wanting to breastfeed more when sick, the infant may be less interested in feedings and may even refuse the breast. Such infants are nose-breathers; blocked airway passages pose the risk of compromising oxygen intake during feeding. To make it easier for the infant to breathe, the mother should feed him in a sitting position, holding him in an upright position as much as possible. For older infants and children, decongestant nose drops can be administered 15 to 20 minutes before breastfeeding. A less satisfactory way to clear nasal secretions is to gently suction them out by using an infant nasal aspirator or rubber ear syringe. Saline nose drops also help to clear nasal passages and to promote feeding. (To prepare saline drops at home, dissolve one teaspoon of salt in one pint of warm water.) For older infants and children who can tolerate nose drops, a vasoconstrictor (e.g., phenylephrine) will shrink the mucous membranes. Two to three drops are gently placed into each of the child's nostrils, but this solution should be used for no longer than three days.

The infant may not act hungry. Anorexia (loss of appetite) and vomiting is often a result of respiratory infections in a toddler or small child, especially if he is coughing. If hydration is not a problem, he should be allowed to determine his own need for food. Once the acute symptoms have passed, his appetite will return, usually in a day or two. Until then, the mother should pump or hand-express her breastmilk. Acetaminophen will reduce the fever and make the child more comfortable. If the infant or child has laryngeal involvement, with hoarseness or a croupy cough, a cool-mist vaporizer in the room or area in which he sleeps is still thought to soothe and moisten mucous membranes, despite lack of evidence that vaporizers are effective (Colombo et al., 1981). An inexpensive, time-honored, and effective method for creating concentrated steam and temporarily relieving croup is for the parent, while safely holding the child, to turn on hot water in an empty shower stall with the bathroom door closed. Fifteen minutes may be all that is necessary for relief. Wrap the infant with a dry blanket or towel afterward to prevent the child from becoming chilled.

Respiratory Syncytial Virus/Bronchiolitis.

Respiratory syncytial virus (RSV) is a respiratory infection that may follow an upper-respiratory-tract infection. It is most common during the winter months, affects young infants, and lasts about two weeks. Breastfeeding has a protective effect against RSV, the primary causative pathogen (Holberg, 1991; Pullan et al., 1980). These viruses cause extensive inflammation that leads to necrosis of bronchiole cells, edema, and increased secretions. The baby can inhale easily because the bronchioles dilate on inspiration and air goes around the obstruction; exhalation, however, is difficult because the airway narrows, trapping air distal to the obstruction. Because bronchiolitis is a viral illness, antibiotics are used only if a secondary bacterial infection develops. Most cases of bronchiolitis are self-limiting, and hospitalization is not necessary unless the child has a preexisting pulmonary condition. The baby is given supportive treatment at home and continues to breastfeed.

Pneumonia. Pneumonia is almost always viral, not bacterial. RSV is responsible for most viral pneumonias in young children. Antibiotic therapy may be given until it is determined that the pneumonia is not bacterial. Hospitalization may be necessary, and the child may need oxygen, intravenous fluids, and corticosteroids.

Although uncommon, bacterial pneumonia is a serious disease and is seen more often in infants than in children. The pneumococcus is the most common organism in bacterial pneumonia (90 percent). Infants with bacterial pneumonia become acutely ill and rapidly develop a high temperature that may be accompanied by seizures. In most cases, these infants are hospitalized and given intravenous antibiotics and other measures to reduce their fever. Antimicrobial therapy has significantly reduced morbidity and mortality from bacterial pneumonia. Discontinuation of breastfeeding was found to be a risk factor for developing severe pneumonia in children living in India (Shah, 1994).

Most infants can receive humidified oxygen through low-flow nasal cannulas and can still breastfeed. Use of a mist tent imposes a necessary (albeit therapeutic) isolation of the child from the parent, but there is no reason for it to interfere with breastfeeding if the child is interested. Taking him out of the tent for brief periods of holding and feeding has more benefits than risks. Another alternative is for the mother to climb into the tent and rezip the side of the tent to prevent loss of cool mist and oxygen. Other than being nontraditional, it has no disadvantages, and the mother's presence may quickly quiet a crying, unhappy infant who has little energy to spare.

Meningitis

Meningitis is an acute inflammation of the meninges caused by a viral or bacterial pathogen. When meningitis occurs in the breastfed infant, it is usually, but not always, aseptic or viral in origin.

Meningitis is also associated with other viral diseases, such as enteroviruses, measles, mumps, or herpes. The range of clinical symptoms and their severity varies widely and may be sudden or gradual in onset. Signs of meningeal irritation include changes in level of consciousness, nausea and vomiting, and a tense anterior fontanel. Other neurological signs are pain when the baby's head is moved and a positive Brudzinski's sign (i.e., lower limbs flex spontaneously when his neck is flexed). An infant who prefers not to be held because of meningeal irritability needs to be seen by a physician as soon as possible.

One mother whose breastfeeding child developed meningitis on a family vacation reported, "We had no idea of just how sick he was, but I had a strong feeling that if we did not get him to a doctor he would die. He didn't have much fever, but he had stopped nursing and he no longer seemed to recognize his older brother and sister. Every time I moved him he would cry."

The child with meningitis should be hospitalized and a lumbar puncture performed to culture cerebrospinal fluid. Intravenous antibiotics may be administered, and the child isolated until bacterial meningitis can be ruled out. The mother will need help in careful handling of the intravenous site when moving her child to her breast. Infants are sometimes uninterested in breastfeeding for a day or two during the acute phase but then resume breastfeeding as eagerly as before.

Bacterial meningitis is a serious disease that may require intensive care. In neonates, the causative organisms are *Escherichia coli* and group B streptococci; in infants, they are *Meningococcus* or *Pneumococcus*. Breastfed infants rarely have bacterial infections of any kind, especially bacterial meningitis (Cochi et al., 1986; Fallot, 1980; Istre et al., 1985; Leventhal, 1986). Meningitis from *Haemophilus influenzae* is now preventable by immunization, and the incidence of this disease has declined. Before *H. influenzae* vaccination was introduced in Sweden, an association of decreased risk for this infection and duration of breastfeeding persisted beyond the period of breastfeeding (Silverdal et al., 1997). This finding supports the hypothesis that breastfeeding has a long-lasting protective effect.

Otitis Media

Inflammation of the middle ear is the second most prevalent childhood disease (after respiratory tract infections). It occurs most often in children from six months to three years of age. It is well established that bottle-feeding increases both the risk of otitis media and the duration of the illness (Aniansson, 1994; Duncan et al., 1993; Saarinen, 1982; Sassen, 1994; Schaefer, 1971; Teele et al., 1989). Harabuchi et al. (1994) suggested that the protective effects of human milk against otitis media may be due in part to inhibition of nasopharyngeal colonization with *H. influenzae,* a frequent cause of otitis media, by specific secretory IgA antibody. Moreover, reflux of milk up the Eustachian tubes is less pronounced in breastfed babies, because the baby is held in an upright position during feedings and, of course, the breast cannot be "propped" as with a bottle (Tully et al., 1995). Smoking and day-care attendance are also risk factors (Alho et al., 1993).

Otitis generally occurs following a respiratory infection when the child suddenly develops a fever and sharp, constant pain in one or both ears. Infants become very irritable, frequently pulling or tugging at the affected ear; a child verbalizes pain. Many middle-ear infections are caused by *H. influenzae* or *Pneumococcus* and are treated with a penicillinase-resistant antibiotic, such as amoxicillin-clavulanate and trimethoprim-sulfamethoxazole. A single intramuscular injection of ceftriaxone (Rocephin), a cephalosporin, is as effective as 10 days of oral amoxicillin for treating uncomplicated otitis media (Green & Rothrock, 1993).

Based on the comfort needs of the child, an analgesic, such as acetaminophen, may be given to relieve pain and fever. An infant with a middle-ear infection will breastfeed more often for solace and will hold his head carefully in an attempt to protect against pressure on the painful ear during breastfeeding. Local heat should be placed over the ear while the child lies on the affected side. This position facilitates drainage if the drum has ruptured (Wong, 1995). If episodes of acute otitis media occur frequently, it may be wise to keep the child on maintenance antibiotic therapy.

Alteration in Neurological Functioning

The suck/swallow reflexes in a full-term, healthy infant are usually neurologically mature at birth, and the infant usually has little difficulty in establishing a pattern of satisfactory suckling. This is not true for the neurologically damaged child, however. Any neurological deficit that affects neuromuscular function carries the risk that the child will have feeding difficulties. Suckling and swallowing, as well as breathing, are integrated under medullary (brainstem) control. When this control is impaired, the normal muscle tension involved in these functions becomes dystonic and flaccid. As a result, feeding by breast or bottle can be difficult and frustrating. As pointed out in Chapter 14, breastfeeding requires less energy than does bottle-feeding. Despite such neuromuscular problems, a number of determined women, with the help of their physicians, nurses, and others, have breastfed these children, developing techniques through trial and error that overcome initial difficulties.

Down Syndrome

The risk of Down syndrome increases with maternal age, which is the only clearly defined factor known to increase the likelihood of faulty chromosome distribution and Down syndrome. A chromosome study can be done early in pregnancy by obtaining amniotic fluid by amniocentesis. Common characteristics include epicanthal folds, flat nasal bridge, broad hands with shortened fingers, a simian crease (single crease across the upper palm), flattened forehead, a small mouth, large tongue, and hypotonicity. In about one-third of these infants, heart development is incomplete (most commonly because of septal defects), and surgery may be required; incomplete development of the GI tract is also common.

In addition to requiring special assistance with feedings (especially when young), these infants need extra stimulation through frequent touching, exercising of extremities in a patterned sequence, carrying, and being spoken to in a varied voice pitch and intonation. In short, the parents should be encouraged to play, laugh, and have fun with the baby. Because the infant with Down syndrome has increased respiratory secretions, the same activities that stimulate the infant's sensory system also help postural drainage, thus preventing the pooling of mucus.

Neural-Tube Defects

Abnormalities along the neural axis occur often enough to warrant their discussion in relation to breastfeeding. With successful surgical interventions, many infants affected by neural-tube defects are able to function and fully participate in life, including being able to breastfeed. In myelomeningocele, a segment of the spinal cord and meninges protrudes through a defect in the bony spine, usually in the lumbosacral region. The infant may have some weakness or complete flaccid paralysis of the legs and later bladder- and bowel-control dysfunction. The important aim of early care is to prevent infection of the sac and to preserve muscular and neurological functions. Surgical correction to close the opening is performed as early as possible, preferably in the first 24 to 48 hours of life. If the defect is extensive, one or more later surgical procedures will be performed using skin flaps.

Because the infant is housed in the intensive care unit during the critical period, the parents should be encouraged to be with their baby and to help in caretaking whenever possible. If the mother is able to feed the infant by breast, the nurse should stay with her during the first several feedings, especially helping her to carefully pick up the infant and use pillows to help position him on the breast while protecting the sac or the surgical site from any pressure. A typical feeding position can be used if the mother's elbow is rotated around a protective device to avoid pressure on his back. The infant can also be fed with the mother lying next to him on a bed. Early feedings should be brief, to conserve the infant's energy. Because the infant cannot be burped or bubbled in the normal way, gently rubbing him between his shoulders or rocking on a firm surface helps to release any ingestion of air. If brainstem impairment is involved, the baby may not be able to breastfeed for a long time, if ever. Yet expressing breastmilk so that it can be given to the infant is immensely rewarding to the mother.

Hydrocephalus

Hydrocephalus, which sometimes occurs with myelomeningocele, is an accumulation of fluid in the intracranial cavity caused by an interference in the flow or absorption of cerebrospinal fluid. In communicating hydrocephalus, the infant maintains normal communication between the ventricles and the subarachnoid space; in the noncommunicating type, the infant's brain experiences a partial or complete blockage between these two areas. Circulation of the cerebrospinal fluid is blocked at some point within the ventricular system, preventing its flow to the subarachnoid spaces.

As the fluid distends the ventricles, the infant's head enlarges, and the sutures begin to separate with bulging fontanels. Hydrocephalus that is already advanced at birth or is allowed to progress is characterized by the ocular "setting sun" sign (the white of the eye showing above the iris and below the upper lid as a result of intracranial pressure), a high-pitched cry, muscle weakness, and severe neurological defects.

Diagnosis of hydrocephalus is confirmed by a computed tomography (CT) scan and by magnetic resonance imaging (MRI). Surgery should be performed as soon as the diagnosis is made. The surgical treatment is a shunt that will bypass the obstruction point and drain the cerebrospinal fluid to another area, usually the peritoneum, where it is absorbed and finally excreted.

The infant with hydrocephalus requires careful nursing care, and the parents need emotional support. Breastfeeding is often possible; with early treatment, many children lead normal lives. Care must be taken in positioning and supporting the infant's head; feeding while lying down with his head supported by a pillow is probably the most comfortable position for the infant with advanced hydrocephalus. To prevent regurgitation, feedings should be frequent and on demand. When there is severe brain damage and breastfeeding is not possible, some mothers of infants with hydrocephalus express their milk, deriving satisfaction from being able to give their baby their milk in a gavage tube or bottle.

Clinical Implications

When an infant is ill, nothing should be assumed without actually putting the baby to breast. Even when a child has a known neurological condition with hypotonia, such as Down syndrome, he may be able to feed effectively. A study of 59 breastfed infants with Down syndrome showed that one-half of the infants had no difficulty in establishing suckling; four were slow to do so for less than one week; eight took one week to establish suckling; and sixteen took longer than one week to do so (Aumonier & Cunningham, 1983).

Mohrbacher and Stock (1997) and McBride and Danner (1987) described suckling disorders in neurologically impaired infants and suggested helpful techniques to improve suckling abilities (Box 20–1). Many of the suggestions for breastfeeding special babies derive from these discussions.

Congenital Defects

Congenital Heart Defects

Infants with congenital heart defects (CHDs) include those who are asymptomatic and those with such severe defects that any exertion, including feeding, can cause cyanosis and early signs of a congestive heart failure. CHDs do not prevent breastfeeding; nurses should encourage breastfeeding for these infants as they would for any other.

Frequently, there are so few symptoms that the problem is not recognized until later in life. A serious difficulty, however, can cause the infant to suckle poorly and to tire easily at the breast. He may begin with vigorous suckling, pulling away after a few minutes to rest. Typically, the hungry infant will again grasp the breast and repeat the cycle. After a time, inadequate intake of breastmilk leads to failure to gain weight. Medical interventions with drug therapy, such as digitalis, can alleviate lack of oxygenation and increase cardiac output. Often corrective surgery is indicated in one or several stages.

With a severe defect, the infant can show early signs of heart failure, becoming cyanotic, with fast respirations (tachypnea) and pulse rate (tachycardia). While the mother is holding her infant, the baby's heartbeat may be so prominent that the mother is aware of it. Any of the symptoms described, along with auscultation of abnormal heart sounds or palpation of a thrill or diminished femoral pulses, should lead the health care worker to suspect a cardiac defect. The child should be immediately referred to a pediatrician for subsequent diagnostic testing to determine whether a defect is present and what type it is.

Infants with CHD gain more weight if they breastfeed than if they are not breastfed. Combs and Marino (1993) compared patterns of weight gain for 45 infants with CHD. More bottle-fed infants significantly fell off their individual growth curves than did breastfed infants. Contrary to conventional wisdom, the severity of the cardiac defect was not a predictor of the infant's ability to breastfeed or of the duration of breastfeeding; rather, it was the mother's commitment to continuing with breastfeeding.

A possible reason for the greater weight gain of the breastfed babies in this study is that they experienced less decrease in tissue oxygenation. Tissue oxygenation during feeding may exert a powerful effect on weight gain in infants with CHD, because they typically eat slowly and often. It was common for the mothers in this study to report that they spent one of every two to three hours feeding their babies. Infants with CHD may spend a significant portion of their lives with poor oxygenation. Box 20–2 contains information for helping the breastfeeding mother.

Oral and Gastrointestinal Defects

Gastroesophageal Reflux. "Spitting up" is a common event for both breastfed and bottle-fed infants. The neonate's small stomach—about the size of a golfball—must accommodate a large volume of milk for its size. The stomach has a capacity of 6 ml on the first day and 12 ml on the second day after birth, whereas the average volume of the mother's colostrum is 25 to 56 ml on the first day and 113 to 185 ml on the second day (Wang et al., 1994). Thus, in the majority of cases, these infants

BOX 20–1

Improving Breastfeeding and Suckling Responses for a Neurologically Impaired Infant

The lactation consultant can help by taking the following actions:

- Arrange for a comfortable and quiet environment (with soft lighting and pillows) for feedings.
- Encourage the mother to find a completely comfortable position for herself and to try different positions for her infant.
- Show the mother how to hold the breast so that it angles slightly upward.
- Teach the mother to use the "dancer-hand" position to help stabilize the infant's lower jaw (Fig. 20–2). While the breast is supported with the last three fingers, the thumb and index finger surround the infant's jaw and rest against his cheeks, applying gentle pressure. The infant is in an upright position, and his chin rests in the web between the thumb and index finger. Swallowing is easier going with the force of gravity rather than against it, and body alignment in a sitting position facilitates the passage of food.

- Teach the mother to hand-express a few drops of milk into the baby's mouth to arouse his interest or brush the nipple on the center of his lower lip to stimulate his rooting reflex. Placing a thumb under the baby's bottom lip or chin encourages bilabial closure and suction.
- Teach the mother to pump her breasts following the feeding. The hindmilk obtained from pumping after feeding has a higher fat content and may be useful for supplementary feedings.
- Encourage the mother to feed the infant frequently.
- Consider providing the mother with a feeding-tube device so that the infant obtains additional milk, thus getting more milk for less effort.

BOX 20–2

Helping the Mother with an Infant with CHD

- Encourage her to feed the baby held in an upright position for short periods.
- Use a feeding-tube device to provide simultaneous supplementation to reduce infant exertion.
- Following surgery, feed at breast as soon as oral feedings can be resumed.

- Enable the mother to remain with her baby, even if he is too ill to hold or feed directly.
- Remind the mother that her milk and breastfeeding are things only she can give to her baby.
- Encourage her to feed the baby frequently.

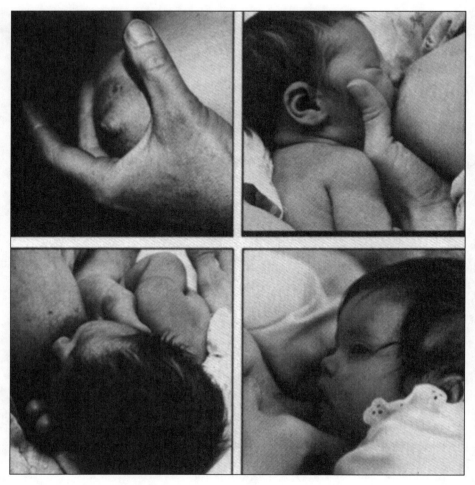

FIGURE 20–2. Mother breastfeeding using the "dancer-hand" position. *A. The mother's hand that supports the breast slides forward so that the breast is supported by three fingers rather than four. The index finger is bent slightly so that the thumb and index finger form a* U. *B. This position helps the baby suckle effectively without using energy to stabilize his jaw. C. The breast is supported with the last three fingers; the thumb and index finger surround the infant's jaw and rest against his cheeks, applying gentle pressure. D. Using a modified "dancer-hand" position to provide chin support only. (From SC Danner, ER Cerutti:* Nursing your baby with Down's Syndrome. *Rochester, NY: Childbirth Graphics, 1989:9.)*

do not experience reflux; they are merely messy babies, and their reflux gradually disappears as they mature. Their parents should be so reassured and advised to

- feed the baby in an upright position to take advantage of the force of gravity
- use one breast per feeding to reduce the amount of each feeding
- feed frequently
- avoid using cereal, a commonly advised treatment, that does not help the condition

A few infants, however, will have persistent reflux, or they will appear to get better for a while; then the regurgitation will reappear and worsen, and the baby will stop gaining weight. This cycle is much more pronounced in formula-fed infants,

presumably because the stomach digests formula or cow's milk more slowly and less completely than breastmilk (Heacock et al., 1992). Such an infant should be referred to a pediatrician for diagnostic workup. Persistent, severe reflux is associated with pyloric stenosis, malrotation of the bowel, Hirshsprung's disease, and some neurological disorders. An esophageal pH probe (a wire inserted in the baby's esophagus to monitor the pH), an upper GI series, and a fibrooptic endoscope are diagnostic tools used to identify the source of the problem.

If the reflux is severe, medications for the infant may be ordered that promote gastric motility, such as metaclopramide (Reglan), a dopamine blocker, cisapride, and ranitidine (Zantac). Cisapride is preferred, because it has fewer side effects. The health care provider is cautioned against prescribing these medications if the reflux appears to be normal spitting up and is not pathological. A common problem with using these medications is overdosing the infant, which can happen when the parents are instructed to give a dose after every meal to a baby who feeds frequently.

The best positioning for these infants is controversial. A 30-degree upright position in an infant seat, a prone position, and an elevated prone position in harness are common recommendations for infants with reflux, but their efficacy is still in question (Wong, 1995).

Pyloric Stenosis. Pyloric stenosis (hypertrophy of the pyloric sphincter) occurs more commonly in male babies and develops about four to six weeks after birth, with regurgitation that becomes progressively more severe and projectile. Rapid dehydration and electrolyte imbalance become a threat. During and after a feeding, it is possible with side lighting to see peristaltic waves that pass from left to right; an olive-shaped tumor (the hypertrophic pylorus) can be palpated in the right upper quadrant of the abdomen. Ultrasound studies confirm the presence of a pyloric mass, and barium studies show the elongated and narrow pyloric canal.

This problem is usually not seen in a breastfed infant; where breastfeeding rates have risen, there has been a decrease in the incidence of pyloric stenosis. Habbick (1989) conducted a case-control study of the hospital charts of 91 infants with pyloric stenosis and matched these infants with a control group. Bottle-feeding was 2.9 times more prevalent among the infants with pyloric stenosis than among the control subjects.

Surgery can be delayed until the infant is rehydrated and electrolyte balance restored. All feedings have to be temporarily interrupted for a day or so after surgery. The mother should be advised to feed with only one breast and for a short time at first to prevent overfilling. These limited feedings of increasing amounts slowly expand the stomach. The infant must be handled very carefully, "as if he were made of crystal." Using an infant seat for a few days may help to stabilize his position during feeding.

Tracheoesophageal Fistula. In the most common form of esophageal anomaly, tracheoesophageal fistula (T-E fistula), the upper end of the esophagus ends in a blind pouch, with a fistula connecting the lower segment of the esophagus to the trachea. An infant who has unexplained episodes of coughing, choking, and cyanosis while feeding and increased mucus secretion may be suspected of having T-E fistula. Feeding at the breast is the optimal way to check for this problem because colostrum is secreted in only small amounts at first; therefore, if a fistula is present, no great amount of fluid can be aspirated.

T-E fistula, a rare defect (1 in 3,000 live births), is suspected when the baby has extreme difficulty in feeding. The conventional diagnostic approach is to pass a catheter into the esophagus to see whether gastric secretions can be aspirated; it is a practice that should not be done routinely. If gastric content cannot be determined and other symptoms are present, medical attention should be obtained at once. If the diagnosis is confirmed by x-ray examination and sonography, surgery is performed in one or two stages to connect the esophagus by end-to-end anastomosis.

Postoperatively, the infant is placed in an isolette with his head elevated. He should have continuous low suction in the esophageal pouch and intermittent low suction to the gastrostomy tube. Until the infant can take oral feedings, the mother can maintain lactation by expressing milk. Her milk should be saved and stored appropriately. If temporary bottle-feeding is required to test for feeding tolerance, breastmilk should be used, because human milk is a physiological fluid.

As soon as the suture line begins to heal, the mother can breastfeed while simultaneously feeding her baby milk through the gastrostomy tube. Oral stimulation, either by feedings or pacifier, is extremely important. To meet the oral needs of the infant, a pacifier may be necessary until breastfeedings can be resumed. Usually, it takes a few days before the baby begins to breastfeed enthusiastically.

Imperforate Anus. The anomaly of imperforate anus ranges from no opening at all to a normal-appearing rectum that ends in a blind rectal pouch just above the opening; it is confirmed only by careful examination and by a diagnostic x-ray examination. Treatment requires surgical reconstruction of the anal opening. In postoperative nursing care, the area around the surgical repair site should be kept clean and dry to promote healing. As soon as peristalsis returns, the infant can be fed from his mother's breast. The normally loose stools of the breastfed infant lessen the risk of constipation with subsequent breakdown of the surgical area and local infection.

Following her infant's surgery for high, imperforate, anal defect that included a temporary colostomy, one mother was encouraged by her physician to resume breastfeeding two days later. When the infant suddenly developed Ritter's disease (toxic epidermal necrolysis) and had to be rehospitalized, she continued to breastfeed and alternately pump her milk for tube feedings. A few months after recovering, the baby underwent pull-through surgery to bring the colon back down to the anal opening with anoplasty. Solids were deliberately delayed to avoid any undue pressure until the colostomy was completely closed at eight months of age. The child continued to breastfeed until he weaned himself at 18 months.

Cleft Lip and Palate. Cleft lip and palate are congenital malformations characterized by incomplete fusing of the central processes around the upper jaw and lip. The clefting may involve only the lip, may extend into the hard and soft palate, and may be unilateral or bilateral. The general classifications include

CL (Lip only)
CLP (Both the lip and palate)
CP (Hard and soft palate only)

Cleft lip and cleft palate each account for 25 percent of the malformations; clefting of both of these structures is found in 50 percent of all cases; therefore, the nurse or lactation consultant will work most frequently with cases involving both the lip and palate. Some cases of cleft palate are discovered when the lactation consultant does a suckling assessment. Breastmilk is recommended for infants with cleft palate because it minimizes the development of otitis media and avoids the necessity for tympanostomy-tube placement. This protection persists well beyond the period of breastmilk feeding (Paradise et al., 1994; Saarinen, 1982; Schaefer, 1971).

The lip is surgically repaired first. Early surgery (during the first days or weeks of life) enhances bonding attachment to a more "normal" infant whose appearance is closer to the ideal baby that

the parents expected; it appears to have no greater risks than does later surgery (Weatherley-White et al., 1987). Surgical closure of the palate between six months and three years of age takes advantage of normal palatal changes in development.

If the infant has unilateral cleft lip with only minor alveolar-ridge deficiency and no palate involvement, he will probably be able to breastfeed before surgery is performed. He must, however, find a way to form a satisfactory seal despite his mouth and nose defect. Mothers of these infants have found that by holding their infant inward, pressing the cleft as tightly to the breast as possible, and placing a thumb or index finger over the cleft, they can create sufficient closure for the infant to effectively milk the breast. When necessity demands, the infant is amazingly adaptive, and the breast is far more flexible than a rigid bottle teat. Radiographic observation of an infant with a bilateral cleft lip showed that during suckling, the tongue is grooved longitudinally, and a peristaltic wave moves backward and obliterates the groove, presses on the nipple, and expresses the milk from it (Jenkins, 1978).

Following surgical repair of the lip, the baby may breastfeed. Early imprinting is of great importance to infants. The infant can move the nipple and areola around in his mouth, against the part of the palate that works and feels best. The mother should express some colostrum each time the infant attempts to latch on (Danner, 1992). Weatherley-White et al. (1987) at Children's Hospital, Denver, CO, offered mothers of 60 infants undergoing surgery for cleft lip the option to breastfeed immediately after surgery. The breastfed infants attained adequate oral intake in a shorter time than did babies fed with a cup. The only surgical complication occurring was a partial separation of the lip on the third postoperative day—in one baby fed by cup. No breastfed infant sustained any gross clinical changes attributable to nursing. At the same time, of the 15 babies with complete cleft lip and palate who attempted breastfeeding, only 1 continued to breastfeed, whereas the other 14 were switched to a bottle by their mothers. The authors failed to mention whether any of these infants wore an artificial palate (Table 20–1). In another study, half of the mothers of neonates with cleft lip or palate attempted to breastfeed. Almost

Table 20–1

WEIGHT GAIN AND COST DIFFERENCES BETWEEN GROUPS

	Breast-feeders*	Cup-Feeders
Weight Gain (%)		
At 1 Month	28	16
At 3 Months	67	50
Hospital		
Length of Stay (in days)	2.1	3.3
Cost (in U.S. dollars)	$2552	$3178

* Only babies with cleft lip.

Source: RCA Weatherley-White, et al: Early repair and breastfeeding for infants with cleft lip. Plast Reconstr Surg 79:879–85, 1987.

all were dissatisfied with the information they had received while in the hospital and with the backup care when they went home (Trenouth & Campbell, 1996).

The ease with which the baby takes the breast is related to the severity and extent of the deficit. When the hard or soft palate is involved in the cleft (CP and CLP), feeding at the breast is more difficult. Because there is a direct space into the nasal cavity, the infant must quickly gulp his food between breaths to prevent regurgitation through his nostrils. This is not possible unless the milk flows easily and quickly into the back of the oral cavity where it can be swallowed rapidly. Danner (1992, p. 625) described in detail the first feedings:

The infant with a unilateral defect does better with the breast entering the mouth from the side on which the defect is located; thus, an infant with a right-sided defect of the lip or the palate should be held so that his right cheek touches the breast. If this position works best, the mother can go from the cradle-hold on one side to the football or "clutch" hold on

the other. In this way, the infant should have an easier time positioning the mother's nipple and areola onto the larger area of the palate.

At the same time, the mother can experiment with positioning and find the way that works best for her. The nipple must stay in the infant's mouth throughout the feeding, and the infant must be held to the breast. Feedings take longer, about 35 to 45 minutes of actual suckling time, with additional time for pauses or nonnutritive suckling. A baby with a bilateral cleft suckles best when straddled on the mother's lap or sitting on one side of her body with his legs under her arm. The breast fills the alveolar-ridge defect and can be moved to one side or the other as needed. As the feedings progress, the mother will gain confidence in her ability to judge position and the patterns of her baby's suckling (Danner, 1992).

One mother started breastfeeding her twins without realizing that one of them had a cleft of the soft palate. The infant cried constantly from hunger and could only drink the milk already let down in the breast. After discovering the cleft, the mother noticed that by milking the breast with her gums and tongue, the child could suckle effectively when the breasts were full and hard (Grady, 1977).

Then we discovered that the only purpose of the suction was to draw in and keep the nipple in her mouth. I found that by placing my index finger on the top edge of my areola and my middle finger on the bottom, I could press my nipple out between these fingers; it would protrude as if it were full of milk. I held the nipple in her mouth during the whole feeding as much as I would a bottle and its nipple.

After four months of using this technique, supplementation was no longer necessary, and the baby was able to breastfeed without additional assistance. Even when this technique is used successfully, the infant must develop strong muscles and jaw capabilities to withdraw the milk (Fig. 20–3).

A palatal obturator, a plastic dental appliance made by a dentist from impressions of the infant's mouth, covers the cleft in the palate and improves the infant's ability to suckle. With early breastfeedings with this artificial palate, the baby does not tire as easily when the feeding is finished or "topped-off"

BOX 20–3

Assisting the Breast-feeding Mother of an Infant with Cleft Lip and Palate

1. First stimulate the milk supply by hand expression or electric pump.

2. Hold the infant in a sitting-up position directly facing the mother, with the infant's legs spread on each side and his head slightly tilted backward.

3. Push the breast into the baby's mouth as far as possible. In this way, the breast helps to seal the cleft.

4. Massage the breast before the feeding to let down the milk. (The mother reported, "When it did, he thought he had done it!")

5. Stimulate suckling motions by placing fingers under his jaw and firmly pushing up and down. The infant soon catches on and initiates the suckling movements him-self, which become stronger.

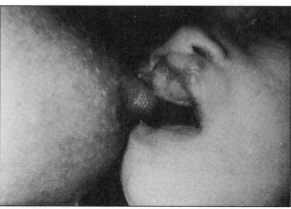

A

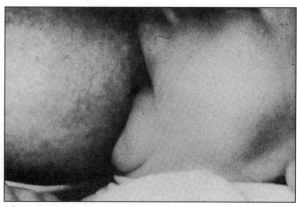

B

FIGURE 20–3. Cleft lip and palate. *A. Infant with cleft lip and complete cleft of hard and soft palates. Palatal obturator in place. B. Same infant at breast .(Both photos courtesy David Barnes, DDS.)*

appropriate growth, the investigators viewed such assisted feeding at the breast as a first step in direct breastfeeding for these babies (Kogo et al., 1997).

Box 20–3 contains another case from the author's practice, highlighting a determined mother who breastfed her infant who had bilateral cleft lip and complete clefts running through the entire hard and soft palates.

In the interval between experimenting with different methods of feeding, breast pumping helps to maintain lactation. Unless the mother is very efficient at hand expression, an electric pump is recommended, particularly one with a double kit for simultaneous pumping of both breasts to save time and energy. Meanwhile, the infant can be fed

with expressed breastmilk using a supplementation device. Sometimes denture powder helps to hold the dental palate firmly in place. One recent study found that of ten babies in whom a Hotz-type palate was used, four infants were able to suckle the breast directly and obtain milk. Although these infants still needed supplemental feeding to sustain

breastmilk by using various methods. Some parents find that a small spouted cup works well. Others favor an eyedropper, a rubber-tipped syringe, or a pipette. Feeding-tube devices (see Chapter 13) have been used successfully for infants with cleft palates. The Beniflex Nurser is another alternative for feeding breastmilk.

Choanal Atresia. Choanal atresia is a narrowing of the posterior nares, which prevents an infant from drawing air through his nose and breathing normally. A rare congenital anomaly, it is a life-threatening emergency in the neonate who develops respiratory distress following birth. Surgery is usually attempted after the second or third week of life, depending on the condition of the infant and his ability to breathe through his mouth. The reconstructive surgery for choanal atresia is highly specialized, and the family will probably have to travel to a regional medical center for the surgery. Surgical placement of nasal stents relieves the baby's respiratory distress.

After the insertion of an oral airway, if the mother desires, she should be encouraged to breastfeed or express her milk for bottle-feeding. The mother will need to be alert for choking during suckling, because the infant is unable to breathe through his nose. Feedings should be interrupted between swallows to allow the infant time to breathe through his mouth (Ledonne, 1986). If the baby is unable to feed from the breast or bottle, breastmilk may be given through a nasogastric tube, but the infant will be expected to take oral feedings before he is allowed to go home.

Ledonne (1986) describes a case in which the mother of a child with choanal atresia gradually switched the baby from formula to breastmilk and continued nursing until he was nine months of age. The mother's desire to breastfeed necessitated cutting down the stents so that they would not be occluded by the breast. In addition, the mother held the baby as upright as possible while feeding to reduce the amount of milk that remained in the rear portion of the nasal stents. The infant needed to be suctioned after every feeding because the stents became plugged, causing difficulty in nasal breathing.

The baby with choanal atresia may resist taking any type of oral feeding at first—breast or bottle—and will curl up his tongue to protect himself against the possibility of choking. After desperately trying "every trick the doctors and nurses knew," a mother tearfully pleaded with her baby that she had tried everything possible to get him to eat and that now it was his turn to do his part. The mother reported: "Then I laid down on the couch with him and for the first time he took my breast and started feeding. It was like he was saying to me, 'OK, Mom, I didn't know it was this bad.'"

Clinical Implications

One of 50 newborns is born with a significant congenital defect, many of which are genetically determined. When the child has myelomeningocele, a cleft palate, or any other abnormality that requires special care over a long period, the parents must adjust psychologically after the birth to the discrepancy between the ideal child visualized during pregnancy and the real child they have. For the mother who intended to breastfeed, the loss of a perfect infant is compounded by the possible loss of being able to feed her infant at her breast; sensitivity to these legitimate feelings is essential. The potential for breastfeeding depends on several variables: the extent of the problem and its short- and long-term implications for feeding, the mother's degree of motivation, and the help she receives.

Surgery may correct congenital defects, enhance quality of life, and prolong life. Preparing the breastfeeding child who is to have surgery depends on his developmental level and his ability to comprehend and reason. Toddlers and preschoolers have vivid imaginations and a strong negative reaction to any procedure in which skin is broken; they may interpret syringes to be knives or daggers. Play interviews encourage children to express their fears and feelings about hospitalization and surgery through play.

Preparing the breastfeeding infant or child for surgery is similar to preparing the nonbreastfeeding child. One or both of the parents should stay with the child as much as possible. Many surgical procedures are now conducted on an outpatient basis, with the family coming to the hospital in the morning and returning home later that day. If the surgery is major and if the baby will be anesthetized, the mother and father should accompany the child to the doors of the surgery suite and then wait in a family waiting area on the pediatric unit for their child to return.

Hospital protocols for pediatric anesthesia are notoriously inconsistent. Some allow breastfeeding up to two hours prior to the induction of anesthesia; others restrict it to from three to six hours before surgery. Breastmilk might be considered a clear liquid if the baby is less than six months of age but not after six months in one hospital; in another, breastmilk might be considered the same as infant formula at any age. Being able to breastfeed an unhappy child going to surgery is an important issue for parents who may turn to the lactation consutant for guidance on this topic.

Clinical research generally supports either two or three hours of fasting before anesthesia for fully breastfed infants. The rate of gastric emptying of breastmilk is twice as fast as that for infant formula but not quite as fast as clear liquids (Cavell, 1981; Husband & Husband, 1969; Littman et al., 1994). Three hours after the test meal, 75 percent of infants fed breastmilk had entered a fasting state, compared with 17 percent of those fed formula (Tomomasa et al., 1987). Littman et al. (1994) found no differences in residual volume and pH between children fed breastmilk and those fed clear liquid before surgery. He recommended that breastfeeding should be terminated three hours prior to induction, compared to two hours prior for clear liquids. In the case of breastfed babies, this distinction raises the question, Why are three hours of fasting before surgery mandated rather than two (Nicholson & Schreiner, 1995)?

The risk of aspiration is as important to the child's surgical recovery as the gastric emptying time, if not greater. In the case of clear liquids, the risk of pneumonitis aspiration is no greater in children allowed clear liquids ad libitum as close as two hours prior to induction of anesthesia (Crawford et al., 1990; Schreiner et al., 1990). When it does occur, lung damage from aspiration of saline solution appears to be less than that of aspirated breastmilk or infant formula (O'Hare et al., 1996).

With the medical technology now available, most infants with congenital abnormalities survive and go on to live relatively normal lives. During the first months after birth, if hospitalization, surgery, or the infant's weakness interfere with normal breastfeeding, the mother must depend on other means to stimulate her milk supply and to remove her milk. To do this, she needs specific information about pumps and other lactation aids available and about how she can obtain the one most suitable for her.

It is best not to offer a rubber teat of any kind to a breastfeeding neonate or young infant to prevent the baby from becoming nipple-confused. However, the question arises: If a rubber nipple is used, what kind is best? There is no special kind of nipple that effectively simulates actual suckling at the breast and thereby prevents nipple confusion. One recent study found that the Playtex nipple set flowed faster with less negative pressure and thus represented an increase in risk of choking and decreased oxygenation because of interrupted breathing patterns, particularly in hypotonic and preterm babies (Fadavi et al., 1997). If the infant is younger than four weeks of age, any oral fluids that are given temporarily may be given using a

- feeding-tube device, such as those described in Chapter 13
- small medicine cup
- spouted cup
- syringe attached to tube
- syringelike device used to give medicine to infants
- periodontal syringe (dental supply store)

In working with a mother whose self-esteem has already been undermined by the loss of the expected "perfect child," the nurse or lactation consultant must make every effort to avoid stimulating any additional feelings of failure. Therefore, all words and actions should be carefully chosen. One mother was devastated after being told, "We've never seen anything like this before" when she was unable to express any milk using an electric pump. Having already given birth to a child who was different from the one she had expected, she could not tolerate being thought of as different in another way, although for another mother the same remark might have gone unnoticed. For this mother, maintaining her milk supply until she could breastfeed directly was a way of retaining normalcy in her relationship with her infant. (Ironically, the pump was later found to be faulty.) Unless proved otherwise, any lactation device should be suspected first when a mother has problems using it.

Metabolic Dysfunction

More than 100 metabolic diseases can be detected in infancy. Of these, only a few cause a health problem, and only a few are suitable for routine screening. Newborn screening for phenylketonuria (PKU) is done in all 50 U.S. states and in more than 30 countries. Direct DNA analysis for PKU is performed to identify the specific mutation and to further define the severity of PKU. Other metabolic disorders for which screening is often performed are hypothyroidism, galactosemia, maple-syrup-urine disease, and homocystinuria. In the United States, where most infants are born in a hospital or clinic, the hospital staff is responsible for obtaining the samples. With early discharge, this is sometimes done after the mother and baby go home. With a home delivery, the responsibility lies with the attending physician or midwife.

Phenylketonuria

PKU is an autosomal recessive inherited metabolic disorder of phenylalanine metabolism, a defect in the enzyme phenylalanine hydroxylase that decreases conversion of phenylalanine to tyrosine. Abnormal metabolites accumulate, and subsequent damage to the brain and nervous system results.

Human milk has lower levels of phenylalanine than does any commercial baby milk (Table 20–2). Breastfeeding along with supplemental use of low-phenylalanine formula (Lofenalac), a casein-free hydrolysate from which 95 percent of the phenylalanine has been removed (Miller & Chopra, 1984), is encouraged. Breastfed infants who receive a daily amount of 362 ml (first month) to 464 ml (fourth month) of breastmilk each day have a lower phenylalanine intake than do infants who are fed exclusively on low-phenylalanine formula during their first six months of life (McCabe et al., 1989). Thus fluctuations in the volume of breastmilk the baby takes are less worrisome than formulas with higher phenylalanine levels.

Parents of children with PKU will be interested in knowing that infants with PKU who are breastfed have significantly higher intelligence quotient scores—a 12.9-point advantage even after adjusting for social and maternal education status ($p = .02$; Riva et al., 1996).

Previous recommendations for breastfeeding included test-weighing of infants before and after breastfeeding to ensure correct dietary intake, a time-consuming task that may not be accurate. Greve et al. (1994) demonstrated a method of eliminating test-weighing by calculating the low-phenylalanine dietary prescription using published estimates of daily volume of human milk consumed by infants who were growing normally. The actual treatment plan for managing PKU is handled by a physician and dietitian specializing in metabolic defects. Each state has at least one medical center designated to serve as a consultant and treatment facility for metabolic defects, including PKU (Duncan & Elder, 1997).

Galactosemia

Another hereditary metabolic condition, galactosemia, occurs once in about every 85,000 births. A rare disorder of the metabolism of galactose-1-phosphate, galactosemia is an enzyme deficiency that is transmitted as an autosomal-recessive trait. With galactosemia, the liver enzyme that changes galactose to glucose is absent; as a result, the infant is unable to metabolize lactose. Any intake of galactose results in liver dysfunction and disease.

These infants appear normal at birth but soon start having feeding difficulties; vomiting and poor weight gain follow. Without treatment, cerebral impairment and lethargy appear, followed by mental retardation. Galactosemia is one of the few cases that demands immediate and total weaning, because breastmilk has a high lactose content. All milk and galactose-containing foods must be eliminated from the diet. The infant is placed on special galactose-free formula, such as Nutramigen. Reassure the mother that by holding and stroking the baby during bottle-feedings, she can meet the emotional and social needs of her infant.

It is possible for mothers with galactosemia to breastfeed. A case study reported that although one mother had galactosemia, her milk was normal in nearly all respects; her well-born baby thrived on exclusive breastfeeding for five months and continued to breastfeed while receiving solids thereafter (Forbes et al., 1988).

Table 20–2

THYROXINE (T$_4$ AND TRIIODOTHYRONINE (T$_3$) LEVELS[a] OF BREASTFED AND FORMULA-FED CHILDREN WITH CONGENITAL HYPOTHYROIDISM

Age (mo)	T$_4$ (nmol/liter)		T$_3$ (nmol/liter)	
	BF	FF	BF	FF
1	161.4 ± 9.4	110.7 ± 9.4[b]	2.7 ± 0.2	3.0 ± 0.2
2	169.6 ± 7.8	128.4 ± 8.0[b]	2.6 ± 0.2	3.1 ± 0.2
3	173.4 ± 7.5	154.5 ± 7.7	3.0 ± 0.1	3.2 ± 0.3
4	176.6 ± 7.6	172.8 ± 8.2	3.2 ± 0.2	3.0 ± 0.2
6	174.2 ± 13.3	169.0 ± 6.3	3.0 ± 0.1	3.0 ± 0.1
9	163.2 ± 9.8	153.9 ± 6.3	2.8 ± 0.1	3.1 ± 0.2
12	161.5 ± 5.2	121.7 ± 4.5	2.4 ± 0.2	2.8 ± 0.1

T$_4$: thyroxine; T$_3$: triiodothyronine; BF: breastfed; FF: formula-fed.
[a] *Mean values plus or minus the standard error of the mean.*
[b] $p < .001$.

Source: JF Rovet: Does breast-feeding protect the hypothyroid infant whose condition is diagnosed by newborn screening? Am J Dis Child *144:319–23, Copyright 1990, American Medical Association.*

Congenital Hypothyroidism

Congenital hypothyroidism is caused by a lack of thyroid secretion, either because the thyroid gland is absent or because there is an inborn enzymatic deficiency in the synthesis of thyroxine. A transient (noncongenital) form of hypothyroidism develops from transfer in utero of antithyroid drugs or use of povidone-iodine on the mother at the time of delivery (Delange et al., 1988). Routine screening results show that congenital hypothyroidism occurs in only one of every 4,000 to 5,000 births.

In the early weeks, parents of an untreated infant may praise their "good baby" because he cries so little. Unless treated, the symptoms of hypothyroidism become noticeable in three to six months. After three months, classic symptoms of myxedema appear: coarse, brittle hair; anemia; a large, protruding tongue; a wide forehead; and lack of skeletal growth. Impairment of the baby's nervous system can lead to severe mental retardation.

Because breastmilk contains small quantities of thyroid hormones, could it interfere with neonatal thyroid screening? Franklin et al. (1985) demonstrated that thyroid hormone concentrations in healthy, term breastfed and formula-fed infants are equivalent. These observations are the same as those found by Misulta et al. (1983) in 1-month-old infants, but they diverge from the results of Hahn et al. (1986), who studied neonates aged 13 to 22 days. Any child with congenital hypothyroidism will need lifelong thyroid replacement therapy regardless of how he is fed. A synthetic levothyroxine sodium (Synthroid or Levothroid) is usually given.

Celiac Disease

Often called *malabsorption syndrome* or *gluten enteropathy,* celiac disease is characterized by changes, in the intestinal mucosa or villi, that prevent the absorption of foods, mainly fat. The mucosal damage appears to stem from a sensitivity to the gluten factor of protein found in wheat, rye, oats, and barley. Formula-feeding and the early introduction of solids accelerate the development of celiac disease (Auricchio, 1983; Greco et al., 1988; Kelly, 1989), which explains why the incidence of celiac disease has declined in the United States as breastfeeding rates have risen and solids are introduced later. Celiac disease is thought to be either an inborn error of metabolism or an immune system disorder. Only recently has a link been made between the mammary tissues and other secretory mucosal sites as part of the immune system (Slade & Schwartz, 1987).

The infant with this disorder will gain adequate weight and show no symptoms until solids containing gluten are introduced into his diet. Then the clinical symptoms are insidious and chronic. Because fat is not absorbed, the child's stools become frothy appearing, foul smelling, and excessive. Deficiencies of the fat-soluble vitamins (A, D, K, and E) appear. If the disease progresses without treatment, abdominal distension and general wasting are evident.

Primary prevention is family teaching and encouraging women with a family history of this disease to breastfeed for a long period and to delay giving their baby solids. The affected child's diet must be modified and vigorously maintained to exclude gluten, thus improving food absorption and preventing malnutrition. Contact with a local support group for gluten-intolerant persons may assist the family in numerous ways.

Cystic Fibrosis

Cystic fibrosis (CF), a congenital disease manifesting itself as a chronic generalized dysfunction of the exocrine (mucus-producing) glands, occurs once in every 1,500 to 2,000 live births. The glands of the affected child produce abnormally thick and sticky secretions that block the flow of pancreatic digestive enzymes, clog hepatic ducts, and impede the movement of cilia in the lungs. The increased sodium chloride in the child's sweat provides an important diagnostic clue: the family reports that the child tastes salty when kissed.

Another early manifestation of CF is intestinal obstruction or ileus. The newborn's meconium blocks the small intestine and gives rise to signs of intestinal obstruction, including abdominal distention, vomiting, and failure to pass stools. In spite of a voracious appetite, the infant fails to gain weight. When he begins to eat cereals and solids, the stools become bulky, more frequent, foul smelling, and frothy. Pulmonary complications are almost always present, and the child suffers persistent, severe respiratory infections because of retained mucus.

Care primarily involves protection from respiratory infection by postural drainage, percussion therapy, aerosol therapy, and medications, such as expectorants and antibiotics. Aerosolized recombinant human DNase is a breakthrough in new CF pharmacotherapy (Jackson & Vessey, 1996). To replace pancreatic enzymes that the child is not producing, pancreatic enzyme replacement (Pancrease) is given, mixed in such soft foods as applesauce.

There is no need to interrupt breastfeeding. In fact, breastfeeding is recommended. Babies with CF produce normal levels of gastric lipase, which is a major digestive enzyme. This enzyme, together with milk lipase in breastmilk, may help the infant with CF to absorb fat efficiently. Human milk contains appreciably greater amounts of lipase than does cow's milk. Pasteurization destroys milk lipase, and rapid loss of activity occurs at room temperature (Ross & Sammons, 1955).

Dodge (1985), diSant'Agnese and Hubbard (1984), and Rooney (1988) suggested that some breastfed infants with CF will develop symptoms only after breastfeeding stops. Moreover, it appears that solely breastfed infants are taller and heavier than are solely formula-fed infants (Holliday et al., 1991). Because the infant with CF is prone to severe respiratory infections, he needs the additional immunological protection conferred by breastmilk. A survey (Luder et al., 1990) of U.S. CF centers found that most centers recommended breastfeeding alone or combined with pancreatic enzyme supplement or hydrolyzed formula. This is a reversal from previous reports, in which breastfeeding was contraindicated.

Allergies and Food Intolerance

It is widely recognized that breastfed infants and children are less susceptible to food allergies (Cunningham et al., 1991). During the past several decades, numerous studies have been published about the relationships between infant feeding and allergies (see Chapter 5). In the majority of these studies, the mode of feeding during the first few months of life affects the incidence of allergies and the risk of allergic disease in subsequent years. This association arises both from the protective effect of breastmilk and from the adverse effect of exposure to cow's milk (and to a lesser extent, other foods).

Nurses, especially those in pediatric settings, know that this advantage of breastfeeding is not to be taken lightly. The unhappy sequence of intolerance to formula starts when the infant becomes fussy and colicky and develops diarrhea. Next, the baby develops eczema while the parents and the physician frantically search for a formula he can tolerate. This experience is an unnecessary emotional and economic burden to the family and a health risk to the infant that may have lifelong consequences.

Food allergy is generally defined as an altered adverse reaction to a foreign substance or antibody accompanied by immunological changes, notably a rise in IgE. The most common offending foods that tend to produce allergic responses in Western cultures are cow's milk, peanuts (and foods derived from them, such as peanut butter), eggs, seafood, and egg whites (Table 20–3). Infants with food allergies are more likely to have families with atopic disease and mothers who were nauseated during pregnancy (Baylis et al., 1983). Food intolerance, on the other hand, is a broad term that includes any adverse response to food and is not limited to a rise in IgE. This term includes food sensitivity. Sensitivities include lactose intolerance, celiac disease, and any condition in which the infant cannot tolerate certain foods (McCarty & Frick, 1983).

The initial exposure is sensitization, which does not usually result in allergic symptoms. With a subsequent exposure, however, allergic symptoms become evident within days. This distinction helps to make it clear why a baby given a routine cow's-milk formula in the hospital may not experience a reaction until the next exposure several days or weeks later. If the mother is not informed of the supplement given in her absence when the baby was in the nursery, she may not recognize that the sensitizing event occurred there. This possibility points up why parents must always be asked for permission before any supplementation is given to their baby during hospitalization.

Cow's-milk allergy is the most common nutritional allergy during infancy. Some infants who are exclusively breastfed develop allergic symptoms following exposure to cow's milk because they have been sensitized to it transplacentally, or in the hospital, or through their mother's milk (Fukushima et al., 1997). Potentially immunogenic proteins in the maternal diet, including cow's milk–derived beta-lactoglobulin can be transferred into the milk and may induce allergic colitis in breastfeeding infants (Host et al., 1988; Odze et al., 1995).

In cow's-milk allergy, vomiting may be accompanied by chronic diarrhea, colic, colitis, excessive crying, a reluctance to feed, and poor sleep patterns. Eczema, urticaria (itching), a severe diaper rash, and excessive pallor may also be present. Individual infants may respond differently to allergenic foods: for instance, from the same food, one infant may develop diarrhea, colic, or GI problems; another may respond through his central nervous system and become irritable or hyperactive; and a third may have dermatological symptoms, such as urticaria or eczema.

The list of allergy symptoms is long: an allergic child may have rhinitis, otitis media, coughing, asthma, conjunctivitis, nausea, vomiting, anorexia, and frequent respiratory infections. Dark circles under the eyes ("allergic shiners") are a common indicator of allergy in the older child. Because foods belonging to the same botanical group have similar antigens, they can trigger a similar allergic response in the same child. Onions, for instance, along with garlic, leeks, and asparagus, all belong to the same botanical family; allergy to one may mean allergy to the others (Suitor & Hunter, 1980).

Allergies While Breastfeeding

A few completely breastfed infants receiving no other foods react to foods passed from the mother to the baby via her breastmilk. The main offender is cow's milk (Host et al., 1988; Jakobsson & Lindberg, 1978; Machtinger & Moss, 1986), and mild bleeding resulting from proctocolitis may be present (Anveden-Hertzberg et al., 1996). Other foods implicated in allergies to breastmilk are eggs (Matsumara et al., 1975), chocolate, fish, citrus (fruits), and peanuts (Cant et al., 1985; Chandra et

Table 20–3

TYPES OF FOODS COMMONLY ASSOCIATED WITH ALLERGIC REACTIONS

Food	Sources
Cow's milk in any form	Butter, bread, pudding, yogurt, cheese, baked goods, sherbet, ice cream, creamed soups, powdered-milk drinks, gravies
Eggs, especially egg whites	Cakes, cookies, custard, baked goods, pancakes, French toast, root beer, mayonnaise, breaded foods, some cake icing, meatloaf, noodles
Wheat	Baked goods, pasta, wieners, bologna, some canned soups, some pudding and gravies, some textured vegetable protein
Peanuts, legumes	Peanut butter, beans, peas, lentils, and foods containing soy protein, soy flour, or oil
Nuts and kola nuts	Candy, granola, baked goods, chocolate, cocoa, cola beverages
Fish or shellfish	Any fish or food fried in same oil as fish, cod liver oil, pizza with anchovies
Corn	Corn cereals, corn chips, Cracker Jacks, corn tortillas and other Mexican foods, popcorn, cornstarch, cornmeal
Citrus fruits	Orange, lemon, lime, grapefruit, fruit desserts, fruit punch
Tomatoes	Juice, meatloaf, stew or other mixed dishes, spaghetti, pizza, catsup
Spices	Cinnamon, catsup, chili, pepper, vinegar

al., 1986; Hattevig et al., 1989). Symptoms in the infants include eczema, diarrhea with foul-smelling stools, vomiting, colic (Host et al., 1988), excessive sleep, screaming (Sutin, 1988), and blood-streaked stools (Klein et al., 1990; Perisic et al., 1988; Wilson et al., 1990).

Eliminating foods from the mother's diet, especially cow's milk, usually solves the problem. If the elimination diet is to be of any value, however, it has to be carefully followed and clearly spelled out: written instructions are the most helpful, and scrupulous reading of labels on packaged foods helps to avoid inadvertent consumption of foods that should be eliminated. Especially if several foods are contributing to the baby's adverse reaction, the mother may find food-elimination plans difficult to implement (de Boissieu et al., 1997). It is necessary in some cases to remove all dairy foods.

The extent of this elimination is described by a mother whose son developed eczema while she was exclusively breastfeeding (Sutin, 1988):

I stopped drinking milk and expected instant miracles, but nothing changed. I cut cheese and yogurt out of my diet and still saw no improvement. Eventually, I had to eliminate all dairy products as well as products containing even trace amounts of milk. Then I could see the improvement.

If the mother removes dairy products from her diet, she must take sufficient calcium from other foods and from calcium supplements.

The most effective prevention of allergies in infants is exclusive breastfeeding for the first several months and gradual introduction of solid foods, one at a time, observing for any symptoms of allergy.

Kajosaari and Saarinen (1983) evaluated the prophylactic effect of six months' total solid food elimination in exclusively breastfed Finnish infants, as compared to infants similarly breastfed who started solid food at about three months of age. At one year, the children who had not received solids until six months of age had atopic eczema and food allergy less frequently than did the early solid groups.

Delaying solids for somewhat longer in infants who are highly allergic to a variety of foods is safe, provided the hemoglobin level is monitored at intervals. Usually, the hemoglobin remains within the normal range because of the efficient absorption of the iron in breastmilk; however, the mother must be prepared to breastfeed often to provide the necessary calories that otherwise would have been provided by solids.

Hypoglycemia

During the last trimester of pregnancy, the fetus builds up his supply of glycogen reserves. After birth, these reserves sustain the full-term infant during the birth process and for the first two or three days afterward. Symptoms of hypoglycemia (low blood glucose) are vague, such as tremors, jitteriness, lethargy, and a weak or high-pitched cry, and are similar to those caused by many other conditions. Severe, persistent hypoglycemia in infants, even after feedings have begun, may be caused by hyperinsulinism, thought to be a familial regulatory defect in beta-cell function (Worden et al., 1994).

According to Hawdon et al. (1993), full-term babies, especially those who are breastfed, are prone to low blood-glucose concentrations in the first two to three days after birth. However, full-term, healthy infants have the ability to generate ketone bodies, which are used as alternative fuels for the brain; thus there should be few occasions on which blood-glucose concentration need be measured. Furthermore, when optimal care is provided, in which mother and baby are roomed together and frequent suckling is encouraged, hypoglycemia occurs very infrequently, even when the definition of asymptomic hypoglycemia is < 40 mg/dl (Yamauchi, 1997). The situation is obviously different for preterm or small-for-gestational-age infants.

Infants considered at risk are screened for hypoglycemia within the first hour after birth with glucose oxidase reagent sticks, which are read after placing blood on the reagent strip or by a glucose reflectance meter. Monitoring blood-glucose values is difficult, because reagent sticks vary greatly and lack reproducibility, especially at levels of less than 50 mg/dl. Glucose reflectance meters are also reported to be unreliable in evaluating capillary blood-glucose concentrations in high-risk infants (Blackburn & Loper, 1992). Readings that indicate a blood-glucose level of less than 45 mg/dl should be confirmed by a laboratory analysis of whole blood.

In the full-term, healthy newborn, hypoglycemia is traditionally defined as a blood-glucose level below 30 mg/dl in the first day of life. Less than 40 mg/dl is the level used on the second day of life (Cornblath, 1976; Heck & Erenberg, 1987). Blood glucose reaches its lowest level between one and two hours after birth, and then it gradually rises. If the infant is not started on feedings until three hours of age, blood-glucose levels still rise and at three hours are significantly higher than one-hour values (Srinivasan et al., 1986).

The medical community is debating the definition of "normal" blood values of neonates. The definition of hypoglycemia used today was derived from early studies that examined whole-blood glucose levels of infant groups by birth weight and were adjusted upward to approximate plasma levels (10 to 15 percent higher). Since then, recognition of gestational age and the common administration of dextrose solution to the mother during labor and delivery has led some physicians to recommend that glucose levels should be maintained at above 40 mg/dl. The level of acceptable serum-glucose concentrations is being revised upward in some hospitals to between 40 and 45 mg/dl, with the result that breastfeeding neonates, who ingest only 25 to 30 percent of the amount of milk ingested by bottle-fed infants (Heck & Erenberg, 1987), are commonly diagnosed as hypoglycemic and given supplements. The use of intravenous dextrose in the mother also increases the incidence of neonatal hypoglycemia. If local obstetric practice requires dextrose to help to prevent maternal exhaustion, its rate of administration should be adjusted so as not to produce maternal hyperglycemia (Mehta, 1994).

Using the classic definition of hypoglycemia (below 30 percent) of Cornblath (1976), incidence rates have ranged from 4 percent (Gutberlet & Cornblath, 1976) to a high of 11.4 percent (Lubchenco & Bard, 1971). However, when the 40 mg/dl criterion is used, about 20 percent, or one-fifth of newborns, regardless of how they are fed, would be diagnosed as hypoglycemic (Sexson, 1984), which seems unreasonably high. In this same study, Sexson measured neonatal hypoglycemia in infants in a level-one nursery. Of the 232 babies, 168 (72 percent) had one or more so-called risk factors for hypoglycemia! This extraordinary incidence probably points to the nonspecific nature of many of the risk factors. Of those infants with a known risk factor, 52 percent did not have hypoglycemia, according to a definition based on a glucose value of less than 40 mg/dl. When neonates are exclusively breastfed on demand, their blood-glucose levels are not significantly different from those infants who receive both breast and formula feedings and those who are completely formula-fed (Wang et al., 1994).

Whether infants with glucose values between 30 and 40 mg/dl are at risk for problems to the same degree as are infants with lower glucose values is not known. In full-term Turkish babies with glucose levels of less than 30 mg/dl, only 9 percent required treatment (Tanzer et al., 1997). Kiovisto (1972), in a study of 66 cases of infants with asymptomatic hypoglycemia and 56 cases without hypoglycemia, found that there was no significant difference in the incidence of central nervous system sequelae. Clearly, using high glucose values as the definition of hypoglycemia for breastfed and formula-fed infants is questionable, particularly because formula and glucose supplements compromise breastfeeding. Weaning to formula can lead to allergies and many other health problems already discussed throughout this book.

Hypoglycemia can be prevented in most cases by putting the baby to breast early and often after delivery. If breastfeedings are poorly tolerated and low serum-glucose levels continue, intravenous glucose or formula (but not oral glucose water) should be given. In addition to its low caloric content, glucose water is stressful to the infant's pancreas and carries the risk of rebound hypoglycemic problems; thus it is a poor nutritional substitute.

Sudden Infant Death Syndrome

Approximately two of every 1,000 live-born infants die suddenly, usually in their sleep and without apparent cause. Put to bed without any indication that something was wrong, except perhaps a minor upper-respiratory infection, the child later is found lifeless. Most deaths from sudden infant death syndrom (SIDS), a major cause of infant death in the Western world, occur between 2 and 6 months of age, with a peak at about 10 weeks of age. The incidence is greater during winter months and in lower socioeconomic groups. SIDS is now diagnosed only for an infant who was previously healthy, and the diagnosis is not confirmed until autopsy. Autopsy finds that total closure of the upper airway seems to be the cause of death; findings include pulmonary congestion, lung hemorrhage, and respiratory inflammation.

In so-called near misses for SIDS, parents report finding the infant apneic, pale, or cyanotic and requiring vigorous stimulation or resuscitation. The infant may be placed on an apnea monitor, because a second apneic episode is not uncommon. It must be pointed out, however, that only a minority of SIDS victims have had documented life-threatening apnea; conversely, most infants with episodes of apnea do not die.

The majority of studies of breastfeeding and SIDS indicate that not breastfeeding is a risk factor for SIDS. It is intuitive to assume that breastfed infants are at lower risk for SIDS than are those not breastfed because of the differences in mothering styles and because of greater immunological protection (Bernshaw, 1991). However, several studies show no such no effect of breastfeeding on SIDS. Such inconsistent results stem from different ways of measuring the type of feedings and the degree to which confounding factors were taken into account (Fleming et al., 1996). Only the most careful studies that accounted for confounding factors are discussed here.

The National Institute of Child Health and Human Development SIDS Cooperative Epidemiological Study conducted in six U.S. cities during the late 1970s showed that only 9.8 percent of SIDS cases were mostly or only breastfed infants, compared to 27.7 percent and 22.3 percent, respectively, of the two nonbreastfed control groups.

The study provides evidence that fewer infants succumbing to SIDS received the benefit of the protective effect of breastfeeding (Hoffman et al., 1988).

Ford et al. (1993) in Canterbury, New Zealand, reported an adjusted odds ratio for SIDS associated with being fully bottle-fed at postnatal discharge from the hospital as 2.45; bottle-fed infants had significantly higher rates of SIDS than did those breastfed, a greater than twofold higher risk. This result led to the promotion of breastfeeding as part of a national cot death prevention program.

Gilbert et al. (1995) conducted a case-control study of British babies succumbing to SIDS in the late 1980s and early 1990s. Compared with being fully breastfed, the odds ratio for SIDS in fully bottle-fed babies was 3.1 and, for mixed breast- and bottle-fed infants, 1.5. After adjustments had been made for smoking, parental employment, preterm gestation, and sleeping position, these odds ratios fell to 1.8 and 1.2, respectively, which was not statistically significant. Sleeping position masked the effect of being bottle-fed on SIDS, because breast-fed babies were more likely than were bottle-fed babies to have slept prone. Although there was a trend for the risk of SIDS to increase with the amount of bottle-feeding, it was not a significant independent risk factor for SIDS in this study.

Also known as *crib death* or *cot death*, SIDS as a subject for research in the last decade has witnessed a resurgence. The major consistent finding has been the sleeping position of the infant (Guntheroth & Spiers, 1992; Irgens et al., 1995). The discovery that merely placing babies in a supine (on-back) position rather than in a prone (on-abdomen) position substantially reduces the frequency of SIDS has spawned public health education programs to inform parents around the world (Skadberg et al., 1998). In addition to breastfeeding and sleeping position, other risk factors include passive smoke inhalation (Klonoff-Cohen et al., 1995; Malloy et al., 1992), fulminating infection, laryngospasm, anaphylactic reaction to cow's milk protein (Coombs & McLaughlan, 1982), sleep disorders, apnea, and botulism (Arnon, 1986). To prevent SIDS, tools have been developed that identify the children at risk (Williams et al., 1995). Once identified, at-risk families are given additional supportive health services. The national SIDS prevention program in New Zealand, which emphasized breastfeeding as a protective factor, resulted in decline in SIDS from 4.2 per thousand in 1987 to 2.5 per thousand in 1991 (Davidson-Rada et al., 1995).

Worldwide, the incidence of SIDS varies considerably among regions. For example, although it is more frequent in Britain, New Zealand, and the United States, SIDS is rare in black Africans in Zimbabawe (Wolf & Ikeogu, 1996). These regional variations suggest environmental causation and the possibility that child-care practices, such as breastfeeding and mother-child sleeping arrangements, play a role in SIDS. Maternal co-sleeping and breastfeeding are covariates, in that breastfeeding women are more likely to co-sleep with their babies than are bottle-feeding mothers. Infants who co-sleep with their mothers breastfeed three times longer during the night than do the infants who sleep separately (McKenna et al., 1997). Because co-sleeping fosters closer monitoring of the infant, the question arises as to whether it is the co-sleeping pattern associated with breastfeeding or the breastfeeding itself that lowers the risk for SIDS. As an example, while sleeping in the same bed, mothers breastfeed their infant three times more frequently than they do with their infants sleeping in an adjacent room and their babies tend to sleep supine rather than prone. Co-sleeping also increases suckling episodes and encourages more light sleep when it is easier for infants to arouse, thus avoiding apnea (McKenna & Bernshaw, 1995; McKenna et al., 1994). Moreover, co-sleeping mothers continuously inspect, visually "check out," and adjust their baby's body position more often. Although McKenna et al. (1994) suggested that face-to-face orientation occurs often during co-sleeping, Gilbert et al. (1995) found that breastfeeding infants were more likely to be placed in the prone position. When this variable was controlled, breastfeeding itself still tended to prevent SIDS but not significantly so. It appears that although prone position, co-sleeping, and breastfeeding are interrelated, each is also an independent factor that can reduce the risk of SIDS.

Community-based health personnel specially trained to work with families who have lost a child through SIDS are an invaluable resource for helping parents. The breastfeeding mother, in addition to bearing her emotional anguish, has painful, engorged breasts, full of milk for the child who is no longer there. One of the many therapeutic actions at this critical time is helping her with physical relief of her engorgement. She should be taught to express as much milk as is necessary for comfort until milk production ceases. A slight fever during this period of milk production may be expected in some cases.

Health care personnel counseling the parents should make them aware that they could not have prevented the events from happening. Often, parents are overwhelmed with guilt; any comments that suggest shirked responsibility (e.g., "Did you check on your baby?") should be avoided. Pamphlets that have helpful information for parents are available from the National Foundation for Sudden Infant Death, Inc. In cases in which women who have lost a baby want to donate their milk to others, getting in touch with a milk bank (see Chapter 24) is an appropriate referral.

Hospitalization

Like any crisis, hospitalization can be a time for learning and growth. Ill children in the United States are now less likely to be hospitalized and, if they are, to return home quickly. Chances for a positive experience increase when the mother stays with her child, who finds security and comfort in breastfeeding. Helping has less to do with using specific techniques than with being sensitive to human beings.

The goal for the hospitalized infant or child is to minimize the discrepancy between self-care provided at home and the care given in the hospital setting. A secondary goal is to maintain and strengthen family unity. Thus, for the child who is breastfed, feeding and nurturing patterns should approximate as closely as possible the normal home situation (Fig. 20–4). Surgery, traction, diagnostic tests, and other therapeutic interventions may represent obstacles, but the goal is still the same.

Collection of both subjective and objective data occurs through interviewing and observation. Only by acquiring information can personalized and individualized care be given to families. One method for gaining a database of normal daily

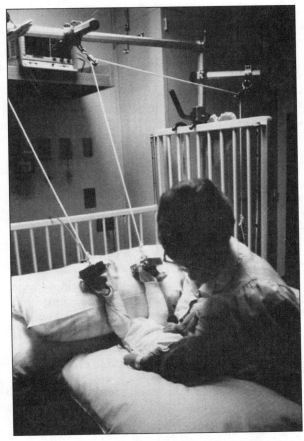

FIGURE 20–4. It is possible to breastfeed while the infant remains in traction.

living patterns before hospitalization is to have the mother or father complete a detailed questionnaire. If the child is breastfeeding, appropriate questions should be asked during the history taking:

- How often does the baby breastfeed at home?
- How do you usually feed him: are you sitting up or lying down?
- Does he take any solids or supplements?
- Is he accustomed to his own bed or does he come to bed with you for night feedings?
- What is his favorite word for breastfeeding?

If the breastfeeding child is old enough to talk, the family may use a "code" word for breastfeeding, such as *nummies, yum-yum, nursie, snugglies, night-night,* or *side.* A family who called breastfeeding *night-night* enjoyed the reaction of relatives and friends when the "good" little girl asked to "night-night" all by herself (Bumgarner, 1980). Keep these code words in mind the next time a breastfeeding toddler keeps demanding a "nursie"–he may not mean the nurse! Acceptance of the normalcy of a walking and talking child who breastfeeds is discussed in Chapter 2.

Parental Stresses

Driving to the hospital and back from their home 100 or more miles away, so as to alternate staying with their sick infant, a breastfeeding mother and her husband try to cope. With three other children at home, they can snatch only a few hours of sleep at a time. It is the third surgical procedure for their infant, who was born with a congenital defect. Although their physician encourages them with the news that the prognosis is good, the worry and strain seem endless. The mother expresses her milk with a pump when necessary, and her baby is able to breastfeed part of the time. Lately she has been able to express only a few drops at a time, and she wonders how long she will be able to continue lactating.

All parents of ill children are under stress, but consider the effects of stress on a parent who must deal with it over many months and perhaps years, such as the family described here. When it becomes apparent that the ill child may have to be hospitalized, one of the first concerns of the mother is whether she will be able to continue breastfeeding. She has already recognized the unique healing effect of putting an irritable, fussy child to breast when he is hurt or ill. Continuing to breastfeed, unless the child refuses, preserves a sense of normalcy in an otherwise highly stressful time. The mother needs reassurance that breastfeeding can continue and that assistance is available if breastfeeding must be temporarily interrupted. Many hospitals now have electric breast pumps available for the mother to use. When the child must undergo a surgical procedure or other intervention, particularly if it will be painful, encourage the mother to breastfeed as soon as possible afterward. It is difficult to say who benefits more, the mother or the baby, when the sobbing child settles into his tearful mother's lap for the comfort of her breast. What is readily apparent is the relief from stress for them

both. A careful explanation of the procedure beforehand will also relieve the mother's anxiety; this relief is in turn transmitted to the child. Parents can handle nearly any treatment if they know what it will be. Of all the nursing interventions, anticipatory guidance is one of the most effective.

What about the father? During the stress of the child's illness, attention is often focused on the mother and the ill child. Because the father's partner is breastfeeding, she will be the one spending most of the time at the bedside. While his child is in the hospital, the baby's father or the mother's partner is expected to be the Rock of Gibraltar, an anchor in a sea of distress. In addition to carrying on job responsibilities, he may also be responsible for keeping things running at home, nurturing and caring for the other children, and spending as much time as possible at the hospital. Fathers are people, too, and the stresses they feel are enormous.

These stresses affect the marriage bond. The divorce rate in families with a child born with a neural-tube defect was nine times greater than the divorce rate for the normal population (Tew et al., 1977). When a sick child becomes the focus of a mother's attention, other relationships and responsibilities become secondary. Some husbands, sensing this, withdraw emotionally until the crisis is over. Yet, for other couples, their mutual concern causes them to grow closer and draw emotional support from each other. Some parents feel guilty about making love while their child lies ill. If it seems appropriate, point out that sexual enjoyment reinforces their bond with each other, a bond that strengthens them during this difficult period.

The family's response to a chronic illness involves not so much the event itself as it does a particular family's definition or perception of the event, and the family's resources to help them to deal with the stress. A family with no health insurance and little or no savings perceives their child's chronic illness as more stressful than would a family with health insurance, sufficient income, and savings on which to draw if necessary.

Unreasonable as such feelings may be, both parents may harbor feelings of guilt for bringing on the illness or for not recognizing how sick the child was in early stages. Such questions as "What have I done?" or "What should I have done?" torment them. It is easier for the breastfeeding mother, who continues to have close contact with her child, to deal with these feelings than it is for the father. Picking up cues about his feelings and encouraging him to talk about them helps; it also provides the opportunity to reassure him that his feelings are normal. The therapeutic value of "talking it out" reduces stress (Foster, 1974). Hearing their own statements aloud releases the parents' tension and speeds resolution of their inner conflicts.

Hospitalization brings about a disruption of lifestyle and environment to the family and is tantamount to culture shock. A barrage of unfamiliar stimuli is thrust on them: infusion pumps that periodically sound an alarm, mist tents, and a constantly rotating staff of new faces all place tremendous stresses on the family. Normally affable parents can be demanding and even hostile when anger becomes a by-product of their stress and guilt. These defensive behaviors are part of the parents' coping strategies for managing their feelings. Defense mechanisms, such as denial and rationalization, help to protect families from painful realities and are not necessarily evidence of maladaptive behaviors. Although it can be difficult and even painful to deal with such parents, the author would far rather work with these concerned parents than with those who are unconcerned or passive. Sympathetic listening and simple, understanding statements, such as "I can see you are upset," or "This is such a difficult time," can help parents through this trying time. If hospital nurses rationally assess parents' behaviors and use of defenses, their interactions with parents will be more therapeutic.

The first response of parents whose children are diagnosed with a chronic illness is shock. This initial disorganization and upheaval does not last long, however. Some time after the diagnosis, the family begins to pull together their resources and develop a support system. Although for many parents their child's diagnosis is the worst problem they have ever faced, they are able to make many adjustments in a short period of time. The family gradually recovers and begins to cope.

Some parents, who are many miles from home during their child's hospitalization, must arrange for sleeping accommodations in the area if both are not allowed to stay overnight at the hospital.

Fortunately, many cities now have Ronald McDonald Houses that shelter these families. Support groups of other parents experiencing a similar life crisis are effective, because each person in the group understands the day-to-day issues and problems of caring for an ill child or rearing one with a chronic disease. Nevertheless, support groups are not for all parents; some are so overwhelmed by their own problems that they are not able to reach out and support others.

Coping with Siblings

Siblings are often the forgotten members of the family when attention and concern is focused on the sick child. In nursing, the concept of family-centered care extends to every person in the family, including the children at home, who frequently react to their brother's or sister's illness with anger, resentment, jealousy, and guilt. The situation is especially difficult when an older child is hospitalized and a younger breastfeeding baby or toddler is at home. The mother is emotionally torn between being with her sick child and attending her breastfeeding baby, who so obviously needs her. If the baby is one of breastfeeding twins or if the mother is breastfeeding both a walking child and a baby, the problem is further compounded. Most hospitals encourage siblings (who are not infectious) to visit their brother or sister in the hospital. Institutions that do not do so may add to the family's stress by enforcing isolation when contact would be most beneficial to all parties. When the ill child is at home, siblings may bear additional responsibilities of child care or helping with household tasks.

Emergency Admission

Staff nursing in emergency situations takes split-second reactions and demands a thorough background of a wide range of nursing knowledge. No single nurse, of course, can be expected to know everything. In addition, patients come and go quickly; they are transferred to other units of the hospital or dismissed without being seen again.

Unless the nurse has had personal experience with a breastfeeding infant or child, she is unlikely to be sensitive to the needs of the family with a breastfeeding child. An example is a situation in which the mother, not the child, became very ill. She overheard the harried nurse say, "If she had given that baby a bottle, we wouldn't be in this mess," when the infant first refused and later vomited bottle-feedings. Because emergencies distort perceptions and magnify emotions, criticism is not always a fair analysis of the situation. This example can serve as a lesson. The registered nurse reacted defensively to a life need. The parents may then have mistrusted that their medical needs would be handled well. How do we avoid insensitivity in care when we are faced with a situation beyond our experience or understanding? Attempt to look at the family's needs through the eyes of each family member and actively seek to support their wishes when an emergency threatens the symbiosis of the breastfeeding relationship.

Home: The Rebound Effect

The child's reactions following hospitalization depend on the extent of trauma he has undergone and his defenses for protecting himself. Almost all hospitals now encourage a parent to stay with the child during hospitalization. Fagin (1966) clearly shows that when parents room-in with the child, very few behavior changes occur on returning home. If the young child has experienced a painful separation, he may at first refuse the breast and show little interest in his mother or family, using withdrawal as a means of coping. He may cry a great deal and want to be held and breastfed exceptionally often, vigorously protesting having his mother out of sight for even a moment. Emotional upheaval, including nightmares and insomnia, is common in the first few weeks following hospitalization.

Short separations during hospitalizations are usually inevitable; however, if a child feels safe and secure in his parent's love, trauma from the illness and temporary separations give way to restoration of trust after being reunited with his family. Helping parents to recognize this is vital to nursing care of the hospitalized child. Inherent in any crisis is the potential for bringing family members closer together with new awareness and appreciation of one another.

Chronic Grief and Loss

When the breastfeeding child is chronically ill or has a disabling defect, the disappointment, sorrow,

and frustration of parents can be overwhelming. Instead of the perfect child expected during the pregnancy, there is an intense feeling of loss. If the child requires indefinite special care and attention, there is a persistent effect described by Olshansky (1962) as *chronic sorrow*. Unlike acute grief, which is limited in time, chronic sorrow is prolonged and recurrent. Through grieving, coping processes evolve, and parents can find satisfaction and even joy from their child: "The shock and numbness linger for days, even months. . . . It is only after you have gotten over that first crisis that you begin to realize a life and soul have been given into your care" (Good, 1980). The onset of chronic sorrow is variable among families and sometimes difficult to identify; however, this condition is a natural outgrowth of parenting and is an adaptive response (Lemons & Weaver, 1986).

Breastfeeding has an ameliorating effect on both the child and the parents when chronic illness is involved. The baby receives added protection from his higher risk of infection and also benefits from close contact and stimulation. Engendered in the parents, especially the mother, is the satisfaction of giving something special to her child, which helps her deal with her feelings of loss. As one mother (Good, 1980) of a baby with Down syndrome said: "As I looked back at Chad's first year, I'm sure that breastfeeding and the closeness that comes with it helped me to love and accept him just as he was. There were still lots of tears sometimes falling on my special baby as we rocked along and I had many anxieties about the future."

The Magic-Milk Syndrome

In the process of grieving, parents move through several stages of adjustment. After the initial shock and emotional numbness, they reach a stage characterized by rationalization, denial, and sometimes a search for a magic cure. If the baby is not being breastfed, a few frightened parents will desperately search for donated breastmilk, hoping that it will cure their child. The unique properties of breastmilk are so well known that it is sometimes perceived by parents to contain magic properties. The health care provider needs to validate the value of human milk while helping the parents to recognize that their baby may need more than breastmilk can offer.

In some cases, breastmilk can help. For example, children with allergies and metabolic disorders may respond well to breastmilk feedings (see Chapter 24). In these situations in which the need is real and substantiated by medical opinion, the child should receive breastmilk from a milk bank if at all possible.

The Empty Cradle

The tremendous task of coping and somehow continuing with life must be faced by parents when their child dies. The first reactions of shock, disbelief, and denial are all the more intense when the death is unexpected, as with SIDS. Parents need to be able to express their feelings by crying, yelling, or quietly talking about how they feel.

Compassionate care assists closure after death. Giving the parents the opportunity to hold their child and to say good-bye helps this process. Afraid at first, one family's members changed their minds and cradled their dead baby in their arms. "Holding him is what helped us most to accept the death of our baby; it made us feel he was really our own. He smelled sweet and felt soft, and we just stroked him and talked with him for a while."

Fathers and mothers grieve differently and have their own ways of coping with grief (Wallerstedt & Higgins, 1996). These differences are called *incongruent grief* and result from societal expectations based on gender; whereas the father may not grieve openly, the mother may be more emotional (Klaus & Kennell, 1982). Moreover, the focus of concern often falls on the mother. The father, who has had a significant, loving relationship with his child, is sometimes forgotten. The cultural stereotype of male stoicism belies his feelings of shock, grief, and pain. Fathers also need to grieve, but their reponse is affected by his responsibilities, such as informing family and friends of the child's death and making funeral arrangements.

As the shock subsides, acute mourning and bereavement are followed by a developing awareness of the full impact of their loss. Parents may feel less than whole, that they have lost a part of themselves. Guilt, silent or expressed, is an almost universal emotion during this period, and the parents often examine their past misdeeds. Questioning the health professional about the possible effects of heredity on the disease is likely as their grief turns inward in the form of self-blame. Explanations of hereditary factors must be honest and factual, tempered with an understanding of what the parents are able to accept.

Physical symptoms, such as sleeplessness or a lack of appetite, often accompany the parents' feelings of loss and pain. Some parents describe feeling "dead inside" or having a "hole inside that nothing can fill." The breastfeeding mother may have to cope with the physical discomfort of breast fullness and leaking for a while and should be advised to express her milk for relief. Occasionally, a mother will continue to pump her milk for several weeks, donating it to a milk bank so that other children may benefit from it. Doing so is her way of coping by maintaining visible evidence of the existence of the lost child. When she offers to do so, the best approach is to put her in touch with a milk bank whose staff members can assist her.

Clinical Implications

Families differ in their response to the birth of a child with a defect or a chronic illness, and they will need support from health care professionals to help them to adjust. Therefore, it is important for the professional to have a working knowledge of grief and crisis theories and the skills to implement them. Although it is not within the scope of this chapter to review all such theories, the nurse or lactation consultant who works with these families will find additional education and study on parental grief helpful. Box 20–4 offers basic care for any breastfeeding child who is ill. Because they are general, these hints may not be applicable to all situations.

When an infant dies, memories that tie the mother to the child must be relived before they can be put aside. Especially important to her is the acknowledgment that her child was special: she should never be denied the right to her sorrow. Remarks such as "It just wasn't meant to be" or "You can always have another baby" are hurtful. They provide no consolation whatsoever regarding her loss of this baby. Statements such as "I'm sorry about your baby" or "If you want to talk, call me" are consoling and show sensitivity. The following suggestions for health care providers who are assisting parents and families through the grief

BOX 20–4

Guidelines for Assisting a Mother in Caring for an Ill Breastfeeding Infant

1. Encourage the mother to breastfeed the baby held in an upright position (generally speaking), because this position facilitates swallowing that may be impaired. Additionally, the mother is able to closely observe her baby during the feeding.

2. Teach the mother alternative feeding methods, such as using a tube-feeding device, small cup, or medicine dropper to supplement with breastmilk. Help her to express her milk, if necessary.

3. Minimize the child's separation from the family. Infants and children should be cared for in their home with the care provider's assistance and monitoring of the family's capabilities.

4. Help the family to mobilize and supplement their resources. Provide them with some of the excellent books available for parents of children with special needs. Refer them to appropriate specialized health professionals and parent support groups.

5. Remind the mother that breastfeeding is less (not more) strenuous than bottle-feeding.

6. Accentuate the child's positive attributes and strengths by making such comments as "What a beautiful child" or "He's so strong!"

7. Praise any progress in breastfeeding, no matter how small.

8. Read the mother's cues that tell you if she wants to continue to lactate or breastfeed. Give permission and assistance to wean if this is her choice.

9. Maintain the family's hope that tomorrow will be better.

process are based on the author's experiences as well as those of other health care professionals:

1. Call the baby by his name. Having a baby is such a joyful experience, and some of that joy is still there, even though the baby might have been stillborn or died shortly after birth.

2. Acknowledge the parent's loss by sending cards or calling. If you do not know the parents well, anything more may be too much.

3. Feel your way through the conversation, getting feedback from the parent; wait for him or her to lead the way. Ensure that they know you are available to talk whenever needed.

4. If the mother was lactating, help her to remain comfortable. Mothers who lose a baby after 20 weeks of gestation may become engorged, which sometimes comes as a complete shock. Often, women are reluctant to relieve their discomfort by expressing milk for fear of stimulating more milk; encourage the mother to express some milk for comfort. Rarely will the discomfort last long.

5. Help the parents to verbalize feelings of anger, fear, guilt, and anxiety by validating them.

For many parents, the peer support system that previously helped them in parenting and breastfeeding changes in significance; seeing other breast-feeding mothers and their babies may be a painful ordeal. The mother may assiduously avoid them, choosing only one or two especially close peers with whom she can privately talk about her feelings and emotional pain. One of the community support systems available for parents during this difficult period is Aiding Mothers Experiencing Neonatal Death. This group has trained counselors to individually help parents work through their grief.

SUMMARY

There are unique considerations for helping the breastfeeding mother and her family when her infant or young child is ill. These special needs can be met by recognizing the developmental stage, assessing family lifestyle, reducing parental stress, involving the parents in direct care of their child, and most of all, minimizing separation between family members. Discontinuing breastfeeding is rarely necessary for the child with a health problem, although feeding patterns may have to be modified. Too often, however, weaning from the breast is assumed to be necessary. It is not; once the infant is weaned, a new cycle of health problems, especially allergies, can appear.

Each family is unique. The experience of one situation can never be duplicated: therefore, care providers helping families with an ill breastfeeding child must use versatility and a firm knowledge of the nature of the health problem. Just as important is recognition of the psychological needs of the breastfeeding child and his family, especially the mother.

Interventions also require awareness of devices that aid lactation and how they can be obtained (see Chapter 13). Support must come from the health care team, not just from one or two of its members; therefore, communication among the staff is essential for continuity of care. Ideally, one individual serves as the case manager and coordinates the entire spectrum of the health care in all its settings, whether in the hospital or out in the community. As needs arise, the nurse not only gives customary hands-on care but acts as a family advocate and broker of additional services (Rogers et al., 1991). This health care worker also informs the parents about every aspect of the health problem and includes them in decision making, creating mutual respect and a working relationship between health care workers and the family.

If the child dies, comprehending the impact of the parents' grief and their stage of adaptive coping requires special sensitivity and crisis-intervention skills to help the bereaved parents in their journey through pain toward an adaptive resolution of their loss, which comes only after a long, slow process of working through their grief. As preoccupation with memories lessens, they are able to establish new interests and to develop new goals. "Time heals all wounds" is true in the sense that healing occurs with time, but the emotional scars and the times of feeling empty and lonely will endure as long as they live. Grieving occurs more normally when the mother feels she has attached to her infant and given all that she can to him while he was alive, including breastfeeding or human milk feeding (Coates & Riordan, 1992).

REFERENCES

Alho OP, et al: Control of the temporal aspect when considering risk factors for acute otitis media. *Arch Otolaryngol Head Neck Surg* 119:444–49, 1993.

Aniansson B, et al: Prospective cohort study on breast-feeding and otitis media in Swedish infants. *Pediatr Infect Dis J* 13:183–8, 1994.

Anveden-Hertzberg L, et al: Proctocolitis in exclusively breast-fed infants. *Eur J Pediatr* 155:464–7, 1996.

Arnon SS: Infant botulism: anticipating the second decade. *J Infect Dis* 154:201–6, 1986.

Aumonier ME, Cunningham CC: Breastfeeding in infants with Down's syndrome. *Child Care Health Dev* 9:247–55, 1983.

Auricchio S, et al: Does breast-feeding protect against the development of clinical symptoms of celiac disease in children? *J Pediatr Gastroenterol Nutr* 2:428–33, 1983.

Bayliss JM, Leeds AR, Challacombe DN: Persistent nausea and food aversions in pregnancy. *Clin Allergy* 13:263–9, 1983.

Beaudry M, Dufour R, Marcoux S: Relation between infant feeding and infections during the first six months of life. *J Pediatr* 126:191–7, 1995.

Bernshaw NJ: Does breastfeeding protect against sudden infant death syndrome? *J Hum Lact* 7:73–9, 1991.

Blackburn ST, Loper DL: *Maternal, fetal and neonatal physiology.* Philadelphia: Saunders, 1992.

Brown KH: Dietary management of acute childhood diarrhea: optimal timing of feeding and appropriate use of milks and mixed diets. *J Pediatr* 118:S92–8, 1991.

Bumgarner NJ: *Mothering your nursing toddler.* Franklin Park, IL: La Leche League International, 1980.

Cant AJ, Marsden RA, Kilshaw PJ: Egg and cow's milk hypersensitivity in exclusively breastfed infants with eczema, and the detection of egg protein in breastmilk. *Br Med J* 291:932–5, 1985.

Cavell B: Gastric emptying in infants fed human milk or infant formula. *Acta Paediatr Scand* 70:639–41, 1981.

Chandra RK, et al: Influence of maternal food antigen avoidance during pregnancy and lactation on incidence of atopic eczema in infants. *Clin Allergy* 16:563–9, 1986.

Chen Y: Relationship between type of feeding and hospitalization for gastroenteritis in Shanghai infants. *J Hum Lact* 10:177–9, 1994.

Chen Y, Yu S, Li W: Artificial feeding and hospitalization in the first 18 months of life. *Pediatrics* 81:58–62, 1988.

Clemens J, et al: Breast-feeding and the risk of life-threatening rotavirus diarrhea: prevention or postponement? *Pediatrics* 92:680–5, 1993.

Coates MM, Riordan J: Breastfeeding during maternal or infant illness. *Clin Iss Perin Wom Health Nurs* 3:683–94, 1992.

Cochi SL, et al: Primary invasive *Hemophilus influenzae* type b disease: a population-based assessment of risk factors. *J Pediatr* 108:887–96, 1986.

Colombo JL, Hopkins RL, Waring WW: Steam vaporizer injuries. *Pediatrics* 67:661–3, 1981.

Combs VL, Marino BL: A comparison of growth patterns in breast and bottle-fed infants with congenital heart disease. *Pediatr Nurs* 19:175–9, 1993.

Coombs RRA, McLaughlan P: The enigma of cot death: Is the modified-anaphylaxis hypothesis an explanation for some cases? *Lancet* 1:1388–9, 1982.

Cornblath M: Diagnosing and treating neonatal hypoglycemia, *Contemp Obstet Gynecol* 8:95, 1976.

Crawford M, et al: Effects of duration of fasting on gastric fluid pH and volume in healthy children. *Anesth Analg* 71:400–3, 1990.

Cunningham AS, Jelliffe BD, Jelliffe EF: Breast-feeding and health in the 1980s: a global epidemiologic review. *J Pediatr* 118:659–6, 1991.

Danner SC: Breastfeeding the infant with a cleft defect. *Clin Iss Perin Wom Health Nurs* 3:634–9, 1992.

Danner SC: Breastfeeding the neurologically impaired infant. *Clin Iss Perin Wom Health Nurs* 3:640–6, 1992.

Danner SC, Cerutti ER: *Nursing your baby with Down's syndrome.* Rochester, NY: Childbirth Graphics, 1989.

Davidson-Rada J, Caldis S, Tonkin SL: New Zealand's SIDS prevention program and reduction in infant mortality. *Health Educ Q* 22:162–71, 1995.

de Boissieu D, et al: Multiple food allergy: a possible diagnosis in breastfed infants. *Acta Paediatr* 86:1042–6, 1997.

Delange F, et al: Topical iodine, breastfeeding, and neonatal hypothyroidism. *Arch Dis Child* 63:106–7, 1988.

Dewey KG, Heinig MJ, Nommsen-Rivers LA: Differences in morbidity between breast-fed and formula-fed infants. *J Pediatr* 126:696–702, 1995.

diSant'Agnese PA, Hubbard VS: The pancreas. In: Taussig LM, ed. *Cystic fibrosis.* New York: Thieme-Stratton, 1984; 278–9.

Dodge JA: The nutritional state and nutrition. *Acta Paediatr Scand* 317 Suppl:31–7, 1985.

Duncan LL, Elder SB: Breastfeeding the infant with PKU. *J Hum Lact* 13:231–5, 1997.

Duncan J, et al: Exclusive breast-feeding for at least 4 months protects against otitis media. *Pediatrics* 91:867–72, 1993.

Fadavi S, et al: Mechanics and energetics of nutritive suckling: a functional comparison of commercially available nipples. *J Pediatr* 130:740–5 1997.

Fagin C: *The effects of maternal attendance during hospitalization on the post hospital behavior of young children.* Philadelphia: Davis, 1966.

Fallot ME, Boyd JL, Oski FA: Breast-feeding reduces incidence of hospital admissions for infection in infants. *Pediatrics* 65:1121–4, 1980.

Fleming PJ, et al: Environment of infants during sleep and risk of the sudden infant death syndrome: results of the 1993–5 case-control study for confidential inquiry into stillbirths and deaths in infancy. *Br Med J* 313(7051)191–5, 1996.

Forbes GB, et al: Composition of milk produced by a mother with galactosemia. *J Pediatr* 113:90–1, 1988.

Ford RPK, et al: Breastfeeding and the risk of sudden infant death syndrome. *Int J Epidemiol* 22:885–90, 1993.

Foster SB: An adrenal measure for evaluating nursing effectiveness. *Nurs Res* 23:118, 1974.

Franklin R, O'Grady C, Carpenter L: Neonatal thyroid function: comparison between breast-fed and bottle-fed infants. *J Pediatr* 106:124–6, 1985.

Fukushima Y, et al: Consumption of cow milk and egg by lactating women and the presence of beta-lactoglobulin and ovalbumin in breast milk. *Am J Clin Nutr* 65:30–5, 1997.

Gilbert RE, et al: Bottle feeding and the sudden infant death syndrome. *Br Med J* 310:88–90, 1995.

Good J: *Breastfeeding the Down's syndrome baby.* Franklin Park, IL: La Leche League International. 1980.

Grady E: Breastfeeding the baby with a cleft of the soft palate. *Clin Pediatr* 16:978–81, 1977.

Greco L, et al: Case-control study on nutritional risk factors in celiac disease. *J Pediatr Gastroenterol Nutr* 7:395–9, 1988.

Green S, Rothrock S: Single-dose intramuscular ceftriaxone for acute otitis media in children. *Pediatrics* 91:23–39, 1993.

Greve L, et al: Breast-feeding in the management of the newborn with phenlketonuria: a practical approach to dietary therapy. *J Am Diet Assoc* 94:305–9, 1994.

Guntheroth WG, Spiers PS: Sleeping prone and the risk of sudden infant death syndrome. *JAMA* 267:2359–62, 1992.

Gutberlet RL, Cornblath M: Neonatal hypoglycemia revisited 1975. *Pediatrics* 58:10–17, 1976.

Habbick BF: Infantile hypertrophic pyloric stenosis: a study of feeding practices and other possible causes. *Clin Commun Stud* 140:401–4, 1989.

Haffejee IE: Cow's milk–based formula, human milk, and soya feeds in acute infantile diarrhea: a therapeutic trial. *J Pediatr Gastroenterol Nutr* 10: 193–8, 1990.

Hahn HB, et al: Breastfeeding and neonatal screening for congenital hypothyroidism. *Tex Med* 82:46–7, 1986.

Harabuchi Y, et al: Human milk secretory IgA antibody to nontypeable *Haemophilus influenzae:* possible protective effects against nasopharyngeal colonization. *J Pediatr* 124:193–8, 1994.

Hattevig G, et al: Effect of maternal avoidance of eggs, cow's milk and fish during lactation upon allergic manifestations in infants. *Clin Exp Allergy* 19:27–32, 1989.

Hawdon JM, Platt MPW, Aynsley-Green A: Neonatal hypoglycaemia-blood glucose monitoring and baby feeding. *Midwifery* 9:3–6, 1993.

Heacock HJ, et al: Influence of breast versus formula milk on physiological gastroesophageal reflux in healthy, newborn infants. *J Pediatr Gastroenterol Nutr* 14:41–6, 1992.

Heck LJ, Erenberg A: Serum glucose levels in term neonates during the first 48 hours of life. *J Pediatr* 110:119–22, 1987.

Hoffman HJ, et al: Risk factors for SIDS: results of the National Institute of Child Health and Human Development SIDS cooperative epidemiological study. In: Schwarz PJ, Sauhall DP, Valdes-Dapnea M, ed. *The sudden infant death syndrome.* New York: New York Academy of Sciences, 1988.

Holberg KJ, et al: Risk factors for respiratory syncytial virus-associated lower respiratory illnesses in the first year of life. *Am J Epidemiol* 133:1135–51, 1991.

Holliday KE, et al: Growth of human milk-fed and formula-fed infants with cystic fibrosis. *J Pediatr* 118:77–9, 1991.

Horta BL, et al: Environmental tobacco smoke and breastfeeding duration. *Am J Epidemiol* 146:128–33, 1997.

Host A, Husby S, Osterballe O: A prospective study of cow's milk allergy in exclusively breast-fed infants. *Acta Paediatr Scand* 77:663–70, 1988.

Howie PW, et al: Protective effect of breastfeeding against infection. *Br Med J* 300:11–16, 1990.

Huffman SL, Combest C: Role of breast-feeding in the prevention and treatment of diarrhea. *J Diar Dis Res* 8:68–81, 1990.

Husband J, Husband, P: Gastric emptying of water and glucose solutions in the newborn. *Lancet* 2:409–11, 1969.

Irgens LM, et al: Sleeping position and sudden infant death syndrome in Norway 1967–91. *Arch Dis Child* 72:478–82, 1995.

Istre GR, et al: Risk factors for primary *Hemophilus influenzae* disease: increased risk from day care attendance and school-aged household members. *J Pediatr* 106:190–5, 1985.

Jackson PL, Vessey KJ: *Child with a chronic condition* (2nd ed). St Louis: Mosby, 1996.

Jakobsson I, Lindberg T: Cow's milk as a cause of infantile colic in breast fed infants. *Lancet* 2:437–9, 1978.

Jenkins GN: *The physiology and biochemistry of the mouth* (4th ed). London: Blackwell, 1978.

Kajosaari M., Saarinen UM: Prophylaxis of atopic disease by six months' total solid food elimination. *Acta Paediatr Scand* 72:411–14, 1983.

Kelly DW, et al: Rise and fall of coeliac disease 1960–1985. *Arch Dis Child* 64:1157–60, 1989.

Kiovisto M, et al: Neonatal symptomatic and asymptomatic hypoglycemia: a follow-up study of 151 children. *Dev Med Child Neurol* 14:603–14, 1972.

Klaus M, Kennell J: *Parent infant bonding.* St Louis: Mosby, 1982.

Klein E, Shvartzman P, Weizman Z: Blood-streaked stools in two breast-fed siblings. *J Fam Pract* 30:713–14, 1990.

Klonoff-Cohen HS, et al: The effect of passive smoking and tobacco exposure through breast milk on sudden infant death syndrome. *JAMA* 273: 795–8, 1995.

Kogo J, et al: Breast feeding for cleft lip and palate patients, using the Hotz-type plate. *Cleft-Palate Craniofac J* 34:351–3, 1997.

Kramer M: Infant feeding, infection and public health. *Pediatrics* 81:164–6, 1988.

Ledonne C: Hospital and home care of the infant with congenital bilateral choanal atresia. *JOGNN* 15:244–8, 1986.

Lemons P, Weaver DD: Beyond the birth of a defective child. *Neon Netw* 5:13–19, 1986.

Leventhal JM, et al: Does breastfeeding protect against infection in infants less than 3 months of age? *Pediatrics* 78:896–903, 1986.

Littman RS, Wu CL, Quinlivan JK: Gastric volume and pH in infants fed clear liquids and breastmilk prior to surgery. *Anesth Analg* 79:482–5, 1994.

Lopez-Alarcon J, Villapando S, Fajardo A: Breast-feeding lowers the frequency and duration of acute respiratory infection and diarrhea in infants under six months of age. *J Nutr* 127:436–43, 1997.

Lubchenco L, Bard H: Incidence of hypoglycemia in newborn infants classified by birth weight and gestational age. *Pediatrics* 47:831–8, 1971.

Luder E, et al: Current recommendations for breast-feeding in cystic fibrosis centers. *Am J Dis Child* 144:1153–6, 1990.

Malloy M, Hoffman H, Peterson, D: Sudden infant death syndrome and maternal smoking. *Am J Public Health* 82:1380–2, 1992.

Machtinger S, Moss R: Cow's milk allergy in breast-fed infants: the role of allergen and maternal secretory IgA antibody. *J Allergy Clin Immunol* 77:341–7, 1986.

Matsumara T, et al: Egg sensitivity and eczematous manifestations in breast-fed newborns with particular reference to intrauterine sensitization. *Ann Allergy* 35:221–9, 1975.

McBride MC, Danner SC: Sucking disorders in neurologically impaired infants. *Clin Perinatol* 14:109–30, 1987.

McCabe L, et al: The management of breastfeeding among infants with phenylketonuria. *J Inherit Metal Dis* 12:467–74, 1989.

McCarty EP, Frick OL: Food sensitivity: keys to diagnosis. *J Pediatr* 102:645–52, 1983.

McKenna J, Bernshaw NJ: In: Stuart-Macadam P, Dettwyler KA, eds. *Breastfeeding: Biocultural perspectives*. New York: Aldine De Gruyter, 1995.

McKenna J, et al: Experimental studies on infant-parent co-sleeping; mutual physiological and behavioral influences and their relevance to SIDS (sudden infant dealth syndrome). *Early Hum Dev* 38:187–201, 1994.

McKenna JJ, Mosko SS, Richard CA: Bedsharing promotes breastfeeding. *Pediatrics* 100:214–19, 1997.

Mehta A: Prevention and management of neonatal hypoglycaemia. *Arch Dis Child* 70:F54–F65, 1994.

Meremikwu MM, Asiudi AA, Antia-Obong OE: The influence of breast feeding on the occurrence of dysentery, persistent diarrhoea, and malnutrition among Nigerian children with diarrhoea. *West Afr J Med* 16:20–3, 1997.

Miller SA, Chopra, JG: Problems with human milk and infant formulas. *Pediatrics* 74(suppl): 639–47, 1984.

Misulta H, et al: Thyroid hormones in human milk and their influence on thyroid function of breast-fed babies. *Pediatr Res* 17:468, 1983.

Mohrbacher N, Stock J: *The breastfeeding answer book* (rev ed). Schaumburg, IL: La Leche League International, 1997.

Nafstad P, et al: Breastfeeding, maternal smoking and lower respiratory tract infection. *Eur Respir J* 12:2623–9, 1996.

Nafstad P, et al: Weight gain during the first year in relation to maternal smoking and breast feeding in Norway. *J Epidemiol Commun Health* 51:261–5, 1997.

Nicholson SC, Schreiner MS: Feed the babies. *Breastfeed Abstr* 15:3–4, 1995.

Odze R, et al: Allergic colitis in infants. *J Pediatr* 126:163–70, 1995.

O'Hare B, et al: Acute lung injury after instillation of human breast milk or infant formula into rabbits' lungs. *Anesthesiology* 84:1386–91, 1996.

Olshansky S: Chronic sorrow: a response to having a mentally defective child. *Soc Casework* 43:190–3, 1962.

Paradise JL, et al: Evidence in infants with cleft palate that breast milk protects against otitis media. *Pediatrics* 94:853–60, 1994.

Perisic VN, Fillpovic D, Kokai G: Allergic colitis with rectal bleeding in an exclusively breast-fed neonate. *Acta Paediatr Scand* 77:163–4, 1988.

Popkin BM, et al: Breast-feeding and diarrheal morbidity. *Pediatrics* 86:874–82, 1990.

Pullan CR, et al: Breastfeeding and respiratory syncytial virus infection. *Br Med J* 281:1034–6, 1980.

Riva E, et al: Early breastfeeding is linked to higher intelligence quotient scores in dietary treated phenylketonuric children. *Acta Paediatr* 85:56–8, 1996.

Rogers M, Riordan J, Swindle D: Community-based nursing case management pays off. *Nurs Man* 22:30–4, 1991.

Rooney K: Breastfeeding a baby with cystic fibrosis. *New Beginnings* 4:43–4, 1988.

Ross CA, Sammons HG: Non-pancreatic lipase in children with pancreatic fibrosis. *Arch Dis Child* 30:428–31, 1955.

Rovet JF: Does breast-feeding protect the hypothroid infant whose condition is diagnosed by newborn screening? *Am J Dis Child* 144:319–23, 1990.

Ruuska T, Vesilkari T: A prospective study of acute diarrhoea in Finnish children from birth to 2-1/2 years of age. *Acta Paediatr Scand* 80:500–7, 1991.

Ruuska T: Occurrence of acute diarrhea in atopic and nonatopic infants: the role of prolonged breastfeeding. *J Pediatr Gastroenterol Nutr* 14:27–33, 1992.

Saarinen UM: Prolonged breastfeeding as a prophylaxis for recurrent otitis media. *Acta Paediatr Scand* 71:567–71, 1982.

Sachdev HPS, et al: Does breastfeeding influence mortality in children hospitalized with diarrhoea? *J Trop Pediatr* 37:275–9, 1991.

Sassen ML, Brand R, Grote JJ: Breast-feeding and acute otitis media. *Am J Otolaryngol* 15:351–7, 1994.

Scariati PD, Brummer-Strawn LM, Fein SB: A longitudinal analysis of infant morbidity and the extent of breastfeeding in the United States. *Pediatrics* 99:e5, 1997.

Schaefer O: Otitis media and bottle-feeding: an epidemiological study of infant feeding habits and incidence of recurrent and chronic middle ear disease in Canadian Eskimos. *Can J Public Health* 62:478–89, 1971.

Schreiner MS, Triebwasser A, Keon TP: Ingestion of liquids compared with preoperative fasting in pediatric outpatients. *Anesthesiology* 72:593–7, 1990.

Sexson WR: Incidence of neonatal hypoglycemia: a matter of definition. *J Pediatr* 105:149–50, 1984.

Shah N, et al: Risk factors for severe pneumonia in children in south Kerala: a hospital-based case-control study. *J Trop Pediatr* 40:201–6, 1994.

Silfverdal SA, et al: Protective effect of breastfeeding on invasive *Haemophilus influenzae:* a case-control study in Swedish preschool children. *Int J Epidemiol* 26:443–50, 1997.

Skadberg BT, Morild I, Markestad T: Abandoning prone sleeping: effect on the risk of sudden infant death syndrome. *J Pediatr* 132:340–3, 1998.

Slade HB, Schwarz, SA: Mucosal immunity: the immunology of breast milk. *J Allergy Clin Immunol* 80:348–58, 1987.

Srinivasan G, et al: Plasma glucose values in normal neonates: a new look. *J Pediatr* 109:114–17, 1986.

Straughn A, English B: Oral rehydration therapy. *MCN* 21:144–7, 1996.

Suitor CW, Hunter MF: *Nutrition: principles and practice.* Philadelphia: Lippincott, 1980.

Sutin R: Eliminating foods worked wonders. *New Beginnings* 4:145, 1988.

Taddio A, et al: Effect of counseling on maternal reporting of adverse effects in nursing infants exposed to antibiotics through breastmilk. *Reprod Toxicol* 9:153–7, 1995.

Tanzer F, et al: Blood glucose levels and hypoglycaemia in full term neonates during the first 48 hours of life. *J Trop Pediatr* 43:58–60, 1997.

Teele DW, Klein JO, Rosner B: Epidemiology of otitis media during the first seven years of life in children in greater Boston: a prospective cohort study. *J Infect Dis* 160:83–94, 1989.

Tew BJ, et al: Marital stability following the birth of a child with spina bifida. *Br J Psychiatry* 131:79–82, 1977.

Tomomasa T, et al: Gastrointestinal motility in neonates: response to human milk compared with cow's milk formula. *Pediatrics* 80:434–8, 1987.

Trenouth MJ, Campbell AN: Questionnaire evaluation of feeding methods for cleft lip and palate neonates. *Int J Paediatr Dent* 6:241–4, 1996.

Tully Bar-Haim SB, Bar-Haim Y, Bradley RL: Abnormal tympanography after supine bottle feeding. *J Pediatr* 126:S105–11, 1995.

Wallerstedt C, Higgins P: Facilitating perinatal grieving between the mother and the father. *JOGNN* 25:389–94, 1996.

Wang YS, et al: Preliminary study on the blood glucose level in the exclusively breastfed newborn. *J Trop Pediatr* 40:187–8, 1994.

Weatherley-White RCA, et al: Early repair and breast-feeding for infants with cleft lip. *Plast Reconstr Surg* 79:879–85, 1987.

Williams SM, et al: Sudden infant death syndrome in New Zealand: are risk scores helpful? *J Epidemiol Commun Health* 49:94–101, 1995.

Wilson NW, Self TW, Hamburger RN: Severe cow's milk induced colitis. *Clin Pediatr* 29:77–80, 1990.

Wolf BHM, Ikeogu MO: Is sudden infant death syndrome a problem in Zimbabwe? *Ann Trop Pediatr* 16:149–53, 1996.

Wong D: *Nursing care of infants and children* (5th ed). St Louis: Mosby, 1995.

Worden FP, Freidenberg G, Pescovitz OH: The diagnosis and management of neonatal hyperinsulinism. *Endocrinology* 4:196–204, 1994.

Yamauchi Y: Hypoglycemia in healthy, full-term, breast-fed neonates during the early days of life: preliminary observation. *Acta Paediatr Japon* 39 Suppl 1:S44–7, 1997.

21

Fertility, Sexuality, and Contraception During Lactation

Kathy I. Kennedy

Fertility, sexuality, and contraception are interrelated aspects of reproduction. Breastfeeding affects each of these entities; thus the reproductive aspects of women's lives are more complex during lactation than during the nonlactating state (Fig. 21–1). Although breastfeeding clearly has a fertility-reducing effect on the nursing mother, the nature of this effect is not fully understood. In general, the child's suckling initiates a cycle of neuroendocrinological events that result in the inhibition of ovulation. One result of this inhibition is the creation of the hypoestrogenic state in the woman. Consequently, the dry, sometimes atrophic, vaginal mucosa may result in pain during intercourse. This and other circumstances result in many breastfeeding women having sexual relationships infrequently, and so they are at reduced risk of pregnancy for behavioral reasons. Emotions related to motherhood, such as intensive (albeit normal) involvement with the infant and feelings of undesirability engendered in a woman who has not recovered her prepregnancy physical appearance, may affect a new mother's sexual behavior as well. Fear of subsequent pregnancy may also play a role in coital behavior. Because some contraceptives

may relieve the vaginal symptoms of hypoestrogenicity and may reduce the fear of pregnancy, coital frequency may be related to family-planning choice. These are but a few examples of the interrelationships among fertility, sexuality, contraception, and lactation. It is fitting that these reproductive issues should be explored together.

This chapter reviews current research in the areas of fertility and contraception and critiques the conventional wisdom and insights from studies in sexuality during breastfeeding. The chapter is divided into three sections, each of which discusses lactation as it relates to fertility, sexuality, or contraception.

Fertility

The Demographic Impact of Breastfeeding

The natural birth-spacing effect of breastfeeding has been recognized for many years. In the past few decades, demographers have been able to quantify, in various ways, the degree of contraceptive protection that results from breastfeeding. In

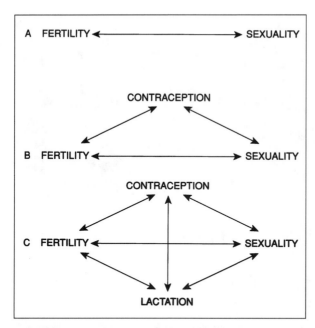

FIGURE 21–1. The interrelationships among fertility, sexuality, contraception, and lactation. *A. In the absence of a family-planning intention, the phenomena of reproduction and sexual behavior (fertility and sexuality) are related in the most simple and direct manner. B. When a family-planning method is used for spacing or limiting pregnancies, it clearly affects fertility and sometimes also sexual behavior (e.g., coitus-dependent methods). C. Lactation can have independent effects on fertility, sexual behavior, and contraceptive decisions and patterns of use.*

the early 1970s, it was determined that, in the developing world, nearly universal breastfeeding provided more woman-months of contraceptive protection than all other modern family-planning methods combined (Rosa, 1975). It is not clear whether this situation still holds in the 1990s. Two more decades of expanding contraceptive choices to women in the developing world have reduced birth rates in countries as diverse as Bangladesh, Thailand, and Kenya (Mauldin & Segal, 1988; United Nations, 1989).

More sophisticated analyses in the early 1980s revealed that, in populations without access to modern methods of family planning, birth spacing is the major determinant of total fertility (the total number of children a woman will bear) and that the birth interval depends for the most part on

breastfeeding (Bongaarts & Menken, 1983; Bongaarts & Potter, 1983).

Demographers have expressed the fertility-suppressing effect of breastfeeding by determining the extent to which contraceptive prevalence would have to increase in order to offset a projected decline in breastfeeding, with its concomitant decrease in natural contraceptive protection (Bongaarts & Potter, 1983). For example, in a country such as Senegal, where contraceptive prevalence is low and breastfeeding prevalence is high, Thapa, Short, and Potts (1988) estimated that an erosion in breastfeeding duration of only 25 percent would require nearly a threefold increase in contraceptive prevalence to prevent an increase in the existing, already high fertility in the country. The authors estimate that total fertility would rise by nearly 12 percent if such a decline in breastfeeding occurred without a simultaneous increase in contraceptive use.

In general, those more developed settings in which the erosion of breastfeeding practices has been profound are the very countries in which contraceptive prevalence is high. Thus in the United States and the United Kingdom, the contraceptive effects of breastfeeding are demographically insignificant.

Mechanisms of Action

During the normal menstrual cycle in the nonlactating woman, the hypothalamus secretes gonadotropin-releasing hormone (GnRH) in a pulsatile fashion, which in turn triggers a pulsatile release of luteinizing hormone (LH) from the anterior pituitary. LH pulses play a major role in follicular growth and estrogen secretion. In the first days of the menstrual cycle, the growing ovarian follicles produce increasing amounts of estrogen, which in turn appear to increase the frequency of LH pulses. When estrogens reach a critical level, there is a surge of LH followed by ovulation in about 17 hours. After ovulation, a corpus luteum is formed that produces estrogens and progesterone, and GnRH and LH secretion declines.

By about four weeks postpartum, plasma levels of LH return to a normal level in nonbreastfeeding women, and cyclical menses begin anew, although the first few cycles are not always normal. In lactating women, LH levels are lower than normal

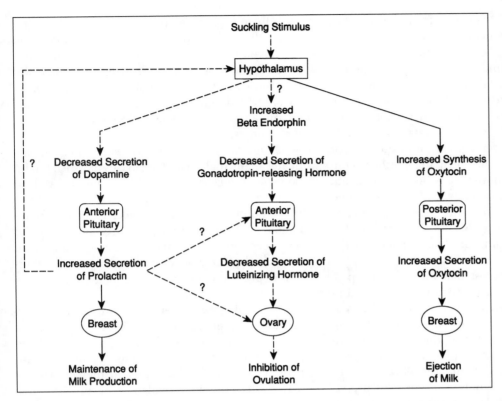

FIGURE 21-2.
The physiological mechanisms involved in lactational infertility. *(Adapted with permission from RV Short: Breast feeding,* Sci Am *250(4):38, 1984.)*

and, more importantly, pulsation is abnormal (Glasier et al., 1983). In fully breastfeeding women, baseline levels of LH remain lower than normal even in the presence of follicular development (Glasier et al., 1984). Presumably, suckling interferes with the normal secretion of GnRH by the hypothalamus, in turn disrupting normal pulsatile LH secretion (Fig. 21-2). Thus normal follicular development does not ensue. Small amounts of estrogen are secreted, but they are insufficient to cause an LH surge and ovulation. An experiment to test this presumption involved the administration of pulsatile GnRH to breastfeeding women, after which follicular development, ovulation, and luteinization were observed (Glasier et al., 1986). (See McNeilly et al. [1994] and McNeilly [1994] for more detailed descriptions of the mechanisms involved in lactational infertility.)

Increased levels of prolactin are clearly associated with breastfeeding patterns (Gross & Eastman, 1985). Inhibitory effects of prolactin on gonadotropin secretion or ovarian function have been postulated. However, the role of prolactin is uncertain, because some lactating women show normal ovula-

tory cycles despite high levels of prolactin (Diaz et al., 1989; 1995), and because pulsatile GnRH infusion can induce follicular development and ovulation in hyperprolactinemic breastfeeding women (Glasier et al., 1986). Possibly, the decline in suckling causes both the decrease in prolactin and the improvement in LH pulsation, and the relationship between prolactin and hypothalamic inhibition is only coincidental (McNeilly, 1983; Tay, 1991).

Our current understanding of the neuroendocrinological mechanisms relative to lactational infertility is by no means complete. In fact, researchers recently summarized existing neuroendocrinological questions and suggested the next generation of studies that are needed (Diaz et al., 1995). The complexity of the process is appreciated, as is the irony that the baby is in charge of it all.

Lactational Amenorrhea

The period of lactational amenorrhea rather than the period of breastfeeding should be considered the phase of natural infertility (Short et al., 1991). Reviews of the international literature have shown that between 3 and 10 percent of women conceive during lactational amenorrhea if they are not otherwise practicing contraception (Badroui & Hefnawi, 1979; Rolland, 1976; Simpson-Hebert & Huffman, 1981; Van Ginnekin, 1974). These percentages are crude indices of the contraceptive efficacy of lactational amenorrhea and are not directly comparable to Pearl pregnancy rates or life-table rates. Also, these percentages are uncontrolled for the postpartum time at which the mothers conceived. (Some women may have become pregnant soon after delivery, but others may have remained amenorrheic for two or more years before they conceived.) They also do not control for the amount of breastfeeding that was ongoing at the time of conception.

Many studies suggest that the expected protection afforded by amenorrhea is significant and competitive with reversible methods of fertility regulation such as pills or intrauterine devices (IUDs). In several retrospective studies, the researchers calculated rates of ovulation or pregnancy during lactational amenorrhea. An analysis of 236 urban women in Chile found only a 0.9 percent probability of pregnancy at six months among amenorrheic women who did not feed their babies any breastmilk substitutes. In contrast, menstruating, breastfeeding mothers who gave milk supplements had cumulative probabilities of pregnancy of 35.6 and 54.7 percent at 6 and 12 months, respectively (Diaz et al., 1991). In a study of 101 Australian women, an estimated cumulative probability of conception during lactational amenorrhea was calculated from the observed rate of the recovery of ovulation. The estimated probabilities of pregnancy were 1.7 percent at six months and 7.0 percent at one year postpartum (Lewis et al., 1991; Short et al., 1991). An analysis of data from 346 amenorrheic women who were not practicing contraception was pooled from nine studies in eight countries; it yielded a 12-month cumulative life-table pregnancy rate of 5.9 percent (Kennedy & Visness, 1992). This study reflects the combined effects of many different breastfeeding patterns and styles or timings of weaning. These three analyses support the assumptions of earlier, cruder estimates of 3 to 10 percent pregnancy rates during lactational amenorrhea, which did not control for postpartum time at which pregnancy occurred.

Obviously, a small proportion of women experience their first normal postpartum ovulation and conceive during the period of lactational amenorrhea. To the best of our knowledge, a woman will have no more than one ovulation during amenorrhea. Ovulation during amenorrhea usually occurs shortly (up to three weeks) before the first postpartum menses.

Some women repeatedly experience "inadequate" menstrual cycles (i.e., cycles in which too little progesterone is produced to sustain a fertilized ovum after the end of lactational amenorrhea). Indeed some women who wish to conceive are unable to do so until after the breastfeeding child has been entirely weaned, because even token breastfeeding may provide enough inhibitory stimulus to prevent ovulation or adequate progesterone production.

Generally, the earlier in the postpartum period that a woman experiences her first menses, the less likely it is that this first bleeding episode will be preceded by ovulation (Howie et al., 1981, 1982b; Perez et al., 1972). The earlier in the postpartum period that the first ovulation occurs, the less likely it is to be characterized by a luteal phase of adequate duration and progesterone production (Howie et al., 1982a).

The Suckling Stimulus

A child's suckling is the stimulus that controls the negative feedback inhibition of normal cycling of the hypothalamic-pituitary-ovarian axis, but accurate measurement or quantification of the suckling stimulus is difficult. In general, researchers have relied on such measures as the frequency of breastfeeding episodes, the duration of each episode, total minutes of suckling, and intervals between suckling episodes, as well as each of these measures classified by day and by night. All of these approaches result in indices of how often suckling occurred but not of other suckling characteristics, such as the strength of the stimulus or the volume of milk obtained. Various creative approaches to measuring suckling strength and milk volume have been attempted, such as breastmilk expression, test weighing of mothers and babies before and after a breastfeeding, isotope dilution, and Moire topography (Arthur et al., 1989). Unfortunately, the methodology required to measure, for example, pounds of pressure per square inch on the nipple or minuscule changes in the baby's weight before and after a feeding, have rendered large-scale measurement of these variables virtually impossible.

A different approach was taken in a study of the recovery of ovulation during lactation in Manila (the Philippines) and in Baltimore, Maryland. Researchers determined that breastfeeding as a proportion of all feedings (a reflection of the relative frequency of breastfeedings) was the best correlate of the risk of ovulation during breastfeeding. Women whose first ovulation occurred before six months had a significantly lower ratio of breastfeedings to total feedings in the first six months (84 percent) than did women whose first ovulation occurred later (88 percent) (Eslami et al., 1990; Gray et al., 1990). Even daily calculation of this simple measure (i.e., whether she is giving more or less than 85 percent of the baby's feedings as breastfeeds), however, may be impractical for mothers. Finally, although the difference in breastfeeds as a proportion of all feedings was statistically significant (84 percent versus 88 percent), this difference is clinically insignificant, so this factor could not be used practically as a sign of impending fertility.

The Manila study (Eslami et al., 1990) is one of a number that sought to develop simple guidelines for the optimal timing for breastfeeding women of modern contraceptive use or of taking full advantage of the natural protection from pregnancy that is provided by breastfeeding. Such guidelines usually involve some simple sign or behavior, such as the number of breastfeedings per day needed to prevent ovulation. To have widespread applicability, the guideline must be based on phenomena that are easily observed or recorded by the woman.

Breastfeeding Frequency and Duration

Studies in Scotland and Denmark showed that no woman ovulated if she breastfed her baby at least six times in 24 hours for a total of at least 65 minutes (Andersen & Schioler, 1982; McNeilly et al., 1983; McNeilly, Glasier, & Howie, 1985). A study in central Africa found that six suckling episodes per day were effective in maintaining levels of pro-

lactin consistent with anovulation (Delvoye et al., 1977). However, subsequent prospective studies on the return of ovulation during lactation found no such minimum value of breastfeeding frequency that could be relied on to suppress ovarian activity (Elias et al., 1986; Israngkura et al., 1989; Rivera et al., 1988; Shaaban et al., 1990). In these studies, some women ovulated despite up to 15 breastfeeding episodes per day (Israngkura et al., 1989), and a case of conception in the face of 12 breastfeedings per 24 hours has been reported (Khan et al., 1989).

The wide range of minimal feeding frequency required to prevent ovulation may be due to measurement differences across studies and among individual women. Additionally, the nature of a breastfeeding changes from setting to setting and from woman to woman. For example, for some women, a breastfeeding is a highly ritualized affair that takes some time to accomplish. It might involve changing the baby's diaper; preparing a beverage for the mother to consume during the feeding; taking the phone off the hook; settling into a particular rocking chair; allowing the baby to suckle for 20 minutes or so; and putting the baby (who may have slipped off to sleep) back into the crib. These breastfeedings occur, for example, five to six times per day and one to two times per night, perhaps with the baby nursing in the parents' bed. By contrast, another woman may identify her baby's cue to feed before the first whimper. She puts the baby to her breast for three to four minutes until he regains serenity, as often as 15 to 20 times per day and night. Not surprisingly, a "magic number" of breastfeedings has not been identified that will keep all women ovulation-free.

Having concluded that there is no universally reliable breastfeeding frequency associated with anovulation, we hasten to note that in studies of a large number of women, frequent breastfeeding remains an important correlate of lactational infertility (Jones, 1988, 1989). In fact, almost any valid measure of the amount of breastfeeding that occurs could be linked to the duration of infertility if the sample studied is large enough, depending on the other variables measured and controlled for.

The relationship between daily suckling frequency and duration (the total number of minutes of suckling) is difficult to generalize across mother-baby pairs. Many investigators assume that because frequent suckling produces higher milk yields than does occasional suckling, mothers who feed their infants frequently will also feed for a longer total time. The more milk there is, the longer it will take for the baby to obtain it. Howie et al. (1981) found this relationship to be so strong that one characteristic could ostensibly be substituted for the other.

Like every other aspect of breastfeeding (and fertility), this generalization needs to be tempered by recognition of normal individual variations. For example, the personal need of the baby to suckle for comfort may affect both breastfeeding frequency and duration. Some babies are efficient sucklers and obtain milk quickly, whereas others are more methodical and unhurried, just as children and adults vary in their speed of food consumption at the dinner table.

Although the Edinburgh study (Howie, et al., 1981) reported a very high positive association between suckling frequency and duration, this association has not been reported in all studies. An investigation of breastfeeding mothers in Manila (Benitez et al., 1992) revealed that the association between suckling frequency and duration at one month postpartum was not significant ($p < .52$). This finding suggests that if such an association exists, it does not hold for all women. Figure 21–3 displays the breastfeeding frequency, minutes of suckling, and their individual correlation coefficients for four women in this study. Across the four panels, the gamut of possibilities can be seen: high-positive, low-positive, high-negative, and low-negative associations.

One of the most promising correlates of the duration of lactational infertility is actually a measure of time *not* spent breastfeeding. The interval between breastfeedings is an inverse expression of both frequency and duration, because the number of intervals will be high if frequency is high, and the length of the average interval will be low if the duration or the frequency of breastfeeds is high. Measuring average intervals between feedings yields no new information or advantage over measuring frequency and duration of feedings. However, the longest interval between feedings reflects a characteristic different from all others mentioned thus far.

Supplemental Feeding

The role that supplementation plays in the return of fertility is anything but straightforward. A prevailing assumption is that anything that decreases the child's suckling behavior or the need to suckle will be a secondary cause of the recovery of fertility. Supplementation may have the effect of decreasing hunger, thirst, and possibly the emotional need for comfort, thereby reducing a child's suckling at the breast.

The pioneering work of the Medical Research Council in Edinburgh found this to be the case (Howie et al., 1981). In a sample of Scottish women, the initiation of supplements to the infant occurred very shortly before the first ovulation. Supplementation was thought to be causally related to the recovery of ovulation because of the close temporal relationship between the two events. By contrast, in studies in developing countries, instances have been observed in which supplements are introduced to the baby without an impact on the underlying maternal ovarian hormone profile (Fig. 21–4). In such cases, the supplements are usually gradual additions to the baby's diet and, like the maternal ovarian hormone levels, the breastfeeding behaviors remain essentially unchanged. A study of well-nourished Australian women who breastfed for an extended period also did not find supplementation to be associated with returning fertility (Lewis et al., 1991), presumably because the introduction of supplements was gradual and quantities small. By contrast, in the Scottish studies, a supplement was generally a milk substitute that was given as a replacement for a breastfeeding, and the suckling stimulus was thus decreased.

Supplementation has also been shown to have an effect on the duration of lactational amenorrhea independent of breastfeeding frequency and duration (Benitez et al., 1992; Jones, 1989). It is possible that supplementation changes some of the more elusive characteristics of breastfeeding, such as suckling strength, rather than just frequency and duration.

The strength and nature of the relationship between infant feeding characteristics (such as breastfeeding frequency and time until supplementation) and the return of fertility changes with the

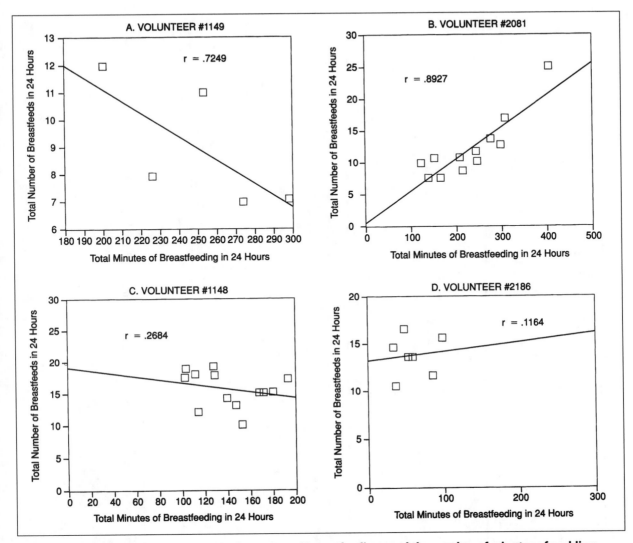

FIGURE 21–3. The association between frequency of breastfeedings and the number of minutes of suckling within the same woman. *This association is sometimes strong (A and B), sometimes weak (C and D), sometimes negative (A and C), and sometimes positive (B and D). (Unpublished data derived from Benitez et al., 1992).*

duration of lactation. For example, if the duration of lactation is short, supplementation is probably more strongly associated with the return of fertility than if lactation extends over a long period.

The Repetitive Nature of the Recovery of Fertility

Unpublished studies in France, the Philippines, Australia, and Canada (reviewed in Kennedy,

1993) found that a significant association exists between the duration of lactational infertility after one pregnancy and the duration in the same woman after her next pregnancy. These and anecdotal observations prompted the secondary analyses of large, existing data sets about the relationship between the durations of lactational amenorrhea reported in consecutive pregnancies.

In a large prospective study of Bangladeshi women, 418 women were observed through two

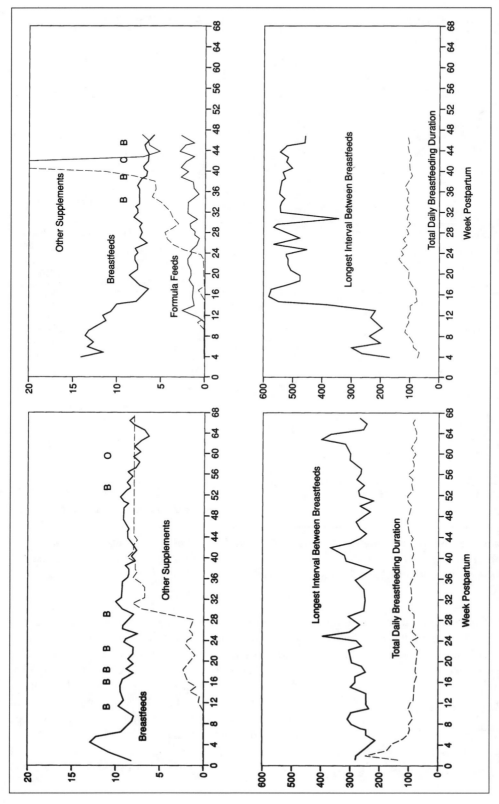

FIGURE 21–4. The effect of supplementation on breastfeeding. *A. In one example, the introduction of supplements at postpartum week 20 had absolutely no effect on breastfeeding frequency, duration, or the interval between feedings. B. In another example, the introduction of supplements at about week 9 coincided with a decrease in breastfeeding frequency and an increase in the longest interval between breastfeedings. Ovulation was still postponed for about 10 months, probably because breastfeeding frequency and duration were high enough. (In-house data from Family Health International, Roberto Rivera, Durango II Study, 1991.)*

consecutive pregnancies, after which the babies were breastfed. The length of the first term of amenorrhea had significant predictive value for the length of the subsequent term of amenorrhea. The author concluded that information about previous experience with lactational amenorrhea should be incorporated into guidelines for the introduction of family planning during lactation (Ford, 1992).

If a woman is to experience the same duration of infertility (or of amenorrhea) while breastfeeding two consecutive babies, the breastfeeding behavior is presumed to be roughly similar in both cases. Hence the amount of neurosensory stimulation received by the mother through suckling would be roughly the same, eliciting roughly the same fertility-repressing effect in the woman. We can suppose that this is likely to happen in many cases because several factors would be roughly the same in both breastfeeding couplets:

- The organism of the woman is the same; that is, her basic physiology is roughly the same. (If many years have passed between the pregnancies, then the woman's organismic responses to reproductive hormones may have changed somewhat with age.)

- The woman's orientation to infant feeding and her ideas and habits about breastfeeding probably remained constant across the two experiences.

- Two infants with markedly different feeding needs and personalities could result in different effects on the mother's return to fertility.

- Differences are also likely to occur if the mother's pattern of breastfeeding also has changed markedly. However, the research to date suggests that women generally can expect a similar pattern of recovery of fertility from one birth to the next, provided that the breastfeeding pattern does not change dramatically.

In a later section of this chapter, the timing of the introduction of postpartum contraception will be addressed. As suggested by Ford (1992), knowledge of the duration of previous lactational amenorrhea may be useful when making an individual decision about the commencement of postpartum contraception. In whole communities, information

about the average duration of lactational amenorrhea may inform programs as to the most effective community approaches to postpartum contraception (Weiss, 1993).

The Bellagio Consensus

By the late 1980s, researchers on five continents had completed prospective studies of the changes in ovarian hormones in breastfeeding women. Many of these researchers assembled in Bellagio, Italy, to determine whether their various findings about women with vastly different patterns of breastfeeding behavior could be synthesized into a statement about how breastfeeding women might predict their recovery of fertility. The conclusions of the group are listed in Box 21–1.

The basis for the consensus in 1988 was a body of published and unpublished studies of the pregnancy rates (3 studies in two countries), as well as data regarding the probability of a recognizable pregnancy from prospective studies of the recovery of ovulation during lactation (10 studies in seven countries). Among these studies, the highest pregnancy rate reported in fully breastfeeding amenorrheic women during the first six months postpartum was lower than 2 percent (Family Health International, 1988; Kennedy et al., 1989).

The Bellagio Consensus states that bleeding in the first 56 days postpartum can be ignored. This claim is supported by a prospective study of postpartum bleeding in 477 experienced breastfeeding women in the Philippines. A median duration of postpartum bleeding of 27 days was reported, which did not vary by age, parity, breastfeeding frequency, or level of supplementation. Further, more than one-fourth of these women experienced a subsequent bleeding episode beginning not later than postpartum day 56. Only 10 women may have had their first cyclic menses before day 56. None became pregnant, although not all were yet sexually active (Visness et al., 1997). A prospective study of 72 fully breastfeeding women in developed countries found that nearly half experienced some bleeding or spotting between the sixth and eighth weeks postpartum. Despite ovarian follicular development in 7 of the 72 cases, there was no ovulation in any woman in the first eight weeks postpartum. (Visness et al., 1997).

Conclusions of the Bellagio Consensus

Breastfeeding should be regarded as a potential family-planning method in all maternal and child health programs in developing and developed countries.

Postpartum women should be offered a choice of using breastfeeding as a means of family planning, either to help achieve optimal birth spacing of at least two years or as a way of delaying the introduction of other contraceptives. They should be informed of how to maximize the antifertility effects of breastfeeding to prevent pregnancy.

Breastfeeding provides more than 98 percent protection from pregnancy during the first six months postpartum if the mother is "fully" or nearly fully breastfeeding and has not experienced vaginal bleeding after the 56th day postpartum.

Source: Family Health International: Breastfeeding as a family-planning method. Derived from Lancet 2(8621): 1204–5, 1988; *and KI Kennedy, R Rivera, AS McNeilly: Consensus statement on the use of breastfeeding as a family planning method.* Contraception 39(5): 477–96, 1989.

The Bellagio consensus is important because it reflects principles that are believed to be applicable cross culturally. Yet this aspect of the consensus is also one of its weaknesses: by making generalizations that apply to a range of breastfeeding patterns and practices, some possible situations could not be accommodated. For example, in societies in which a child is breastfed for two years or more, or among La Leche League mothers in industrialized countries who choose to breastfeed for these longer periods, lactational amenorrhea alone may be a viable marker of returning fertility. Cognizant of this, Kennedy et al. (1989, p. 485) cautioned:

Guidelines specific to a particular country or population for using breastfeeding as a postpartum family planning method can be developed based on this consensus. Local infant feeding practices, the average duration of amenorrhea and the ongoing changes in women's status and health practices should be considered in adapting these general guidelines.

The consensus is also important because it represents the framework for the actual use of lactational amenorrhea as a method of contraception. Guidelines on how to integrate the Lactational Amenorrhea Method (LAM) into family-planning and breastfeeding support programs have been developed based on the Bellagio consensus (Labbok et al., 1994).

During the eight years after the Bellagio Consensus, a new body of research was undertaken to test the consensus prospectively. Four clinical trials of the contraceptive efficacy of LAM were conducted in Chile (Perez et al., 1992), Pakistan (Kazi et al., 1995), the Philippines (Ramos et al., 1996), and in a multinational study (Labbok et al., 1997). These studies found, during correct use of the method, cumulative six-month life-table rates of pregnancy of 1.0, 0.5, 1.5, and 0.6 percent, respectively. These studies observed women who chose to use LAM as their postpartum contraceptive method and who were taught and actually used the method (Visness et al., 1997). Other researchers conducted secondary data analyses on existing data sets (Rojnik et al., 1995; Short et al., 1991; Weiss, 1993) and found that the protection from pregnancy under the LAM conditions can outlast the parameters set in the Bellagio Consensus. On the basis of these studies, as well as unpublished research from a variety of sources, scientists who reconvened at Bellagio in 1995 were able to conclude that: ". . . the Bellagio Consensus has clearly been confirmed" (Kennedy, Labbok, & Van Look, 1996).

Having accumulated data and experience from prospective clinical trials, the group at the second Bellagio conference was able to draw conclusions about the modification of LAM on a local level:

1. *"It is not possible to eliminate the amenorrhea criterion. . . ."* (Kennedy et al., 1996). Once menstruation has resumed, fertility is returning or already has returned. Menses is an absolute indication of the need for another contraceptive method if continued protection is desired.

2. *"It may be possible to relax the full or nearly full breastfeeding criterion. . . ."* (Kennedy et al., 1996). If breastfeeding behaviors are sound and the introduction of weaning foods is not accompanied by a decline in any breastfeeding parameter, then theoretically the full or nearly full breastfeeding criterion may be relaxed. However, this possibility requires more research, because the breastfeeding stimulus is what causes lactational amenorrhea, and supplementation can (but does not always) affect that stimulus.

3. *"It may be possible to extend LAM beyond six months postpartum"* (Kennedy et al., 1996). In the clinical trials and the secondary analyses, the protection provided by lactational amenorrhea beyond the sixth postpartum month—and hence during supplemented breastfeeding—was found to be relatively low in some settings (e.g., 4–9 percent in the multinational study [Labbok et al., 1997] and 0–5 percent in the Philippine clinical trial [Ramos et al., 1996]). These rates are not surprising, given that decades of retrospective research (reviewed earlier) showed that 3–10 percent of women conceive during lactational amenorrhea. Although these rates indicate significant protection among successfully breastfeeding women using LAM, many other modern contraceptives used correctly can provide better protection in the second six

months postpartum. Programmatic experience with the extension of LAM beyond six months has produced some useful observations (Cooney et al., 1996; Wade, Sevilla, & Labbok, 1994), but no rigorous, prospective data are yet available on extended LAM from clinical trials.

Sexuality

Human sexuality in the 1990s promises to be no less complex than in previous decades. The variety of living arrangements in combination with various sexual orientations makes for new circumstances in which sexuality is expressed. Although the following discussion will presuppose a marriage or stable union between a breastfeeding woman and her male partner, this presupposition is simply for convenience. Nevertheless, the majority of lactating mothers are heterosexual; there is virtually no information in the scientific literature about the sexuality of breastfeeding single and lesbian women. It is likely that much of the following discussion will apply to these women also.

This discussion is also based on the assumption that libido or sexual desire is the main driving force or motivation for sexual expression (although the desire to please one's partner is also recognized as a motivation). Yet we acknowledge that many women have intercourse against their will or without sexual desire. This chapter does not consider the role of breastfeeding in coercive or indifferent sexual relationships.

Libido

At least five categories of factors may influence sexual drive or desire during lactation:

1. Common situational factors unrelated to breastfeeding
2. Libido-inhibiting influences related to parturition
3. Libido-inhibiting influences of lactation
4. Libido-enhancing factors related to pregnancy, birth, and lactation
5. Factors related to the breastfeeding woman's partner

Common Situational Factors Unrelated to Breastfeeding. Many preexisting factors that either facilitated or inhibited sexual arousal before pregnancy or birth will remain a part of one's living experience, family routine, or personal preference after the birth of the child. Preexisting factors that inhibit libido—such as the chronic illness of one of the partners, fear of pregnancy, or lack of privacy—persist and are unrelated to breastfeeding. A dysfunctional or unsatisfying sexual rapport in a couple is no more likely to be spontaneously remedied by lactation than a faltering marriage is to be saved by adding a child to the family chemistry.

Conversely, there is no reason to assume that individualized stimuli per se, such as a preferred cologne, a special song, or candlelight, should lose their excitatory effects because a baby joins the family. Opportunity to attend to the old stimuli, however, is another matter. Some of the preexisting sexual stimuli or circumstances associated with sexual opportunity may be decreased because of having a young baby in the home. For example, the couple may find that they now lack time alone and that they endure constant interruptions—especially, it seems, at night. The quiet evening at home may seem gone forever.

Libido-Inhibiting Influences Related to Parturition. Most of the natural process of physical recovery from vaginal delivery takes about six weeks, although there is some variation across women. Postpartum abstinence is sensible until the woman decides that she has sufficient physical comfort to resume sexual intercourse.

The tenderness from episiotomy or vulvovaginal or perineal damage after vaginal delivery usually lasts for several months. Although the mother's stitches may have healed, she may still experience discomfort with intercourse. In a study of 93 parturients in New South Wales, Australia, the median time required to achieve comfort during intercourse was 3 months, with a range of from 1 to more than 12 months. Whether the women had episiotomies (58 of 93 did) did not affect the time until pain-free intercourse was experienced, but this may be because of the commonness of tearing of the vulval tissues (69 percent), which required sutures in the women who did not have an episiotomy (Abraham et al., 1990). In a longitudinal study of 119 primiparous women attended at a London teaching hospital, 40 percent complained of soreness and occasionally painful intercourse at three months postpartum (Robson et al., 1981). Another study of British women reported dyspareunia during the first postpartum intercourse in 40 percent of mothers; of these, 64 percent refrained from further coitus after the initial distressing event (Grudzinskas & Atkinson, 1984). The anticipation of pain during intercourse may cause a woman to avoid sexual suggestion. A clear understanding of her feelings and communication with her partner may help the couple to defer intercourse until some future time and to express their love and caring in other ways.

Soon after delivery, women experience a precipitous decline in ovarian steroid levels. This drastic hormonal change is sometimes associated with noticeable mood changes. The immediate effect is usually temporary and probably overlaps with the period of postpartum abstinence. In some women, postpartum depression can follow delivery immediately or occur after a few days or weeks. Although the etiology of postpartum depression is not well understood, this depression probably has both endogenous and exogenous sources. Some women experience emotional vulnerability when their progesterone levels are low, such as during the postpartum period. (By way of analogy, the symptoms of premenstrual syndrome in the nonpregnant woman are often relieved by progesterone administration.) The overwhelming needs of the new baby plus other familial and extrafamilial responsibilities seem enough to make a normal person weary; exogenous sources of postpartum depression should not be underestimated (Fig. 21–5). Depression is commonly characterized by a lack of sexual drive, and the "postpartum blues" is no exception.

Even if the mother does not experience postpartum depression, she will probably be spending most of her emotional energy caring for and bonding with her newborn. This process is sometimes likened to a love affair in which infatuation with one's beloved appears obsessive: it is difficult to refrain from thinking about and doing things for the person who is the object of one's affection. Between mother and child, this bonding serves exceedingly important functions by creating an

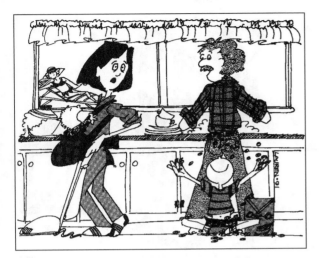

FIGURE 21–5. *The overwhelming needs of the new baby plus other familial and extrafamilial responsibilities are enough to make any person weary. When one has children, there are lots of other things to do.*

enduring parental talent and commitment in the mother and a sense of trust and security in the infant. However, this process can interfere with the mother's emotional availability for her partner.

Psychological factors unrelated to hormones or to attachment can also be strong inhibitors of libido. Fear of pregnancy can be an important inhibitor of sexual drive. If the new baby was unplanned, especially if a contraceptive failure occurred, sexual inhibition could understandably be great. Parents of a firstborn sometimes have trouble synthesizing the roles of lover and parent, because the parental role was previously understood subconsciously to be asexual. Colic or minor or major problems with the infant can decrease sexual interest by either partner and, if a difficult parenting challenge is faced by a mother who has had no previous parenting experience, she may be even less emotionally available to her partner. Preexisting marital difficulties may manifest themselves in an exclusive emphasis on the child and neglect of the adult love relationship. One mother suggested that the factors contributing to a decrease in the frequency of sexual relations were not very complex or deeply rooted and were probably unrelated to any particular psychological construct. She declared simply, "Our priorities changed! When you have kids, there are lots of other things to do, and your values change."

Libido-Inhibiting Influences of Lactation. Libido is thought to be elevated during the middle of the menstrual cycle in normal, nonlactating women. The mid-cycle is the period during which peaks in follicle-stimulating hormone (FSH), LH, and estrogen are observed. Accordingly, libido in the breastfeeding woman may be linked to one or more of these substances, or to a drop in prolactin which, during breastfeeding, is elevated above the levels in normally cycling women. The study of parturients in New South Wales showed that breastfeeding duration longer than five months was associated with longer duration of discomfort during intercourse and longer periods of lactational amenorrhea (Abraham, 1990). This finding supports an association between the hormonal milieu during breastfeeding and sexual activity. Alder and Bancroft (1988) found that women who bottle-fed their infants tended to resume coitus earlier and had intercourse more frequently than did breastfeeders, which similarly supports a hormone-libido association. However, these same researchers had earlier found no relationship between basal prolactin levels, estrogen levels, or even the return of follicular development with measures of sexuality in breastfeeding women (Alder et al., 1986). Some design problems could account for these results, namely the retrospective nature of the data collected, the small number of women being studied, and the infrequent intervals of data collection. A possible explanation is that hormones may in fact exert some influence over sexual desire but factors other than the hormonal milieu exert greater influence over sexual behavior.

Nonbreastfeeding postpartum women produce low levels of estrogen until they begin to recover fertility at one to two months postpartum. Among breastfeeding women, this period of hypoestrogenemia can endure for the entire lactation course. As in menopause, lactation-related hypoestrogenemia can cause the vaginal epithelium to be very thin and to secrete little fluid during arousal. Dryness and pain are experienced during intercourse, and vaginal tears are possible. Atrophy of the vaginal mucosa can be relieved quickly and easily by the use of inert, water-based lubricants. Estrogen cream is sometimes prescribed for vaginal application and yields satisfactory results in many cases (Wisniewski & Wilkinson, 1991). However, the vagina is so absorptive that users should be alert to the possible consequences of estrogen administration, such as the recovery of ovulation and a decrease in breastmilk production.

As if the emotional demands of parenthood are not enough, breastfeeding adds another dimension of complexity. Exhaustion may be the most pervasive inhibitor of sexual desire. The London study of primiparous women mentioned earlier reported that 25 percent of mothers indicated that tiredness reduced their libido or enjoyment of sex (Robson et al., 1981). Of course, the nonbreastfeeding woman with a new infant is also vulnerable to exhaustion, especially if she has other small children. Yet breastfeeding women may be more vulnerable if frequent night feeding disturbs their sleep. Allowing the breastfeeding child to sleep in the parents' bed may afford the mother a better night's sleep (McKenna et al., 1997). Conversely, the presence of the child could inhibit sexual expression, unless the parents choose another site for lovemaking.

Emotional attachment between the mother and child is thought to be more intense if the dyad is breastfeeding rather than bottle-feeding (Bottorff, 1990; Virden, 1988; Wrigley & Hutchinson, 1990). The emotional availability of the mother to her sexual partner may be correspondingly reduced. One mother, in describing her feelings during lactation, gave the following report (Riordan, 1983):

When you are home and you touch, hold, hug, and nurse all day, you're not so interested in it when your husband walks through the door. But then his day has been all talk all day and no touch, and he's ready. It creates a problem.

Some men may feel that they are in competition with the baby not only for the breastfeeding woman's attention but for her breasts. The woman's breasts are often an important aspect of eroticism for the couple. If either or both partners feel that the breasts are "off limits" for sexual play because the woman is producing milk, then the couple's sexual expression may be negatively affected. Even if the couple feels no taboo about the woman's breasts,

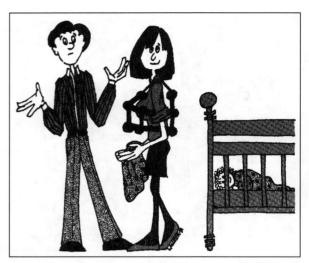

FIGURE 21–6. *If the breasts are "off limits," sexual expression may be negatively affected.*

there may be a dislike of milk leakage and thereafter a fear of eliciting it. The breasts may be tender, and the new mother may be tired of having her breasts "handled" (Fig. 21–6). Conversely, there is little harm in breast stimulation and even suckling by the woman's partner, especially after the baby has had his fill. The partner may actually help to prevent or relieve engorgement by periodically stimulating breast leakage.

Libido-Enhancing Factors Related to Pregnancy, Birth, and Lactation. Especially in the context of a planned pregnancy, the birth can be a positive and fulfilling experience, and many couples express this mutual happiness in lovemaking. Childbirth is a major life event and, when this occurs under emotionally and physically healthy conditions, sexual expression can be particularly joyful and rewarding.

In contrast to the possible inhibitors just mentioned, pregnancy, childbirth, and breastfeeding can also have the effect of magnifying a partner's appreciation of the womanliness of the mother. For example, to some men and women, the shape or fullness of the lactating breasts is particularly arousing.

The breastfeeding woman may feel more interested in sexual relations after a few months postpartum because of the interaction of some of the factors mentioned. Her perineum is less tender, she may be experiencing some ovarian activity, she no longer has the body shape of a pregnant woman, and she feels more normal. One mother described it this way (Kenny, 1973):

To me, sex is best of all during the later breastfeeding period because (1) I feel physically better than at any other time, (2) no fear of pregnancy and no contraceptives are needed because for me breastfeeding is a 100% effective contraceptive for at least one year after the birth of a baby, and (3) there is something about nursing a little baby that gives you an "all's right with the world" kind of feeling. I feel so happy and loving toward my whole family, husband, and other children as well as the baby. Sex just seems to be a nice, natural expression of this good feeling.

Human sexual expression can be a creative, as well as a procreative, activity. It is also obviously a personal endeavor for the lovers as individuals and as a couple. For this reason, some potentially inhibiting factors might actually be arousing factors that add to the likelihood that the couple will have sexual intercourse. For example, one couple may make love more frequently in times of stress, whereas another couple may experience a paucity of emotional reserve for lovemaking under the same circumstances. The former pattern may be quite functional, because orgasm helps to release tension and promotes relaxation and a feeling of well-being, thus providing one or both partners with more psychic energy with which to cope with the causes of stress. For some couples, pregnancy itself often stimulates erotic responses. Therefore, to some people, having given birth and becoming nonpregnant again may be less sexually stimulating than being "great with child." Because each person and each couple is unique, any discussion between health care professionals and clients of sexuality during lactation must be couched in generalities, recognizing that individual expression varies widely.

Factors Related to the Breastfeeding Woman's Partner.
The possibility of role conflict has already been mentioned and is a reminder that men also experience psychological adjustments in accommodating to the major life event of birth. No doubt the experience is most profound the first time that a man becomes a father. Although the male partner is often assumed to be ever ready and willing to and desirous of engaging in sex, this is an overgeneralization, possibly reflecting the relative lack of a cycle in the male capacity to fertilize. Men are subject to libidinal influences in everyday life and, analogous to the female perspective discussed earlier in this section, these facilitating and inhibiting influences do not disappear with the birth of his child or during the lactation course of his partner.

Witnessing his pregnant partner's metamorphosis into a lactating mother may affect a man's perception of her as a sex partner, either because of her body's obvious changes or because of the meaning he ascribes to her maternity. Motherhood may make his partner more or less sexually appealing to him.

Fear of hurting a postpartum woman during vaginal intercourse may inhibit male sexual expression. A man may feel guilty for desiring his breastfeeding partner if he perceives that she has more important maternal matters. Identifying and talking about their sexual feelings, desires, and inhibitions, while earnestly caring for the welfare of each other can help the couple through this sometimes awkward period.

Sexual Behavior During Lactation

To measure a level of sexual functioning or behavior in breastfeeding women, researchers have studied the resumption of postpartum intercourse and coital frequency. First intercourse and coital frequency are relatively easy variables to quantify, although they certainly do not yield a complete understanding of sexual functioning during lactation. Unfortunately, little qualitative information about sexual behavior during lactation is reported in the scientific literature. Few studies of sexual behavior during lactation contain large numbers of subjects, and the results of the studies are sometimes contradictory.

First Postpartum Intercourse.
In one study in the postnatal hospital clinic of an English city, 328 women were interviewed. By the time of the postnatal visit, 51 percent had already resumed intercourse, most frequently (the mode) during the fifth week postpartum (Grudzinskas & Atkinson, 1984). An intensive study of 25 breastfeeding women in Edinburgh, Scotland, found that six to seven weeks

was the mean time preceding initial postpartum intercourse. In a prospective study of 130 breastfeeding women in Santiago, Chile, the participants had "usually" resumed sexual relations by the beginning of the second month (Diaz et al., 1982). In a probability sample of U.S. women taken from 1979 to 1982, 66 percent of breastfeeding women reported that they were sexually active in the first month postpartum, and only 4.3 percent were not sexually active at three months postpartum (Ford & Labbok, 1987). Thus, in those few developed countries studied, the first postpartum intercourse generally occurred between about the fourth and seventh weeks.

A population-based survey of 3,080 parturients was conducted in Cebu, the Philippines, where breastfeeding is the norm. The study included all identified pregnancies in 27 administrative districts in and around metropolitan Cebu. Sixty percent of women returned to coitus by eight weeks postpartum (Udry & Deang, 1993). A study of 485 LAM users in Manila, the Philippines, reported a median time to the resumption of coitus of seven weeks (Ramos et al., 1996). In a study involving 27 breastfeeding women in Bangkok, Thailand, the mean time until the first postpartum coitus was 7.8 weeks, although the range of time until the first coitus was from 3 weeks to more than 21 weeks postpartum (Israngkura et al., 1989). (Although this is a small and nonrepresentative study, the women recorded coitus data prospectively, unlike the methodology used in population-based surveys.) In a study of 399 LAM users in Pakistan, three-fourths of the volunteers were from the city of Karachi. By the end of the second month, 80 percent reported that they were sexually active, up from 14 percent in the first month (Kazi et al., 1995). The Cebu, Manila, Bangkok, and Karachi studies show that the postpartum resumption of sexual activity in urban areas of Asian developing countries typically occurs by seven to eight weeks.

Whether the average time to resumption of sexual relations during breastfeeding is four weeks or eight weeks, large numbers of women are sexually active before the traditional time of the postpartum checkup (i.e., six weeks postpartum). As will be discussed later, an argument can be made to schedule the postpartum visit on the basis of the time that the woman needs a provider to deliver her chosen contraceptive method. Of course the new mother should always have access to care in the event of unexpected pain, vaginal discharge, or other physical concerns.

Postpartum Coital Frequency. An analysis of retrospective and prospective data on coital frequency was performed using information provided by 91 nonpregnant, nonlactating women in North Carolina who were married or living with a male partner as if married. First the women reported from memory their usual weekly frequency of sexual intercourse. Then they recorded each morning, for one to three months, whether they had intercourse during the previous 24 hours. The women reported a significantly higher frequency of coitus for the period prior to the first interview (2.5 times per week) compared with their later prospective recordings (1.7 times per week)—an average decrease of 0.8 episodes per week. This overestimate occurred uniformly in subgroups of women and was thought to be caused by the women's tendency to report a frequency that would exist in the absence of travel, illness, menses, and other influencing factors. The prospective data showed trends toward decreased coital frequency with increasing age, education, income, and duration of relationship. Also, women currently using an IUD or who had had a tubal ligation had intercourse twice as often (2.0 times per week) as did women who did not use any contraceptive (1.1 times per week) (Hornsby & Wilcox, 1989). Although the North Carolina analysis is a study of the methodology for obtaining information about coital frequency, it offers a clear example of the potential bias incurred with the use of retrospective data. Although it is a study of normally cycling women, it provides a good context in which to view studies of coital frequency during lactation.

In the aforementioned study in Santiago, Chile, the reported coital frequency ranged from one to six times per week in the first six months postpartum among breastfeeding women (Diaz et al., 1982). Conversely, the Cebu study found a remarkable lack of variance in coital frequency in the first six months postpartum. These women were asked every two months about the frequency of intercourse in the previous week. After controlling for a large number of potentially influential factors, coital frequency of 0.5 to 0.6 times per week did not vary meaningfully with any of the demographic or situational factors observed.

The variability in coital frequency in the Cebu study could not be well explained by factors such as age and education. Other factors, such as fear of pregnancy, may be stronger correlates of sexual behavior, as may psychological factors, such as perceived locus of control (the perception that one is in control of one's life and fate rather than the victim of forces outside oneself).

In a study conducted in Manila, the Philippines, coital frequency averaged three times per month among LAM users (Visness & Kennedy, 1997). In this study of breastfeeding women, the number of living children was unrelated to coital frequency, whereas maternal age was related in two ways: younger women reported an increase in frequency with time postpartum, and their overall frequency was greater than that reported by older women (Visness & Kennedy, 1997).

On an individual basis, postpartum coital frequency may be an important fact to know, so that it may be compared with frequency before the pregnancy or the birth. The Edinburgh study mentioned earlier prospectively measured coital frequency during weeks 12 to 24 postpartum and found a mean frequency of 1.2 times per week. The recalled prepregnancy frequency was 2.6 times per week ($p < .01$) (Alder et al., 1986). In light of the findings of Hornsby and Wilcox (1989), it is possible that the retrospectively generated prepregnancy frequency was an overestimate. Also, it is not clear whether the prepregnancy period being recalled is a time in which pregnancy was actively sought, which could inflate sexual frequency above previous or later levels for the couple.

Does breastfeeding affect the resumption of sexual activity or coital frequency? Survey data from Bangladesh (Islam & Khan, 1993) and the Philippines show lower coital frequencies among breastfeeding than nonbreastfeeding women. Alder and Bancroft (1988) reported that, when compared with bottle-feeders, breastfeeding women showed a lower preferred frequency of intercourse; delayed the resumption of coitus for a longer period; had a greater reduction in sexual interest and enjoyment compared with prepregnancy levels; experienced more pain during inter-

course; and were slightly more depressed at three months postpartum. All of these differences except for dyspareunia disappeared by six months postpartum.

By contrast, works by Masters and Johnson (1966) and by Kenny (1973) reported a more prompt return of sexual desire and a return to higher levels of sexual functioning among breastfeeding women than among bottle-feeders. These earlier works were conducted during a time and at locations in which breastfeeding was not popular. It is unknown whether women who were less sexually inhibited were the ones who breastfed.

In 1981, Robson, Brant, and Kumar reported that breastfeeding showed no influence over several indices of maternal sexuality in 119 primiparas in London. Grudzinskas and Atkinson (1984) reported that breastfeeding was not related to the resumption of coitus in their sample of 328 women. Nationally representative data from Thailand show that there is no overall difference in coital frequency between breastfeeders and nonbreastfeeders, except for a reduced frequency among women who breastfeed six or more times at night (Knodel & Chaynovan, 1991).

What do these conflicting results mean? Does breastfeeding stifle sexual experience, accelerate it, or neither? Conflicting results can derive differences in research methodology or to cultural norms. In addition, psychologically, behaviorally, and biologically based hypotheses are needed to clarify this issue. Can breastfeeding have either an inhibiting or a stimulating effect? Perhaps breastfeeding is a swing factor, sometimes enhancing sexual feelings and sometimes acting as the obstacle to their expression.

Contraception

During lactation, the choice of whether to practice contraception and, if so, the choice of method requires different considerations as compared with the same choices during the nonlactating state (Fig. 21–7). The array of available family-planning methods has been arranged in a hierarchy according to the general advisability for use of such methods during breastfeeding (Labbok et al., 1994). The hierarchy of family-planning options (Table 21–1) places nonhormonal methods first,

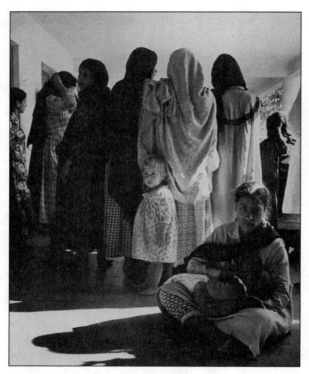

FIGURE 21-7. *In the WHO perspective, family planning is concerned with the quality of life. It is a way of thinking and living that promotes the health and welfare of the family group and thus contributes to economic and social development. In an Egyptian health center, family-planning care is included in maternal and child health services.*

progestin-only methods second, and methods containing estrogen a distant third, to be used only when other methods are unavailable. This hierarchy is consistent with guidelines recently published by the World Health Organization (1996), the International Planned Parenthood Federation (1996), and the Technical Guidance Working Group (1994).

Contraceptive Methods

The following discussion describes the advantages and disadvantages of various contraceptive methods used during lactation. It is not intended to be an exhaustive exposition of the methods. Instead it emphasizes the implications of use of the methods for the breastfeeding mother and baby. A fully detailed discussion of instructions for use, as well as the contraindications for each method that are unrelated to breastfeeding, can be found in the most recent edition of *Contraceptive Technology* (Hatcher et al., 1998).

Almost every method of family planning can be used during breastfeeding, but the timing of the introduction of the methods can vary profoundly. The question of when to initiate contraceptive use will be revisited at the end of this section and is also an integral aspect of LAM. It bears repeating that hormonal methods containing estrogen should be avoided during breastfeeding to the degree possible and reasonable.

Nonhormonal Methods. The permanent methods of family planning—now the most popular category of methods in the United States—are all nonhormonal methods. They are highly appropriate methods, provided that a couple wishes to prevent any future pregnancy, has been properly counseled, fully appreciates the irreversibility of the procedure, and is fully satisfied with the decision to use a permanent method.

When a permanent method is indicated, *vasectomy* is one of the most appropriate alternatives available, because it is safe and effective and should have no effect whatever on lactation. After the vasectomy, the male reproductive tract continues to clear itself of sperm during about 20 ejaculations. If the woman is not pregnant, the couple needs to use a second method of contraception for some time in order to be fully protected. The couple may feel that the vasectomy is ideally timed either during the pregnancy itself or in the first few months postpartum, especially if the current pregnancy was unplanned. In an era of only one or two children per family, however, the presumed final pregnancy is often highly planned. If so, couples may feel more comfortable postponing vasectomy until after the pregnancy, in case a miscarriage should occur, or even until after the child's infancy.

Female sterilization carries several advantages. It is safe, effective, and relatively convenient, because it can be performed in hospital, even on the delivery table. Contrary to previous assumptions, a small risk of female sterilization failure can persist for at least a decade, but this risk is smallest after partial salpingectomy as compared with other methods of tubal occlusion (Peterson et al., 1996).

Table 21–1

FAMILY-PLANNING OPTIONS AS THEY RELATE TO THE SPECIFIC CONCERNS OF BREASTFEEDING WOMEN

Method	Advantages	Disadvantages	Comments
First choice: nonhormonal methods			
Condoms	No effect on breastfeeding. Can be very effective if used correctly.	May be irritating to vagina and may require additional lubrication.	Offers some protection against sexually transmitted diseases. No risks to mother or child.
Diaphragms	No effect on breastfeeding. Can be very effective if used correctly.	Diaphragm must be refitted postpartum after the uterus has returned to prepregnancy size.	May not be widely available. Effectiveness depends on use with a spermicide.
Spermicides	No effect on breastfeeding. Can be very effective if used correctly.	May be irritating to the genital area. May be irritating to the male partner.	Small amounts may be absorbed into maternal blood, and there may be some passage into milk; there is no known effect on the infant.
Intrauterine devices (nonhormonal IUDs)	No effect of IUD itself, or of the copper in some IUDs, on breastfeeding. Very effective.	Possible risk of expulsion and uterine perforation if not properly placed or if inserted prior to six weeks postpartum.	Insertion may need to be delayed until after six weeks postpartum to reduce the possibility of expulsion or perforation of the uterus.
Natural family planning (periodic abstinence)	No effect on breastfeeding. Can be very effective if used correctly.	May require extended periods of abstinence. May be difficult to interpret fertility signs during breastfeeding.	Additional training of method users may be necessary to accurately interpret signs and symptoms of fertility during breastfeeding. Calendar rhythm method alone has limited value prior to first ovulation.
Vasectomy (male voluntary surgical sterilization)	No effect on breastfeeding. Nearly 100 percent effective.	Minor surgery with chance of side effects for father. It is irreversible.	A recommended method if no more children are desired. Counseling necessary for couples. No risk to mother or child.

Table 21–1 *(cont.)*

Tubal ligation (female voluntary sterilization)	No direct effect on breastfeeding. Nearly 100 percent effective.	May involve short-term mother-infant separation. Anesthesia can pass into breastmilk and sedate the infant. Surgery, in general, has risks. It is irreversible.	A recommended method if no more children are desired. General anesthesia is not recommended. Counseling necessary for couples.

Second choice: progestin-only methods

Progestin-only methods (mini-pill, injectables, implants)	Can be very effective. May increase milk volume. Effectiveness during breastfeeding approaches that of combined pill.	Some hormone may pass into breastmilk.	There is no evidence of adverse effects on the infant from the very small amount of hormone that passes into the milk.

Third choice: methods containing estrogen

Combined oral contraceptives (estrogen and progestin)	Very effective.	Estrogens may reduce milk supply. Some hormone may pass into breastmilk.	There is no evidence of a direct negative effect on infants; however, in some women, suppression of milk supply appears to lead to earlier cessation of breastfeeding. If these methods cannot be avoided, *breastfeeding can and should continue,* as it offers important health and nutritional benefits for the infant or toddler.

Source: M Labbok, et al. 1994: Guidelines: breastfeeding, family planning, & the lactational amenorrhea method. Adapted with permission of the Institute for Reproductive Health, Georgetown University.

There is a potential negative effect of the sterilization procedure on lactation, in that any general anesthesia used may synergistically interfere with the early breastfeeding pattern. The mother needs time to recover from the anesthesia, and during this period she is not breastfeeding. By the time she begins to breastfeed, the anesthetic agent has passed into her milk, contributing to the baby's drowsiness and causing difficulty in feeding effectively. In addition, any pain the mother feels may temporarily reduce her ability or desire to breastfeed, and it may limit her options for comfortably positioning herself or her infant for breastfeeding. If the mother is experienced or well counseled, and if hospital staff does not interfere by bottle-feeding the baby, this interruption of early breastfeeding should not have serious consequences for lactation. Regional or local anesthesia is preferable to general anesthesia and should be sought when reasonable. The mother should breastfeed just before the administration of the anesthetic and delay somewhat the breastfeeding after the procedure to minimize the infant's exposure to the anesthetic agent (American ~~demy~~ of Pediatrics, 1994; Burkman, 1993).

~~dies~~ reviewed in the early 1980s have ~~d~~ that up to 7 percent of women express ~~out~~ tubal sterilizations (Divers, 1984; ~~al.,~~ 1985). In general, regret over the pro- ~~r~~ desire for reversal has been associated ~~with~~ ~~unger~~ age (e.g., younger than 30) or low parity at the time of the procedure, as well as remarriage, the death of a child after the proce- dure, and undergoing the procedure with a con- current cesarean section or during the puerperal or postabortion period. Occasionally, lower socioeco- nomic class and desire for a child of a specific gen- der have also been associated with regret over undergoing a tubal ligation. It is possible that regret is intensified when pre-, post-, and intraprocedural factors interact, such as when a young woman with few children is sterilized immediately postpartum, and she later remarries.

Of more than 5,000 women in the Collabo- rative Review of Sterilization, a U.S. multicenter prospective observational study, 2.0 and 2.7 percent reported that they regretted their sterilization one and two years after the procedure, respectively. The preoperative risk factors for experiencing regret after two years were identified as an age of less than 30 and (for whites) concurrent cesarean section (Grubb et al., 1985). Chi et al. (1989c) also reported that women whose tubal ligations were combined with the cesarean procedure were more likely to have characteristics associated with later regret.

Counseling is crucially important when help- ing women or couples to select the best family- planning approach for them. When a permanent method is a serious consideration, counseling must begin long before the procedure and must be repetitive. This may be especially important when younger women of low parity express an interest in the procedure during the puerperium, as well as when young men under the same conditions con- sider vasectomy.

The *lactational amenorrhea method* (LAM) is the proactive use of lactational infertility as a contra- ceptive method during the period of lactational amenorrhea, under very specific circumstances: (1) the woman is breastfeeding her child exclu- sively or nearly exclusively (i.e., no supplemental feedings); (2) the woman has experienced no vagi-

nal bleeding or spotting after lochia ends (all bleeding, spotting, or bloody vaginal discharge before postpartum day 56 can be ignored); and (3) the child is less than six months of age. LAM is based on the Bellagio consensus (Kennedy et al., 1989; Labbok et al., 1994). It is a temporary method of family planning. For continued preg- nancy protection, another contraceptive method should begin immediately when LAM expires (Kennedy et al., 1996; Van Look, 1996). Experi- ence with LAM is growing but still limited in the United States. LAM may prove to be a useful stop- gap method for women who are delaying the use of a hormonal or a permanent method, but access to continuing protection should be assured.

Nonhormonal *intrauterine devices* (IUDs) have been shown to have either no effect or a positive effect on lactation (Koetsawang, 1987). One study found Copper T-380A IUD insertion easier and less painful during lactation, with possibly higher continuation rates than in nonlactating women (Chi et al., 1989a, b). IUDs inserted during the postpartum period tend to be expelled more fre- quently than IUDs inserted at other times. However, insertion immediately after delivery of the placenta (within 10 minutes) by an experienced person who places the device high in the fundus significantly reduces the chance of expulsion (Chi & Farr, 1989). Breastfeeding has not been found to increase the risk of expulsion when the device is inserted at this time or after the postpartum period (Chi et al., 1989a; Cole et al., 1983). Ideally, the IUD should be inserted immediately after placen- tal delivery, within 48 hours, after six to eight weeks, or with care and infection prophylaxis after four to six weeks, in this order (O'Hanley & Huber, 1992). An IUD can also be inserted after a cesare- an delivery through the uterine incision.

Because of the advantages of immediate postplacental insertion, contraceptive counseling should take place and informed consent to IUD insertion should be obtained long before labor and delivery. Counseling on postinsertion care is also important. Women should be encouraged to have early postpartum checkups and to return if the IUD thread is missing, because expulsion, if it occurs, often does so soon after insertion.

A U.S. study found the risk of uterine per- foration to be significantly elevated in women who were breastfeeding at the time of insertion (Heartwell & Schlesselman, 1983), although large studies have been unable to confirm this (Chi et al., 1984; Farr & Rivera, 1992). Insertion by an experienced person is thought to minimize the risk of perforation.

Little research has been conducted on the effectiveness of *barrier methods* used during lactation. Clinical trials of contraceptive efficacy have deliberately excluded breastfeeding women because their naturally subfertile state may influence pregnancy rates. The relative effectiveness of the various barrier methods vis-à-vis each other is probably maintained during lactation.

Barrier or spermicidal methods are the most widely used contraceptives among lactating U.S. women (Ford & Labbok, 1987). Several characteristics of these methods make them particularly attractive during the breastfeeding period. Condoms, diaphragms, sponges, and spermicides are all coitus-dependent methods. Even if couples prefer other methods, they may find these methods useful if they are having intercourse less frequently than before the pregnancy. The lubricating effect of the spermicide can be welcome if the woman experiences vaginal symptoms from estrogen suppression. The contraceptive sponge, the diaphragm, and the cervical cap should not be used in the first six weeks postpartum, to avoid postpartum endometritis and toxic shock syndrome (Faich et al., 1986) and because it may not be possible earlier to fit the latter two properly. The condom is a good barrier-method choice during the early postpartum period. Condoms with or without a lubricant coating or a spermicide in the reservoir can be purchased. A condom used with a spermicide, whether applied by the user or as part of the condom itself, offers better contraceptive efficacy than does the condom alone.

The diaphragm that a woman used prior to her pregnancy is apt to be an unsuitable size after childbirth. A new diaphragm can usually be properly fitted at six weeks postpartum (and in some cases sooner), but some breastfeeding women may find the fitting process to be too uncomfortable for many weeks. In this case the couple may wish to abstain or to use lubricated condoms, LAM, or a spermicide until vaginal lubrication is more normal. If the woman will be sexually active before her diaphragm

can be sized, she should use another method (e.g., condoms or LAM) in the interim. With the gain or loss of every 10 pounds, a new diaphragm may need to be fitted to achieve effective protection, and a clinical gynecological visit should be sought for this purpose. The diaphragm should always be used with a spermicidal cream or jelly.

The vaginal contraceptive sponge is a safe and convenient barrier method. It can be purchased over the counter and is perceived to be less messy than the diaphragm to use because the sponge comes with spermicide already in it. However, the contraceptive efficacy of the sponge used by parous women has been found to be significantly lower than among women who have never had a child, with up to 28 pregnancies per 100 parous women in the first year of use (McIntyre & Higgins, 1986).

Spermicidal cream, jelly, foam, or foaming tablets used alone are not as effective in preventing pregnancy as is a spermicide used with a barrier, such as a sponge, diaphragm, or condom. However, spermicides used during breastfeeding, especially during the period of LAM protection, should result in a higher level of effectiveness owing to double protection. They also represent a significant improvement over unprotected intercourse and have the advantage of being widely available over the counter.

The Billings' ovulation method and the symptothermal method are considered to be modern *natural family-planning* (NFP) *methods* because they are based on sound scientific research. The methods require abstinence from intercourse during the fertile period, which is identified by observing the woman's physical signs and symptoms (e.g., cervical mucus volume, color, stretchiness, sensation, and clarity; basal body temperature; cervical position; and breast tenderness). The modern natural methods are highly effective when used correctly, but most studies observe a great deal of incorrect use. Incorrect use is usually the failure to abstain from intercourse during the fertile period rather than a misunderstanding of the method or how to apply it. Knowledge of the fertile period is also useful for achieving pregnancy.

Modern NFP methods have been adapted for use during lactation. A Basic Infertile Pattern (BIP) of fertility symptoms (such as cervical mucus) is established during a two-week period of abstinence. Thereafter, every other night is available for intercourse unless there is a change in the BIP, which then requires additional abstinence according to method-specific rules (Parenteau-Carreau & Cooney, 1994).

The effectiveness of NFP methods during breastfeeding has seldom been systematically evaluated. As with the study of other contraceptives, most previous efficacy research has excluded all but ostensibly normally cycling women. One study of breastfeeding women observed a poor association between estrogen metabolite excretion and women's reports of the cervical mucus symptom, which is regulated by estrogen (Brown et al., 1985). Basal body temperature is unknowable unless the woman has at least six hours of uninterrupted sleep; this requirement excludes many fully breastfeeding women, particularly in the early months of lactation. One prospective study of the symptothermal method used during breastfeeding found that the method is highly sensitive although not very specific in its ability to determine which days are fertile: that is, fertile days are identified very well, but the method also requires abstinence on many days that probably are not fertile. Thus correct use of the method during breastfeeding should result in a high degree of protection from pregnancy but requires more abstinence than is necessary to prevent pregnancy (Kennedy et al., 1995). The requirement for somewhat more abstinence than is absolutely necessary is intentionally built into the method to err on the side of pregnancy avoidance. It is not at all clear whether the amount of abstinence required by NFP methods used during breastfeeding is a hardship on couples. If coital frequency is low at this time anyway, and if the BIP is clear and consistent, abstinence may not be a problem. Under opposite circumstances, abstinence may be difficult. Thus NFP leaders recommend that breastfeeding users of this method first apply the rules of LAM to eliminate the need for abstinence for up to six months postpartum (Parenteau-Carreau & Cooney, 1994).

Although NFP methods can be taught and learned in simple terms (and illiterate women in many countries have learned to use the modern NFP methods), learning is apparently easier during normal cycles, as compared with the hypoestrogenic period of lactation. There may be an excess risk of unplanned pregnancy after the first postpartum menses in new users, because the changing fertility symptoms may be especially difficult to interpret (Labbok et al., 1991). Therefore, couples who wish to use natural methods to space or limit pregnancies during lactation are at an advantage if they have learned how to use their NFP method of choice prior to conception and subsequent lactation. However, one ovulation method study in Chile found a 12-month pregnancy rate of 11.1 percent during breastfeeding, but only 2 percent at 12 months were determined to be method failures (Perez et al., 1988).

Hormonal Methods. Hormonal contraceptive methods are not the category of first choice for breastfeeding women. The main reason is that all steroid hormones, natural or synthetic, are detectable in milk to some degree (Johansson & Odlind, 1987). The effect of the infant's exposure to exogenous hormones is presumed to be minor, because very small amounts of hormone are excreted in the milk or absorbed by the infant. Because the fetus is exposed to very high levels of progesterone in utero, exposure to small quantities of progestins in breastmilk may be of no consequence. Nevertheless, the degree to which exogenous hormones can be cleared by the neonate is unknown. Plasma does not bind steroids well, the immature liver does not metabolize them well, and newborn kidneys are assumed to excrete inefficiently (Diaz & Croxatto, 1993; Fraser, 1991). Excess steroids or their metabolites may attach to receptor sites in the brain or reproductive organs (Harlap, 1987). The long-term effects of consumption of exogenous steroid hormones on development are as yet unknown. Although the concern about infant exposure to exogenous hormones is theoretical, avoidance of exposure in the early weeks or months is urged, because its effects are unknown, and other contraceptive methods are available (Diaz & Croxatto, 1993).

Progestin-only hormonal methods include progestin-only pills, which are marginally less effective than combined estrogen-progesterone formulations but are still highly effective when taken consistently and correctly. Progestin-only pills, however, are somewhat unforgiving of incorrect use (e.g., missing a pill). Their lower effectiveness can be reasonably compensated for by good counseling on method use (Chi, 1993).

Progestin-only pills, injections, and subdermal implants have not been associated with reduced milk volume or impaired infant growth in studies in which the method was begun at six weeks postpartum (McCann & Potter, 1994; WHO, 1994a, b).

Little is known about the degree to which the infant absorbs the progestin it ingests, although one study found that maternal use of medroxyprogesterone (Depo-Provera) did not cause abnormalities in infant hormone regulation in male offspring (Virutamasen et al., 1996). Progestin transfer to the infant probably varies across formulations of progestin-only methods. Norplant subdermal implants maintain a level of serum levonorgestrel that is lower than the levels achieved with progestin-only pills; thus Norplant should have no effect on milk production or infant growth. However, progestin-only injectable contraceptives such as Depo-Provera create much higher circulating levels of steroid than either the oral pills or the implants.

It is generally recommended that the use of progestin-only hormonal methods be delayed for at least six weeks postpartum (International Planned Parenthood Federation, 1996; Technical Guidance Working Group, 1994; WHO, 1996) to avoid neonatal exposure to artificial progestins. Because other temporary methods, such as barriers and LAM, should be available to the breastfeeding woman, and because coital frequency can be low during the first six weeks postpartum, the use of a stop-gap method in the early postpartum period is a reasonable approach.

Although progestin-only methods should not interfere with breastfeeding (and may actually enhance lactation) anecdotal accounts of lactation failure associated with the very early use of progestin-only contraceptives are of concern. Despite the caution of experts to delay initiating progestin use for at least six weeks, some women receive progestin injections on the delivery table or within 72 hours of delivery, prior to hospital discharge. It seems likely that this early bolus of exogenous progestin could interfere with the establishment of lactation, because the physiological trigger for lactogenesis is the precipitous withdrawal of natural progesterone, which does not occur in humans until two to three days postpartum (Cowie

et al., 1980). Accordingly, progestin contraceptive initiation should be delayed for at least three full days (Kennedy et al., 1997) and preferably until after the mature milk has come in and lactation is rather well established. Two studies of the initiation of progestin-only pills during the first week postpartum found no deleterious effect on milk production (McCann et al., 1989; Moggia et al., 1991). However, the pill dose is relatively small compared with the injected amount, and pill consumption may have begun later than three days postpartum.

Combined estrogen-progestin hormonal method. Hormone formulations containing estrogen have been observed to decrease the milk supply in several studies (Koetsawang, 1987; WHO, 1988). Therefore, combined estrogen-progesterone methods (usually in the form of combined oral contraceptive pills) should not be used unless there is no other acceptable alternative. If combined pills (including low-dose formulations) are the only choice, they should begin no earlier than 8 to 12 weeks postpartum (Technical Guidance Working Group, 1994), although the WHO (1996) recommends that they be avoided or postponed for at least six months and the International Planned Parenthood Federation (1996) suggests that they be avoided altogether during lactation. Due to the elevated risk of thrombosis in the first few weeks postpartum, methods containing estrogen should be avoided for about three weeks, regardless of breastfeeding status (WHO, 1996).

Clinical Implications

When a woman or couple makes a legitimate family-planning decision or chooses a method for achieving their family-planning ideal based on full and accurate information and reflection, that woman or couple has maximized the likelihood of being satisfied with the decision or choice and of using the chosen method correctly and effectively.

Informed choice—which has been defined as "effective access to information on reproductive choices and to the necessary counseling, services and supplies to help individuals choose and use an appropriate method of family planning, if desired" (Piotrow, 1989, p. 2)—should be viewed as a continuing process that parallels changing procreative desire and phase of life as well as personal changes over time. It is naive to think that family-planning intentions will remain fixed throughout life and equally naive to suggest that one type of contraceptive is appropriate for the same person throughout all the reproductive years. An appropriate range of available methods includes both male- and female-user methods and permanent and long- and short-acting temporary methods. If only a limited range of methods is available to the health care provider, he or she should be prepared to offer referrals to help meet a given patient's needs.

Information can be shared with patients in various ways, using the written word through pamphlets, books, and posters, or the spoken word through videotapes, audiovisual presentations, or "class-style" (part lecture, part participatory) discussions. Providing information, however, is not sufficient. An interpersonal exchange is necessary to ensure that effective communication of information has been achieved and to provide clarification and counseling. The desired result of counseling is a patient or couple who has made a choice based on full understanding of the alternatives and who has made that choice freely, unaffected by the counselor. Information should flow freely between the provider or counselor and the woman or couple. This circumstance exists, ideally, between the lactation consultant and the breastfeeding woman. Accordingly, the lactation consultant must be well versed in available family-planning services and alternatives in her community; perhaps most importantly, the health care provider should be aware of the possible interaction of various contraceptives with breastfeeding, as discussed in this chapter.

A study in Scotland showed that postpartum counseling about family planning during the hospital stay after delivery is ineffective (Glasier et al., 1996). Conversely, counseling is essential before delivery for the immediate postpartum insertion of an IUD or for postpartum sterilization. Ideally, a plan for postpartum contraception is decided before delivery, with postpartum follow-up timed to match the requirements of the chosen method. A postpartum checkup with the mother's obstetrician/gynecologist is advised but can probably occur at any time from the third to the eighth week after delivery. The longer the consultation is delayed, the more comfortable a pelvic examination is likely to be for a breastfeeding woman, but the woman should also insist on seeing her clinician earlier than the traditional six weeks in the event of abnormal vaginal discharge or pain or if she needs a contraceptive method before the sixth week. All women who wish to avoid pregnancy should be assured of a method for doing so before hospital discharge, preferably before delivery. If a woman's choice of method is not one that can be appropriately delivered in the hospital, then condoms or progestin-only pills—and clear instructions for their use—should be distributed generously at hospital discharge, and LAM should be taught prior to delivery and reinforced at hospital discharge. Some kind of family-planning follow-up (e.g., by phone) should occur in the third to fourth week postpartum to revisit and support the chosen contraceptive strategy. Because the lactation consultant is one of the most likely health care providers to interact with parents in the first month postpartum, the lactation consultant should check that a plan is in place and should facilitate or support the parents in procuring a contraceptive method.

Accurate information is an essential tool for the lactation consultant, and posing the questions in Box 21–2 will help her ascertain some essential information. Additionally, such accurate information will influence the ability of the woman or couple to make a decision without undue influence from the consultant. When the couple freely makes informed choices, the lactation consultant is better able to support the woman and her family in their choices.

BOX 21–2

Issues to Consider when Discussing Family Planning with the Lactating Mother

QUESTIONS

1. Does the mother wish to limit or space any future pregnancies? If so, what method(s) of family planning does she prefer?

2. If she has breastfed a previous child, how long did she remain amenorrheic? What factors may have influenced the duration of her lactational amenorrhea?

3. If she has not breastfed before, how does she plan to do so? Is she familiar with the factors that can reduce the duration of lactational amenorrhea?

4. If she wishes to have no more children, how will her family be affected if a temporary method of contraception fails and she becomes pregnant before she had planned to, or in the face of a desire to have no more children?

INFORMATION TO SHARE

1. Discuss the effectiveness of the mother's preferred method(s) and offer additional information about other contraceptives. Include information about the effect of each method on lactation and on the suckling child.

2. This information may predict the degree of double protection that the mother may experience by using both a contraceptive and breastfeeding to reduce the risk of an unplanned pregnancy.

3. Review the factors that reduce the duration of lactational amenorrhea and increase the early resumption of fertility. Pay particular attention to what is meant by exclusive or nearly exclusive breastfeeding, the impact of pacifier use, regular use of solid foods in the infant's diet, and supplementary bottle-feedings.

4. When the reproductive intention is to prevent any future pregnancies, it is especially important that a highly effective contraceptive method be chosen. Double protection is not an issue under this circumstance.

SUMMARY

Fertility, sexuality, and contraception are normally related, but each of these aspects of reproduction also affects or is affected by lactation. A clear understanding of the interrelationships of these elements is essential if the health care provider is to discuss issues and concerns of the lactating mother as she seeks to determine her fertility in concert with her sexual self. The health care provider will benefit from an understanding of the relationship between physiological responses to suckling stimulation and the resumption of fertility. Additionally, the breastfeeding woman needs to be prepared for the ways in which her own breastfeeding experience may alter her sexual feelings as well as her fertility—in the early weeks postbirth as well as when her breastfeeding child is weaning.

Nearly all modern contraceptive methods can be used during breastfeeding, but the timing of the introduction of the methods can vary profoundly. Permanent, long-term, short-term, nonhormonal, and hormonal methods are all viable options when introduced appropriately. Temporary stop-gap methods, such as condoms and LAM, may comprise a suitable bridge in the early weeks or months of breastfeeding, especially if coital frequency is low, until another method of the couple's choosing is appropriate. All breastfeeding women who wish to avoid pregnancy can be helped to do so and should plan to do so from the first postpartum coitus. Lactation consultants are well positioned to ensure that a family-planning strategy is in place within the first few weeks postpartum. To best serve the breastfeeding family, the health care provider who is assisting the lactating mother should be thoroughly familiar with how lactation, fertility, sexuality, and contraception are intertwined threads in the cord of life experience.

REFERENCES

Abraham S: Recovery after childbirth. *Med J Aust* 152:387, 1990.

Abraham S, et al: Recovery after childbirth: a preliminary prospective study. *Med J Aust* 152:9–12, 1990.

Alder E, Bancroft J: The relationship between breastfeeding persistence, sexuality, and mood in postpartum women. *Psychol Med* 18:389–96, 1988.

Alder EM, et al: Hormones, mood and sexuality in lactating women. *Br J Psychiatry* 148:74–9, 1986.

American Academy of Pediatrics, Committee on Drugs: The transfer of drugs and other chemicals into human milk. *Pediatrics* 93:137–50, 1994.

Andersen AN, Schioler V: Influence of breastfeeding pattern on pituitary-ovarian axis of women in an industrialized community. *Am J Obstet Gynecol* 143:673–7, 1982.

Arthur PG, et al: Measuring short-term rates of milk synthesis in breastfeeding mothers. *Q J Exp Physiol* 74:419–28, 1989.

Badroui MHH, Hefnawi F: Ovarian function during lactation. In: Hafez ESE, ed. *Human ovulation*. Amsterdam: Elsevier-North Holland Biomedical, 1979:233–41.

Benitez I, et al: Extending lactational amenorrhea in Manila: a successful breast-feeding education program. *J Biosoc Sci* 24:211–31, 1992.

Bongaarts J, Menken J: *Determinants of fertility in developing countries.* New York: Academic, 1983: 27–60.

Bongaarts J, Potter RG: *Fertility, biology and behavior.* New York: Academic, 1983.

Bottorff JL: Persistence in breastfeeding: a phenomenologic investigation. *J Adv Nurs* 15:201–9, 1990.

Brown JB, Harrison P, Smith MA: A study of returning fertility after childbirth and during lactation by measurement of urinary estrogen and pregnanediol excretion and cervical mucus production. *J Biosoc Sci* 9(suppl):5–23, 1985.

Burkman RT: Puerperium and breast-feeding. *Curr Opin Obstet Gynecol* 5:683–7, 1993.

Chi IC: The safety and efficacy issues of progestin-only oral contraceptives–an epidemiologic perspective. *Contraception* 44:1-21, 1993.

Chi IC, Feldblum PJ, Rogers SM: IUD-related uterine perforation: an epidemiologic analysis of a rare event using an international dataset. *Contracept Deliv Syst* 5:123–30, 1984.

Chi IC, et al: Insertional pain and other IUD insertion-related rare events for breastfeeding and non-breastfeeding women–a decade's experience in developing countries. *Adv Contraception* 5:101–19, 1989a.

Chi IC, et al: Performance of the Copper T-380A intrauterine device in breastfeeding women. *Contraception* 39:603–18, 1989b.

Chi IC, et al: Tubal ligation at cesarean delivery in five Asian centers: a comparison with tubal ligation soon after vaginal delivery. *Int J Gynecol Obstet* 30:257–65, 1989c.

Chi IC, Farr G: Postpartum IUD contraception–a review of an international experience. *Adv Contraception* 5:127–46, 1989.

Cole LP, et al: Effects of breastfeeding on IUD performance. *Am J Public Health* 73:384–8, 1983.

Cooney KA, et al: An assessment of the nine month lactational amenorrhea method in Rwanda. *Stud Fam Plann* 27:162–71, 1996.

Cowie AT, Forsyth IA, Hart IC: *Hormonal control of lactation.* Berlin: Springer-Verlag, 1980:164–5.

Delvoye P, et al: The influence of the frequency of nursing and of previous lactation experience on serum prolactin in lactating mothers. *J Biosoc Sci* 9:447–51, 1977.

Diaz S, et al: Circadian variation of basal plasma prolactin, prolactin response to suckling and length of amenorrhea in nursing women. *J Clin Endocrinol Metab* 68:946–55, 1989.

Diaz S, et al: Contraceptive efficacy of lactational amenorrhea in urban Chilean women. *Contraception* 43:335–52, 1991.

Diaz S, et al: Fertility regulation in nursing women: I. The probability of conception in full nursing women living in an urban setting. *J Biosoc Sci* 14:329–41, 1982.

Diaz S, et al: Neuroendocrine mechanisms of lactational infertility in women. *Biol Res* 28:155–63, 1995.

Diaz S, Croxatto HB: Contraception in lactating women. *Curr Opin Obstet Gynecol* 5:815–22, 1993.

Divers WA: Characteristics of women requesting reversal of sterilization. *Fertil Steril* 41:233–6, 1984.

Elias MF, et al: Nursing practices and lactational amenorrhea. *J Biosoc Sci* 18:1–10, 1986.

Eslami SS, et al: The reliability of menses to indicate the return of ovulation in breastfeeding women in Manila, the Philippines. *Stud Fam Plann* 21:243–50, 1990.

Faich G, et al: Toxic shock syndrome and the vaginal contraceptive sponge. *JAMA* 255:216–8, 1986.

Family Health International: Breastfeeding as a family planning method. *Lancet* 2(8621):1204–5, 1988.

Farr G, Rivera R: Interactions between IUD and breast-feeding status at time of IUD insertion: analysis of PCU 380A acceptors in developing countries. *Am J Obstet Gynecol* 167:2027–31, 1992.

Ford K: Correlation between subsequent lengths of postpartum amenorrhea in a prospective study of breastfeeding women in rural Bangladesh. *J Biosoc Sci* 24:89–95, 1992.

Ford K, Labbok M: Contraceptive usage during lactation in the United States: an update. *Am J Public Health* 77:79–81, 1987.

Fraser IS: A review of the use of progestogen-only minipills for contraception during lactation. *Reprod Fertil Dev* 3:245–54, 1991.

Glasier AF, Logan J, McGlew TJ: Who gives advice about postpartum family planning. *Contraception* 53:217–20, 1996.

Glasier A, McNeilly AS, Baird DT: Induction of ovarian activity by pulsatile infusion of LHRH in women with lactational amenorrhea. *Clin Endocrinol* 24:243–52, 1986.

Glasier A, McNeilly AS, Howie PW: Fertility after childbirth: changes in serum gonadotrophin levels in breast and bottle feeding women. *Clin Endocrinol* 19:493–501, 1983.

Glasier A, McNeilly AS, Howie, PW: Pulsatile secretion of LH in relation to the resumption of ovarian activity postpartum. *Clin Endocrinol* 20:415–26, 1984.

Gray RH, et al: Risk of ovulation during lactation. *Lancet* 335:25–9, 1990.

Gross BA, Eastman CJ: Prolactin and the return of ovulation in breastfeeding women. *J Biosoc Sci* 9(suppl):25–42, 1985.

Grubb GS, et al: Regret after decision to have a tubal sterilization. *Fertil Steril* 44:248–53, 1985.

Grudzinskas JG, Atkinson L: Sexual function during the puerperium. *Arch Sex Behav* 13:85–91, 1984.

Harlap S: Exposure to contraceptive hormones through breast milk–are there long-term health and behavioral consequences? *Int J Gynaecol Obstet* 25(suppl):47–55, 1987.

Hatcher RA, et al: *Contraceptive technology* (17th rev ed). New York: Irvington Publishers, 1998.

Heartwell SF, Schlesselman S: Risk of uterine perforation among users of intrauterine devices. *Obstet Gynecol* 61:31–6, 1983.

Hornsby PP, Wilcox AJ: Validity of questionnaire information on frequency of coitus. *Am J Epidemiol* 130:94–9, 1989.

Howie PW, et al: Effect of supplementary food on suckling patterns and ovarian activity during lactation. *Br Med J* 283:757–9, 1981.

Howie PW, et al: Fertility after childbirth: adequacy of postpartum luteal phases. *Clin Endocrinol* 17:609–15, 1982a.

Howie PW, et al: Fertility after childbirth: postpartum ovulation and menstruation in bottle and breastfeeding mothers. *Clin Endocrinol* 17:323–32, 1982b.

International Planned Parenthood Federation: IMAP statement on breastfeeding, fertility and postpartum contraception. *IPPF Med Bull* 30:1–3, 1996.

Islam MM, Khan HTA: Pattern of coital frequency in rural Bangladesh. *J Fam Welfare* 39:38–43, 1993.

Israngkura B, et al: Breastfeeding and return to ovulation in Bangkok. *Int J Gynaecol Obstet* 30: 335–42, 1989.

Johansson E, Odlind V: The passage of exogenous hormones into breastmilk: possible effects. *Int J Gynaecol Obstet* 25(suppl):111–4, 1987.

Jones RE: Breastfeeding and postpartum amenorrhea in Indonesia. *J Biosoc Sci* 21:83–100, 1989.

Jones RE: A hazards model analysis of breastfeeding variables and maternal age on return to menses postpartum in rural Indonesian women. *Hum Biol* 60:853–71, 1988.

Kazi A, et al: Effectiveness of the lactational amenorrhea method in Pakistan. *Fertil Steril* 64:717–23, 1995.

Kennedy KI, et al: Breastfeeding and the sympto-thermal method. *Stud Fam Plann* 26:107–15, 1995.

Kennedy KI: Fertility, sexuality and contraception during lactation. In: Riordan J, Auerbach KG: *Breastfeeding and human lactation,* Chap. 16. Boston: Jones & Bartlett, 1993:435–7.

Kennedy KI, Labbok MH, Van Look PFA: Consensus statement–lactational amenonorrhea method for family planning. *Int J Gynecol Obstet* 54:55–7, 1996.

Kennedy KI, Rivera R, McNeilly AS: Consensus statement on the use of breastfeeding as a family planning method. *Contraception* 39:477–96, 1989.

Kennedy KI, Short RV, Tully MR: Premature introduction of progestin-only contraceptive methods during lactation. *Contraception* 55:347–50, 1997.

Kennedy KI, Visness CV: Contraceptive efficacy of lactational amenorrhoea. *Lancet* 339(8787): 227–30, 1992.

Kenny JA: Sexuality of pregnant and breastfeeding women. *Arch Sex Behav* 2:215–29, 1973.

Khan T, et al: A study of breastfeeding and the return of menses and pregnancy in Karachi, Pakistan. *Contraception* 40:365–76, 1989.

Knodel J, Chaynovan N: Coital activity among married Thai women. In: *Demographic and Health Surveys World Conference Proceedings,* vol 2. Columbia, MD: IRD/Macro International, 1991:925–45.

Koetsawang S: The effects of contraceptive methods on the quality and quantity of breastmilk. *Int J Gynaecol Obstet* 25(suppl):115–28, 1987.

Labbok M, et al: *Guidelines: breastfeeding, family planning and the lactational amenorrhea method–LAM.* Washington, DC: Institute for Reproductive Health, 1994.

Labbok MH, et al: Multicenter study of the lactational amenorrhea method (LAM): efficacy, duration and implications for clinical guidance. *Contraception* 55:327–36, 1997.

Labbok MH, et al: Ovulation method use during breastfeeding: is there increased risk of unplanned pregnancy? *Am J Obstet Gynecol* 165:2031–6, 1991.

Lewis PR, et al: The resumption of ovulation and menstruation in a well-nourished population of women breastfeeding for an extended period of time. *Fertil Steril* 55:529–36, 1991.

Masters WH, Johnson VE: *Human sexual response.* Boston: Little, Brown, 1966.

Mauldin WP, Segal SJ: Prevalence of contraceptive use: trends and issues. *Stud Fam Plann* 19:335–53, 1988.

McCann MF, et al: The effects of a progestin-only oral contraceptive (levenorgestrel 0.03 mg) on breastfeeding. *Contraception* 40:635–48, 1989.

McCann MF, Potter LS: Progestin-only oral contraception–a comprehensive review. *Contraception* 50:S1–S198, 1994.

McIntyre SL, Higgins JE: Parity and use–effectiveness with the contraceptive sponge. *Am J Obstet Gynecol* 155:796–801, 1986.

McKenna J, Mosko S, Richard C: Bedsharing promotes breastfeeding. *Pediatrics* 100:214–19, 1997.

McNeilly AS: Suckling and the control of gonadotropin secretion. In: Knobil E, Neill J, et al, eds. *The physiology of reproduction* (2nd ed). New York: Raven, 1994:1179–212.

McNeilly AS, et al: Fertility after childbirth: pregnancy associated with breastfeeding. *Clin Endocrinol* 18:167–73, 1983.

McNeilly AS, Glasier A, Howie PW: Endocrine control of lactational infertility, I. In: Dobbing J, ed. *Maternal nutrition and lactational infertility.* New York: Raven, 1985:1–24.

McNeilly AS, Tay CCK, Glasier A: Physiological mechanisms underlying lactational amenorrhea. *Ann NY Acad Sci* 145–55, 1994.

Moggia AV, et al: A comparative study of a progestin-only oral contraceptive versus non-hormonal methods in lactating women in Buenos Aires, Argentina. *Contraception* 44:31–43, 1991.

O'Hanley K, Huber DH: Postpartum IUDs: keys for success. *Contraception* 45:351–61, 1992.

Parenteau-Carreau S, Cooney KA: *Breastfeeding, lactational amenorrhea method and natural family planning interface: teaching guide.* Washington, DC: Institute for Reproductive Health, 1994.

Perez A, et al: Use-effectiveness of the ovulation method initiated during postpartum breastfeeding. *Contraception* 38:499–508, 1988.

Perez A, et al: First ovulation after childbirth: the effect of breastfeeding. *Am J Obstet Gynecol* 114:1014–47, 1972.

Perez A, Labbok MH, Queenan JT: Clinical study of the lactational amenorrhoea method for family planning. *Lancet* 339:968–70, 1992.

Peterson HB, et al: The risk of pregnancy after tubal sterilization. *Am J Obstet Gynecol* 174:1161–70, 1996.

Piotrow PT: *Informed choice: report of the Cooperating Agencies Task Force.* Baltimore: Johns Hopkins University, Center for Communication Programs, 1989:i, 2–68.

Ramos R, Kennedy KI, Visness CM: Effectiveness of lactational amenorrhea in prevention of pregnancy in Manila, the Philippines: non-comparative prospective trial. *Br Med J* 313:909–12, 1996.

Riordan J: *A practical guide to breastfeeding.* St Louis: Mosby, 1983:339.

Rivera R, et al: Breastfeeding and the return to ovulation in Durango, Mexico. *Fertil Steril* 49: 780–7, 1988.

Robson KM, Brant HA, Kumar R: Maternal sexuality during first pregnancy and after childbirth. *Br J Obstet Gynaecol* 88:882–9, 1981.

Rojnik B, Kosmelj K, Andolsek-Jeras, L: Initiation of contraception postpartum. *Contraception* 51:75–81, 1995.

Rolland R: Bibliography (with review) on contraceptive effects of breastfeeding. *Biblio Reprod* 28:1–4, 93, 1976.

Rosa FW: The role of breastfeeding in family planning. *WHO Protein Advisory Group Bull* 5:5–10, 1975.

Shaaban MM, et al: The recovery of fertility during breastfeeding in Assiut, Egypt. *J Biosoc Sci* 22:19–32, 1990.

Short RV: Breast feeding. *Sci Am* 250:3541, 1984.

Short RV, et al: Contraceptive effects of extended lactational amenorrhea: beyond the Bellagio consensus. *Lancet* 337:715–7, 1991.

Simpson-Hebert M, Huffman SL: The contraceptive effect of breastfeeding. *Stud Fam Plann* 12:125–33, 1981.

Tay CCK: Mechanisms controlling lactational infertility. *J Hum Lact* 7:15–18, 1991.

Technical Guidance Working Group: *Recommendations for updating selected practices in contraceptive use: results of a technical meeting,* vol 1. Chapel Hill, NC: Program for International Training in Health (INTRAH), School of Medicine, University of North Carolina at Chapel Hill, 1994.

Thapa S, Short RV, Potts M: Breastfeeding, birthspacing and their effects on child survival. *Nature* 335(6192):679–82, 1988.

Udry JR, Deang L: Determinants of coitus after childbirth. *J Biosoc Sci* 25:117–25, 1993.

United Nations: *Levels and trends of contraceptive use as assessed in 1988.* New York: United Nations, 1989:17–28.

Van Ginnekin JK: Prolonged breastfeeding as a birth spacing method. *Stud Fam Plann* 5:201–6, 1974.

Van Look PFA: Lactational amenorrhea method for family planning. *Br Med J* 313:893–4, 1996.

Virden SF: The relationship between infant feeding method and maternal role adjustment. *J Nurse Midwif* 33:31–5, 1988.

Virutamasen P, et al: Pharmacodynamic effects of depo-medroxyprogesterone acetate (DMPA) administered to lactating women on their male infants. *Contraception* 54:153–7, 1996.

Visness CM, Kennedy KI: The frequency of coitus during breastfeeding. *Birth* 24:253–7, 1997.

Visness CM, et al: Fertility of fully breast-feeding women in the early postpartum period. *Obstet Gynecol* 89:164–7, 1997.

Visness CM, Kennedy KI, Ramos R: The duration and character of postpartum bleeding among breast-feeding women. *Obstet Gynecol* 89:159–63, 1997.

Wade KB, Sevilla F, Labbok MH: Integrating the lactational amenorrhea method into a family planning program in Ecuador. *Stud Fam Plann* 25:162–74, 1994.

Weiss P: The contraceptive potential of breastfeeding in Bangladesh. *Stud Fam Plann* 22:294–307, 1993.

Wisniewski PM, Wilkinson EJ: Postpartum vaginal atrophy. *Am J Obstet Gynecol* 165:1249–54, 1991.

World Health Organization: Effects of hormonal contraceptives on breast milk composition and infant growth. *Stud Fam Plann* 19:361–9, 1988.

World Health Organization: *Improving access to quality care in family planning—medical eligibility criteria for initiating and continuing use of contraceptive methods.* Geneva: World Health Organization, Family and Reproductive Health Division, 1996.

World Health Organization: Progestin-only contraceptives during lactation: I. Infant growth. *Contraception* 50:35–53, 1994a.

World Health Organization: Progestin-only contraceptives during lactation: II. Infant development. *Contraception* 50:55–68, 1994b.

Wrigley EA, Hutchinson SA: Long-term breast-feeding: the secret bond. *J Nurse Midwif* 35:35–41, 1990.

CONTEMPORARY ISSUES

The increasing visibility and acceptance of lactation consulting as an allied health profession offers opportunities for persons who seek to practice in hospitals and clinics as well as privately. The presence of lactation consultants in large institutions and in the community highlights the special needs of breastfeeding babies and their lactating mothers. Caring for breastfeeding mothers and infants also means measuring clinical outcomes as the trend continues toward evidence-based health care. Thus knowledge of research methods is a necessary skill for lactation consultants. In addition, we need more research to expand our knowledge of the lactation process and the variations in breastfeeding behavior. Only with such research will myths about breastfeeding be put to rest. Milk banks represent a means of obtaining a scarce resource, yet fewer of them remain in operation in light of fears about the spread of AIDS through breastmilk. The political implications of the continued use of human milk from banks is an ongoing story that continues to unfold.

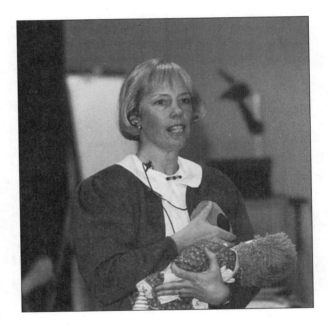

22

WORK STRATEGIES AND THE LACTATION CONSULTANT

Kathleen G. Auerbach and Jan Riordan

A lactation consultant (LC) is a specialist trained to focus on the needs and concerns of the breastfeeding mother-baby pair and to prevent, recognize, and solve breastfeeding difficulties. The LC's services do not replace those of the physician or nurse or any other health care worker; instead, the LC is an extender of maternal-child services. LCs work with the public in many settings: hospitals, clinics, private medical practices, community health departments, home health agencies, and private practices. Almost all LCs are women; many have educational and clinical backgrounds in the health professions. The majority of LCs are also registered nurses.

The LC designation is a new occupational category under the broad umbrella of allied health workers. Prior to recognition of the LC as a paid specialist in 1985, individuals serving breastfeeding women did so as volunteers or as unrecognized private practitioners. The lack of standardization of skills and minimal competencies led to formal development of the occupation. This occurred, in part, through a certification examination and through the establishment of the International Lactation Consultant Association (ILCA), which publishes a journal on issues relating to breastfeeding and a document identifying the competencies

that can be expected of the LC in any practice setting. La Leche League International and the Nursing Mothers Association of Australia also publish professional materials that teach and support the LC. This chapter traces the historical roots of LCs and discusses work-related issues.

History

In a cultural setting in which nearly all mothers breastfed, help with breastfeeding was available through the shared knowledge of other family members, neighbors, and friends. As childbirth came to be managed by health professionals in hospital settings, however, knowledge of lactation, which a mother formerly shared with her daughters or a sister with her younger siblings, was set aside.

Thus, during the 1960s, at the nadir of breastfeeding in the United States and, shortly thereafter, in other countries (including Australia and the Scandinavian countries in Europe), volunteer breastfeeding support groups became a major source of assistance and information about how to breastfeed (Phillips, 1990b). As the numbers of breastfeeding mothers increased, health care providers at first denounced these groups; later they came to appreciate them for the important role they played in helping mothers and in forcing the medical profession to consider lactation as an integral part of prenatal and postpartum care (Gerrard, 1975; Jelliffe & Jelliffe, 1977, Shea, 1992). In a salute to La Leche League International, Lee Forest Hill, editor of the *Journal of Pediatrics,* praised, "A dedicated women's organization has taken on the task of attempting to restore what is called by some, 'the lost art of breastfeeding.' Certainly, their efforts deserve the commendation of the medical and nursing professions" (Hill, 1968).

As these volunteers relearned the art of breastfeeding, they also sought more knowledge of the science of lactation. La Leche League responded by providing research information to their group leaders, who serve as mother-to-mother helpers, and by publishing a quarterly newsletter, *Breastfeeding Abstracts,* which focuses exclusively on the scientific literature. Through La Leche League's professional liaison department, key individuals seek to cultivate and maintain communication links to health providers in local communities.

Out of this context, some experienced breastfeeding support group members began to look beyond what they could accomplish as volunteers. Many of these women sought to apply in a paid work setting what they had learned from many years of helping breastfeeding mothers. From this small beginning grew the notion of the need for a new health care worker.

Certification

In 1981, experienced La Leche League leaders JoAnne Scott and Linda Smith were asked to develop a certification and training program for LCs. This need derived from (1) an awareness that many health care providers discredited the accomplishments of the volunteer because she was unpaid, and (2) a need to establish minimum standards for individuals who were already providing lactation-consultant services for a fee. A certification program was viewed as a way to recognize the important role of the volunteer and to provide a recognized credential that identified a certain level of competence (Scott, 1990).

Scott and Smith assembled a small group of breastfeeding experts who had come to the field of lactation through voluntary service, mostly through La Leche League. In 1984, these individuals gathered and concluded that legitimacy of the field would be heightened if minimal standards of knowledge and skills were recognized through a certification examination.

The first examination was administered in July 1985 under the International Board of Lactation Consultant Examiners, Inc. (IBLCE).* Since 1985, a certification examination has been given annually in eight languages in 38 countries on every continent except Antarctica. To date, nearly 10,000 candidates have been certified, approximately 76 percent of whom live in the United States and Canada. Periodic recertification as an LC is required through the acquisition of continuing-education credits and by reexamination (Scott, 1994). This dual-recertification option increases the likelihood that the LC will remain current in a rapidly changing field.

Early candidates for the certification examination had a baccalaureate degree and were originally trained through La Leche League leadership accreditation. After the first year, candidate affiliation with La Leche League declined, and affiliation with a hospital or clinical setting increased. Although there was no correlation between educational attainment and test scores in the first year of the examination, in subsequent years a baccalaureate (or higher) degree was significantly related to higher test scores. Among nonnurses, however, an inverse relationship exists between education and test performance. People with a master's degree (or greater) do not obtain higher scores than do those with a lower level of educational attainment (Riordan, 1990). The authors of the first evaluation of certification candidates (Riordan & Auerbach, 1987) speculated that the pass rate would decline as the backgrounds of the candidates broadened to include individuals with fewer years of clinical experience prior to their taking the examination. As can be seen in Table 22–1, this did not happen. In the United States, certification is respected and popular. More than 40 specialty certifications exist

---

The International Board of Lactation Consultant Examiners, Inc., can be reached at PO Box 2348, Falls Church, VA 22042-0348. Telephone: 703-560-7330; Fax: 703-560-7332; e-mail: iblce@erols.com.

Table 22–1

IBLCE Examination Summary Data, 1985–1997

Year of Examination	Number of Candidates	Mean Score	Pass-Fail Score	Pass Rate (%)
1985	259	72.8	61.8	94.6
1986	222	72.6	62.9	93.2
1987	281	72.5	63.8	90.7
1988	281	74.0	64.6	91.1
1989	306	76.1	67.5	92.5
1990	428	72.1	64.6	89.3
1991	683	72.9	63.6	91.1
1992	834	71.9	64.0	88.0
1993	1,171	76.4	64.0	93.0
1994	1,198	73.4	63.8	87.3
1995	1,556	73.8	61.8	94.1
1996	1,764	74.8	63.0	92.0
1997	1,670	71.8	64.0	83.7

Source: International Board of Lactation Consultant Examination (IBLCE).

in the field of nursing alone, despite the fact that certification is a voluntary credential. Some state laws limit clinical service in hospitals to licensed medical or nursing staff only, often for legal reasons. However, awarding credentials by certification evidence of their competency to practice enables LCs with other educational prerequisites to see clients under medical supervision.

Educational Offerings

The Lactation Institute in Encino, CA, affiliated with Pacific Oaks College, was the first organization to offer a specialization in lactation as part of a degree program (see Chapter 8 for more information). The Continuing Education Department of the Health Sciences Division at Douglas College (New Westminster, BC, Canada) offers a breast-feeding counselor certificate course requiring 90 hours of instruction and clinical activities with uni-

versity credit. Rush University (Chicago, IL, USA) also offers a 30-hour (three-credit) graduate course in human lactation through its school of nursing.

Breastfeeding Support Consultants' Center for Lactation Education, with offices in Chalfont, PA, USA, is a home-study course approved for college credits by the Accrediting Commission of the Distance Education and Training Council. Another self-study program is offered under the auspices of the Australasian Lactation Courses (Mt. Barker, SA, Australia). Participants are expected to complete a series of 12 workshops within seven months.

By means of the Internet, a three-credit course for graduate students (open to those with a nursing or nonnursing background) is offered at the School of Nursing, Wichita State University, Wichita, KS, USA. These offerings will probably increase as the demand for evidence-based care requires completion of college-level credits to receive a credential in lactation science.

Hospital Lactation Programs

The 1990s could be characterized as the decade for the emergence of in-hospital and private-practice breastfeeding programs or clinics in the United States and other countries. In 1991, of 293 surveys returned from hospital-based nurses, only 12 percent reported having a lactation consultant in their institution, although 80 percent had a breastfeeding protocol (Anderson & Geden, 1991). Most nurses learned about breastfeeding on the job rather than as part of their educational experience (89 percent versus 28 percent, respectively), and only a minority received in-service programs about breastfeeding, relying instead on journals or books to remain current. Freed et al. (1996) reported that nursing students relied most on their previous breastfeeding experience, which was often inadequate. Clinical activities rarely included demonstrations of helping skills for assisting breastfeeding mothers or instruction on how to do so.

In New York state, a 1984 law mandated that any institution providing care for new mothers and babies had to have at least one person on staff who was designated to serve as a resource for other staff members and to provide breastfeeding assistance to patients. Initially, many hospitals met the letter of the law by assigning someone already on staff, most often a nurse, to be the lactation person (Fig. 22–1). Often, these individuals were no more prepared than were other staff members to provide assistance to breastfeeding mothers or to serve as a resource for their colleagues. However, since the law was enacted, many of these individuals have chosen to become more informed about breastfeeding. Still others have sought certification as LCs.

Only a small number of hospitals in the United States had a lactation program in the early 1990s. As the decade comes to a close, most large medical centers and managed-care organizations employ LCs. In the past decade, the LC discipline and the number of persons practicing it has grown in numbers and visibility. One example of such visibility occurred in the October 27, 1997, issue of *US News and World Report,* which listed LC second in a list of "hot track" occupations in the health care field. Opportunities for paid positions have increased to the point that hospitals now advertise for such posi-

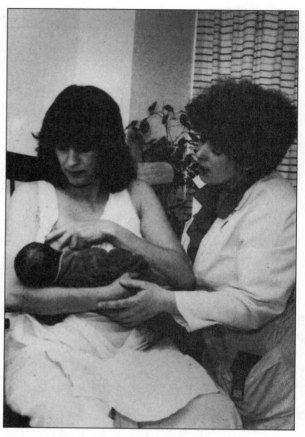

FIGURE 22–1. Early assistance promotes maternal confidence.

tions. Box 22–1 identifies the elements most often found in hospital-based programs.

A lactation program may take many guises. A breast-pump rental depot, because it is so likely to generate revenue, may serve as a first kind of service for breastfeeding women (Rago, 1987). A lactation service may be part of a community health program already in place but funded for a breastfeeding clinic or promotion program (Dublin, 1989). Such programs often require that the LC become cognizant of both the political and social climates, not only of the particular agency for whom she works but of the larger community that it serves. For example, in a community in which health care workers are already well versed in assisting breastfeeding mothers and babies, the presence of a lactation clinic may simply be part of an environment supportive of lactation. In another

BOX 22–1

Hospital-Based Lactation Programs and Services

- Telephone hotline or "warmline" (which may serve as a referral source, in addition to offering assistance without requiring an office visit)
- Prenatal education about breastfeeding (breastfeeding classes)
- In-hospital postbirth assistance with breastfeeding (one-to-one) (see Fig. 22–1)
- At-home postbirth assistance with breastfeeding
- Pump rental and sales (Fig. 22–2)

- Breastfeeding problem-solving clinic (often both inpatient and outpatient service)
- Education: seminars, classes, clinical experience
- Preceptorship (usually requiring a medical or nursing license)
- Research about lactation and breastfeeding issues (most often at a tertiary-care medical center)
- Evaluation of lactation products and devices and services

community in which breastfeeding is not seen as part of regular health care, establishing such a clinic may represent a threatening but potentially exciting departure from previous care patterns.

A lactation program may also develop out of a patient-education program that began with childbirth preparation and other classes designed to meet the many needs of pregnant and postpartum women and their families. From clientele who have already developed rapport with the patient educator, additional classes may be provided, including prenatal breastfeeding classes and follow-up services after the babies are born. Also some programs began in neonatal intensive care units (NICUs) and expanded to include the rest of the hospital.

Other programs are the outcome of patient surveys, often pertaining to satisfaction with care they received as new mothers. In one case, a survey included questions relating to the mothers' interest in using the services of a lactation clinic, a phone hotline, and a prenatal or postpartum breastfeeding class (Wilton, 1989). Still others have developed from an identified need of a hospital to "keep up with the medical Joneses" (i.e., when a competing hospital provides and then publicizes its LC services, other hospitals compete by providing

similar services, such as the lactation clinic seen in Figure 22–3).

How those services are structured varies by the institution. In some programs, the LC sees all new mothers who indicate that they plan to breastfeed. In other cases, she sees all new mothers, identifying her clients when they tell her how they are feeding, or planning to feed, their babies. A few LCs counsel both breastfeeding and bottle-feeding mothers. Other institutions restrict the LC's contact only to those breastfeeding mothers for whom the referring physician has asked for a consultation and follow-up care.

Whatever system is used, it is wise to estimate the anticipated workload prior to the start of the lactation service. The actual number of work hours is based on the number of births in the institution and the percentage of mothers who are breastfeeding. Daily rounds of breastfeeding women may be feasible in a hospital in which the LC sees fewer than 10 patients per day; it may not be possible if more than 10 breastfeeding mothers are housed in the maternity unit on a given day, unless there is more than one LC in the service or staff members providing other care are trained to provide optimal lactation-related care as well, thus reserving the LC for mothers and babies needing additional help

Sample Time Expended to Provide LC Services in a Hospital

Assume three visits per mother per day (to coincide with recommended frequency of offering the breast in an eight- to nine-hour period).

Time per visit: 20 minutes – average length of first visit + 15 minutes × 2 (average length of each of the next two visits) × 10 breastfeeding mothers in the mother-baby unit = 8.3 hours of work for the LC

This does not count time spent entering information in the chart(s), lunch, meeting with colleagues to discuss the mother's or baby's needs, plans for their discharge, follow-up care, prenatal education classes, staff in-services, and the like.

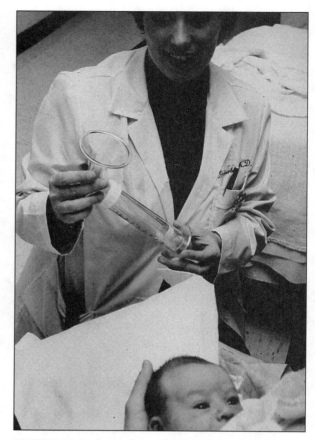

FIGURE 22–2. Lactation consulting sometimes requires knowing how to teach appropriate use of a breast pump.

and as a resource for the staff. Thus, in a hospital with 200 births per month and with an 80 percent breastfeeding rate, the LC will see about 6 to 8 patients on weekdays (and fewer on the weekend). A hospital with 3,000 deliveries each year should have at least three full-time LC positions to avoid burnout (Box 22–2) and get the job done. In addition, the service—to be effective—should be available seven days a week, on all shifts. Most hospital lactation programs, based on the 1:1,000 ratio, are woefully understaffed and only provide part-time

service as a result of partial shift coverage or coverage for fewer than seven days a week.

The lactation program at Georgetown University (Washington, DC) began with a "hotline" service for mothers (Kim, 1997), prenatal breastfeeding classes, and breastfeeding classes on the maternity unit. A grant from the March of Dimes established a Community Human Milk Bank at the hospital in 1976. Later, an LC training program was developed to provide both class lectures (40 hours) and a clinical site for hands-on training. This program, including the milk bank and the lactation center (which began with three and a half FTEs), has since been downsized to two individuals working part time. The training program continues independently of its original university affiliation.

The Beth Israel Medical Center Lactation Program in New York City was developed by pedi-

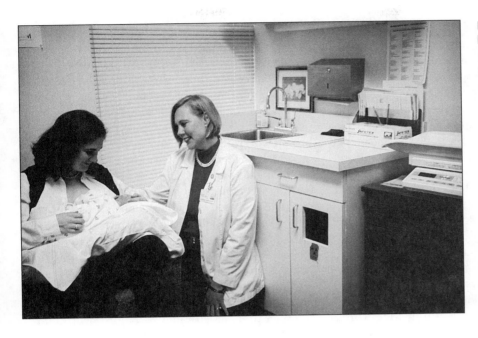

FIGURE 22–3. A hospital-based lactation clinic . *(With permission of Carolinas Lactation Center, Charlotte, NC, USA.)*

atrician Marvin Eiger. A nurse-LC and a nonnurse-LC provide prenatal and postpartum teaching to breastfeeding mothers. They perform an integral function in educating prospective LCs and other health care workers through regularly sponsored seminars, grand rounds, and other teaching courses. Additionally, hands-on training opportunities are offered and enable the prospective LC to gain valuable experience under supervision.

Playing Politics

In proposing a lactation program, it is essential to realize that such a service will overlap with the interests of several ongoing departments or programs. As a result, it is both politic and appropriate to involve all such departments in the early stages of the proposal process. "Touching base" and developing a working relationship with hospital decision makers is critical. Without it, any hope of establishing and maintaining a program will be seriously undermined, and the likelihood of the program becoming and remaining an integral part of the institution will remain low.

No new program will be implemented without someone in power pushing it, especially in a downsizing environment. A sponsor with "clout" is needed to lend momentum beyond the actions of the innovators and to commit resources from the

institutional budget. This person can be a high-level administrator, a chief of staff, or a department chairman. Kantor (1983) calls this individual the "prime mover" or an "idea sponsor": "prime movers push in part by repetition by mentioning the new idea or practice on every possible occasion in every speech and at every meeting."

Department heads particularly critical to securing support for the new program include the director of maternity nursing (who may oversee labor and delivery, postpartum and nursery units, and sometimes the intensive-care nursery); the director of the pediatric unit, the chairman or medical director for obstetrics and gynecology, pediatrics, and family medicine, and (in some cases) internal medicine; and the director of the emergency department. If the institution has a midwifery service, the support of its director should also be sought. Usually, department heads meet as a committee to review requests and attempt to solve problems. These committees should be approached in proposing a new lactation service (Bachman, 1987).

If the institution has an employee health department or a women's health clinic, the supervisors of such units should be informed of the proposal and asked for their support. Written proposals or documents that highlight how the new program will assist and support the services that are already being provided helps to build their acceptance. For example, the head of employee health may be particularly interested in learning that the lactation program will include services to employees, such as a special place in which employees returning to work after the birth of a baby can express milk or pump their breasts or nurse their babies during work hours (Dodgson & Duckett, 1997). The women's health service may want to know how to refer clients to the lactation service and how they can take advantage of the resources of the lactation service as it relates to information pertaining to the use of medication during lactation.

Experienced LCs who have started a lactation service point out the importance of not taking for granted that everyone knows about the service and what it offers (Williams, 1986). Being as visible as possible around the hospital helps to get the word out. The LC is a member of the staff and thus able to attend staff meetings for the departments (nursing service, family practice, pediatrics, obstetrics) in which the lactation service will have the greatest impact. In all cases, each contact and presentation must focus on the ways in which the department and institution will benefit from the service. Although improved patient care is an obvious item to mention, most hospital administrators also expect that any new service will generate income for the institution or at least pay for itself.

Hospital administrators choose new programs from dozens of new possibilities for hospital investment (e.g., another magnetic resonance imager versus a new diabetes center). Administration looks at two "bottom-line" factors—revenue and marketing potential—of proposed services before selecting which to offer. In deciding on any new health program, money speaks loudest. For example, although it appears obvious that premature infants should receive follow-up home care, it was not taken seriously by health officials until Brooten et al. (1986) at the University of Pennsylvania School of Nursing showed that postdischarge home visits for very-low-birth-weight infants could save as much as $334 million annually in the United States.

Although lactation services will generate minimal revenue compared to "high-tech" machines, such services are an effective marketing tool for the hospital. Women make most of the decisions about health care services for all family members. Health strategists claim that if the mother uses a certain hospital for her baby's birth and she likes the service she received there, she will probably use that same hospital again for the family's future health care needs. In the United States and many other developed countries, the women most likely to breastfeed are educated and in middle- to higher-income brackets; thus a lactation service increases the hospital's visibility and credibility with young, educated families who have a high earning potential. The income-generating nature of patient care makes such a service attractive, particularly in settings in which several local hospitals are competing for the same patient dollars. The new trend in hospitals is product-line management, an approach that markets a product-line of services: lactation services are a new "product" that medical centers can offer to their "customers" (Sonstegard, 1988).

Support for a lactation program must come from various areas, including nursing services, medical services (particularly family practice, internal medicine, obstetrics and gynecology, and pediatrics), and ancillary services, such as those pertaining to billing and supplies. If the health professionals running the lactation service are part of a major teaching medical center, they should have faculty status, particularly if they are expected to teach medical or nursing students (Best, 1987).

Just as the lack of physicians' support can prevent a program's being added to the array of services already offered, physicians' support can pave the way for the addition of a lactation program. Such support is most likely to be obtained if the key physicians—often chiefs of service or department heads—see that a lactation program will meet needs that they feel are important. In some cases, the need for such a service is highlighted through either a female physician's personal breastfeeding experience and subsequent greater interest and support or a male physician's spouse's experiences. In other cases, the comments of patients often highlight a need and generate the physician's initial interest in such a service.

Physicians are powerful figures in the hospital; therefore, maintaining positive relations with physicians, both staff and attending, is critical. Even with managed care, the physician as "gatekeeper" plays a major role in the fiscal health of a hospital. If the physician's patients do not want to go to a particular hospital because it lacks certain amenities, such as a lactation service, the hospital administrator, with the backing of several physicians, may choose to back such a program rather than lose patients to a competing institution in an adjoining community or even within the same city. Physicians have the influence to make or break the program, and physician support should be encouraged and nurtured. Standing orders for lactation consultations creates a ready-made demand (Shrago, 1996). Supportive physicians are more likely to be mothers who breastfed, fathers of breastfed children, those building a new practice, and those from countries in which breastfeeding is the norm.

Mothers who are satisfied with the help they received with infant feeding are very likely to stay with the physician for other aspects of care. It is advisable to get input on all important plans from the physicians who will most influence the success of the program. For example, before putting forth a breastfeeding protocol for a unit or agency, advocates are advised to distribute it to the appropriate physicians with a note asking for their input.

Some health care workers will not support lactation services; they may feel that their turf has been invaded. The best way to handle the situation is to "hang tough"–be courteous but make it clear that you intend to continue with your plans with or without their help. Health providers who are consistently antagonistic to the program usually have had a personal (negative) family experience with breastfeeding. If the resisting physician is male, chances are that his partner chose not to breastfeed or had an unhappy experience with breastfeeding.

The first several months of the existence of a lactation service, as with any new service, are usually characterized by generalized good will. The team approach, which involves several different areas within the institution, becomes important in providing continued support for the lactation service. This is particularly true if the lactation service has neither a medical director on a daily basis nor one whose reputation within the medical community is well established. Potential antagonists usually hold their tongues and bide their time; they are willing to allow the lactation-service personnel to "make a mistake." During this honeymoon period, the LC often finds that her enthusiasm carries her further than she

imagined. This experience encourages confidence that many short-term goals will be met.

After the lactation service has been in existence 9 to 18 months, unresolved problems become more noticeable. For example, if in-service programs have been provided for all areas of the hospital except the emergency room and the NICU, this lack of coverage may become an issue. At this time, antagonists to the service may begin to make their opinions known to their peers. Sometimes, this takes the form of a direct challenge to the lactation-service personnel to prove their worth, both monetarily and in terms of quality of service. Failure to support the service may take the guise of structuring the service in such a way that it cannot develop a financial base sufficient to support itself or of removing its financial or administrative underpinnings and thereby killing it (Eiger, 1991). This is particularly likely if physicians must write an order for lactation services to be provided and the physicians remain unconvinced that such a service is necessary.

Changing well-established routines is a major source of conflict between other health care workers and the lactation-service personnel, even when the change is supported by research. Because few people like to do things differently and most health professionals tend to provide service as they were taught to in medical or nursing school (Auerbach & Walburn, 1987a, b), recommendations from the LC can cause resentment and irritation among the nursing and medical staff.

When any change in protocols or routines, however small, is contemplated, the wise LC will enlist the assistance of those most likely to be affected by such change. Such preplanning can go a long way toward defusing potential antagonism and reducing resistance to change. Nearly always, this means consulting with the physicians who write orders and the nurses who are expected to carry them out. Even something so apparently insignificant as the removal of supplemental water bottles from the cribs of neonates will require meetings and discussions, often with a committee mandated to initiate the change.

In addition, in-service programs are needed to explain the change. When a team approach is used, change is more likely to be accomplished, and compliance is more likely to occur. After change is instituted, additional in-servicing is often necessary to ensure that all staff members are following the new protocol and to iron out any difficulties that may arise as the new protocol is put into effect.

The Unique Characteristics of Breastfeeding Counseling

There are unique aspects of working with breastfeeding women that differ from other areas of health care:

1. Breastfeeding is an emotion-laden subject; it may be viewed as an integral part of human sexuality, not just an infant feeding method. It touches deep-seated feelings that people have about themselves and their bodies that reach back to childhood. This makes breastfeeding counseling, like sex counseling or childbirth education, unusually sensitive. Health care workers assisting breastfeeding families must be especially intuitive, caring listeners and advisors. It was probably because of these necessary traits that the term *lactation counselor* is sometimes used.

2. Working with new mothers and babies is a popular, and thus competitive, activity. Everyone loves taking care of babies. Not only are newborns adorable but the mothers and fathers are healthy and (generally) happy. By working on the hospital maternity unit or in a birth center, the nurse gets to play a paid, starring, ongoing role in the usually joyous family dramas of birthing. As a result, nurses compete to work there, and the mother-baby unit tends to have a low rate of staff turnover. Thus introducing change in maternal care nursing may be difficult, because the same nurses continue to work in the maternity area for many years. Gardner (1978) described competition to "play the mother" as an unconscious conflict between nurses and new mothers.

3. Breastfeeding counseling is almost exclusively provided by women who must daily interact and work with other women: mothers and other female health workers. Women interact in the work place differently than men do. Awareness and understanding of the typical ways that women interact with women and

compete with each other gives the nurse or LC who comes onto the unit or into the community agency as a "new kid on the block" an advantage (Gilligan, 1982). See Table 22–2 regarding how women tend to work together and how they *need* to work together.

Three characteristics—the emotional quality of breastfeeding, the popularity of caring for babies, and the dysfunctional, covert games that women bring to the work environment—set the stage for potential difficulties between the LC and the nurse, the nurse and the breastfeeding mother, the volunteer counselor and the LC, and the female physician and the LC.

Although workplace standards of behavior tend to follow men's rules, it does not negate feminine elements. Feminine, nurturing qualities help us in working with breastfeeding families. Our best qualities have to do with becoming attached and developing close relationships and friendships with others. These attributes are critical for all health care workers, including LCs, if they are to empathize with breastfeeding mothers. However, when women personalize the business or professional setting, it is counterproductive to their professional or business goals.

Survival in the workplace requires that we learn to operate within two concurrent cultures: the culture of nurturing and caring and the culture of the profession's business, which is about accomplishing tasks efficiently. Virginia Woolf noted that the values of women differ from the values of men; yet, she added, "it is the masculine values that prevail" (Woolf, 1929). Women succeed in the workplace when they use their womanly strengths of compassion and intuitiveness in their work while playing by men's rules.

A primer entitled "How to Swim with Sharks" (Box 22–3) is offered for consideration by all those who, by virtue of their occupation, find that they must swim and that the water is sometimes infested with sharks.

Assertiveness

To be assertive is to be self-confident and to feel comfortable when presenting oneself and one's views to another (Clark, 1984). When women act

Table 22–2

WHAT WOMEN TEND TO DO AND WHAT THEY NEED TO LEARN TO DO

What Women Tend to Do	What Women Need to Learn to Do
• *Women tend to express anger covertly* behind their coworkers' backs rather than openly and confrontationally. Girls learn that they should be "nice" to everyone, not to fight, and especially not to hit anyone. These concepts are called *Mommy's Rules* (Davidson-Crews, 1989), and they are deeply embedded female behaviors, especially in white, middle-class, American women.	Be overt, not covert. If there's a problem, confront, forget, and move on.
• *Women try to avoid being criticized;* they often take it personally. Women are socialized to derive their self-worth from external, rather than internal, sources; therefore, they tend to react excessively to others' opinions, whether positive or negative. Women are more likely to hold grudges for long periods.	Communicate. Do not make scenes or public outbursts.
• *Women are less likely than men to have used the give-and-take team concept* of "you help me and I'll help you and we'll both get ahead." Women operate on a higher utopian level: what is RIGHT and JUST is more important than any other consideration. Women act as police officers of one another, making sure that what their coworker does is right and correct and "trashing" them to keep them in their place.	Be friendly, but do not strive to be close friends.
• *Women tend to become overfriendly,* one-to-one. Women who work together and become fast friends tell each other their deepest secrets, which are sometimes used against them when the friendship dissolves. Women give away power by giving away too much of themselves. Women are more likely to work for social rewards; men work for money.	Accept and love yourself. Accept (and appreciate) that some people are not your friends, now or ever.

assertively, they may be accused of being aggressive, an attack on their use of actions that would not be viewed as negative were the same tactics employed by men. Women who have been taught that it is appropriate for men to be aggressive and for women to be passive are hesitant to act assertively. The assertive person

- takes an active rather than a passive orientation toward work
- works constructively and collaboratively
- is able to give and take criticism and assistance
- deals with anxiety and fear to continue to function effectively

BOX 22–3

How to Swim with Sharks*

Swimming with sharks is like any other skill; it cannot be learned from books alone; the novice must practice in order to develop the skill. The following rules simply set forth the fundamental principles which, if followed, will make it possible to survive while becoming expert through practice.

Rule 1. *Assume unidentified fish are sharks.* Not all sharks look like sharks, and some fish that are not sharks sometimes act like sharks. Unless you have witnessed docile behavior in the presence of shed blood on more than one occasion, it is best to assume an unknown species is a shark.

Rule 2. *Do not bleed.* It is a cardinal principle that if you are injured, either by accident or by intent, you must not bleed. Experience shows that bleeding prompts an even more aggressive attack. The control of bleeding has a positive protective element for the swimmer. The shark will be confused as to whether or not his attack has injured you, and confusion is to the swimmer's advantage. On the other hand, the shark may know he has injured you and be puzzled as to why you do not bleed or show distress. This also has a profound effect on sharks. They begin questioning their own potency or, alternatively, believe the swimmer to have supernatural powers.

Rule 3. *Counter any aggression promptly.* Sharks rarely attack a swimmer without warning. Usually there is some tentative, exploratory aggressive action. It is important that the swimmer recognizes that this behavior is a prelude to an attack and takes prompt and vigorous remedial action. The appropriate countermove is a sharp blow to the nose. Almost invari-

ably this will prevent a full-scale attack, for it makes it clear that you understand the shark's intentions and are prepared to use whatever force is necessary to repel his aggressive actions. Some swimmers mistakenly believe that an ingratiating attitude will dispel an attack under these circumstances. Those who hold this erroneous view can usually be identified by their missing limb.

Rule 4. *Get out if someone is bleeding.* If a swimmer (or shark) has been injured and is bleeding, get out of the water promptly. The presence of blood and the thrashing of water will elicit aggressive behavior even in the most docile of sharks. No useful purpose is served in attempting to rescue the injured swimmer. He either will or will not survive the attack, and your intervention cannot protect him once blood has been shed.

Rule 5. *Use anticipatory retaliation.* A constant danger to the skilled swimmer is that the sharks will forget that he is skilled and may attack in error. Some sharks have notoriously poor memories in this regard. This memory loss can be prevented by a program of anticipatory retaliation. The skilled swimmer should engage in these activities periodically, and the periods should be less than the memory span of the shark. Thus, it is not possible to state fixed intervals. The procedure may need to be repeated frequently with forgetful sharks and need be done only once for sharks with total recall.

The procedure is essentially the same as described under Rule 3—a sharp blow to the nose. Here, however, the blow is unexpected and serves to remind the shark that you are both alert and unafraid. Swimmers should take care not to injure the shark and draw blood during this exercise for two reasons: First, sharks often bleed profusely, and this leads to the chaotic situation described under Rule 4. Second, if swimmers act in this fashion, it may not be possible to distinguish swimmers from sharks.

Rule 6. *Disorganize an organized attack.* Usually sharks are sufficiently self-centered that they do not act in concert against a swimmer. This lack of organization greatly reduces the risk of swimming among sharks. However, upon occasion the sharks may launch a coordinated attack upon a swimmer or even upon one of their number.

The proper strategy is diversion. Sharks can be diverted from their organized attack in one of two ways. First, sharks as a group are especially prone to internal dissension. An experienced swimmer can divert an organized attack by introducing something, often something minor or trivial, which sets the sharks to fighting among themselves. Usually by the time the internal conflict is settled, the sharks cannot even recall what they were setting about to do, much less get organized to do it.

A second mechanism of diversion is to introduce something that so enrages the members of the group that they begin to lash out in all directions, even attacking inanimate objects in their fury.

What should be introduced? Unfortunately, different things prompt internal dissension or blind fury in different groups of sharks. Here one must be experienced in dealing with a given group of sharks, for what enrages one group will pass unnoted by another.

It is unethical for a swimmer under attack by a group of sharks to counter the attack by diverting them to another swimmer. It is, however, common to see this done by novice swimmers and by sharks when they fall under a concerted attack.

---

*The author, Voltaire Cousteau, died in 1812. He is thought to be a descendant of François Voltaire and an ancestor of the late Jacques Cousteau. The essay was originally written for sponge divers but may have broader implications. It was translated from the French by Richard J. Johns, a French scholar and Massey Professor and director of the Department of Biomedical Engineers, The Johns Hopkins University and Hospital, 720 Rutland Avenue, Baltimore, MD 21205.

Assertiveness and aggressiveness are not the same thing, although many people think they are. The goal of aggressive behavior is to win, the price of which is not only negative feelings, such as humiliation and resentment, but a consequent sense of loss by all parties. Aggressive behavior is reactive and may result in an attempt to get back at the aggressor through sarcasm, defiance, passive resistance, and other behavior that does not deal with the original behavior in a straightforward manner. Assertive behavior is initiating and enables the person to participate in active learning experiences. Ultimately, such active learning supports continued assertive behavior.

Assertiveness is neither manipulative nor does it imply an uncaring attitude toward other people. When challenged, an assertive person identifies the strengths and limitations of what she has proposed. She will say "I don't know" if she doesn't have an answer to a question. She does not become

BOX 22–4

Assertiveness Scenario

Problem to be solved: Postpartum patients are becoming confused about breastfeeding because different staff members are providing conflicting information. The LC has asked for a meeting with the postpartum nursing manager (NM) to discuss the issue.

LC: I have observed some problems that are contributing to patient confusion about breastfeeding. [factual statement]

NM: What is that? [asking for information]

LC: Mrs. A, Mrs. B, and Ms. D were all told to give the baby water instead of breastfeeding during the night shift, to nurse every two hours on the morning shift, and every three to four hours on the PM shift. [additional information]

NM: Do you know who gave them that information?

LC: The charts were signed by . . . [additional information; no accusations]

NM: Do you want me to talk with them?

LC: That might be helpful. I was also wondering whether we should schedule another group of in-services and go over the basic information all the patients need to hear. [offers suggestion]

NM: Will you take responsibility for setting it up?

LC: If you can tell me what the best times would be.

NM: (laughter) Pushy, pushy. Okay, Thursday is good.

LC: (checking her calendar) That's not good for me. I have several meetings that day. Can we schedule it next week?

NM: (shutting her calendar forcefully) That's not good. We'll have to put it off until next month.

LC: I'd really prefer that we get at this problem sooner. How about next week? [focuses on the effect of the problem for them as a group]

NM: (opening her calendar again) Wednesday looks good–if you can come in a bit early to get the night shift before they leave? I'll tell their unit leader to start reports earlier than usual.

LC: (Writing times in her calendar) Sure. Thanks so much. I knew you would help to solve this problem.

---

defensive or give up in the face of such a challenge. Box 22–4 contains an example of a situation in which all parties acted assertively. In this scenario, the positive elements included

- avoiding personal attacks
- providing factual information
- asking for assistance and support in a straightforward manner

In addition, each person displayed a willingness to work around other responsibilities to produce a solution (additional in-services). The discussion focused on the need for consistent information without accusing or humiliating any staff member. The LC was not defensive when the nursing manager (NM) laughingly implied that she was "pushy." Had she done so, the discussion could have degenerated into a match of one-upping, which would have solved nothing. Assertive communication avoided antagonism, accusations, or a passive refusal. This encounter was a win-win situation for both the NM and the LC; they came to a joint agreement about the legitimacy of the problem and how best to attempt to resolve it.

Roles and Responsibilities

The LC is responsible to the mothers she sees to provide up-to-date and accurate information and appropriate assistance (Marmet & Shell, 1990). In a medical-center setting, however, such service will be molded by the other services also provided there. Said one hospital-based lactation consultant:

When I started this [job], I went through culture shock. I had been a childbirth educator and had no experience on the postpartum floor. My impression was that I'd walk in the patient's room and help with breastfeeding. I didn't expect to walk in and find babies being fed with glucose water and supplemental formula and babies being discharged without weights. I expected to learn from the nursing staff, but they either did not know about breastfeeding or did not keep up. Somehow, I thought the staff nurses would already have the theory behind the practice, but they didn't, so I had to start from square one. I have in my mind ideas of how it should be up there on the floor; I need to know more about how to validate what I do.

This LC's shock is not an uncommon experience and reinforces the importance of in-servicing health care workers in the maternal-child area of the hospital. From such an experience, as well, come the seeds of burnout, if the lactation consultant does not have a support network of people who, like herself, are knowledgeable about lactation but who may work with many people who are not.

Staff in-services on breastfeeding increase the likelihood that the staff will give breastfeeding mothers consistent breastfeeding information. According to Cohen (1987), "the patient usually takes for granted that the person they spoke to knows exactly what should be done. If confusion or controversy is found among the staff, we cannot expect the patient to become knowledgeable and comfortable with learning mother-infant tasks."

Although in-servicing is an important, perhaps even essential, role of the LC, like the proverbial horse brought to a watering hole, one can offer but not impel other health care workers to drink from the pool of knowledge. One cause of the reluctance of others to avail themselves of formal or informal in-service opportunities is the dependence of other staff members on the LC to "take care of" all breastfeeding issues. Those issues may involve highly complex problems requiring the teamwork of many individuals from an array of disciplines, or they may involve simply providing basic assistance in putting the baby on the breast and teaching basic breastfeeding information. Moreover, in a situation in which an LC is not available on all shifts or on all days, this person cannot possibly always be there. Rather than being expected to do it all, it is more effective for her to teach the staff, so that all health care workers are operating from the same frame of reference in how they assist breastfeeding mothers and when they will intervene to resolve a difficulty (Shrago, 1995).

Another function of the LC, whether she is located in a hospital or has a private practice, is to evaluate products related to lactation and to share her evaluations with others (Shrago, 1988). Evaluation of pumps and other technologies sometimes results in other benefits: assessment forms identify the special needs of the new mother or her baby (Dodgson, 1989); seeking feedback from patients ensures that quality service is being provided (Turner, 1996); and consent forms enable the breastfeeding mother to make a clear, informed choice (Bull, 1986; Kutner, 1986).

The roles of health professionals have been extensively studied and shown to progress through stages of development (Hickey et al., 1996). Benner (1984), for example, used the Dreyfus (1980) model of skill acquisition to describe the progression of skills and competencies of nurses in the clinical setting. This model, a structure for the metamorphosis that occurs as nurses persevere in their practice, can also apply to lactation consultants The stages of role acquisition according to Benner (1984) are

1. *Novice:* develops technical skills; has narrow scope of practice; needs a mentor

2. *Advanced beginner:* enhances clinical competencies; develops diagnostic reasoning and clinical decision-making skills; begins to incorporate research findings into practice

3. *Competent:* expands scope of practice; becomes competent in diagnostic reasoning and clinical skills; senses nuances; develops organizational skills

4. *Proficient:* achieves highest level of clinical expertise; conducts or directs research projects; acts as change agent; uses holistic approach; interprets nuances

5. *Expert:* global scope of practice; consults widely; empowers patients and families; serves as mentor

Benner derived these insights from the stories nurses told about their practice and applied them into a logical, orderly progression of skill development. Joel (1997, p. 7) painted a vivid picture of the journey from novice to expert.

At first we see situations as tidbits of equal significance; later we move to the idea of a highly complex integrated whole where some pieces are just more important to solving the problem. And finally, the nurse becomes as one with the clinical situation. Rather than looking from the outside in, at the zenith of your practice you are indivisible from the puzzle you are challenged to solve. You move right to the heart of the matter without responding to distraction.

Lactation consultants may also work as case managers in the maternal-child service area of a hospital or health care organization (HCO). Case management is a byproduct of managed care and

- applies during the client's entire course of pregnancy, childbearing, and early parenting, regardless of the location in which the service is provided;

- is organized around a system of interdisciplinary services and resources; and

- is coordinated by clinical and financial management of coordinators, not direct caregivers, who have a financial incentive to manage risk

and maximize the quality of care (Ethridge & Lamb, 1989).

LCs who work as case managers are responsible not only for breastfeeding but for all aspects of the educational and clinical needs of the family. The nurse case manager removes the barrier of the hospital walls (Rogers et al., 1991). Her role also benefits the managed-care company, in that she refers the family to the various services and providers that are within the managed-care health system, thus boosting their productivity and profits. At the same time, she is saving money for the HCO, because she anticipates problems before they occur and prevents the unnecessary use of resources that reduce company profits. A case in point is the common situation of uncertain new parents coming to the emergency room concerned that their infant is "not getting enough milk." In a large managed-care system, preventing this situation alone from happening would save tens of thousands of dollars. Case managers are also responsible for maintaining databases regarding individuals enrolled in the HCO and for collecting data on outcomes of care, including costs of care.

Lactation Consultants and Voluntary Counselors

The relationship between LCs and voluntary breastfeeding counselors has been discussed and debated. Gardiner et al. (1986) note that the client is apt to obtain more complete services when lactation consultants maintain a congenial, reciprocal relationship with volunteer counselors and with other health care professionals in their community.

When the volunteer counselor and the LC work together, each contributes valuable skills toward the same end: a mother's positive breastfeeding experience and her baby's optimal start in life (Table 22–3).

Because the role of the LC is new, many other health providers are unclear about what to expect of this new allied health care worker. If their experience has been with community-based voluntary breastfeeding counselors, they may assume that *lactation consultant* is simply a new title for a resource with which they may be familiar. To clarify areas of expertise that can be expected of such

Table 22–3

WAYS IN WHICH THE VOLUNTEER COUNSELOR AND THE LACTATION CONSULTANT SUPPORT THE BREASTFEEDING MOTHER

	Volunteer Counselor	Lactation Consultant
Setting	Her home Mother's home	Health care clinic Hospital Doctor's office LC's office Mother's home
Communication	Telephone	Face-to-face
Timing of contact	Prenatally After hospital discharge	Prenatally In hospital and after hospital discharge
Type of assistance	Lifestyle-oriented Mother-to-mother Ongoing follow-up Preventive	Problem-oriented Inpatient assistance Short-term Episodic
Referral	To LC, MD, other specialists	To volunteer, M.D., other specialists, including other LCs

an individual, the ILCA has developed a set of recommendations and related competencies for LC practice (Appendix H).

The volunteer counselor and the LC provide similar services. They most often differ about where such service is provided, the nature of clinical assistance, and the degree of follow-up care. For example, volunteer breastfeeding counselors are an excellent source of preventive health care information pertaining to breastfeeding and lactation. They also spend more time giving long-term assistance than does the LC, particularly if the latter sees clients in a clinic or hospital setting. It is not uncommon for a mother to continue to receive assistance and caring concern from a volunteer breastfeeding counselor through the entire lactation course; only rarely will a LC meet with a client regularly through that entire period. Instead, she is more apt to have sporadic contact, initiated by the client when a specific question or concern arises.

The LC is more apt to assist a mother when specific clinical skills are needed to assess or to resolve a problem. One recent report of mothers who sought assistance at a lactation clinic identified several factors, many related to breastfeeding initiation in hospital or early feeding practices, that may have contributed to the mothers' difficulties. Such findings can be highlighted in in-service presentations when hospital staff seek feedback regarding the recommendations they are offering or the practices they know to be routine (Mukasa, 1992).

Volunteer breastfeeding helpers and LCs can assist one another. The volunteer may have seen a certain mother in her own home and thus may be able to alert the LC working in a hospital, doctor's office, or clinic to elements about the mother's home life that may bear on her lactation course. The LC may serve as a referral source for women with complex problems. When the LC works in a medical center in which ongoing research is part of her role, she helps to generate new knowledge. Both the volunteer and the paid LC can review written materials for clients. The volunteer may be sensitive to ongoing issues that surface after the mother has left the hospital or does not choose to mention to her health care providers. The LC may be aware of aspects of the health care system that influence breastfeeding. At Via Christi Medical Center in Wichita, KS, for example, the LCs and community La Leche League leaders have an ongoing professional relationship and share information and resources.

Perhaps because their roles overlap, some LCs and some voluntary breastfeeding counselors view the other as competitors rather than as partners with the same goals (Shrago, 1995). Phillips (1990a) notes that the new LC often expects understanding and moral support from the volunteer counselors with whom she initially worked; instead, she may encounter overt or covert resentment toward her decision to take on a paid professional role after having learned much of her craft in an unpaid capacity. Rather than identifying with one another as related sources of assistance for the breastfeeding mother, both the volunteer and the paid breastfeeding specialist may choose not to work with one another, erecting barriers that contribute to additional misunderstanding (Auerbach, 1989). As Phillips (1990a) points out, each would do well to remember what other health care providers also often forget: "No one owns breastfeeding; except, properly, the mother/baby dyad."

Marketing

Marketing is a "discipline used by business to convert people's needs into profitable company opportunities" (Kotler, 1984). Marketing is still poorly understood and appreciated by health workers; either they need to learn marketing techniques themselves or seek assistance from marketing experts. Some nurse-entrepreneurs visit small-business centers at state universities, which help small-business people at no cost. Also, books on marketing are available, as are classes at various educational institutions.

Following are several basic marketing techniques that LCs may find useful:

- Collect data (demographics, attitudes) on potential clients; a marketing-research example that the LC might use as a guide is one compiled by Shamansky et al. (1985) about the attitudes of consumers toward the services of nurse practitioners.

- Analyze strengths and weaknesses of competitors and focus on service needs not currently being met.

- Establish a small niche within the health care market that is ignored by large health care providers (Tinari, 1986).

- Promote the practice by advertising and public relations: brochures, newsletters, letterhead stationery, business cards, fact sheets, and radio and TV interviews all help to inform clients and other health workers about the LC's services (Gardner & Weinrauch, 1988).

The independent health practitioner is more likely to survive if she markets her specific skills to compete with other health care professionals who are covered by health insurance. A later section of this chapter discusses what LCs themselves have to say about effective methods of marketing their services.

Networking

Networking is an established mechanism used by members of groups to exchange information, to assist others, and to get help in solving problems (Harter et al., 1987). Most people think first of networking with physicians and others from whom referrals are sought and to whom reports are sent (Williams, 1995). However, LCs also network with other lactation consultants and with volunteer breastfeeding counselors—a "good ole girl" network (Fig. 22–4). Generally, these contacts are with LCs who work in a similar setting, such as a hospital or in a private practice or with LCs who belong to city- or countywide task forces or other groups of like-minded individuals.

Networking serves several purposes. It offers people an opportunity to learn from one another. When a difficult case arises, many LCs feel more comfortable if they can use the telephone to work through the situation with another LC. Additional assessment of the problem and how to begin mov-

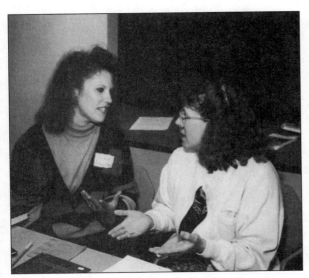

FIGURE 22–4. Making their "net" work for them, two lactation consultants share experiences. *(Courtesy Via Christi Health System.)*

ing toward a solution might offer new insights or creative alternatives to the plan of action already considered. Networking also identifies job possibilities, colleagues who will cover for others, and referrals for clients needing equipment or specialized help. Networks may also be used to change systems and to improve methods of providing care. Harter et al. (1987) described how networking connected people with information and skills in a successful breastfeeding promotion project at Ohio State University.

Opportunities to communicate with others also abound via the Internet. Foremost among these electronic offerings is LACTNET. LACTNET began with fewer than 10 LCs. In less than six months, more than 1,000 individuals were subscribing; to date, nearly 2,000 people receive the daily digests. LACTNETers represent more than 27 different countries, including every U.S. state, nearly every Australian state, and every Canadian province. Other networks have started, including one for Spanish-speaking individuals and one exclusively set up for and run by private-practice LCs. The benefit of electronic contact is ease of communication with persons for whom telephone contact would be too expensive and postal contact would be too slow. In addition, being able to vent

and obtain sympathetic electronic "clucks" within minutes or hours or to seek assistance for a troubling case supports the private LC in a way that can be duplicated only by the existence of as many knowledgeable professionals in the local area. It is the rare setting in which so many colleagues would be gathered in a single place; therefore, such electronic networking is here to stay.

In addition to e-mail discussion groups, Web pages (available through multiple linkages) also provide information about items of interest to LCs. An example is LACTNEWS On-Line, which offers updated information about conferences, educational materials, and breastfeeding courses. Exploring the Internet can take hours, and new links are created daily. For example, La Leche League International and the Nursing Mothers' Association of Australia have Web sites that describe their purpose, services, and coming events. The ability to access such disparate resources as the National Library of Medicine, Web pages created by proprietary companies, and the like means that LCs can now quite easily electronically "reach out and touch someone," or something, at any time of the day or night, by means of a computer and modem.

Reporting and Charting

It is the responsibility of the LC, regardless of where she practices, to chart each contact with her clients and to provide complete reports to referring physicians and other health care providers (Williams, 1995). Almost all record keeping involves using a computer. Computer skills are rapidly becoming a necessity for health care workers. As for other health providers, computers can be used to generate records, reports, and charts to

- provide other health workers with valuable information
- reflect quality of care delivered (quality assurance and utilization review organize care)
- highlight sometimes subtle observations or findings
- validate health services for insurance companies to determine reimbursement payment
- provide data that can be used for research
- serve as evidence in a legal dispute

In the hospital, the mother's and infant's charts are a clinical record that contains information about the hospital stay and all contacts with everyone involved in their care. Because the mother and infant usually have separate charts, it is sometimes necessary to "double-chart." At the same time, care plans tend to be geared to the mother, because it is she who is taught and the baby who is the recipient of her learning.

Nursing Diagnosis

Nursing diagnosis is a way to identify and describe problems and concerns related to breastfeeding. Nursing diagnoses validate special skills and experience, pave the way for third-party reimbursement for client care, and enhance professional autonomy. Unlike medical diagnoses based on disease groupings, nursing diagnoses are based on how the problem affects the daily life of a person; thus a nursing diagnosis is more appropriate to use for breastfeeding (Orlando, 1991).

Use of the term *nursing diagnosis* began in the 1950s. The First National Conference on the Classification of Nursing Diagnosis was held in 1973; at that time, a list of 34 diagnoses was developed. Since then, the concept has been tested, expanded, and refined and is now defined as "a clinical judgement about an individual, family, or community response to actual or potential problems or life processes that is derived through a systematic process of data collection and analysis, and provides the basis for prescription for definitive therapy for which the nurse is accountable" (Shoemaker, 1984).

The first breastfeeding diagnosis, ineffective breastfeeding, was accepted by the North American Nursing Diagnoses Association (NANDA) in 1987. Three years later in 1990, NANDA met in Orlando, FL, and adopted the nursing diagnosis effective breastfeeding (Appendix D). Gorrie (1989) suggested other nursing diagnoses that may relate to breastfeeding and lactation:

- Alteration in comfort
- Alteration in nutrition (less than body requirements)
- Anxiety
- Disturbance in self-concept
- Knowledge deficit
- Potential for infection

Methods for Charting

The most commonly used methods of charting are narrative charting and problem-oriented charting. Flow sheets and standard-care plans that are individualized are becoming more popular. They reduce paper work and save time (and money).

Narrative Charting. Narrative documentation uses a diary or story format to document client-care events. A simple paragraph describes the client's status and the care that was given. Narrative notes, sometimes called *progress notes,* are used less now, with the advent of flow sheets and clinical care plans, which capture the routine aspects of care. Narrative notes can be easily combined with flow sheets or any other client record.

An example of a narrative note follows:

Date	Time	Progress note
6/11/91	0730	**Alert, oriented, and in good spirits. Infant latches onto breast effectively. Baby breast-fed for 15 minutes until asleep.**

Problem-Oriented Charting. Charting based on a problem uses a structured problem list and logical format for each entry in the medical record. The format used in problem-oriented charting is called the *SOAP* or *SOAPIE method.* Each letter stands for a different phase of the nursing process: assessment (using subjective and objective data), plan, interventions, and evaluation of care (Box 22–5).

For the independent contractor, the completeness of reports also assists the referring health care worker to understand the hows and the whys of an LC's practice and methods. Reporting provides a database for all types of information (e.g., an increase in the number of referrals from a particular physician's practice). Early referrals may be for one or two common problems, whereas tracking over a time may show that later referrals are for a wider variety of problems.

BOX 22–5

Problem-Oriented Medical Records

S = *subjective data:* What the mother herself tells you (example: "My nipples feel sore"). (*Note:* If the charting relates to only the infant, there will be no subjective data.)

O = *objective data:* Concrete data you can observe (examples: infant position at breast, temperature, infant weight).

A = *assessment and nursing diagnosis:* An assessment of physical and psychosocial factors based on subjective and objective data; what you think is going on (examples: infant poorly positioned on the breast, breastfeeding at margin of nipple). Nursing diagnosis: ineffective breastfeeding. An alternative is ineffective suckling.

P = *plan:* Organized plan for care, based on the assessment, what you plan to do about the problem to help the breastfeeding mother and baby (example: will reposition infant on breast at next feeding).

I = *interventions:* What you have done about the problem or what you plan to do; includes teaching, referrals, finding the right pump (example: infant repositioned on mother's breast so that adequate breast tissue is being grasped by infant during suckling).

E = *evaluation:* Review of outcomes: What happened? Was it effective? (examples: infant appears to be suckling effectively at the breast; baby breastfed four times during shift, three times following repositioning, infant had bowel movement during feeding, appears well hydrated) In some cases in which a nursing care plan with diagnoses is used, evaluation may reflect only the presenting problem. Outcomes are then charted in the flow sheet.

Clinical Care Plans

A clinical care plan provides basic information about client assessment, diagnosis, and planned interventions. It also offers a guide for care, establishes a continuity of care, and represents a means of communication among all caregivers. There are two types of care plans: individual and standard. Individual care plans are developed "from scratch" for each client on the basis of her specific needs. A standard care plan is a preprinted plan of care* for a group of patients within the same diagnosis-related group (DRG)† or nursing diagnosis. Because each standard care plan must be tailored according to the needs of a particular client,

they are designed to include space for adding information.

The Joint Commission on Accreditation of Healthcare Organizations requires a care plan for each patient in the hospital as a necessity for

---

Samples of clinical records that relate to lactation and breastfeeding are found in the Lactation Consultant Series (see especially Units 3 and 8), the Journal of Human Lactation, *in the* Resource Guide *that accompanies this text, and lactation forms available from a variety of sources, such as Breastfeeding Support Consultants, the Lactation Institute, and Lactation Seminars, Inc.*

†*See glossary in the accompanying* Study Guide *for other terminologies.*

accreditation; however, the plan of care can be computer generated, preprinted, or appear in progress notes or standards of care (American Nurses Association, 1991b). Care plans are legal requirements of practice and may also serve as protocols or standards of care.

Traditionally, individual care plans are divided into three or four columns. Column headings change over the years to reflect new ideas in nursing, and some column labels are preferred over others. In this book, for instance, the clinical care plans include the heading *assessment/interventions/rationale*. Other commonly used labels are *problems/nursing goals/evaluation, nursing diagnosis/patient outcomes/nursing action,* or simply *intervention/evaluation*. The critical care path or clinical path is a new type of care plan used in hospitals. These paths are abbreviated care plans that focus on the client's length of stay in the hospital.

Legal Considerations

Whenever an LC offers advice or touches a mother or baby, she is risking a potential legal action. The action that is most likely to be brought includes battery (when a client does not consent to be touched by another person), breach of warranty (meaning that a service promised verbally or in writing is not provided); or the infliction of emotional distress (usually through a reckless, intentional, or negligent act resulting in a negative outcome, such as bodily harm of some kind (Bornmann, 1986). People usually sue health care workers not because of their clinical actions but because they are angry with them or for some other reason. Therefore, the most effective protection against such actions is establishing a mutually respectful relationship and rapport. The lactation consultant's pattern of practice should include the following standards:

1. Obtain permission (at least verbal, but preferably written) before touching the client or her infant. In different cultures, how one touches a baby may be important. For example, in some cultures, use of the left hand to do a digital assessment of the baby's mouth is a highly offensive action and would be deeply resented by the mother. One way to avoid inadvertent-

ly offending a client is to ask *whether* the baby may be touched and to explain how the baby *will* be touched before doing so.

2. Make no promise or guarantee you cannot fulfill. If the LC says she will make a home visit, such a visit should be provided. Generally, breach of warranty is considered an actionable offense when one party guarantees a particular outcome that is not forthcoming. The wise LC does not guarantee that the baby will be nursing fully on the breast, without needing other nutriment, within a specified number of breastfeeding episodes, hours, days, or weeks. Because each mother and baby is unique, as is their breastfeeding relationship, it is generally not possible to guarantee an outcome for one such couple based on the outcome of another pair. Although similarities exist among mother-baby pairs, the LC should confine her comments to encouragement, without providing a guarantee, particularly one involving a specific time or similar frame of reference.

3. Avoid causing the mother, the baby, or any other member of the client's family emotional distress as a result of words said, reports written, or other actions that reflect the LC's relationship with the mother and baby. Judicious choice of words and actions is usually sufficient to avoid this problem.

4. Maintain confidentiality about the mother, baby, and family. To fail to do so is an invasion of privacy, a tort (wrongful act) that involves confidential information that is revealed without permission to someone not entitled to know it.

A clearly written, detailed record of the health provider's actions, initial recommendations, and follow-up assistance (by phone and in person) is one of the most effective ways of avoiding legal action. Referrals increase following a well-written, complete report sent in a timely and professional manner. Client records are considered business records of the agency and are admissible as such under legal (court) rules of evidence. Records will often prevent cases from going to court; lawsuits are often won and lost on the basis of what is in the record. Although testimony is another form of evidence, the written health chart is viewed as more accurate and reliable.

The LC who works in a doctor's office, clinic, or hospital is very apt to be part of the staff who are covered in an "umbrella" professional liability policy. The LC in private practice must determine for herself how much coverage she needs and what she can afford. It is the rare LC in private practice who "goes bare" (i.e., without insurance coverage) when she works in a country where litigation is a frequent occurrence. Although legal action against an LC has not yet been reported, it could occur; therefore, every practitioner needs to consider how she will protect herself and her family against a judgment that could ruin her financially.

Reimbursements

Physicians and hospitals are major providers recognized by third-party payers. Third-party payers can be divided into three categories: private health insurance companies (e.g., Blue Cross/Blue Shield), government or public health insurance, and independent health plans (e.g., health maintenance organizations or HMOs). Reimbursement to the health care provider can be either direct or indirect. Indirect payment usually involves billing by or through a health agency or physician. Major barriers to third-party reimbursement for nonphysician health care workers have been third-party payers who fear expansion of provider eligibility, state licensure laws, and opposition by the medical profession (Caraher, 1988). The 1997 passage of a provision contained in the budget bill Public Law 105-33 to expand Medicare reimbursement for advanced-practice nurses (nurse practitioners and clinical nurse specialists) allows greater access to services of LCs who are advanced-practice nurses (American Nurses Association, 1997a).

More than 80 percent of Americans are covered by some form of medical-care insurance. Insurance policies usually spell out by title who may be reimbursed. Payment to nurses and allied health workers is usually done only under a physician's referral. Health services delivered by nurse practitioners and clinical nurse specialists (including certified nurse midwives) can often be directly reimbursed. Lactation consulting is rarely covered (Calhoun,

1993), unless it is from an advanced-practice nurse (a midwife, for example). A special claim form, the so-called lactation super-bill developed at the University of California, Los Angeles, may be helpful, because it lists procedure code numbers relating to breastfeeding and thus saves time and effort.*

In private practice, payment for services rendered or for equipment is usually requested from the client at the time of the service. The client, in turn, seeks reimbursement from the insurance company and provides the third-party payer with the needed information. If breastfeeding assistance is given as a part of routine home health care or as a postpartum visit, the employing agency usually requests the third-party reimbursement. In preparation for this edition, one of this chapter's authors surveyed nearly two dozen LCs to learn about their practice patterns and programs. The following discussion summarizes the findings from these interviews with lactation consultants practicing in various settings.

The LC in Hospital-Based Practice

The hospital-based LC often creates her own position when hospital administrative personnel respond to patient demands for lactation services. Most LCs working in hospitals develop a plan for providing lactation services and then present a proposal to administration for approval.

Most hospital-based programs surveyed had been in existence for four or five years and employed two or three LCs who mostly worked part time. Thus one must measure full-time equivalent (FTE) hours to determine the completeness of coverage. For example, in one hospital, three part-time LCs shared seven-day-per-week coverage. In all programs surveyed, the primary job requirement was certification by the IBLCE.

Not all of the LCs working in the hospital were paid nurses; half provided care for breastfeeding mothers as volunteers. Of those who were nurses, several mentioned that their nursing education was not what they relied on in their work. When income was generated from inpatient care, it was

---

* *"Lactation super-bills" may be ordered from UCLA Lactation Alumni Association, 2021 Grismer, #17, Burbank, CA 91504. Fax: 818-848-2882.*

managed through the regular accounting or finance office and submitted for insurance coverage, as occurs for other hospital-based charges.

Hospital size did not predict the existence of a lactation program. The range of births per year in each institution was broad: 750 to 15,000, although most hospitals had 1,500 to 2,000 births annually. Warmer months were busier than were the cooler months. The most comprehensive programs had personnel providing varied care 85 to 90 hours per week:

- One-to-one rounds of new mothers and babies seven days a week, including holidays
- Primary visits in the NICU, pediatric unit, and medical and surgical floors
- Breastfeeding classes as part of the childbirth-education program
- Inpatient consultations
- Outpatient consultations
- Rental and sale of breast pumps and other devices
- Phone assistance and "warm-milk lines"
- An employee pumping station
- Regular in-services for staff
- Self-instructional learning packet for staff
- Networking opportunities with the volunteer breastfeeding support groups in the community.

Many LCs who are employed in a hospital also volunteer additional time in an effort to meet patient needs—time for which they are unpaid, time that is not recognized as part of the effort of making an LC program a going concern. Almost all of the hospitals charged for some lactation services, especially if special consults were involved.

Lactation services are usually provided in a single room serving as the home base for telephone follow-up, inpatient services, and record keeping, and as a site for professional resources. LCs also saw mothers in an empty patient room for those women who returned for outpatient care. Although many in-hospital programs had outpatient services as a result of patient expectations or requests, few provided home visits.

The most frequently mentioned positive outcomes of a hospital-based lactation program were more positive physician support for breastfeeding, more consistent assistance for breastfeeding mothers by nonphysician hospital personnel, and increased community support for the hospital.

The most difficult hurdle was obtaining continued funding of the program, followed by resistance to change by key hospital personnel, and "dumping" all breastfeeding patients on the LC, thus creating overload and burnout. The respondents often felt thwarted by being asked to do too much in too little time with too few personnel. Then why choose to work in the hospital? Said one, "I love working with mothers and the institution—seeing the changes that I have envisioned come about is quite rewarding. I suggested a comprehensive lactation center more than 10 years ago and was quite thoroughly rebuffed. Now our center is considered a great idea."

Although many hospitals now provide in-hospital care and some have expanded to provide outpatient care as well, a few also offer home visits. Most private LCs see mothers both in their own homes and in the office. Therefore, it behooves LCs in different settings to see how they might work together, providing a coordinated package of care or making appropriate referrals to ensure ongoing care or follow-up assistance when it is necessary. For example, if the LC in the hospital sees a mother whose baby has difficulty latching onto the breast, that person might benefit from follow-up on hospital discharge from an LC in the community who is informed of these early difficulties. Referral to the community LC would then generate a report to the hospital LC. In this way, the hospital-based LC is better able to anticipate what to suggest to another mother in the hospital whose baby presents with a similar difficulty. At the same time, the hospital-based LC learns which private practice LCs are most skilled in helping mothers with particular difficulties.

The LC in Private Practice

Driven by managed care, nurses, LCs, and other health care providers are offering alternative services to meet the demands of a population needing more care outside the hospital setting. LCs set up

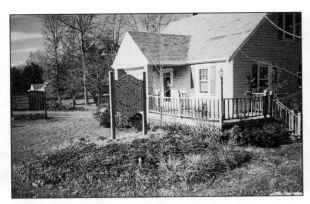

FIGURE 22–5. One free-standing lactation consultant clinic whose sign invites mothers to obtain help there. *(With permission from Jane Bradshaw.)*

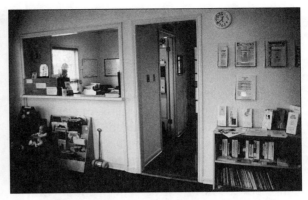

FIGURE 22–6. The lobby and products area of a lactation consultant office is both welcoming and a place in which business is conducted. *(With permission from Barbara Wilson-Clay.)*

and operate practices in various ways. The LCs in private practice who were surveyed for information about their experiences lived in a variety of settings: rural, suburban, medium to large cities, and major metropolitan areas in Canada and all across the United States–the Atlantic and Pacific coasts, the South, northern states, and the Midwest–and two in countries outside North America. Most had been in practice for an average of seven years. More than two-thirds of these women had served in a volunteer breastfeeding support capacity, most as La Leche League leaders, prior to opening their private practice. The remainder indicated that they began helping breastfeeding mothers as part of their professional nursing role. One LC reported, "In the early days, [other people] laughed. 'Who needs credentials to help with breastfeeding?!' Now the local hospitals will only hire lactation consultants who are certified by IBLCE. It [certification] has become more important."

Most of these LCs began their practices with offices in their homes; however, one-fourth now maintain office space in commercial settings (Figs. 22–5, 22–6). Of those LCs who have secured space outside their homes, all had been in private practice for at least seven years. Of those practicing from their homes, most devote one room to their business. The majority would prefer a separate entrance to this space, to make a clearer distinction between home space and work space, between activities relating to their children and home behaviors and to those relating to their world of work.

Women who used their homes as a business site tended not to have employees other than themselves. Of those who did, the additional person usually managed rental and pump deliveries, answered the phone when the LC was seeing a mother, and handled filing and other paperwork. Private-practice LCs with offices external to their homes were more likely to hire assistants. These individuals not only took care of the aforementioned chores but often served as receptionist-assistants, taught classes or led support groups, and sometimes also provided phone assistance. It was rare for the LC in private practice in her home to have incorporated her business; by contrast, those in external offices were more likely to have incorporated, often on the advice of an attorney or accountant. Partnerships tended to be loose rather than governed by a legal contract. Most typical is providing coverage for one another when one person is out of town, rather than sharing the same office space and clientele.

Most of these private-practice LCs reported that they worked four to five hours per day, qualifying for part-time status when seeking professional liability coverage, which all maintained. The number of clients seen in a given week or month varied widely and was related to several factors, including how long the LC had been in practice, whether she limited herself to home visits (more time-consuming and thus less frequent), and whether her practice was located in a rural or more densely populated metropolitan area.

Where did these LCs get their clients? In descending order of frequency, they listed women who self-referred (100 percent); other mothers who had used the service (95 percent); referral from local physicians (86 percent) or from the local hospital (81 percent); from other LCs, childbirth educators, prenatal breastfeeding classes taught by the LC, or from volunteer breastfeeding groups in the community (67 percent each); from nurses in doctor's offices (62 percent); from nurses or midwives in the hospital (57 percent); and from prenatal childbirth classes (33 percent), among others. Practices in existence for only two to three years reported seeing the fewest number of clients, reflecting how practices grow over time as one satisfied customer makes referrals to her friends, relatives, and colleagues.

Some LCs started by opening a breast-pump rental depot. Others set up a private practice after receiving numerous calls from mothers who requested their help with breastfeeding. Several LCs who had been hospital nurses wanted to do more to help breastfeeding mothers than could be accomplished in the hospital. Still others found that a private practice in lactation consulting was an extension of their previous work as volunteer La Leche League leaders.

Many of these women noted a gap in service between hospital discharge and the first well-baby check-up. For one LC, the poor quality of the local hospital's breast-pump rental service motivated her to set up a pump-rental depot, out of which developed a full-service practice (see Fig. 22–3). Most of the private-practice LCs rent or sell breast pumps. The number of breast pumps carried ranges from 3 to more than 100. In some cases, breast-pump rental income represents a substantial percentage of their income. Finally, those women with growing children at home found that a lactation consultant practice—particularly when it was conducted from the LC's home—offered an ideal way to provide income and meet family needs.

Most of the LCs interviewed recommended that the practice should be located in her own home if a room could be devoted exclusively to her practice. Such a space carries with it a minimum of overhead and financial outlay; however, the U.S. Internal Revenue Service (IRS) will not allow a tax deduction on this space (including utilities, rent or mortgage, and cleaning fees) unless the room is used exclusively for business. Seeing clients in the living room, storing files in the bedroom closet, answering the phone in the kitchen, and keeping breast pumps in the basement does not a home business make—at least in the eyes of the IRS.

If the LC plans to obtain a business loan, the cost of renting commercial space has to be a factor in determining the size of the loan. One LC who still dreams of a practice location outside her home said, "If I had to do it over again, I would bite the bullet and go for commercial property right from the beginning. I think it reflects on one's professionalism." Another LC, with an office in a commercial setting, noted that physicians and others viewed her as a professional much more than they had when her office was in her home; her business has grown since she moved out of her home. Still another practitioner with an office in a building she purchased found that the overhead became too much after so much competition was introduced in her area that she returned to offering home visits and working from her home to turn a profit. The same difficulties that assail any business can also make a nightmare of a lactation-consulting business.

Secondary to the LC's own home, the next best beginning location may be space in a clinic, physician's office, or hospital where the LC receives referrals from the staff members of these organizations. A location that is easy to find and reach is another factor if clients are to frequent the LC in private practice. Some residential neighborhoods have restrictive covenants that prevent home business or signage that a business is located in a home. A post office box for an address avoids neighborhood zoning restrictions. These details must be checked in advance of opening such a facility. Inadequate road signs in suburban settings or in rural areas will make maps on the backs of flyers and other advertisements a necessity. In North American practices, busy periods clustered in March, April, and May, reflecting the higher birth rates during the warmer months, whereas slower periods tended to occur in November, December, and January.

The commitment of the clientele is another important consideration in job satisfaction. As one LC bluntly put it,

If you are working in private practice or with a physician's office, you will be working with patients who have already decided to breastfeed. This is much less likely in the hospital; there is something to be said for not having to beat your head against the wall every day working with mothers who say they will 'try' and then don't even do that.

In spite of this, most stated that they went into the business to help others and that this orientation kept them going through even the roughest periods.

The Business of Doing Business

One of the hardest lessons for a new LC to learn is that a private practice is a business; if she has no business experience, she must learn about it (Auerbach, 1995). Advertising is essential in establishing and maintaining a client pool. Generally, the best advertising is word-of-mouth referral from clients who are satisfied with the LC's services. Other successful advertising includes distributing business cards and flyers and sending personal letters to hospital staff, local physicians (pediatricians, family physicians, obstetricians), community women's groups, childbirth educators, and La Leche League leaders. Teaching a prenatal breastfeeding class is a form of advertising. At the same time, the LC has to make it clear that she charges for later visits. Additional techniques include listings in the telephone book (white or yellow pages), newspaper articles, and press releases for new activities or special events relating to the business.

Lactation consultants disagree about whether to advertise in local newspapers or on the radio. Several people said that such visibility "attracts the crazies." Newspaper articles, radio, or television interviews may provide name recognition, but they rarely result in generating clients. The choice of words in advertisements or signs should be considered carefully. In one case, an LC posted a large sign with her name but not the words *breast* or *lactation* to alert passersby to her business. Said she, "The sign advertising your service must fit the place where you work. In my community, it would not be wise for me to advertise my services using the word *breast*. I chose the name of my practice very carefully with this in mind." Using family-, parenting-, or mother-related phrases works well in lieu of more obvious words. In other communities, inclusion of the words *breastfeeding* or *breast* may not be controversial.

More effective marketing techniques include meeting face-to-face with local physicians, their office staff, and hospital nurse managers and attending professional meetings, such as hospital grand rounds and continuing-education programs for nurses. See Box 22–6 for ways to generate referrals. Presenting a case history to hospital physicians, midwives, doulas, childbirth educators, and other health providers raises the visibility of the LC practice and generates referrals.

Incorporating the private practice should be considered only after carefully reviewing the advantages and disadvantages (Box 22–7). A list of resources that apply to incorporation and other business considerations of private practice is included in the bibliography at the end of this chapter.

Lactation consultants harbor a strong streak of idealism. Although they may need to run their business as a business, all those surveyed said that they have, on occasion, refrained from charging a client for their services when it was clear that the client could not pay. In every case, the LC provided the services in a spirit of goodwill, either forgoing even writing a bill or writing it off after the client left. Some LCs have established an informal sliding scale to assist people for whom a total payment at the time of service is not possible. One LC noted that she has received payment as much as 18 months after the service was provided; others reported that only rarely are their bills not paid. Most people prefer to pay something rather than nothing. Even when clients pay only a very small amount for the care they receive, they are more inclined to follow through with the suggestions that the LC has offered. The average length of time LCs are in business before they are no longer putting all of their profits back into the practice is three years.

Those LCs in business the longest were not necessarily making the most money, and several reported sustaining a loss. Two major factors in losing income were competing with discount stores for sale of breast pumps and new LC practices. Another factor is how hard you want to work. One LC noted that she would have been earning a

BOX 22–6

Ways to Generate Referrals

METHOD	TARGET AUDIENCE
Teach a prenatal breastfeeding class	Mothers
One-to-one contacts	Physicians
	Hospital nurses
	Perinatal educators
	Postpartum and nursery managers
	Physicians' office nurses
A flyer describing the LC service	Anyone who is unfamiliar with what an LC does
Contacts with community groups geared to new, inexperienced mothers	Future referral sources
Informal relationships with physicians (or their spouses) who have had new babies and want to breastfeed	A satisfied customer is often the best advertisement
Providing pump rentals (use free advertising often provided by the company)	Such referrals may generate other nonpump business
Displays at baby fairs, community activities	The community unfamiliar with the services of an LC

profit sooner had she not limited the number of clients she sees.

In nearly all cases, those practices seeing the greatest number of clients also had free-standing sites. Most clients paid in full for their visits by cash or check at the time of service; only about one-third of these practices offered a payment option by credit card. About one-third reported having received insurance coverage for some portion or all of their client's bills. The most frequently mentioned U.S. national insurance company for which payment for LC services was covered was Aetna. Most offered a payment plan for those who could not pay in full at the time of the visit, and many had accepted in-kind payment, such as printing of brochures, in exchange for LC services.

Another aspect of doing business is setting fees. This issue seems to generate the greatest concern when LCs first go into practice. Anxiety about how much to charge for their services may stem from having been a volunteer breastfeeding support person for many years and coming to value the helping relationships with the mothers without thinking of charging for the service. This problem is not confined to LCs. Women tend to be reluctant to charge what their services are worth. This undervaluing of skills or services is part of a woman's socialization when she is growing up. In addition, lack of familiarity with running a business results in undervaluing the service provided.

The prospective private-practice LC needs to set her fees on the basis of what other comparable

---

BOX 22–7

Advantages and Disadvantages of Incorporation

Advantages

- Life of the business is perpetual.
- Stockholders have a limited liability.
- Ownership transfer is easy.
- It is easy to raise capital and expand.
- Efficiency of management is maintained.
- The corporation is a legal entity.
- Possible tax advantages may be found.
- A corporation is adaptable to both small and large businesses.
- Other professionals may view the corporation as a sign that the business is a business rather than a "toy."

Disadvantages

- It is closely regulated and subject to many state and federal controls.
- It is more difficult and more expensive to organize.
- The corporate charter restricts the type of business activity one engages in.
- Extensive record keeping is necessary.
- Double taxation may apply.

---

professionals in her community are charging for similar services (e.g., other LCs in private practice, nurses who make home health visits, and pediatricians who make house calls). Another factor to consider in setting fees is the length of visits. Although well-baby visits to a physician's office may last only 15 to 20 minutes, the usual first LC visit may run 60 to 90 minutes. If the visits take place in the mother's home, travel time is included: one LC adds one hour to account for travel time to and from the client's home when she bills for the visit. Still others charge a set fee for the number of miles or kilometers they travel to provide a home visit in addition to their usual visit fee. In doing so, it is important to carry all the tools one might have at one's fingertips if the client came to the office (Hatcher, 1994).

Nearly all of the LCs surveyed have raised their fees since first going into business, which helps to keep the number of clients to a reasonable level and to take inflation into account. Saturdays and Sunday visits are sometimes charged at double the usual rate, which reduces the number of clients asking to be seen on Sunday.

Phone consultations also should be considered in establishing a fee structure. Some LCs do not charge for phone consultations at all, preferring instead to limit calls to no more than 10 minutes. If more time is needed, they suggest that a visit for which they will be paid is in order. LCs bill differently for phone consultations. Some bill for a specific amount of time within a set framework, such as up to one hour of calls within a week after the first visit. Others bill for each call separately. Still others provide free phone consultation for minor issues.

Collaboration with Other Health Care Workers

Lactation consultants are most successful when they have an ongoing, mutually respectful relationship with physicians and nurses in the community who refer clients to them. The physicians may also act as mentors and are invaluable in helping the LC to understand medical problems that occur in breastfeeding families.

In some cases, clinics and physicians' offices serve as a point of distribution for an LC's flyers or business cards. In other cases, office staff give this information to the physician's patients. Other referral sites are childbirth-education classes, midwifery practices and obstetrics-gynecology offices, where LCs may teach prenatal breastfeeding classes. Relationships with physicians have established rules, one of which is that if a baby is thought to have a medical problem, before proceeding with lactation assistance, the LC refers the family to their baby's own pediatrician or family physician. One lactation consultant cautioned, "Never take responsibility that is beyond your expertise. Always counsel mothers to go back to their doctor to resolve a medical problem." When in doubt, LCs often call the physician to inquire about medical concerns while the mother and baby are in the LC's office.

If the family does not have an attending physician, the lactation consultant has the responsibility of referring them to a reputable care provider who is knowledgeable about breastfeeding. Some LCs require that the baby be under a physician's care before they will offer their services. Such a requirement ensures that any medical problems can be referred. It also offers a measure of legal protection for the LC against a charge that she is practicing medicine without a license. Referral is usually to a physician with whom the LC has a collaborative, trusting relationship. Said one LC, "I'm not a doctor and I'm not interested in being a doctor. I market myself as a breastfeeding management consultant, working with mother and baby and how they go together. Most problems I see aren't medical. I refer her back to her doctor or her baby's doctor if I spot something that is beyond my expertise to handle." Another LC reported that the next most frequent referral after the pediatrician-family physician is to a psychologist or psychiatrist who specializes in helping women with postpartum depression. She also encourages every private-practice LC to know about local crisis hotlines in her community and to be prepared to refer women to them.

Essential to developing a professional reputation and high ethical standards is sending a written report to the referring physician or calling the physician after the patient has been seen. Referrals increase following a well-written, complete report sent in a timely and professional manner (Williams, 1995).

Being a professional requires that the lactation consultant present herself professionally: in her demeanor, the clothing she wears, the reports she writes, and the phone calls she makes. The professional LC knows her potential client population and how the professional system works in her area. "Don't go barging in there expecting to change things instantaneously," warned one LC. "Otherwise, you will speak to brick walls. When you offer services, do it professionally. Do what you do well; that establishes your reputation. The referrals will follow."

Partnerships

Partnerships vary in how they are structured. In some cases, each partner sees all clients, and income that is generated is shared equally. In other practices, each partner maintains her own client group. Covering for a partner when the other's duties take precedence or the LC is out of town is automatic, as long as the partner is available. Going into a partnership requires that each LC be clear about what she wants from the arrangement at the outset. Complementary ways of working are a plus; it is not necessary for each partner to be a "clone" of the other. However, when very different philosophies exist about how to provide client services, conflicts that cannot be resolved are more likely to arise. Like a marriage, a partnership has its high and low points, and several LCs reported that conflict between partners was particularly difficult. "Getting a partner doesn't always solve problems. Sometimes, partners can simply create a whole new set of problems." Still another wrote that she had ended her partnership because too many conflicts cut into the ability of each to meet their clients' needs. Box 22–8 describes the pros and cons of partnerships.

Private practice is clearly not something for every lactation consultant to consider. However, those who have done so and weathered the first five years report that it can provide rewards that are rarely found in another occupation. The independence, which is most frightening to persons who are used to a guaranteed salary and set

BOX 22–8

Solo Practice Versus Partnerships: Advantages and Disadvantages

SOLO PRACTICE

Advantages

- Simple to organize
- Low start-up costs
- Relative freedom from regulation
- Direct control by owner
- Owner free to make all decisions
- Minimal working-capital requirements
- Possible tax advantages for the small-business owner
- All profits to the owner
- Easy to dissolve

Disadvantages

- Unlimited liability
- Necessity to arrange for coverage when out of town
- Skills limited to those of the solo practitioner
- Possibly difficult to raise capital

PARTNERSHIPS

Advantages

- Easy to organize
- Low start-up costs
- Greater financial strength
- Broader management base
- Additional sources of venture capital
- Combines managerial skills and judgments
- A legally recognized business entity
- Equal partner interest in the business
- Possible tax advantages
- Limited outside regulation
- Time off possible without closing the business
- Ongoing networking

Disadvantages

- Unlimited liability
- Lack of authority for individual decision making
- Difficulty in raising additional capital
- Difficulty in finding a suitable partner
- Disagreements about workload, responsibility, income
- Need for coordinating time-off activities

Source: Derived in part from materials devised by Janet N. Repucci and Jacki R. Shina, Cofounders, Galatea Lactation Consultants, 1989.

working hours, also offers an opportunity to structure one's work in a way that may allow family involvement that is simply not possible otherwise.

Burnout

Failure to control an increase in demand for services can lead to burnout. Although restructuring work can guard against burnout, the LC may need to sit down with someone who has a sympathetic and objective ear and make decisions about how many clients she can comfortably handle in a given space of time—and refuse to take on more. In some cases, LCs reported that changes in the needs of their families often contributed to a sense of running in place even while the work piled up. (See Box 22–9 for burnout symptoms.)

Because advertising influences growth, one LC suggested limiting advertising so as to be able to handle the influx of patients that advertising

BOX 22–9

Symptoms of Burnout, Why It Occurs, and Ways to Avoid It

Symptoms of Burnout

- You are always thinking of the problems you are encountering.
- You are (more) accident-prone (than usual).
- You are (or feel) disorganized.
- You are unable to get things done, unable to make decisions.
- You are unable to sleep.
- You feel cynical, depressed, disappointed, disinterested, drained, emotional, exhausted, frustrated, helpless, inadequate, lethargic, overloaded, overwhelmed, resentful, tired, and unappreciated.
- You feel that everyone is against you.

Why (or When) Burnout Occurs

- At your work site, there is inadequate continuity of care, lack of debriefing among colleagues, lack of help and support, and lack of motivation to help one another.
- Attitudes of others toward you (or your work) are not supportive.
- Others expect you to solve all breastfeeding problems.
- The level of complexity of the work has heightened.
- The mothers you care for seem to be too dependent on you.
- There is inadequate funding to support your position.
- There is no balance between work and play.
- You are assuming responsibilities that belong to others.
- You are engaged in emotionally demanding work.

- You are experiencing conflicts between family and work roles.
- You are not seeing your goals realized.
- You are unable or unwilling to delegate responsibilities to others.
- You are unable to say no.
- You feel isolated.
- You encounter ongoing WHO Code breaches in the care offered at your work site.
- You feel that no one else can do the job as well as you can.
- You feel that there is too much work to do.
- You feel pressure to provide quick resolution to all problems.
- You (or others) feel that your work is never quite good enough.
- You have unrealistic expectations of yourself.
- You have unresolved personal issues.
- You receive no formal recognition as an LC.
- You receive no thanks or appreciation for what you do.

How to Avoid Burnout

- Acknowledge your limitations.
- Attempt to achieve balance in all that you do.
- Attend breastfeeding conferences and seminars; they will buoy your spirits, teach you new skills, affirm what you already know, and enable you to network with like-minded individuals.
- Attend meetings to discuss local concerns.
- Be good to yourself with healthful food, rest, exercise, meditation, fun, massage, and adequate sleep.

- Manage your workload by pacing yourself and referring to colleagues.
- Delegate responsibilities.
- Establish clear boundaries regarding what you can and cannot do, will and will not do.
- Find a mentor.
- Focus on the magic of the moment.
- Keep a diary; write down frustrations and clarify your thoughts and feelings.
- Learn to say no.
- Learn to say "I don't know."
- Learn to let go of the problem.
- Make a list of what needs to be done, however small.
- Network with others in the field.
- Pause between activities, assess your performance, and praise yourself for what you have achieved.
- Prioritize your activities.
- Love and appreciate yourself.
- Set goals and know where you are heading (i.e., have a vision).
- Set time for your family and your partner.
- Set time for yourself to do something that reduces stress.
- Treat everyone you meet as you would like to be treated.
- Try not to assume guilt for something that you cannot control.

Source: Derived from Ellen McIntyre, unpublished presentation at New Zealand Lactation Consultant's Association Conference, Christ Church, New Zealand, March 1996.

generates. "Be realistic about the time you have to give and your other responsibilities and commitments. Don't expect too much; there is no way to know how quickly your practice will build."

Going slowly reduces burnout. One LC's recommendation was, "Don't feel like you are the breastfeeding 'goddess' of the community, the only one who can make or break a particular situation. Empower the mother and let her take over her experience. Burnout comes from trying to 'own' the situation." Advised another, "Lay the groundwork of your practice with an eye to the future. Try not to grow too quickly without realizing the implications, and complete the [paperwork] before you deposit the check." Still other LCs have attempted to reduce the risk of burnout by going into partnership with one or more LCs or by limiting their practice to a specialized area. They refer some cases to nearby LCs who, in turn, refer more complicated cases to the LC who has chosen to specialize.

Given the difficulties just mentioned, what do these lactation consultants advise others regarding pitfalls? Nearly all the LCs, in one way or another, urged tempering enthusiasm with an acceptance of reality and being willing to accept very slow change. One LC noted that after several years, her state now has a breastfeeding task force that meets regularly. "This snail is jogging. You have to be happy with tiny incremental improvements." Avoiding being thought of as radical was also mentioned. To illustrate her point, one LC said, "Don't use cabbage leaves to reduce engorgement on someone you've never seen before—even when you know it has worked for other mothers in similar circumstances."

Do's and Don'ts of Lactation Consulting

People already in the field are the best sources of information on what others entering the field should know. Box 22–10 lists do's and don'ts suggested by LCs in practice—either when establishing a private practice or when initiating an office-, clinic-, or hospital-based LC service.

BOX 22–10

Do's and Don'ts of Lactation Consulting

Do . . .

- Insist on gaining credibility for the profession by passing the IBLCE examination. Ensure that people know this is the minimum credential for any person practicing as an LC in the community.
- From the very first client, behave with the utmost professionalism.
- Charge what you are worth; do not apologize for your fees.
- Set limits immediately, so that people know the boundaries of your availability. Know your own knowledge and skills boundaries. Do not be afraid to ask for help.
- Develop a network of LCs in the community; they can serve as a sounding board for problem situations and as backup when you are not available.
- Avoid repeating problems other LCs have experienced by learning from those with more experience than you have.
- Know what you are doing if you rent or sell equipment. Learn how the equipment works and who should and shouldn't use it. Be aware that its availability from you may influence what you tell a client to do.
- Be aware of the marketing of artificial formula and what makes it attractive to mothers. Says one LC, "Don't let the medical folklore interfere with mothers' decisions to breastfeed; go armed with the facts."
- Learn how to use a computer, recommends another LC, "It can be a godsend, not just for working up practice notes, but also for maintaining the business end of things."
- Learn as much as possible about running a business. It takes years to break even. Be prepared for that.
- Get a competent business advisor for accounting, marketing, and taxes. Ensure that those advisors understand exactly what you are trying to do.
- Bill the client directly for the service. The client then files a claim to her insurance company. Use a "lactation super-bill," standard forms for billing, and a letter that the client can use to seek insurance coverage.
- Develop a specialization within the field. Said one LC who has established induced lactation as her specialty area, "Get very good at what you do. This will help you build a reputation for good care."
- Always document what you have done and send the original to the primary care provider, whether or not this individual made the initial referral. Such documentation can help to legitimize the service, particularly when repeated problems are resolved to the client's satisfaction and when references supporting care provided are shared with the primary care provider.
- Recognize that this business is a labor of love. Do not expect to get rich. Often the biggest competition is the grocery store that sells artificial baby milk.

Don't . . .

- Don't make rounds at a hospital by announcing that you are the LC without having first obtained permission to see the client through the powers that be in that hospital.
- Don't get heavily involved in phone consultations, paid or unpaid. You are on shaky ground legally giving out such advice without having seen the mother and baby. Often the information may not be accurate. Also, such information is usually incomplete without an overall assessment.
- Don't give away your time without reimbursement.
- Don't waste your money on a lot of expensive advertising. Advertise judiciously and be patient. Put everything you make back into the business for the first two years.
- Don't give away free advice with breast pump or other equipment rentals; this sets a poor precedent for obtaining fees for other services.

- Don't use someone else's opinion as a reason for doing something. Experiment; be creative. What works in one practice may not work in another one.
- Don't begin a private practice if you are working full time elsewhere. Your availability is important; if you aren't available, your practice won't grow.
- Don't get too many partners at the beginning. Knowing how each partner works as an individual will not necessarily predict how each works as part of a group. The more partners one has, the greater the number of problems that can arise. One LC laughingly posed the following rhetorical question: "Would you take on more than one husband at the same time?"
- Never forget that a happy mother and thriving baby are your best advertisements–and apt to generate more referrals than anything else.
- Don't forget to document what you have done with a mother; send the original form with this information on it to the primary care provider.

SUMMARY

The field of lactation as a health care specialty has grown rapidly in recent years. The opportunity to work with healthy families and adorable babies and to enhance early parenting and child health has made it a popular, satisfying field. Although growth is welcomed, rapid growth causes growing pains. Some health professionals feel threatened by the emergence of new practitioners who expect to share their turf.

The experiences of the lactation consultant in this decade are similar to those of the childbirth educator in the 1960s and 1970s. Then it was the childbirth educator who was the innovator and change agent who flew against the prevailing wind and traditional practices in birthing. These two disciplines share more than a common history: both empower mothers and act as change agents for women and for families during an age in which technology and defensive medicine rule medical practice.

Those working with breastfeeding families cannot expect to become wealthy. However, they reap the reward of personal fulfillment as they assist other women in becoming empowered by their own breastfeeding experiences. This outcome has no price.

REFERENCES

American Nurses Association: ANA hails passage of Medicare reimbursement. *Am Nurse* 1997a:11.

American Nurses Association: Has JCAHO eliminated care plans? *Am Nurse* 1991b:6.

Anderson E, Geden E: Nurses' knowledge of breastfeeding. *JOGNN* 20:58–64, 1991.

Auerbach KG: Record-keeping: making the business end of doing business work for you. *J Hum Lact* 11:220–1, 1995.

Auerbach KG: A we/they dichotomy [editorial]. *J Hum Lact* 5:121, 1989.

Auerbach KG, Walburn J: Nebraska family practitioners' infant feeding recommendations. *Fam Pract Res J* 6:189–99, 1987a.

Auerbach KG, Walburn J: Nebraska physicians' infant feeding recommendations. *Neb Med J* 72:168–74, 1987b.

Bachman MC: The lactation consultant in a hospital setting. *J Hum Lact* 3:104–5, 1987.

Benner P: *From novice to expert: Excellence and power in clinical nursing practice.* Menlo Park, CA: Addison-Wesley, 1984.

Best LJ: An option for LCs–adjunct staff member status. *J Hum Lact* 3:157–9, 1987.

Bornmann PG: *Legal considerations and the lactation consultant–USA,* Unit 3 (Lactation Consultant Series). Garden City Park, NY: Avery Publishing, 1986.

Brooten D, et al: A randomized clinical trial of early hospital discharge and home follow-up of very-low-weight infants. *N Engl J Med* 315:934–9, 1986.

Bull P: Consent form to supplement newborns. *J Hum Lact* 2:27–8, 1986.

Calhoun DM: Applying for provider status with insurance companies. *J Hum Lact* 9:41–2, 1993.

Caraher MT: The importance of third-party reimbursement for NPs. *Nurse Pract* 13:50–4, 1988.

Clark CC: Assertiveness issues for nursing administrators and managers. In: Stone S, et al. *Management for nursing: a multidisciplinary approach.* St Louis: Mosby, 1984:74–5.

Cohen SP: High tech-soft touch: breastfeeding issues. *Clin Perinatol* 4:187–96, 1987.

Davidson-Crews E: Women working with women [seminar]. St. Joseph Medical Center, Wichita, KS, August 11, 1989.

Dodgson J: Early identification of potential breastfeeding problems. *J Hum Lact* 5:80–1, 1989.

Dodgson JE, Duckett L: Breastfeeding in the workplace: building a support program for nursing mothers. *AAOHN J* 45:290–8, 1997.

Dreyfus SE, Dreyfus HO: *A five-stage model of the mental activities involved in directed skill acquisition* (USAF Contract No. F49620-79-C-0063). Berkeley, CA: University of California, 1980.

Dublin P: Options for lactation consultants: the public health arena. *J Hum Lact* 5:19–20, 1989.

Eiger MS: "For one brief shining moment . . ." [editorial]. *J Hum Lact* 7:169–70, 1991.

Ethridge P, Lamb G: Professional nursing case management improves quality access and cost. *Nurs Manage* 20:30–5, 1989.

Freed GL, et al: Methods and outcomes of breastfeeding instruction for nursing students. *J Hum Lact* 12:105–10, 1996.

Gardiner J, et al: *Relationships and roles: the lactation consultant and lay breastfeeding groups,* Unit 7 (Lactation Consultant Series). Garden City Park, NY: Avery Publishing, 1986:6–8.

Gardner KL, Weinrauch D: Marketing strategies for nurse entrepreneurs. *Nurse Pract* 13:46–9, 1988.

Gardner SL: Mothering: the unconscious conflict between nurses and new mothers. *Keep Abreast J* 3:193–205, 1978.

Gerrard JW: Breast-feeding: should it be recommended? *Can Med Assoc J* 113:138–9, 1975.

Gilligan C: *In a different voice.* Cambridge: Howard University Press, 1982.

Gorrie TM: *A guide to the nursing of childbearing families.* Baltimore: Williams & Wilkins, 1989.

Harter C, et al: Networking to implement effective health care. *MCN* 14:387–92, 1987.

Hatcher S: The 'home bag': a must for lactation consultants on the go. *J Hum Lact* 10:191–2, 1994.

Hickey JR, Ouimette RM, Venegoni SL: *Advanced Practice Nursing: Changing roles in clinical application.* Philadelphia: Lippincott, 1996:42–43.

Hill LF: A salute to La Leche League International [letter]. *J Pediatr* 73:161–2, 1968.

Jelliffe DB, Jelliffe EFP: 'Breast is best': modern meanings. *N Engl J Med* 297:912–15, 1977.

Joel LA: An epiphany in retrospect [editorial]. *Am J Nurs* 97(11):7, 1997.

Kantor MB: *The change masters: innovation for productivity in the American corporation.* New York: Simon & Schuster, 1983:409.

Kim H: Support of breastfeeding through telephone counseling in Korea. *J Hum Lact* 13:29–32, 1997.

Kotler P: *Marketing management: analysis, planning, and control* (5th ed). Englewood Cliffs, NJ: Prentice-Hall, 1984.

Kutner L: Nipple shield consent form: a teaching aid. *J Hum Lact* 2:25–7, 1986.

Marmet C, Shell E: The role of the lactation consultant. In: Coates MM, ed. *The lactation consultant's topical review and bibliography of the literature on breastfeeding.* Franklin Park, IL: La Leche League International, 1990:169–73.

Mukasa GK: A 12-month lactation clinic experience in Uganda. *J Trop Pediatr* 38:78–82, 1992.

NANDA: *Nursing diagnosis,* Washington, DC: NAACOG, 1989:2.

Orlando R: *Breastfeeding care plans for the hospital-based lactation consultant.* Presentation at the La Leche League Conference, Miami Beach, FL, July 1991.

Phillips V: Lactation consultants and voluntary breastfeeding counselors: complementary roles or conflict? *Breastfeed Rev* 2:92–4, 1990a.

Phillips V: The Nursing Mother's Association of Australia as a self-help organization. In: Katz AH, Bender EL: *Helping one another: Self-help groups in a changing world.* Oakland, CA: Third Party Publishing, 1990b.

Rago JL: Breast pump rental depot: a way to bridge the gap. *J Hum Lact* 3:156–7, 1987.

Riordan J: A statistical overview of IBLCE certification exams. *J Hum Lact* 6:90–2, 1990.

Riordan J, Auerbach KG: Lactation consultant certification candidates: the influence of background characteristics on test scores. *Birth* 14:196–8, 1987.

Rogers M, Riordan J, Swindle D: Community-based nursing case management pays off. *Nurs Manage* 22:30–4, 1991.

Scott J: The importance of certification. In: Coates MM, ed. *The lactation consultant's topical review and bibliography of the literature on breastfeeding.* Franklin Park, IL: La Leche League International, 1990:175.

Scott JW: Recertification by examination. *J Hum Lact* 10:294–6, 1994.

Shamansky S, et al: Determining the market for NP services: the New Haven experience. *Nurs Res* 34:242–7, 1985.

Shea E: La Leche League: more than just breastfeeding support. *Can Fam Phys* 38:1221–4, 1992.

Shoemaker JK: Essential features of a nursing diagnosis. In: Kim MJ, McFarlane G, McLane A, eds. *Classification of nursing diagnosis.* St Louis: Mosby, 1984:109.

Shrago LC: Fostering collegial relationships among lactation consultants [editorial]. *J Hum Lact* 11:1–2, 1995.

Shrago LC: Product evaluation: nipple shields. *J Hum Lact* 4:169, 1988.

Shrago L: A standing order for in-hospital lactation consultation. *J Hum Lact* 12:236–8, 1996.

Sonstegard L: A better way to market maternal-child care. *MCN* 13:395–402, 1988.

Tanis AL, Coleman AB, Gross L: I.B.C.L.C. *Pediatrics* 86:149, 1990.

Tinari MA: Lactation consultant job proposal. *J Hum Lact* 2:114–15, 1986.

Turner MR: Twenty questions for the consumer: a quality assurance tool for the lactation consultant. *J Hum Lact* 12:50–2, 1996.

Williams EL: Increasing your credibility with physicians: strategies for lactation consultants [editorial]. *J Hum Lact* 11:3–4, 1995.

Williams N: Creating a lactation consultant position. *J Hum Lact* 1:86–8, 1986.

Wilton JM: Development of a hospital breastfeeding center. *J Hum Lact* 5:132–4, 1989.

Woolf V: *A room of one's own*. New York: Harcourt, Brace, 1929.

RESEARCH AND BREASTFEEDING

Roberta J. Hewat

Are intuition, gut reaction, or tradition the bases of breastfeeding practice and education? Or are practice and education founded on a body of knowledge generated or validated from data gathered and interpreted by systematic methods that practitioners continually question, study, and expand? Research is a process for developing a knowledge base for accountable and responsible practice that legitimizes professional care.

The intent of this chapter is to assist breastfeeding practitioners in developing an interest in–and understanding of–breastfeeding research and in becoming research consumers. This entails reading articles to learn about current practices, understanding research methods to evaluate and determine whether study findings are relevant, incorporating appropriate findings into their practices, and consistently investigating practices to develop questions for further research.

Approaches to Research Methods

There are many approaches to research methods. The research question, topic, existing research related to the topic, and the philosophical perspective of the inquiry direct the approach that is used. Qualitative and quantitative methods are major approaches for conducting research. Traditionally, quantitative methods are the most commonly used, but since the 1980s, breastfeeding studies using qualitative methods are increasing. This chapter describes these approaches, as well as observational, historical, and feminist approaches that are suitable for breastfeeding research.

Qualitative Approaches

Qualitative methods generate an understanding of the meaning that human values, beliefs, practices, or life experiences and events have for individuals. The aim is to discover new information or to gain a new perspective on a familiar topic. Generally conducted in naturalistic settings, all possible variables that influence individuals' perspectives are considered data; these data are broad and frequently complex. This humanistic approach is congruent with a holistic philosophy of providing health care.

The outcomes of qualitative studies are mainly twofold: theory generation and rich descriptions that provide a deeper understanding of the meaning of the experiences, events, and practices of individuals. Theory is generated primarily by the process of inductive reasoning, which means that specific ideas progress to more generalized statements. Thus, from the study of an everyday life phenomenon, variables and the ways that they relate are identified. Further interpretation of the data can lead to conceptualization of an experience from which theories are developed (Morse & Field, 1995). In some studies, a rich, linguistic construction of an interpretation of the essence of a human experience, which shows the meaning or significance of the experience in a deeper manner and so provides a greater understanding of a phenomenon, may be the outcome (van Manen, 1984).

Types of Qualitative Methods

The origins of qualitative methods are inherent in philosophy and the social sciences. Three types of qualitative methods commonly used are phenomenology, ethnography, and grounded theory. Phenomenology and grounded-theory methods emanate from philosophy and sociology, whereas ethnographic methods originate from anthropology. Depending on the origin, variations of each method exist, as do specific practices and procedures for conducting the research.

Phenomenology. *Phenomenology* is a philosophy, a research method, and a humanistic scientific approach. The objective is to understand the meaning or nature of everyday life experiences or events from the perspective of those living the experiences. As the science developed, variations in phenomenological methods emerged. Two approaches are illustrated by the following studies.

Three studies using a phenomenological approach are described by van Manen (1990): "Woman to mother: A transformation" (Bergum, 1989); "Persistence in breastfeeding: A phenomenological investigation" (Bottorff, 1990); and "The experience of living with an incessantly crying infant" (Hewat, 1992). In all three studies, the meaning of lived experiences are captured through articulation of content, form, and language specific to phenomenological writing. These rich descriptions attempt to show how these experiences are lived in the everyday world. The deeper understanding that practitioners gain from reading these studies should contribute to more humanistic care in working with individuals who are living these experiences.

A more structured process for conducting phenomenological research is one proposed by Giorgi (1970). A study using this method addresses women's perceptions of the breastfeeding experience (Hewat & Ellis, 1984). Findings describe similarities and differences among women who breastfeed for short and long duration (Hewat &

Ellis, 1986) and discuss a conceptualization of the mother-infant breastfeeding relationship (Hewat & Ellis, 1984). These findings explain the complexity of the breastfeeding experience and provide direction for breastfeeding practitioners.

Ethnography. Ethnography is a method used to understand the beliefs, practices, and patterns of behavior from the perspective of individuals of a culture or subculture within the context of their environment. A "traditional" ethnography describes the many facets of an entire culture or subculture, whereas a "focused" ethnography portrays one aspect of a culture (Morse, 1991a). The purpose is to come to understand the cultural meanings people use to organize and interpret their experiences (Spradley, 1979).

Neander and Morse (1989) conducted a focused ethnography. The authors describe and compare infant-feeding practices of the Northern Alberta Woodlands Cree when infants were born at home with practices followed when childbirth was relocated to the hospital. The decline in breastfeeding that occurred is associated with the mothers' loss of social support from native women and the lack of understanding by health professionals about Cree cultural beliefs and practices.

Grounded Theory. Grounded theory is a research method for ". . . generating explanatory theory that furthers the understanding of social and psychological phenomena" (Chenitz & Swanson, 1986). Using a rigorous and structured process, data based on individuals' realities are simultaneously collected and analyzed to develop theoretical constructs (Glaser, 1978; Strauss & Corbin, 1990). The emerging theory represents reality, because it is "grounded" in the data. From this new understanding, relevant interventions for clinical practice can evolve.

Using a grounded theory approach, Locklin (1993a) and Locklin & Napier (1995) conducted indepth interviews among educated, low-income women to examine their breastfeeding experiences. An outcome of this study was that the mother's positive perception of breastfeeding can have an empowering effect on these women.

Wrigley and Hutchinson (1990) also used this method in a study examining the mother-infant breastfeeding relationship for dyads breastfeeding for more than one year. Two key processes were identified: *synchronization,* in which the mother proceeded in step with her infant, and *reorientation,* in which the mother rearranged her life to meet the needs of her infant. For women breastfeeding for more than one year, the authors suggest that a "secret bond" develops between mother and child that limits intrusion and protects the breastfeeding relationship from a society that disapproves of long-term breastfeeding.

Quantitative Approaches

Quantitative methodologies are traditional research methods advanced by the biological, physical, and social sciences. Key characteristics are objectivity, measurement, and control. Studies examine specific variables and control intervening variables. Data collection and analysis are conducted as objectively as possible to control prejudice on the part of the investigator and other sources of potential bias. Statistical procedures and principles of measurement determine relationships and examine cause and effect among variables.

Theories, principles, or conceptualizations are a common source of the variables or hypotheses for study. The process of studying components and their relationships deduced from a general premise is known as *deductive reasoning.*

The goal of quantitative studies is to determine relationships that are predictable and can be generalized to populations larger than the study sample. This may take many years of ongoing study by many independent investigators. The decades in which numerous studies were conducted before scientists declared that smoking is related to the development of lung cancer is an example.

Types of Quantitative Methods

The major types of quantitative methods are descriptive, correlational, quasi-experimental, and experimental (Burns & Grove, 1993). The type of inquiry chosen depends on the amount of knowledge of the study topic and the purpose of the research.

Descriptive Studies. Descriptive studies are appropriate when there is little knowledge about a topic of interest and specific information is desired. For example, the research questions may address characteristics, influencing factors, or knowledge deficits related to a topic. Findings describe the studied phenomenon and may identify relationships among variables.

The descriptive study conducted by Lazzaro et al. (1995) examined the breastfeeding attitudes of health professionals working with pregnant women or new mothers. Of 464 survey questionnaires mailed to health professionals in one county in the United States, 138 (30 percent) provided information for the analysis. Respondents were categorized into five groups; physicians, hospital nurses, community nurses, licensed practical nurses and medical assistants, and nutritionists. Using descriptive statistics, the responses of the five groups were compared. Significant differences in knowledge or attitudes among the groups were identified in regard to breastfeeding advocacy, supplementation of breastfed infants, the importance of specific factors on a mother's decision to breastfeed, and reasons for early discontinuance of breastfeeding. Although this convenient sample represents a limited number of health professionals in one county, it identifies their similarities and differences in attitudes toward breastfeeding. Findings of some descriptive studies may identify relationships between variables that form the basis for further study.

Correlational Studies. Correlational studies examine the relationships among two or more variables and the type (negative or positive) and strength of the relationship(s). These studies require a greater type of control than do descriptive studies. Structuring the collected data is necessary to allow for numerical translation and correlational analysis for determining whether the relationships between variables are statistically significant. In quantitative studies, the term *significant* is used only when a relationship is statistically significant.

Richardson and Champion's (1992) investigation of variables, previously identified in the literature as influencing breastfeeding duration, is an example of a correlational study. One hundred and two mothers who initiated breastfeeding in hospital were prospectively followed for one year after their infants' birth to determine the relationship among the mothers' perceived attitudes about benefits of and barriers to breastfeeding, perceived social support, knowledge, and experiential and demographic characteristics and the length of time that they breastfed their infants. For the women participating in this study, findings indicate significant and positive relationships between longer breastfeeding and the following variables: perceptions that nursing is natural, easy, and satisfies an emotional need; strong encouragement from a mother's extended family and coworkers; mothers who are older, married, and have more education; and mothers who have previously breastfed. Supplementation at four months was associated positively with longer breastfeeding, whereas supplementation in the first month following delivery was related negatively to length of breastfeeding. A mother's knowledge about breastfeeding was not related to breastfeeding duration.

Findings from this study provide direction for further investigations. For example, more in-depth study of the association of breastfeeding duration and the influence of extended family members, particularly those who are female, the role of coworkers when a mother returns to work, and mothers' knowledge about breastfeeding is warranted. A study with a larger sample size could examine the combined influence of variables on breastfeeding duration, using multivariate analysis.

Experimental Studies. Experimental studies examine hypothesized relationships between variables to determine cause (often an intervention or treatment) and effect (the outcome). Rigorous control of variables is integral to conducting these studies. Three criteria are essential for a true experimental study (Burns & Grove, 1997):

- *manipulation* of an experimental intervention or treatment (the independent variable) by the investigator

- *control* of the experimental situation to eliminate interference or confounding effect of extraneous variables (additional influencing factors) on the outcome (dependent variable)

- *randomization,* which is a process of systematically allocating subjects so that all have an equal chance of participating in the experimental or control study groups

Schy et al. (1996) used an experimental design to determine the effect of an in-hospital lactation-

education session (the treatment or independent variable) on the duration of breastfeeding and satisfaction among postpartum women (the dependent or outcome variables). One hundred and fifty subjects were randomly assigned to experimental or control groups. During their hospital stay, those in the experimental group participated in one lactation-education session and received daily visits from a lactation specialist. Those in the control group received routine hospital care. A seven-day-a-week breastfeeding telephone help-line was a follow-up service offered to all study participants. Continuance of breastfeeding was followed for six months postpartum, at which time the women completed a satisfaction questionnaire. Study findings revealed no statistical differences between the control and experimental groups. As a result, Schy et al. (1996) were unable to infer that the lactation session prolonged breastfeeding duration or mothers' satisfaction.

The results of the Schy et al. study may seem disappointing, but these findings are important for contributing knowledge about one method of providing breastfeeding support. These findings highlight further questions for study that may produce different outcomes. Examples are: What is the effect on breastfeeding duration when assistance from a lactation consultant is provided during hospital stay and for four weeks following hospital discharge? What is the effect of breastfeeding assessment and information from a lactation consultant–during pregnancy, in the hospital, and throughout the breastfeeding period? Many additional studies are needed before the relationship between support and breastfeeding duration is understood. Research is an ongoing process; many experimental studies about a topic are necessary before definitive conclusions can be drawn.

The involvement of human subjects does not always permit the rigor necessary for a true experiment. For example, it is not always practical, ethical, or feasible to randomly select subjects or to expose them to a specific treatment or experience. When these criteria for controlling the influence of extraneous variables are not met, but an experimental procedure is used, the research design is considered quasi-experimental (Christensen, 1991). Many breastfeeding studies can be classified as quasi-experimental: one example is the study examining the effect of peer counselors on breast-feeding initiation, exclusively, and duration among low-income women (Kistin et al., 1994). Two groups of women–those receiving breastfeeding assistance from a peer counselor and those not receiving this type of assistance–were compared, but the intervention (peer counseling) was not randomly assigned to the study participants.

Additional Approaches

Other research methods that are suitable for breastfeeding research but do not fit within the qualitative or quantitative classification are observational, historical, and feminist research.

Observational Research. Observational research is important for studying overt human behavior or events (Booth & Mitchell, 1985). Some behaviors of a study interest such as mother-infant behaviors during breastfeeding cannot be captured through interviews or self-report questionnaires. The origin of observational research is biology, specifically ethology, which is the study of animal behaviors within natural settings. Behavioristic psychology has also contributed to developing structured methods of observational research.

If knowledge of the behaviors of interest is limited, the researcher may be initially inductively learning about the behaviors by making detailed descriptions of observations. From these descriptions, referred to as an *ethogram,* a guide is developed for coding behaviors for further examination, quantification, and statistical analysis. Study outcomes can include frequencies of behavioral occurrences, timing of specific behaviors, and sequences of behaviors. Although observational research is rigorous and complex, it has particular potential for contributing to the development of a practice profession (Morse & Bottorff, 1990).

In an observational study, Conway (1989) videotaped bottle-feeding sessions of infants between one and four months of age while they had an acute respiratory infection and while they were well. Using behavioral checklists, suck/pause and suck/swallow patterns, nipple seal, and respiration patterns were examined. Differences in the feeding behaviors and respiration patterns were identified and described when infants were ill and when they were well.

Historical Research. Historical research methods are valuable for exploring past practices, examining patterns and trends during specific periods, discovering relationships, and drawing inferences. Past revelations can increase understanding of traditions and practices and guide decision making. Historical inquiry entails identifying, collecting, categorizing, and determining validity of evidence, critical analysis, synthesis, and writing to present meaningful discussion of the subject (Shafer, 1980).

Millard's work (1990) illustrates the value of historical research. Examination of the pediatric literature between 1897 and 1987 shows that although breastfeeding was advocated, advice centered on regimens and schedules. Even as flexibility in feeding times became more acceptable, advice including time limitations continued. Millard's study findings suggest that emphasis on time in regard to breastfeeding and the allocation to medical experts of control of breastfeeding practices has undermined breastfeeding during the 90-year period.

Feminist Research. Feminist research is an approach that is congruent with, but not overtly evident in, current breastfeeding research. Whether there is a "feminist method" or whether any research method can be conducted from a feminist perspective is an issue (Kelly et al., 1994). Feminist research is guided by the following principles: it is about women, for women, and done *with* (not *to*) women; it should be empowering for participants; it is directed toward positive social change; and it generally uses qualitative methods. A feminist perspective encourages the researcher to focus on women in a societal and political context and to consider cultural influences and attitudes within society as central to the experience of the women involved (Harding, 1987). Feminist researchers recognize the negotiated social act between the researcher and the participants. The researcher defines the study and interprets the findings, and the participants decide what information they will share with the researcher (Maynard & Purvis, 1994).

Multiple Approaches

In developing a scientific base for breastfeeding practice, all research approaches generate knowledge. Most studies use one approach; the choice depends on the research question addressed and whether theory is generated inductively or tested deductively. Simultaneous use of multiple approaches is called *triangulation* (Denzin, 1989). Types of triangulation include the use of different theoretical perspectives, data sources, research methods, investigators with expertise in different methods, and different analysis techniques for the same data set (Burns & Grove, 1997). Triangulation is used, particularly in complex studies, to enhance the comprehensiveness of data or to confirm or validate results. When using multiple approaches, researchers must be clear about the purpose of each and the separate strategies employed for collecting, analyzing, and interpreting data (Knafl & Breitmayer, 1991).

Elements of Research

The elements of research are essential to writing proposals and reports, conducting research, and evaluating studies. The major elements are the research problem and purpose, review of the literature, protection of human subjects, method (including identification of variables, their operational definitions, and the variables examined), analysis, and results and discussion. Although the elements are similar for both qualitative and quantitative research approaches, the content and processes vary. The following sections describe the elements and discuss the differences between qualitative and quantitative methods.

Research Problem and Purpose

The research problem is a critical component of a study. It identifies what is being studied and with whom. The purpose delineates why the study is conducted. There are many sources for generating research problems. Questioning clinical practice, observing clinical and societal patterns and trends, building on findings from previous studies, and examining theoretical propositions are ways of developing research questions.

A problem that is suitable for study should be important to the topic of breastfeeding and amenable to investigation by scientific inquiry. It should be meaningful to many individuals or have

a distinct influence on a few. A descriptive survey conducted by Buxton et al. (1991) regarding predictors of early infant-feeding experiences among women intending to breastfeed illustrates importance to many. In contrast, a study about the effect of sequential and simultaneous breast pumping on milk volume and prolactin levels among women who express milk for a prolonged period (Hill et al., 1996) has important implications for a few. Criteria that render a problem appropriate for scientific inquiry include

- suitability of the research design for the research question
- accessibility of study participants
- feasibility of the study with regard to time, funding, and equipment
- potentiality of adhering to ethical requirements throughout all study phases

Reviewing the literature about a study topic provides direction for asking a relevant question and selecting an appropriate method. A qualitative method is indicated when literature about a phenomenon is limited or when more in-depth knowledge is desired. However, when many studies about a topic have been undertaken, these study findings often provide a base and focus for further study, and a quantitative method is generally appropriate.

Research problems can be written as questions or declarative statements. Clearly identifying the topic, population, and variables for study is essential for quantitative methods. In qualitative studies, less is known about the topic of interest; therefore, the research question is broader. The purpose is to describe and interpret the meanings of a phenomenon, to gain an in-depth understanding of an experience or situation, or to discover variables relevant to a topic rather than to examine variables previously identified. Examples of research questions that are applicable to specific research methods are shown in Table 23–1. All questions pertain to breastfeeding preterm infants, but for quantitative methods the questions are more specific and address social network and breastfeeding preterm infants, a topic and population studied by Kaufman and Hall (1989).

Table 23–1

EXAMPLES OF RESEARCH QUESTIONS AND METHODS

Question	Research Method	Variables for Study
Qualitative Methods		
Topic of interest: Breastfeeding preterm infants		
What are mothers' experiences of breastfeeding a preterm infant?	Phenomenology	
What are the cultural factors influencing feeding patterns of preterm infants among Chinese women?	Ethnography	
What is the experience of learning how to breastfeed a preterm infant?	Grounded theory	
Quantitative Methods		
Topic: Social support and breastfeeding*		
Population: Mothers of preterm infants		
What kinds of social support are most useful to breastfeeding mothers of preterm infants?	Descriptive	Social support
Is there a relationship between social network and choice of feeding method and duration of breastfeeding for mothers of preterm infants? (Kaufman & Hall, 1989)	Correlational	Social network Feeding method choice Breastfeeding duration
What is the effect on breastfeeding duration of scheduled visits by a lactation consultant to breastfeeding mothers of preterm infants?	Experimental	Breastfeeding duration (dependent variable) Scheduled visits by a lactation consultant (independent variable)

*The topic and variables for study are usually more specifically identified in quantitative studies.

Variables, Hypotheses, and Operational Definitions

Variables. Variables are defined as "qualities, properties, or characteristics of persons, things, or situations that change or vary and are manipulated or measured in research" (Burns & Grove, 1997). Qualitative studies may aim to discover indicators that influence the study phenomenon, whereas quantitative studies identify specific variables for investigation. Experimental studies have at least one dependent and one independent variable. The *dependent variable,* also called the *outcome variable,* is what the investigator is most interested in understanding, explaining, or predicting. In the example of an experimental study cited in Table 23–1, the dependent variable is breastfeeding duration. The *independent variable* is thought to affect or change the dependent variable. It is the treatment or intervention that affects the outcome; in this example, it is the scheduled visits by a lactation consultant.

Uncontrolled, confounding, or extraneous variables are those elements in quantitative studies that may affect the dependent or outcome variable. Sometimes such variables come between the occurrence of the treatment (independent variable) and the measurement of the outcome variable. For example, if mothers with preterm infants view a television documentary on the advantages of breastmilk for preterm infants, the television program–rather than the scheduled visits by the lactation consultant–may be the motivating factor for prolonging breastfeeding. To "control" the effect of these variables on experimental study outcomes, study participants are randomly assigned to an experimental group receiving visits from a lactation consultant or to a control group receiving existing care but no such visits from a lactation consultant. The random placement of subjects in each group is expected to ensure that each group is similar in regard to background characteristics, practices, and opportunities. Therefore, if the participants of the experimental group breastfeed longer than those of the control group (as determined by statistical procedures), the increased breastfeeding duration is attributed to the visits by the lactation consultant that occurred in the experimental group.

Hypotheses. "A hypothesis is the formal statement of the expected relationship(s) between two or more variables in a specified population" (Burns & Grove, 1997). Qualitative studies may generate hypotheses, whereas correlational and experimental studies examine and test relationships among identified variables.

Hypotheses for correlational studies focus on the association of variables. For the study by Kaufman and Hall (1989), a hypothesis may be written as follows: "For mothers of preterm infants, there is a positive relationship between the mothers' perceptions of their social network and breastfeeding duration."

In experimental studies, a hypothesis represents a prediction of how an intervention or independent variable specifically influences an identified outcome or dependent variable. The written hypothesis includes these components and names the study groups. For the experimental study in Table 23–1, a research hypothesis is written as follows: "Mothers of preterm infants who receive scheduled visits from a lactation consultant

will breastfeed longer than mothers of preterm infants who do not receive scheduled visits from a lactation consultant." The experimental and control groups, the dependent and independent variables, and the predictor (longer breastfeeding duration) are identified.

For statistical purposes, some investigators prefer to write hypotheses in the null form. For example: "There will be *no* difference in the duration of breastfeeding between mothers of preterm infants who receive scheduled visits from a lactation consultant and mothers of preterm infants who do not receive scheduled visits from a lactation consultant." In using the null hypothesis, outcomes for the groups are considered the same until it is established that they are statistically different. When this occurs, the null hypothesis is rejected, and an inference is made that the visits by a lactation consultant are the reason for the different outcomes for the groups. The visits are then considered an effective intervention.

Operational Definitions. Operational definitions are explicit descriptions of how the major variables are observed and measured and of how they are integral to correlational and experimental studies. In the Kaufman and Hall (1989) study, both major variables are defined so that numerical comparisons can be made. *Breastfeeding duration* is specified as "the number of postnatal days of any breastfeeding or expression," and *social network* is defined as a mother's perception of influence from social referents as measured by the Influence of Specific Referents (ISR) scale.

In experimental studies, the independent variable must be clearly defined. In the fictitious experimental study described in Table 23–1, a definition of the intervention regimen–the scheduled visits from a lactation consultant–could be operationally defined in many ways. One example is that a lactation consultant will visit a mother once weekly from birth until four weeks after hospital discharge.

Operational definitions of breastfeeding are extensive. Table 23–2 illustrates differences in definitions used in studies. As the number of possible feeding categories increases, data regarding the variability of infant feeding patterns is more precise. The selection of definitions depends on the purpose of the study and can influence sample size. A large number of categories generally requires large samples.

Table 23–2

OPERATIONAL DEFINITIONS OF BREASTFEEDING

Study	No. of Categories	Breastfeeding Groups Defined
Maternal characteristics associated with the duration of breastfeeding (Jones et al., 1986)	1	Breastfeeder: anyone who breastfed her baby at least once Nonbreastfeeder: all others
Factors predicting breastfeeding success (Hellings, 1984)	4	1 = total breastfeeding 2 = breastfeeding with less than 4 oz. of supplementation 3 = breastfeeding with more than 4 oz. of supplementation 4 = total formula feeding
Evaluation of the efficacy of a breastfeeding clinic in prolonging the duration of breastfeeding (Ellis et al., 1991)	6	Exclusive = total breastfeeding Primarily = breastfeeding or expressed breastmilk (EBM), plus a maximum of one alternate milk feeding per week Mainly = more than one breastfeeding or EBM feeding per day, plus more than one alternate milk feeding per week to a maximum of one alternate milk feeding per day Partial = more than one breastfeeding or EBM feeding per day, plus more than one alternate milk feeding per day Minimal = one or no breastfeeding or EBM feeding per day to one breastfeeding or EBM feeding per week Weaned = having stopped breastfeeding or EBM feeding for one week or more

How breastfeeding is operationally defined is of particular interest when evaluating and comparing study results, because imprecise definitions of breastfeeding categories affect data analysis and interpretation of study outcomes. Readers of research articles and reports must be cognizant of how breastfeeding is defined when determining the merits of a study. For example, infants who are only breastfed may be grouped with infants who are breastfed *once*. Likewise, exclusive or total breastfeeding may mean that the infant has ingested only breastmilk, or it may also include one formula feeding per week and supplements of water, glucose water, or juice. This has implications when comparing published studies and examining relationships between "patterns of breastfeeding and their effects on infant nutrition, health, and fertility" (Labbok & Coffin, 1997). Auerbach et al. (1991) state that "research purporting to compare breastfeeding with artificial feeding is seriously flawed," and illustrate their contention by providing reviews of breastfeeding definitions and outcomes of 43 studies. The authors outline guidelines for defining feeding categories that should be considered by investigators when designing studies that compare different feeding groups. These include detailed information about all types, combinations, volume, and frequency of any substance ingested by an infant; the method of feeding (e.g., gavage, bottle, or type of nipple used); and identification of the feeder (e.g., nurse or mother); and whether the infant is in a hospital or clinic.

In 1988 the Interagency Group for Action on Breastfeeding (IGAB), an international organization, began developing standard definitions for breast-feeding patterns that are internationally recommended for use (Armstrong, 1991; Labbok & Coffin, 1997). The definitions, published by Labbok and Krasovec (1990), include the following classifications: *full* breastfeeding, which is further delineated into subcategories of exclusive and almost exclusive breastfeeding; *partial* breastfeeding, with suggested (but not yet discretely differentiated) groupings of high, medium, and low; and *token* breastfeeding, which is described as minimal, occasional, and irregular breastfeedings. These definitions are a beginning; however, all subcategories of the classifications require further specification. Such definitions must reflect cultural practices and meanings and must satisfy the precision required for careful and rigorous investigations. Further refining of the definitions is essential for more consistent and valid outcomes from breastfeeding research.

Review of the Literature

Reviewing the body of literature on a study topic provides knowledge and understanding about the phenomenon. Findings from studies help to formulate the research problem and provide direction for research methods. The purpose of a literature review can be different for qualitative and quantitative approaches. In qualitative studies, an initial review of literature is done for investigator awareness and knowledge of the studies conducted. Because the goal of qualitative methods is discovery, literature should not influence the mind-set of the investigator during initial data collection. In the analysis stage, study findings reported in the literature are used to compare, contrast, and verify findings of the current study. Findings from a new study may even be combined with those of a pre-

vious study to identify new insights and expand current knowledge about a phenomenon.

In quantitative studies, the existing literature will help to clarify the research problem and identify theories or concepts on which the study is based. Identification of key concepts and their relationships provides a conceptual framework or structure for the study. Literature is also useful in assisting with selection of a research design, providing strategies for data collection and analysis, and interpreting findings (Woods & Catanzaro, 1988).

Protection of the Rights of Human Subjects

Most breastfeeding research involves human subjects. To protect the rights of study participants throughout the research process, investigators must adhere to ethical guidelines. The first international ethical standard was the Nuremberg Code, developed in 1949. The impetus was disclosure of inhumane acts, described by the Nazis as scientific research, during the post–World War II crime trials held in Nuremberg, Germany. This code is the basis of ethical standards developed by medicine and the behavioral science disciplines. The Declaration of Helsinki, adopted in 1964 and revised in 1975 by the World Medical Assembly, provides further guidelines for investigators conducting clinical research (Levine, 1986). Ethical requirements for funded research are stipulated by governments and institutions, and individual codes have been developed by professional associations that represent researchers who conduct human research. Disciplines have developed specific ethical guidelines for research. For nursing research, guidelines have been adopted by the American Nurses Association (ANA, 1985), the Canadian Nurses Association (CNA, 1983), and the Royal College of Nursing of the United Kingdom (RCN, 1977). Four basic rights of human subjects are recognized (Wilson, 1989):

1. freedom from risk or injury from physical, emotional, financial, or social harm

2. full knowledge of the study purpose, procedures to be used, time commitments expected of the participants, and any other factors that may affect the subjects

3. the assurance of subjects' right to self-determination, which means that they may refuse to participate or withdraw from a study *at any time* without any effect on the care they are receiving or will receive

4. the affirmation of subjects' privacy, anonymity, or confidentiality throughout all phases of the research

Mechanisms developed to ensure that research is ethically conducted include the investigator's use of an informed-consent document and review of the proposed study by human subjects or ethical review boards. An informed-consent document describes the study, addresses how the rights of subjects will be maintained, and explains how the investigator may be contacted. It is presented to subjects when they are recruited. A subject's signature on the informed-consent document indicates an understanding of the study and willingness to participate. Ethical review boards–established by universities and many health care agencies, school boards, or organizations that are resources for human subjects–review study proposals to ensure that the research process protects the rights of study participants. The investigators are bound by the recommendations of these review boards during the research process.

Method

Each study method addresses setting, sample, data collection, and data analysis.

Setting. A study setting is the location of the study or source of participating subjects or sample. In all studies, the setting must be clearly described.

Population and Sample. A population, which is often called the *target population,* is the group of individuals in which the researcher is interested. For example, it could be all breastfeeding mothers, primiparas who breastfeed, mothers who work and breastfeed, or mothers of preterm infants. In some cases, an object, such as breastmilk, rather than individuals, may be the phenomenon of interest. Because it is difficult to study an entire population, researchers generally study a subgroup of the larger population; this is the sample.

Sampling. Sampling is a process for selecting the sample from the population. Two basic types are probability and nonprobability sampling.

Probability sampling involves quantitative studies that seek to generalize to larger populations findings from the sample studied; therefore, it is important that the sample be representative of the target population. This is accomplished by the *random selection* of subjects from the population, a process requiring that every individual in the population of interest have an equal and independent chance of being chosen. Several distinct methods of probability sampling are identified.

Simple random sampling is achieved by numbering all members of the population and then selecting subjects by using a table of random numbers available in many quantitative research books. Other procedures include drawing subjects' names from a hat or flipping a coin.

Systematic sampling follows the procedure of choosing every *n*th (e.g., every eighth, tenth, or one hundredth) subject from a list of the population. To ensure that all possible subjects have an equal chance, the names on the list must not be grouped in any special way, such as alphabetical order or age of subjects. For example, in a study of the effect of hospital routines on early breastfeeding experience, selecting every *n*th case from the list of mothers admitted to a particular postpartum unit would be an appropriate sampling technique.

Stratified random sampling is a process of identifying subgroups of a population and selecting numbers of subjects that represent the distribution of the subgroups in the population. For example, if a researcher wishes to study a population of all mothers giving birth in a specific geographical location and learns that the population distribution is 40 percent primiparas and 60 percent multiparas, then the investigator will randomly select the numbers for each subgroup (or stratum) that reflects the population distribution.

In studies that involve human subjects, probability sampling is frequently not possible, because all subjects in a population (e.g., all breastfeeding mothers) cannot be identified. Depending on the purpose of the study, random assignment of women to feeding groups may be unethical or, for qualitative studies, it is undesirable. Therefore, many breastfeeding studies employ nonprobability sampling.

Nonprobability sampling is the nonrandom selection of subjects for a study. In qualitative studies, subjects are generally known as *informants* or *participants*. Individuals who provide rich descriptions enhance the quality of the data. They are called *key informants* and are sought by investigators. Methods for selecting the study participants or informants vary.

Convenience sampling is a common method used for both qualitative and quantitative studies. The sample consists of consenting subjects from a readily available source–for example, all mothers giving birth at a hospital or attending a particular clinic.

Network, nominated, or snowball sampling is a strategy that bases recruitment on asking current study participants to identify other individuals, similar to themselves, who may also consent to be study subjects. This method is useful in the study of an ethnic group or individuals with a specific condition for which a support group has been established, such as parents who are experiencing a perinatal loss.

Purposive sampling occurs when the investigator selects participants "according to the needs of the study" (Morse, 1991b). Participants are selected because they are thought to be "good informants" about the study topic. As the study progresses, additional participants are chosen to enrich the data and expand the developing theory.

Solicited or volunteer sampling is used when the investigator wishes to broaden the sample. Advertisements in newspapers and notices on bulletin boards regarding the research often entreat interested participants (Morse, 1991b).

Methods of Data Collection. Data are collected by asking questions, observing, or measuring key variables identified in the research question. The data-collection method must be appropriate to the research methodology and the study population.

Self-report questionnaires are an effective and common way of obtaining specific information from a large sample. However, the construction of questionnaires that can be understood by all participants and are sufficiently broad in scope to reflect "true" meanings can be time-consuming and expensive to develop. If questionnaires are too long or repeated frequently throughout a study, participants may not complete all of them. This

results in study attrition and may lower the response rate to the extent that the sample does not represent the potential whole of the population.

Interviews elicit more in-depth information than do questionnaires, but they are more time-consuming and expensive to administer. A skilled interviewer is required to ensure explicit and valid collection of data. When more than one interviewer is used, varying degrees of bias on the part of the interviewer must be considered as a potential limitation of the data.

Observations are useful for collecting data about events, patterns of behavior, activities, or interactions. Observations can be unstructured and recorded as field notes, or they can be structured for specific recording on checklists. Developing a coding scheme that is congruent with the research question and specific to the level of behaviors that are of interest is essential; however, the process must be precise and is time-consuming. Methods of recording data can be paper and pencil, a digital data-acquisition system consisting of a hand-held keyboard for entering coded behaviors as they occur, or videotaping (Morse & Bottorff, 1990). The latter is a means for recording observations that can be coded more precisely and in greater detail at a later time.

Biophysiological measurements, such as infant weight, length, head circumference, respirations, oxygen consumption, and heart rate, as well as the mother's temperature, prolactin levels, and milk composition, have been used in breastfeeding research. However, measurements are only as accurate as the equipment used and the investigator responsible for measuring and recording.

Data Analysis

Data analysis is the process of examining, summarizing, and synthesizing the data collected to determine whether study findings answer the research question. Strategies for data analysis depend on the research question, sample selection and size, and method and type of data collection.

Results, Discussion, and Conclusions

Study results or findings should be clear, concise, and congruent with the research question(s) asked and the methodology used. The presentation of results varies for the type of study conducted. Qualitative studies are descriptive narratives that include participants' verbatim accounts, providing evidence of the researcher's data interpretations. The results may be rich descriptions of the study phenomenon, hypothetical propositions generated from the data, or a theory.

Quantitative studies frequently use tables and graphs to display results. Variables examined in descriptive studies should be precisely described, and responses should be numerically reported. Relationships of variables investigated in correlational studies and the procedures used to determine relationships must be clear. In studies that test hypotheses, the statistical procedures used, the results, and the decision for supporting or not supporting the hypothesized relationships must be evident for each hypothesis stated. Significant, nonsignificant, and unexpected results must be reported. Findings in studies that are not what the investigator anticipates also contribute knowledge about the study topic; they can be an impetus for asking more relevant or more detailed research questions.

Interpreting study results is an intellectual process that gives meaning to the study (Burns & Grove, 1997). The investigator considers both the study results with regard to the study process and findings from other studies that support or contradict current results. These can be addressed with the presentation of the results or separately in a section discussing the findings.

The limitations of a study are acknowledge factors that may affect study outcomes. Compromises are often necessary in the study process for pragmatic and ethical reasons. These can create weaknesses in design, sampling process, sample size, methods of data collection, or data-analysis techniques. The extent to which study findings can be generalized to populations beyond the study sample should also be discussed. Stating limitations helps readers to evaluate the scientific merits of the study and enhances the credibility of the investigator.

Conclusions are concise statements that synthesize the findings; they provide an overall account of the importance of the study and an understanding of the phenomenon in question. The conclusions must be pertinent to the findings and not expanded beyond the study parameters. Following the con-clusions, the implications of the findings for clinical practice are generally described, and suggestions for further research are identified.

Application of Methods to Qualitative Approaches

Specific methodological procedures, based on the philosophical base of each qualitative method, have been developed. Investigators should use the qualitative method and ascribed procedure that is most appropriate to the study problem. An issue in qualitative research is that an increasing number of studies are combining qualitative methods. However, as use of qualitative methods has proliferated, some methods have blended. A current debate among qualitative researchers is whether this enhances a study or whether mixing methods transgresses assumptions of data-collection procedures and analysis, resulting in unrealistic outcomes and compromising the science (Morse, 1990, 1991a). As the use of qualitative research increases, it is inevitable that new or altered methods will be advanced. However, alterations should be done by experienced investigators who are explicit about the philosophical base of the study and methods used.

Reliability and Validity

Ensuring reliability and validity requires ongoing examination by the investigator throughout the research process. Sources of error can occur in sampling, data collection, and analysis. The following factors should be evaluated:

- the credibility of key informants providing accurate data
- the interviewer's skill in obtaining the participants' true perspectives
- the accuracy of field observations
- the generation of codes or units of analysis that represent data accurately within a social context
- interpretations of the data to determine whether they represent true meanings

The longitudinal nature of most qualitative studies can enhance reliability and validity of data, because checks are often built into the process. The following factors should be considered:

- the number of kinds of data collection used (one method can validate another)
- the frequency with which data are collected from subjects using the same method
- the number of investigators collecting data
- rigor of the analytical process

Sampling and Sample Size

All nonprobability sampling methods are suitable for recruiting study participants, but a frequently used procedure is purposive or theoretical sampling. Purposive sampling permits the investigator to select participants thought to be the best informants for providing data about the population and the topic of interest. Sample size is determined through a process called *theoretical sampling*. This means that as data are simultaneously collected and analyzed from initial participants and as descriptions of experiences are revealed, additional informants are recruited on the basis of expanding the developing knowledge base. Participants are recruited until no new information is disclosed, and data are fully explored (Chenitz & Swanson, 1986; Glaser, 1978). Sample size depends on the scope of the topic explored, but samples are generally small for qualitative studies.

Data Collection

Methods of data collection include interviews, field observations and review of documents. In-depth, unstructured interviews that explore participants' perceptions and, in many studies, validate the investigator's subjective interpretation of the data remain the most common method for the three qualitative methods described. The interviews are usually taped on audiocassette and then transcribed for detailed analysis. Participant observation, another common method, is particularly suitable for ethnographic research. For the circumstance under study, the investigator observes the activities, people, and physical aspects of the situation while engaging, either passively or actively, in the activities (Spradley, 1980). Field notes of the observations are recorded for later analysis. In

phenomenological studies, data resources may be expanded to include movies, pictures, poetry, stories, or any medium that portrays the nature of the meaning of the study topic.

Data Analysis

Data analysis is ongoing throughout the period of data collection. Each datum, whether from transcriptions of interviews, detailed field notes, documents, or photographs, is compared and contrasted with the other data. As the study progresses, interpretations are made by the investigator. Descriptions or theoretical propositions are frequently validated by study participants to ensure that findings represent true meanings.

In phenomenological studies, several processes of analysis have evolved. An investigator should identify the procedure used in the study. For example, Giorgi (1985) outlines a specific structure for data analysis. It includes compiling and examining descriptions about the meaning of a phenomenon; identifying common elements or units of meaning; delineating themes; naming abstract meanings; and generating what are called *structural descriptions* that embrace the meaning of the lived experience from the participants' perspectives. In contrast, van Manen (1990, pp. 30–31) describes methodological themes of phenomenological research as "the dynamic interplay of six research activities." These are:

1) turning to a phenomenon which seriously interests us and commits us to the world; 2) investigating experience as it is lived rather than conceptualized; 3) reflecting on essential themes which characterize the phenomenon; 4) describing it through the art of writing and rewriting; 5) maintaining a strong and oriented pedagogical relation to the phenomenon; and 6) balancing the research context by considering parts and whole.

The lived experience is represented through language. This is achieved by writing and rewriting until the written word portrays a deep understanding of the meaning of a lived experience.

In ethnographic studies, observational field notes of and interviews with individuals within a specific culture (e.g., society, community, or institution such as a hospital or clinic) are analyzed. Ethnographies may be descriptive or analytical. Descriptive ethnographies generally identify and describe social patterns or actions within a specific culture, whereas analytical ethnographies examine social meanings and cultural biasis or norms that guide the actions of individuals within the identified culture (Morse & Field, 1995).

Grounded-theory research follows an exceptionally systematic analytical process. Data from transcribed interviews are coded and categorized, and connections between categories are made; a tentative conceptualization or theory is formulated, and examination continues until a core variable emerges that is the focus of the theory. Concept modification and integration continue through two processes called *memoing* and *theoretical coding*. The process of analysis is not linear. Throughout the data analysis, codes, categories, conceptualizations, and theory are constantly compared, and the researcher moves between inductive and deductive reasoning. Conceptualizations of relationships are deductively proposed, and these are inductively examined for verification. The analytical process in ongoing until a theory, substantiated by the data, is generated (Glaser, 1978; Strauss & Corbin, 1990).

Application of Methods to Quantitative Approaches

Sampling and Sample Size

Probability sampling methods, particularly for correlational and experimental studies, are preferred for quantitative approaches, so that the study findings can be generalized to a larger population. However, as previously discussed, many studies involving human subjects must employ nonprobability sampling methods. The most common method is convenience sampling.

Deciding on the sample size can be a critical issue in quantitative studies. There are no established guidelines. Factors to consider include the study purpose, level of inquiry, design, and type of analysis, as well as the availability of subjects and research funds and the time frame of the study. Generally, samples should be as large as possible, and sample size should increase as the number of variables and groups to be studied increases (Burns & Grove, 1993).

For descriptive studies that identify and describe characteristics of a population, sample size will generally not affect study outcomes to the same degree that it will for other quantitative methods. Recommendations are to recruit as large a sample as possible after considering the previously described factors.

Correlational studies and those using survey questionnaires generally require large samples. The size is reflected in the number of variables to be examined or subgroups to be compared. As each of these factors increases, so must the sample size. If numbers are insufficient, statistical analyses and study findings can be compromised.

Epidemiological studies that examine associations between variables such as exposure (risk factors) and a disease or health condition are case-control and cohort studies. In case-control studies, subjects identified as having a specific condition are compared with a control group of subjects who do not have the condition. Differences between the two groups in subjects' past experiences or life events are examined to identify factors that may lead to the onset of the condition. During the past decade, there has been increased interest in the relationship of breastfeeding duration and exclusivity and diseases such as childhood leukemia, diabetes, and upper respiratory infections.

Cohort studies are similar to case-control studies but are generally follow-up studies of subjects who are exposed or not exposed to a risk factor that is assumed to be associated with the onset of an identified health problem. An example is a study by Wright et al. (1989) regarding breastfeeding and lower respiratory tract illness during the first year of life. Infants in a pediatric practice were followed from birth through their first year of life, and comparisons were made between infants who were breastfed and those not breastfed and of the durations of breastfeeding in regard to lower respiratory tract illnesses. Findings showed that breastfeeding for any duration was related to a decreased incidence of wheezing illnesses during a infant's first four months of life.

Case-control studies are frequently retrospective (data collected about past events), whereas cohort studies are generally prospective (data collected as it happens), though these types of data collection are applicable to both methods of study (Hennekens et al., 1987). If subjects are asked to respond retrospectively, their recall bias is a research issue that must be considered. Mechanisms for examining accuracy of responses can be included in the study design. Examples are studies identifying infant-feeding practices and breastfeeding duration in Malaysia (Haaga, 1988) and Brazil (Huttley et al., 1990). In each study, retrospective data were collected at three intervals, and responses to similar questions asked at each interval were compared. Although both studies found that consistency of responses decreased over longer periods, factors considered more important were the characteristics of subjects; increased years of education and higher socioeconomic class were associated with more accurate responses. Haaga (1988) also reported that urban, as opposed to rural, populations and Chinese, as opposed to the Malaysian, ethnic groups were more consistent. Huttley et al. (1990) found that 70 percent of the subjects were accurate between the first and second interviews in their recall of how long they breastfed. For the 30 percent who were inconsistent in their responses, women with more education tended to increase the duration of time they breastfed, whereas those with less education increased or decreased their breastfeeding durations equally.

Sample size is critical in experimental studies or hypotheses testing, because numbers of subjects can influence study outcomes. If the sample size is too small, group differences may not be detected when they actually exist, and a null hypothesis (no difference between groups) is not rejected. Statistically, this is known as a type II error. The result is that an intervention or treatment that is effective is not recognized as making a difference.

For the studies described in the preceding paragraphs, a sample size that is adequate to show true differences between groups can be estimated using a *power analysis* (Cohen, 1988; Kramer & Thiemann, 1987). Computer software programs are available for computing this statistical procedure. When a research proposal is being developed, researchers frequently consult with a statistician for advice about sample size.

In experimental or quasi-experimental studies, *random assignment* of subjects to experimental and control groups is advised. This technique serves two purposes: all subjects have an equal and independent chance of receiving the treatment, and the probability that each group is similar in regard to background characteristics is increased. The latter purpose serves as a control of extraneous variables that may influence the effect of treatment. Random assignment should not be confused with random selection (previously discussed), which allows findings to be generalized to the population from which the sample was selected.

Data Collection

All methods of data collection previously described are applicable to quantitative studies *if* they are applied consistently and objectively. Descriptive studies gather data that are broader in scope or more subjective than in correlational or experimental studies. However, questionnaires, interview schedules, and observation criteria must be structured so that the same data are collected in the same manner from all subjects. Measurement studies, such as correlational, quasi-experimental, and experimental studies, require data that can be reduced to numbers in order to apply statistical procedures. Reliable and valid questionnaires and observation checklists used for measuring variable relationships often take years to develop. Once established, they may be used in numerous studies.

Questionnaires and assessment tools specific to breastfeeding have been developed, though studies to determine reliability and validity estimates of these measures are limited. Table 23–3 presents an overview of current breastfeeding questionnaires and assessment tools and indicates what is known about their reliability and validity. For correlational and experimental studies, it is recommended that the questionnaires or measures used for data collection be reliable and valid.

Reliability and Validity

Reliability and validity are central issues concerned with error in research. The occurrence of error "anywhere during the research process compromises the outcomes of the study and limits the usability of the data" (Brink, 1991). *Reliability* refers to the accuracy, consistency, precision, and stability of measurement or data collection. *Validity*

Table 23–3

BREASTFEEDING QUESTIONNAIRES AND ASSESSMENT TOOLS

Title	Purpose	Reliability	Validity
Breastfeeding Attrition Prediction Tool (BAPT) (Janke, 1992, 1994; Riordan et al., 1994; Riordan & Koehn, 1997)	To identify women at risk for early, unintended weaning. Four factors measure negative and positive breastfeeding attitude, perceived maternal control, and social and professional support.	Cronbach alphas for all scales, 0.79–0.85 (Janke, 1992, 1994) and 0.80–0.93 (Riordan et al., 1994; Riordan & Koehn, 1997).	Known group comparison: two scales distinguished between women with prior successful experience and those with no experience. Prediction validity: three of four scales related to 8-week feeding outcome (Janke, 1992), and negative sentiment scale predicted early unintended weaning (Janke, 1994).
Maternal Breastfeeding Evaluation Scale (MBFES) (Leff et al., 1994b; Riordan et al., 1994)	To measure a mother's overall evaluation of the breastfeeding experience using a 30-item Likert scale.	Test-retest correlations: 0.82–0.93. Cronbach alphas for subscales: 0.80–0.93 (Leff et al., 1994b) and 0.84–0.94 (Riordan et al., 1994).	Items developed from qualitative study interviews (Leff et al., 1994a). Significant positive correlation of total scale and subscales with intent and duration of breastfeeding (Leff et al., 1994b).
Infant Breastfeeding Assessment Tool (IBFAT) (Matthews, 1988, 1991)	To assess and measure infant breastfeeding competence. Four subscales measure readiness to feed, rooting, fixing, and sucking. Score range, 0–12.	Interrater reliability: 91% agreement in coassessed feeds (Matthews, 1988). Pairwise correlations of raters' scores, 0.58 (Riordan & Koehn, 1997).	Content validity and observation in clinical practice (Matthews, 1988).
Mother/Baby Assessment Score (MBA) (Mulford, 1992)	To assess maternal and infant breastfeeding behaviors. For both, breastfeeding is rated using five steps: signaling, positioning, fixing, milk transfer, and ending. Score range, 0–10.	Unknown.	Observations in clinical practice (Mulford, 1992).

Table 23–3 *(cont.)*

Title	Purpose	Reliability	Validity
Systematic Assessment of the Infant at the Breast (SAIB) (Shrago & Bocar, 1990)	To document breast-feeding techniques and problems and plan interventions. Measures alignment, areolar grasp and compression, and audible swallowing. Not scored.	Unknown.	Unknown.
Breast Engorgement (BESS) and Nipple Tenderness Scales (NTSS) (Storr, 1988)	To measure breast engorgement and nipple tenderness. Five levels of engorgement and nipple tenderness are each scored on a scale of 0–4.	Unknown.	Unknown.
The Baby Weigh Scale (Meier et al., 1994)	To determine accuracy of a scale for use in the home.	Reliable with standard scale to 0.02 gm.	

reflects truth, accuracy, and reality. To be valid, measures and methods of data collection must also be reliable.

Reliability. Accuracy and consistency in the method of data collection, as well as the tools or instruments used, are essential in quantitative studies. Several types of reliability should be addressed.

Interrater reliability refers to the accuracy and consistency of data collection. When more than one individual observes phenomena, or when more than one instrument (such as a thermometer) is used for data collection, the probability of error between the instruments or interviewers increases. To control this aspect, checks are made. Similar instruments should be calibrated until measurement is consistent. For individuals making similar observations, the degree of accuracy can be statistically determined. Acceptable levels of reliability depend on the statistical method used: for example, for interobserver reliability, an agreement of

0.90 (90 percent) is adequate. When a Cohen's kappa statistic, a procedure that corrects for level of chance agreement, is used, an acceptable level is 0.70 (Bakeman & Gottman, 1986). For the Infant Breastfeeding Assessment Tool described in Table 23–3, interrater reliability was determined by comparing agreement of the mother's and the investigator's breastfeeding assessments. Overall, agreement was 91 percent accurate, although it was noted that infants who fed well or poorly were easier to assess than were those who rated in the middle range and were classified as moderate feeders (Matthews, 1988, 1991).

Intrarater reliability refers to accuracy and consistency over time. When data are collected for more than six months, investigators may want to check the accuracy of the individual who is making the observations–and of the instrument(s) used–every few months. An acceptable intrarater reliability coefficient reported for longitudinal observational studies is also in the range of 0.85 to 0.95.

Test-retest reliability indicates the stability of a measure, such as a questionnaire, over time. Results of two administrations to the same subjects, occurring approximately three weeks apart, are statistically compared. A coefficient reported as 0.80 or higher is generally acceptable for measurement questionnaires that reflect attitudes or feelings that should be constant. However, for some events, such as postpartum adjustment, a low correlation coefficient (such as 0.40 or 0.50) may be desired, because differences in individual scores over time reflect inconsistency, a possible indication that the individual is changing or adjusting to a different lifestyle. The Maternal Breastfeeding Evaluation Scale presented in Table 23–3 has test-retest correlations of 0.82 to 0.93.

Internal consistency refers to the statistical agreement of several items on a questionnaire that reflect the meaning of a concept (e.g., satisfaction with breastfeeding). Similarity in meaning or internal consistency of the items can be statistically determined. Cronbach's alpha is a reliability coefficient frequently computed to determine internal consistency. A coefficient of 0.70 to 0.80 is generally acceptable for a questionnaire measuring a construct (Nunnally, 1978). Therefore, the Breastfeeding Attrition Prediction Tool and the Maternal Breastfeeding Evaluation Scale described in Table 23–3 are both internally consistent questionnaires for data collection.

Validity. Validity addresses the extent to which a questionnaire or measurement instrument reflects the meaning of the concept that is being measured (Woods & Catanzaro, 1988). Types of validity cited in quantitative studies are content, concurrent, and construct validity. Questionnaires and interview schedules used for descriptive studies should have *content* validity, meaning that the questions reflect the study concepts. In developing questionnaires, investigators review the literature to include dimensions of the concept being studied and then submit the questionnaire for review to individuals who are considered experts on the research topic. This validation of content with literature and experts is known as *content validity.*

Questionnaires used to measure concepts should also be subjected to *concurrent* and *construct* validation. Both require psychometric testing or statistical validation of the meaning of concepts used in a specific context. Use of questionnaires shown to have either concurrent or construct validity enhances the validity of a study.

Data Analysis

Data analysis is the process of organizing, summarizing, examining, and synthesizing the data collected in order to reach conclusions about the research question. Numerical analysis of data is central to quantitative studies. The data collected is converted to numerical values in a variety of ways. Table 23–4 defines levels of measurement and provides examples. The level of measurement has implications for the statistical procedures applied.

Statistical procedures used for correlational and experimental or quasi-experimental studies can be classified as parametric or nonparametric. Parametric tests are more powerful and preferred, because they permit inferences to be made from findings of the study sample to the larger population. Use of parametric procedures requires

- random selection of the sample
- variables that are normally distributed among the study groups
- measurement of the dependent variable(s) at an interval level

Nonparametric statistics are used in situations in which

- sample size is small
- normal distribution of variables in the sample cannot be assumed
- parameters of the population are unknown
- the level of measurement of variables is at a nominal or ordinal level

The selection of an appropriate statistical procedure depends on the type of study, sample size, sampling procedure, and the type of data for analysis. Table 23–5 indicates commonly used procedures for study type and level of data. In experimental or quasi-experimental studies, the level of data of concern is the dependent variable. The purpose of Table 23–5 is to assist research novices to recognize the appropriate use of statistics for reviewing studies.

Table 23–4

LEVELS OF MEASUREMENT

Type	Definition	Examples
Nominal	Discreet categories of data that do not have any implied order.	Gender: male–female Breastfed/not breastfed Marital status
Ordinal	Assigned categories of data that can be ranked in order. Intervals between categories are not equal.	Most Likert-type scales Infant Breastfeeding Assessment Scale (IBFAT) (Matthews, 1991)
Interval or ratio	Categories of data that are ordered and are equal distances apart. Ratio also has a known zero point.	Body temperature Blood pressure Weight or length Duration of breastfeeding measured in specified days, weeks, months, or years

Extensive knowledge about statistical procedures is beyond the scope of this chapter.

Controversy exists regarding the use of interval and ordinal data. Human feelings and perceptions do not fit the interval scale, because most psychosocial variables can only be superimposed on ordinal scale. Therefore, statistical procedures that traditionally require interval data are often used in human research with ordinal data.

Descriptive Studies. Data collected to describe variables and their relationships are generally subjected to content analysis and descriptive statistics. Content analysis consists of examining the data, identifying similar content or meanings, and classifying those that are classified in mutually exclusive categories. These nominal data can then be used with the descriptive statistics identified in Table 23–5. Findings may be reported as frequencies, percentages, or modes; they may be displayed in graphs, histograms, or contingency tables.

Correlational Studies. Correlational coefficients are statistical procedures for determining the relationship between two variables. The type of relationship is reported as positive (i.e., as one variable increases, so does the other), negative (i.e., both

variables decrease), or inverse (i.e., as one variable increases, the other decreases). The strength of the relationship is reported as a number between 1 and −1; stronger relationships are near 1 (positive) or −1 (negative), and 0 indicates no relationship. (See Table 23–5 for specific procedures.)

Associations in epidemiological studies are estimated using relative risk (RR) or risk ratio and odds ratio (OR). Cohort studies use RR, which indicates the probability that a group exposed to an identified factor will develop a specific disease or condition in relation to a group not exposed to the factor. The RR is expressed as the incidence rate of the disease in the exposed group to the incidence rate in the unexposed group (Harness, 1995). It is calculated using the formula

$$\mathbf{RR} = [a/(a + b)]\Big/[c/(c + d)]$$

(see representations in Table 23–6). In case-control studies, subjects have developed the disease or condition of interest, and the RR is then estimated by calculating the ratio of the odds of exposure among the cases to that among the controls (Hennekens et al., 1987). In a hypothetical case, the OR for estimating the association of disease X to exposure to a factor such as being fed only milk

Table 23–5

APPROPRIATE STATISTICS FOR TYPE OF STUDY AND LEVEL OF DATA

Type of Study	Nonparametric Tests and Level of Data	Parametric Tests and Level of Data
Descriptive		
One variable	Frequency, *nominal* Percentage, *ordinal* Mode, *nominal* Median, *ordinal* Mean, *interval* Standard deviation, *interval*	
Two or more variables	Contingency table, *nominal* Cross-tabulation, *nominal* Chi-square, *nominal*	
Correlational	Spearman's rho, *ordinal* Kendall's tau, *ordinal*	Pearson-*r*, *ordinal*
Experimental or Quasi-experimental		
Two independent groups	Median test, *ordinal* Mann-Whitney U, *ordinal*	*t*-test (pooled), *interval* *
Two dependent or paired groups	Wilcoxon signed-rank, *ordinal* McNemar chi-square, *nominal*	*t*-test (paired), *interval* *
Two or more groups	Chi-square, *nominal* Kruskal-Wallis, *ordinal* Friedman test, *ordinal*	ANOVA (F test), *interval* *

*Level of data of dependent variable.

substitutes in the first six months of life can be calculated using the formula

$$OR = ad/bc$$

These variables are represented in a 2 × 2 table (Table 23–6).

An RR or OR of 1.0 suggests that the incidence rate of disease is the same for both the exposed and nonexposed groups; however, a value exceeding 1 (e.g., 1.5) indicates an increased risk of one and a half times (that is, 50 percent higher) among those exposed to the factor. Ratios of less than 1 indicate decreased risk among those exposed. ORs are often reported with confidence intervals, which "represent the range within which the true magnitude of effect lies with a certain degree of assurance" (Hennekens et al., 1987).

Experimental and Quasi-Experimental Studies. The statistical procedure used to determine differences between groups depends on the number of groups and the level of measurement of the dependent variable, as shown in Table 23–5. Statistical differences are calculated using probability theory. Before analysis, the investigator decides on a level of significance, a *p* value, that will be used to accept that a statistically significant result indicates true

Table 23–6

CALCULATION OF RISK RATIO AND ODDS RATIO

Factor	Disease X	
	Cases	**Controls**
With milk substitutes	*a*	*b*
No milk substitutes	*c*	*d*

differences between groups. The *p* value reflects the probability that the statistical result can occur by chance. In most breastfeeding research, a *p* value of .05 is used. This indicates that the probability of a chance occurrence is 5 of 100 (or 1 of 20).

Multivariate Analysis. Multivariate analysis is the concurrent analysis of three or more variables to determine patterns of relationships between variables (Roberts & Burke, 1989). These advanced statistical procedures are suitable for analyzing complex correlational and experimental studies that have several independent or dependent variables (Tabachnick & Fidell, 1989). Generally, large sample sizes are required to accommodate analysis of increasing numbers of variables. Procedures commonly used include multiple regression; path analysis; analysis of covariance (ANCOVA), factor analysis; discriminate analysis; canonical correlation; and multivariate analysis of variance (MANOVA). As research becomes more sophisticated, the use of multivariate statistics in studies increases. This is a dilemma for beginning researchers and research consumers because studies using complex analytical procedures are more difficult to evaluate.

The Evaluation of Research Reports and Articles for Use in Practice

Evaluation is an analytical appraisal that makes judgments about the scientific merits of a study (Wilson, 1989). The analysis objectively addresses the study's strengths and weaknesses, poses questions about the research, and makes constructive

recommendations. Purposes for evaluating studies include determining whether study findings are useful for clinical decision making, deciding whether clinical practice should change, or concluding whether further study of a topic is indicated.

Evaluation begins with reading the research report or journal article several times, to become familiar with the study. Analysis of the research elements can then proceed. This chapter can serve as a base for understanding the research process and expectations for research approaches and specific methodologies. A key issue in evaluation is congruency. In a congruent study, the design is consistent with the research question; sampling procedures and methods of data collection are compatible with the design; analysis is suitable for the type of data collected; and the findings answer the research question. Table 23–7 lists questions that ought to be asked in evaluating qualitative and quantitative studies. Although not exhaustive, the guidelines will assist with the systematic review of studies.

Following examination of the research elements, the reviewer identifies the strengths and weaknesses of the study. All studies have flaws (Burns & Grove, 1997); therefore, weaknesses are considered in relation to how they affect outcomes and the overall meaning of the study. Judgments are made regarding the relevancy of knowledge generated and the usefulness of findings to clinical practice. Legitimate criticisms of a study should be presented with rational and constructive recommendations. Evaluating studies is a skill that develops with practice, increased knowledge and understanding of the research process, and awareness of studies related to a specific topic.

Research articles published in professional journals are the most common source of research reports. The limitations, particularly the length of the report, must be considered in the appraisal. Journal articles lack the detail of accounts of full research reports. Studies in refereed journals are subject to review before publication. Members of journal review boards, generally considered to be experts in the field, critique articles to judge them for their scientific merit and make recommendations regarding whether they should be published. The beliefs that members of review boards have regarding the scientific value of qualitative research can influence the publication of research reports.

Table 23–7

GUIDELINES FOR EVALUATING QUANTITATIVE AND QUALITATIVE STUDIES

General Guidelines	Quantitative Studies	Qualitative Studies
1. Problem and purpose Clearly stated? Amenable to scientific investigation? Significant to breastfeeding knowledge?	Provides direction for study?	Broadly stated? Exploratory?
2. Review of literature Pertinent? Well organized?	Includes recent and classic references? Theoretical base or conceptual framework evident?	Acknowledged the existence of (or lack of) literature on the topic?
3. Protection of human rights Subject's protection from harm ensured? Subjects suitably informed by written informed consent? Study reviewed by ethics board or committee? Means for ensuring privacy, confidentiality, or anonymity are explained?		
4. Method Design congruent with research question? Sampling procedure appropriate for research method? Method of data collection relevant for design?	Deductive approach used? Variables identified and defined? Sample representative of population and adequate size? Measuring tools suitable, reliable, and valid? Control of extraneous variables evident?	Inductive approach used? Key informants selected? Theoretical sampling addressed? Data collection and analysis concurrent? Process for data collection and analysis described? Data saturated? Reliability and validity explained?
5. Results and discussion Analysis suitable for method and design? Results clearly presented? Interpretations clear and based on data? Research question answered? Limitations of study identified? Conclusions based on results? Implications for practice and research described?	Statistical procedures used suitable for data and sample size? Tables clear and representative of data? Successful and unanticipated results reported?	Examples of informants' accounts displayed? Rich descriptions or theory presented? Findings compared with literature? Theory logical and complete?

Recognition of qualitative research is recent, and publication of these studies is gradually increasing.

Because breastfeeding encompasses many disciplines in the natural, social, and health sciences, breastfeeding practitioners should consult numerous journals to remain aware of current research. Although a challenging task, staying up to date is essential for professional practice.

Using Research in Clinical Practice

Bridging the gap between knowledge production and knowledge utilization is an ongoing process that requires motivation, commitment, persistence, and patience. Implementing research findings in clinical practice is a challenge for both researchers and practitioners. The process is facilitated when researchers and practitioners work together to achieve the goal of implementing evidence-based practice (Polit & Hungler, 1993). Responsibilities of researchers in assisting this process are

- disseminating study findings directly to practitioners as soon as a study is completed, through informal discussions; local, regional, and national presentations; and publications

- replicating studies that may improve clinical practice, as changes are seldom made on the basis of the outcomes from one small study

- encouraging and assisting practitioners to participate in research to develop interest and awareness

- listening to concerns about practice in order to generate problems for study that are relevant to a specific practice area

- collaborating with practitioners in research projects

- assisting practitioners with evaluation of research articles, to increase their knowledge and competence in judging research findings

Among the responsibilities of practitioners in translating research findings to the practice field are:

- developing a questioning attitude and openness to change

- sharing concerns about practice with researchers to develop pertinent clinical studies

- collaborating with researchers and participating in research projects

- critically reading and evaluating research articles and using relevant findings in practice

- attending professional conferences at which research is presented and discussed

- telling other clinicians about study findings that reflect, assist, or may alter practice

Scientific knowledge related to breastfeeding practice is in an early stage of development; most published studies are descriptive, exploratory, and correlational. Few studies test interventions specific to clinical practice. Findings from many current studies are relevant, however, and can be applied to practice. It is important to adopt new methods and approaches, to question their effect, and to develop new studies. Through such an ongoing process knowledge will be expanded, optimum practice will be facilitated, and mothers, infants, families, and society will all benefit.

SUMMARY

Research is a process for developing knowledge that serves as a base for accountable and responsible practice. Approaches to conducting research include qualitative, quantitative, observational, historical, and feminist methodologies. The research question that is asked–and whether knowledge is generated inductively or deductively–directs the approach used.

Qualitative methods generate an understanding of the meaning that reflects human values, beliefs, practices, and life experiences or events. Three types of qualitative methods are phenomenology, ethnography, and grounded theory. Characteristics of quantitative methods are objectivity, measurement, and control. Descriptive, correlational, experimental, and quasi-experimental studies use quantitative methods. Simultaneous use of qualitative and quantitative methods in one study is known as *triangulation*.

The major elements of research are the research problem and purpose, the review of the literature, protection of human subjects, method, and results and discussion. The research problem identifies what is studied and with whom, whereas the purpose delineates why the study is conducted. Research questions for quantitative methods are more specific than those of qualitative studies. In quantitative studies, variables are delineated and operationally defined. For example, how breastfeeding and the duration of breastfeeding are defined is of particular importance when conducting or evaluating studies.

Reviewing the body of literature about a study topic assists in formulating the research problem and directs the research method. Qualitative methods are frequently used when little is known about a topic.

Research that involves human subjects must assure the study participants of four basic rights. Mechanisms that assist in protecting subjects include use of an informed-consent form and evaluation of studies, before they are conducted, by ethical review boards or committees.

Study methods address setting, sample, data collection, and data analysis. The setting indicates the location of the study or the source of the participants. The sample is a subset of a larger population or group of individuals in whom the investigator is interested. Sampling is a process for selecting the sample from the population; two types are probability and nonprobability. Nonprobability sampling is used in all qualitative studies, whereas probability sampling is preferred in quantitative studies, because findings can then be generalized from the study sample to the target population. The latter method requires random selection of subjects, which is not always possible; therefore, many quantitative studies involving human subjects also use nonprobability sampling.

Data are collected by the researcher asking questions, makes observations, or measures key variables identified in the research question. In-depth interviews and observations are the most common methods used for qualitative studies, and data collection and analysis occur simultaneously. Systematic and rigorous methods for collecting and analyzing data are developed for all qualitative methods. Methods for data collection in quantitative studies are highly structured and must be the same for every subject.

Reliability and validity issues must be addressed for all research. Reliability refers to accuracy, consistency, precision, and stability of data collected; validity reflects the true meaning of data. In qualitative studies, checks are built into the data-collection-and-analysis process. In quantitative studies, reliability of measurement tools and investigators who are collecting data can be statistically estimated, as can the validity of the measurements used.

Data analysis is the process of organizing, summarizing, examining, and synthesizing the data collected to identify study findings. Qualitative studies generate rich descriptions and posit hypotheses or a theory. Descriptive narratives of participants' verbatim accounts support the investigator's interpretations. In quantitative studies, data are translated into numerical terms for statistical analysis. Depending on the type of study and the level of measurement of the data collected, a variety of statistical procedures can be employed. Results are displayed in tables and graphs.

Study results must be clear, concise, and congruent with the method used and answer the research question(s). Significant, nonsignificant, and unexpected results are reported. Limitations of the study and the extent to which findings can be generalized to additional populations must also be addressed. Study conclusions should reflect only the study findings.

Research reports or articles are evaluated to make judgments about their scientific merit and the usefulness of findings for clinical practice. A key issue in evaluation is study congruency.

Implementing research findings in clinical practice is a challenge for researchers and practitioners. This process can be expedited when both groups work together. Although findings from current studies are not generally definitive and further study is frequently recommended, using relevant findings in practice often serve to question effects and generate new studies. Our specific area of interest is breastfeeding research, which is an ongoing process that expands knowledge and facilitates optimal practice for the benefit of mothers, infants, families, and society.

REFERENCES

American Nurses Association: *Human rights guidelines for nurses in clinical and other research*. Kansas City: American Nurses Association, 1985.

Armstrong HC: International recommendations for consistent breastfeeding definitions. *J Hum Lact* 7:51–4, 1991.

Auerbach KG, Renfrew MJ, Minchin MA: Infant feeding comparisons: a hazard to infant health? *J Hum Lact* 7:63–71, 1991.

Bakeman R, Gottman JM: *Observing interaction: an introduction to sequential analysis*. Cambridge, UK: Cambridge University Press, 1986.

Bergum V: *Woman to mother: a transformation*. Granby, MA: Bergin & Garvey, 1989.

Booth CL, Mitchell SK: Observing human behavior. In: Woods NF, Catanzaro M (eds). *Nursing research: theory and practice*. St Louis: Mosby, 1985:278–99.

Bottorff J: Persistence in breastfeeding: a phenomenological investigation. *J Adv Nurs* 15:201–9, 1990.

Brink PJ: Issues of reliability and validity. In: Morse JM (ed). *Qualitative nursing research: a contemporary dialogue*. London: Sage Publications, 1991:164–86.

Burns N, Grove SK: *The practice of nursing research: conduct, critique and utilization* (3rd ed). Philadelphia: Saunders, 1997.

Buxton KE, et al: Women intending to breastfeed: predictors of early infant feeding experiences. *Am J Prev Med* 7:101–106, 1991.

Canadian Nurses Association: *Ethical guidelines for nursing research involving human subjects*. Ottawa: Canadian Nurses Association, 1983.

Chenitz WC, Swanson JM: *From practice to grounded theory*. Menlo Park, CA: Addison-Wesley, 1986: 96–98.

Christensen LB: *Experimental methodology* (5th ed). Boston: Allyn and Bacon, 1991:267–325.

Cohen J: *Statistical power analysis for the behavioural sciences* (2nd ed). New York: Academic Press, 1988.

Conway AE: Young infants' feeding patterns when sick and well [monograph 19]. *MCN* 18(4): 225–353, 1989.

Denzin NK: *The research act* (3rd ed). New York: McGraw-Hill, 1989.

Ellis DJ, Hewat RJ: Factors related to breastfeeding duration. *Can Fam Phys* 30:1479–84, 1984.

Ellis DJ, Hewat RJ, Livingstone V: *Report of an evaluation of the efficacy of a breastfeeding clinic in prolonging the duration of breastfeeding*. Vancouver, BC: University of British Columbia, School of Nursing and Department of Family Practice, 1991.

Giorgi A: Sketch of a psychological phenomenological method. In: Giorgi A (ed). *Phenomenology and psychological research*. Pittsburgh: Duquesne University Press, 1985:8–22.

Glaser BG: *Theoretical sensitivity*. Mill Valley, CA: The Sociology Press, 1978.

Haaga JG: Reliability of retrospective survey data on infant feeding. *Demography* 25:307–15, 1988.

Harding S, (ed). *Feminism and methodology*. Bloomington: Indiana University Press, 1987.

Harkness GA: *Epidemiology in nursing practice*. St Louis: Mosby, 1995:86–95.

Hellings PJ: *Factors predicting breastfeeding success*. Doctoral dissertation, University of Oregon, 1984.

Hennekens CH, Buring JE, Mayrent S: *Epidemiology in medicine*. Boston: Little, Brown, 1987:77–82, 93–5, 132-77, 252-7.

Hewat RJ: Living with an incessantly crying infant. *Phenomenol Pedagogy* 10:160–71, 1992.

Hewat RJ, Ellis DJ: Breastfeeding as a maternal-child team effort: women's perceptions. *Health Care Wom Int* 5:437–52, 1984.

Hewat RJ, Ellis DJ: Similarities and differences between women who breastfeed for short and long duration. *Midwifery* 2:1–7, 1986.

Hill PD, Aldag JC, Chatterton RT: The effect of sequential and simultaneous breast pumping milk volume and prolactin levels: a pilot study. *J Hum Lact* 12:193–99, 1996.

Huttley SRA, et. al: Do mothers overestimate breast feeding duration? An example of recall bias from a study in southern Brazil. *Am J Epidemiol* 132:572–5, 1990.

Janke J: Development of the breast-feeding attrition prediction tool. *Nurs Res* 34:100–4, 1994.

Janke J: Prediction of breast-feeding attrition: instrument development. *Appl Nurs Res* 5:48–63, 1992.

Jones DA, West RR, Newcombe RG: Maternal characteristics associated with the duration of breast-feeding. *Midwifery* 2:141–6, 1986.

Kaufman KJ, Hall LA: Influences of the social network on choice and duration of breast-feeding in mothers of preterm infants. *Res Nurs Health* 12:149–59, 1989.

Kelly L, Burton S, Regan L: Researching women's lives or studying women's oppression? Reflections on what constitutes feminist research. In: Maynard M, Purvis J (eds). *Researching women's lives from a feminist perspective.* London: Taylor & Francis, 1994:27–48.

Kistin N, Abramson R, Dublin P: Effect of peer counselors on breastfeeding initiation, exclusivity, and duration among low-income urban women. *J Hum Lact* 10:11–5, 1994.

Knafl KS, Breitmayer J: Triangulation in qualitative research: issues of conceptual clarity and purpose. In: Morse JM (ed). *Qualitative nursing research: a contemporary dialogue.* London: Sage Publications, 1991:226–39.

Kramer HC, Thiemann S: *How many subjects? Statistical power analysis in research.* Newbury Park, CA: Sage, 1987.

Labbok MH, Coffin CJ: A call for consistency in definition of breastfeeding behaviors. *Soc Sci Med* 44:1931–2, 1997.

Labbok M, Krasovec K: Toward consistency in breastfeeding definitions. *Stud Fam Plann* 21:226–30, 1990.

Lazzaro E, Anderson J, Auld G: Medical professionals' attitudes toward breastfeeding. *J Hum Lact* 11:97–101, 1995.

Leff EW, Jefferis SC, Gagne MP: Maternal perceptions of successful breastfeeding. *J Hum Lact* 10:99–104, 1994a.

Leff EW, Jefferis SC, Gagne MP: The development of the maternal breastfeeding evaluation scale. *J Hum Lact* 10:105–111, 1994b.

Levine RJ: *Ethics and regulation of clinical research* (2nd ed). Baltimore: Urban & Schwarzenberg, 1986.

Locklin MP: Telling the world: low income women and their breastfeeding experiences. *J Hum Lact* 11:285–91, 1995.

Locklin MP, Naber SJ: Does breastfeeding empower women? Insights from a select group of educated low-income, minority women. *Birth* 20:30–5, 1993.

Matthews MK: Developing an instrument to assess infant breastfeeding behaviour in the early neonatal period. *Midwifery* 4:154–65, 1988.

Matthews MK: Mothers' satisfaction with their neonates' breastfeeding behaviours. *JOGNN* 20:49–55, 1991.

Maynard M, Purvis J: *Researching women's lives from a feminist perspective.* London: Taylor & Francis, 1994.

Meier PP, et al: A new scale for in-home test weighing for mothers of preterm and high risk infants. *J Hum Lact* 10:163–8, 1994.

Millard AV: The place of the clock in pediatric advice: rationales, cultural themes, and impediments to breastfeeding. *Soc Sci Med* 31:211–21, 1990.

Morse JM: Qualitative nursing research: a free-for-all? In: Morse JM (ed). *Qualitative nursing research: a contemporary dialogue.* London: Sage Publications, 1991a:14–22.

Morse JM: Strategies for sampling. In: Morse JM (ed). *Qualitative nursing research: a contemporary dialogue.* London: Sage Publications, 1991b:127–44.

Morse JM, Bottorff JL: The use of ethology in clinical nursing research. *Adv Nurs Sci* 12:53–64, 1990.

Morse JM, Field PA: *Qualitative research methods for health professionals.* (2nd ed). London: Sage Publications, 1995.

Mulford C: The mother-baby assessment (MBA): an "apgar score" for breastfeeding. *J Hum Lact* 8:79–82, 1992.

Neander WL, Morse JM: Tradition and change in the northern Alberta Woodlands Cree: implications for infant feeding practices. *Can J Public Health* 80:190–4, 1989.

Nunnally JC: *Introduction to psychological measurement.* Toronto: McGraw-Hill, 1978:245.

Polit DF, Hungler BP: *Essentials of nursing research: methods, appraisal, and utilization* (3rd ed). Philadelphia: Lippincott, 1993:415–21.

Richardson V, Champion V: Variables related to length of breast-feeding. *Issues Comp Pediatr Nurs* 183–97, 1992.

Riordan JM, Koehn M: Reliability and validity testing of three breastfeeding assessment tools. *JOGNN* 26:181–7, 1997.

Riordan JM, Woodley G, Heaton K: Testing validity and reliability of an instrument which measures maternal evaluation of breastfeeding. *J Hum Lact* 10:231–5, 1994.

Roberts CA, Burke SO: *Nursing research: a quantitative and qualitative approach.* Boston: Jones and Bartlett, 1989:293.

Royal College of Nursing of the United Kingdom: *Ethics related research in nursing.* London: Royal College of Nursing, 1977.

Schy DS, et al: The effects of in-hospital lactation education on breastfeeding practice. *J Hum Lact* 12:119–22, 1996.

Shafer RJ: *A guide to historical method* (3rd ed). Belmont, CA: Wadsworth Publishing, 1980.

Shrago L, Bocar D: The infant's contribution to breastfeeding. *JOGNN* 19:209–15, 1990.

Spradley JP: *The ethnographic interview.* New York: Holt, Rinehart and Winston, 1979:3–5.

Spradley JP: *Participant observation.* New York: Holt, Rinehart and Winston, 1980.

Strauss A, Corbin J: *Basics of qualitative research: grounded theory procedures and techniques.* Newbury Park, CA: Sage Publications, 1990:24–32.

Storr GB: Prevention of nipple tenderness and breast engorgement in the postpartal period. *JOGNN* 17:203–9, 1988.

Tabachnick BG, Fidell LS: *Using multivariate statistics* (2nd ed). New York: HarperCollins, 1989:1–10.

van Manen M: Practicing phenomenological writing. *Phenomenol Pedagogy* 2:37–69, 1984.

van Manen M: *Researching lived experience: human science for an action sensitive pedagogy.* Ann Arbor: Althouse Press, 1990.

Wilson HS: *Research in nursing* (2nd ed). Redwood City, CA: Addison-Wesley, 1989:56–81, 163–84.

World Medical Association: *Declaration of Helsinki: Recommendations guiding doctors in clinical research.* New York: World Medical Association, 1964.

Woods NF, Catanzaro M: *Nursing research: theory and practice.* St Louis: Mosby, 1988:246–56.

Wright AL, Holberg CJ, Martinez FD, et al: Breast feeding and lower respiratory tract illness in the first year of life. *Br Med J* 299:946–9, 1989.

Wrigley EA, Hutchinson SA: Long-term breastfeeding. *J Nurse Midwif* 35:35–41, 1990.

RELATED READINGS

Denzin NK, Lincoln YS (ed): *Handbook of qualitative research.* Thousand Oaks, CA: Sage Publications, 1994.

Walker, LO: *Parent-infant nursing science: paradigms, phenomena, methods.* Philadelphia: Davis, 1992.

Waltz CF, Strickland OL, Lenz ER: *Measurement in nursing research* (2nd ed). Philadelphia: Davis, 1991.

Donor Human Milk Banking: More Than Nutrition

Lois D.W. Arnold

In 1980, the World Health Organization (WHO) and UNICEF issued a joint resolution stating that the "first alternative" when a mother is unable to breastfeed should be banked donor milk (WHO/UNICEF, 1980). More recent support for donor milk banking was issued in 1992 with the inclusion of banked donor milk as an acceptable feeding alternative when the biological mother tests positively for the human immunodeficiency virus (WHO/UNICEF, 1992).

A small population of infants and children depend on banked donor milk for health and even survival. Therefore, health professionals must know about banked donor milk: its clinical uses, its availability, its safety, its standardization as a product, and its merits and limitations.

A significant portion of the milk-banking literature refers to the banking of a mother's milk

for her infant. The reader needs to take careful note when perusing the literature to determine whether a study is concerned with donor milk banking or mother's-own-milk banking. Donor milk banking and wet-nursing are also not synonymous because of the processing that occurs in donor milk banking. This chapter deals only with donor milk banking.

The History of Human Milk Banking

The roots of donor milk banking may be found in wet-nursing. In ancient civilizations, wet nurses (women who breastfed a biologically unrelated child) were essential to the survival of infants whose mothers died in childbirth or postpartum or whose mothers were unable or unwilling to breastfeed them for any reason. The quality of milk from the nonbiological mother was of concern from earliest times. Rules governing wet-nursing can be found in the Code of Hammurabi (1800 BC). Wet nurses were carefully chosen both for their physical attributes and personality characteristics, because these were presumed to be transmitted through the milk to the nursing infant (Fildes, 1986; Lawrence, 1994; see also Chapter 1 of this text).

Note: The author expresses appreciation to members of the Human Milk Banking Association of North America, Inc., for their assistance in writing this chapter; to Richard J. Schanler, MD, for his thoughtful review of the content of this chapter; and to John C. Wallingford, PhD, Susie Buchter, MD, and Lisa Wright, MS, RD/LD, CNSD, for their comments on selected portions of this chapter.

In eighteenth-century Europe, foundling hospitals with a policy of routine dry-nursing (i.e., hand- or artificially feeding) their infants had much higher rates of mortality than did those hospitals that either provided wet-nurses for the infants in their care or sent them out to supervised wet nurses in the countryside (Fildes, 1988). Without exception, studies showed that during the late nineteenth and early twentieth centuries in Europe and the United States, infants breastfed by their own mothers or wet nurses had mortality rates lower than those of artificially fed infants (Cunningham, 1981). The clear benefits of breastfeeding for infant health and the difficulties of formulating artificial infant milk spurred the development of donor human-milk banks.

In the United States during the early twentieth century, wet nurses were difficult to find. Consequently, two Boston physicians, Denny and Talbot, developed the idea of stockpiling human milk. Both were aware of a Boston study that showed that bottle-fed babies were six times more likely to die of diarrhea and enteritis during the first year of life than were breastfed babies (Davis, 1913). Both were medical directors of the Massachusetts Infant Asylum, which employed wet nurses to feed sick foundlings and were concerned about the quality of the stored product (Golden, 1988). Before milk was banked, donors were screened for tuberculosis, syphilis, and other contagious diseases (Talbot, 1911; see also Arnold & Erickson, 1988). Advances in dairy technology also benefited early milk banks. Freezing, pasteurization, sterilization, and lyophilization (freeze-drying) were used with varying success to lengthen storage time so that a steady supply of uncontaminated milk could be guaranteed (Emerson & Platt, 1933; Scheuer & Duncan, 1936; Smith, 1942; Smith & Emerson, 1924). In 1943, the American Academy of Pediatrics (AAP) published its first recommendations for operating donor human milk banks (AAP, 1943).

After World War II, milk banking fell out of favor in the United States as the acceptance and use of formula increased. In the 1970s, with rapid advances in neonatal intensive care and recognition that human milk provided special properties that improved survival and decreased complications, milk banking once again became popular, and milk banks were established in many hospitals across the country. In the mid- to late 1980s, milk banking once again declined in North America because of concerns about viral transmission, particularly the human immunodeficiency viruses, and because of the development of special formulas for premature infants. In 1985, the Human Milk Banking Association of North America Inc. (HMBANA) was formed to facilitate communications among North American milk banks, act as a liaison with governmental regulatory agencies, formulate standards for donor milk-banking operations, educate health professionals and the public, and influence nutritional policy for ill infants and children (Box 24–1).

Current Trends in the United States and Canada

Since 1990, the number of donor milk banks in the United States and Canada has remained relatively stable, with seven distributing milk banks in the United States and one in Canada. These milk banks have dispensed an increasing volume of milk each year since 1991 (Table 24–1). The increase in use is partially due to publicity about the safety of donor milk and the establishment of guidelines for establishing and operating a donor milk bank, developed in consultation with the U.S. Food and Drug Administration (FDA) and the Centers for Disease Control and Prevention (CDC).

Regionalization is the key to economically operating donor milk banks. It is not cost effective for every hospital or even every state to have a donor milk bank, because production costs on a per-ounce basis decrease with an increase in volume. It is vital to the continuing safety and quality of donor milk that new milk banks become members of the HMBANA. Such membership provides informational support and assistance in establishing a milk bank and in remaining current with the latest changes in the standards and protocols for operating donor-milk banks.

Despite attempts to educate health care providers about the benefits of donor milk for the premature or ill infant, donor milk banking still has its detractors. The Canadian Paediatric Society Nutrition Committee published a statement in 1995

BOX 24–1

HMBANA Member Donor Milk Banks in North America

CANADA		UNITED STATES	
Lactation Support Service	Vancouver, British Columbia	Mothers' Milk Bank	San Jose, CA
		Mothers' Milk Bank	Denver, CO
		Triangle Mothers' Milk Bank	Raleigh, NC
MEXICO		Community Human Milk Bank*	Washington, DC
Banco de Leche	Xalapa, Vera Cruz, Mexico (Dr. Rafael Lucio)	Mothers' Milk Bank	Wilmington, DE
		Human Milk Bank*	Syracuse, NY
		Regional Milk Bank	Worcester, MA

In-house-only milk banks; they do not accept outside donors or dispense to recipients outside their own neonatal intensive care unit.

expressing the opinion that donor milk banking should not be practiced in industrialized countries. The statement equates donor milk banking with wet-nursing, ignores the precautions taken by HMBANA milk banks to prevent disease transmission, and claims that disease transmission rates for pasteurized donor milk are the same as those for blood transfusions (Canadian Paediatric Society, 1995). Canada is the only country in the world in which a pediatric professional society has issued a negative statement about donor milk banking.

Donor Milk Banking Outside North America

Although this chapter focuses primarily on donor milk banking as it is practiced in the United States and Canada, it also thrives in many other countries. Information about milk banking in other countries is often difficult to obtain, because there is no parent organization to which all milk banks belong, nor is there a central repository for data

about existing milk banks. Often there is little or no government support for, or policy regarding, donor milk banking. Many milk banks exist solely as a result of the commitment of a particular individual or group of individuals.

Donor milk banking is a common practice in much of Europe, although in some countries it has encountered difficulties. For example, in 1952, the German Democratic Republic (East Germany) decreed that every city with a population over 55,000 was required to have its own milk bank. In both East and West Germany, great interest in donor milk banking existed until the early 1970s, when collection reached its lowest point. At that time, West Germany closed all its milk banks, largely due to the aggressive marketing of manufactured specialty milks meant for premature infants. In East Germany, where the country's economy dictated that formula could not be purchased in large amounts and where pediatric chiefs of staff supported the preservation of existing milk banks, donor milk banks increased in number, and the volume dispensed rose, despite predictions to

Table 24–1

COMPARISON OF TOTAL OUNCES DISPENSED BY HMBANA MILK BANKS DURING SELECTED YEARS

Year	No. of Ounces	No. of MBs
1986	266,000	14
1989	177,000	8
1991–1992	133,716	9
1992–1993	144,156	8
1993–1994	162,950	8
1994–1995	182,392	8
1995–1996*	203,537	8

Source: HMBANA: Human Milk Banking Association of North America, Inc.

*Figures incomplete for one milk bank.

the contrary. In 1989, there were 60 milk banks in East Germany. With reunification of the two Germanys in 1990, many of these milk banks closed. In 1996, only 18 milk banks still existed, all in the former East Germany. They supply milk not only for the hospitals with which they are associated but also for hospitals whose milk banks have been closed (Springer, 1997).

Other European countries have developed standards for milk-banking practices. In France, for instance, standards for operation are incorporated into the body of public health law. These laws and regulations dictate donor-screening procedures, pasteurization methods, and bacteriology standards (Arnold, 1994; Arnold & Courdent, 1994; see also Roy & Lescop, 1979). England also has developed its standards for operation based on those developed by HMBANA and, though not part of the body of law per se, they are used by every milk bank in the country and have the support of the government and the British Paedi-

atric Association, which publishes the guidelines (Balmer, 1995; Balmer & Wharton, 1992; Baum, 1989; British Paediatric Association, 1994). Donor milk banks have existed for many years in Scandinavian countries (Siimes & Hallman, 1979; Tully, 1991). Poland also has a large milk bank in Lodz, the main purpose of which is to increase the number of premature infants receiving human milk as first feedings (Penc, 1996).

Developing countries appear to see the economy and advantages of donor milk banking. Countries in Central America and the Caribbean have developed donor milk banks as part of national campaigns to promote breastfeeding and the benefits of human milk. Help with funding for equipment has come from UNICEF in many cases. However, it is unclear how universally these milk banks are used and whether there are trained personnel to staff them. Brazil's milk-bank system of 78 donor milk banks is a ". . . key part of its 15-year-old federal program to promote breastfeeding. At a time of new discoveries of the benefits of breast milk, some experts contend it's a program with cost-cutting—and perhaps life-saving—implications for the United States" (Ellison, 1996).

In the People's Republic of China, a 1996 People-to-People International delegation of breastfeeding experts found that donor milk banking is considered a logical extension of step 6 of the Baby-Friendly Hospital Initiative (i.e., to "give newborn infants no food or drink other than breastmilk, unless *medically* indicated"). Donor milk is collected from postpartum mothers while they are in the hospital. The milk is then processed and dispensed to healthy newborns whose mothers are too ill to nurse immediately or who have insufficient milk to meet the infants' needs in the first five to seven days of life (Arnold, 1996a).

Issues for milk banks in emerging nations may be different, and the establishment of milk banks in these countries according to the standards of milk banks in industrialized countries presents a number of problems. For a more detailed discussion of these issues and guidelines based on practical experience, the reader is referred to Fernandez et al. (1993), Narayanan (1982), and Narayanan et al. (1982). Clinical uses and the rationales for donor milk use may also vary.

Cultural Issues

Even when health care providers accept the use of donor milk, there may be opposition to donor milk on the part of both prospective donors and parents of recipients. Among Africans, it is widely believed that diseases and genetic traits can be transferred through breastmilk. In a survey conducted in Nigeria, 70 percent of mothers were unwilling to accept donated breastmilk for their infants because of these fears and of sociocultural and religious beliefs (Ighogboja et al., 1995). The other 30 percent of mothers surveyed would accept donor milk only if it came from a close relative. Similar reasons would prevent 40 percent of women surveyed from donating milk.

Narayanan et al. (1980) noted that Muslim women object to their babies receiving milk from Hindu women, although Hindu mothers report no similar objections to donor milk from mothers practicing other religions. The Koran treats milk as altered blood; children suckled by the same woman become blood relations or milk siblings, and they are forbidden to marry each other to avoid the possibility of incest from a consanguineous marriage (Baumslag, 1987; Ighogboja et al., 1995; Kocturk, 1989). Donor milk banking is not an option in the Arab world.

The Benefits of Donor Milk

The benefits of donor milk are similar to those for breastfeeding in general: species specificity; ease of digestion; promotion of growth, maturation, and development of organ systems; allergy prophylaxis; and immunological benefits. All are related to the unique composition of human milk and the dual functions of many milk components.

Species Specificity

Occasional references appear in the literature to the theoretical potential for a graft-versus-host (GVH) reaction to donor milk by the recipient when fresh breastmilk is used (AAP, 1980; Xanthou, 1987). Young animals fed breastmilk white cells from a different species exhibit this type of reaction. However, this has not been shown to occur in humans, when human milk is given to members of the same species. In Toronto, fresh breastmilk was dispensed for many years within 24 hours of collection, without freezing or pasteurizing, and no ill effects were observed (Xanthou, 1987). The successful wet-nursing and cross-nursing that have occurred throughout human history also negate the GVH theory. The 1980 AAP statement on donor milk banking flatly states that GVH reactions are not an issue with human milk.

Ease of Digestion

Donor milk is advantageous to premature infants and to infants and children with certain digestive and metabolic conditions, because it is so easy to digest and creates less stress to organs and tissues during metabolism. Even though some enzymes in human milk are heat sensitive and are destroyed during processing (e.g., bile salt–stimulated lipase), most infants with immature digestive systems can handle donor milk as easily as their own mother's milk. Every effort is made to match the lactational stage of the donated milk with the age of the infant to further improve digestibility through the appropriate whey-casein ratio. Efforts are also made to provide premature infants with milk donated by mothers of other premature infants, especially the early milk, in which protein levels are higher.

Promotion of Growth, Maturation, and Development of Organ Systems

Many components of human milk are heat stable. They include growth factors and essential fatty acids that have been shown to improve neurological development in the infant. In the case of a premature infant who has been deprived of the full complement of developmental factors in utero, the presence of these factors in donor milk is extremely advantageous. These factors do not appear in commercial formulas.

In situations in which infants and children have suffered actual tissue damage (e.g., damage to the mucosal epithelial lining of the digestive tract as a result of allergies to formulas), donor milk allows healing of these tissues and maturation of the tissues and enzyme systems so that other foods can be tolerated as the child matures.

Allergy Prophylaxis

For infants with a family history of allergy, use of donor milk, especially when organs and tissues are still immature and developing, can prevent long-term allergic consequences. When infants have been shown to have allergies to particular components of formulas, donor milk can provide an alternative to other allergenic feedings. Milk from donors who have dairy-free diets may often be procured on special request.

Immunological Benefits

The immune factors, such as IgA, lactoferrin, and lysozyme, are very important to infants and children whose immune systems are either too immature to function or have been compromised in some way by disease or genetics. Equally important are the nutrients in human milk that have anti-infective roles in addition to their nutrient role. For example, human milk is the optimal source of IgA for the IgA-deficient patient. Other antiinfective factors include the mucin complexes, lipids with antiviral properties, carbohydrates that prevent bacterial and parasitic adhesion, and the like. Donor milk is an ideal way to acquire many of these factors, because they are not present in formulas or other animal milks.

Clinical Uses of Donor Milk

The clinical uses of banked donor milk may be arbitrarily divided into nutritional, medicinal or therapeutic, and preventive uses (Box 24–2). In practice, however, donor milk may serve several purposes for the same recipient. For example, a preterm infant receives not only nourishment from donor milk but medicinal therapy in the form of immune substances and growth factors. Simultaneously, necrotizing enterocolitis and feeding intolerances are also prevented through the use of donor milk.

Donor milk can be used in any case in which it is necessary to buy time while a diagnosis is made. Donor milk will "first do no harm" and is frequently part or all of the solution to a problem. The use of donor milk is meant to be temporary, although the definition of *temporary* varies according to the needs of the individual. Several case histories are presented later in this chapter.

Donor milk is never used when a mother's own milk is available but may be used to supplement a mother's supply. Donor milk is primarily used when the infant is ill or has some medical indication; however, donor milk may be provided if the mother is HIV positive, has miliary tuberculosis, or is undergoing chemotherapy, situations in North America in which use of the mothers own milk is contraindicated.

Distribution of Donor Milk: Neonates Versus Older Infants

In 1986, approximately 72 percent of donor milk dispensed went to infants in neonatal intensive care units (NICU), 23 percent to infants at home, and 2 percent to patients in pediatric units of hospitals (Arnold, 1988). In 1994, an unpublished survey of seven of the eight HMBANA milk banks indicated that the distribution pattern had shifted, with only 40 percent going to premature or ill infants in the NICU and 60 percent going to older infants.

Some NICUs use banked milk routinely for first feedings when a mother's own milk is unavailable (Arnold, 1991). At the Triangle Lactation Center and Mothers' Milk Bank in Raleigh, NC, where 70 to 80 percent of the mothers of premature infants express their own milk, the donor milk bank is a psychologically reassuring entity. Mothers relax when they know that the option of donor milk is available should their supply falter and thus are more successful in producing adequate amounts of their own milk. The presence of the donor milk bank and the use of donor milk also makes a strong statement that human milk is important to the welfare of these tiny infants (MR Tully, personal communication, 1996).

Nutrition

Donor milk is most commonly used for its nutritional properties and has been used in cases of malabsorption and feeding-intolerance conditions (Asquith et al., 1987). Malabsorption is a well-recognized complication of neonatal surgery. Banked milk is beneficial following surgery to repair damage from necrotizing enterocolitis and following surgery for congenital anomalies of the gastrointestinal tract,

BOX 24–2

Clinical Uses of Donor Human Milk

Nutritional

Prematurity

Malabsorption syndromes

Renal failure

Inborn errors of metabolism

Cardiac problems

Pediatric burn cases

Failure to thrive

Short-gut syndrome

Feeding intolerance

Postsurgical nutrition

Bronchopulmonary dysplasia

Medicinal or Therapeutic

Infectious diseases (intractable diarrhea, gastroenteritis, infantile botulism, sepsis, pneumonia, hemorrhagic conjunctivitis)

Postsurgical healing (omphalocele, gastroschisis, intestinal obstruction or bowel fistula, colostomy repair)

Immunodeficiency diseases (severe allergies, IgA deficiencies)

Inborn errors of metabolism

Solid-organ transplantations (including adults)

Noninfectious intestinal disorders (ulcerative colitis, irritable bowel syndrome)

Preventive

Necrotizing enterocolitis

During immunosuppressive therapy

Allergies to bovine and soy milks

Crohn's disease

Colitis

Feeding intolerance

---

such as gastroschisis, tracheoesophageal fistulas, intestinal atresia, intestinal obstruction, anorectal abnormalities, and diaphragmatic hernias (Rangecroft et al., 1978; Riddell, 1989).

Infants who fail to thrive may benefit greatly from the use of donor milk, which allows them to heal, gain weight, and then gradually wean to foods that they can tolerate without adverse effects (Arnold, 1995b). Subtle and sometimes unrecognized feeding intolerances may lead to failure to thrive or slow weight gain. Other feeding intolerances are more overt, with gastrointestinal bleeding, projectile vomiting, wheezing, and skin rashes as symptoms. Donor milk has been used in several cases of feeding intolerance in which gastrointestinal bleeding was severe. Within 24 hours

of starting exclusive donor-milk feedings, bleeding ceased, and the infant began to show improvement (MR Tully, personal communication, 1996).

Other conditions that lend themselves to the use of donor milk for nutritional purposes are those in which the infant cannot tolerate the additional metabolic stress of digesting formula. Cardiac problems (A Radcliffe, personal communication, 1995), chronic renal failure (Anderson & Arnold, 1993), and bronchopulmonary dysplasia (BPD) are examples. For a case history of renal abnormality that included donor milk, see Box 24–3. In the case of BPD, in which energy requirements are high to compensate for the extra work by respiratory muscles, infants need greater protection from respiratory infections, and fatty acids are important to the

BOX 24–3

Case History 1

A female infant was born at 36 weeks' gestation weighing 2,760 gm. She had numerous renal abnormalities, including hydronephrosis, hydrometrocolpos, bilateral cystic dysplastic kidneys, other urogenital abnormalities, and minor coarctation of the aorta, all of which combined to significantly impair renal function. At day 2 of life, she vomited a cow's-milk-based formula, displaying cow's-milk protein intolerance that two older siblings had also exhibited during infancy. Casein hydrolysate formulas were considered, but these formulas are higher in protein, calcium, and potassium and would have worsened the infant's renal failure. Soy-based formulas were similarly not an appropriate option because of their higher solute load. The infant's mother was breastfeeding but unable to meet the infant's demands for growth, so banked donor milk was used to supplement the mother's supply, beginning at one month (corrected age). At three months (corrected age), her length and weight had increased on donor milk, but she was still below the fifth percentile. At eight months, daily intake remained low and was insufficient to meet protein and energy requirements. At that time, donor milk (60 percent) was supplemented with a hypoallergenic formula (40 percent) to provide more protein and phosphorus without worsening the uremia. Glucose polymers were also added for extra energy. She gained weight well on this diet. By manipulating her feedings in this manner, her renal function was improved, and dialysis during infancy was avoided. She will still need a kidney transplant at some point in childhood.

Source: Anderson A, Arnold LDW: Use of donor breastmilk in the nutrition management of chronic renal failure: three case histories. J Hum Lact 9:263–4, 1993.

metabolism of surfactant. Donor milk can be supplemented and fortified to provide adequate calories for the extra expenditure of energy, although caution is needed not to oversupplement or overfortify. The infant would receive from the donor milk immune substances to prevent respiratory or other infections that might affect further nutritional status, growth factors to help the lungs and other organ systems to mature, and fatty acids. For a BPD case history that used donor milk, see Box 24–4 (Buchter & Wright, 1996).

Donor milk has also been used in cases of inborn errors of metabolism. For example, symptoms of the fatal molybdenum cofactor deficiency are eased when donor milk is used because of its 1:1 ratio of methionine to cystine and the occurrence of these two amino acids in lesser amounts than in formula (S Yannicelli, personal communication, 1991). A glycolytic pathway defect has also been an appropriate nutritional use of donor milk (Arnold, 1995c).

Donor milk is a metabolically ideal feeding medium for severely burned infants. Animal models show that complications from stress ulcers are fewer when elemental formulas (e.g., formulas that have fats, proteins, and carbohydrates broken down into their simplest elements) are added to the diet of burn victims (Young et al., 1981). However, elemental formulas are hyperosmolar and formulated for adults and are not meant for long-term

BOX 24–4

Case History 2

A male infant was born at 28 weeks' gestation to a 32-year-old HIV-positive mother who abused cocaine and alcohol and had no prenatal care. At birth he weighed 900 gm and had Apgar scores of 6 and 9. He was HIV negative by polymerase chain reaction (PCR) testing. He developed severe bronchopulmonary dysplasia (BPD) and failure to thrive. At two months of age, he had *Staphylococcus aureus* sepsis and his BPD worsened. Weight gain was a serious problem because he was working so hard to breathe, frequently took nothing by mouth because of medical procedures (54 days of 149 days of life), and suffered from periodic bouts of diarrhea. Nutrition was a medical emergency of its own. To treat this medical emergency, he was pharmacologically paralyzed and placed on a ventilator with bronchodilators. He was weaned from the ventilator only when all the nutritional problems had been solved.

Nutritionally, he presented with a number of signs of malabsorption, including guaiac-positive stools. He did not tolerate the formulas tried, and it was concluded that he had lost much of the villous surface of the intestines, along with the enzyme systems needed for digestion and absorption. Donor milk was first given at four months of age, starting with 1 ml/hour to allow for intestinal healing. As the amount of donor milk gradually increased, total parenteral nutrition (TPN) was gradually decreased. He achieved full enteral feedings of donor milk spiked with added calories after 40 days. Thirty kilocalorie-per-ounce feedings were achieved by adding fortifiers and medium-chain triglyceride (MCT) oil. Anthropometric measures were used to evaluate growth. Head circumference was the first measure to correct and, at nine months of age, his growth was correct for his age.

The infant was on donor milk for a total of 122 days and was discharged to foster care at 15 months of age on Pediasure fed by a G-tube. He had an open tracheotomy tube. At 26 months of age, he had had no hospital readmissions and was performing age-appropriate tasks, walking, waving, scribbling, and talking through a Passy-Muir valve.

Why did donor milk work? It provided enzymes to aid digestion; it contained increased bioavailability of nutrients; it provided trophic factors, such as long-chain fatty acids and intact protein to foster growth and maturation; and it provided antiinfective properties (lipids, immunoglobulins, polysaccharides) and antiinflammatory agents to prevent illness.

Source: Buchter S, Wright L: Use of donor milk for the treatment of severe formula intolerance in a preterm infant with chronic lung disease and failure to thrive: a case presentation. *Presentation at the annual meeting of the Human Milk Banking Association of North America, Raleigh, NC, March 1, 1996.*

pediatric use (Brady et al., 1986). Burn victims have an increased metabolism and therefore greater energy requirements, but they do not metabolize glucose efficiently. They also have a high risk of sepsis and would benefit from more immune factors. Finally, they lose nitrogen through their open wounds and need higher amounts of protein (Young et al., 1981). Human milk provides lactose as a more easily metabolized energy source, immunoglobulins and bacteriostatic protection, and growth factors for wound healing.

Nutrition and Disease Prevention for Premature Infants

In their large prospective multicenter study of the effect of early diet on the development of premature infants, Lucas and Cole (1990) found that necrotizing enterocolitis (NEC) was 6 to 10 times more likely to develop in exclusively formula-fed infants than in those infants fed only human milk, and NEC was 3 times more common when the exclusively formula-fed infants were compared to those receiving both human milk and formula. Furthermore, pasteurized donor milk was as protective as was unheated maternal milk.

Eibl et al. (1988) found that giving oral immunoglobulin to formula-fed infants was prophylactic against NEC. Lucas and Cole (1990) believed that human milk may protect against NEC by providing IgA to the lumen of the intestine. Most IgA remains intact in donor milk during the heat-treatment process, and banked milk continues to be effective prophylaxis. With the decrease in the use of human milk—both maternal and donor—in British neonatal units, Lucas and Cole estimated that exclusive formula-feeding could account for approximately 500 cases of NEC each year and 100 additional infant deaths per year in the United Kingdom.

Lucas and Cole's study also found that delay in starting feedings was associated with a significant reduction in the incidence of NEC among formula-fed infants. This was not the case with infants fed human milk. These infants could start enteral feedings much earlier without serious consequences. Neonatologists at the University of Leipzig attributed their low rate of NEC (0.2 percent) to early enteral feedings of fresh human milk, either mother's own or banked donor milk, at one, two, and three days postpartum (Springer, 1997).

Other benefits of donor milk for the premature infant can be found in the presence of growth factors that encourage maturation of tissue and organ systems, such as the gastrointestinal, respiratory, and nervous systems. Additionally, fatty acids, such as docosahexanoic acid (DHA) and arachidonic acid (AA), which are present in human milk and are not affected by pasteurization, are known to improve visual acuity in premature infants, probably by promoting better development of neurological synapses and impulse conduction. These fatty acids and other as-yet-undetermined components of human milk are considered to be possible important factors in the IQ differences found in human milk-fed versus formula-fed infants in Lucas's multicenter prospective study (Lucas et al., 1992). Finnish neonatologists have concluded that the use of banked donor milk is preferable to formula, because it is a good source of the long-chain polyunsaturated fatty acids (Luukkainen et al., 1995).

Milk Fortification

Low-birth-weight (LBW) and very low-birth-weight (VLBW) infants have nutritional requirements different from those of full-term infants because of nutrient malabsorption secondary to immaturity of their digestive systems. The composition of milk from preterm mothers differs from that of term mothers for about the first two weeks postpartum. There has also been a long-standing debate on whether LBW and VLBW infants can achieve proper growth on banked milk obtained from mothers of term infants, often several months postpartum (AAP, 1985).

There are several mechanisms by which donor milk can better meet the nutritional needs of the premature infant:

1. *Efforts are always made by donor milk banks to match gestationally appropriate milk to the recipient.* Milk banks define milk that is collected by the mother of a preterm infant within the first month postpartum as *preterm* milk. When preterm milk is donated, most milk banks separate it from the milks of mothers of term infants, labeling it as such, so that it is available for younger, premature infants. The Vancouver, British Columbia, milk bank can also supply colostrum separately.

2. *There are a number of physical manipulations that can improve the nutritional content or availability of nutrients in donor milk.* The Milk Bank at Hvidovre Hospital in Hvidovre, Denmark, uses infrared analysis to measure protein, fat, and carbohydrate content of donor milk (Michaelsen et al., 1990). Individual milk donations can then be analyzed and pooled to

produce milks with the desired levels of proteins, fats, and carbohydrates to meet the requirements of premature infants. Martinez et al. (1987) used ultrasonic homogenization of expressed milk to prevent fat from adhering to feeding tubes. Premature Brazilian infants with an average birthweight of 1,400 gm were fed pasteurized, ultrasonically homogenized banked milk; they gained an average of 5 gm/day more than did their counterparts receiving the same milk that had not been ultrasonically homogenized (Martinez, 1989). The group receiving the homogenized donor milk also had significantly greater gains in length, tricipital skinfold, and subscapular skinfold (Raiol et al., 1993). Furthermore, they achieved intrauterine growth rates, and hospital stays were shortened (Martinez, 1989).

3. *Fortifiers can be added to or used separately from donor milk.* Enfamil Human Milk Fortifier (powder), vegetable oils (a good source of essential fatty acids) and Polycose (carbohydrates in liquid form) can be added directly to the human milk or, in the case of Similac Natural Care (liquid), fed alternately with human milk.

There is a downside to the use of such commercial preparations. These nutritional additives can impair the antiinfective properties of the donor milk. Quan et al. (1994) found significant decreases in lysozyme content and specific IgA to *E. coli* when fortifiers were added to fresh frozen milk. Jocson et al. (1996) also noted a slight increase in bacterial growth during 24 hours of refrigeration when commercial fortifier was added to human milk, although this increase was not statistically significant. Differences were significant, however, when fortified milk was refrigerated for 72 hours. Schanler (1996) and Shulman and Lau (1996) found that premature infants fed fortified human milk had a lower incidence of infection and NEC compared to formula-fed infants and infants who received alternate feedings of fortified human milk and preterm formula.

Commercial fortifiers for human milk have a whey-to-casein ratio of 60:40, whereas human milk in the early stages of lactation has a whey-to-casein ratio of approximately 80:20, a more appropriate ratio for the immature digestive system (Brady et al., 1986). Moreover, these fortifiers are derived from cow's milk, which always carries the risk of triggering an allergic response.

Some work is being done currently in Italy using fractionated and lyophilized (i.e., freeze-dried) donor milk to fortify either mother's own or donor milk (A Moro, personal communication, 1996). Other European milk banks also have the ability to lyophilize human milk and to fractionate it. However, there are no clinical studies comparing lyophilized human milk fortifier with bovine-derived fortifier. The process of lyophilization requires a very large volume of milk, much larger than is currently being collected and dispensed by milk banks in North America, which still tally milk dispensed in ounces rather than in liters, as do European milk banks.

In Athens, Greece, mothers of healthy term newborns express their milk while they are still in the hospital (average hospital stay, four to five days). This milk is pooled, pasteurized, and fed to premature infants. Mothers of premature infants express their milk as well. The milk that is fed to premature infants consists primarily of colostrum and transitional milk from term mothers and milk from mothers of premature infants. This milk is unfortified. In a study of 44 infants born weighing less than 1,500 gm, a comparison was made between infants fed the pooled pasteurized donor milk, their own mothers' milk, or preterm formula. No significant differences were found between groups in how rapidly they regained their birthweight or achieved a weight of 2,000 gm. All groups gained more than the intrauterine daily weight gain. The investigator concluded that the quality of the banked milk determines appropriate growth (Zachou, 1996).

Medicinal Therapy

Donor milk also has been used in the treatment of IgA deficiencies. Marinkovich (1988; see also Tully, 1990) used as little as 4 oz./day of fresh donor milk to provide IgA to patients deficient in this immunoglobulin to combat allergic reactions. When milk was heat-treated, additional volume was prescribed to compensate for the partial loss of IgA during heat treatment. Merhav et al. (1995) used an empirically chosen 12 oz. of donor milk a day with an adult liver-transplant patient who is IgA deficient. The number of organs available for transplant each year is far lower than the number of patients who need them. It is, therefore, crucial that organs not be "wasted" either through rejection or through death of the recipient from other causes, such as sepsis or pneumonia. Because donor milk is a readily available source of IgA, it is being used to protect the transplant recipient from pneumonia and other infections. The insurer in this case has chosen to cover this supply of donor milk for the lifetime of the recipient because it is more cost-effective to pay for the donor milk than to pay for hospitalization in a critical-care unit if the recipient becomes ill (Wright, 1996; see also Arnold, 1996b). Donor milk has also been used in patients with immunodepressed states related to bone-marrow transplants or leukemia therapy (Asquith et al., 1987).

Asquith also reports the use of banked milk in the treatment of such diseases as intractable diarrhea, gastroenteritis, ulcerative colitis, infantile botulism, sepsis, and pneumonia. Other uses of donor milk have been noted as well (e.g., as treatment for conjunctivitis and as food for the aged) (Baumslag, 1987, 1991). The CDC reported the use of human milk as a medical therapeutic in American Samoa during an outbreak of hemorrhagic conjunctivitis when the supply of antibiotics ran out (CDC, 1982). Historically, expressed human milk was used in ancient India during eye and ear surgeries and in eleventh-century Turkey for the treatment of ophthalmia.

Current Practice

The HMBANA (1996), in consultation with the FDA, has developed guidelines to standardize donor-milk-banking operations. These guidelines follow the United States Public Health Service recommendations for tissue and organ transplant banks (CDC, 1991, 1994) and are reviewed and revised annually, with a new edition being published each year.*

Donor Selection and Screening

In the early days of milk banking, mothers were paid by the ounce for their milk. They were also sometimes provided with transportation funds so that they could come to the milk bank to express their milk. In this way, milk banks retained control over the cleanliness of the mother and her expression technique and could ensure that the milk was not adulterated in any way (Chapin, 1923; Jones, 1928). The earliest guidelines (AAP, 1943; MacPherson & Talbot, 1939) include payment to mothers. MacPherson and Talbot's guidelines also included a test using a 0.25 percent aqueous solution of Nile blue sulfate to detect dilution or substitution of cow's milk by determining chloride content (MacPherson & Talbot, 1939; Talbot, 1927). Jones wrote that the Detroit milk bank checked the specific gravity of the milk to test for adulteration.

The current guidelines do not allow payment of donors. Although some countries in Europe allow payment of donors (Tully, 1991), Williams et al. (1985) offer two reasons why mothers should not be paid: (1) to avoid the need for surveillance of milk for water dilution or addition of cow's milk, and (2) to assure that the mother's own infant is receiving adequate nutrition and is not being deprived of milk so that the mother can earn more money. Concern about the health of the donor's infant has been seen in the literature since Talbot's time. Patient-information forms are sent to the donor's primary care provider and to the infant's care provider to ensure that donating milk is appropriate for the mother-baby dyad.

Donors must be healthy, lactating women, usually of healthy full-term infants (Arnold & Borman, 1996). Mothers of premature infants often donate their excess pumped milk, although some milk banks do not use this milk until the donor's infant is either discharged or is nursing well. Occasionally, a mother whose baby has died will donate milk that she has pumped, working through the grieving process by helping another infant.

Donors are recruited by word of mouth from childbirth classes, breastfeeding support groups,

---

*Guidelines for the Establishment and Operation of a Donor Human Milk Bank, *HMBANA, PO Box 370464, West Hartford, CT 06137-0464 USA.*

BOX 24–5

Reasons for Excluding a Donor

The following conditions exclude women from donating their milk to a human milk bank:

- Receipt of a blood transfusion or blood products within the last 12 months
- Receipt of an organ or tissue transplant within the last 12 months
- Regular use of more than 2 oz. of hard liquor or its equivalent in a 24-hour period
- Regular use of over-the-counter medications or systemic prescriptions (Replacement hormones and some birth-control hormones are acceptable.)
- Use of megadose vitamins or pharmacologically active herbal preparations
- Total vegetarian diet (vegan) without vitamin supplementation
- Use of illegal drugs
- Use of tobacco products
- Use of silicone breast implants
- A history or hepatitis, systemic disorders of any kind, or chronic infections (e.g., human immunodeficiency virus, human T-lymphotropic virus, tuberculosis)

---

and physicians' offices and by newspaper articles or television and radio public service announcements publicizing a need for milk. In Germany, many donors are second- and third-generation donors (Springer, 1997).

Donor human milk is the only human donor tissue with three layers of protection for the recipient. All prospective donors are verbally screened for health history and risk behaviors, as with blood donations (Box 24–5). Donors are then screened serologically for a panel of viruses:

- HIV-1 and HIV-2 antibody and antigen
- antibody to human T-lymphotropic virus types 1 and 2
- hepatitis B surface antigen
- hepatitis C antibody, and
- syphilis

Because the heterosexual population is increasingly at risk for HIV, it is critical that potential donors be serum-screened for HIV (WHO, 1987, 1992). If a donor has a reactive test later found on repeat testing to be a false reactive, she is still not accepted as a donor.

Heat Treatment

The third level of protection is heat treatment of donor milk. Fresh-frozen milk may be provided under special circumstances for patients whose conditions necessitate milk that has not been heat-treated.

When a milk bank heat-treats milk, the frozen milk is first thawed, and the contents of several containers are pooled. Most milk banks pool milks from up to five donors to make up a batch. Pooling mixes milks of various fat concentrations to ensure a more even concentration of fat from one batch to another (AAP, 1980). After aliquoting the pooled milk, the containers are submerged in a constant-temperature, agitating water bath set for the desired temperature. A control bottle is also submerged to monitor the actual temperature of the milk. Once the control reaches the desired temperature, the batch is held for 30 minutes at that temperature, then is removed, chilled rapidly, tested bacteriologically, and refrozen for dispensing. In some countries, pasteurizers specifically designed for human milk are used for this process.

Standard practice among milk banks has been holder pasteurization (heating the milk to 62.5°C and holding it at that temperature for 30 minutes).

The goal of research commissioned by the FDA in 1989 was to find the optimal temperature for heat-treating donor milk to ensure destruction of harmful bacteria and viruses while preserving as many of the beneficial properties of human milk as possible. Human milk was spiked with various concentrations of either HIV-free cells or HIV-infected cells. Samples were heated for 30 minutes at 56°C or at 62.5°C, using the protocol in the HMBANA guidelines. Destruction of the virus was rapid at both temperatures, and no virus could be recovered through reculturing after processing at either temperature (Orloff et al., 1993). These results confirm those of Eglin and Wilkinson (1987). As new viruses are identified, it will be important to assess each virus individually for its viability in heat-treated banked milk.

Heat treatment does have an effect on the beneficial components of human milk. Again using the HMBANA protocol for heat treatment, Eitenmiller (1990) looked at the effects of heat treatment on IgA, lactoferrin, lysozyme, and folic acid in samples of banked milk spiked with *E. coli* and *S. aureus* as bacterial markers (Table 24–2). If lysozyme is not denatured prior to heat treatment, it becomes activated. The increase in activity is due to conformational changes in the shape of the protein. Lysozyme is a very heat-stable protein. Eitenmiller (1990) found that enzymes and vitamins are much more stable than are bacterial cells. His results are in general agreement with the results of other earlier studies. Eitenmiller found that the majority of vitamins are relatively stable at 56°C and 62.5°C; he also found that the loss rate depends much more on oxidation than on temperature. However, if milk is deaerated to preserve vitamins, more IgA and lactoferrin are lost. Because vitamin supplements are routinely given in NICU nurseries, opting for more lactoferrin and IgA is the wiser choice. Based on the results of these studies commissioned by the FDA, the guidelines were changed to designate 56°C as the lowest acceptable temperature for heat treatment. Some bacteriostatic properties will continue to be sacrificed in favor of being assured of viral and bacterial decontamination.

Wallingford (1987) extensively reviewed studies looking at the effects of various heat-treatment methods on the components of human milk. The general rule is that the higher the temperature to which milk

---

Table 24-2

EFFECTS OF HEAT TREATMENT ON HUMAN MILK COMPONENTS

EXPRESSED AS PERCENTAGE RETAINED AFTER 30 MINUTES AT TEMPERATURE

Component	56°C	62.5°C
Bacterial markers		
S. aureus	100% killed	100% killed
E. coli	100% killed	100% killed
Components		
Lactoferrin	72%	22%
IgA	84%	51%
Folic acid	72%	57%
Lysozyme	132%	100%
Phosphatase	23%	1.4%

Source: Eitenmiller R: An overview of human milk pasteurization. *Presentation at the annual meeting of the Human Milk Banking Association of North America, Lexington, KY, October 15, 1990.*

---

is exposed, the greater will be the loss of beneficial components. At high temperatures, much of the bacteriostatic effect of human milk is destroyed, decreasing the benefit to the patient and making it more susceptible to later contamination (Bjorksten et al., 1980; Ford et al., 1977; Wills et al., 1982). The Wilmington, DE, milk bank still autoclaves its donor milk, as it has done since opening in 1947.

The effects of freezing, heating, and handling of human milk are cumulative. For example, Garza et al. (1986) reported that freezing affects lipids in human milk by breaking down fat-globule membranes, decreasing the size of the fat globules, and thereby increasing the surface available for lipase activity. This may lessen the digestibility and availability of fat to the patient. Heat treatment additionally alters other nutrients. Some immunological potency is lost during freezing, which destroys living cells in the milk. When previously frozen milk is heat-treated, further loss of immunoglobulins occurs. Even with this loss of bacteriostatic activity, some of the antiinfective properties remain intact, and the nutrients provided are still the most appropriate for the human infant.

The use of lyophilization and irradiation to reduce bacterial and viral contamination has been explored. However, early reports indicated that both these methods also lower the concentration of immune substances (Liebhaber et al., 1977; Raptopoulou-Gigi et al., 1977). Oxtoby (1988) reports that they may not be effective in destroying HIV.

Collection, Handling, and Storage

Donors are carefully instructed in methods for clean collection, handling, storage, and transportation of their milk. Milk banks may supply donors with sterile glass or plastic containers for milk collection, or they may accept milk stored in containers that the donor has provided (Fig. 24–1). The type of container used for collection may also have an effect on milk components. Disposable plastic bottle liners are not generally recommended because they puncture and tear easily, thereby increasing the risk of contamination during processing. Greater loss of fat, certain vitamins, and secretory IgA specific for *E. coli* polysaccharides is also reported when polyethylene bags are used. Donors are instructed to freeze their milk immediately after expressing it to preserve the immunological and nutritional elements (Arnold, 1996). Comprehensive instructions for storage and handling of expressed human milk are found in Box 24–6.

Differences in collection methods can also affect the nutrient content, especially the amount of fat. Milk that is passively collected from one breast while the infant feeds at the other (drip milk) is basically skim milk; it lacks the fat content of milk from a breast that is obtained by nursing or expressing. Drip milk also tends to be more contaminated (Lawrence, 1994). In general, drip milk is no longer used in most milk-banking situations around the world, but older studies in which donor milk was used may very well have used "drip milk" including Lucas's prospective longitudinal study of diet in preterm infants (Lucas, et al., 1984). Lack of sufficient fat may explain some of the less-than-favorable outcomes in studies using "drip milk."

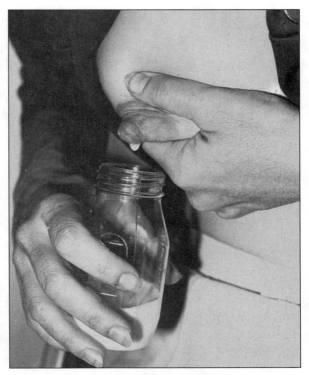

FIGURE 24–1. Hand-expressing breastmilk into a sterile container for the milk bank.

Packaging and Transport

Milk can be shipped over great distances by bus or airline. For long-distance shipping of milk, dry ice should be used. Containers may be insulated boxes used to transport blood, or styrofoam coolers, or the type of insulated box used by chemical companies for shipping frozen chemicals. Milk packed in dry ice can be successfully sent from one area of the country to another by overnight shipping companies, as are other frozen medical supplies.

Quality Assurance

To ensure the safety of donor human milk beyond the donor screening and heat-treatment processes, bacteria counts are performed after heat treatment. Milk banks also sample and test for bacteria prior to heat treatment or dispensing if the milk is to be used fresh-frozen. This can indicate whether a donor needs further education in clean collection techniques, including methods of pump sterilization. When more than one donor's milk is pooled, the sample of milk to be tested for bacteria may be

BOX 24–6

Storage and Handling of Expressed Human Milk

Depending on the health and age of the infant, expressed human milk should be handled with different degrees of safety precautions. Banked donor milk requires the highest level of safety precautions, because it is used to feed and treat infants who are biologically unrelated to the donor and who are already extremely ill. An intermediate level of safety should be observed in handling a mother's milk for her hospitalized or ill infant. For milk that is expressed for a healthy full-term infant or older baby in child care, less stringent precautions are necessary. The goal in all cases is to minimize the losses involved in storing and handling expressed milk to supply a feeding that (1) will not make the infant sick and (2) will provide milk that is as close in quality as possible to that nursed directly from the breast.

It is important for mothers in any setting to realize that their milk is extremely valuable to their infant's well-being and development. It is truly "liquid gold." For this reason, expressed milk should be treated with respect and provided with proper storage facilities. Subtle messages given to mothers are very important for efficient milk expression.

Viewing expressed human milk as a potential disease-transmission vector and a danger to the person feeding the expressed milk is incorrect. The question should be not how to protect the person handling the milk but how to protect the milk from the person doing the handling! Although human milk is considered a tissue that requires disease-transmission precautions when being used as a donor tissue (to protect the tissue recipient), it has been purposely omitted from guidelines on handling of blood and body fluids published by the Occupational Safety and Health Administration (OSHA, 1991). The hysteria surrounding expressed human milk is unwarranted and may be a result of misinformation or conflicting information (Calder, 1994). Some hospitals have hand-written addenda to OSHA guidelines, treating spilled milk like a toxic spill. There are also reports of group day-care providers refusing to accept breastfed infants because of fears of HIV transmission from the expressed milk. There is no known case of transmission of HIV through occupational exposure to human milk (Jones & Rogers, 1990). A second goal, therefore, is to reduce perceived risk of disease transmission, whether warranted or not, to the day-care provider or other individual handling milk.

The more one "handles" milk, the more one loses individual milk components and overall quality. Most research looking at the issues of milk storage and handling is outdated. Few studies have used similar methodologies; thus comparisons and generalizations are difficult. The information in this box examines storage and handling issues for both the ill or hospitalized infant and for the healthy term infant. For a more complete discussion of handling milk for the hospitalized infant, see *Recommendations for Collection, Storage, and Handling of a Mother's Milk for Her Own Infant in the Hospital Setting* (HMBANA, 1993). Recommendations for the healthy term infant or day-care setting are part of a Wellstart International work group consensus found in Hamosh (1994).

I. The Hospital Setting for the Ill or Preterm Infant

A. Use of Communal Equipment

1. *Each mother should have her own collecting kit or hand pump. She should be responsible for cleaning her own equipment.*

Rationale: Sharing collecting kits may be a source of cross-contamination. Cleaning their own kits gives mothers an investment in keeping their milk safe for the baby. Autoclaving kits give the mother the message that she cannot be trusted to clean her equipment properly and that her expressed milk is "dirty." There is no research evidence to support the hospital practice of periodically autoclaving kits.

2. *Electric breast pumps should be monitored regularly for spills, milk backup, and suction levels and should be cleaned and serviced appropriately.*

Rationale: Hospitals that do not provide mothers with closed-system kits for hospital-grade pumps need to check pumps frequently for milk backup. Hospital pumps can malfunction and be misused, and they can be ignored as a possible source of milk contamination. External spills can be cleaned up with 70% isopropanol, a 10% bleach solution, or a similar disinfectant. Internal contamination requires servicing by either the manufacturer or the hospital biomedical engineering department.

3. *Freezers should be set aside for the storage of expressed human milk. Freezers should be non-self-defrosting and should maintain –20°C (–4°F). Individual storage bins or boxes within the freezer should be provided for each mother's use. Labeling of containers should be clear and waterproof.*

Rationale: Providing large waterproof labels and separate storage bins for each mother within the freezer reduces the risk of staff feeding errors.

B. *Containers*

1. *Mothers should have access to an ample supply of clean containers with lids that provide an airtight seal.*

Rationale: Containers should not be closed with bottle nipple units because the nipple hole could allow contamination of milk and oxidation of milk components. Solid lids reduce the risk of contamination and oxidation of nutrients. In some settings, mothers are being asked to reuse their containers. Nurses set aside empty containers under the infant's bed, and mothers take them home, clean and sterilize them, and then refill them (Kuhnly, personal communication, 1996). This reportedly has not had any adverse effects on sepsis rates in NICU settings (N Wight, personal communication, 1995). See Arnold (1995a) for container options and their advantages and disadvantages.

2. *Glass or hard plastic containers (polycarbonate or polypropylene) are preferred for storage of expressed milk. Use of any polyethylene bag for milk storage is strongly discouraged.*

Rationale: Glass and hard plastic containers show the least loss of immunological factors during storage. In the case of fresh milk, live white cells tend to adhere to container surfaces when milk is placed in the container. White cells tend to fall back into solution faster when stored in glass containers over a 24-hour period (Goldblum et al., 1981). According to Hamosh (1994), glass is the preferred container for human milk storage but may not always be practical in terms of breakage.

Titers of secretory IgA antibody specific for *E. coli* polysaccharides is decreased by as much as 60 percent when milk is stored in polyethylene bags. Some vitamins are lost in greater amounts when polyethylene is used for storage. A considerable amount of fat is also lost to the polyethylene surface (Hamosh, 1994) and may affect delivery of fat-soluble nutrients to the infant. Furthermore, bags may be difficult to seal (providing opportunities for oxidation), may puncture

BOX 24–6 *(cont.)*

easily, and increase the risk of contamination. Some brands of storage bags are also extremely costly on a per-unit basis.

  C. Duration of Storage

  1. Expressed milk should be refrigerated immediately on expression unless it will be used within one hour.

Rationale: For the ill or preterm infant, caution is appropriate. Although numerous studies have looked at "safe" storage durations at room temperature, study designs vary considerably and may be inappropriate for the ill infant.

  2. Milk that will not be or has not been used within 48 hours of expression should be frozen.

Rationale: Several studies have addressed storage at 4°C (39°F) for periods of up to eight days and have found no appreciable bacterial growth over these storage times. In a majority of samples, bacterial colony counts either decreased or remained the same over time (Pardou et al., 1994). The 48-hour time limit for the ill infant is conservative enough to cover variations in home-refrigeration and -collection techniques.

  3. Frozen milk should be used by oldest date first to ensure use within three months of expression.

Rationale: Milk enzymes continue to be active at the commonly used freezing temperature of –20°C (–4°F). Milk components, especially fats, continue to be hydrolyzed or denatured over long periods of storage, (resulting in a "soapy" smell to the milk). For premature infants, this hydrolysis is felt to be a disadvantage. However, use of older milk is preferred to formula use. (Most home freezers and some hospital freezers do not approach –20°C, and milk composition may change more rapidly in these cases.)

  4. Thawed milk that has not been warmed for consumption should be stored in the refrigerator and used within 24 hours.

Rationale: Many bacteriostatic properties are lost during freezing, and the milk's ability to counteract bacterial growth is weakened after freezing (Pardou et al., 1994). Storage after thawing should therefore be limited.

  D. Thawing Procedures

  1. Thawing should be done in lukewarm water in a small bowl, and water should be prevented from touching the lid of the container. Thawing should not occur in a sink in which hand washing occurs.

Rationale: Thawing under running water may introduce contamination if the container lid becomes wet or if milk is thawed in a pan of water in the sink. Lukewarm water should be used to avoid damage to components from excessive heat.

  2. Thawing should never be done in a microwave oven.

Rationale: Microwaving significantly reduces levels of IgA in milk, decreases the activity of lysozyme, and allows greater coliform growth (Nemethy & Clore, 1990; Quan et al., 1992; Sigman et al., 1989). There is also a potential for hot spots with uneven heating. Milk should not be heated but merely brought to body temperature to avoid loss of milk components.

  E. Bacteriological Assessment of Expressed Milk

  Routine bacteriological culturing of expressed milk is unnecessary in most cases.

Rationale: Routine screening is not cost effective and does not always prevent exposure to potential pathogens (Law et al., 1989). Mothers should never be made to feel that their milk is "dirty" and that they cannot be trusted to follow directions and to express their milk safely for their infant. Screening may preclude using fresh milk because of delays in obtaining culture results.

  II. The Home Use or Day-Care Setting for the Healthy Full-Term Infant

  A. Use of Communal Equipment

1. *Work sites providing employee lactation services and shared electric breast pumps should have protocols in place for training employees in pump and work-surface cleanup and for ensuring that cleanups occur between individual users.*

Rationale: Cleanups reduce the potential risk of cross-contamination.

2. *Mothers should place containers of expressed milk inside more packaging with their name clearly labeled.*

Rationale: In work settings in which refrigerators may also be used for employee lunches, putting the container of expressed milk into another clearly labeled package (e.g., lunch box or plastic storage bin) will prevent milk from being used or contaminated.

3. *Refrigerators in day-care settings should contain clearly labeled bins for each infant's feedings. Only day-care providers should have access to refrigerators.*

Rationale: Limiting access to refrigerators lessens the risk of milk being fed to the wrong infant. Individual bottles should also be labeled with the child's full name, in case the mother and child have different last names.

B. Containers

1. *Regardless of the container type, feedings should arrive at the day-care center prepackaged, in feeding-size portions, thawed, and ready to feed.*

Rationale: Feedings that are already premeasured and prepackaged reduce the amount of spillage, avoid the risk of contamination by the day-care provider, and minimize exposure to the day-care provider.

2. *Hard plastic containers are recommended for day-care settings.*

Rationale: Glass containers cause breakage problems, and state regulations may prohibit their use in day-care settings. Storage bags are also not recommended because of their fragility and the loss of milk components, particularly the loss of IgA antibody specific for *E. coli* polysaccharides. Coliform infections may be easily contracted in day-care settings.

C. Universal Precautions

Universal precautions are not necessary when feeding expressed milk to infants.

Rationale: The CDC has stated on three separate occasions that gloves do *not* need to be worn when feeding a child or handling bottles of expressed milk. (CDC, 1988, 1994; Simonds & Chanock, 1993).

D. Duration of Storage at Different Temperatures

1. *Freshly expressed breastmilk may be safely stored at room temperature (77°F) for four hours.*

Rationale: Bacterial growth was low at 25°C (77°F) for four to eight hours, according to a study by Hamosh et al. (1996). When temperatures were lower (15°C; 59°F), bacterial growth was reduced, and storage at room temperature was safe for a longer period. The recommendation of four hours at room temperature is considered a conservative and safe time span.

2. *Expressed milk may be safely stored in the refrigerator (4°C; 39°F) for use within 72 hours. Milk that is not to be used within that time frame should be frozen.*

Rationale: See rationale for hospitalized infants.

3. *Expressed milk may be frozen for three to six months, depending on the freezer temperature and the type of freezer.*

Rationale: Using a thermometer to monitor freezer temperature is recommended. For freezers that are opened frequently and are frost-free (i.e., cycling a warm-up period in

BOX 24–6 *(cont.)*

each 24 hours to remove frost), milk should be stored away from the door and fan and should be stored for shorter periods than that stored in a freezer that is opened infrequently and needs manual defrosting. In a regular refrigerator freezer with its own external door (e.g., side by side) and temperatures in the range of –5°C to –15°C (5°F to 21°F), three months is the suggested storage duration. For deep freezers that must be defrosted by hand and have temperatures approximating –20°C (–4°F), milk may be safely stored for up to six months. In either instance, it is wisest to use the oldest stores of milk first to minimize the effects of long-term storage. It is preferable to use slightly outdated milk rather than formula.

taken from the pool, so that it represents what is actually being dispensed. Prior to heat treatment, the total bacterial count must be less than 10^6 colony-forming units per milliliter for milk to be considered for use. After heat treatment, there must be no bacterial growth. Milk samples are sent to either hospital laboratories or state or city health departments for analysis.

Environmental Contaminants

There is little information available to guide administrators of milk banks regarding acceptable levels of environmental contaminants. When contaminants are found in banked milk, each exposure has to be considered on a case-by-case basis and in consultation with experts from the FDA, the Environmental Protection Agency (EPA), and the AAP.

In Hawaii in 1981, cow's milk became contaminated with the pesticide heptachlor. Pregnant or lactating mothers were exposed through their consumption of cow's milk and local dairy products. It was necessary for Hawaii Mother's Milk, Inc., to test all donor milk for heptachlor before dispensing it to ensure that the pesticide content was within safe limits set by the EPA. Testing continued until banking operations ceased in 1988. Acceptable levels for dispensing were set well below those considered safe for the general population, because the recipient population was primarily ill, low-birth-weight infants for whom the body burden of pesticide would have been unacceptable if higher limits had been used.

Policies and Procedures

Most milk banks are affiliated with hospitals and, as part of the hospital, must have written policies and procedures governing their operations. These policies are reviewed and updated frequently. Consent forms allow the milk bank to dispense the donated milk to patients in need or to release it for research purposes if the milk is unacceptable for human use. Consent and release forms and publicity and appeals for new donors must also pass an institutional approval process. Milk banks must establish advisory boards, whose members are called on for their expertise and advice in such areas as infection control, nutrition, and the law. Milk banks that are part of a hospital or medical research facility are legally covered by the umbrella of that facility's insurance.

Costs of Donor Milk

All U.S. donor milk banks charge a processing fee for milk, which averages $2.50 an ounce. This fee is not for the milk but rather for the labor, supplies, and equipment costs involved in screening donors and collecting and processing the milk. Third-party reimbursement sometimes covers the processing fee. The WIC program has covered the processing fee in a number of states, and Medicaid has covered the fee for eligible babies in other states. Some private insurers pay reimbursement, but they are more likely to do so when the banked milk is used as part of in-hospital patient care.

Processing fees do not begin to cover the actual expense involved in getting milk from a donor to a recipient. Methods of raising money to meet this shortfall include sales and rentals of pumps and supplies, lactation consulting fees, grants, membership dues, and fund-raisers.

SUMMARY

The availability of donor human milk is essential to a small but needy population. Without it, some patients would not survive. For others, banked donor milk may help to prevent long-term medical problems. Although many experts agree on the efficacy of donor milk as therapy, much of the data are still in anecdotal form and are not well documented. Too often, breastmilk is tried as a last resort when damage is already severe. When the child dies, it is seen as a failure of the breastmilk, not as a failure of previous therapy that has placed the child in a condition from which recovery is unlikely.

The challenge in North America is to educate the health care provider who will be writing the prescription for this valuable fluid so that any patient who needs banked human milk can have speedy access to it. Banked human milk should be considered more frequently by physicians in the treatment plan for certain infants and adults to prevent further trauma, disease, and suffering. Although banked human milk as a therapeutic agent may not be the whole answer in all cases, in the absence of the biological mother's own milk, it will "first do no harm."

REFERENCES

American Academy of Pediatrics, Committee on Mother's Milk: Recommended standards for the operation of mothers' milk bureaus. *J Pediatr* 23:112–28, 1943.

American Academy of Pediatrics, Committee on Nutrition: Human milk banking. *Pediatrics* 65:854–7, 1980.

American Academy of Pediatrics, Committee on Nutrition: Nutritional needs of low-birth-weight infants. *Pediatrics* 75:976–86, 1985.

Anderson A, Arnold LDW: Use of donor breastmilk in the nutrition management of chronic renal failure: three case histories. *J Hum Lact* 9:263–4, 1993.

Arnold LDW: Donor milk banking in China: the ultimate step in becoming Baby Friendly. *J Hum Lact* 12:297–9, 1996a.

Arnold LDW: The lactariums of France: Part 1. The Lactarium Docteur Raymond Fourcade in Marmande. *J Hum Lact* 10:125–6, 1994.

Arnold, LDW: Milk bank survey–preliminary report of findings and discussion. *HMBANA Newsl* 3:7–9, 1988.

Arnold LDW: Possibilities for donor milk use in adult clinical settings–a largely unexplored area. *J Hum Lact* 12:59–60, 1996b.

Arnold LDW: The statistical state of human milk banking and what's in the future. *J Hum Lact* 7:25–7, 1991.

Arnold LDW: Storage containers for human milk: an issue revisited. *J Hum Lact* 11:325–8, 1995a.

Arnold LDW: Use of donor human milk in the management of failure to thrive: case histories. *J Hum Lact* 11:137–40, 1995b.

Arnold LDW: Use of donor milk in the treatment of metabolic disorders: glycolytic pathway defects. *J Hum Lact* 11:51–3, 1995c.

Arnold LDW, Borman LL: What are the characteristics of the ideal human milk donor? *J Hum Lact* 12:143–5, 1996.

Arnold LDW, Courdent M: The lactariums of France: Part 2. How association milk banks operate. *J Hum Lact* 10:195–6, 1994.

Arnold LDW, Erickson M: The early history of milk banking in the USA. *J Hum Lact* 4:112–3, 1988.

Asquith MT, et al: Clinical uses, collection, and banking of human milk. *Clin Perinatol* 14:173–85, 1987.

Balmer SE: Donor milk banking and guidelines in Britain. *J Hum Lact* 11:221–3, 1995.

Balmer SE, Wharton BA: Human milk banking at Sorrento Maternity Hospital, Birmingham. *Arch Dis Child* 67:556–9, 1992.

Baum JD: *Milk banking in the UK*. Presentation at the annual meeting of the Human Milk Banking Association of North America, Vancouver, British Columbia, October 15, 1989.

Baumslag N: Breastfeeding: cultural practices and variations. In: Jelliffe DB, Jelliffe EFP, eds. *Advances in international maternal and child health,* vol. 7. Oxford: Oxford University Press, 1987:36–50.

Baumslag N: *The mystery of the velvet bean*. Presentation at the Nineteenth Annual Seminar for Physicians, La Leche League International, Miami Beach, FL, July 23, 1991.

Bjorksten B, et al: Collecting and banking human milk: to heat or not to heat? *Br Med J* 281:765–9, 1980.

Brady MS, et al: Specialized formulas and feedings for infants with malabsorption or formula intolerance. *J Am Diet Assoc* 86:191–200, 1986.

British Paediatric Association, Committee on Nutrition: *Guidelines for the Establishment and Operation of Human Milk Banks in the UK*. London: British Paediatric Association, 1994:28.

Buchter S, Wright L: *Use of donor milk for the treatment of severe formula intolerance in a preterm infant with chronic lung disease and failure to thrive: a case presentation*. Presentation at the annual meeting of the Human Milk Banking Association of North America, Raleigh, NC, March 1, 1996.

Calder J: Occupational health and safety issues for child-care providers. *Pediatrics* 94:S1072–4, 1994.

Canadian Paediatric Society, Nutrition Committee: *Human milk banking and storage* [statement no. 95-03]. Toronto: Canadian Paediatric Society, 1995.

Centers for Disease Control: Acute hemorrhagic conjunctivitis–American Samoa. *MMWR* 31:21, 1982.

Centers for Disease Control: Guidelines for preventing transmission of human immunodeficiency virus through transplantation of human tissue and organs. *MMWR* 43(RR-8):1–17, 1994.

Centers for Disease Control and Prevention: Bloodborne pathogens–interpretive quips of the Federal Register. *Fed Reg* 56(235), December 6, 1991.

Centers for Disease Control and Prevention: Update: universal precautions for prevention of transmission of human immunodeficiency virus, hepatitis B virus, and other bloodborne pathogens: I. Health-care settings. *MMWR* 37:376–88, 1988.

Chapin HD: The operation of a breast milk dairy. *JAMA* 81:200–2, 1923.

Cunningham AS: Breast-feeding and morbidity in industrialized countries: an update. In: Jelliffe DB, Jelliffe EFP, eds. *Advances in international maternal and child health*. Oxford: Oxford University Press, 1981:128–68.

Davis WH: Statistical comparison of the mortality of breast-fed and bottle-fed infants. *Am J Dis Child* 5:234–47, 1913.

Eglin RP, Wilkinson AR: HIV infection and pasteurisation of breast milk. *Lancet* 1:1093, 1987.

Eibl MM, et al: Prevention of necrotizing enterocolitis in low-birth-weight infants by IgA-IgG feeding. *N Engl J Med* 319:1-7, 1988.

Eitenmiller R: *An overview of human milk pasteurization*. Presentation at the annual meeting of the Human Milk Banking Association of North America, Lexington, KY, October 15, 1990.

Ellison, K: Banking milk. *Miami Herald,* March 1, 1996:F–1, 2.

Emerson PW, Platt W: The preservation of human milk: VI. A preliminary note on the freezing process. *J Pediatr* 2:472–7, 1933.

Fernandez A, Mondkar J, Nanavati R: The establishment of a human milk bank in India. *J Hum Lact* 9:189–90, 1993.

Fildes V: *Breasts, bottles and babies: a history of infant feeding*. Edinburgh: Edinburgh University Press, 1986.

Fildes V: *Wet-nursing: a history from antiquity to the present*. Oxford: Basil Blackwell, 1988:144–89.

Ford JE, et al: Influence of the heat treatment of human milk on some of its protective constituents. *J Pediatr* 90:29–35, 1977.

Garza C, Hopkinson J, Schanler RJ: Human milk banking. In: Howell RR, Morriss RH, Pickering LK, eds. *Human milk in infant nutrition and health.* Springfield, IL: Thomas, 1986:225–55.

Goldblum RM, et al: Human milk banking: I. Effects of container upon immunologic factors in mature milk. *Nutr Res* 1:449–59, 1981.

Golden J: From wet nurse directory to milk bank: the delivery of human milk in Boston, 1909–1927. *Bull Hist Med* 62:589–605, 1988.

Hamosh M: *Breastmilk storage: renew of the literature and recommendations for research needs.* San Diego: Wellstart International/WHO/USAID, 1994, 31 pp.

Hamosh M, et al: Breastfeeding and the working mother: effect of time and temperature of short-term storage on proteolysis, lipolysis, and bacterial growth in milk. *Pediatrics* 97:492–8, 1996.

Human Milk Banking Association of North America, Inc: *Guidelines for the establishment and operation of a donor human milk bank.* West Hartford, CT: HMBANA, 1996:1–23.

Human Milk Banking Association of North America, Inc.: *Recommendations for collection, storage, and handling of a mother's milk for her own infant in the hospital setting.* West Hartford, CT: Human Milk Banking Association of North America, Inc., 1993.

Ighogboja IS, et al: Mothers' attitudes towards donated breastmilk in Jos, Nigeria. *J Hum Lact* 11:93–6, 1995.

Jocson M, et al: Human milk properties and nutrient fortification [abstract]. *FASEB J* 10:A554, 1996.

Jones DS, Rogers MF: Human immunodeficiency virus infection in children in daycare. *Sem Pediatr Infect Dis* 1:280–6, 1990.

Jones K: The mothers milk bureau of Detroit. *Public Health Nurs* March 142–3, 1928.

Kocturk T: Breast-feeding in Islam [letter]. *Acta Paediatr Scand* 78:777–9, 1989.

Law BJ, et al: Is ingestion of milk-associated bacteria by premature infants fed raw human milk controlled by routine bacteriologic screening? *J Clin Microbiol* 27:1560–6, 1989.

Lawrence RA: *Breastfeeding: a guide for the medical profession.* St Louis: Mosby, 1994:6–9, 599–619.

Liebhaber M, et al: Alterations of lymphocytes and of antibody content of human milk after processing. *J Pediatr* 91:897–900, 1977.

Lucas A, Cole TJ: Breast milk and neonatal necrotising enterocolitis. *Lancet* 336:1519–23, 1990.

Lucas A, et al: Breast milk and subsequent intelligence quotient in children born preterm. *Lancet* 339:261–4, 1992.

Lucas A, et al: Multicentre trial on feeding low birthweight infants: effects of diet on early growth. *Arch Dis Child* 59:722–30, 1984.

Luukkainen P, Salo MK, Nikkari T: The fatty acid composition of banked human milk and infant formulas: the choices of milk for feeding preterm infants. *Eur J Pediatr* 154:316–9, 1995.

MacPherson CH, Talbot FB: Standards for directories for mother's milk. *J Pediatr* 15:461–8, 1939.

Marinkovich V: *IgA deficiency and allergies.* Presentation at the annual meeting of the Human Milk Banking Association of North America, San Jose, CA, September 30, 1988.

Martinez FE: *Growth of premature neonates fed banked pasteurized human milk homogenized by ultrasonication.* Presentation at the annual meeting of the Human Milk Banking Association of North America, Vancouver, British Columbia, October 15, 1989.

Martinez FE, et al: Ultrasonic homogenization of expressed human milk to prevent fat loss during tube feeding. *J Pediatr Gastroenterol Nutr* 6:593–7, 1987.

Merhav HJ, et al: Treatment of IgA deficiency in liver transplant recipients with human breast milk. *Transpl Int* 8:327–9, 1995.

Michaelsen KM, et al: Variation in macronutrients in human bank milk: influencing factors and implications for human milk banking. *J Pediatr Gastroenterol Nutr* 11:229–39, 1990.

Narayanan I: Human milk in the developing world: to bank or not to bank? *Indian Pediatr* 19:395–9, 1982.

Narayanan I, Prakash K, Gujral VV: Management of expressed human milk in a developing country– experiences and practical guidelines. *J Trop Pediatr* 28:25–8, 1982.

Narayanan I, et al: Partial supplementation with expressed breast-milk for prevention of infection in low-birth-weight infants. *Lancet* September 13, 561–3, 1980.

Nemethy M, Clore ER: Microwave heating of infant formula and breast-milk. *J Pediatr Health Care* 4:131–5, 1990.

Occupational Safety and Health Administration, Department of Labor: Occupational Exposure to Bloodborne Pathogens; Final Rule. Fed Register 56(235):64175–82, December 6, 1991.

Orloff SL, Wallingford JC, McDougal JS: Inactivation of human immunodeficiency virus type I in human milk: effects of intrinsic factors in human milk and of pasteurization. *J Hum Lact* 9:13–7, 1993.

Oxtoby MJ: Human immunodeficiency virus and other viruses in human milk: placing the issues in broader perspective. *Pediatr Infect Dis J* 7:825–35, 1988.

Pardou A, et al: Human milk banking: influence of storage processes and of bacterial contamination on some milk constituents. *Biol Neonate* 65:302–9, 1994.

Penc B: Organization and activity of a human milk bank in Poland. *J Hum Lact* 12:226–9, 1996.

Quan R, et al: Effects of microwave radiation on anti-infective factors in human milk. *Pediatrics* 89:667–9, 1992.

Quan R, et al: The effect of nutritional additives on anti-infective factors in human milk. *Clin Pediatr* 33:325–28, 1994.

Rangecroft L, de San Lazaro C, Scott JES: A comparison of the feeding of the postoperative newborn with banked breast-milk or cow's-milk feeds. *J Pediatr Surg* 13:11–2, 1978.

Raptopoulou-Gigi M, Marwick K, McClelland DBL: Antimicrobial proteins in sterilized human milk. *Br Med J* 1:12–4, 1977.

Raiol MRS, et al: Feeding premature infants banked human milk homogenized by ultrasonic treatment. *J Pediatr* 123:985–8, 1993.

Riddell DG: *Use of banked human milk for feeding infants with abdominal wall defects*. Presentation at the annual meeting of the Human Milk Banking Association of North America, Vancouver, British Columbia, October 15, 1989.

Roy CC, Lescop J: Human milk banking: high rate of interest for a still uncertain credit balance. *Am J Dis Child* 133:255–6, 1979.

Schanler RJ: Human milk fortification for premature infants. *Am J Clin Nutr* 64:249–50, 1996.

Schanler RJ, Shulman RJ, Lau C: Fortified human milk improves the health of the premature infant [abstract]. *Pediatr Res* 40:548, 1996.

Scheuer LA, Duncan JE: A method of preserving breast milk: a study of its clinical application. *Am J Dis Child* 51:249–54, 1936.

Sigman M, et al: Effects of microwaving human milk: changes in IgA content and bacterial count. *J Am Diet Assoc* 89:690–2, 1989.

Siimes MA, Hallman N: A perspective on human milk banking, 1978. *J Pediatr* 94:173–4, 1979.

Simonds RJ, Chanock S: Medical issues related to caring for human immunodeficiency virus-infected children in and out of the home. *Pediatr Infect Dis J* 12:845–52, 1993.

Smith CA: Human milk technology. *J Pediatr* 20:616–26, 1942.

Smith LW, Emerson PW: Notes on the experimental production of dried breast milk. *Boston Med Surg J* 191:938–40, 1924.

Springer S: Human milk banking in Germany. *J Hum Lact* 13:65–8, 1997.

Talbot FB: Directory for wet-nurses. *Boston Med Surg J* 196:653–4, 1927.

Talbot FB: A directory for wet-nurses: its experiences for twelve months. *JAMA* 56:1715–7, 1911.

Tully MR: Banked human milk in the treatment of IgA deficiency and allergy symptoms. *J Hum Lact* 6:75, 1990.

Tully MR: Human milk banking in Sweden and Denmark. *J Hum Lact* 7:145–6, 1991.

Wallingford J: *Nutritional and anti-infective consequences of pasteurization of breast milk.* Presentation at the annual meeting of the Human Milk Banking Association of North America, Raleigh, NC, October 15, 1987.

Williams AF, et al: Human milk banking. *J Trop Pediatr* 31:185–90, 1985.

Wills ME, et al: Short-time low-temperature pasteurization of human milk. *Early Hum Dev* 7:71–80, 1982.

World Health Organization: Breast-feeding/breast milk and human immunodeficiency virus (HIV). *Wkly Epidemiol Rec* 62:245–6, 1987.

World Health Organization/United Nations Children's Fund: Concensus statement from the WHO/UNICEF consultation on HIV transmission and breast-feeding, Geneva, April 30–May 1, 1992.

World Health Organization/United Nations Children's Fund: Meeting on infant and young child feeding. *J Nurse Midwif* 25:31–8, 1980.

Wright HI: *The use of donor milk in solid organ transplantation.* Presentation at the annual meeting of the Human Milk Banking Association of North America, Inc., Raleigh, NC, March 1, 1996.

Xanthou M: Immunology of breast milk. In: Stern L, ed. *Feeding the sick infant* (Nestle Nutrition Workshop Series, vol. 11). New York: Raven, 1987:101–7.

Young VR, Motil KJ, Burke JF: Energy and protein metabolism in relation to requirements of the burned pediatric patient. In: Suskind RM, ed. *Textbook of pediatric nutrition.* New York: Raven, 1981:309–40.

Zachou T: *Growth in preterm infants fed different types of feedings.* Presentation at the annual meeting of the Human Milk Banking Association of North America, Raleigh, NC, March 1, 1996.

APPENDIXES
A–L

Composition of Human Colostrum and Mature Breast Milk

Constituent (per 100 mL)		Colostrum 1–5 days	Mature milk >30 days
Energy	kcal	58	70
Total solids	g	12.8	12.0
Lactose	g	5.3	7.3
Total nitrogen	mg	360	171
Protein nitrogen	mg	313	129
NPN	mg	47	42
Total protein	g	2.3	0.9
Casein	mg	140	187
α-Lactalbumin	mg	218	161
Lactoferrin	mg	330	167
IgA	mg	364	142
Amino acids (total)			
Alanine	mg	—	52
Arginine	mg	126	49
Aspartate	mg	—	110
Cystine	mg	—	25
Glutamate	mg	—	196
Glycine	mg	—	27
Histidine	mg	57	31
Isoleucine	mg	121	67
Leucine	mg	221	110
Lysine	mg	163	79
Methionine	mg	33	19
Phenylalanine	mg	105	44
Proline	mg	—	89
Serine	mg	—	54
Threonine	mg	148	58
Tryptophan	mg	52	25
Tyrosine	mg	—	38
Valine	mg	169	90
Taurine (free)	mg	—	8
Urea	mg	10	30
Creatine	mg	—	3.3
Total fat	g	2.9	4.2
Fatty acids (% total fat)			
12:0 lauric		1.8	5.8
14:0 myristic		3.8	8.6
16:0 palmitic		26.2	21.0
18:0 stearic		8.8	8.0
18:1 oleic		36.6	35.5
18:2, n-6 linoleic		6.8	7.2
18:3, n-3 linolenic		—	1.0
C_{20} and C_{22} polyunsaturated		10.2	2.9

APPENDIX A *(cont.)*

Constituent (per 100 mL)		Colostrum 1–5 days	Mature milk >30 days
Cholesterol	mg	27	16
Vitamins			
Fat soluble			
Vitamin A (retinol equivalents)	μg	89	47
β-Carotene	μg	112	23
Vitamin D	μg	—	0.04
Vitamin E (total tocopherols)	μg	1280	315
Vitamin K$_1$	μg	0.23	0.21
Water soluble			
Thiamine	μg	15	16
Riboflavin	μg	25	35
Niacin	μg	75	200
Folic acid	μg	—	5.2
Vitamin B$_6$	μg	12	28
Biotin	μg	0.1	0.6
Pantothenic acid	μg	183	225
Vitamin B$_{12}$	ng	200	26
Ascorbic acid	mg	4.4	4.0
Minerals			
Calcium	mg	23	28
Magnesium	mg	3.4	3.0
Sodium	mg	48	15
Potassium	mg	74	58
Chlorine	mg	91	40
Phosphorus	mg	14	15
Sulphur	mg	22	14
Trace elements			
Chromium	ng	—	39
Cobalt	μg	—	1
Copper	μg	46	35
Fluorine	μg	—	7
Iodine	μg	12	7
Iron	μg	45	40
Manganese	μg	—	0.4,1.5
Nickel	μg	—	2
Selenium	μg	—	2.0
Zinc	μg	540	166

Source: CE Casey, KM Hambidge: Nutritional aspects of human lactation. In: MC Neville, MR Neifert (eds.), Lactation: physiology, nutrition and breastfeeding. *New York: Plenum, 1983:203–4.*

APPENDIX B

Via Christi Health System, St. Joseph Campus

BREASTFEEDING POLICIES

DEFINITION AND PURPOSE

To promote a philosophy of maternal and infant care which advocates breastfeeding and supports the normal physiologic functions involved in this maternal-infant process. The goal is to assure that all families who elect to breastfeed their infants will have a successful and satisfying experience. These polices apply to the full term, normal newborn and may not apply to infants with certain clinical conditions, i.e., intra-uterine growth retardation (IUGR), prematurity, infant of diabetic mother.

I. GENERAL POLICIES

1. All pregnant women should receive information regarding the availability of classes on the benefits and management of breastfeeding.
2. Mothers who are undecided about feeding method will be encouraged to breastfeed.
3. Mothers expressing desire to breastfeed will have nipples examined for degree of eversion during admission procedures.
4. Educational pamphlets on breastfeeding shall be provided following birth, well before discharge.
5. Infants are to be put to breast as soon after birth as feasible for both mother and infant, with 20 minutes post-birth ideal and within the first 2 hours whenever possible.
6. Every mother is to be instructed in proper breastfeeding technique and re-evaluated before discharge. (See II: Functional Assessment of Infant at Breast.)

7. The infant is to be encouraged to nurse *at least* every 2 to 3 hours, for a minimum of 8 feedings per 24 hours.
8. Infants should feed from both breasts at all feedings, with a minimum of 6 minutes per breast. An infant may be returned to the first breast for continued suckling, if positioning is correct and nursing is comfortable.
9. If within the first 24–48 hours post-birth feedings at breast are incomplete or ineffective, the mother should be instructed to begin regular expression of her breasts, with continued assistance by an experienced staff member. The colostrum or milk obtained by expression should be given to the baby.
10. Supplementary water or formula is given for certain clinical conditions as ordered by the physician, but not on a routine basis. If prolonged supplementation is necessary, the physician will be contacted regarding formula choice and amount.
11. Mothers who wish to feed by both breast and bottle will be educated about breastfeeding and encouraged to breastfeed without supplement.
12. Pacifiers should not be used on a routine basis for the breastfeeding infant as a hunger satiety measure.
13. Breastfeeding mothers are to have their breasts examined for evidence of lactation or breastfeeding problems at least once every 24 hours.
14. Infants should remain at the mothers' bedside

Used with permission of Via Christi Health System, St. Joseph Campus, Wichita, Kansas, 1991.

APPENDIX B *(cont.)*

both day and night. The nurse should plan with the mother and family for periods of rest/sleep both day and night. If the mother chooses to have the infant in the nursery, she will be encouraged to feed the baby on demand.

15. Commercial discharge packs containing water or formula are not to be given unless specifically ordered by the physician or requested by the mother.

16. At discharge, each mother is to be given a phone number to call for breastfeeding assistance.

17. Mothers who are separated from their infants will be instructed on the proper use of breast pumps as well as the storage and transportation of breast milk.

II. FUNCTIONAL ASSESSMENT OF THE INFANT AT BREAST (FAIB) POLICY*

A. Functional assessment of the infant at breast should be completed:
   1. Within first 24 hours of life AND
   2. Before discharge from birth setting.
   3. Additional assessments should be performed anytime a breastfeeding problem is suspected (i.e., slow weight gain, persistent sore nipples, etc.).

B. Direct observation of breastfeeding is critical.

C. Assessment should be as nonobtrusive as possible.

D. Assessment is NOT necessary during the first breastfeeding experience. The first breastfeeding should be a "getting acquainted" session with lots of enthusiasm and little intervention from health care providers.

E. If the FAIB indicates difficulties with breastfeeding, the infant's physician will be notified prior to discharge.

Procedure

A. Four A's help guide assessment and documentation

1. Alignment

- Infant is in flexed position—relaxed, no muscular rigidity
- Infant's head is aligned with trunk
- Infant's head is at breast level (no traction exerted on breast or nipple)
- Infant's head is straight on breast (not turned or hyperextended)
- Imaginary line drawn from ear to shoulder to iliac crest
- Mother is in comfortable position, supported with pillows

2. Areolar Grasp

- Mouth is opened widely, lips not pursed
- Lips are visible and flanged outward
- Tongue covers lower gum, curved (troughed) around areola
- Approximately 1/2 to 1 inch of areola is drawn SYMMETRICALLY into mouth
- Complete seal and strong vacuum is formed by infant's mouth
- No clicking or smacking sounds during feeding
- No drawing in or dimpling of cheek pads

3. Areolar Compression

- Mandible moves in a rhythmic motion
- Initially, approximately two sucks per second (non-nutritive sucking, "flutter" sucking); as milk/colostrum becomes available post Milk Ejection Reflex (M.E.R.), sucking slows to approximately one suck per second (nutritive sucking)
- Wavelike motion of tongue compresses lactiferous sinuses against hard palate (milk sprays from nipple pores)
- Confirmed by previous digital exam (exam not routinely performed at time of feeding)
- Tongue, jaw, lips move in single rhythmic unit

4. Audible Swallowing

- Quiet sound of swallowing is heard
- May be preceded by several sucking motions
- May increase in frequency and consistency after M.E.R.

B. Functional Assessment of Infant at Breast (FAIB) should be included in patient education to assure adequacy of breastfeeding upon discharge.

C. Document feedings on the newborn flow sheet

---

* *L Shrago, D Bocar:* JOGNN *19:209–15, 1989.*

in the "Feeding" section utilizing the following abbreviations:

BO—Breastfeeding attempted

BAS—Breastfeed with audible swallowing

D. Document FAIB on mother's chart as a narrative notation:

"Mother and infant positioned correctly, unable to arouse sleepy baby, latch-on not accomplished."

"Infant accomplished latch-on with several bursts of 3–4 sucks."

"Audible swallowing at both breasts."

Above examples are more helpful than "breastfed well." Overemphasis on "number of minutes" of breastfeeding teaches clock watching rather than responding to infant behavior.

III. BREASTFEEDING ROUNDS POLICY:

In response to the Amercian Academy of Pediatrics, American College of Obstetricians and Gynecologists, and the World Health Organization's promotion of breastfeeding as the preferred method of infant feeding, and the Surgeon General's Health Promotion/Disease Prevention objective which states "by 2000, 75% of mothers will breastfeed when discharged and 35% will continue for the first 6 months," the Family Birthplace will provide "Breastfeeding Rounds"—an average length visit of 20 minutes is provided free of charge during the hospital stay. Women who have a short length of stay may not be seen by a consultant.

Procedure

A. A Certified Breastfeeding Educator or Certified Lactation Consultant who is a R.N. visits mothers who have chosen to breastfeed, in order to provide:

1. Information consistent with current research on practices relevant to successful lactation.

2. One-to-one patient education assisting mothers in identifying:
   - Infant's hunger cues and readiness to feed
   - Proper positioning and "latch-on" of the infant
   - Satiety cues of the infant, adequacy of milk supply
   - Problem signs indicating need for follow-up care

Breastfeeding rounds are charted on the "Breastfeeding Assessment" form, kept on clipboard with other mother/baby forms. Upon discharge, the original stays on mother's chart, copy to baby chart and copy to department.

3. When the Functional Assessment of the Infant at Breast (FAIB) indicates a dysfunction unrelated to maternal causes, a suck assessment will be performed. When a suck assessment reveals a dysfunction requiring intervention, the plan will be noted on the Care Plan and charted on the "Breastfeeding Assessment" form.

Procedure

a. Wash hands and don sterile glove or finger cot.

b. Perform digital oral motor exam.

c. Chart findings in "Breastfeeding Assessment" and discuss plan with physician and mother.

d. Add interventions to nursing care plan

4. Babies in NICU:

Mothers of babies in NICU will be visited by the Breastfeeding Educator/Lactation Consultant for the purpose of instructing the mother on the proper use of breast pumps as well as the storing and transporting of breast milk.

When the infant is deemed medically stable and able to be put to breast, the breastfeeding consultant will be available to perform one-time assessment of the infant at breast, if prior notification is received. The mother will be informed of the breastfeeding consultant's observations, and the session will be charted in the infant's record. Continued consultations must be noted as a physician's request in the infant's record and proper notification received.

5. Follow-up Phone Contact

The Breastfeeding Educator/Lactation Consultant will provide a one-time phone contact to breastfeeding mothers within 1 week of discharge. If the need for continued consultation/support or problems is identified, the physician will be contacted.

IV. USE OF BREASTFEEDING AIDS POLICY

A. Medela Nipple Shield

To be used only when the *cause* of the infant's

inability to achieve latch-on has been identified and documented. Nipple shields treat only the *symptom* of ineffective latch-on and *not the cause.*

Procedure

1. The shield will be initiated by the Breastfeeding Educator/Lactation Consultant.
2. The shield should be used as a tool for training an infant in developing an effective suckling pattern. Any patient discharged with a nipple shield must be referred to the Breastfeeding Educator/Lactation Consultant for follow-up care as shields have been shown to reduce milk volume by 22–58%.
3. Rubber bottle nipples over the mother's own nipple are not to be used.
4. Obtain the nipple shield from the supply cart, initiate appropriate charges, document use, obtain physician order for reimbursement as necessary.

B. Medela Breast Shells

Policy: Indications

1. Flat nipples causing difficult latch-on.
2. Inverted nipples.
3. Treatment of severely sore nipples after cause of soreness has been identified.

Procedure: Use to Erect Nipples

1. Obtain one package of breast shells (contains two shells) from supply cart.
2. Wash shells in soap-water before each use.
3. Instruct mother to wash her hands before handling shells.
4. Snap together dome and cone to form a shell.
5. Mother is to place shell inside her bra with the cone centered over nipple.
6. Shells are to be worn constantly between feedings when treatment is initiated after birth. Document use.
7. A physician order is necessary to obtain third party reimbursement.

Procedure: Use for Sore Nipples

1. Wash shells before each use.

2. Instruct mother to wash hands and snap together the dome and ring to form a shell.
3. Instruct mother to wear the shield inside bra between feedings, allowing nipples to dry and keeping clothing off sore nipple.
4. Bra pads may be necessary at lower border of shells if milk leakage is occurring.
5. Instruct mother to discard any milk that collects in the shells as this is not safe for the baby.

V. BREASTFEEDING CONSULTATION

Policy: To provide a mechanism for patients to receive consultation from a Breastfeeding Educator or Lactation Consultant.

1. Appropriate conditions for consultations include:
   a. Special situations (twins, premature infants, reluctant nursers, relactation).
   b. Patients at high risk for lactation failure (flat/inverted nipples, teenagers, uncommitted mothers, persistent sore nipples, use of nipple shield).
   c. Infants with a sucking disorder, slow weight gain, nipple confusion, anomalies.
   d. Breast/nipple problems (mastitis, abscess, clogged duct).

Procedure: Consult protocols approved by the Breastfeeding Committee; they will serve as guidelines for assessment and care and will be updated yearly and as needed.

1. Inpatient Visits
   a. Ideally, every breastfeeding mother is visited free of charge during her stay at the hospital (see Breastfeeding Rounds III.A). The average length of a visit is 20 minutes.
   b. Nursing staff identify mothers with questions or breastfeeding problems and make referrals to the Breastfeeding consultant.
   c. When problems exist, an order for a consultation is written by either the OB-GYN, family physician, or the baby's physician. Visits lasting more than 20 minutes are considered consults. Documentation of a diagnosis of "Infant Feeding Difficulties" in the medical record is helpful in obtaining third party reimbursement.

d. A breastfeeding consultation fee of $30.00 is initiated upon receiving the written order.

e. The Breastfeeding Assessment Record and/or progress notes are utilized for documentation of the consult.

2. Outpatient Visits. The breastfeeding consult does not take the place of routine pediatric health care visits; it is meant to assist the mother and infant in this special area only.

a. Routine appointments are made during regular working hours. Brief follow-up visits occur as needed. All patients need to check in at admissions either in the main lobby or the Emergency Room entrance.

b. During each visit both the mother and the nursing infant are evaluated. The infant is weighed, and a history is obtained to determine appropriate management. These routine appointments normally take one to two hours.

c. Documentation is made on the Clinical Progress Note. The original is sent to Medical Records along with physician orders, outpatient registration form and other documentation as needed. One copy of the Clinical Progress Note is sent to the referring physician and one copy for the department file.

d. An order for each consultation and a diagnosis of "Infant Feeding Difficulties" in the medical record are necessary for third party reimbursement.

e. A Breastfeeding Consultation fee of $30.00 is made for each routine appointment. If follow-up visits last longer than 20 minutes, the consult fee is initiated.

VI. EMPLOYEE BREASTFEEDING SUPPORT: "THE WHEY STATION"

Policy

1. To provide positive support for St. Joseph employees wishing to continue breastfeeding while coming back to work by providing a private area and an electric breast pump for their use.

Equipment and Supplies

1. Employees may use their own manual breast pump. All employees wishing to use the electric pump must first obtain their own accessory parts. These may be purchased at the PK Pharmacy located at 3305 East Harry or at any medical supply store.

2. If you deliver at SJMC, a Universal Pumping System can be obtained and charged to your inpatient account. The Universal System includes a manual breast pump, tubing and accessories to use for single and double pumping with the electric pump. Double pumping can be accomplished in about 10 minutes.

3. The employee will be responsible for cleaning her own manual breast pump and accessory breast pump parts.

Procedure

1. The breastfeeding pump room will be located on 4 North.

2. A sign-in book will be located in the room, in order to track frequency of usage.

3. Each employee will be responsible for spraying the breast pump and tubing with the hospital approved disinfectant after using the pump. Please wipe excess disinfectant off with clean washrags provided. Washrags may then be placed in laundry hamper. A bottle of dishwashing detergent will be provided to wash the breast pump parts.

4. Maintenance of the pump will be handled by the staff of The Family Birthplace or the Neonatal Intensive Care Unit. For problem solving please call 4 East, extension 5490 or NICU, extension 5475.

5. Employee is responsible for labeling and storing her own breastmilk. Containers for milk will not be provided. Infection Control has asked that any breastmilk being stored in a St. Jospeh refrigerator be placed in a plastic bag. The plastic bags will be provided.

6. Assistance in choosing and using a pump, maintaining your milk supply or any breastfeeding concerns may be directed to the Breastfeeding Educator/Lactation Consultants by calling 689–5404 and leaving a message.

APPENDIX C

Via Christi Health System, St. Joseph Campus

Breastfeeding Education Protocol*

INTERVENTION/MANAGEMENT	RATIONALE	
POLICY #1: All pregnant women should receive information regarding the availability of classes on the benefits and management of breastfeeding.		
Mothers identified as choosing breastfeeding during prenatal contacts will be informed of the breastfeeding class in the childbirth education series. Childbirth education class schedules will be available on the labor-delivery-recovery-postpartum (LDRP) unit and at physicians' offices.	Breastfeeding success and performance is improved by specific knowledge and the support of significant others.	
POLICY #2: Mothers who are undecided about feeding method will be encouraged to breastfeed.		
Family Birthplace and perinatal education staff will inform mothers of the benefits of breastfeeding and human milk.	Demonstrates compliance with the American Academy of Pediatrics policy statement on breastfeeding and the Surgeon General's goal for the nation. Provides optimal nutritional composition for CNS development. Serves as standard for commercial infant formula.	

Developed March 1991 by the Breastfeeding Committee: Gina Woodley, R.N., A.C.C.E., IBCLC; Rachel Lewis, R.N., C.B.E.; Pat Rierson, R.N.C., C.B.E.; Judy Angeron, R.N., IBCLC; Sharon Foster, R.N.C., M.N.; Jan Riordan, R.N., Ed.D.; Howard Whiteside, M.D.; Jean Broberg, R.N., M.N.

Source: Adapted from Arizona Healthy Mothers/Healthy Babies Wellstart–San Diego Lactation Program.

INTERVENTION/MANAGEMENT	RATIONALE	
	Decreases incidence of diarrhea, upper respiratory infections and some allergies; recent studies show decreased incidence in otitis media.	
	Promotes bonding and mother/infant closeness.	
	Promotes uterine involution due to increased oxytocin secretion.	
	Economical and convenient.	
	Mother can always change her mind and discontinue breastfeeding.	

POLICY #3: Mothers expressing desire to breastfeed will have nipples examined for degree of eversion during admission procedures.

Admitting nurse or resident will perform nipple palpation/pinch test during standard admissions procedures. Gently squeeze one inch behind the nipple base on the areola with thumb and forefinger. The nipple should protrude from the breast.	Identify mothers with non-protruding nipples prior to birth so the appropriate nursing care plan can be implemented. Infants may have difficulty latching on to non-protruding nipples. The pinch test can assist in determining how the nipple will react in the infant's mouth.	

POLICY #4: Educational pamphlets on breastfeeding shall be provided following birth, well before discharge.

Breastfeeding Educator or Primary Care Nurse provides appropriate pamphlet post-birth.	Literature can be used by breastfeeding educator and nursing staff for one-to-one patient education. Provides consistency of information given by nursing staff and provides a frame of reference. Mother may refer to literature during hospital stay to reinforce learning.	

POLICY #5: Infants are to be put to breast as soon after birth as feasible for both mother and infant, with 20 minutes post-birth ideal and within the first 2 hours whenever possible.

The baby will be given to the mother to nurse during the first two hours, and preferably within the first 20 minutes. This includes the alert, stable, post-cesarean birth, mother and baby.	Suck reflex is strongest 20–30 minutes post-birth; delaying gratification can make it difficult for infant to learn sucking process later on.	

APPENDIX C *(cont.)*

INTERVENTION/MANAGEMENT	RATIONALE	
	Infant promptly receives immunologic benefits of colostrum and digestive peristalsis is stimulated.	
	Suckling stimulates uterine involution and inhibits bleeding.	
	Post-cesarean mothers may still be comfortable from epidural medications and interested in breastfeeding.	
	Mothers should be permitted to engage in this normal, physiologic process regardless of birth method, as long as medically stable.	
Contraindications to immediate breastfeeding: 1. Heavily medicated mother. 2. Infant with Apgar <6. 3. Premature infant <36 weeks gestation.		

POLICY #6: Every mother is to be instructed in proper breastfeeding technique and re-evaluated before discharge.

Nurse assists mother with breastfeeding and provides guidelines and support when indicated.	Assistance should support mother's efforts and be unobtrusive.	
Nurse gives positive reinforcement of mother and baby's efforts and success. Pillows may be needed to support mother's arms and bring baby to breast level.	Nipple trauma can be prevented with proper attachment and nipple soreness minimized. Support and comfort of mother and baby prevent fatigue and facilitate proper positioning of the baby at breast. Pillow under baby prevents nipple trauma by raising baby to nipple height.	
Functional assessment of infant at breast performed by nurse/breastfeeding educator within 24 hours of birth by utilizing the FAIB tool.	Provides for early identification of latch-on difficulties.	
	Direct observation of infant at breast assures adequacy of breastfeeding prior to discharge.	
	Provides opportunity for positive reinforcement of breastfeeding and assuring "baby getting something."	

INTERVENTION/MANAGEMENT	RATIONALE	
Infant's mouth should be at nipple level. Mother supports the breast using a "C" hold. The thumb is placed on top of the breast and the four fingers support the breast underneath. (All fingers should be well back from the areola.)	The "C" hold provides breast support and control and allows the infant to grasp the areola without interference.	
Mother tickles the center of the infant's bottom lip with her nipple until the infant opens his mouth as wide as possible. The infant may take several minutes to do this.	Tickling the bottom lip causes the baby to open his mouth and assume a position wide enough to get well behind the nipple onto the areola.	
When infant's mouth is open very wide, mother should center her nipple quickly and draw the baby in close to her body.	Bringing baby in close to mother causes the jaws to bypass the centered nipple and come together on the areola.	
Infant's nose and chin should be touching the breast. There is no need to create an air space for most infants. Mother may be taught to lift baby's buttocks if needed.	Infant's nose touching the breast assures proper positioning and latch-on. Baby will not suffocate if close to the breast.	
Infant's mouth and lips should form a flanged seal around the breast tissue. The tongue should be curved around the breast, cupping it and extending over the gum line.	Negative pressure created by the flanged seal acts synergistically with positive pressure in the duct system to ensure transport of milk.	

POLICY #7: The infant is to be encouraged to nurse at least every 2 to 3 hours, for a minimum of 8 feedings/24 hours.

Breastfeeding shall be initiated as soon as possible post-birth.	Baby is more alert within the first 2 hours.	
Feeding every 2–3 hours will be supported by the nursing staff. Mothers will be assisted in identifying infant's hunger cues and readiness to feed, i.e., R.E.M., hand to mouth movement.	Breastmilk digests in 90 minutes. Eight feedings/24 hours has been associated with increased meconium passage and lower serum bilirubin levels of the infant.	
Mother will be educated on the "supply and demand" principle of milk production.	Maternal prolactin levels fall after 3 hours. Every three hour feedings enhance milk production.	
	Understanding of *basic* physiology enhances lactation success.	

APPENDIX C *(cont.)*

INTERVENTION/MANAGEMENT	RATIONALE	
POLICY #8: Infants should feed from both breasts at all feedings, with a minimum of 6 minutes per breast. An infant may be returned to the first breast for continued suckling, if positioning is correct and nursing is comfortable.		
Babies put to breast every 2–3 hours with at least 6 minutes active swallowing time/breast.	Feeding from both breasts provides regular breast stimulation and allows for greater volume of milk consumption. It often takes 2–3 minutes for milk to let down and may take as long as 6–10 minutes for oxytocin release with the onset of sucking.	
Mothers instructed on listening for quiet sounds of swallowing.	Audible swallowing is the most reliable indicator of intake.	
Mothers instructed to burp baby after first breast and put baby to second breast to complete feeding.	Limiting suckling time has not been shown to reduce nipple soreness. Breastfeeding is biphasic with larger volume of milk obtained when nursed from both breasts.	
Mothers will be instructed on observing baby's early cues for hunger (crying is a late hunger cue) and changes in suck/swallow patterns.	Restricting breastfeeding may increase degree of physiologic engorgement which occurs during transitional milk phase.	
Responding to infant's hunger cues takes priority over other events which may be delayed, i.e., infant "waiting" in nursery for lab work.		
POLICY #9: If within the first 24–48 hours post-birth, feedings at the breast are incomplete or ineffective, the mother should be instructed to begin regular expression of her breasts, with continued assistance by an experienced staff member. The colostrum or milk obtained by expression should be given to the baby.		
The primary care nurse/breastfeeding educator will instruct the mother on pumping techniques using the electric breast pump, when infant consistently demonstrates inadequate suckling.	Piston electric pumps most closely imitate the suck cycle of the infant.	
	Electric system is time saving for the mother.	
	Breast stimulation and breast emptying are necessary to initiate and maintain lactation.	

INTERVENTION/MANAGEMENT	RATIONALE	
Expressed colostrum and breastmilk will be given to the infant in addition to any other supplement which may be indicated and prescribed by the physician.	Incomplete breast emptying may lead to insufficient milk due to pressure involution of glandular tissue. Validates mother's pumping efforts as valuable and provides added benefits to baby.	

POLICY #10: Supplementary water or formula is given for certain clinical conditions as ordered by the physician, but not on a routine basis. If prolonged supplementation is necessary, the physician will be contacted regarding formula choice and amount.

Neonatal assessment completed as per nursing protocol.	Preterm or medically compromised infants may need additional nutritional support during the colostral phase of milk production.	
Sterile water, glucose water or formula feedings are to be given only with specific written order of the attending physician.	Initial water feedings became standard for formula fed infants as formula and glucose water are irritating to the respiratory tree if aspirated. Colostrum is a physiologic substance and readily passes through the respiratory tree if aspirated.	
	Colostrum and breastmilk will completely meet the newborn's nutritional and fluid needs (provides 17–20 cal./oz.).	
	Alteration of the flora of the baby's gut occurs with supplemental feedings.	
	Infants may be confused by a rubber nipple which requires a different tongue and jaw motion.	
	Water supplements have not been shown to prevent or cure hyperbilirubinemia in the neonatal period.	
	Higher protein levels in colostrum have a more stabilizing effect on blood glucose levels than glucose water.	
	Formula has a longer gut transit time than breastmilk and may decrease the infant's interest in nursing.	

APPENDIX C *(cont.)*

INTERVENTION/MANAGEMENT	RATIONALE	
	Glucose water with 6 cal./oz. can give infant sense of fullness without providing adequate nutrition (colostrum and breastmilk provide 17–20 cal./oz.).	
	Encouraging supplementation communicates that mother's milk is inadequate or inappropriate for her infant.	

POLICY #11: Mothers who wish to feed by both breast and bottle will be educated about breastfeeding and encouraged to breastfeed without supplement.

INTERVENTION/MANAGEMENT	RATIONALE	
Primary care nurse/breastfeeding educator (PCN/BE) will educate mother on rationale for encouraging exclusive breastfeeding during the first weeks, and teach recommended time for introducing bottles.	Reduces mother's anxiety about "insufficient milk" by teaching how to establish and maintain adequate supply.	
	Exclusive breastfeeding during the first two weeks aids in the establishment of an adequate milk supply and appropriate breastfeeding technique.	
	Three to four weeks of age is the recommended age for introducing a bottle. Expressed breastmilk may be used for bottle feedings as well as infant formula.	

POLICY #12: Pacifiers should not be used on a routine basis for the breastfeeding infant as a hunger satiety measure.

INTERVENTION/MANAGEMENT	RATIONALE	
Mothers shall be educated to respond to baby's cues for readiness to feed, and identify nutritive and non-nutritive sucking.	Pacifiers should be used for non-nutritive sucking needs.	
Pacifiers are not given to prolong length of time between breastfeedings in order to "get baby on a schedule."	Frequently needing a pacifier may be a sign of inadequate milk intake.	
	Infants with a weak or ineffective suck may be content to suck on a pacifier for both nutritive and non-nutritive sucking needs.	

INTERVENTION/MANAGEMENT	RATIONALE	
POLICY #13: Breastfeeding mothers are to have breast examined for evidence of lactation or breastfeeding problems at least once every 24 hours.		
PCN examines breast during daily nursing assessments.	Provides appropriate maternity nursing care.	
BE/PCN examines nipples whenever concerns or complaints of sore nipples are expressed by mother.	Physiologic nipple tenderness occurs during the first few minutes of a feeding and eases up during the same feed. Pathologic nipple soreness is considered whenever mother complains of nipple pain throughout entire feeding or between feedings.	
POLICY #14: Infants should remain at the mother's bedside both day and night. The nurse should plan with the mother and family for periods of rest/sleep both day and night. If the mother chooses to have the infant in the nursery, she will be encouraged to feed the baby on demand.		
Babies are cared for at the mothers' bedside as per Family Birthplace philosophy.	Infant's presence facilitates bonding and the attachment process. The infant's adaptation to extra-uterine life is aided by the mother's presence.	
	Provides opportunity for individualized teaching. Aids mother in learning cues and behaviors of her baby.	
The nurse shall plan with the mother for 1–2 hours of undisturbed rest twice daily.	Rest is an important physiologic and psychologic need for all post-partum mothers.	
	Adequate rest is essential to lactation.	
	With liberalized visiting hours, there is no time for mothers to rest unless naps are planned.	
Infants will be cared for at night in the nursery at the request of the mother, but brought to the mother for demand feeding when exhibiting hunger cues or every 3 hours.	Prolactin levels are highest at night and may contribute to successful breastfeeding. Provides additional opportunities for mother and baby to establish effective nursing pattern prior to discharge.	
POLICY #15: Commercial discharge packs containing water or formula are not to be given unless specifically ordered by the physician or requested by the mother.		
Mothers are not refused formula sample when requested.		

APPENDIX C *(cont.)*

INTERVENTION/MANAGEMENT	RATIONALE	
Nurses who are concerned infant will not be adequately nourished at the breast due to poor latch-on shall inform the attending physician.	Assists in the development and implementation of a discharge plan which can meet both the infant's nutritional needs and the mother's breastfeeding goals.	
Discharge formula packs are not routinely given to breastfeeding mothers.	Endorses supplementation. Implies that breastmilk is inadequate to meet infant's needs.	

POLICY #16: At discharge, each mother is to be given a phone number to call for breastfeeding assistance.

Patients contacting physician office for mother/baby concerns reinforced and SJMC Lactation Program #689–5404 stamped on BF pamphlet; Ask-A-Nurse number 685–5700 for after-hours information.	Early discharge often occurs before lactation and breastfeeding well established. Reassurance can be given for transient breastfeeding difficulties (i.e., engorgement, sore nipples) and differentiated from situations requiring medical intervention.	

POLICY #17: Mothers who are separated from their infant will be instructed on the proper use of breast pumps as well as the storing and transportation of breast milk.

When prolonged separation of mother and infant is expected (i.e., prematurity, ill infant), the mother will be provided the opportunity for pumping as soon after birth as medically feasible.	Involves mother in care for her infant. Allows her to make "unique" contribution.	
Pumping *may* need to be delayed if maternal cause for separation—i.e., pregnancy induced hypertension (P.I.H.).	Pumping may be regarded as additional stressor on already vulnerable patient. Certain medications used to treat P.I.H. and other medical conditions may be contraindicated.	
Breastfeeding Educator/PCN shall instruct the mother on use of the electric breast pump and pumping technique as per protocol.	Following protocol maintains consistency of information given. Parents may need to have instructions repeated frequently.	
Breastfeeding Educator/PCN provides parents with written guidelines.	Parents want specific, concrete guidelines.	
Discharge planning of the mother shall include pumping/expression options, with method decided upon noted in the record.	Emphasizes the importance of regular breast expression in maintaining lactation. Pumping sessions need to be part of daily routine. Pumping frequency and length guidelines are based on the method of expression.	

APPENDIX D

Nursing Diagnosis Related to Breastfeeding

Approved diagnostic labels of the North American
Nursing Diagnosis Association (NANDA)

Effective Breastfeeding

Definition:
The state in which a mother-infant dyad/family exhibits adequate proficiency and satisfaction with breastfeeding process

Defining Characteristics

- Mother able to position infant at breast to promote a successful latch-on response
- Signs and/or symptoms of oxytocin release (let-down or milk ejection reflex)
- Adequate infant elimination patterns for age
- Eagerness of infant to nurse
- Maternal verbalization of satisfaction with the breastfeeding process

Related Factors

- Basic breastfeeding knowledge
- Normal breast structure
- Normal infant or structure

Ineffective Breastfeeding

Definition:
The state in which a mother or child experiences difficulty with the breastfeeding process

Defining Characteristics

- Mother unable to position infant at breast to promote a successful latch-on response
- Maternal reluctance to put infant at breast
- Inadequate infant elimination
- Maternal verbalization of dissatisfaction with breastfeeding
- Non-sustained suckling at the breast
- Infant does not receive nourishment at the breast for some or all of feedings
- Separation of mother and infant
- No signs or symptoms of oxytocin release (let-down)
- Nursing less than 7 in 24 hours (First month)

Related Factors

- Prematurity
- Maternal breast anomaly
- History of previous breastfeeding failure

Interrupted Breastfeeding

Definition:
A break in the continuity of the breastfeeding process as a result of inability or inadvisability to put baby to breast for feeding.

Defining Characteristics

- Infant does not receive nourishment at the breast for some or all of feedings
- Maternal desire to maintain lactation and provide (or eventually provide) her breastmilk for her infant's nutritional needs.
- Separation of mother and infant
- Lack of knowledge regarding expression and storage of breastmilk

Related Factors

- Maternal or infant illness
- Prematurity
- Maternal employment

APPENDIX D *(cont.)*

- Infant gestation; age greater than 34 weeks
- Support source
- Maternal confidence

- Infant receiving supplemental feedings with artificial nipple
- Poor infant sucking reflex
- Non-supportive partner/family
- Knowledge deficit
- Maternal anxiety
- Delayed initiation of breast-feeding

- Contraindications to breastfeeding (e.g. drugs, true breastmilk jaundice)
- Need to abruptly wean infant

Courtesy of NANDA

APPENDIX E

New York State Code in Support of Breastfeeding (Added 1984)*

(10(i) The hospital, with the advice of the maternity staff, shall formulate a program of instruction and provide assistance for each maternity patient(s) in the fundamentals of (normal) infant care including infant feeding choice and techniques, post-pregnancy care and family planning.

(ii) The hospital shall provide instruction and assistance to each maternity patient who has chosen to breastfeed and shall provide information on the advantages and disadvantages of breastfeeding to women who are undecided as to the feeding method for their infants. As a minimum:

(a) the hospital shall designate at least one person who is thoroughly trained in breastfeeding physiology and management to be responsible for ensuring the implementation of an effective breastfeeding program; and

(b) policies and procedures shall be developed to assist the mother to breastfeed which shall include but not be limited to:

(1) prohibition of the application of standing orders for antilactation drugs;

(2) placement of the infant for breastfeeding immediately following delivery, unless contraindicated;

(3) restriction of the infant's supplemental feedings to those indicated by the medical condition of the infant or of the mother;

(4) provision for the infant to be fed on demand; and

(c) assurance that an educational program has been given as soon after admission as possible which shall include but not be limited to:

(1) the nutritional and physiological aspects of human milk;

(2) the normal process for establishing lactation, including care of breasts, common problems associated with breastfeeding and frequency of feeding;

(3) dietary requirements for breastfeeding;

(4) diseases and medication or other substances which may have an effect on breastfeeding;

(5) sanitary procedures to follow in collecting and storing human milk; and

(6) sources for advice and information available to the mother following discharge.

---

* *Chapter V Subchapter A Article 2 Part 405 Hospitals—minimum standards (Statutory authority: Public health law § 2803) 405.8 Maternal, child health and newborn services*

APPENDIX F

American Academy of Pediatrics

Work Group on Breastfeeding

Breastfeeding and the Use of Human Milk

ABSTRACT. This policy statement on breastfeeding replaces the previous policy statement of the American Academy of Pediatrics, reflecting the considerable advances that have occurred in recent years in the scientific knowledge of the benefits of breastfeeding, in the mechanisms underlying these benefits, and in the practice of breastfeeding. This document summarizes the benefits of breastfeeding to the infant, the mother, and the nation, and sets forth principles to guide the pediatrician and other health care providers in the initiation and maintenance of breastfeeding. The policy statement also delineates the various ways in which pediatricians can promote, protect, and support breastfeeding, not only in their individual practices but also in the hospital, medical school, community, and nation.

ABBREVIATION. AAP, American Academy of Pediatrics.

HISTORY AND INTRODUCTION

From its inception, the American Academy of Pediatrics (AAP) has been a staunch advocate of breastfeeding as the optimal form of nutrition for infants. One of the earliest AAP publications was a 1948 manual, *Standards and Recommendations for the Hospital Care of Newborn Infants.* This manual included a recommendation to make every effort to have every mother nurse her full-term infant. A major concern of the AAP has been the development of guidelines for proper nutrition for infants and children. The activities, statements, and recommendations of the AAP have continuously promoted breastfeeding of infants as the foundation of good feeding practices.

THE NEED

Extensive research, especially in recent years, documents diverse and compelling advantages to infants, mothers, families, and society from breastfeeding and the use of human milk for infant feeding. These include health, nutritional, immunologic, developmental, psychological, social, economic, and environmental benefits.

Human milk is uniquely superior for infant feeding and is species-specific; all substitute feeding options differ markedly from it. The breastfed infant is the reference or normative model against which all alternative feeding methods must be measured with regard to growth, health, development, and all other short- and long-term outcomes.

Epidemiologic research shows that human milk and breastfeeding of infants provide advantages with regard to general health, growth, and development, while significantly decreasing risk for a large number of acute and chronic diseases. Research in the United States, Canada, Europe, and other *developed* countries, among predominantly middle-class populations, provides strong evidence that human milk feeding decreases the incidence and/or severity of diarrhea,[1-5] lower respiratory infection,[6-9] otitis media,[3,10-14] bacteremia,[15,16] bacterial meningitis,[15,17] botulism,[18] urinary tract infection,[19] and necrotizing enterocolitis.[20,21] There are a number of studies that show a possible protective effect of human milk feeding against sudden infant death syndrome,[22-24] insulin-dependent diabetes mellitus,[25-27] Crohn's disease,[28,29] ulcerative colitis,[29] lymphoma,[30,31] allergic diseases,[32-34] and other chronic digestive diseases.[35-37] Breastfeeding has also been related to possible enhancement of cognitive development.[38,39]

There are also a number of studies that indicate possible health benefits for mothers. It has long been acknowledged that breastfeeding increases levels of oxytocin, resulting in less postpartum bleeding and more rapid uterine involution.[40] Lactational amenorrhea causes less menstrual blood loss over the months after delivery. Recent research demonstrates that lactating women have an earlier return to prepregnant weight,[41] delayed resumption of ovulation with increased child spacing,[42-44] improved bone remineralization postpartum[45] with reduction in hip fractures in the postmenopausal period,[46] and reduced risk of ovarian cancer[47] and premenopausal breast cancer.[48]

In addition to individual health benefits, breastfeeding provides significant social and economic benefits to the nation, including reduced health care costs and reduced employee absenteeism for care attributable to child illness. The significantly lower incidence of illness in the breastfed infant allows the parents more time for attention to siblings and other family duties and reduces parental absence from work and lost income. The direct economic benefits to the family are also significant. It has been estimated that the 1993 cost of purchasing infant formula for the first year after birth was $855. During the first 6 weeks of lactation, maternal caloric intake is no greater for the breastfeeding mother than for the nonlactating mother.[49,50] After that period, food and fluid intakes are greater, but the cost of this increased caloric intake is about half the cost of purchasing formula. Thus, a saving of >$400 per child

APPENDIX F *(cont.)*

for food purchases can be expected during the first year.[51,52]

Despite the demonstrated benefits of breastfeeding, there are some situations in which breastfeeding is not in the best interest of the infant. These include the infant with galactosemia,[53,54] the infant whose mother uses illegal drugs,[55] the infant whose mother has untreated active tuberculosis, and the infant in the United States whose mother has been infected with the human immunodeficiency virus.[56,57] In countries with populations at increased risk for other infectious diseases and nutritional deficiencies resulting in infant death, the mortality risks associated with not breastfeeding may outweigh the possible risks of acquiring human immunodeficiency virus infection.[58] Although most prescribed and over-the-counter medications are safe for the breastfed infant, there are a few medications that mothers may need to take that may make it necessary to interrupt breastfeeding temporarily. These include radioactive isotopes, antimetabolites, cancer chemotherapy agents, and a small number of other medications. Excellent books and tables of drugs that are safe or contraindicated in breastfeeding are available to the physician for reference, including a publication from the AAP.[55]

THE PROBLEM

Increasing the rates of breastfeeding initiation and duration is a national health objective and one of the goals of Healthy People 2000. The target is to "increase to at least 75% the proportion of mothers who breastfeed their babies in the early postpartum period and to at least 50% the proportion who continue breastfeeding until their babies are 5 to 6 months old."[59] Although breastfeeding rates have increased slightly since 1990, the percentage of women currently electing to breastfeed their babies is still lower than levels reported in the mid-1980s and is far below the Healthy People 2000 goal. In 1995, 59.4% of women in the United States were breastfeeding either exclusively or in combination with formula feeding at the time of hospital discharge; only 21.6% of mothers were nursing at 6 months, and many of these were supplementing with formula.[60]

The highest rates of breastfeeding are observed among higher-income, college-educated women >30 years of age living in the Mountain and Pacific regions of the United States.[60] Obstacles to the initiation and continuation of breastfeeding include physician apathy and misinformation,[61–63] insufficient prenatal breastfeeding education,[64] disruptive hospital policies,[65] inappropriate interruption of breastfeeding,[62] early hospital discharge in some populations,[66] lack of timely routine follow-up care and postpartum home health visits,[67] maternal employment[68,69] (especially in the absence of workplace facilities and support for breastfeeding),[70] lack of broad societal support,[71] media portrayal of bottle-feeding as normative,[72] and commercial promotion of infant formula through distribution of hospital discharge packs, coupons for free or discounted formula, and television and general magazine advertising.[73,74]

The AAP identifies breastfeeding as the ideal method of feeding and nurturing infants and recognizes breastfeeding as primary in achieving optimal infant and child health, growth, and development. The AAP emphasizes the essential role of the pediatrician in promoting, protecting, and supporting breastfeeding and recommends the following breastfeeding policies.

RECOMMENDED BREASTFEEDING PRACTICES

1. Human milk is the preferred feeding for all infants, including premature and sick newborns, with rare exceptions.[75–77] The ultimate decision on feeding of the infant is the mother's. Pediatricians should provide parents with complete, current information on the benefits and methods of breastfeeding to ensure that the feeding decision is a fully informed one. When direct breastfeeding is not possible, expressed human milk, fortified when necessary for the premature infant, should be provided.[78,79] Before advising against breastfeeding or recommending premature weaning, the practitioner should weigh thoughtfully the benefits of breastfeeding against the risks of not receiving human milk.

2. Breastfeeding should begin as soon as possible after birth, usually within the first hour.[80–82] Except under special circumstances, the newborn infant should remain with the mother throughout the recovery period.[80,83,84] Procedures that may interfere with breastfeeding or traumatize the infant should be avoided or minimized.

3. Newborns should be nursed whenever they show signs of hunger, such as increased alertness or activity, mouthing, or rooting.[85] Crying is a *late* indicator of hunger.[86] Newborns should be nursed approximately 8 to 12 times every 24 hours until satiety, usually 10 to 15 minutes on each breast.[87,88] In the early weeks after birth, nondemanding babies should be aroused to feed if 4 hours have elapsed since the last nursing.[89,90] Appropriate initiation of breastfeeding is facilitated by continuous rooming-in.[91] Formal evaluation of breastfeeding performance should be undertaken by trained observers and fully documented in the record during the first 24 to 48 hours after delivery and again at the early follow-up visit, which should occur 48 to 72 hours after discharge. Maternal recording of the time of each breastfeeding and its duration, as well as voidings and stoolings during the early days of breastfeeding in the hospital and at home, greatly facilitates the evaluation process.

4. No supplements (water, glucose water, formula, and so forth) should be given to breastfeeding newborns unless a medical indication exists.[92–95] With sound breastfeeding knowledge and practices, supplements rarely are needed. Supplements and pacifiers should be avoided whenever possible and, if used at all, only after breastfeeding is well established.[93–98]

5. When discharged <48 hours after delivery, all breastfeeding mothers and their newborns should be seen by a pediatrician or other knowledgeable health care practitioner when the newborn is 2 to 4 days of age. In addition to determination of

infant weight and general health assessment, breastfeeding should be observed and evaluated for evidence of successful breastfeeding behavior. The infant should be assessed for jaundice, adequate hydration, and age-appropriate elimination patterns (at least six urinations per day and three to four stools per day) by 5 to 7 days of age. All newborns should be seen by 1 month of age.[99]

6. Exclusive breastfeeding is ideal nutrition and sufficient to support optimal growth and development for approximately the first 6 months after birth.[100] Infants weaned before 12 months of age should not receive cow's milk feedings but should receive iron-fortified infant formula.[101] Gradual introduction of iron-enriched solid foods in the second half of the first year should complement the breast milk diet.[102,103] It is recommended that breastfeeding continue for at least 12 months, and thereafter for as long as mutually desired.[104]

7. In the first 6 months, water, juice, and other foods are generally unnecessary for breastfed infants.[105,106] Vitamin D and iron may need to be given before 6 months of age in selected groups of infants (vitamin D for infants whose mothers are vitamin D-deficient or those infants not exposed to adequate sunlight; iron for those who have low iron stores or anemia).[107–109] Fluoride should not be administered to infants during the first 6 months after birth, whether they are breast- or formula-fed. During the period from 6 months to 3 years of age, breastfed infants (and formula-fed infants) require fluoride supplementation only if the water supply is severely deficient in fluoride (<0.3 ppm).[110]

8. Should hospitalization of the breastfeeding mother or infant be necessary, every effort should be made to maintain breastfeeding, preferably directly, or by pumping the breasts and feeding expressed breast milk, if necessary.

ROLE OF PEDIATRICIANS IN PROMOTING AND PROTECTING BREASTFEEDING

To provide an optimal environment for breastfeeding, pediatricians should follow these recommendations:

1. Promote and support breastfeeding enthusiastically. In consideration of the extensive published evidence for improved outcomes in breastfed infants and their mothers, a strong position on behalf of breastfeeding is justified.

2. Become knowledgeable and skilled in both the physiology and the clinical management of breastfeeding.

3. Work collaboratively with the obstetric community to ensure that women receive adequate information throughout the perinatal period to make a fully informed decision about infant feeding. Pediatricians should also use opportunities to provide age-appropriate breastfeeding education to children and adults.

4. Promote hospital policies and procedures that facilitate breastfeeding. Electric breast pumps and private lactation areas should be available to all breastfeeding mothers in the hospital, both on ambulatory and inpatient services. Pediatricians are encouraged to work actively toward eliminating hospital practices that discourage breastfeeding (eg, infant formula discharge packs and separation of mother and infant).

5. Become familiar with local breastfeeding resources (eg, Special Supplemental Nutrition Program for Women, Infants, and Children clinics, lactation educators and consultants, lay support groups, and breast pump rental stations) so that patients can be referred appropriately.[111] When specialized breastfeeding services are used, pediatricians need to clarify for patients their essential role as the infant's primary medical care taker. Effective communication among the various counselors who advise breastfeeding women is essential.

6. Encourage routine insurance coverage for necessary breastfeeding services and supplies, including breast pump rental and the time required by pediatricians and other licensed health care professionals to assess and manage breastfeeding.

7. Promote breastfeeding as a normal part of daily life, and encourage family and societal support for breastfeeding.

8. Develop and maintain effective communications and collaboration with other health care providers to ensure optimal breastfeeding education, support, and counsel for mother and infant.

9. Advise mothers to return to their physician for a thorough breast examination when breastfeeding is terminated.

10. Promote breastfeeding education as a routine component of medical school and residency education.

11. Encourage the media to portray breastfeeding as positive and the norm.

12. Encourage employers to provide appropriate facilities and adequate time in the workplace for breast-pumping.

CONCLUSION

Although economic, cultural, and political pressures often confound decisions about infant feeding, the AAP firmly adheres to the position that breastfeeding ensures the best possible health as well as the best developmental and psychosocial outcomes for the infant. Enthusiastic support and involvement of pediatricians in the promotion and practice of breastfeeding is essential to the achievement of optimal infant and child health, growth, and development.

WORK GROUP ON BREASTFEEDING, 1996 TO 1997
Lawrence M. Gartner, MD, Chairperson
Linda Sue Black, MD
Antoinette P. Eaton, MD
Ruth A. Lawrence, MD
Audrey J. Naylor, MD, DrPH
Marianne E. Neifert, MD
Donna O'Hare, MD
Richard J. Schanler, MD

APPENDIX F *(cont.)*

LIAISON REPRESENTATIVES
Michael Georgieff, MD
  Committee on Nutrition
Yvette Piovanetti, MD
  Committee on Community Health Services
John Queenan, MD
  American College of Obstetricians and
  Gynecologists

REFERENCES

1. Dewey KG, Heinig MJ, Nommsen-Rivers LA. Differences in morbidity between breast-fed and formula-fed infants. *J Pediatr.* 1995;126:696–702
2. Howie PW, Forsyth JS, Ogston SA, et al. Protective effect of breast feeding against infection. *Br Med J.* 1990;300:11–16
3. Kovar MG, Serdula MK, Marks JS, et al. Review of the epidemiologic evidence for an association between infant feeding and infant health. *Pediatrics.* 1984;74:S615–S638
4. Popkin BM, Adair L, Akin JS, et al. Breast-feeding and diarrheal morbidity. *Pediatrics.* 1990;86:874–882
5. Beaudry M, Dufour R, Marcoux S. Relation between infant feeding and infections during the first six months of life. *J Pediatr.* 1995;126:191–197
6. Frank AL, Taber LH, Glezen WP, et al. Breast-feeding and respiratory virus infection. *Pediatrics.* 1982;70:239–245
7. Wright AI, Holberg CJ, Martinez FD, et al. Breast feeding and lower respiratory tract illness in the first year of life. *Br Med J.* 1989;299:945–949
8. Chen Y. Synergistic effect of passive smoking and artificial feeding on hospitalization for respiratory illness in early childhood. *Chest.* 1989;95:1004–1007
9. Wright AL, Holberg CJ, Taussig LM, et al. Relationship of infant feeding to recurrent wheezing at age 6 years. *Arch Pediatr Adolesc Med.* 1995;149:758–763
10. Saarinen UM. Prolonged breast feeding as prophylaxis for recurrent otitis media. *Acta Paediatr Scand.* 1982;71:567–571
11. Duncan B, Ey J, Holberg CJ, et al. Exclusive breast-feeding for at least 4 months protects against otitis media. *Pediatrics.* 1993;91:867–872
12. Owen MJ, Baldwin CD, Swank PR, et al. Relation of infant feeding practices, cigarette smoke exposure, and group child care to the onset and duration of otitis media with effusion in the first two years of life. *J Pediatr.* 1993;123:702–711
13. Paradise JL, Elster BA, Tan L. Evidence in infants with cleft palate that breast milk protects against otitis media. *Pediatrics.* 1994;94:853–860
14. Aniansson G, Alm B, Andersson B, et al. A prospective cohort study on breast-feeding and otitis media in Swedish infants. *Pediatr Infect Dis J.* 1994;13:183–188
15. Cochi SL, Fleming DW, Hightower AW, et al. Primary invasive *Haemophilus influenzae* type b disease: a population-based assessment of risk factors. *J Pediatr.* 1986;108:887–896
16. Takala AK, Eskola J, Palmgren J, et al. Risk factors of invasive *Haemophilus influenzae* type b disease among children in Finland. *J Pediatr.* 1989;115:694–701
17. Istre GR, Conner JS, Broome CV, et al. Risk factors for primary invasive *Haemophilus influenzae* disease: increased risk from day care attendance and school-aged household members. *J Pediatr.* 1985;106:190–195
18. Arnon SS. Breast feeding and toxigenic intestinal infections: missing links in crib death? *Rev Infect Dis.* 1984;6:S193–S201
19. Pisacane A, Graziano L, Mazzarella G, et al. Breast-feeding and urinary tract infection. *J Pediatr.* 1992;120:87–89
20. Lucas A, Cole TJ. Breast milk and neonatal necrotising enterocolitis. *Lancet.* 1990;336:1519–1523
21. Covert RF, Barman N, Domanico RS, et al. Prior enteral nutrition with human milk protects against intestinal perforation in infants who develop necrotizing enterocolitis. *Pediatr Res.* 1995;37:305A. Abstract
22. Ford RPK, Taylor BJ, Mitchell EA, et al. Breastfeeding and the risk of sudden infant death syndrome. *Int J Epidemiol.* 1993;22:885–890
23. Mitchell EA, Taylor BJ, Ford RPK, et al. Four modifiable and other major risk factors for cot death: the New Zealand study. *J Paediatr Child Health.* 1992;28:S3–S8
24. Scragg LK, Mitchell EA, Tonkin SL, et al. Evaluation of the cot death prevention programme in South Auckland. *N Z Med J.* 1993;106:8–10
25. Mayer EJ, Hamman RF, Gay EC, et al. Reduced risk of IDDM among breast-fed children. *Diabetes.* 1988;37:1625–1632
26. Virtanen SM, Rasanen L, Aro A, et al. Infant feeding in Finnish children <7 yr of age with newly diagnosed IDDM. *Diabetes Care.* 1991;14:415–417

27. Gerstein HC. Cow's milk exposure and type 1 diabetes mellitus. *Diabetes Care.* 1994;17:13–19
28. Koletzko S, Sherman P, Corey M, et al. Role of infant feeding practices in development of Crohn's disease in childhood. *Br Med J.* 1989;298:1617–1618
29. Rigas A, Rigas B, Glassman M, et al. Breast-feeding and maternal smoking in the etiology of Crohn's disease and ulcerative colitis in childhood. *Ann Epidemiol.* 1993;3:387–392
30. Davis MK, Savitz DA, Graubard BI. Infant feeding and childhood cancer. *Lancet.* 1988;2:365–368
31. Shu X-O, Clemens J, Zheng W, et al. Infant breastfeeding and the risk of childhood lymphoma and leukaemia. *Int J Epidemiol.* 1995;24:27–32
32. Lucas A, Brooke OG, Morley R, et al. Early diet of preterm infants and development of allergic or atopic disease: randomised prospective study. *Br Med J.* 1990;300:837–840
33. Halken S, Host A, Hansen LG, et al. Effect of an allergy prevention programme on incidence of atopic symptoms in infancy. *Ann Allergy.* 1992;47:545–553
34. Saarinen UM, Kajosaari M. Breastfeeding as prophylaxis against atopic disease: prospective follow-up study until 17 years old. *Lancet.* 1995;346:1065–1069
35. Udall JN, Dixon M, Newman AP, et al. Liver disease in α_1-antitrypsin deficiency: retrospective analysis of the influence of early breast- vs bottle-feeding. *JAMA.* 1985;253:2679–2682
36. Sveger T. Breast-feeding, α_1-antitrypsin deficiency, and liver disease? *JAMA.* 1985;254:3036. Letter
37. Greco L, Auricchio S, Mayer M, et al. Case control study on nutritional risk factors in celiac disease. *J Pediatr Gastroenterol Nutr.* 1988;7:395–399
38. Morrow-Tlucak M, Haude RH, Ernhart CB. Breastfeeding and cognitive development in the first 2 years of life. *Soc Sci Med.* 1988;26:635–639
39. Wang YS, Wu SY. The effect of exclusive breastfeeding on development and incidence of infection in infants. *J Hum Lactation.* 1996;12:27–30
40. Chua S, Arulkumaran S, Lim I, et al. Influence of breastfeeding and nipple stimulation on postpartum uterine activity. *Br J Obstet Gynaecol.* 1994;101:804–805
41. Dewey KG, Heinig MJ, Nommsen LA. Maternal weight-loss patterns during prolonged lactation. *Am J Clin Nutr.* 1993;58:162–166
42. Kennedy KI, Visness CM. Contraceptive efficacy of lactational amenorrhoea. *Lancet.* 1992;339:227–230
43. Gray RH, Campbell OM, Apelo R, et al. Risk of ovulation during lactation. *Lancet.* 1990;335:25–29
44. Labbock MH, Colie C. Puerperium and breast-feeding. *Curr Opin Obstet Gynecol.* 1992;4:818–825
45. Melton LJ, Bryant SC, Wahner HW, et al. Influence of breastfeeding and other reproductive factors on bone mass later in life. *Osteoporos Int.* 1993;3:76–83
46. Cumming RG, Klineberg RJ. Breastfeeding and other reproductive factors and the risk of hip fractures in elderly woman. *Int J Epidemiol.* 1993;22:684–691
47. Rosenblatt KA, Thomas DB, WHO Collaborative Study of Neoplasia and Steroid Contraceptives. *Int J Epidemiol.* 1993;22:192–197
48. Newcomb PA, Storer BE, Longnecker MP, et al. Lactation and a reduced risk of premenopausal breast cancer. *N Engl J Med.* 1994;330:81–87
49. Heck H, de Castro JM. The caloric demand of lactation does not alter spontaneous meal patterns, nutrient intakes, or moods of women. *Physiol Behav.* 1993;54:641–648
50. Butte NF, Garza C, O'Brien Smith JE, et al. Effect of maternal diet and body composition on lactational performance. *Am J Clin Nutr.* 1984;39:296–306
51. Montgomery D, Splett P. Economic benefit of breast-feeding infants enrolled in WIC. *J Am Diet Assoc.* 1997;97:379–385
52. Tuttle CR, Dewey KG. Potential cost savings for Medi-Cal, AFDC, food stamps, and WIC programs associated with increasing breast-feeding among low-income Hmong women in California. *J Am Diet Assoc.* 1996;96:885–890
53. Wilson MH. Feeding the healthy child. In: Oski FA, DeAngelis CD, Feigin RD, et al., eds. *Principles and Practice of Pediatrics.* Philadelphia, PA: JB Lippincott; 1990:533–545
54. Rohr FJ, Levy HL, Shih VE. Inborn errors of metabolism. In: Walker WA, Watkins JB, eds. *Nutrition in Pediatrics.* Boston, MA: Little, Brown; 1985:412
55. American Academy of Pediatrics, Committee on Drugs. The transfer of drugs and other chemicals into human milk. *Pediatrics.* 1994;93:137–150
56. American Academy of Pediatrics, Committee on Pediatric Aids. Human milk, breastfeeding, and transmission of human immunodefi-

ciency virus in the United States. *Pediatrics.* 1995;96:977–979

57. Centers for Disease Control and Prevention. Recommendations for assisting in the prevention of perinatal transmission of human T-lymphotropic virus type III/lymphadenopathy-associated virus and acquired immunodeficiency syndrome. *MMWR.* 1985;34:721–732

58. World Health Organization. Consensus statement from the consultation on HIV transmission and breastfeeding. *J Hum Lactation.* 1992;8: 173–174

59. *Healthy People 2000: National Health Promotion and Disease Prevention Objectives.* Washington, DC: Government Printing Office; 1990: 379–380. US Dept of Health and Human Services publication PHS 91-50212

60. Ryan AS. The resurgence of breastfeeding in the United States. *Pediatrics.* 1997;99(4). URL: http://www.pediatrics.org/cgi/content/full/99/4/e12

61. Freed GL, McIntosh Jones T, Fraley JK. Attitudes and education of pediatric house staff concerning breast-feeding. *South Med J.* 1992;85: 484–485

62. Freed GL, Clark SJ, Sorenson J, et al. National assessment of physicians' breast-feeding knowledge, attitudes, training, and experience. *JAMA.* 1995;273:472–476

63. Williams EL, Hammer LD. Breastfeeding attitudes and knowledge of pediatricians-in-training. *Am J Prev Med.* 1995;11:26–33

64. World Health Organization. *Protecting, Promoting and Supporting Breast-Feeding: The Special Role of Maternity Services.* Geneva, Switzerland: WHO; 1989:13–18

65. Powers NG, Naylor AJ, Wester RA. Hospital policies: crucial to breast-feeding success. *Semin Perinatol.* 1994;18:517–524

66. Braveman P, Egerter S, Pearl M, et al. Problems associated with early discharge of newborn infants. *Pediatrics.* 1995;96:716–726

67. Williams LR, Cooper MK. Nurse-managed postpartum home care. *J Obstet Gynecol Neonatal Nurs.* 1993;22:25–31

68. Gielen AC, Faden RR, O'Campo P, et al. Maternal employment during the early postpartum period: effects on initiation and continuation of breast-feeding. *Pediatrics.* 1991;87:298–305

69. Ryan AS, Martinez GA. Breast-feeding and the working mother: a profile. *Pediatrics.* 1989;83:524–531

70. Frederick IB, Auerback KG. Maternal-infant separation and breast-feeding: the return to work or school. *J Reprod Med.* 1985;30:523–526

71. Spisak S, Gross SS. Second Followup Report: *The Surgeon General's Workshop on Breastfeeding and Human Lactation.* Washington, DC: National Center for Education in Maternal and Child Health; 1991

72. World Health Assembly. *International Code of Marketing of Breast-milk Substitutes. Resolution of the 34th World Health Assembly.* No. 34.22, Geneva, Switzerland: WHO; 1981

73. Howard CR, Howard FM, Weitzman ML. Infant formula distribution and advertising in pregnancy: a hospital survey. *Birth.* 1994;21:14–19

74. Howard FM, Howard CR, Weitzman ML. The physician as advertiser: the unintentional discouragement of breast-feeding. *Obstet Gynecol.* 1993;81:1048–1051

75. Gartner LM. Introduction. Gartner LM, ed. Breastfeeding in the hospital. *Semin Perinatol.* 1994;18:475

76. American Academy of Pediatrics, Committee on Nutrition. Nutritional needs of low-birth-weight infants. *Pediatrics.* 1985;75:976–986

77. American Dietetic Association. Position of the American Dietetic Association: promotion of breast feeding. *Am Diet Assoc Rep.* 1986;86: 1580–1585

78. Schanler RJ, Hurst NM. Human milk for the hospitalized preterm infant. *Semin Perinatol.* 1994;18:476–486

79. Lemons P, Stuart M, Lemons JA. Breast-feeding the premature infant. *Clin Perinatol.* 1986;13:111–122

80. Righard L, Alade MO. Effect of delivery room routines on success of first breast-feed. *Lancet.* 1990;336:1105–1107

81. Widstrom AM, Wahlberg V, Matthiesen AS, et al. Short-term effects of early suckling and touch of the nipple on maternal behavior. *Early Hum Dev.* 1990;21:153–163

82. Van Den Bosch CA, Bullough CHW. Effect of early suckling on term neonates' core body temperature. *Ann Trop Paediatr.* 1990;10:347–353

83. Wiberg B, Humble K, de Chateau P. Long-term effect on mother–infant behavior of extra contact during the first hour post partum v follow-up

at three years. *Scand J Soc Med.* 1989;17:181–191

84. Sosa R, Kennell JH, Klaus M, et al. The effect of early mother–infant contact on breast feeding, infection and growth. In: Lloyd JK, ed. *Breast-feeding and the Mother.* Amsterdam: Elsevier; 1976:179–193

85. Gunther M. Instinct and the nursing couple. *Lancet.* 1955;:575–578

86. Anderson GC. Risk in mother–infant separation postbirth. *IMAGE: J Nurs Sch.* 1989;21:196–199

87. De Carvalho M, Klaus MH, Merkatz RB. Frequency of breast-feeding and serum bilirubin concentration. *Am J Dis Child.* 1982;136:737–738

88. De Carvalho M, Robertson S, Friedman A, et al. Effect of frequent breast-feeding on early milk production and infant weight gain. *Pediatrics.* 1983;72:307–311

89. Klaus MH. The frequency of suckling—neglected but essential ingredient of breast-feeding. *Obstet Gynecol Clin North Am.* 1987;14:623–633

90. Mohrbacher N, Stock J. *The Breastfeeding Answer Book.* Schaumburg, IL: La Leche League International; 1997:60

91. Procianoy RS, Fernandes-Filho PH, Lazaro L, et al. The influence of rooming-in on breastfeeding. *J Trop Pediatr.* 1983;29:112–114

92. The American Academy of Pediatrics and the American College of Obstetricians and Gynecologists. *Guidelines for Perinatal Care.* 3rd ed. Washington, DC: ACOG, AAP; 1992:183

93. American Academy of Pediatrics, Committee on Nutrition. *Pediatric Nutrition Handbook.* 3rd ed. Elk Grove Village, IL: AAP; 1993:7

94. Shrago L. Glucose water supplementation of the breastfed infant during the first three days of life. *J Human Lactation.* 1987;3:82–86

95. Goldberg NM, Adams E. Supplementary water for breast-fed babies in a hot and dry climate—not really a necessity. *Arch Dis Child.* 1983;58: 73–74

96. Righard L, Alade MO. Sucking technique and its effect on success of breastfeeding. *Birth.* 1992;19:185–189

97. Neifert M, Lawrence R, Seacat J. Nipple confusion: toward a formal definition. *J Pediatr.* 1995;126:S125–129

98. Victora CG, Tomasi E, Olinto MTA, et al. Use of pacifiers and breast-feeding duration. *Lancet.* 1993;341:404–406

99. The American Academy of Pediatrics, Committee on Practice and Ambulatory Medicine. Recommendations for preventive pediatric health care. *Pediatrics.* 1995;96:373

100. Ahn CH, MacLean WC. Growth of the exclusively breast-fed infant. *Am J Clin Nutr.* 1980;33:183–192

101. The American Academy of Pediatrics, Committee on Nutrition. The use of whole cow's milk in infancy. *Pediatrics.* 1992;89:1105–1109

102. Saarinen UM. Need for iron supplementation in infants on prolonged breast feeding. *J Pediatr.* 1978;93:177–180

103. Dallman PR. Progress in the prevention of iron deficiency in infants. *Acta Paediatr Scand Suppl.* 1990;365:28–37

104. Sugarman M, Kendall-Tackett KA. Weaning ages in a sample of American women who practice extended breastfeeding. *Clin Pediatr.* 1995; 34:642–647

105. Ashraf RN, Jalil F, Aperia A, et al. Additional water is not needed for healthy breast-fed babies in a hot climate. *Acta Paediatr Scand.* 1993;82: 1007–1011

106. Heinig MJ, Nommsen LA, Peerson, JM, et al. Intake and growth of breast-fed and formula-fed infants in relation to the timing of introduction of complementary foods: the Darling study. *Acta Paediatr Scand.* 1993;82:999–1006

107. American Academy of Pediatrics, Committee on Fetus and Newborn, and American College of Obstetricians and Gynecologists. Maternal and newborn nutrition. In: *Guidelines for Perinatal Care.* 4th ed. Washington, DC: ACOG, AAP; 1997

108. Pisacane A, De Visia B, Valiante A, et al. Iron status in breast-fed infants. *J Pediatr.* 1995;127:429–431

109. American Academy of Pediatrics, Committee on Nutrition. Vitamin and mineral supplement needs in normal children in the United States. *Pediatrics.* 1980;66:1015–1021

110. American Academy of Pediatrics, Committee on Nutrition. Fluoride supplementation for children: interim policy recommendations. *Pediatrics.* 1995;95:777

111. Freed GL, Clark SJ, Lohr JA, et al. Pediatrician involvement in breast-feeding promotion: a national study of residents and practitioners. *Pediatrics.* 1995;96:490–494

APPENDIX G

Prototype Lactation Consultant Job Proposal or Description

NOTE TO READER: In all cases, a job proposal or description should reflect those specific elements that are relevant to the setting and the individual offering to provide the service in question. This prototype job proposal/description is more inclusive than would be necessary in most settings.

QUALIFICATIONS NEEDED

1.0 Certification by the International Board of Lactation Consultant Examiners (I.B.L.C.E.)

2.0 Minimum five years experience working with childbearing families or maternal health nursing.

OBJECTIVES

1.0 Document the need for a lactation consultant.

1.1 Establish base-line data on the numbers and percentages within the institution's patient base of mothers who initiate breastfeeding and the length of time they continue to breastfeed after hospital discharge.

1.2. Collect and analyze data to determine when and what kind of support the breastfeeding mother would like to receive prior to her baby's birth, while she is in the hospital, and after she returns home.

1.3. Survey other health-care providers who staff the institution and/or who work in the community which the hospital serves regarding their perceived need for the assistance and resources that a lactation consultant could provide. [N.B.: In settings where the profession of lactation consultant is unknown, this goal may need to be changed to determine the degree to which health providers—if given access to the resources of a lactation consultant—might choose to use such a service.]

2.0. Promote breastfeeding beyond the first few weeks of life and assist the mother to reach her own goals for breastfeeding.

2.1. Develop and implement guidelines and standards of care for assisting breastfeeding mothers in all areas of the institution where they might be served (emergency room, obstetrics/gynecology, family medicine, the midwifery service, employee health, women's health service, pediatrics, and internal medicine).

2.2. Clarify roles of and perceptions about breastfeeding support among all health providers in the hospital, paying particular attention to those care providers who are most likely to serve lactating women and their breastfeeding infants.

2.3. Develop a reference library of breastfeeding materials appropriate for both health-care providers and mothers interested in learning more about lactation. Particular attention should be paid to maintaining and regularly updating a file of journal articles and to obtaining reference works that include the latest information on lactation in a variety of contexts and circumstances.

2.4. Provide regular in-service education for all relevant medical, nursing, and ancillary staff. In some cases, hospital policies may determine the frequency with which such in-servicing must be offered and attended. In other cases, invitations may need to be secured from the administrative offices of the services in question.

Source: Derived in part from MA Tinari: Lactation consultant job proposal. J Hum Lact *2:114–15, 1986.*

2.5. Offer case conferences that highlight the particular needs of lactating mothers and/or their breastfeeding infants. Such case conferences may serve as a springboard for reexamining care routines and/or other aspects of the hospital experience of the mother-baby couple in question.

2.6. Set up a telephone warmline/hotline to provide continuing contact between the lactation consultant and the clients she has assisted in the hospital and others who may be referred to her for out-patient assistance.

2.7. Establish a regular follow-up system of continuing care for mothers first seen in the hospital. Such a system may be part of the hotline/warmline service, or it may consist of communication by postcard or letter, the incorporation of home visits by the hospital-based LC, or referral to a community-based breastfeeding counselor who makes home visits and reports back to the hospital LC. When such referral continues without reports, continuity of care is lost, although continued support for the breastfeeding mother may continue.

2.8. Provide an out-patient service for persons who were not initially seen in the hospital and/or who are not in the immediate postpartum period.

2.9. Offer regularly scheduled prenatal breastfeeding classes to inform prospective mothers of the services available in the institution that support the breastfeeding course and to provide them with sufficient information to make an informed choice about infant feeding.

2.10. Offer regularly scheduled postpartum breastfeeding classes to mothers who give birth in the institution prior to their return home.

2.11. Provide access to breastfeeding equipment and devices when their use is appropriate to the lactating mother and her breastfeeding infant. In most cases, such equipment will include breast pumps, breast shells, tube feeding devices, and the like. In some cases, such devices are available for purchase; in other cases, they are rented. In situations where the lactation consultant is unable or unwilling to provide such rental or purchase options, she needs to develop an ongoing relationship with those businesses in the community that do offer such a service, in order that she may assist the mother who needs such devices with a minimum of disruption to the lactation course.

3.0. Coordinate the services of the professional staff to the benefit of the lactating mother and her breastfeeding baby.

3.1. Document teaching and progress of the mother and baby on patient charts. In some cases, this may necessitate completing separate charts for the mother and the baby, a time-consuming duplication of effort. In other cases, lactation assessment charts have been developed whose copies can be appended to each patient's chart and/or sent to the physician seeing the mother and/or baby.

3.2. Confer regularly with the relevant obstetrician, pediatrician, mother-baby, and postpartum or nursery nursing staff member on each patient's progress, special needs, and continuity of care.

3.3. Develop and/or review all literature relating to infant feeding that is distributed to patients in the hospital and related to their discharge home.

3.4. Initiate and maintain contact with all relevant medical staff, particularly pediatric and obstetric/family medicine physicians regarding the policies and programs that affect their patients in order to effect a team approach to promoting successful breastfeeding.

3.5. Participate in a committee charged with evaluating relevant hospital policies that may influence the breastfeeding course of mothers and babies receiving care in the institution.

4.0. Participate in scholarly activities: research, publications, grants.

4.1. Maintain statistics on breastfeeding initiation and duration of all clients seen in the hospital or assisted in the out-patient clinic in order to periodically assess the effectiveness of the lactation consultant service within the institution.

4.2. Participate in the development, implementation, and dissemination of the results of research in which lactating mothers and/or their breastfeeding babies were subjects.

4.3. Write and submit articles for publication in the health-profession journals and maternal-child literature.

4.4. Apply for grants to support new clinical care procedures, research protocols evaluating some aspect of the maternal lactation course, and/or infant breastfeeding patterns.

A P P E N D I X G *(cont.)*

5.0. Serve as a speaker/participant in public and professional forums providing programs relating to lactation and breastfeeding.

5.1. Participate in continuing education through seminars, workshops, conferences, and network with others in the field.

RESOURCES NEEDED

1. Office space and supplies, including lockable file cabinets in which to store client information forms and other records relating to the performance of the LC's duties.

2. Secretarial assistance in keeping with the needs of the LC or the LC practice.

3. Telephone with at least two lines. An answering machine and beeper system in order that the LC may be reached when she is not at her desk.

4. Small reference library.

5. Financial support for the LC to participate in regular continuing education at annual conferences and the purchase of books and other resource materials relevant to the practice of lactation consulting.

6. Computer with word processing and spreadsheet software*.

---

* *"Rental Manager" spreadsheet software for reports and breast pump rental information is available from Medela, Inc., 4610 Prime Parkway, McHenry, IL 60050 USA; (815) 363-1166; or 1-800-435-8316; TELEX (815) 353-1246.*

APPENDIX H

Standards of Practice for Lactation Consultants*

INTERNATIONAL LACTATION CONSULTANT ASSOCIATION

Philosophy

ILCA believes it is the right of every woman to breastfeed her children and the right of every child to receive human milk. Further, we believe it is the right of every woman to receive accurate and consistent information and positive support for breastfeeding and lactation. The lactation consultant respects these rights regardless of age, race, religion, ability, economic or social status.[2]

Statement of Purpose

The purposes of the International Lactation Consultant Association are to:

1. provide for education, communication, networking and mutual support among lactation consultants and other health workers concerned with breastfeeding and related issues;
2. aid lactation consultants in the provision of effective breastfeeding support and services;
3. uphold high standards of professional practice;
4. promote appropriate certification for lactation consultants;
5. foster awareness of breastfeeding and human milk feeding as important measures for health promotion and disease prevention;
6. heighten recognition of the hazards of artificial feeding;
7. encourage research in all aspects of human lactation, the work of the lactation consultant and the feeding of infants and young children;
8. support the implementation of the World Health Organization's International Code of Marketing Breast-Milk Substitutes and other initiatives and recommendations which are consistent with the goals and objectives of the Association;
9. advise relevant authorities on issues of concern to lactation consultants;
10. cooperate with other organizations that have aims and objectives, in whole or in part, similar to those of the Association.

Introduction

Breastfeeding has proven benefits for mothers, infants, children, families, and societies. It is an instinctive survival behavior which most mothers and children around the world practice without any need for formal instruction or assistance. Breastfeeding also is a learned art and skill; as such it often benefits from the assistance and support of another experienced and skilled individual, especially in environments where the intergenerational transfer of information and skill has been weakened or interrupted. The lactation consultant is a health care professional who is knowledgeable, skilled and experienced in lactation and breastfeeding management and whose primary focus is the provision of education, assistance and support to breastfeeding women and children. Lactation consultants function as members of the health care team to promote, support, and protect breastfeeding by:

- empowering women to make informed infant feeding decisions acting as advocates for and with the breastfeeding family
- fostering family support for the breastfeeding mother
- assisting women to learn the skills to successfully initiate and maintain lactation and to overcome obstacles to breastfeeding, thus enhancing maternal role satisfaction.

Lactation consultants throughout the world are linked by the work they do, by the knowledge and skills they possess, and by the way they use these skills to promote and protect the health and well-being of women, infants, children, and the family.

Quality practice and service constitute the core of a profession's responsibility to the public. Standards of practice have been defined as "stated measures or levels of quality" that serve as models for the conduct and evaluation of practice.[3] Standards promote consistency by encouraging a common systematic approach among lactation consultants. They must be global to address the diversity of backgrounds, educational preparation, and settings in which lactation consultants work; they also must be specific in content to meet the demands of daily practice. These standards are presented as a recommended framework for the development of policies and protocols, educational programs, and quality improvement efforts. They are intended for use in diverse settings, institutions, and cultural contexts to allow for innovation and the development of programs best suited to consumers and communities.

---

* *These standards are based upon and supersede the ILCA Recommendations and Competencies for Lactation Consultant Practice. Copyright © 1998. International Lactation Consultant Association. The Standards are current at the time of printing.*

APPENDIX H (cont.)

Standard 1. CLINICAL PRACTICE

The clinical practice of the lactation consultant focuses on helping breastfeeding women and families define and achieve their breastfeeding goals. This is best accomplished within the framework of systematic problem solving in cooperation with the client. Lactation consultants are responsible for decisions and actions undertaken as a part of their professional role, including the:

- assessment, planning, intervention, and evaluation of care in a variety of situations, both simple and complex
- prevention of problems whenever possible by acting to enhance the knowledge and strengths of the breastfeeding woman and her support system
- establishment of priorities based on the individual needs of each breastfeeding mother, infant, child and family
- demonstration of competence in lactation consultant practice
- complete, accurate, and timely documentation of care
- communication and collaboration with other health care professionals
- procurement of the mother's written consent prior to initiating care

1.1 ASSESSMENT

1.1.1 The lactation consultant will obtain and document an appropriate history of the breastfeeding mother and child, which may include, but is not limited to:

- family history related to breastfeeding
- health history of mother and child, past and present
- pregnancy and birth history
- lactation and breastfeeding history, past and present
- mother's perception of her breastfeeding status and that of her child
- health practices, e.g. diet, sleep
- mother and child medication use
- mother's support system
- breastfeeding goals
- sociocultural factors
- attitudes, values and beliefs

1.1.2 The lactation consultant will systematically collect objective and subjective information, including but not limited to:

- physical appearance and health status of the mother
  - emotional status and related behaviors
  - appearance and condition of mother's breasts and nipples
- physical appearance and health status of the infant or child
  - oro-facial structure
  - state related behaviors, e.g., consolability, irritability, alerting, and clarity of cues
  - intake and output
  - weight gain or loss
  - behavior, including feeding, sleeping, crying, and excretion patterns
    - growth and development
- interaction of mother and child
- dynamics of the feeding process
- transfer of breastmilk from mother to child
  - latch-on
  - suck

1.1.3 Assessment information will be discussed with the mother, documented in the client record, and communicated to the primary health care provider(s) as appropriate.

1.2 PLAN

The lactation consultant will:

1.2.1 analyze assessment information to identify concerns and/or problems

1.2.2 develop a plan of care based on identified concerns or problems and the mother's breastfeeding goals

1.2.3 formulate expected outcomes of suggested interventions

1.2.4 arrange for follow-up evaluation

1.2.5 document the plan of care in the client record.

1.3 IMPLEMENTATION

The elements of implementation include:

- intervening and instructing as appropriate
- communicating effectively with the mother and significant others
- discussing benefits and risks associated with recommended interventions
- demonstrating procedures, techniques, equipment, and devices
- providing written instructions and information to reinforce and enhance verbal and demonstrated teaching
- documenting interventions and related outcomes in the client record.

The lactation consultant will:

1.3.1 implement the plan of care in a manner appropriate to the situation and acceptable to the mother

1.3.2 exercise principles of safety, hygiene, infection control, and universal precautions

1.3.4 provide a written report to the primary health care provider as appropriate, including:
- assessment information
- suggested interventions
- instructions given

1.3.5 facilitate referrals to other health professionals, community services, and support groups as needed.

1.4 EVALUATION

The lactation consultant will:

1.4.1 evaluate outcomes of planned interventions and teaching

1.4.2 modify the plan based on the evaluation of outcomes

1.4.3 document in the client's record and communicate to the primary health care provider(s) as appropriate:
- evaluation of outcomes
- modifications in the plan
- follow-up

Standard 2. BREASTFEEDING EDUCATION AND COUNSELING

Breastfeeding education and counseling are integral parts of the care provided by the lactation consultant. They encourage participation by the breastfeeding mother and shared responsibility for decision making.

2.1 Breastfeeding education may include, but is not limited to:
- benefits and risks of breastfeeding and human milk
- benefits and risks of artificial feeding
- breast anatomy
- physiology of lactation
- basic management and techniques such as positioning, achieving latch-on, and evaluating intake
- prevention and management of simple and complex problems
- breastfeeding during employment or return to school
- expression, storage, and transportation of human milk
- correct use of equipment and devices
- management of special situations
- nutritional guidelines
- effects of medications, environmental toxins/contaminants, drugs of abuse, herbs and home remedies
- resources for support

- safe suppression of lactation in situations where breastfeeding or human milk feeding is impossible.

The lactation consultant will:

2.2 educate parents and families to encourage informed decision making about infant and child feeding

2.3 provide anticipatory teaching to:
- promote ideal breastfeeding practices
- minimize the potential for breastfeeding problems or complications

2.4 provide emotional support for continued breastfeeding in difficult or complicated circumstances

2.5 educate other health care professionals by sharing current research-based information and demonstrating skills, thereby empowering those professionals to provide informed and appropriate guidance to the breastfeeding family.

Standard 3. PROFESSIONAL RESPONSIBILITIES

The lactation consultant has a responsibility to maintain professional conduct and to practice in an ethical manner. The lactation consultant is clinically competent and accountable for professional actions and legal responsibilities inherent in that professional role.

3.1 Professional responsibility and accountability include:
- respecting the primacy of the mother-child relationship
- maintaining awareness of changing practices and of professional or ethical issues
- recognizing limitations in one's knowledge or skills
- obtaining clients' written consent prior to providing care
- communicating relevant information to primary health care provider(s)
- collaborating with and referring to other health care professionals as appropriate
- participating in appropriate professional organizations
- lending support to colleagues.

The lactation consultant will:

3.2 adhere to these Standards of Practice

3.3 become familiar with the ILCA *Position Paper on Infant Feeding*[4] and the World Health Organization's *International Code of Marketing of Breast-Milk Substitutes*[5]

3.4 act as an advocate for breastfeeding women, infants, and children

APPENDIX H (cont.)

3.5 assist the mother in maintaining an intact breastfeeding relationship with her child

3.6 maintain and expand knowledge and skills for lactation consultant practice by participating in continuing education programs and professional development activities and by reading current literature

3.7 undertake periodic and systematic appraisal for evaluation of one's clinical practice

3.8 use breastfeeding equipment and devices appropriately by:
- refraining from unnecessary or excessive use
- discussing the risks and benefits of recommended use
- evaluating safety and effectiveness
- assuring cleanliness and good operating condition
- maintaining an awareness of conflict of interest when/ if profiting from their rental or sale

3.9 support and promote well-designed research in human lactation and breastfeeding, and base clinical practice, insofar as possible, on such research.

Standard 4. LEGAL CONSIDERATIONS

Lactation consultants are obligated to practice within the laws of the geopolitical region in which they reside. They must practice with consideration for clients' rights of privacy and with respect for matters of a confidential nature.

4.1 The lactation consultant's legal responsibilities extend to:
- established parameters of professional practice
- legislation that affects practice
- institutional standards
- policies, procedures, and protocols within the practice environment.

The lactation consultant will:

4.2 clearly state applicable fees prior to providing care

4.3 obtain the client's written informed consent prior to:
- performing a physical assessment of the mother or child which requires touching
- reporting relevant information to the primary health care provider or other health care professional(s)
- taking photographs for any purpose
- seeking publication of information associated with the consultation

4.4 protect client confidentiality at all times

4.5 maintain records for a reasonable period.

GLOSSARY

Client—the party for whom professional services are rendered;[6] the breastfeeding woman employing the services of the lactation consultant.

Lactation Consultant—a health care professional whose scope of practice is focused upon providing education and management to prevent and solve breastfeeding problems and to encourage a social environment that effectively supports the breastfeeding mother/infant dyad.

Primary health care provider—a health professional such as a physician or midwife, who manages, directs and coordinates the health care of a client.

Protocol—a standardized written plan focusing on an aspect of care or a breastfeeding problem, e.g., Protocol for Breastfeeding Premature Infants.

Universal precautions—a method of infection control involving the use of personal protective equipment, e.g., gloves, gown, goggles, for the handling of blood and selected body fluids.

REFERENCES

1. *Recommendations and Competencies for Lactation Consultant Practice.* International Lactation Consultant Association, 1991.

2. *Australian Lactation Consultants' Association (ALCA) Standards of Practice.* ALCA, 1993.

3. *Standards for the Nursing Care of Women and Newborns* (4th edition). Association of Women's Health, Obstetric and Neonatal Nursing (AWHONN), 1991.

4. *Position Paper on Infant Feeding* (2nd edition). International Lactation Consultant Association, 1994.

5. WHO/UNICEF. *International Code of Marketing Breast-Milk Substitutes.* World Health Organization, Geneva: 1981.

6. *American Heritage Dictionary of the English Language* (3rd edition) Boston: Houghton Mifflin Co., 1992.

APPENDIX I

Tables of Equivalencies and Methods of Conversion

METRIC

1 liter (L) = 10 deciliters (dl) = 1000 milliliters (ml) or 1000 cc

1 dl = 100 ml

1 ml = 0.001 L = 10^{-3} L = 1 cc = 1 gm (water)

1 kilogram (kg) = 1000 grams (gm)

1 gm = 100 milligrams (mg) = 0.001 kg

1 mg = 1000 micrograms (µg or mcg) = 0.001 gm = 10^{-3} gm

1 µg = 0.001 mg = 10^{-6} gm

1 nanogram (ng) = 0.001 µg = 10^{-9} gm

1 picogram (pg) = 0.001 ng = 10^{-12} gm

VOLUME

Household Measure	*Fluid Ounces (Fl oz)*	*Metric Equivalent** (ml)	
1 cup (C)	8	240	1 C = 16 Tbsp
2 Tablespoons (Tbsp)	1	30	1 Tbsp = 3 tsp
1 Tbsp	not used	15	
1 teaspoon (tsp)	not used	5	
1 quart (qt)	32	960 ($\cong$ 1 L)	1 qt = 4 C = 2 pt
1 pint (pt)	16	480 ($\cong$ 500 ml)	1 pt = 2 C

WEIGHT

1 pound (1 lb or #) = 0.45 kg   1 oz = 28 gm $\cong$ 30 gm

1 kg = 2.2 lb

To convert lb to kg, divide lb by 2.2 *or* multiply lb times 0.45

To convert kg to lb, multiply kg times 2.2

LINEAR MEASURE

1 inch (in. or ") = 2.54 centimeters (cm) ($\cong$ 2.5)

1 cm = 0.4 in.

To convert in. to cm, multiply in. times 2.5.

To convert cm to in., multiply cm times 0.4 *or* divide cm by 2.5.

TEMPERATURE

To convert Celsius (C) to Fahrenheit (F), $°C = \frac{5}{9}(°F - 32)$

(Subtract 32, then multiply times $\frac{5}{9}$)

To convert Fahrenheit to Celsius, $°F = \frac{5}{9}°C + 32$

(Multiply times $\frac{5}{9}$, then add 32)

---

*Equivalent is given to nearest multiple of five. Number given in parentheses may sometimes be used to simplify calculations.
$\cong$ *means* approximately equals.

APPENDIX J

Patient History

WELLSTART INTERNATIONAL℠

Patient History

Name:	☐ Boy	Birthday: _____	Date of Visit: _____

Baby: _____ ☐ Girl Age of Baby: _____ Birthplace (Hosp.): _____

Mother: _____ Age: _____ Home Phone: _____

Father: _____ Age: _____

Obstetrician: _____ Phone: _____

Pediatrician: _____ Phone: _____

Mother's race/ethnicity (optional) _____ Mother's marital status _____

Reason for visit: | **For office use only**

MATERNAL HISTORY

1. Are you allergic to any medication?   ☐ Yes   ☐ No   If yes, please list: _____

2. Have you ever had any of the following? Please check (✔) all that apply.
   - ☐ Abnormal pap smear
   - ☐ Allergy/asthma
   - ☐ Anemia
   - ☐ Cancer
   - ☐ Constipation/hemorrhoids
   - ☐ Depression/blues
   - ☐ Diabetes
   - ☐ Diarrhea (chronic)
   - ☐ Heart disease
   - ☐ High blood pressure
   - ☐ Infertility
   - ☐ Kidney disease/bladder infection
   - ☐ Liver disease/hepatitis
   - ☐ Thyroid disorders
   - ☐ Tuberculosis
   - ☐ Venereal disease
   - ☐ None known
   - ☐ Other: _____

3. Have you ever had any of the following problems or procedures related to your breasts? Please check (✔) all that apply.
   - ☐ Biopsy
   - ☐ Lumps
   - ☐ Nipple problems: _____
   - ☐ Surgery: _____
   - ☐ None

4. Are you taking the following medications? Please check (✔) all that apply.
   - ☐ Prenatal vitamin-mineral
   - ☐ Other vitamins
   - ☐ Iron
   - ☐ Other minerals
   - ☐ Diet pills
   - ☐ Antihistamines/cold remedies
   - ☐ Laxatives/antacids
   - ☐ Diuretics/water pills
   - ☐ Aspirin/pain pills
   - ☐ Birth control pills
   - ☐ Antibiotics
   - ☐ None of the above
   - ☐ Other drugs _____
   - _____

PERINATAL HISTORY   List all pregnancies:

5.

Date Preg. Ended	Weeks Gesta-tion	Sex	Birth Weight	Complications of Pregnancy	Complications of Labor and Delivery	*Type of Anes-thesia	Type of Delivery		Breast-feeding Duration
							Vag.	C/S	

___/___/___/___/___

*Anesthesia: ① None   ② Local   ③ Epidural   ④ Spinal   ⑤ General (asleep)
            ⑥ Other _____

6. Did you have any of the following during this pregnancy? Please check (✔) all that apply.
   - ☐ Anemia (low iron level)
   - ☐ Fever
   - ☐ Gestational diabetes
   - ☐ High blood pressure
   - ☐ Nausea/vomiting (severe)
   - ☐ Premature labor
   - ☐ Urinary tract infection
   - ☐ Medication
   - ☐ None of the above
   - ☐ Other: _____

For office use only

7. Did you have any of the following during this labor and delivery? Please check (✔) all that apply.
- ☐ Drugs to induce or speed labor: If yes, for how long during labor was this drug administered?

  _____ hours
- ☐ Premature rupture of membranes
- ☐ Drugs to control high blood pressure
- ☐ Drugs to control pain
- ☐ Fever
- ☐ Antibiotics
- ☐ Hemorrhage
- ☐ None of the above
- ☐ Other:_____

  _____

8. With this labor and delivery, did you have any of the following? Please check (✔) all that apply.
- ☐ Total labor longer than 30 hours
- ☐ Pushing stage longer than 2 hours
- ☐ Episiotomy or vaginal tear
- ☐ Tear that involved the rectum (a "third or fourth degree" laceration)
- ☐ Breech presentation
- ☐ Forceps delivery
- ☐ Vacuum extraction
- ☐ None of the above

9. How would you rate your labor and delivery experience? Please check (✔) all that apply.
- ☐ Easy
- ☐ Difficult
- ☐ Painful
- ☐ Long
- ☐ Short
- ☐ Average length
- ☐ Just what I'd expected
- ☐ Not what I'd expected
- ☐ Other_____

10. Postpartum complications? Please check (✔) all that apply.
- ☐ Urinary/other infection
- ☐ Excessive bleeding (hemorrhage)
- ☐ High blood pressure
- ☐ Low blood pressure (shock)
- ☐ None of the above
- ☐ Other_____

11. Did the baby have any of the following shortly after birth? Please check (✔) all that apply.
- ☐ Breathing problems
- ☐ Fever
- ☐ High hematocrit
- ☐ Jaundice
- ☐ Low blood sugar
- ☐ Meconium aspiration
- ☐ None of the above

☐ Medications:_____

☐ Other:_____

12. How soon after delivery did you first put your baby to your breast? _____

13. Were you and your baby separated for more than 2 hours while in the hospital?   ☐ Yes   ☐ No

14. While in the hospital, how many times in 24 hours did you breastfeed your baby?
- ☐ Less than 8 times
- ☐ 8-12 times (every 2-3 hours)
- ☐ More than 12 times

15. While in the hospital, what was the longest time between breastfeeding?   Day:_____   Night:_____

16. Did you have any of the following problems with your breasts or with breastfeeding your baby while in the hospital? Please check (✔) all that apply.
- ☐ Attachment difficulties
- ☐ Engorgement
- ☐ None
- ☐ Sleepy baby
- ☐ Sore nipples
- ☐ Other:_____
- ☐ Preference for one breast
- ☐ Not enough milk

17. While in the hospital, was your baby given any supplements?   ☐ Yes   ☐ No
If yes, please check (✔) all that apply.
- ☐ Formula
- ☐ Water (plain)
- ☐ Sugar water

How were supplements given?   ☐ Bottle   ☐ Syringe   ☐ Dropper   ☐ Other:_____

18. While in the hospital, was your baby given a pacifier?   ☐ Yes   ☐ No

19. Did you and your baby go home at the same time?   ☐ Yes   ☐ No

20. How old was the baby at discharge? _____

21. Are you currently having vaginal bleeding?   ☐ Yes   ☐ No
Have your menstrual periods returned?   ☐ Yes   ☐ No   Date of last menstrual period:_____

22. Which of the following family planning methods are you using or do you plan to use?   ☐ None
- ☐ Birth control pills
- ☐ Other:_____

FEEDING HISTORY

23. How many times in 24 hours are you currently breastfeeding your baby?
- ☐ Less than 8 times
- ☐ 8-12 times (every 2-3 hours)
- ☐ More than 12 times

APPENDIX J *(cont.)*

24. What is the longest time between breastfeedings? Day:_____   Night:_____   **For office use only**

25. How long does your baby nurse on each breast? _____

26. While nursing, do you sense any of the following in your breasts?
   ☐ Filling   ☐ Burning   ☐ Milk dripping from other breast
   ☐ Tingling   ☐ Emptying   ☐ None of the above
   ☐ Other_____

27. Who decides when the feeding is over?   ☐ Mother   ☐ Baby

28. At home, has your baby received:
   ☐ Water   ☐ Formula   ☐ Liquids, other than formula   ☐ Any solids

29. How many times in 24 hours has your baby had: Wet diapers:_____   Bowel movements:_____

30. Does your baby spit up?   ☐ Never   ☐ Occasionally   ☐ Often

31. Is the baby content or sleeping between feedings?   ☐ Never   ☐ Occasionally   ☐ Often

32. Has your baby had any prolonged crying spells?   ☐ Never   ☐ Occasionally   ☐ Often

33. Is your baby given a pacifier?   ☐ Never   ☐ Occasionally   ☐ Often

34. Have you had any of the following problems with your breasts or with breastfeeding since coming home?
   ☐ Baby always hungry   ☐ Cracked/bleeding nipples   ☐ Painfully full breast(s)
   ☐ Baby prefers one breast   ☐ Nipple pain   ☐ Not enough milk
   ☐ Baby not interested   ☐ Breast pain   ☐ None of the above
   ☐ Other:_____

35. Have you used any of the following? Please check (✔) all that apply.
   ☐ Hand expression   ☐ Nursing bra (no underwire)   ☐ Breast or nipple shield
   ☐ Breast pump   ☐ Nursing bra (with underwire) ☐ None of the above
   ☐ Breast cream
   ☐ Other:_____

36. Your bra size: before pregnancy_____   now_____

FAMILY HISTORY

37. Does anyone on either side of the baby's family have any of the following?
   ☐ Allergy (food)   ☐ Allergy (hay fever)   ☐ Genetic disease
   ☐ Allergy (asthma)   ☐ Cancer (breast)   ☐ Thyroid disease
   ☐ Allergy (eczema)   ☐ Diabetes   ☐ None of the above
   ☐ Other:_____

38. How are members of your family adjusting to the new baby?
   ☐ Very well   ☐ Reasonably well   ☐ Poorly   ☐ Very poorly

39. Was your baby planned?   ☐ Yes   ☐ No

40. When did you decide to breastfeed this baby?
   ☐ Before pregnancy   ☐ During pregnancy   ☐ After delivery

41. How did you prepare for breastfeeding?
   ☐ Classes   ☐ Reading   ☐ Other:_____

42. Were you breastfed?   ☐ Yes   ☐ No   ☐ Not known

43. Was your baby's father breastfed?   ☐ Yes   ☐ No   ☐ Not known

44. How many previous babies have you breastfed?_____
   How long? _____   Why did you stop? _____

45. Why do you wish to breastfeed your baby? _____

46. Is there anyone in your household/family who feels you should **not** breastfeed this baby?   ☐ Yes   ☐ No

47. For how long do you plan to breastfeed this baby?_____

48. Why do you think you will discontinue breastfeeding at that time?_____

For office use only

49. What was the highest grade or year of regular school you have completed?
- [ ] Less than 6 years
- [ ] High school (12 years)
- [ ] 4-year college (16 years)
- [ ] Elementary school (6 years)
- [ ] 2-year college (14 years)
- [ ] Graduate school (17+ years)
- [ ] Junior high school (9 years)

50. Usual occupation? Mother:_____ Father:_____
When does mother plan to return to work? _____

NUTRITION

51. Did you see a nutritionist during your pregnancy? [ ] Yes [ ] No

52. Are there any foods that you avoid eating? [ ] Yes [ ] No If yes, what: _____
Why? _____

53. Are you now on any of these special diets?
- [ ] Diabetic
- [ ] High protein
- [ ] Low salt
- [ ] No special diet
- [ ] Low fat
- [ ] Weight loss
- [ ] Other:_____

If yes, who suggested the diet?_____

54. Are you trying to lose weight at this time? [ ] Yes [ ] No If yes, how much?_____
How? [ ] Less food/more exercise [ ] Program:_____ [ ] Other:_____

55. Are you a vegetarian? [ ] Yes [ ] No
If yes, do you consume: [ ] Milk products (milk, cheese, yogurt) [ ] Eggs?

56. How would you rate your appetite presently? [ ] Good [ ] Fair [ ] Poor

57. How would you describe the type and amount of food in your household?
- [ ] Enough of the kind you want
- [ ] Enough, but not always the kind you want
- [ ] Sometimes not enough
- [ ] Often not enough

58. Are you receiving any of the following?
- [ ] Food stamps
- [ ] Medi-Cal
- [ ] Donated food/meals
- [ ] WIC
- [ ] AFDC/welfare
- [ ] None of the above
- [ ] Other:_____

59. Do you have someone to help you shop and prepare meals? [ ] Yes [ ] No

60. How many times a day do you eat meals:_____ and snacks:_____

61. How many cups (8 oz.) of the following liquids do you usually drink per day?
- _____ Water
- _____ Sodas with sugar
- _____ Coffee
- _____ Juice
- _____ Diet soda, diet punch
- _____ Tea
- _____ Milk
- _____ Punch, Kool-Aid, Tang
- _____ Other:_____

LIFESTYLE

62. How often are you now drinking beer, wine, hard liquor, or mixed drinks?
- [ ] Daily
- [ ] Weekly
- [ ] Monthly
- [ ] Never
When you drink, how many drinks do you have? [ ] One [ ] Two [ ] Three [ ] More

63. How many cigarettes do you smoke each day?
- [ ] Do not smoke
- [ ] Fewer than 10 cigarettes
- [ ] 11-20 cigarettes
- [ ] More than 20 cigarettes

64. How often are you currently exercising (besides housework, child care)? _____
What types of exercise do you do? _____

65. Do you feel you are getting adequate rest? [ ] Never [ ] Occasionally [ ] Often

66. Having a new baby can be a stressful time for the family. What other stresses are present in your home?
- [ ] Relationship difficulties
- [ ] Moving
- [ ] Illness/death in the family
- [ ] Lack of help with home/child care
- [ ] Financial concerns
- [ ] Other: _____
- [ ] Drug or alcohol use
- [ ] None of the above

67. Who lives with you in your home? _____

68. Do you have any other concerns about yourself, your baby, or your family's health that you would like to discuss during your appointment? [ ] Yes [ ] No
If yes, what?_____

MATERNAL ANTHROPOMETRY

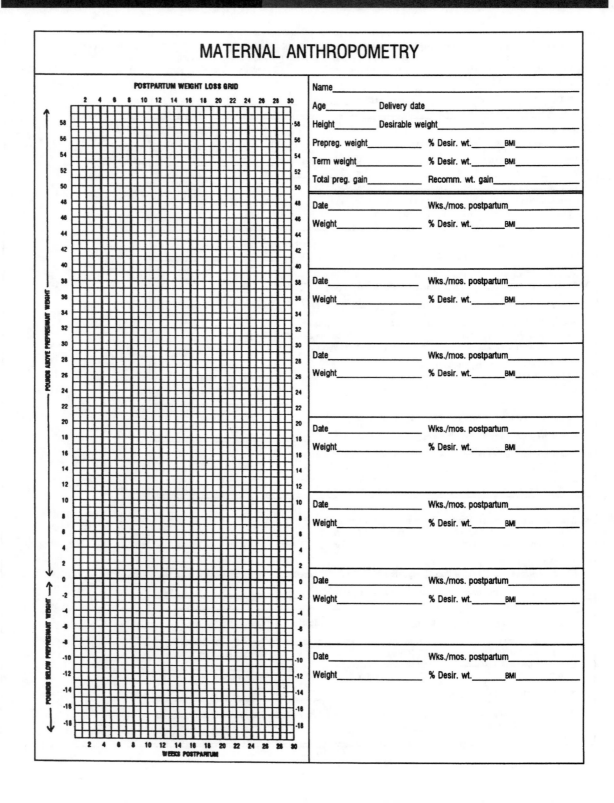

POSTPARTUM WEIGHT LOSS GRID

POUNDS ABOVE PREPREGNANT WEIGHT

POUNDS BELOW PREPREGNANT WEIGHT

WEEKS POSTPARTUM

Name_____

Age_____ Delivery date_____

Height_____ Desirable weight_____

Prepreg. weight_____ % Desir. wt._____BMI_____

Term weight_____ % Desir. wt._____BMI_____

Total preg. gain_____ Recomm. wt. gain_____

Date_____ Wks./mos. postpartum_____

Weight_____ % Desir. wt._____BMI_____

Date_____ Wks./mos. postpartum_____

Weight_____ % Desir. wt._____BMI_____

Date_____ Wks./mos. postpartum_____

Weight_____ % Desir. wt._____BMI_____

Date_____ Wks./mos. postpartum_____

Weight_____ % Desir. wt._____BMI_____

Date_____ Wks./mos. postpartum_____

Weight_____ % Desir. wt._____BMI_____

Date_____ Wks./mos. postpartum_____

Weight_____ % Desir. wt._____BMI_____

Date_____ Wks./mos. postpartum_____

Weight_____ % Desir. wt._____BMI_____

MOTHER'S PHYSICAL EXAM

Postpartum days/weeks	Height	Prepreg. wt.	Term wt.	Current wt.	Temperature	Blood Pressure
General Appearance			Thyroid			

BREASTS	RIGHT			LEFT		
AREOLA						
NIPPLES						
SECRETION						
OTHER						

INFANT'S PHYSICAL EXAM

DATE	AGE	WEIGHT (pounds)	(kg.)	HEIGHT (inches)	(cm.)	H.C. (inches)	(cm.)
	Birth						
Discharge:							
Today:							

GENERAL/BEHAVIOR		Temp.

Head		Heart	
Eyes		Pulses	
Ears		Abdomen	
Nose		Genitalia	
Mouth		Extremities	
Thorax		Neuro	
Lungs		Skin	

A P P E N D I X   J   *(cont.)*

ORAL-MOTOR EXAMINATION/FUNCTION

MOUTH	☐ Normal	☐ Small	☐ Large		
JAW	☐ Normal	☐ Receding	☐ Asymmetrical	☐ Thrusting	☐ Tight/poor opening
LIPS	☐ Normal	☐ Cleft	☐ Passively pulled in	☐ Pursed/tight	
GUMS	☐ Normal	☐ Asymmetrical	☐ Excessive clenching/bite		
TONGUE	☐ Normal resting position ☐ Behind gum line	☐ Flat ☐ Thrust/protruding	☐ Clicking ☐ Sucking	☐ Elevated	☐ Up in back
FRENULUM	☐ Normal	☐ Tight			
PALATE	☐ Normal	☐ High arch	☐ Cleft		

BREASTFEEDING OBSERVATION

Position used: ☐ Cradle   ☐ Side-sitting   ☐ Other:_____

Infant interest:
☐ Hungry, eager; goes easily to breast   ☐ Willing, falls asleep quickly   ☐ Awake, will not attach
☐ Willing but not insistent   ☐ Sleepy, totally disinterested   ☐ Awake, hungry, vigorously refuses
☐ Willing but distractable

Rooting:
☐ Normal   ☐ Depressed/absent   ☐ Tongue back/flat
☐ Frantic, disorganized

Attachment:
☐ Adequate   ☐ Lips retracted   ☐ Refuses
☐ Drops back   ☐ Arches   ☐ Other:_____
☐ Tongue malposition   ☐ Cries   _____

Milk ejection reflex:
☐ Prior to attachment   ☐ After attachment, _____ sec / min   ☐ Not apparent after _____ sec / min
☐ Hyperactive

Effectiveness:
☐ Good suck/rhythm   ☐ Starts/stops repeatedly   ☐ Excessive vertical movement
  suck:swallow _____:_____   ☐ Persistent flutter sucking only   ☐ Clenching/biting
☐ Becomes ineffective   ☐ Disorganized   ☐ Other:_____
☐ Weak suction   ☐ Cheeks dimple during suckling   _____
☐ Attached, not suckling   ☐ Tongue clicking   _____

Swallow: ☐ Normal   ☐ Uncoordinated

Comments:_____

Condition of nipple after nursing: (Right)   (Left)
Color_____ Shape_____   Color_____ Shape_____

Infant stress
Mellow, relaxed — Disturbed slightly, not screaming — Screaming, resists positioning

Maternal stress:
At ease, relaxed — Anxious — Extremely tense

Maternal interaction with infant:
☐ Hovering   ☐ Attentive   ☐ Harsh
☐ Over-stimulating   ☐ Affectionate   ☐ Detached

COMMENTS:

	ASSESSMENT	PLAN
MOTHER		
INFANT		
BREASTFEEDING		

COUNSELING	☐ Attachment ☐ Bras ☐ Burping ☐ Expression/storage ☐ Family adjustment ☐ Feeding frequency, duration	☐ Hand expression ☐ How to tell if baby is getting enough ☐ Hydration ☐ Maternal nutrition ☐ Nipple care	☐ Positioning ☐ Rapid growth period ☐ Waking ☐ Other_____ _____ _____
HANDOUTS	☐ Blocked Duct ☐ Breastfeeding Record ☐ Calcium Rich Foods ☐ Candidiasis ☐ Daily Food Guide	☐ Engorgement ☐ Hand Expression ☐ How Much is Enough ☐ Is Baby Getting Enough ☐ Mastitis	☐ Mechanical Expression ☐ Increasing Milk Supply ☐ Milk Storage ☐ Nipple Trauma ☐ Other_____
Date		**Clinician**	
Letter sent:_____			

APPENDIX K

Conversion Tables

TABLE K–1. CONVERSION OF POUNDS TO KILOGRAMS FOR PEDIATRIC WEIGHTS

Pounds →

	0	1	2	3	4	5	6	7	8	9
0	0.00	0.45	0.90	1.36	1.81	2.26	2.72	3.17	3.62	4.08
10	4.53	4.98	5.44	5.89	6.35	6.80	7.25	7.71	8.16	8.61
20	9.07	9.52	9.97	10.43	10.88	11.34	11.79	12.24	12.70	13.15
30	13.60	14.06	14.51	14.96	15.42	15.87	16.32	16.78	17.23	17.69
40	18.14	18.59	19.05	19.50	19.95	20.41	20.86	21.31	21.77	22.22
50	22.68	23.13	23.58	24.04	24.49	24.94	25.40	25.85	26.30	26.76
60	27.21	27.66	28.12	28.57	29.03	29.48	29.93	30.39	30.84	31.29
70	31.75	32.20	32.65	33.11	33.56	34.02	34.47	34.92	35.38	35.83
80	36.28	36.74	37.19	37.64	38.10	38.55	39.00	39.46	39.91	40.37
90	40.82	41.27	41.73	42.18	42.63	43.09	43.54	43.99	44.45	44.90
100	45.36	45.81	46.26	46.72	47.17	47.62	48.08	48.53	48.98	49.44
110	49.89	50.34	50.80	51.25	51.71	52.16	52.61	53.07	53.52	53.97
120	54.43	54.88	55.33	55.79	56.24	56.70	57.15	57.60	58.06	58.51
130	58.96	59.42	59.87	60.32	60.78	61.23	61.68	62.14	62.59	63.05
140	63.50	63.95	64.41	64.86	65.31	65.77	66.22	66.67	67.13	67.58
150	68.04	68.49	68.94	69.40	69.85	70.30	70.76	71.21	71.66	72.12
160	72.57	73.02	73.48	73.93	74.39	74.84	75.29	75.75	76.20	76.65
170	77.11	77.56	78.01	78.47	78.92	79.38	79.83	80.28	80.74	81.19
180	81.64	82.10	82.55	83.00	83.46	83.91	84.36	84.82	85.27	85.73
190	86.18	86.68	87.09	87.54	87.99	88.45	88.90	89.35	89.81	90.26
200	90.72	91.17	91.62	92.08	92.53	92.98	93.44	93.89	94.34	94.80

TABLE K–2. CONVERSION OF POUNDS AND OUNCES TO KILOGRAMS FOR PEDIATRIC WEIGHTS

Pounds	Kilograms	Ounces	Kilograms	Pounds	Kilograms	Ounces	Kilograms
1	0.454	1	0.028	9	4.082	9	0.255
2	0.907	2	0.057	10	4.536	10	0.283
3	1.361	3	0.085	11	4.990	11	0.312
4	1.814	4	0.113	12	5.443	12	0.340
5	2.268	5	0.142	13	5.897	13	0.369
6	2.722	6	0.170			14	0.397
7	3.175	7	0.198			15	0.425
8	3.629	8	0.227				

APPENDIX L

Standardized Height and Weight Growth Charts

BOYS: BIRTH TO AGE 36 MONTHS—PHYSICAL GROWTH (LENGTH, WEIGHT), NCHS PERCENTILES

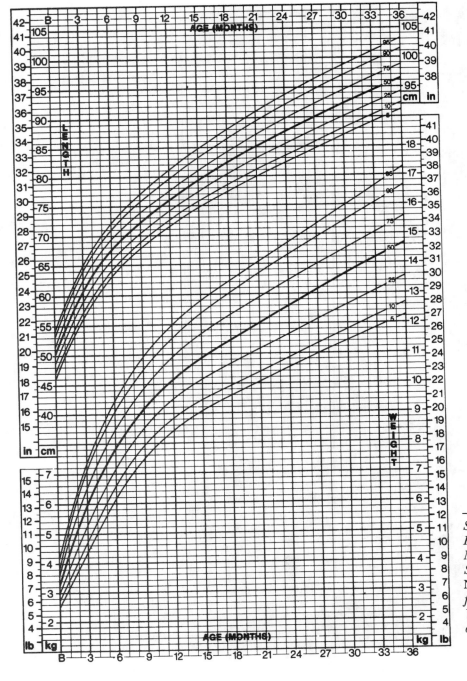

Source: Modified from PVV Hamill et al: Physical growth: National Center for Health Statistics percentiles. Am J Clin Nutr *32: 607–29, 1979. Data from the Fels Research Institute, Wright State University School of Medicine, Yellow Springs, OH.*

APPENDIX L *(cont.)*

Standardized Height and Weight Growth Charts

GIRLS: BIRTH TO AGE 36 MONTHS—PHYSICAL GROWTH (LENGTH, WEIGHT), NCHS PERCENTILES

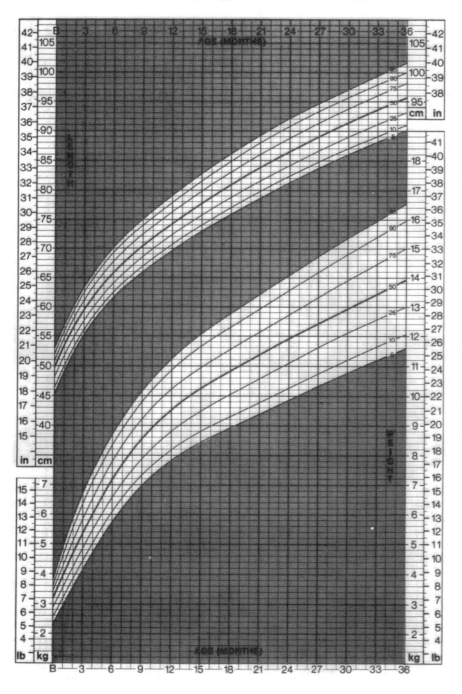

Acinus Smallest division of a gland; a group of secretory cells arrayed around a central cavity. In the breast, an acinus secretes milk. Acini (pl). *See also* alveolus.

Aerobic Requiring air for metabolic processes (e.g., aerobic bacteria). Normal skin, including the breast, is colonized with aerobic bacteria.

Afferent Being conducted toward an organ or gland. Suckling produces afferent impulses which travel from the nipple to the pituitary gland, which then incites oxytocin release, causing milk to let down. The opposite of *efferent*.

Allergen Any substance causing an allergic response. Foods, drugs, or inhalants may be allergens. Cow's milk protein is a common allergen of infants.

Allopathic medicine A form of medical care characterized by a focus on the cure of disease presenting in a given organ or organ system; also called *Western medicine;* nonallopathic medicine is sometimes called *traditional* or *folk medicine* to distinguish it from the allopathic form.

Alphalactalbumin The principal protein found in the whey portion of human milk; it assists the synthesis of lactose. The dominant whey protein in cow's milk and most artificial infant milks, betalactoglobulin, is not found in human milk. *See also* Noncasein protein.

Alveolar ridge The ridge on the hard palate immediately behind the upper gums. Movement of the infant's jaw during nursing compresses the areola between his tongue and alveolar ridge.

Alveolus In the mammary gland, a small sac at the terminus of a lobule in which milk is secreted and stored. Alveoli (pl). Groups of alveoli, organized in lobes, give the mammary gland the appearance of a "bunch of grapes." *See also* Acinus.

Ampulla A normally dilated portion of a duct. Ampullae (pl). Ampullae in the lactiferous ducts underlie the areola near the base of the nipple. *See also* Lactiferous sinuses.

Anorectal abnormalities Anomalies of the rectum, the lower few inches of the large intestine, and the anus, the opening in the skin at the distal end of the rectum. An example is imperforate anus, in which the rectum ends in a blind pouch.

Antibody An immunoglobulin formed in response to an antigen, including bacteria and viruses. Antibodies then recognize and attack those bacteria or viruses, thus helping the body resist infection. Breastmilk contains antibodies to antigens to which either the mother or the infant has been exposed.

Antigen A substance that stimulates antibody production. It may be introduced into the body (as dust, food, or bacteria) or produced within it (as a by-product toxin).

Antigenemia The state of having an antigen of interest in the blood.

Applied research Research that focuses on solving or finding an answer to a clinical or practical problem.

Areola Pigmented skin surrounding the nipple that overlies the ampullae or lactiferous sinuses. In order to suckle effectively, an infant should have his gums placed well back on the areola.

Artificial infant milk Any milk preparation, other than human milk, intended to be the sole nourishment of human infants.

Atopic eczema An inherited allergic tendency to rashes or inflammation of the skin. Exclusively breastfed infants are less likely to manifest this condition, as cow's-milk protein is a common allergen.

Atresia, intestinal Congenital blockage or closure of any part of the intestinal tract.

Axilla The underarm area; in it lies the uppermost extent of the mammary ridge or milk line. Deep breast tissue (the axillary tail or tail of Spence) extends toward and sometimes into the axilla. This tissue may engorge the axilla along with the rest of the breast in the early postpartum period.

B cell A lymphocyte produced in bone marrow and peripheral lymphoid tissue and is found in breastmilk. It attacks antigens and is one type of cell that confers cell-mediated immunity.

Bactericidal Capable of destroying bacteria. Breastmilk contains so many bactericidal cells that the bacteria count of expressed milk actually declines during the first 36 hours following milk expression.

Bacteriostatic Capable of inhibiting the proliferation of bacterial colonies.

BALT/GALT/MALT Bronchus/gut/mammary-associated immunocompetent lymphoid tissue. A lymphocyte pathway that causes IgA antibodies to be produced in the mammary gland after a lactating woman is exposed to an antigen on her intestinal or respiratory mucosa. These antibodies are then transferred through breastmilk to the breastfeeding infant, who thus may possess antibodies to antigens to which he has not been directly exposed.

Banked human milk *See* Donor milk.

Basic research Research that generates knowledge for the sake of knowledge.

Betalactoglobulin The dominant protein present in the whey fraction of the milk of cows and other ruminants; it is absent from human milk.

Bias Any factor, action, or influence that distorts the results of a study.

Bioavailable That portion of an ingested nutrient actually absorbed and used by the body. Because the nutrients in breastmilk are highly bioavailable, low concentrations may actually result in more nutrients being absorbed by the infant than do the higher, less bioavailable concentrations in cow's milk or artificial infant milks.

Bivariate Statistics derived from the analysis of the relationship between two variables.

Buccal pads Fat pads sheathed by the masseter muscles in young infants' cheeks. The buccal pads touch and provide stability for the tongue, which enhances the tongue's ability to compress breast tissue during suckling. Breastfed infants typically have a plump-cheeked appearance because of well-developed buccal pads.

Candidiasis A fungal infection caused by *Candida albicans;* also called "thrush." Common in the maternal vagina, it may inoculate the infant during delivery and be transferred from the infant's mouth to the mother's nipple. Candidiasis of the nipple and breast may produce intense nipple and breast pain. In the infant, it may produce white spots on the oral mucosa and a bright red, painful rash ringing the anus. Formerly termed moniliasis.

Casein The principal protein in milks of all mammals. Human milk has a ratio of soluble whey proteins to casein of about 65:35. Casein of human milk forms soft, easily digested curds in the infant stomach. The whey-to-casein ratio in cow's milk is 20:80; artificial infant milks have whey-to-casein ratios that vary from those of cow's milk to 40:60. Cow's-milk casein forms firm curds that require a high expenditure of energy to digest.

Centers for Disease Control (CDC) An agency of the U.S. Public Health Service established in 1973 to protect the public health of the nation by providing leadership and direction in the prevention and control of diseases and other preventable health conditions, and to respond to public health emergencies.

Certification The process by which a nongovernmental professional association attests that an individual has met certain standards specified by the association for the practice of that profession.

Chi-square A statistical procedure that uses nominal level data and determines significant differences between observed frequencies in relation to the data and expected frequencies.

Colostrum The fluid in the breast at the end of pregnancy and in the early postpartum period. It is thicker and yellower than mature milk, reflecting a higher content of proteins, many of which are immunoglobulins. It is also higher in fat-soluble vitamins (including A, E, and K) and some minerals (including sodium and zinc).

Concept A word, idea, or phenomenon that generally has abstract meaning.

Conceptual framework A structure of interrelated concepts that may be generated inductively by qualitative research or provide a base for a quantitative study.

Congenital infection An infection existing at birth that was acquired transplacentally. Infections that may be so acquired include HIV and TORCH organisms. *See also* Human immunodeficiency virus; TORCH.

Conjunctivitis Inflammation of the mucous membrane that lines the eyelid. In many traditional and some modern societies, fresh breastmilk is instilled into the eyes to alleviate this condition.

Construct A cluster of several concepts that has abstract meaning.

Contraception Preventing conception. Breastfeeding provides significant contraceptive protection during the first few months postpartum–as long as the infant is fully breastfed and feeds during the night, and maternal menses have not resumed.

Cooper's ligaments Triangular, vertical ligaments in the breast that attach deeper layers of subcutaneous tissue to the skin.

Cord blood Blood remaining in the umbilical cord after birth.

Correlation coefficient A statistic that indicates the degree of relationship between two variables. The range in value is +1.00 to –1.00; 0.0 indicates no relationship, +1.00 is a perfect positive relationship, and –1.00 is a perfect inverse relationship.

Creamatocrit The proportion of cream in a milk sample, determined by measuring the depth of the cream layer in a centrifuged sample. An indicator of caloric content of milk, which must be used with care; the fat (and thus caloric) content of human milk varies between breasts, within a feeding, diurnally, and over the entire course of lactation.

Cross-nursing Occasional wet-nursing on an informal, short-term basis, usually in the context of child care.

Cultural relativism Recognition of the wide variation in beliefs and actions that pertain to given behaviors in different cultures.

Culture The values, beliefs, norms, and related practices of a given group that are learned and shared by the group members and that guide both the thoughts and behaviors of that group.

Cytoprotective Any condition or factor that protects cells from inflammation or death.

Deductive reasoning The process of reasoning from a general premise to the concrete and specific.

Dependent variable The variable the investigator measures in response to the independent or treatment variable; the outcome variable that is affected by the independent variable.

Design The blueprint or plan for conducting a study.

Diagnostic-related grouping (DRG) A group of diagnoses for health conditions that result in similar intensity of hospital care and similar length of hospital stay for patients hospitalized with those conditions.

Diffusion The process by which the molecules of one substance (e.g., a drug) are spread uniformly throughout a given substance (e.g., blood or plasma). *Passive diffusion* refers to movement from a higher to a lower concentration; *active diffusion* refers to movement from a lower to a higher concentration.

Disaccharide A carbohydrate composed of two monosaccharides. The principal sugar in human milk is lactose, a disaccharide; its constituent monosaccharides are glucose and galactose.

Donor milk Human milk voluntarily contributed to a human milk bank by women unrelated to the recipient.

Donor milk, fresh-frozen Fresh-raw milk that has been stored frozen at –20°C for less than 12 months.

Donor milk, fresh-raw Milk stored continuously at 4°C for not longer than 72 hours after collection.

Donor milk, heat-treated Fresh-raw milk or fresh-frozen milk that has been heated to a minimum of 56°C for 30 minutes.

Donor milk, pooled A batch of milk containing milk from more than one donor.

Dopamine The prolactin-inhibiting factor (PIF), or a mediator of PIF, secreted in the hypothalamus. It blocks the release of prolactin into the bloodstream.

Drip milk Milk that leaks from a breast that is not being directly stimulated. Because its fat content is low, this milk should not be used regularly for infant feedings.

Ductules Small ducts in the mammary gland that drain milk from the alveoli into larger lactiferous ducts that terminate in the nipple.

Dyad A pair (e.g., the breastfeeding mother and her infant).

Eczema Skin inflammation or rash. *See also* Atopic eczema.

Elemental formula Artificial infant milks containing fats, proteins, and carbohydrates in their simplest (most elemental) forms.

Eminences of the pars villosa Tiny swellings on the inner surfaces of infant's lips that help the infant to retain a grasp on the breast during suckling.

Energy density The number of calories per unit volume; caloric density. Mature human milk averages 65 calories/dl, controlled largely by the fat content of the milk.

Envelope virus A virus that cannot infect other cells without its coat (envelope). If the envelope is destroyed (e.g., by heat or soap and water), the ability of the virus to produce infection is destroyed. Cytomegalovirus and the human immunodeficiency virus are envelope viruses.

Epidemiology The study of the frequency and distribution of disease and the factors causing that frequency and distribution.

Epiglottis Cartilaginous structure of the larynx. An infant's epiglottis lies just below the soft palate. It closes the larynx when the infant swallows, ensuring passage of milk to the esophagus.

Estrogen A hormone that causes growth of mammary tissue during part of each menstrual cycle and assists in the secretion of prolactin during pregnancy; one of the hormones whose concentration falls sharply at parturition.

Ethnocentrism A view that one's own culture and how it defines appropriate behavior is used as the basis for assessing all other cultures and behaviors.

Ethnography One research method that attempts to support an understanding of the beliefs, practices, and behavioral patterns within a (sub)culture from the perspective of the people living in that culture.

Exogenous Derived from outside the body—e.g., iron supplements that provide the infant with exogenous iron.

External validity The extent to which study findings can be generalized to samples different from those studied.

Extraneous variable Variables that can affect the relationship of the independent and dependent variables, i.e., interfere with the effect of treatment. In experimental studies, strategies for controlling these variables are built into the research design.

Foremilk The milk obtained at the beginning of a breastfeeding. Its higher water content keeps the infant hydrated and supplies water-soluble vitamins and proteins. Its fat content (1–2 gm/dl) is lower than that of hindmilk.

Frenulum Fold of mucous membrane, midline on the underside of the tongue, that helps to anchor the tongue to the floor of the mouth. A short or inelastic frenulum, or one attached close to the tip of the tongue, may restrict tongue extension enough to inhibit effective breastfeeding. Called also the frenum.

Fructose A carbohydrate present in small quantities in human milk.

Galactagogue Any food or group of foods thought to possess qualities that increase the volume or quality of milk produced by the lactating woman who eats such foods.

Galactopoiesis The maintenance of established milk synthesis that is controlled by the autocrine system of supply and demand.

Galactorrhea Abnormal production of milk. It may occur under psychological influences or be a sign of pituitary tumor.

Galactose A monosaccharide present in small quantities in human milk. It is derived from lactose and, in turn, helps to produce elements essential for the development of the human central nervous system.

Gastroenteritis Inflammation of the stomach and intestines resulting from bacterial or viral invasion. Breastfed infants are at lower risk for this illness, as compared to nonbreastfed infants.

Gastroschisis An opening in the wall of the abdomen; a congenital malformation.

Gestational age An infant's age since conception, usually specified in weeks. Counted from the first day of the last normal menstrual period.

Half-life The length of time for half of a drug dosage to be eliminated; generally, it takes four to five half-lives for a drug to be considered completely or nearly completely eliminated. *Example:* Half-life of drug A is 12 hours, so 50 percent of the original drug dosage is eliminated in 12 hours; 25 percent of the drug is remaining after 24 hours; 12.5 percent of the original dosage is remaining after 36 hours; 6.25 percent of the original dosage is present after 48 hours, and only 3.12 percent is present after 60 hours (five half-lives from time of original dosage).

Hindmilk Milk released near the end of a breastfeeding, after active let-down of milk. Fat content of hindmilk may rise to 6 percent or more, two or three times the concentration in foremilk.

Horizontal transmission Transmission of pathogens through direct contact. *See also* Vertical transmission.

Human immunodeficiency virus (HIV) A retrovirus that disarms the body's immune system, causing death from an opportunistic infection. First identified in 1981. The virus may be transmitted to unborn infants, and it is carried in the breastmilk, although not all breastfed infants born to HIV-positive mothers become ill themselves. The greatest risk to the infant is posed when a woman experiences her initial HIV-related illness while pregnant or breastfeeding.

Human milk Milk secreted in the human breast.

Human milk bank A service that collects, screens, processes, stores, and distributes donated human milk to meet the needs of those, usually infants, for whom human milk has been prescribed by a physician.

Human milk fortifiers Nutrients added to expressed human milk to enhance the growth and nutrient balances of very low-birth-weight infants. Added protein may be derived from protein components of donor human milk or from cow's-milk-based products. *See also* Lactoengineering.

Hydration The water balance within a body. Adequate hydration is necessary to maintain normal body temperature and for most other metabolic functions. Breastmilk is 90 percent water. Therefore, even in hot or dry climates, a fully breastfed infant obtains all the water he requires through breastmilk.

Hyperalimentation The intravenous feeding of an infant, commonly a very premature infant, with a solution of amino acids, glucose, electrolytes, and vitamins.

Hyperosmolar A fluid that is of higher osmotic pressure than the reference fluid. Elemental formulas are hyperosmolar; breastmilk is isoosmolar with human serum.

Hyperprolactinemia Higher-than-normal prolactin levels, which may result in spontaneous breastmilk production and amenorrhea. Causes include pituitary tumors and some pharmaceuticals. *See also* Prolactin.

Hypothalamus A gland that controls postpartum serum prolactin levels through release of dopamine. Inhibition of dopamine permits the release of prolactin, which controls the secretion of milk.

Immunity, active Immunity conferred by the production of antibodies by one's own immune system.

Immunity, passive Immunity conferred on an infant by antibodies manufactured by the mother and passed to the infant transplacentally or in breastmilk. Passive immunity is temporary but very important to the young infant.

Immunoassay Any method for the quantitative determination of chemical substances that uses the highly specific binding between antigen or hapten and homologous antibodies (e.g., radioimmunoassay, enzyme immunoassay, and fluoroimmunoassay).

Immunogen A substance that stimulates the body to form antibodies. *See also* Antigen.

Immunoglobulin Proteins produced by plasma cells in response to an immunogen. The five types are IgG, IgA, IgM, IgE, and IgD. IgG is transferred in utero and provides passive immunity to infections to which the mother is immune; IgA is the principal immunoglobulin in colostrum and mature milk; IgM is produced by the neonate soon after birth and is also contained in breastmilk. *See also* Noncasein protein.

Incidence How much a particular behavior is practiced at a given time. *Example:* How many women are initiating breastfeeding from time A to time B?

Incubation period The period between exposure to infectious pathogens and the first signs of illness.

Independent variable The experimental or treatment variable that is manipulated by the investigator to influence the dependent variable.

Inductive reasoning The process of reasoning from specific observations or abstractions to a general premise.

Infection control Practices—in hospitals formalized by protocols—that reduce the chance that infection will be spread between patients or between patients and staff. Hand washing and wearing of rubber gloves are two such practices.

Internal validity The extent to which manipulation of the independent variable really makes a significant difference on the dependent variable rather than on extraneous variables.

International Code of Marketing of Breast-Milk Substitutes A set of resolutions that regulate the marketing and distribution of any fluid intended to replace breastmilk, certain devices used to feed such fluids, and the role of health care workers who advise on infant feeding. Developed by members of a joint commission convened in 1979 by WHO and UNICEF, it was approved in 1981 by members of the WHO (only the United States dissented). Intended as a voluntary model that could be incorporated into the legal code of individual nations in order to enhance national efforts to promote breastfeeding. Also referred to as the *WHO Code* or the *WHO/UNICEF Code.*

Intracellular Occurring within cells. Viruses live within other cells during part of their reproductive lives. Although virus within cells may be passed to the infant in breastmilk, other cells in breastmilk enhance the destruction of these infected cells.

Intrauterine Within the uterus; in utero.

Intrauterine growth rate The normal rate of weight gain of a fetus. It is considered by many, but not all, physicians to be the ideal growth rate for premature infants.

Involution Refers to the return of the mammary gland to a nonproductive state of milk secretion.

Lactase Enzyme needed to convert lactose to simple sugars usable by the infant. Present from birth in the intestinal mucosa, its activity diminishes after weaning.

Lactase deficiency *See* Lactose intolerance.

Lactiferous ducts Milk ducts; 15 to 24 tubes that collect milk from the smaller ductules and carry it to the nipple. They appear similar to stems on a bunch of grapes, the alveoli being the "grapes." The ducts open into nipple pores.

Lactiferous sinuses Dilations in the lactiferous ducts under the areola that act as small milk reservoirs. To nurse effectively, an infant must take enough breast into his mouth to be able to strip milk from these sinuses.

Lactobacillus bifidus Principal bacillus in the intestinal flora of breastfed infants. Low intestinal pH (5–6) of fully breastfed infants discourages the colonization of *Streptococcus faecalis, Bacteroides sp.* and *E. coli,* which are common in feces of infants fed cow's-milk-based infant milks.

Lactoengineering The process of fortifying human milk with nutrients (especially protein, calcium, and phosphorus) derived from other batches of human milk, in order to meet the special nutritional needs of very low-birth-weight infants. *See also* Human milk fortifiers.

Lactoferrin A protein that is an important immunological component of human milk. It binds iron in the intestinal tract, thus denying it to bacteria that require iron to survive. Exogenous iron may upset this balance. *See also* Noncasein protein.

Lactogenesis The initiation of milk secretion. The initial synthesis of milk components that begins late in pregnancy may be termed *lactogenesis I;* the onset of copious milk production two or three days postpartum may be termed *lactogenesis II.*

Lactose The principal carbohydrate in human milk; about 4 percent of colostrum and 7 percent of mature milk. A disaccharide, it metabolizes readily to glucose, which is used for energy, and galactose, which assists lipids that are laid down in the brain. Lactose also enhances calcium absorption, thus helping prevent rickets in the breastfed infant, and it inhibits the growth of pathogens in the breastfed infant's intestine.

Lactose intolerance The manifestation of lactase deficiency; the inability of the intestines to digest lactose, the principal carbohydrate in human milk. More common beyond early childhood because of diminished activity of intestinal lactase, especially in cultures that do not use milk or milk products as foods after early childhood.

Larynx The region at the upper end of the trachea (windpipe) through which the voice is produced. In the infant, the larynx lies close to the base of the tongue; during swallowing, it rises and is closed off by the epiglottis.

Lesion Circumscribed area of injured or diseased skin.

Let-down The milk-ejection reflex. Caused by contraction of myoepithelial cells surrounding the alveoli in which milk is secreted. It is under the control of oxytocin released during nipple stimulation and, sometimes, of psychological influences.

Leukocytes Living cells, including macrophages and lymphocytes, that inhabit breastmilk and combat infection.

Licensure The process by which an agency of state government grants permission to an individual, who is accountable for the practice of a profession, to engage in that profession. The corollary of licensure is that unlicensed individuals are prohibited from legally practicing licensed professions. The purpose of licensure is to protect the public by ensuring professional competence.

Ligand A small molecule that binds specifically to a larger molecule (e.g., the binding of an antigen to an antibody, or of a hormone to a receptor).

Likert scale A scale that primarily measures attitudes by asking respondents their degree of agreement or disagreement for a number of statements.

Lipase Enzyme that aids in the digestion of milk fats by reducing them to a fine emulsion.

Low-birth-weight Term applied to infants weighing less than 2,500 gm at birth.

Lymphadenopathy Abnormal swelling of lymph nodes.

Lymphocyte A mature leukocyte; a lymph cell that is bactericidal.

Lyophilization A process of rapid freeze-drying of a fluid under a high vacuum. This process is used on human milk to obtain nutrient fractions used to fortify expressed human milk.

Lysozyme Enzyme in breastmilk that is active against *Escherichia coli* and *Salmonella. See also* Noncasein protein.

Mammary bud A clump of embryonic epithelial cells formed along the mammary ridge that extend into the underlying mesenchyme. It develops about 49 days postconception. From this bud sprout the precursors of the milk ducts.

Mammary ridge Milk line; the linear thickening of epithelial cells to each side of the midline of the embryo. Develops during weeks 5 through 8. Later this ridge differentiates into breast and nipple tissue.

Mammogenesis The development of the mammary gland and related structures within the breast.

Mandible The lower jaw. Strong, rhythmic closing of the mandible during breastfeeding drives the compression of the lacteriferous sinuses, one component of the infant's milking process.

Mature milk Breastmilk commonly produced after about two weeks postpartum and containing no admixture of colostrum. It is higher in lactose, fat, and water-soluble vitamins. Its exact composition varies in response to infant needs.

Median The middle number in a series of numbers; the number on either side of which exist an equal amount of numbers.

Mesenchyme The embryonic mesoderm.

Milk-plasma ratio The quantity of a given drug or its metabolite in human milk in relation to its quantity in the maternal plasma or blood. Generally, if the M/P ratio exceeds 1.00, the drug is found in lesser quantities in milk than in plasma. If the M/P ratio is less than 1.00, the drug is found in lower quantities in milk than in plasma.

Mitosis A type of cell division in which each daughter cell contains the same DNA as the parent cell.

Morbidity   The number of ill persons or instances of a disease in a specific population.

Mortality   The number of deaths in a specific population.

Mucocutaneous   Involving both mucous membranes and skin. Herpes blisters, for example, can form on both sites.

Multiparous   Having carried two or more pregnancies to viability.

Myelination   The process by which conducting nerve fibers develop a protective fatty sheath. The long-chain polyunsaturated fats that are important to myelination are abundant in human milk; they are much less abundant in cow's milk or cow's-milk-based infant milks. Loss of myelin is a characteristic of the disease multiple sclerosis.

Myoepithelial cells   Contractile cells. In the breast, these cells surround the milk-secreting alveoli; their contraction forces milk into the milk ducts. When many of these cells contract at the same time, a let-down occurs. *See also* Let-down.

Necrotizing enterocolitis   Inflammation of the intestinal tract that may cause tissue to die. Premature infants not receiving human milk are at markedly greater risk for this serious complication of premature birth.

Neurotransmitter   A chemical that is selectively released from a nerve terminal by an action potential and then interacts with a specific receptor on an adjacent structure to produce a specific physiologic response.

Nipple   Cylindrical pigmented protuberance on the breast into which the lactiferous ducts open. The human nipple contains 15 to 20 nipple pores through which milk flows. The mammary papilla.

Nipple, inverted   A nipple that is retracted into the breast both when at rest and when stimulated.

Noncasein protein   The protein in the whey portion of milk. Noncasein proteins in human milk include alphalactalbumin, serum albumin, lactoferrin, immunoglobulins, and lysozyme.

Nongovernmental organization (NGO)   Title conferred by UNICEF on private organizations that command expertise valuable to UNICEF; such organizations are permitted to comment on and

attempt to influence UNICEF activities. La Leche League International and the International Lactation Consultant Association are NGOs.

Nonparametric statistics   Statistical procedures used when required assumptions for using parametric procedures are not met.

Nonprotein nitrogen (NPN)   About one-fourth of the total nitrogen in human milk is derived from sources, such as urea, other than protein. NPN contains several free amino acids, including leucine, valine, and threonine, which are essential in the young infant's diet because he cannot yet manufacture them.

Nutriment   Any nourishing substance.

Oligosaccharide   Carbohydrate, comprised of a few monosaccharides, present in human milk. Some oligosaccharides promote the growth of *Lactobacillus bifidus,* thus increasing intestinal acidity, which discourages the growth of intestinal pathogens.

Operational definition   Explicit description of a concept or variable of interest in measurable terms.

Oral rehydration therapy (ORT)   The administration by mouth of a solution of water, salt, and sugar in order to replace body fluids lost during severe diarrhea. The proportions of elements in an oral rehydration solution are essentially the same as they are in breastmilk. Artificially fed infants are much more susceptible than those who are breast-fed to the diarrhea that may lead to severe dehydration and the need for ORT.

Oxytocin   A lactogenic hormone produced in the posterior pituitary gland. It is released during suckling (or other nipple stimulation) and causes ejection of milk as well as uterine contractions.

Palate, hard   The hard, anterior roof of the mouth. A suckling infant uses his tongue to compress breast tissue against the hard palate.

Palate, soft   The soft, posterior roof of the mouth, which lies between the hard palate and the throat. It rises during swallowing to close off nasal passages. Also called the velum.

Parametric statistics   Statistical procedures used when a sample is randomly selected, represents a normal distribution of the target population, and is considered sufficiently large in size and interval level data are collected.

Parenchyma The functional parts of an organ. In the breast, the parenchyma include the mammary ducts, lobes, and alveoli.

Parenteral Introduction of fluids, nutrients, or drugs into the body by any avenue other than the digestive tract.

Pasteurization The heating of milk to destroy pathogens. Milk banks commonly heat donor milk to 56° for 30 minutes.

Pathogen Substance or organism capable of producing illness.

Peristalsis Involuntary, rhythmic, wavelike action. Commonly thought of in relation to food and waste products moving along the gastrointestinal tract. In order to strip milk from the breast, an infant's tongue uses a peristaltic motion that begins at the tip of the tongue and progresses toward the back of the mouth.

Pharynx The muscular tube at the rear of the mouth, through which nasal air travels to the larynx and food from the mouth travels to the esophagus. During infant feeding, contraction of pharyngeal muscles moves a bolus of fluid into the esophagus.

Pituitary An endocrine gland at the base of the brain that secretes several hormones. Prolactin, which is essential for production of milk, is secreted by the anterior lobe; oxytocin, which is essential for milk let-down, is secreted by the posterior lobe.

Placenta The intrauterine organ that transfers nutrients from the mother to the fetus. The expulsion of the placenta at birth causes an abrupt drop in estrogen and progesterone, which in turn permits the secretion of milk.

Polymastia The presence of more than two breasts. These additional structures, which usually contain only a small amount of glandular tissue, may occur anywhere along the milk line from axilla to groin.

Population The total set of individuals that meet the study criteria from which the sample is drawn and about whom findings can be generalized.

Power The probability that a statistical test will reject a null hypothesis when it should be rejected, or in other words, detect a significant difference that does exist.

Premature infant One born before 37 weeks' gestational age, regardless of birth weight.

Prevalence How much a given behavior is occurring at a given time as well as how long that behavior is practiced. *Example:* the combined effect of breastfeeding initiation rates and breastfeeding continuance and duration rates.

Primary infection The first incidence of illness after exposure to a pathogen.

Primiparous Having carried one pregnancy to viability.

Progesterone Hormone produced by the corpus luteum and placenta that maintains a pregnancy and helps develop the mammary alveoli.

Prolactin Hormone that is produced in the anterior pituitary gland. It stimulates development of the breast and controls milk synthesis. Normal concentrations are 10–25 ng/ml in a nonpregnant woman; 200–400 ng/ml at birth.

Prone Lying on one's stomach.

Reliability The degree to which collected data are accurate, consistent, precise, and stable over time.

Respiratory syncytial virus (RSV) Organism causing a respiratory illness; breastfed infants are at less risk for this illness than are nonbreastfed infants.

Rickets Abnormal calcification of the bones and changes in growth plates that lead to soft or weak bones. Rarely seen in breastfed children; exceptions include those not exposed to the sun.

Rotavirus A class of viruses that are a major cause of diarrheal illness leading to hospitalization of infants. Breastfed infants are at less risk for illness caused by this organism, as compared to breastfed infants.

Rugae Corrugations on the hard palate behind the gum ridge that help the infant to retain a grasp on the breast during suckling.

Sample A subset of the population selected for study.

Sampling The procedure of selecting the sample from the population of interest.

Sebaceous glands Glands that secrete oil. Those on the areola are called the *tubercles of Montgomery;* the oil they secrete is presumed to lubricate and provide bacteriostatic protection to the areola.

Secretory IgA An immunoglobulin abundant in human milk that is of immense value to the neonate. It is synthesized and stored in the breast; after ingestion by the infant, it blocks adhesion of pathogens to the intestinal mucosa.

Secretory immune system The system that produces specific antibodies or thymus-influenced lymphocytes in response to specific antigens.

Sepsis The presence of bacteria in fluid or tissue.

Seroconvert A process by which serum comes to show the presence of a factor that previously has been absent, or vice versa. When antibodies to an infecting agent, such as cytomegalovirus, become present the person is said to have seroconverted.

Serological tests Tests performed on blood samples to ascertain the presence or absence of pathogens.

Seronegative Serum that does not demonstrate the presence of a factor for which tests were conducted; "tests negative."

Seropositive Serum that demonstrates the presence of a factor for which tests were conducted; "test positive."

Serum Clear fluid portion of blood that remains after coagulation.

Serum albumin A protein in serum. *See also* Noncasein protein.

Smooth muscle The type of muscle that provides the erectile tissue in the nipple and areola.

Somatic Pertaining to the body, especially nonreproductive tissue.

Spontaneous lactation Secretion and release of milk unrelated to a pregnancy or to nipple stimulation intended to stimulate milk production.

Suck, Suckle Used in this textbook interchangeably to mean the baby's milking action at the breast. In traditional usage, a baby at the breast "sucked," whereas a mother "suckled."

Sucking, nonnutritive Sucking not at the breast (e.g., as on a pacifier or on baby's own tongue); or sucking at the breast characterized by alternating brief sucks and long rest periods during minimal milk flow. However, insofar as any milk is transferred, even this latter pattern of sucking may, in fact, be nutritive. *See also* Sucking, nutritive.

Sucking, nutritive Steady rhythmic sucking during full, continuous milk flow. Insofar as any milk is transferred, other sucking patterns also may be nutritive. *See also* Sucking, nonnutritive.

Supine Lying on one's back.

Symbiosis The intimate association of two different kinds of organisms. The breastfeeding dyad is considered by many to exemplify a mutually beneficial symbiosis.

Systemic immune system The nonspecific immune responses of the body.

T cells Any of several kinds of thymic lymphoid cells or lymphocytes that help to regulate cellular immune response. A subset of these cells (T_4 cells) are preferentially attacked by the human immunodeficiency virus.

Target population The population that is of interest to the investigator and about which generalizations of study results are intended.

Teleological Describing the belief that all events are directed toward some ultimate purpose.

Thrombocytopenia Low levels of platelets in blood.

TORCH Acronym for organisms that can damage the fetus: toxoplasmosis, rubella, cytomegalovirus, herpes simplex.

Tracheoesophageal fistula (T-E fistula) An abnormal opening between the trachea and esophagus; this congenital malformation occurs in about 1 in 3,000 births. T-E fistula may cause a neonate to aspirate fluids. Colostrum, a physiologic fluid, is much less irritating to the lungs than water, glucose water, or artificial infant milks.

Transcutaneous bilimeter A device that estimates bilirubin concentrations in the blood by measuring intensity of yellowish skin coloration.

Transitional milk Breast fluid of continuously varying composition produced in the first two to three weeks postpartum as colostrum decreases and milk production increases.

Transplacental Transferred from mother to fetus through the placenta. Nutrients and certain immunoglobulins are, and some infections may also be, transferred to the fetus transplacentally.

United Nations Children's Fund (UNICEF) Originally established in 1946 as the United Nations International Children's Emergency Fund. An agency of the United Nations charged with protecting the lives of children and enabling children to lead fuller lives. It assists member nations in providing health care, safe water, sanitation, nutrition, housing, education, and training to accomplish these goals.

Univariate Statistics derived from analysis of a single variable, e.g., frequencies.

Universal precautions Guidelines for infection control based on the assumption that every person receiving health care carries an infection that can be transmitted by blood, body fluids, or genital secretions.

Vaccine An infectious agent, or derivatives of one, given to a person so that his or her immune system will produce antibodies to that infection without a preceding illness.

Validity The degree to which collected data are true and represent reality; the extent to which a measuring instrument reflects what it is intended to measure.

Variable Attributes, properties, and/or characteristics of persons, events, or objects that are examined in a study.

Vertical transmission Transmission of infection from mother to child transplacentally or through breastmilk.

Very low-birth-weight Term applied to infants weighing less than 1,500 gm at birth.

Virus Very small organisms that rely on material in invaded cells to reproduce. Viruses identified in breastmilk include cytomegalovirus, *herpes zoster, herpes simplex,* hepatitis, and rubella.

Water-soluble vitamins The B vitamins and vitamin C, pantothenic acid, biotin, and folate. These vitamins are present in serum; concentrations in breastmilk approximate those in serum. Concentrations reflect current maternal diet more directly than do fat-soluble vitamins (A, D, E, K).

Wet nurses Women who, for pay, breastfeed infants who are not their own.

Whey The liquid left after curds are separated from milk. Alphalactalbumin and lactoferrin are the principal whey proteins. Because human milk has a whey-to-casein ratio of about 65:35, it forms soft, easily digested curds in the infant stomach. *See also* Casein, Noncasein protein.

Witch's milk Colostrum, formed under the influence of maternal hormones, which may be expressed from temporarily enlarged mammary tissue in the neonate's breasts.

World Health Organization (WHO) An agency of the United Nations charged with planning and coordinating global health care and assisting member nations to combat disease and train health care workers.

Xerophthalmia Disease of the eyes caused by vitamin A deficiency; endemic in parts of Africa. Human milk is a preventive.

Abscess, breast, 486–487
  clinical implications of, 504–507
Abrupt weaning, 179–180
Abusive families, 68–69, 71
Accessory nipple, 97
Acebutolol, 174
Acetaminophen, 170, 178, 194, 640
Acquired immune deficiency syndrome, 222. *See also* HIV
Active diffusion, 166
Active immunity, and breastfeeding, 138
Acute infections, 550–551
Acyclovir, 229
A&D Ointment, 322, 490
Adenitis, 487
Adolescent family functioning, 61–62
Adolescents, and breastfeeding, 263–264
Adoption, induced lactation and, 555–557
Adult
  education, 242–243
  family functioning, 62
  learning principles, 242–244
Advertising
  for artificial milk, 9–10, 19
  and breastfeeding promotion, 76, 81
  formula marketing, 11, 19, 225–226
  International Code for Marketing Breastmilk Substitutes, 19
  LC services, 726, 735, 741
Advocacy
  and breastfeeding promotion, 73, 76–81
  deliberative approach, 76, 78
Affiliation, in families, 55
Agricultural revolution and hand-fed foods, 6–7
AIDS, 222. *See also* HIV
Alcohol, effect of, 167, 181, 194
Allegra, 173
Allergies
  to bovine milk, 147–148
  and donor milk, 780
  protection against, 147–149, 655–658
  to solid foods, 628
Allopathic medicine, 30
Alprazolam, 566, 568
Alternate Breast Massage, 315
Alternatives to breastfeeding
  hand-feeding, 6–8
  wet-nursing, 5–6, 7, 37–38, 775–776
Alveoli, 94
Ameda/Egnell breast pumps, 400, 404, 411, 412, 415, 417–418, 421, 422, 425
Ameliorating properties of breastmilk, 136–137
Amenorrhea
  consecutive pregnancies and, 681, 683
  infertility and, 677–678, 684
  ovulation during, 678
  supplemental feeding and, 680–681
American Academy of Pediatrics statement on transfer of drugs to breastmilk, 190–207
Amitriptyline, 172, 193, 568
Amoxicillin, 195, 642

Amphetamines, 181
Ampicillin, 178
Ampullae, 95
Amylase, 145
Anafranil, 172
Analgesics, 170, 178
Anderson Behavioral State Scale, 606, 608
Anesthetics, 170, 287, 292
Ankyloglossia, 357–358
Animal milks, 6, 128, 131, 132, 133, 142, 143, 145, 146, 147, 183, 324, 655, 656
Antiallergenic properties of breastmilk, 147–149, 655–658
Antianxiety drugs, 566, 568
Antiasthmatic medications, 569
Antibacterial factors in breastmilk, 139–143
Antibiotics, 173, 178
  and breastfeeding, 551
  and development of candidiasis, 488
  for mastitis, 487
Antibodies in breastmilk, 139, 231
Anticholinergic effects in nurslings, 172
Anticoagulants, 170
Anticonvulsants, 170, 562
Antidepressants, 178, 193, 568
  effect on breastmilk, 172–173
  for postpartum depression, 566, 568
Antiepileptic drugs, 171, 178
Antifungal drugs
  interaction with Seldane, 490
  for treatment of candidiasis, 173, 174, 489, 490, 491
Antihistamines, 173, 178, 293–294, 358
Antihypertensives, 174
Antiinfective properties of breastmilk, 133–137
Antiinflammatory properties of breastmilk, 142–143
Antimicrobials, 173
Antiparasite factors in breastmilk, 145
Anti-retroviral therapy, 221
Antiviral factors in breastmilk, 144
Aprazolam, 568
Arta Plast breast pump, 400
Asian cultural beliefs and practices, 14, 35–36
Aspirin, 170, 178, 194
Assertiveness, 719, 721–723
Assessment
  breast, 104–106
  breastfeeding, 113, 150, 298–300, 318, 334, 356, 763–764
  child growth and development, 619
  cultural, 32–34, 45
  infant growth, 342, 349, 359, 368–373
  infant temperament, 617–618
  maternal diet, 522–524, 526
  nipple, 320–321
  lactation history and risk factors, 334–335
  suckling, 113–115, 355, 356, 357
Astemizole, 173
Asthma and lactation, 569
Atenolol, 174
At-home vs. employed mothers, 587–588
Atopic eczema, 148–149, 488

At-risk populations and breastfeeding education, 262–264
Attachment
   clinical implications of, 619
   father-infant, 58–59, 68
   mother-infant, 611–613, 615–616, 617, 687
Attending communication skills, 257
Audiovisual aids in breastfeeding education, 258–260
Autocrine control of lactation, 102
Autoimmune diseases
   multiple sclerosis, 558
   rheumatoid arthritis, 558–559
   systemic lupus erythematosus, 557–558
Autoimmunization, 15
Automatic electric breast pumps, 403, 407–408, 410–411,
   414–15
Avent breast pump, 401, 404, 412, 421
Axi-Care Nursing Supplementer, 433
Axillary enlargement technique, 494
Axillary tail, 95
AZT and risk of HIV transmission, 221, 223, 226, 227

Baby care guidelines for physically impaired mothers,
   561–562
Baby food. *See* Solid food
Baby-Friendly Hospital Initiative (BFHI), 20, 21, 77–79, 80, 778
Baby Weigh Scale, The, 764
Bacteremia and breastmilk, 409
Bag Balm, 322
BALT (bronchus–associated lymphoid tissue), 139
Barum breast pump, 401, 404, 412
Basal Infertile Pattern (BIP), 697
Battery-operated breast pumps, 402, 406, 413–414
B cells, 138
Behavioral objectives and breastfeeding education, 269
Bellagio consensus, 683–685
Belly band, 33, 40
Benadryl, 173, 294
Best Start program, 82–83
Beta-agonists, 569
Beta-blockers, 174
Betapace, 174
Bicycle-horn breast pumps, 393, 401, 404
Bifidus factor, 141
Bilirubin, 375, 376–377. *See also* Jaundice
Binter breast pump, 400
Bioactive components of breastmilk, 143–147
Biopsy methods, 496–497
Biotinidase, 145
Birth weight and neonatal jaundice, 378
Bleeding
   breast, 498–499
   postpartum hemorrhage, 314–315, 359
   uterine, dysfunctional, 552–553
   See also hemorrhage
Blocadren, 174
Blood, white cells, 130
Blue light therapy, 380
Body language, 255–256
Body-substance precautions, 226, 234
Bonding, 613, 615–616, 619, 687
Bone loss, 519–520, 534
Bottle-feeding
   and colic, 323–324
   and illness, 135, 137, 642, 644

   and malocclusion, 621, 624
   and SIDS, 660
   and weaning interval, 8
   introduction of, 585
   versus breastfeeding, 111–112, 114, 224, 289, 325, 342–344,
     466, 601–602, 776
Bovine milk
   allergy to, 147, 656
   and infant colic, 324
   versus breastmilk, 128, 131, 132, 133, 142, 143, 145, 146, 147,
     183, 655
Bras, and breastfeeding, 104–105, 331, 561
Breach of warranty, and LC practice, 730–731
Breast
   abscess, 486–487
   assessment of, 104–106, 483
   bleeding from, 498–499
   cancer, 499–502
   emotional significance of, 483
   engorgement, 294–295. *See* Engorgement
   fibrocystic disease of, 497–498
   immunity, 140
   implants, 494–496, 498
   insufficient tissue and FTT, 358–359
   lobes, 95
   lumps and surgery, 496–502
   massage, 296, 315, 394, 395, 484, 485, 492
   mastitis in, 176, 485–487, 501, 502–504, 543
   milk blister on, 493
   pads, 330–331
   pain, 492
   palpation of, 106
   physiology, 102
   preparation for nursing, 280–281, 484
   pumps. *See* Breast pumps, brand names
   refusal of, 328–329
   shells, 429, 432–433, 438, 484, 493, 498
   skin rashes and lesions on, 487–488, 489, 493
   stimulation, 280–281, 394
   storage capacity, 124–126
   structure of, 94–96
   surgery, 493–496, 504–507
   vasospasm, 492–493
Breast Engorgement (BESS) and Nipple Tenderness Scales
   (NTSS), 764
Breastfeeding
   abuse and, 68–69, 70
   active immunity and, 138
   alcohol consumption and, 167, 181, 194
   alternatives to, 5–8, 652
   assessment, 113, 150, 298–300, 334, 356, 763–764
   behaviors, 16–17, 614–616
   benefits of, 224
   bioactive components of, 143–147
   breast cancer and, 499–502
   breast surgery and, 105, 314, 493–496, 496–502, 504–507
   chemotherapy and, 502
   chickenpox and, 229
   child development and, 601–602
   childhood diarrhea and, 133–134, 133–135, 137
   clinical research on, 335
   cluster feedings, 283, 314
   co-sleeping and, 660
   cultural context of, 29–49. *See* Culture

cystic fibrosis and, 550
decision process, 67, 74–75, 225, 452, 456
definitions of, 755–756
delay of, 7
dental health and, 621, 624
in developing regions, 12–13, 14, 16
devices, 393–439, 472
drugs and, 163–185, 190–207. *See also* Drugs, Maternal medications
duration of, 73, 77–79, 80, 102, 106, 284, 349, 353, 594–595, 679–680
early, 4–5, 18, 21, 77, 106–107, 249, 281–287, 466
education about. *See* Breastfeeding education
environmental contaminants and, 182–184
evaluation of, 266–268, 349
evidence about, 3–4
fathers and, 59–60, 68
fertility-reducing effect of, 675, 679–680, 683–685
flowchart, 287
foods and, 40–42, 200
frequency of, 126, 353–354, 679–680, 681
headaches and, 563
herbs and, 43, 176–177
herpes viruses and, 228, 229–231
hindmilk to preterm infants, 464
HIV transmission and, 221–223, 226
hospital practices and, 66, 77, 77–79, 245, 281, 316, 385
HTLV-1 transmission and, 233–234
immunological effects of, 133–137, 138, 139–143, 144, 145, 283, 620, 637
in mid-1990s, 14
infant illnesses and, 355, 637–667, 644
infant mortality and, 223
influential person in, 66, 73
initiation of, 281–283, 466–467
insufficient milk supply and, 312–315
interruption of, 180, 382, 388
isotope use and, 545–548
jaundice and, 379, 386
log and questionnaire, 266–268
low-income families and, 64–68
mastitis and, 485–487
maternal nutrition and health and, 515–536, 541–572
medication, 179. *See also* Drugs, Maternal medications
mismanagement of, 350, 358
multiple infants and, 326–328
obstacles to, in low-income families, 64–68
oral contraceptives and, 175
otitis media and, 135, 137
pain during, 331
peer counselors and, 22, 65, 71, 262, 262–263, 264
physical impairments and, 559–560, 561–562
positions. *See* Positions for breastfeeding
postpartum hemorrhage and, 314–315
practices, 3–22
pregnancy and, 331–332
preparation for, 279–280, 279–281
preterm infants, 449–474
prevalence of, 3, 12–14
process, 279–305
promotion of, 16–22. *See also* Breastfeeding promotion
questionnaires about, 763–764
regulation of, 10–11
respiratory infections and, 135

risk factors, 299–300
seizure disorders and, 562–563
signs of needed intervention, 303–304
smoking and, 569–570
supplemental feeding and, 359–363, 682
support groups, 22, 262, 270–271, 271–272, 280, 562, 709–710
techniques, 302–303
teenage attitudes about, 62–64
thyroid disease and, 543–544
trends in, 3–23
tuberculosis and, 551
uterine contractions and, 103, 332
versus bottle-feeding, 111–112, 114, 126, 289, 325, 342–344, 466, 601–602
Western cultures and, 12, 14
See also Breastmilk, Breast pumps
Breastfeeding Attrition Prediction Tool (BAPT), 763
Breastfeeding education, 241–272
adolescents and, 263–264
after birth, 249
at-risk groups and, 262–264
before hospital discharge, 264–265, 300–303, 312, 332, 333, 418
change process and, 244–246
communication skills in, 255–256
continuing support and, 249–250, 252–253
in early pregnancy, 248–249
effectiveness of, 253–255, 256
on expressing breastmilk, 418
materials for, 260–262, 263, 280
follow–up, 304, 333
on feeding techniques, 302–303
and health-care professionals, 241–242, 245–246, 253–254, 259–260, 261–262, 265, 268–270
long-distance, 242
multimedia presentations and, 258–260
Internet and, 242
outcomes of, 269–270
purposes of, 248
sample teaching plans, 250, 251–252, 254, 269
self-care and, 279
self-help groups, 241
small-group dynamics and, 258
strike, 328–329
support system for, 248, 250, 251–252, 253, 262, 271–272, 280
teaching strategies, 242–244, 255, 258
team approach to, 270–272
transition to parenthood, 247–248
and WIC program, 254
Breastfeeding promotion, 18–23
advertising in, 76, 81
advocacy and counseling, 76–81
checklist of factors, 82
exhortation and, 18
government agencies and, 18–19, 80–81
health organizations and, 18
legislation and, 21–22
peer counselors and, 22, 71
successful programs, 81–83
support systems, 22, 72–73
WIC program, 18–19
Breastfeeding Support Consultants of Philadelphia, 242

Breastmilk, 91
  abnormal secretion of, 104
  advantages of, for preterm infant, 451
  allergies from, 656–657
  amelioration of disease and, 133–137
  analysis of contaminants in, 184
  antiallergenic properties of, 147–149, 655–658
  antibacterial factors in, 139–143
  antiinfective properties of, 133–137
  antiinflammatory components of, 142–143
  antiparasite factors in, 145
  antiviral factors in, 144
  bacteria in expressed, 409, 416–418
  caloric density of, 123, 127, 349, 464
  changes during pregnancy, 331
  collecting, transporting, storing, and feeding of, 453–455,
    789, 790–794
  components of, 133, 134
  drugs and, 163–185, 190–207. *See also* Drugs, Maternal
    medications
  environmental contaminants and, 182–184
  expression of. *See* Expression of breastmilk
  fat content of, 127–128
  food flavorings in, 522, 625
  foods for increasing, 40–42
  fortifiers and, 784–785
  gavage feeding and, 461
  growth factors in, 145–146
  half-life of chemicals in, 183
  herbs and, 175–177
  hormones in, 146–147
  IgA antibodies in, 140
  immunoglobulins in, 138, 139–140
  insufficient supply of, 312–315, 341
  jaundice. *See* Jaundice, late-onset
  lactose in, 128–129
  leaking of, 330
  let-down, 103
  maternal health and, 541–550
  maturation of, 121–122, 127
  minerals in, 131–133
  nonantibody antibacterial factors in, 141–143
  nonprotein nitrogen of, 129
  nuclear pollution and, 183
  nucleotides in, 129–130
  nutrients in, 123, 126–133
  output and prolactin receptor theory, 100–101
  overproduction of, 329–330
  preterm versus full-term, 129, 130, 449–450
  prolactin in, 98–101, 292, 396, 398, 400, 542, 557
  protein in, 129–130
  renal solute load in, 133
  storage of, 417, 465–466
  supply-demand response, 102
  synthesis of, 102, 124, 125, 126
  taurine in, 147
  transfer for preterm infants, 467–468
  transmission of viruses and, 221–234
  versus bovine milk, 128, 131, 132, 133, 142, 143, 144, 146,
    147, 183, 655
  versus formulas, 123, 126, 128, 129, 132, 133, 134, 135, 142,
    143, 146, 147, 149, 783
  viruses in, 233
  vitamins and micronutrients in, 130–131
  volume ingested, 123–124, 126
  volume produced, 17, 124–126, 167, 175, 181, 355, 356, 360,
    395, 461
  white cells in, 138
  See also Donor milk; Lactation; Milk banking
Breast pumps, 297, 325
  backflow risk, 401, 404, 417–418
  battery-operated, 395–396, 402, 406, 413–414
  clinical implications regarding, 409, 416–418
  comparison of, 400–403, 407
  consumer rights and, 408, 416
  disinfection of, 409, 417–418
  double pumping, 400, 403–407
  electric, 396, 402–403, 407–408, 410–411, 414–415, 423–425
  flanges in, 403, 407
  guidelines for selecting, 418–419, 582, 583
  hand-operated, 399–402, 404–405, 412–413, 420–421
  history of, 393, 399
  hormonal considerations with, 396, 398–399
  infections from, 409
  mechanical, 399
  milk contamination and, 408, 409, 417–418
  milk stimulation and, 400
  mothers' concerns about, 393–394
  mothers of preterm infants and, 409, 416–417, 456–457, 470
  nipple cups on, 407
  problems from, 419, 425–426
  reimbursement for, 456–458
  semiautomatic, 402–403, 410, 414–415
  squeeze-handle, 401, 404, 412, 421
  technical data on, 400–403, 407, 410–415
  types of, 401–403, 407
  use of, 394–395, 418–419
  water-powered, 408
  working mothers and, 419
  See also Brand names
Breast surgery
  augmentation, 494–496, 506–507
  clinical implications of, 504–507
  effect on breastfeeding, 105, 314, 493–496, 496–502,
    504–507
  mastopexy, 494
  reduction, 493–494, 495, 506
Breathing, suckling and, 113, 466, 467, 468
Breeder-feeder-producer role, 586–587
Bromocriptine, 167, 296
Brompheniramine, 173
Bronchiolitis, 641
Bronchodilators, 174, 178, 569
Burnout, 740–742
Burrow's solution, 229

Cadogan, William, 10, 11
Caffeine and breastfeeding, 522, 534
Calcium
  breastmilk and, 132
  channel blockers, 174
  lactation and, 519–521, 528, 531
Caloric density of breastmilk, 123, 127, 349, 464
Caloric intake, insufficient
  clinical implications of, 359
  disorganized suckling and, 355–357
  feeding supplementation, 359–364
  infant factors in, 355–358

maternal factors in, 358–359
risk factors for, 349, 352–353
Cancer, breast, 499–502
Candidiasis, 173, 174, 319, 488–492
Carbamazepine, 170, 195, 562
Carbohydrates, 525–526
Cascara, 175, 195
Casein, 129
Case managers, 724
CCK (cholecystokinin), 147, 150
CD ROMs and breastfeeding education, 259–260
Celiac disease and breastfeeding, 136, 654–655
Cell-mediated immunity, 138
Cellulitis, 487
Central nervous system, immaturity of, 357
Cephalexin, 173
Cephalothin, 173
Cesarean birth
    breastfeeding and, 291–294
    HBV transmission and, 232
    HIV transmission and, 223
    mother-child antibodies transmission and, 231
Change process
    breastfeeding education and, 244–246
    lactation programs and, 715–718
    theory of, 244–246
Chaotic family functioning, 61
Charting, 728–729
CHDs. *See* Congenital heart defects
Chemotherapy and breastfeeding, 502
Chemstrips, 289
Chickenpox, mother-child transmission, 229, 233
Child
    abuse, 181
    attachment and bonding of, 611–613, 615–616, 619
    development and infant feeding, 601–602, 604, 605, 607
    intellectual maturation of, 607–608, 609
    intelligence, studies of, 602, 603
    language and communication process, 608–613
    psychosocial and breastfeeding behaviors, 614–615
    social development of, 608, 611–613, 615–619
    temperament style of, 616–618
    theories of development of, 606–608
    See also Infant(s)
Childbirth
    cultural practices, 38
    educators, 271
    father's response to, 689
    regulation of, 10
    and sexuality, 688–689
Child health, 601–630
    allergic disease, 147–149
    breastmilk and, 126–151, 637–638
    dental care, 621, 624
    immunizations and, 619–620, 622
    obesity and, 628–629
    orofacial development of, 621, 624
    solid foods and, 624–628
    See also Ill child
Childhood family functioning, 61
Chlopheniramine, 178
Chloramphenicol, 173
Chlorpromazine, 363, 566, 568
Choanal atresia and breastfeeding, 651

C-hold, 285
Cholecystokinin (CCK), 147, 150
Cholesterol challenge hypothesis, 128
Chronic illness, breastmilk and, 664–665
Chronic sorrow, 664
Cipro, 173
Ciprofloxacin, 173, 551
Cisapride, 646
Claritin, 173
Cleft lip and palate, 648–651
Clinical care
    for sore nipples, 320–321
    plans, 730
Clinical research. *See* Research
Clomipramine, 172, 196
Closet nursing, 47
Clothing, when breastfeeding, 331
Clotrimazole, 174, 489, 490, 491
CLP. *See* Cleft lip and palate
Cluster feedings, 283, 314
Clutch position, 292, 302, 303
CMV, 229–231, 233
Cocaine, 180–181
Codeine, 170, 196
Colic, 323–324
Colostrum, 7, 10, 94, 102, 124, 280, 542
    and bacterial growth, 417
    components of, 122, 123, 129, 131, 132, 139, 145–147
    cultural beliefs about, 33, 37
    See also Breastmilk
Comfort nursing, 110
Comfort Plus breast pump, 404
Commercial milk fortifiers, 463–464, 785
Communication
    infant-mother, 611–613
    skills, 255–256
Components of breastmilk, 133–137
Computer technology and breastfeeding education, 258–259
Condoms, 693, 696
Congenital defects and breastfeeding
    celiac disease, 654–655
    choanal atresia, 651
    cleft lip and palate, 648–651
    clinical implications of, 651–653
    cystic fibrosis, 655
    gastroesophageal reflux, 644, 646–647
    heart defects, 644, 645
    hypothyroidism, 654
    imperforate anus, 647–648
    pyloric stenosis, 647
    tracheoesophageal fistula, 647
Constructive confrontation, 246
Constructive feedback, 257
Continuing education programs, 265, 268–270
Contraception, 693–694
    barrier methods, 693, 696
    during lactation, 691–699, 691–700, 691–701
    hormonal methods, 697
    Lactational Amenorrhea Method (LAM), 684–685
    nonhormonal methods, 692–697
    regulation of, 11
    See also Oral contraceptives; specific methods
Contraceptives
    barrier methods, 693, 696

breastfeeding and, 175
    clinical implications, 698–699
    hormonal methods, 697–698
    nonhormonal methods, 692–697
    See also specific methods
Control, endocrine-autocrine, 102
Corgard, 174
Correlational studies, 749–750
Corticosteroids, 569
Cortisol, 101, 146–147
Corzide, 175
Co-sleeping, 660
Cost of not breastfeeding, 14–16, 149, 601
Cot death. *See* Sudden infant death syndrome
Coumadin, 170
Counseling HIV-infected women, 227
Cow's milk. *See* Bovine milk
Cradle position, 292, 301, 303
Creamatocrit, 464
Crib death. *See* Sudden infant death syndrome
Cromolyn, 174
Cross-chest position, 301, 303
Cross-nursing. *See* Wet-nursing
Crotamiton, 178
Crying, 321, 323–324, 609
Cultural context of breastfeeding, 29–49. *See also* Culture
Cultural relativism, 31–32
Culture
    assessment of, 32–34
    breastfeeding beliefs and practices, 31, 73, 79, 313
    characteristics of, 29–31
    childbirth practices and, 38
    defined, 29
    effects of, on breastfeeding, 35–38, 126
    effects of, on milk banking, 778–779
    implications for practice, 47–48
    infant care and, 38–40
    language barriers and, 34–35
    maternal foods and, 40–44
    yin-yang, 31, 43
    See also Ethnicity; Ethnography
Cup-feeding, 287, 289, 359, 471, 585–586
Curriculum development for breastfeeding education, 244
Custody and breastfeeding, 68
Cyanosis, 113
Cylinder breast pumps, 401–402, 404
Cystic fibrosis, 355, 550, 655
Cystic mass, aspiration of, 496
Cytomegalovirus, 221, 229–231, 233

Dancer-hand position, 645, 646
Darvon, 170
Data collection methods, 758, 762
Davol breast pump, 400, 401, 404, 412
Day care, 592–593, 596
DDT in breastmilk, 182, 200
Declaration of Helsinki, 756
Dehydration, 638–639
    and FTT, 348, 349, 359
Deliberative approach, 76, 78
Delivery, infection transmission during, 221
Demerol, 170
Demographics of lactation, 675–676
Dental care of children, 621, 624

Depakene, 170
Depomedroxyprogesterone (DMPA), 175
Depo-Provera, 175, 698
Depositions, giving, 70
Descriptive studies, 749
Desipramine, 172, 568
Dextrostix, 289
DHA (docosahexanoic acid), in breastmilk, 127–128
Diabetes, 541–543
Diaphragms, 693, 696
Diarrhea
    and breastfeeding, 638–639
    breastmilk and, 133–135, 137
Diazepam, 173, 193, 568
Diet
    Food Guide Pyramid, 525
    macronutrients in, 525–527
    maternal, 40–44, 128, 131, 150, 184, 200, 326, 355, 515–528, 550
    micronutrients in, 527–528
    supplements, 521–522
    vegetarian, 44, 521, 527, 535
    See also Maternal diet; U.S. Dietary Guidelines
Dietary
    counseling, 522–524
    supplements, 521–522
Dieticians, and breastfeeding education, 271
Diflucan, 174, 491
Digoxin, 174, 196
Dilantin, 170, 562
Dimetane, 173
Dindevan, 170
Dioxin, 182
Diphenhydramine, 173, 178, 294
Disabilities, mothers with, 559–560, 561–562
Discharge. *See* Hospital discharge
Diseases and breastfeeding
    autoimmune, 557–559
    acute infections, 550–551
    asthma, 569
    celiac, 136, 654–655
    cystic fibrosis, 355, 550, 655
    diabetes, 136, 541–543
    eczema, 136, 488
    galactosemia, 653
    gastrointestinal, 638–639
    hyperthyroidism, 544, 549
    hypothyroidism, 146, 358, 544, 654
    meningitis, 641
    multiple sclerosis, 558
    pituitary dysfunction, 549–550
    pneumonia, 641
    postpartum depression, 172, 176, 564–568, 686
    rheumatoid arthritis, 558–559
    seizure disorders, 562–563
    systemic lupus erythematosis, 558
    tuberculosis, 551
    urinary tract, 551
Diuretics, 175
D-I-Y Nursing Supplementer, 433
DMPA, 175
DNase, 655
Docosahexanoic acid (DHA), 127–128, 784
Domperidone, 167

Donor milk
  benefits of, 779–780
  clinical uses of, 780
  collection, handling, and storage of, 789, 790–794
  costs of, 794
  distribution of, 780
  environmental contaminants in, 794
  fortification of, 784–785
  heat treatment of, 787–789
  homogenized, 784–785
  medicinal therapeutic uses of, 781, 785–786
  nutritional uses of, 780–782
  preventive uses of, 781, 783–785
  shipping of, 789
  uses of, 780–786
  See also Milk banking
Doula, 44
Down syndrome, 642–643, 664
Doxepin, 172
Drip milk, 789
Drugs
  breastmilk and, 163–185, 190–207
  compatible with breastfeeding, 194, 486, 562–563, 566, 569
  contraindicated in breastfeeding, 191, 192, 359
  FTT and, 363–364
  generic and trade names, 178, 201–203
  illegal, 180–182
  mastitis and, 486
  milk volume and, 167
  nurslings and, 194
  transfer of, to breastmilk, 166–167, 190–207
  See also Maternal medications; specific drug or drug type
Ductules, 94
Dulcolax, 175

Eczema, 136, 488
Educational materials and breastfeeding education, 260–262
Effexor, 566, 568
EGF (epidermal growth factor), 146
Egnell breast pumps, 399, 400, 403
Elavil, 568
Employment and breastfeeding, 577–598
  at-home vs. employed mothers, 587–588
  barriers to, 589
  clinical implications of, 593, 596
  company benefits of, 590
  day-care issues, 579, 581, 592–593, 596
  decisions about, 594–596
  duration of, 594–595
  expressing milk, 581–583, 595
  feeding options, 585–586, 593
  job-sharing, 587
  length of workday, 587
  milk storage, 584
  prenatal planning, 579
  research results on, 597
  returning to work, 580–581, 594
  reverse-cycle nursing, 583, 586
  sleep pattern changes, 586, 593
  social support for, 588–590
  telecommuting, 587
  use of milk substitutes, 595–596
  See also Breast pumps; Expression of breastmilk
Endocrine control of lactation, 102

Endogenous hormonal response, 146
Energy
  infant intake of, 123, 352–353, 355–364
  needs during lactation, 524–525, 527
Enfamil Human Milk Fortifier, 785
Engorgement, 504
  breast pumping and, 396, 398
  early breastfeeding and, 283
  mastitis and, 486, 504
  risk factors for, 296, 298
  treatment of, 167, 175, 296, 431, 630
  versus breast fullness, 294–295
Entrainment, 616, 617
Environmental contaminants, 182–185, 200
Enzymes in breastmilk, 143–144
Ephedrine, 174, 178
Epidural anesthesia and breastfeeding, 286–287, 292, 295
Epinephrine, 174
Epithelial cells, and mammary growth, 93–94
Ergonovine maleate, 167
Ergot alkaloids, 167
Ergotrate, 167
Erikson's psychosocial theory, 606–607, 609
Erythromycin, 173, 486
  interaction with Seldane, 490
Estrogen-progestin hormonal contraceptive methods, 698
Ethnocentrism, 31
Ethnography, 4, 32, 748
Ethogram, 751
Ethosuximide, 170
Eucerin Cream, 322
Evenflo breast pumps, 400, 401, 404, 406, 411, 412, 413, 420, 422
Evil eye *(mal de ojo)*, 33, 39–40
Exercise and lactation, 519, 528, 535
Experimental studies, 750–751
Expressed mothers' milk (EMM)
  collection and storage of, 453–455, 462, 463
  deficiencies of, 463–464
  contamination of, 409, 416–418, 461
  gavage feeding of, 461–463
  maternal employment and, 581–584, 590–591, 593
  minimizing bacteria in, 463
  volume of, 456
  warming of, 463
Expression of breastmilk, 364
  educating mothers about, 419
  hand, 295, 296–298, 395, 399, 400
  hand pumps, 399–402
  mechanical, 399
  milk-ejection reflex and, 394–395
  mothers' attitudes toward, 426–427
  principles of, 456
  problems arising from, 419, 426–427
  by pump, 327, 393–439, 456–457, 582
  schedule and technique for, 458–459, 582
  See also Breast pumps

Failure to thrive, 346–349
  clinical implications of, 359
  conditions contributing to, 348, 355–359
  feeding supplementation, 359–364
  lack of support system and, 349
  risk factors for, 349, 352–355

See also Slow weight gain
Family, 53–84
    abuse in, 68–69, 71
    costs of formula to, 15–16
    effect of baby on, 56–57
    effect of ill child on, 662–663
    extended, 53–54, 72
    fathers in, 58–59
    functioning, 61–62
    influential person on breastfeeding, 66, 73
    low-income, 64–68, 71
    mature, 62
    nuclear, 53
    of orientation, 54
    -planning counseling, 699–700
    of procreation, 54
    teenage mother, 62–64
    traditional, 53
Fat, 527
Fathers
    attachment to infant, 58–59
    breastfeeding and, 59–61, 68, 252–253
Fatigue, maternal, 331–332, 688
Fat-soluble vitamins, 130–131, 528, 655
Fatty acids in breastmilk, 127–128
Faultless breast pump, 400
Fecal flora, breastfed vs. bottle-fed infants, 142
Feeding, 354. *See also* Breastfeeding; Food(s)
    early, 281–287
    length of, 349, 353
    nests, 561
    patterns, 353, 380
    plan, 281, 282, 435, 436
    techniques, 302–303
    vessels, 6–7
Feeding-tube devices
    clinical implications of, 435
    description of, 433–434
    finger-feeding with, 290–291, 329, 434–435, 471
    situations for use, 353–354, 357, 388, 434–435, 436–437, 645
    slow weight gain and, 359–360
    use of, 290–291, 360, 361–362, 433–434, 437–438
Female sterilization. *See* Tubal ligation
Feminist research, 751
Fennel, 175
Fenugreek, 175
Fertility
    lactation and, 675–685
    prolactin and, 100
Fetal hemoglobin, 375–376
Fibroadenomas, 498
Fibrocystic breast disease, 497–498
Finger-feeding, 290–291, 329, 434–435, 471
Flagyl, 173
Flowchart of breastfeeding process, 287
Floxin, 173
Fluconazole, 174, 490, 491, 493
Fluoxetine, 172, 193, 566, 568
Focus groups, in cultural assessment, 32–33
Folate, 531, 534
Folk medicine, 30
Folkways and nursing practice, 47
Follow-up care, 299–300, 304

Fontanel, 39
Food Guide Pyramid, 525
Food(s)
    affecting breastfeeding, 40–42, 200
    allergies and breastfeeding, 147–149, 655–656, 657
    behavior and culture, 40–44
    flavorings in breastmilk, 522, 625
    hand-fed, 6–7
    "hot" and "cold," 43
    mixed, 7–8
    postpartum restrictions, 42–43
    prelacteal, 7
    sensitivities, 656
    serving sizes of, 528
    solid. *See* Solid infant foods
    that pass through milk, 522
    See also Nutrition basics
Foodways, and culture, 40–44
Football position, 292, 302, 303, 330
Formulas, 9
    economic costs of, 15–16
    health risks of, 14–15, 581, 654–655
    hospital-based marketing of, 66–67
    International Code for Marketing, 19
    intolerance to, 656
    manufacturers of, and physicians, 11–12
    marketing of, 11, 19, 66–67, 225–226
    versus breastmilk, 123, 126, 128, 129, 132, 133, 134, 135, 142, 143, 146, 147, 149, 783
    and WIC program, 18–19
    See also Bottle-feeding
Free amino acids, 129
Free-nipple technique, 494
Frenulum, 108, 115, 357–358
FTT. *See* Failure to thrive

Galactocele, 496, 497
Galactogogues, 40–42, 167, 175, 176
Galactopoiesis, 93, 99, 102–103
Galactorrhea, 104
Galactosemia, 653
GALT (gut-associated lymphoid tissue), 139
Gastroesophageal reflux, 136, 644, 646–647
Gastrointestinal infections, 136, 638–639
Gavage feeding of preterm infant, 461–463
Generic
    equivalents of trade names, 204–207
    versus trade names, 200–203
Gentian violet, 490, 491
Gentle Expressions breast pump, 400, 406, 413, 423
Gerber breast pumps, 400, 401, 404, 407, 410, 414
Ginseng, 176
Glandular tissue, insufficient, 358–359
Glucocorticoids, 101
Glucose administration, 288–289
Gluten enteropathy. *See* Celiac disease
Gomco breast pump, 400, 410
Gonadotropin-releasing hormone (GnRH), 676–677
Goodyear breast pump, 401
Grand mal epilepsy. *See* Seizure disorders
Graves disease, 544
Grief, support for parents in, 665–667
Grounded theory, 748
Growth

charts, 343–344, 345, 346, 347
factors in breastmilk, 145–146
normal, 126, 341–343
Growth and development
attachment, 611–613, 615–616, 619
cognitive, 607–609
language, 608–609
length, 604
oro-facial, 621, 624
outcomes of, 601–602
physical, 602, 604
reflexes, 606, 607
sensory, 604–606
social, 608–619
theories of, 606–608
weight, 313, 341–346, 604
Gruels, 6
Gyne-Lotrimin, 489, 490

Half-life of chemicals in breastmilk, 183
Hand expression of breastmilk, 295, 296–298, 395, 399, 400
Hand feeding, 7–8
Hand pumps, 399–402
See also Breast pumps; Expression of breastmilk
Happy Family breast pumps, 401, 405, 412, 420
HBV. *See* Hepatitis B
HCV. *See* Hepatitis C
Headaches, and breastfeeding, 563
Health-care professionals
application of child development theories, 619
breastfeeding education of, 265, 268–270, 712, 723
as breastfeeding educators, 271, 283, 284–286, 328
breastfeeding in the workplace, 591–592
as family-planning counselors, 698–699, 700, 701
handling families in emergencies, 663–664
and hospital-based lactation programs, 715–718
stages of role acquisition, 724
Health-care system
change process in, 244–246
dominant culture and, 30
in initiation of breastfeeding, 17
See also Medical community
Health risks of formulas, 14–15, 581, 654–655
Hedulin, 170
Hemoglobin, 375–376
Hemorrhage
postpartum, 314–315
vitamin K and, 131
Hepatitis B, 221, 231–232, 233, 620
Hepatitis C, 232, 233
Herbicides, 182
Herbs
breastfeeding and, 175–177
medicinal, 43
Heredity, and growth rates, 342, 345
Herpes simplex virus (HSV), 227–229
neonatal infection, 228
transmission of, 228, 233
treatment of, 229, 230, 488
Hexofenadine, 173
Hindmilk feeding, 464
Hismanal, 173
Historical research, 751
History of infant feeding, 4–8

HIV
counseling, 225, 226–227, 227
high-risk practices, 223, 226
mother-child transmission, 221–227, 233
prevention of, in women, 224
testing infants and pregnant women for, 222, 226–227
HMGF (human milk growth factors) I, II, and III, 146
Hollister Ameda/Egnell breast pumps, 401, 402, 404, 407, 411, 412, 415, 417–421
Hormonal contraceptive methods, 697–698
Hormones
breastmilk and, 146–147
estrogen, 676, 677
follicle-stimulating, 677, 687
gonadotropin-releasing, 676–677
lactation and, 98–102, 103–104, 396, 398–399, 676–677
libido and, 687–688
luteinizing, 676–677
mammary growth and, 94, 98
oxytocin, 103–104, 398–399, 426, 577
pregnancy and, 100
prolactin, 98–101, 292, 396, 398, 400, 542, 557
thyroid and, 543–544
Hospital-based lactation programs, 712–714
establishment of, 715–718
LCs in, 732–733
Hospital discharge
breastfeeding education and, 264–265, 304
early, advantages and disadvantages of, 311
follow-up to, 304, 312–315
planning, 301–304, 333
Hospitalization
breastfeeding child and, 661–662
breastfeeding mother and, 570–571
effect on siblings, 663
emergency admission, 663–664
parental stresses of, 662–663
returning home from, 664
Hospital practices
breastfeeding a presurgical child, 652
effect on breastfeeding, 66, 77–79, 80, 245, 316
effects on neonates, 385
formula marketing, 66–68
infant feeding plans and, 281, 298
neonatal jaundice and, 378–380
See also NICU
"Hot" and "cold" foods, 43
Hot-cold system, 43
"How to swim with sharks," 720–721
HPL, 101
HSV. *See* Herpes simplex virus
HTLV-1, 221, 233–234
Human growth hormone, 167
Human immunodeficiency virus. *See* HIV
Human lymphotropic virus. *See* HTVL-1
Human milk. *See* Breastmilk; Milk banking; Donor milk
Human Milk Banking Association of North America, 776, 777, 779
Human Placental Lactogen. *See* HPL
Human T-cell lymphotropic virus type I. *See* HTLV-1
Hydration, infant, 312, 313, 349, 638–639
Hydrocephalus, 643–644
Hygroton, 175
Hyperbilirubinemia. *See* Jaundice

Hypoestrogenicity, 675, 687–688
Hypoglycemia, 288–289, 291
    and breastfeeding, 658–659
Hypothesis, 754
Hypothyroidism, 146, 358, 544, 654

Ibuprofen, 170, 178, 197, 493
IDDM (Insulin–dependent diabetes mellitus). *See* Diabetes
IgA deficiency and human milk, 785–786
IgE system, 148, 628, 656
IGF-I (insulinlike growth factor), 146
Ill child
    with celiac disease, 654–655
    with chronic illness, 664–665
    with congenital defects, 644, 646–653
    with heart defects, 644
    with hypothyroidism, 654
    with cystic fibrosis, 655
    with Down syndrome, 642–643
    with food allergies, 655–658
    with galactosemia, 653
    with gastrointestinal infections, 638–639
    guidelines in caring for, 666
    hospitalization and, 661–664
    with hydrocephalus, 643–644
    with hypoglycemia, 658–659
    with meningitis, 641
    with metabolic dysfunction, 653–655
    with neural-tube defects, 643
    with neurological dysfunction, 642–644, 645
    with otitis media, 642
    with phenylketonuria, 653
    with respiratory infections, 640–641
    siblings of, 663
    and SIDS, 659–661, 665
    See also specific illnesses
Illness
    acute infant, 638–642
    chronic maternal, 664–665
    failure to thrive, 355
    See also specific illnesses
Illegal drugs, and breastfeeding, 180–182, 192
"Illustrated Multi-Language Pocket Glossary," 262
Imipramine, 171, 172, 193, 566, 568
Immune system, 137–143
Immunity, cell-mediated and passive, 138
Immunizations, 619–620
    recommended schedule of, 622
Immunoglobulins, 138, 139–140
Impaired mobility, mothers with, 559–560, 561–562
Imperforate anus, 647–648
Implants. *See* Silicone breast implants
Imprinting, 613, 615–616
IMS. *See* Insufficient Milk Supply
Incipient vulnerable child syndrome, 381–382
Induced lactation, 555–557
Infa breast pump, 405, 413, 421
Infancy level of family functioning, 61
Infant(s)
    adaptive-social development of, 611
    breastfed versus bottle-fed, 123, 234
    care, cultural differences in, 38–40
    carriers, 39
    effect of, on family, 56–57

energy-intake patterns of, 124, 349, 352–358, 624–625
failure to thrive in, 346–349, 352–353
father's attachment to, 58–61
feeding and development of, 601–602. *See also*
    Breast-feeding
feeding plan for, 281
formulas. *See* Bottle-feeding; Formulas
growth and development of, 126, 341–344, 601–606
growth charts for, 343–344, 345, 346, 347
health risks of formulas, 14–15, 581, 654–655
hydration and nutrition of, 312, 313
hypoglycemia in, 288–289, 291
illness and slow weight gain in, 355
levels of arousal in, 606
maternal medications and, 165–166, 180–182, 194–199
mortality, 13, 223
-mother bonding, 611–613, 615–616, 619
oral development of, 107–108
orofacial development of, 621, 624
positioning for breastfeeding. *See* Positioning
postmature, 289
psychosocial and breastfeeding behaviors, 614–615
reasons for having, 56–57
reflexes of, 606, 607
sensory development in, 604–606
separation anxiety of, 619
sleep patterns of, 294, 610–611
slow weight gain in, 344–346, 348, 350–351
stranger distress in, 618–619
suckling process of, 108–113
temperament of, 616–618
thinking: sensorimotor state, 610
viral infections in, 234
weaning of, 629–630
weight patterns, 313, 341–346, 604
    See also Preterm infants; Child; Child health; Ill child
Infant Temperament Questionnaire (ITQ), 617, 618
Infection control, universal precautions, 226
Infections
    ear, infant, 642
    gastrointestinal, infant, 638–639
    respiratory, infant, 640–641
    urinary tract, maternal, 137, 551
Informed choice, 699
Informed consent
    for IUD insertion, 695, 695–696
    for nipple shields, 430
    for research subjects, 757
Informed decision to breastfeed, 452, 455
Infrasubmammary procedure, 494
Innocenti Declaration, 20
Insufficient milk supply, 312–315, 316
Intal, 174
Intercourse
    first postpartum, 689–690
    frequency of, 690–691
International Board of Lactation Consultant Examiners, Inc.,
    710
International Code for Marketing Breast-milk Substitutes, 19,
    77, 226, 261
International Lactation Consultant Association, 265, 709
Internet
    breastfeeding education via, 242, 711
    LC networking via, 727–728

See also LACTNET, LACTNEWS
Intervention
  signs of needed, 303–304
  when neonates do not latch on, 288
Intraductal papilloma, 499
Intrauterine devices (IUDs), 693, 695–696
Intrpartum period, breastfeeding process in, 279–304
Inverted nipples, 98
Iodine, 533
Iron, 132, 533, 534, 624
ITQ. *See* Infant Temperament Questionnaire
Itraconazole, 173, 490, 491
Ixbut, 175

Japan, breastfeeding in, 48
Japanese breast massage, 317
Jaundice
  birth weight and, 378
  and breastfeeding, 283, 321, 378, 379, 382, 386, 388, 389
  clinical care plan and implications of, 385–386, 387, 388
  early-onset (neonatal), 375–377, 380, 381
  hospital practices and, 379–380, 382
  incipient vulnerable child syndrome and, 381–382
  late-onset, 382–384, 388
  pathological, 377–380
  racial/ethnic tendency toward, 377–378
  stool patterns and, 378
  supplemental feeds, 379–380, 388
  therapy for, 380–381, 382
  weight loss and, 378
Juice-jar breast pump, 408

Kadan breast pump, 414
Kaneson breast pumps, 400, 401, 404, 413, 421
Kangaroo care, 39
Keflex, 173
Keflin, 173
Ketoconazole, 178, 490, 491
Ketoralac, 170
Korea, breastfeeding in, 49
Kwashiorkor, 45–46

Labetolol, 174, 197
Lact-Aid feeding-tube, 433
Lactation
  after radiation therapy, 502
  bone loss and, 519–521
  breast cancer and, 499–500
  breast surgery and, 493–496
  contraception and, 691–700
  drugs that affect, 167
  endocrine-autocrine control, 102
  environmental contaminants and, 182–184
  exercise and, 519
  fertility and, 675–685
  fibroadenomas and, 497–498
  fibrocystic disease and, 497–498
  herbs and, 176–177
  history, 334–335
  illegal drug use and, 180–182
  initiation and continuance of, 17, 283
  intercourse during, 689–691
  isotope use during, 545–548
  leaking, 330

  maternal health and, 541–572
  nursing diagnoses and, 728
  nutrition and, 516–517, 519–522, 526, 529–532, 534–535
  oral contraceptives and, 175
  programs, 590–591, 712–714, 715–718
  prolactin and other hormones in, 98–101
  pseudo-induced, 555–557
  restimulating, 553–555
  sexuality and, 685–691
  smoking and, 569–570
  stages of, 93, 94
  surgery and, 552–553, 552–555
  tubal ligation and, 694
  vitamin and mineral intake during, 529–532
  weight loss and, 518–519
Lactational amenorrhea. *See* Amenorrhea
Lactational Amenorrhea Method (LAM), 684–685, 695
Lactational infertility
  amenorrhea and, 677–678
  breastfeeding frequency and, 679–680
  in consecutive pregnancies, 681, 683
  physiology of, 677
Lactation consultants, 271
  burnout and, 740–742
  as case managers, 724
  certification of, 710–711
  collaboration with physicians, 738
  do's and don'ts for, 742–743
  fees and payment policies of, 736–738
  hospital-based programs and, 713–714, 715, 732–733
  legal considerations of practice, 730–731
  liability insurance and, 731
  marketing skills for, 726
  networking process and, 727–728
  partnerships among, 738–740
  in private practice, 731, 733–738
  reporting and charting, 728–729
  roles and responsibilities of, 701, 707, 709, 714, 723–724
  stages of role acquisition, 724
  third-party reimbursement to, 731–732
  training of, 265, 711
  and volunteer counselors, 725–726
Lactation history and risk assessment form, 334
Lactiferous duct. *See* Mammary duct
Lactiferous sinuses, 95, 106
LACTNET, 242, 727
LACTNEWS On-Line, 727
Lactobacillus bifidus, 129, 141
Lactoferrin in breastmilk, 129, 141
Lactogenesis, 93, 94, 98, 121–122, 698
  for mothers with IDDM, 542
Lactoperoxidase, 141–142
Lactose
  intolerance, 129
  in breastmilk, 128–129
La Leche League, 22, 271–272
  breastfeeding education and, 262, 280, 562, 710
  certification of LCs, 710
Language
  barriers, 34–35
  development of, 608–609
Lanolin, 184
Lansinoh, 323
Lasix, 175

Latch-on, 285–286
Late-onset jaundice. *See* Jaundice
Laxatives, 175
LCs. *See* Lactation consultants
Lead in breastmilk, 183–184, 200
Learning principles, 242
Legal considerations for LCs, 730–731
Let-down reflex, 103
Lever pump, 393, 395
Levothroid, 654
Levothyroxine sodium, 654
Libido
    -enhancing factors, 688–689
    -inhibiting effects of lactation, 687–688
Licorice, 177
Lihi ritual, 36–37
Lindane, 177–178
Lipase, 145
Listening skills, 257
Lithium, 173, 566
LLLI. *See* La Leche League
Lobes, 95
Loratidine, 173
Lotrimin, 174, 491
Low-income families
    Best Start program for, 82–83
    maternal energy intake in, 517
    obstacles to breastfeeding in, 64–68, 71
Loyd-B breast pump, 400, 401, 404, 412, 421
Lupus. *See* Systemic lupus erythemetosis
Luteinizing hormone (LH), 676–677
Lymphocytes, 138
Lysine, 229
Lysozyme, 144–145

Macronutrients
    carbohydrates, 525–526
    fats, 527
    protein, 526–527
Macrophages in breastmilk, 138
Madonna position, 301, 303
Mag Mag breast pumps, 400, 406, 414, 422
Magnesium, 531
Magnesium sulfate, 171, 197
Malabsorption syndrome. *See* Celiac disease
Mal de ojo (evil eye), 39–40
Malocclusion, 137, 621, 624
Mammaplasty, 493–496, 505, 506–507. *See also* Breast surgery
Mammary structures, 93–96
Mammogenesis, 93–94
Mammol Ointment, 322
Manufactured infant milks. *See* formulas
Marcalan, 323
Marijuana, 180
Marketing
    of LC services, 726, 735, 736
    See also Advertising
Massage, 315
Massee Cream, 322
Mastitis, 485–487
    classifications of, 487
    clinical implications of, 502–504
    diabetes and, 543
    herbs and, 176

similarities to breast cancer, 501
    teaching plan, 503
Mastopexy, 494, 496
Maternal
    behaviors affecting infant growth, 345–346
    employment, 577–598. *See also* Employment
    exercise, 519
    fatigue, 331–332, 688
    health, 541–572
    hospitalization and breastfeeding, 570–571
    seropositivity, 223
    virus load, 223
Maternal Breastfeeding Evaluation Scale (MBES), 763
Maternal diet, 40–44, 200
    assessment of, 522–524
    breastmilk and, 128, 131, 355, 515, 522, 527, 528
    caloric intake from, 515–517, 524–525
    and colic, 324
    and cystic fibrosis patients, 550
    fluids in, 517
    frequently asked questions about, 534–536
    for mother of multiples, 326
    macronutrients in, 525–527
    micronutrients in, 527–528
    potential allergens in, 150
    safeguards against pollution, 184
    supplements in, 521–522
    in treatment of candidiasis, 490
    vegetarian, 521
    weight loss and, 518–519
    See also Nutrition basics; U.S. Dietary Guidelines
Maternal-Infant History Form, 349, 368–373
Maternal medications, 165, 180–182, 194–199
    milk production and, 171, 358
    in breastmilk, 164–167, 168–169, 170–180, 190–207, 562–563, 569
    preterm infants and, 465
    mastitis and, 486
    See also Drugs; specific drug or type of drug
Maturation index of colostrum and milk. *See* MICAM
Mature family functioning, 62
Medela breast pumps, 400, 403, 411, 413, 414, 415, 417–418, 425
    hand, 420
    Little Hearts, 401, 405, 406, 413, 414
    Manualectric, 400, 401, 402, 403, 413
    Mini-Electric, 406, 423
    pedal pump, 408
    Spring Express, 405, 413
Medical community, role of, 10–12
    See also Health-care entries
Medications. *See* Maternal medications
Medicinal herbs, 43
Medicine, allopathic, 30
MEDwatch, 416
Mellaril, 167, 171, 568
Meningitis, 641
Menstrual cycle, 676–677
Meperidine, 170
Mephyton, 170
Mercury and breastfeeding, 182, 200
Mesoridazine, 568
Metabolic disorders
    cystic fibrosis, 550
    diabetes, 541–543

pituitary dysfunction, 549–550
thyroid disease, 543–549
Metabolic dysfunction
galactosemia, 653
phenylketonuria, 653
Metaclopramide, 646
Metamucil, 175
Methadone, 181–182, 197
Methergine, 167, 552
Methyldopa, 174
Methylergonovine maleate, 167, 552
Metoclopramide, 167, 315, 364, 470
Metoprolol, 174
Metronidazole, 173
MICAM method, 123, 150
Miconazole, 174, 490, 491
Micronutrients
minerals, 528
vitamins, 527–528
Micronutrients in breastmilk, 130–131
Migraine headaches, 563
Milk
blister, 493
drip, 791
hill stage, 93
preterm, 417, 450
See also Breastmilk; Donor milk
Milk banks, 661, 665
collection and storage procedures, 789, 790–794
donor selection process, 786–787
fees, 794
heat treatment of donor milk, 787–789
history of, 775–776
in North America, 776, 778, 786–794
outside North America, 777–779
policies and procedures of, 794
preterm milk, 784
quality assurance in, 789
ultrasonic homogenization, 784–785
See also Donor milk
Milk-ejection reflex, 408
breast pain and, 492
oxytocin and, 398–399
stimulation of, 394–395, 419, 426
Milk transfer
estimating, 468–469, 472
facilitating, 469–470, 470–471, 472
Minerals
in breastmilk, 131–133
intake during lactation, 531–532
Mini-Manual breast pump, 405
Minocycline, 173
Mites, treatment for, 177–178
Mixed feeds, 7–8
Modesty, and breastfeeding, 36, 63
Molla caida, 39
Mommy's rules, 719
Monistat, 174, 490, 491
Monoamine oxidase (MAO) inhibitors, 566, 568
Mother-infant bonding, 613, 615–616
Mother of preterm infant
breastfeeding and, 450, 452, 464
breastfeeding devices and, 472
lactoengineering and, 464

milk expression and collection, 453–454, 456–457, 458, 463, 470
milk volume of, 459, 460–461, 469–470
nipple shields and, 470–471
nonnutritive suckling and, 460
postdischarge breastfeeding plans for, 473–474
skin-to-skin care and, 459–460
transporting and storing milk, 454, 462, 463
See also Maternal medications
Motilium, 167
Motrin, 170
MS. *See* Multiple sclerosis
Multimedia presentations in breastfeeding education, 258–260
Multiple infants, breastfeeding, 326–328
Multiple sclerosis, breastfeeding and, 558
Mutual caregiving, 612
Mycelex, 174, 491
Mycostatin, 173, 174, 491
Myoepithelial cells, 94
Mysoline, 170, 562

Nadolol, 174, 198
Narcotics, 170, 178
following cesarean birth, 293–294
Nardil, 568
National Center for Health Statistics, 3
National Fertility Studies of 1965 and 1970, 3
National Institute of Child Health and Human Development, 3
SIDS Cooperative Epidemiological Study (1970s), 659–660
National Natality Surveys, 3
National Surveys of Family Growth of 1973 and 1976, 3
Natural family planning, 693, 696–697
Natural Mother hand pumps, 420
Necrotizing enterocolitis (NEC), 133, 137
and preventive properties in milk, 783–784
Neonatal jaundice. *See* Jaundice
Neonates. *See* Infant(s)
Networking, 727–728
Neural-tube defects, 643
Neurological dysfunction, 642–644
clinical implications of, 644
and inadequate caloric intake, 357
Newborns' and Mothers' Health Protection Act, 311
NFP. *See* Natural family planning
Niacin, 530
NICU
breastfeeding services in, 452–456, 458
discharge from, 472
milk storage and handling in, 454, 455, 462, 463, 465–466
postdischarge breastfeeding plans, 473–474
test weighing, 468–469
Nifedipine, 174, 493
Nipple
anatomy, 96
assessment, 105
autotransplantation, 494
blanching of, 492–493
classification of, function, 106, 107
cups on breast pumps, 402
elongated, 484
glasses, 428, 432
inverted or flat, 98, 281, 431, 432, 483–484
milk blister on, 493
nuzzling of, 284

ointments and creams, 184, 318–319, 321, 322–323, 335
  pain, 492
  plugged ducts, 484–485
  protractility, 97
  rolling, 280–281
  shields. *See* Nipple shields
  soreness, 315–321, 331, 354, 357, 419, 431, 504
  stimulation and lactation, 99, 315
  supernumerary, 97
  vasospasm in, 174, 492–493
Nipple shields, 287–288, 296, 427–432, 438
  alternatives to, 431
  effects on milk transfer rates, 428, 470
  informed consent for, 430
  professional responsibilities and, 430–431
  purposes of, 427
  risks of, 428–430
  use of, with preterm infants, 470–471
  weaning from, 431–432
Nizoral, 491
NMA. *See* Nursing Mothers Association
Nonhormonal contraceptive methods, 692–697
Nonnutritive suckling (NNS), 110, 460
Nonprotein nitrogen in breastmilk, 129
Nonsteroidal antiinflammatory drugs, 170. *See also* NSAIDs
Norfloxacin, 551
Norplant, 175, 698
Norpramine, 172, 568
Nortriptyline, 172, 566, 568
NSAIDs, 170, 553, 558–559, 563
Nuclear pollution, and breastmilk, 183
Nucleotides in breastmilk, 129–130
Nuremburg Code, 756
Nursing-bottle caries, 621
Nursing diagnosis, 728
Nursing Mothers Association, 280, 562
Nurture III breast pump, 410, 414, 424
Nutrition, frequently asked questions, 534–536
Nutritional values of breastmilk, 127–133
Nutrition basics
  carbohydrates, 525–526, 525–527
  energy, 524–525
  fat, 527
  minerals, 528
  protein, 526–527
  vitamins, 527–528
Nuzzling behavior, 294
Nystatin, 173, 174, 490, 491

Observational research, 751
Office of Population, USAID, 3
Ofloxacin, 173
Oligosaccharides in breastmilk, 142
Ora'lac breast pump, 400, 408
Oral contraceptives (OCs), 698
  effect on breastmilk, 11, 167, 175, 461, 697–698
  Raynaud's syndrome and, 493
Oral development, in children, 107–108
Organohalogen compounds, 182
OTC (over-the-counter) drugs, 178–179
Otitis media, 135, 137, 642
Overactive letdown reflex, 329
Ovulation
  and lactation, 677, 678, 679

  and supplemental feeding, 680–681
Oxacillin, 173
Oxycodone, 170
Oxytocin
  expression of breastmilk and, 426
  in lactation, 103–104, 398–399, 557

Pacifiers, 302, 355
Palatal obturator, 649
Pamelor, 566, 568
Pancrease, 655
Panhypopituitarism, 549–550
Papilloma, intraductal, 499
Papyrus Ebers, 4
Parenthood, and breastfeeding education, 247–248
Parlodel, 167
Parnate, 568
Paroxetine, 172, 566, 568
Passive diffusion, 166
Passive immunity, 138, 140, 229, 230, 234
Pasteurization, 226, 231
Pathological jaundice. *See* Jaundice
Paxil, 172, 566, 568
PBBs, 182, 200
PCBs, 182
Pedicle technique for breast reduction, 494
Pediculicides, 177–178
Peer counselors, 22, 71, 262, 262–263, 264, 265, 272
Penicillin, 179
Pentobarbital, 171
Percentile rank, growth charts, 344
Percodan, 170
Periareolar technique, 494
Peri-Colace, 175
Perinatal nurses and breastfeeding education, 271
Perinatal period and breastfeeding, 279–304
Perphenazine, 566, 568
Pesticides, 182
Phagocytes in breastmilk, 138
Phenelzine, 568
Phenindione, 170
Phenobarbital, 170, 171, 194, 562
Phenomenology, 748
Phenothiazines, 167, 566, 568
Phenylketonuria and breastfeeding, 653
Phenytoin, 170, 171, 562
Philippines, *lihi* ritual, 36–37
Phosphorus, 531
Phototherapy, 380–381, 385, 388
Physicians
  accommodation with formula manufacturers, 11–12
  breastfeeding education and, 271, 280
  breastfeeding in the workplace, 591–592
  in hospital-based lactation programs, 716–717
Piaget's cognitive theory, 607–608
PIF, 101
Pinch test, 99, 106
Pituitary dysfunction and lactation, 549–550
PKU. *See* Phenylketonuria
Plugged ducts, 484–485, 486, 504
Pneumonia, 641
"Pocket Guide to Breastfeeding," 262
Polybrominated biphenyls. *See* PBBs
Polychlorinated dibenzodioxins (PCDDs), 182